N. EDWARD ROBINSON, Ph.D., M.R.C.V.S.

Professor, Departments of Large Animal
Clinical Sciences and Physiology,
Michigan State University College of Veterinary Medicine,
East Lansing, Michigan

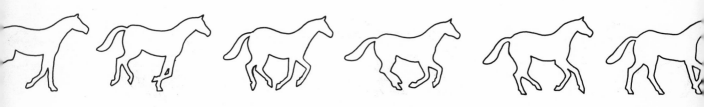

PHILADELPHIA/LONDON/TORONTO/MEXICO CITY/RIO DE JANEIRO/SYDNEY/TOKYO

CURRENT THERAPY IN EQUINE MEDICINE

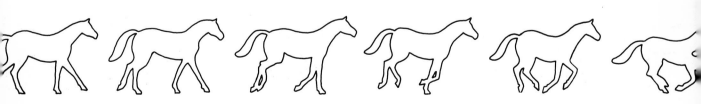

W. B. SAUNDERS COMPANY

W. B. Saunders Company: West Washington Square
Phildelphia, PA 19105

1 St. Anne's Road
Eastbourne, East Sussex BN21 3UN, England

1 Goldthorne Avenue
Toronto, Ontario M8Z 5T9, Canada

Apartado 26370–Cedro 512
Mexico 4, D.F., Mexico

Rua Coronel Cabrita, 8
Sao Cristovao Caixa Postal 21176
Rio de Janeiro, Brazil

9 Waltham Street
Artarmon, N.S.W. 2064, Australia

Ichibancho, Central Bldg., 22-I Ichibancho
Chiyoda-Ku, Tokyo 102, Japan

Library of Congress Cataloging in Publication Data
Main entry under title:

Current therapy in equine medicine.

1. Horses—Diseases.   I. Robinson, N. E.
SF951.C93 1983   636.1′089   81-48620
ISBN 0-7216-7617-0 (v. 1)

Current Therapy in Equine Medicine   ISBN   0-7216-7617-0

Last digit is the print number: 9   8   7   6   5   4   3   2

To

W. B. BOUCHER, V.M.D.

Emeritus Professor of Medicine
School of Veterinary Medicine
University of Pennsylvania

High standards of personal and professional integrity, careful clinical observation, humane concern for the patient, an awareness of the owner's requirements of the animal, and a broad knowledge of medicine make Bill Boucher an outstanding role model for all of us fortunate enough to have been his students.

Current Therapy in Equine Medicine

CONSULTING EDITORS

CONTRIBUTORS

STEPHEN B. ADAMS, D.V.M., M.S.,
Diplomate, A.C.V.S.

Associate Professor of Large Animal Surgery, Purdue University School of Veterinary Medicine, West Lafayette, Indiana.

Cribbing

ALEX A. ARDANS, D.V.M., M.S.

Director, Virology/Immunology Diagnostic Laboratory, University of California School of Veterinary Medicine, Davis, California.

Immunologic Diseases

A. C. ASBURY, D.V.M.

Associate Professor of Reproduction, University of Florida College of Veterinary Medicine, Gainesville. Theriogenologist, Veterinary Medical Teaching Hospital, University of Florida, Gainesville, Florida.

Bacterial Endometritis; Obstetrics

GORDON J. BAKER, B.V.Sc., Ph.D.,
M.R.C.V.S.

Professor and Chief, Equine Medicine and Surgery, University of Illinois College of Veterinary Medicine, Urbana, Illinois.

Strangles; Laryngeal Hemiplegia

WARWICK M. BAYLY, B.V.Sc., M.S.

Associate in Veterinary Medicine, Washington State University College of Veterinary Medicine, Pullman, Washington.

Pharyngitis

RALPH E. BEADLE, D.V.M., Ph.D.

Associate Professor of Equine Medicine, Veterinary Clinical Sciences, Louisiana State University School of Veterinary Medicine, Baton Rouge. Equine Clinician, Veterinary Teaching Hospital, Louisiana State University, Baton Rouge, Louisiana.

Summer Pasture–Associated Obstructive Pulmonary Disease

CAROLYN R. BEAL, B.S.

Research Technologist, University of Florida College of Veterinary Medicine, Gainesville, Florida.

Cerebrospinal Fluid Collection and Analysis

JAMES L. BECHT, D.V.M., M.S.

Assistant Professor of Medicine, University of Pennsylvania School of Veterinary Medicine, New Bolton Center, Kennett Square, Pennsylvania.

Gastric Diseases

JILL BEECH, V.M.D.

Assistant Professor of Medicine, University of Pennsylvania School of Veterinary Medicine, Kennett Square. Attending Clinician in Internal Medicine, University of Pennsylvania School of Veterinary Medicine, Kennett Square, Pennsylvania.

Tumors of the Pituitary Gland (Pars Intermedia); Antimicrobial Treatment of Respiratory Disease

G. MARVIN BEEMAN, D.V.M.

Associate Instructor of Biomedical Sciences, Colorado State University College of Veterinary Medicine, Fort Collins, Colorado. President, Littleton Large Animal Clinic, P.C., Littleton, Colorado.

Care of the Teeth

DWIGHT G. BENNETT, D.V.M., Ph.D.

Professor of Equine Medicine, Colorado State University College of Veterinary Medicine, Fort Collins. Equine Internal Medicine, Veterinary Teaching Hospital, Colorado State University, Fort Collins, Colorado.

Medical Management of Colic

ROY V. BERGMAN, V.M.D.

Practitioner, Cochranville, Pennsylvania.

Retained Meconium

LARRY C. BOOTH, D.V.M., M.S.

Assistant Professor, Equine Medicine and Surgery, University of Minnesota College of Veterinary Medicine, St. Paul, Minnesota.

Rabies

CHRISTOPHER M. BROWN, B.V.Sc., Ph.D., M.R.C.V.S.

Associate Professor, Large Animal Clinical Sciences, Michigan State University College of Veterinary Medicine, East Lansing, Michigan.

Examination of the Cardiovascular System; Congenital Cardiac Lesions; Thrombophlebitis; Diseases of the Great Vessels; Examination of the Urinary System; Renal Diseases; Bladder Diseases

MURRAY P. BROWN, D.V.M., M.Sc.

Associate Professor of Surgery, Department of Surgical Sciences, University of Florida College of Veterinary Medicine, Gainesville. Large Animal Surgeon, Veterinary Medical Teaching Hospital, University of Florida, Gainesville, Florida.

Surgical Treatment of Equine Sarcoid

T. D. BYARS, D.V.M.

Associate Professor, Large Animal Medicine, University of Georgia College of Veterinary Medicine, Athens. Large Animal Clinic, Veterinary Medical Teaching Hospital, University of Georgia, Athens, Georgia.

Flatulent Colic; Disseminated Intravascular Coagulation; Behavioral Abnormalities

CHARLES C. CAPEN, D.V.M., M.Sc., Ph.D.

Professor of Pathobiology, Ohio State University College of Veterinary Medicine, Professor of Endocrinology, Ohio State University College of Medicine, Columbus. Consulting Clinician, Veterinary Teaching Hospital, Ohio State University, Columbus, Ohio.

Nutritional Secondary Hyperparathyroidism

GARY P. CARLSON, B.S., D.V.M., Ph.D.

Associate Professor, Department of Medicine, University of California School of Veterinary Medicine, Davis. Large Animal Medicine Service, Veterinary Medical Teaching Hospital, University of California, Davis, California.

Evaluation of the Hematopoietic System; Blood Loss Anemia; Fluid Therapy; Medical Management of the Exhausted Horse; Hemolytic Anemia

HILARY M. CLAYTON, B.V.M.S., Ph.D., M.R.C.V.S.

Associate Professor, Department of Veterinary Anatomy, Western College of Veterinary Medi-

cine, University of Saskatchewan, Saskatoon, Saskatchewan.

Lung Parasites

LEROY COGGINS, D.V.M., Ph.D.

Professor of Virology, North Carolina State University School of Veterinary Medicine, Raleigh. Head, Department of Microbiology, Pathology, and Parasitology, North Carolina State University, Raleigh, North Carolina.

Equine Viral Arteritis; Equine Infectious Anemia

MORTIMER COHEN, V.M.D., Diplomate, A.C.V.I.M.

Sunol Valley Animal Hospital, Sunol, California.

Anthrax; Malignant Edema; Tetanus; Ulcerative Lymphangitis

MICHAEL A. COLLIER, D.V.M.

Assistant Professor of Surgery, New York State College of Veterinary Medicine, Cornell University, Ithaca, New York.

Renal Diseases; Bladder Diseases

WENDELL L. COOPER, V.M.D.

Veterinarian, Almahurst Farm, Lexington, Kentucky.

Artificial Breeding of Horses

FREDERIK J. DERKSEN, D.V.M., Ph.D.

Assistant Professor of Large Animal Clinical Sciences, Michigan State University, East Lansing. Equine Clinician, Veterinary Medical Teaching Hospital, Michigan State University, East Lansing, Michigan.

Actinobacillosis; Chronic Airway Disease

STEPHEN G. DILL, D.V.M.

Resident in Medicine, Department of Clinical Sciences, New York State College of Veterinary Medicine, Cornell University, Ithaca, New York.

Acute Hepatitis

THOMAS J. DIVERS, D.V.M.

Assistant Professor of Medicine, University of Pennsylvania School of Veterinary Medicine, New Bolton Center, Kennett Square, Pennsylvania.

Thromboembolic Colic

MAARTEN DROST, D.V.M.

Professor of Reproduction, University of Florida College of Veterinary Medicine, Gainesville. Theriogenologist, Veterinary Medical Teaching Hospital, Gainesville, Florida.

Obstetrics

J. H. DRUDGE, D.V.M., Sc.D.

Professor of Veterinary Science, University of Kentucky, Lexington, Kentucky.

Ascariasis; Strongylosis; Strongyloidosis; Bots; Cestode Infection; Oxyuris Infection

ROLF M. EMBERTSON, D.V.M.

Resident, Large Animal Surgery, Veterinary Medical Teaching Hospital, University of Florida, Gainesville, Florida.

Parturient Perineal and Rectovestibular Injuries

BERNARD F. FELDMAN, D.V.M., Ph.D.

Associate Professor of Veterinary Clinical Pathology, Department of Clinical Pathology, University of California School of Veterinary Medicine, Davis. Head, Bone Marrow Cytology Service, Veterinary Medical Teaching Hospital, Clinical Pathology Service, University of California, Davis, California.

Anemia as a Result of Insufficient Erythropoiesis; Hemostasis

GREGORY L. FERRARO, D.V.M.

Assistant Clinical Professor of Surgery, University of California, Davis, California. President, Southern California Equine Foundation, Inc., Arcadia, California.

The Diagnosis and Treatment of Coughing

DONALD D. FLEMMING, D.V.M.

Lecturer, University of California School of Veterinary Medicine, Davis, California.

BCG Therapy for Equine Sarcoid

DAVID E. FREEMAN, M.V.B., M.R.C.V.S.

Assistant Professor of Surgery, University of Pennsylvania School of Veterinary Medicine, New Bolton Center, Kennett Square, Pennsylvania.

Guttural Pouch Disease; Nutrition of the Sick Horse

DENNIS R. GEISER, D.V.M.

Assistant Professor, Equine Medicine and Surgery, Department of Rural Practice, University of Tennessee, Knoxville. Anesthesiologist, Veterinary Teaching Hospital, University of Tennessee, Knoxville, Tennessee. Consultant to Anheuser Busch Clydesdale Operation.

Soft Palate Displacement; Diseases of the Epiglottis

JOHN S. GILMOUR, B.V.M., B.V.S., F.R.C.V.S.

Principal Veterinary Research Officer, Animal Diseases Research Association, Moredun Institute, Edinburgh, United Kingdom.

Grass Sickness

MARY B. GLAZE, D.V.M., M.S., Diplomate, Amer. Coll. Vet. Ophthalmologists

Assistant Professor of Veterinary Ophthalmology,

Veterinary Clinical Sciences, Louisiana State University School of Veterinary Medicine, Baton Rouge. Veterinary Ophthalmologist, Veterinary Teaching Hospital and Clinic, Louisiana State University, Baton Rouge, Louisiana.

Red, Painful Eyes (Equine Uveitis)

DALLAS O. GOBLE, D.V.M., Diplomate, A.C.V.S.

Associate Professor, University of Tennessee College of Veterinary Medicine, Knoxville. Director, Equine Clinic, Veterinary Teaching Hospital, University of Tennessee, Knoxville, Tennessee.

Sinusitis

DEAN E. GOELDNER, D.V.M.

Practitioner, Van Nuys, California.

Western Equine Encephalomyelitis

CRAIG E. GRIFFIN, D.V.M., A.C.V.I.M.

Animal Dermatology Clinic, San Diego, California.

Nodular Collagenolytic Granuloma (Nodular Necrobiosis)

JEFFREY B. GRIMMETT, B.V.Sc., M.R.C.V.S.

Resident, Department of Reproduction, Veterinary Medical Teaching Hospital, University of Florida, Gainesville, Florida.

Behavioral Anestrus

ROBERT M. GWIN, D.V.M., M.S.

Director, Animal Ophthalmic Research Facility, McGee Eye Institute, Adjunct Associate Professor, University of Oklahoma, Oklahoma City, Oklahoma.

Corneal Opacities

GEORGE K. HAIBEL, D.V.M.

Resident, Department of Reproduction, University of Florida College of Veterinary Medicine, Gainesville, Florida.

Disorders of the Cervix

RICHARD C. HALLIWELL, Vet. M.B., Ph.D.

Professor, Department of Medical Sciences, University of Florida College of Veterinary Medicine, Gainesville, Florida.

Urticaria and Angioedema

DAN L. HAWKINS, D.V.M., M.S.

Hagyard-Davidson-McGee Hospital, Lexington, Kentucky.

Progesterone Therapy

J. PIERRE HELD, D.M.V., F.V.H.

Assistant Professor, University of Tennessee School of Veterinary Medicine, Knoxville. Equine

Clinics, University of Tennessee, Knoxville, Tennessee.

Retained Placenta

ROBERT B. HILLMAN, D.V.M., M.S.

Senior Clinician, New York State College of Veterinary Medicine, Cornell University, Ithaca, New York.

Induction of Parturition

RONALD W. HILWIG, D.V.M., M.Sc., Ph.D.

Associate Professor of Veterinary Science, University of Arizona, Tucson, Arizona.

Cardiac Arrhythmias

H. F. HINTZ, Ph.D.

Professor of Animal Nutrition, Cornell University, Ithaca, New York.

Energy and Protein; Minerals; Vitamins; Feeding Programs; Sample Rations and Commercial Foods; Hoof Growth and Nutrition; Eclampsia

STEVEN M. HOPKINS, D.V.M., Diplomate, Amer. Coll. of Theriogenologists.

Assistant Professor, Department of Theriogenology, Iowa State University College of Veterinary Medicine, Ames. Staff, Department of Veterinary Clinical Sciences, Veterinary Teaching Hospital, Iowa State University, Ames, Iowa.

Ovulation Induction

JOHN P. HURTGEN, D.V.M., M.S., Ph.D.

Assistant Professor, Section of Reproduction, University of Pennsylvania School of Veterinary Medicine, New Bolton Center, Kennett Square, Pennsylvania.

Evaluation of Stallion Fertility; Disorders Affecting Stallion Fertility

PETER J. IHRKE, V.M.D.

Assistant Professor of Dermatology and Allergy, Department of Medicine, University of California College of Veterinary Medicine, Davis. Staff Dermatologist, Veterinary Medical Teaching Hospital, University of California, Davis, California.

Diseases of Abnormal Keratinization; Contact Dermatitis

THOMAS J. KERN, D.V.M. Diplomate, Amer. Coll. Vet. Ophthalmologists

Assistant Professor of Ophthalmology, New York State College of Veterinary Medicine, Cornell University, Ithaca, New York.

Ocular Fundus and Central Nervous System Causes of Blindness

JAMES P. KLYZA, D.V.M.

Practitioner, Paris, Kentucky.

Botulism Syndromes

CATHERINE W. KOHN, V.M.D.

Assistant Professor, Equine Medicine and Surgery, Ohio State University School of Veterinary Medicine, Columbus, Ohio.

Colitis-X

ANN A. KOWNACKI, D.V.M.

El Camino Veterinary Hospital, Atascadero, California.

Plant Toxicities

JANVER D. KREHBIEL, D.V.M., Ph.D.

Professor and Assistant Chairman, Department of Pathology, Michigan State University College of Veterinary Medicine, East Lansing. Director, Clinical Pathology Laboratory, Veterinary Clinical Center, Michigan State University, East Lansing, Michigan.

Normal Clinical Pathology Data

D. S. KRONFELD, B.V.Sc., Ph.D.

Professor of Clinical Nutrition, School of Veterinary Medicine, University of Pennsylvania, New Bolton Center, Kennett Square, Pennsylvania.

Hyperlipemia

DOLORES J. KUNZE, D.V.M., M.S.

Assistant Professor, Department of Food Animal and Equine Medicine, North Carolina State University School of Veterinary Medicine, Raleigh, North Carolina.

Endotoxemia; Cataracts

IRWIN K. M. LIU, D.V.M., Ph.D.

Assistant Professor, Department of Reproduction, University of California School of Veterinary Medicine, Davis. Veterinary Medical Teaching Hospital, University of California, Davis, California.

Equine Influenza; Equine Herpesvirus; Equine Adenovirus; Equine Rhinovirus; Vesicular Stomatitis; Ovarian Tumors; Pyometra

EDMOND C. LOOMIS, Ph.D.

Parasitologist, Extension Lecturer, Department of Microbiology, University of California School of Veterinary Medicine, Davis, California.

Common Ectoparasites and Their Control

J. E. LOWE, D.V.M., M.S.

Associate Professor of Surgery, New York State College of Veterinary Medicine, Cornell University, Ithaca, New York.

Founder; Heat Bumps, Sweet Feed Bumps, Sweet Itch; Thyroid Diseases

ROBERT G. LOY, Ph.D.

Professor of Veterinary Science, University of Kentucky, Lexington, Kentucky.

Control of Ovulation

E. T. LYONS, Ph.D.

Professor of Veterinary Science, University of Kentucky, Lexington, Kentucky.

Ascariasis; Stronglylosis; Strongyloidosis; Bots; Cestode Infection; Oxyuris Infection

ROBERT J. MᴀᴄKAY, B.V.Sc.

Instructor, Medical Sciences, University of Florida College of Veterinary Medicine, Gainesville, Florida.

Equine Herpesvirus 1 Myeloencephalitis

JOHN E. MADIGAN, D.V.M., M.S.

Ackerman Creek Large Animal Clinic, Ukiah, California.

Equine Ehrlichiosis

THOMAS O. MANNING, D.V.M.

Assistant Professor of Medicine, New York State College of Veterinary Medicine, Cornell University, Ithaca. Dermatologist, Department of Clinical Sciences, Cornell University, Ithaca, New York.

Pemphigus Foliaceus

R. J. MARTENS, D.V.M.

Associate Professor, Large Animal Medicine and Surgery, Texas A&M University College of Veterinary Medicine, College Station, Texas.

Foal Pneumonia and Lung Abscesses

M. G. MAXIE, D.V.M., Ph.D.

Veterinary Pathologist, Veterinary Services Branch, Ontario Ministry of Agriculture and Food, Guelph, Ontario, Canada.

Aortoiliofemoral Arteriosclerosis

IAN G. MAYHEW, B.V.Sc., Ph.D.

Associate Professor, Department of Medical Sciences, University of Florida College of Veterinary Medicine, Gainesville. Service Chief, Large Animal Medicine, Veterinary Medical Teaching Hospital, University of Florida, Gainesville, Florida.

Cerebrospinal Fluid Collection and Analysis; Seizure Disorders

JILL JOHNSON McCLURE, D.V.M., M.S., Diplomate, A.C.V.I.M., A.B.V.P.

Associate Professor, Equine Medicine, Department of Veterinary Clinical Sciences, Louisiana State University School of Veterinary Medicine, Baton Rouge, Louisiana.

Anterior Enteritis

CHERYL McCULLOUGH, D.V.M.

Resident, Equine Medicine, Veterinary Medical Teaching Hospital, University of California, Davis, California.

Mycotic Diseases

WILLIAM C. McMULLAN, D.V.M., M.S.

Professor, Large Animal Medicine and Surgery, Texas A&M University College of Veterinary Medicine, College Station, Texas.

Scratches; Phycomycosis; Habronemiasis

A. M. MERRITT, D.V.M., M.S.

Professor of Medicine, University of Florida College of Veterinary Medicine, Gainesville. Assistant Chief of Staff, Large Animal Clinic, Veterinary Medical Teaching Hospital, University of Florida, Gainesville, Florida.

Diabetes Mellitus; Chronic Diarrhea; Gastrointestinal Neoplasia

DEBRA DEEM MORRIS, D.V.M.

Lecturer, Large Animal Internal Medicine, University of Pennsylvania School of Veterinary Medicine, Kennett Square. Clinician, Cytologist, University of Pennsylvania School of Veterinary Medicine, New Bolton Center, Kennett Square, Pennsylvania.

Salivary Gland Disease; Chronic Pancreatitis

PAUL G. MORRIS, D.V.M., M.S.

Assistant Professor, Equine Medicine and Surgery, Kansas State University, Manhattan, Kansas.

Blood Transfusion; Sporotrichosis

JOYCE M. MURPHY, D.V.M., M.S., Diplomate, Amer. Coll. Vet. Ophthalmologists

Alaska Animal Eye Clinic, Anchorage, Alaska.

Administration of Ocular Therapy

JONATHAN M. NAYLOR, B.V.Sc., M.R.C.V.S., Diplomate, A.C.V.I.M.

Associate Professor, University of Saskatchewan School of Veterinary Medicine, Saskatoon, Saskatchewan, Canada.

Hyperlipemia; Nutrition of the Sick Horse; Bilirubinemia

DEAN P. NEELY, V.M.D., Ph.D.

Associate Professor, Michigan State University College of Veterinary Medicine, East Lansing. Equine Theriogenologist, Michigan State University, East Lansing, Michigan.

Causes and Prevention of Abortion

A. W. NELSON, D.V.M., Ph.D.

Professor of Clinical Sciences, Colorado State University College of Veterinary Medicine and Biomedical Sciences, Fort Collins. Professor and Head, Small Animal Surgery, Veterinary Teaching Hospital, Colorado State University, Fort Collins, Colorado.

Cleft Palate

FREDERICK W. OEHME, D.V.M., Ph.D.

Professor of Toxicology, Medicine and Physiology,

Kansas State University College of Veterinary Medicine, Manhattan. Director, Comparative Toxicology Laboratories, Kansas State University, Manhattan, Kansas.

Toxicoses Commonly Observed in Horses; General Principles in Treatment of Poisoning; Insecticides; Rodenticides; Snakebite; Blister Beetle Poisoning; Carbon Tetrachloride; Phenothiazine; Petroleum Products; Lead; Selenium; Water Quality

JAMES A. ORSINI, D.V.M.

Lecturer in Surgery, University of Pennsylvania School of Veterinary Medicine, New Bolton Center, Kennett Square, Pennsylvania.

Large Bowel Obstruction

JONATHAN E. PALMER, V.M.D.

Lecturer in Medicine, University of Pennsylvania School of Veterinary Medicine, Kennett Square. Section of Medicine, University of Pennsylvania George D. Widener Hospital, New Bolton Center, Kennett Square, Pennsylvania.

Malabsorption Syndromes

B. W. PARRY, B.V.Sc.

Research Associate, Department of Veterinary Clinical Medicine and Surgery, Washington State University College of Veterinary Medicine, Pullman, Washington.

Indirect Blood Pressure Measurement

JOHN R. PASCOE, B.V.Sc.

Department of Surgery, University of California School of Veterinary Medicine, Davis, California.

Exercise-Induced Pulmonary Hemorrhage

REGINALD R. R. PASCOE, B.V.Sc., M.V.Sc., F.R.C.V.S., F.A.C.V.Sc.

Senior Partner, Oakey Veterinary Hospital, Oakey, Queensland, Australia.

Dermatophilosis

WALDIR M. PEDERSOLI, D.V.M., M.S., Ph.D.

Associate Professor of Pharmacology, Department of Physiology and Pharmacology, Auburn University School of Veterinary Medicine, Auburn, Alabama.

Antibiotics

JOHN E. PEEL, B.V.Sc.

Resident, Large Animal Medicine, University of California School of Veterinary Medicine, Davis. Veterinary Medical Teaching Hospital, University of California, Davis, California.

Brucellosis; Tuberculosis

P. W. PHYSICK-SHEARD, B.V.Sc., M.Sc., M.R.C.V.S.

Assistant Professor of Large Animal Internal Medicine, Ontario Veterinary College, University of Guelph, Ontario, Canada.

Limitations of Electrocardiography; Cardiac Murmurs; Bacterial Endocarditis; The ECG and Performance Prediction: Heart Scores; Aortoiliofemoral Arteriosclerosis

CORINNE F. RAPHEL, D.V.M.

Lecturer in Medicine, University of Pennsylvania School of Veterinary Medicine, New Bolton Center, Kennett Square, Pennsylvania.

Bacteremia

STEPHEN M. REED, D.V.M.

Assistant Professor of Equine Medicine, Washington State University College of Veterinary Medicine, Pullman, Washington.

Head Trauma; Spinal Cord Trauma; Pleuritis

VIRGINIA REEF, D.V.M.

Lecturer in Large Animal Medicine, University of Pennsylvania School of Veterinary Medicine, Kennett Square. Attending Cardiologist, Large Animal Heart Station, University of Pennsylvania School of Veterinary Medicine, New Bolton Center, Kennett Square, Pennsylvania.

Glossitis

DEAN W. RICHARDSON, D.V.M.

Lecturer in Large Animal Surgery, University of Pennsylvania School of Veterinary Medicine, New Bolton Center, Kennett Square, Pennsylvania.

Rectal Tears

THOMAS W. RIEBOLD, D.V.M. Diplomate, Amer. Coll. Vet. Anesthesiologists

Assistant Professor, Oregon State University School of Veterinary Medicine, Corvallis. Anesthesiologist, Veterinary Teaching Hospital, Oregon State University, Corvallis, Oregon.

Emergency Ventilation; Oxygen Therapy

N. EDWARD ROBINSON, Ph.D., M.R.C.V.S.

Professor, Department of Large Animal Clinical Sciences and Physiology, Michigan State University College of Veterinary Medicine, East Lansing, Michigan.

Onchocerciasis; Sweet or Queensland Itch (Culicoides Hypersensitivity); Table of Common Drugs: Approximate Doses; Aging the Horse

GARY E. RUMBAUGH, D.V.M. Diplomate, A.C.V.I.M.

Assistant Professor, Department of Medicine, University of California School of Veterinary Medicine, Davis. Equine Field Service, Veterinary Medical Teaching Hospital, University of California, Davis, California.

Internal Abscesses; Vaccination Programs; Foal Heat Diarrhea; Immunologic Diseases

W. KENT SCARRATT, D.V.M.

Assistant Professor, Large Animal Medicine, University of Florida College of Veterinary Medicine, Gainesville, Florida.

Equine Protozoal Myeloencephalitis

GRETCHEN M. SCHMIDT, D.V.M.

Associate Professor, Michigan State University College of Veterinary Medicine, Veterinary Clinical Center, East Lansing, Michigan. Animal Eye Associates, Berwyn Veterinary Hospital, Berywn, Illinois.

Approach to Ophthalmic Problems

H. F. SCHRYVER, D.V.M., Ph.D.

Equine Research Program, New York State College of Veterinary Medicine and New York State College of Agriculture and Life Sciences, Cornell University, Ithaca, New York.

Energy and Protein; Minerals; Vitamins

DANNY W. SCOTT, D.V.M.

Associate Professor of Medicine, New York State College of Veterinary Medicine, Cornell University, Ithaca, New York.

Folliculitis and Furunculosis

EDWARD A. SCOTT, D.V.M., M.S.

Professor of Large Animal Clinical Sciences, Michigan State University College of Veterinary Medicine, East Lansing, Michigan.

Esophageal Disease

W. L. SCRUTCHFIELD, D.V.M., M.S., Diplomate, A.C.V.I.M.

Associate Professor, Large Animal Medicine and Surgery, Texas A&M University College of Veterinary Medicine, College Station, Texas.

Peritonitis; Foal Pneumonia and Lung Abscesses

GAY WILES SENK, D.V.M.

Practitioner, Brookville, New York.

Ocular Discharge in Young Horses

DAN C. SHARP, Ph.D.

Associate Professor of Physiology, Animal Science Department, University of Florida, Gainesville, Florida.

The Effects of Artificial Lighting on Reproduction

ROBERT K. SHIDELER, D.V.M.

Professor, Equine Medicine, Colorado State University College of Veterinary Medicine, Fort Collins. Equine Ambulatory Service, Head Equine Section, Veterinary Teaching Hospital, Colorado State University, Fort Collins, Colorado.

Medical Management of Colic

BRADFORD P. SMITH, D.V.M.

Associate Professor, Department of Medicine, University of California School of Veterinary Medicine, Davis. Chief, Large Animal Medicine Service, Veterinary Medical Teaching Hospital, University of California, Davis, California.

Rotavirus Infection; Salmonellosis; Enteric Salmonellosis; Chronic Liver Disease

T. S. STASHAK, D.V.M., M.S.

Associate Professor of Surgery, Department of Clinical Sciences, Colorado State University College of Veterinary Medicine and Biomedical Sciences, Fort Collins, Colorado.

Cleft Palate

JOHN A. STICK, D.V.M.

Assistant Professor of Surgery, Michigan State University College of Veterinary Medicine, East Lansing. Equine Staff Surgeon, Veterinary Clinical Center, Michigan State University, East Lansing, Michigan.

Rectal Prolapse

BUD C. TENNANT, D.V.M.

Professor and Chief of Medicine, Department of Clinical Sciences, New York State College of Veterinary Medicine, Cornell University, Ithaca, New York.

Acute Hepatitis

GORDON H. THEILEN, D.V.M.

Professor, University of California School of Veterinary Medicine, Davis. Chief, Oncology Service, Veterinary Medical Teaching Hospital, Davis, California.

Papillomatosis (Warts)

THOMAS TOBIN, D.V.M.

Professor, Department of Veterinary Science, University of Kentucky, Lexington, Kentucky.

Plant Toxicities

ERIC P. TULLENERS, D.V.M.

Lecturer, Large Animal Surgery, University of Pennsylvania School of Veterinary Medicine, New Bolton Center, Kennett Square, Pennsylvania.

Small Bowel Obstruction

STEVEN D. VAN CAMP, D.V.M.

Associate Professor, Mississippi State University College of Veterinary Medicine, Theriogenologist, Mississippi State University, Starkville, Mississippi

Prolonged Distress

PAMELA C. WAGNER, D.V.M., M.S.

Assistant Professor, Large Animal Surgery, Oregon State University College of Veterinary Medicine,

Corvallis. Clinician, Veterinary Teaching Hospital, Oregon State University, Corvallis, Oregon.

Pericarditis; Cervical Vertebral Malformation

ANGELINE WARNER, D.V.M., M.S.

Resident, Large Animal Medicine, University of Pennsylvania School of Veterinary Medicine, New Bolton Center, Kennett Square, Pennsylvania.

Anhidrosis

KARL K. WHITE, D.V.M., Diplomate, A.C.V.S.

Assistant Professor of Surgery, Director, Large Animal Hospital, New York State College of Veterinary Medicine, Cornell University, Ithaca, New York.

Exertional Myopathy

NATHANIEL A. WHITE, D.V.M., M.S.

Associate Professor of Surgery, University of Georgia College of Veterinary Medicine, Athens, Georgia.

Thromboembolic Colic; Postanesthesia Myopathy-Neuropathy

ROBERT H. WHITLOCK, D.V.M., Ph.D., Diplomate, A.C.V.I.M.

Associate Professor of Medicine, Chief of Medicine, University of Pennsylvania School of Veterinary Medicine, New Bolton Center, Kennett Square, Pennsylvania.

Clinical Signs of Some Disorders of the Gastrointestinal Tract

MARTIN WIERUP, D.V.M., Ph.D.

Associate Professor of Bacteriology and Epizootiology, Faculty of Veterinary Medicine, Swedish University of Agricultural Sciences, Uppsala, Sweden. Associate Professor, Department of Epizootiology, National Veterinary Institute, Uppsala, Sweden.

Intestinal Clostridiosis

JULIA H. WILSON, D.V.M.

Resident, Large Animal Medicine, Department of Medical Sciences, University of Florida College of Veterinary Medicine, Gainesville, Florida. Associate, Loudoun Veterinary Service, Purcellville, Virginia.

Eastern Equine Encephalomyelitis

WALTER W. ZENT, D.V.M.

Hagyard-Davidson-McGee Hospital, Lexington, Kentucky

Postpartum Complications

JOSEPH G. ZINKL, D.V.M., Ph.D.

Associate Professor, Department of Clinical Pathology, University of California School of Veterinary Medicine, Davis. Hematology and Cytology Service, Veterinary Medical Teaching Hospital, University of California, Davis, California.

Evaluation of the Hematopoietic System; Blood Loss Anemia; Lymphoproliferative and Myeloproliferative Diseases; Hemolytic Anemia

PREFACE

This is the first edition of what I hope will be a continuing series of books designed to provide the practicing veterinarian and veterinary student with the most recent information on the therapy of the common medical diseases of the horse. The style of the book is similar to that used in other current therapy texts published by W. B. Saunders Company. In general, each article contains a brief description of the disease and confirmatory tests. Therapy and prevention are emphasized, and we have attempted to provide specifics of doses and routes of administration. Each article represents the author's opinion of the therapy he or she would use in treating the condition. The dosages of drugs suggested by authors are generally within recommended guidelines. At times dosages may be greater than is recommended because in the author's opinion there is good evidence for the use of the higher dose. It is assumed that veterinarians using this book will read the latest information available from the drug manufacturer before prescribing a treatment. The use of a drug at doses outside those recommended by the manufacturer is then dependent on the veterinarian's own clinical judgment.

In preparing this text I have relied heavily on section editors for advice on the content of each section, the selection of authors, and the initial review of manuscripts. The enthusiasm of both authors and section editors has been gratifying. The success of this book will be in large part due to them.

We were all shocked by Dr. Humphrey Knight's death during book production. As a leader in equine medicine, he had given me a great deal of advice throughout planning of the book. I owe special thanks to Drs. Brad Smith, Gary Rumbaugh, Mort Cohen, Waldir Pedersoli, Fred Derksen and Corinne Raphel, who at short notice agreed to write Dr. Knight's articles.

Many individuals have been involved in the production of the book. I particularly want to acknowledge the staff of W. B. Saunders, who have been extremely encouraging and have responded immediately to all my concerns; Shirley Goodwin and Linda Friedsburg, who retyped all the edited manuscripts with superb attention to detail; Bob Ingersoll and Rick Hill, who checked all the references; and Dr. Chris Brown in the Department of Large Animal Surgery and Medicine, who has an encyclopedic knowledge of the world literature in equine medicine and who was always available for discussion of controversial points in manuscripts. Finally, I must thank my wife Pat, who initially encouraged me to undertake the task and who held up my flagging spirits when there were delays or problems.

N. Edward Robinson

NOTICE

Extraordinary efforts have been made by the authors, the editors, and the publisher of this book to insure that dosage recommendations are precise and in agreement with standards officially accepted at the time of publication.

It does happen, however, that dosage schedules are changed from time to time in the light of accumulating clinical experience and continuing laboratory studies. This is most likely to occur in the case of recently introduced products.

It is urged, therefore, that you check the manufacturer's recommendations for dosage, especially if the drug to be administered or prescribed is one that you use only infrequently or have not used for some time.

In addition, some drugs mentioned have been used by the authors as experimental drugs. Others have been used in dosages greater than those recommended by the manufacturer. In these cases the authors have reported on their own considerable experience, but readers are urged to view the recommendations with discretion and precaution. Finally, within the United States, please check government regulations for U.S.D.A. approved drugs.

THE PUBLISHER

CONTENTS

Section 1 INFECTIOUS DISEASES

H. D. Knight, *Consulting Editor*

EQUINE INFLUENZA *Irwin K. M. Liu*	3
EQUINE HERPESVIRUS *Irwin K. M. Liu*	4
EQUINE ADENOVIRUS *Irwin K. M. Liu*	5
EQUINE RHINOVIRUS *Irwin K. M. Liu*	6
EQUINE VIRAL ARTERITIS *Leroy Coggins*	6
EQUINE INFECTIOUS ANEMIA *Leroy Coggins*	7
RABIES *Larry C. Booth*	9
ROTAVIRUS INFECTIONS *Bradford P. Smith*	11
VESICULAR STOMATITIS *Irwin K. M. Liu*	12
EQUINE EHRLICHIOSIS *John E. Madigan*	13
ACTINOBACILLOSIS *Frederik J. Derksen*	14
ANTHRAX *Mortimer Cohen*	17
BRUCELLOSIS *John E. Peel*	19
MALIGNANT EDEMA *Mortimer Cohen*	21
SALMONELLOSIS *Bradford P. Smith*	22
STRANGLES *Gordon J. Baker*	24
TETANUS *Mortimer Cohen*	27
TUBERCULOSIS *John E. Peel*	29
ULCERATIVE LYMPHANGITIS *Mortimer Cohen*	31
MYCOTIC DISEASES *Cheryl McCullough*	32
BACTEREMIA *Corinne F. Raphel*	36
INTERNAL ABSCESSES *Gary E. Rumbaugh*	38
VACCINATION PROGRAMS *Gary E. Rumbaugh*	40
ANTIBIOTICS *Waldir M. Pedersoli*	43
ENDOTOXEMIA *Dolores J. Kunze*	57

Section 2 NUTRITION

H. F. Hintz, *Consulting Editor*

ENERGY AND PROTEIN *H. F. Hintz and H. F. Schryver* **65**

MINERALS *H. F. Schryver and H. F. Hintz* **71**

VITAMINS *H. F. Schryver and H. F. Hintz* **84**

FEEDING PROGRAMS *H. F. Hintz* **91**

SAMPLE RATIONS AND COMMERCIAL FEEDS *H. F. Hintz* **97**

HOOF GROWTH AND NUTRITION *H. F. Hintz* **100**

EXERTIONAL MYOPATHY *Karl K. White* **101**

FOUNDER *J. E. Lowe* **104**

HYPERLIPEMIA *Jonathan M. Naylor* **107**

HEAT BUMPS, SWEET FEED BUMPS, SWEET ITCH *J. E. Lowe* **110**

ECLAMPSIA *H. F. Hintz* **111**

NUTRITION OF THE SICK HORSE *Jonathan M. Naylor and D. E. Freeman* **111**

BILIRUBINEMIA *Jonathan M. Naylor* **116**

Section 3 CARDIOVASCULAR DISEASES

Christopher M. Brown, *Consulting Editor*

EXAMINATION OF THE CARDIOVASCULAR SYSTEM *Christopher M. Brown* **121**

LIMITATIONS OF ELECTROCARDIOGRAPHY *P. W. Physick-Sheard* **125**

INDIRECT BLOOD PRESSURE MEASUREMENT *B. W. Parry* **128**

CARDIAC ARRHYTHMIAS *Ronald W. Hilwig* **131**

CARDIAC MURMURS *P. W. Physick-Sheard* **141**

CONGENITAL CARDIAC LESIONS *Christopher M. Brown* **146**

BACTERIAL ENDOCARDITIS *P. W. Physick-Sheard* **147**

THE ECG AND PERFORMANCE PREDICTION: HEART SCORES *P. W. Physick-Sheard* ... **148**

PERICARDITIS *Pamela C. Wagner* **149**

THROMBOPHLEBITIS *Christopher M. Brown* **151**

DISEASES OF THE GREAT VESSELS *Christopher M. Brown* **152**

AORTOILIOFEMORAL ARTERIOSCLEROSIS *P. W. Physick-Sheard and M. G. Maxie* **153**

Section 4 ENDOCRINE DISEASES

V. K. Ganjam, *Consulting Editor*

THYROID DISEASES *John E. Lowe* **159**

NUTRITIONAL SECONDARY HYPERPARATHYROIDISM *Charles C. Capen* **160**

TUMORS OF THE PITUITARY GLAND (PARS INTERMEDIA) *Jill Beech* **164**

DIABETES MELLITUS *A. M. Merritt* **169**

ANHIDROSIS *Angeline Warner* **170**

Section 5 GASTROINTESTINAL DISEASES

Robert H. Whitlock, *Consulting Editor*

CLINICAL SIGNS OF SOME DISORDERS OF THE GASTROINTESTINAL TRACT
Robert H. Whitlock 175

CLEFT PALATE *A. W. Nelson and T. S. Stashak* 177

CRIBBING *Stephen B. Adams* 181

SALIVARY GLAND DISEASE *Debra Deem Morris* 183

GLOSSITIS *Virginia Reef* 185

CARE OF THE TEETH *G. Marvin Beeman* 186

ESOPHAGEAL DISEASE *Edward A. Scott* 192

GASTRIC DISEASES *James E. Becht* 196

COLITIS-X *Catherine W. Kohn* 200

ENTERIC SALMONELLOSIS *Bradford P. Smith* 207

INTESTINAL CLOSTRIDIOSIS *Martin Wierup* 210

FOAL HEAT DIARRHEA *Gary E. Rumbaugh* 213

ANTERIOR ENTERITIS *Jill Johnson McClure* 214

CHRONIC DIARRHEA *A. M. Merritt* 216

MEDICAL MANAGEMENT OF COLIC *R. K. Shideler and D. G. Bennett* 220

SMALL BOWEL OBSTRUCTION *Eric P. Tulleners* 224

LARGE BOWEL OBSTRUCTION *James Orsini* 231

FLATULENT COLIC *T. D. Byars* 236

THROMBOEMBOLIC COLIC *Thomas J. Divers and Nathaniel A. White* 238

PERITONITIS *W. Leon Scrutchfield* 241

GRASS SICKNESS *John S. Gilmour* 244

MALABSORPTION SYNDROMES *Jonathan E. Palmer* 245

ACUTE HEPATITIS *Bud C. Tennant and Steve Dill* 249

CHRONIC LIVER DISEASE *Bradford P. Smith* 251

CHRONIC PANCREATITIS *Debra Deem Morris* 253

RECTAL PROLAPSE *John A. Stick* 254

RECTAL TEARS *Dean W. Richardson* 256

GASTROINTESTINAL NEOPLASIA *A. M. Merritt* 259

RETAINED MECONIUM *Roy V. Bergman* 260

ASCARIASIS *J. H. Drudge and E. T. Lyons* 262

STRONGYLOSIS *J. H. Drudge and E. T. Lyons* 267

STRONGYLOIDOSIS *J. H. Drudge and E. T. Lyons* 281

BOTS *J. H. Drudge and E. T. Lyons* 283

CESTODE INFECTION *J. H. Drudge and E. T. Lyons* 287

OXYURIS INFECTION *J. H. Drudge and E. T. Lyons* 288

Section 6 DISEASES OF THE HEMATOPOIETIC AND LYMPHATIC SYSTEMS

Gary P. Carlson, *Consulting Editor*

EVALUATION OF THE HEMATOPOIETIC SYSTEM *Joseph G. Zinkl and Gary P. Carlson*   293

BLOOD LOSS ANEMIA *Gary P. Carlson and Joseph G. Zinkl* 297

HEMOLYTIC ANEMIA   *Gary P. Carlson and Joseph A. Zinkl* 299

ANEMIA AS A RESULT OF INSUFFICIENT ERYTHROPOIESIS   *Bernard F. Feldman* 303

LYMPHOPROLIFERATIVE AND MYELOPROLIFERATIVE DISEASES   *Joseph G. Zinkl* 305

HEMOSTASIS   *Bernard F. Feldman* 306

DISSEMINATED INTRAVASCULAR COAGULATION   *T. D. Byars* 309

FLUID THERAPY   *Gary P. Carlson* 311

MEDICAL MANAGEMENT OF THE EXHAUSTED HORSE   *Gary P. Carlson* 318

IMMUNOLOGIC DISEASES   *Gary E. Rumbaugh and Alex A. Ardans* 321

BLOOD TRANSFUSION   *Paul G. Morris* 325

Section 7   NEUROLOGIC DISEASES

I. G. Mayhew, *Consulting Editor*

CEREBROSPINAL FLUID COLLECTION AND ANALYSIS   *Carolyn R. Beal
   and Ian G. Mayhew* 331

BEHAVIORAL ABNORMALITIES   *T. D. Byars* 335

HEAD TRAUMA   *Stephen M. Reed* 339

SEIZURE DISORDERS   *Ian G. Mayhew* 344

EASTERN EQUINE ENCEPHALOMYELITIS   *Julia H. Wilson* 350

WESTERN EQUINE ENCEPHALOMYELITIS   *Dean E. Goeldner* 352

SPINAL CORD TRAUMA   *Stephen M. Reed* 355

CERVICAL VERTEBRAL MALFORMATION   *Pamela Carroll Wagner* 359

EQUINE HERPESVIRUS-1 MYELOENCEPHALITIS   *Robert J. MacKay* 362

EQUINE PROTOZOAL MYELOENCEPHALITIS   *W. Kent Scarratt* 365

BOTULISM SYNDROMES: SHAKER FOALS AND FORAGE POISONING   *James P. Klyza* 367

POSTANESTHESIA MYOPATHY-NEUROPATHY   *N. A. White* 370

Section 8   OCULAR DISEASES

Gretchen M. Schmidt, *Consulting Editor*

APPROACH TO OPHTHALMIC PROBLEMS   *Gretchen M. Schmidt* 377

ADMINISTRATION OF OCULAR THERAPY   *Joyce M. Murphy* 378

RED, PAINFUL EYES (UVEITIS)   *Mary B. Glaze* 382

OCULAR DISCHARGE IN YOUNG HORSES   *Gay Wiles Senk* 385

CORNEAL OPACITIES   *Robert M. Gwin* 388

CATARACTS   *Dolores J. Kunze* 390

OCULAR FUNDUS AND CENTRAL NERVOUS SYSTEM CAUSES OF BLINDNESS
   Thomas J. Kern 393

Section 9   REPRODUCTION

A. C. Asbury, *Consulting Editor*

THE EFFECTS OF ARTIFICIAL LIGHTING ON REPRODUCTION   *Dan C. Sharp* 399

BEHAVIORAL ANESTRUS   *Jeffrey B. Grimmett* 400

PROLONGED DIESTRUS   *Steven D. Van Camp* 401

OVULATION INDUCTION   *Steven M. Hopkins* 402

CONTROL OF OVULATION   *Robert G. Loy* 404

PROGESTERONE THERAPY   *Dan L. Hawkins* 405

OVARIAN TUMORS   *Irwin K. M. Liu* 408

DISORDERS OF THE CERVIX   *George K. Haibel* 409

BACTERIAL ENDOMETRITIS   *A. C. Asbury* 410

PYOMETRA   *Irwin K. M. Liu* 414

CAUSES AND PREVENTION OF ABORTION   *Dean P. Neely* 415

OBSTETRICS   *Maarten Drost and A. C. Asbury* 422

RETAINED PLACENTA   *J. Pierre Held* 425

POSTPARTUM COMPLICATIONS   *Walter W. Zent* 428

PARTURIENT PERINEAL AND RECTOVESTIBULAR INJURIES   *Rolf M. Embertson* 431

INDUCTION OF PARTURITION   *Robert B. Hillman* 438

EVALUATION OF STALLION FERTILITY   *John P. Hurtgen* 442

DISORDERS AFFECTING STALLION FERTILITY   *John P. Hurtgen* 449

ARTIFICIAL BREEDING OF HORSES   *Wendell L. Cooper* 456

Section 10   RESPIRATORY DISEASES

N. E. Robinson, *Consulting Editor*

THE DIAGNOSIS AND TREATMENT OF COUGHING   *Gregory L. Ferraro* 463

ANTIMICROBIAL TREATMENT OF RESPIRATORY DISEASE   *Jill Beech* 467

EMERGENCY VENTILATION   *Thomas W. Riebold* 475

OXYGEN THERAPY   *Thomas W. Riebold* 478

SINUSITIS   *Dallas O. Goble* 481

GUTTURAL POUCH DISEASE   *David E. Freeman* 485

PHARYNGITIS   *Warwick M. Bayly* 490

SOFT PALATE DISPLACEMENT   *Dennis R. Geiser* 493

DISEASES OF THE EPIGLOTTIS   *Dennis R. Geiser* 494

LARYNGEAL HEMIPLEGIA   *Gordon J. Baker* 496

FOAL PNEUMONIA AND LUNG ABSCESSES   *W. L. Scrutchfield and R. J. Martens* 501

CHRONIC AIRWAY DISEASE   *Frederik J. Derksen* 505

SUMMER PASTURE–ASSOCIATED OBSTRUCTIVE PULMONARY DISEASE   *Ralph E. Beadle* ... 512

EXERCISE-INDUCED PULMONARY HEMORRHAGE   *John R. Pascoe* 516

LUNG PARASITES   *Hilary M. Clayton* 520

PLEURITIS   *Stephen M. Reed* 523

Section 11   SKIN DISEASES

A. A. Stannard, *Consulting Editor*

COMMON ECTOPARASITES AND THEIR CONTROL   *Edmond C. Loomis* 529

URTICARIA AND ANGIOEDEMA   *Richard C. Halliwell* 535

PAPILLOMATOSIS (WARTS)   *Gordon H. Theilen* 536

SURGICAL TREATMENT OF EQUINE SARCOID   *Murray P. Brown* 537

BCG THERAPY FOR EQUINE SARCOID   *Donald D. Flemming* 539

PEMPHIGUS FOLIACEUS *Thomas O. Manning* **541**

FOLLICULITIS AND FURUNCULOSIS *Danny W. Scott* **542**

NODULAR COLLAGENOLYTIC GRANULOMA (NODULAR NECROBIOSIS) *Craig E. Griffin* **545**

DISEASES OF ABNORMAL KERATINIZATION (SEBORRHEA) *Peter J. Ihrke* **546**

CONTACT DERMATITIS *Peter J. Ihrke* **547**

SCRATCHES *William C. McMullan* **549**

PHYCOMYCOSIS *William C. McMullan* **550**

HABRONEMIASIS *William C. McMullan* **551**

DERMATOPHILOSIS *Reginald R. R. Pascoe* **553**

SPOROTRICHOSIS *Paul Morris* **555**

ONCHOCERCIASIS *N. E. Robinson* **557**

SWEET OR QUEENSLAND ITCH (CULICOIDES HYPERSENSITIVITY) *N. E. Robinson* **558**

Section 12 URINARY TRACT DISEASES

Christopher M. Brown, *Consulting Editor*

EXAMINATION OF THE URINARY SYSTEM *Christopher M. Brown* **561**

RENAL DISEASES *M. A. Collier and Christopher M. Brown* **564**

BLADDER DISEASES *Christopher M. Brown and M. A. Collier* **567**

Section 13 TOXICOLOGY

F. W. Oehme and T. Tobin, *Consulting Editors*

TOXICOSES COMMONLY OBSERVED IN HORSES *Frederick W. Oehme* **573**

GENERAL PRINCIPLES IN TREATMENT OF POISONING *Frederick W. Oehme* **577**

INSECTICIDES *Frederick W. Oehme* **580**

RODENTICIDES *Frederick W. Oehme* **584**

SNAKE BITE *Frederick W. Oehme* **587**

BLISTER BEETLE POISONING *Frederick W. Oehme* **588**

CARBON TETRACHLORIDE *Frederick W. Oehme* **590**

PHENOTHIAZINE *Frederick W. Oehme* **590**

PETROLEUM PRODUCTS *Frederick W. Oehme* **591**

LEAD *Frederick W. Oehme* **592**

SELENIUM *Frederick W. Oehme* **593**

PLANT TOXICITIES *Ann A. Kownacki and Thomas Tobin* **595**

WATER QUALITY *Frederick W. Oehme* **607**

THE ETIOLOGIC DIAGNOSIS OF SUDDEN DEATH *Frederick W. Oehme* **611**

Section 14 APPENDICES

NORMAL CLINICAL PATHOLOGY DATA *J. D. Krehbiel* **619**

TABLE OF COMMON DRUGS: APPROXIMATE DOSES *N. Edward Robinson* **621**

AGING THE HORSE *N. Edward Robinson* **625**

INDEX **627**

Section 1
INFECTIOUS DISEASES
Edited by H. D. Knight

The content of this section was organized by Dr. Knight prior to his death.

EQUINE INFLUENZA 3

EQUINE HERPESVIRUS 4

EQUINE ADENOVIRUS 5

EQUINE RHINOVIRUS 6

EQUINE VIRAL ARTERITIS 6

EQUINE INFECTIOUS ANEMIA 7

RABIES 9

ROTAVIRUS INFECTIONS 11

VESICULAR STOMATITIS 12

EQUINE EHRLICHIOSIS 13

ACTINOBACILLOSIS 14

ANTHRAX 17

BRUCELLOSIS 19

MALIGNANT EDEMA 21

SALMONELLOSIS 22

STRANGLES 24

TETANUS 27

TUBERCULOSIS 29

ULCERATIVE LYMPHANGITIS 31

MYCOTIC DISEASES 32

BACTEREMIA 36

INTERNAL ABSCESSES 38

VACCINATION PROGRAMS 40

ANTIBIOTICS 43

ENDOTOXEMIA 57

EQUINE INFLUENZA

Irwin K. M. Liu, DAVIS, CALIFORNIA

Equine influenza is an acute infectious disease of the respiratory tract characterized by fever, depression, anorexia, and a hacking cough. Signs suggesting myalgia have also been reported. Variations in clinical signs are common, and often secondary complications may be the first presenting sign.

Two subtypes of equine influenza virus are recognized: A/Equi 1/Prague/56 and A/Equi 2/Miami/63. The virus noticeably affects two- and three-year-olds in training or where horses congregate, for example, sales, shows, and racetracks. Crowding and stress are often considered to be predisposing factors. Secondary complications include bronchopneumonia, myositis, and myocarditis. An association with chronic obstructive pulmonary disease has been suggested.

Diagnosis is based upon clinical signs and hemagglutination inhibition (HI) or serum neutralization (SN) tests. Isolation of the virus from nasal secretions constitutes a positive diagnosis, however; evaluation of acute and convalescent serum samples may also serve as confirmatory evidence of active infection.

TREATMENT

Complete rest for at least two weeks is necessary for an uncomplicated recovery. In cases in which fever is abnormally high (104° F or higher), antipyretics such as phenylbutazone, 4 mg per kg per day, or flunixin meglumine,* 1 mg per kg per day have been successfully used to reduce fevers. Aspirin (acetylsalicylic acid) 125 to 250 mg per kg, although effective, requires frequent doses in order to maintain its effectiveness in the horse. Expectorants, such as ethylene-diamine dihydriodide† at the rate of 0.5 to 1 ounce per animal per day, or glyceryl guaicolate‡ have been used to stimulate secretions of the respiratory epithelium. Use of expectorants is primarily palliative but in selected cases may be beneficial.

The routine use of antibiotics and combination antibiotic and corticosteroid preparations in uncomplicated influenza, while it may appear to be clinically effective, is not wise. This practice may lead to the development of an infection by resistant bacteria with no effect on the viral agent. Antibacterial therapy should be reserved for secondary bacterial

complications as a result of viral infections. The choice of antibacterial drugs should be made following transtracheal aspirations with growth and sensitivity tests of the isolated organism(s) from the aspirate.

The use of specific antiviral drugs against equine influenza virus is in the experimental phase of study. The successful use of amantadine in controlling replication of influenza virus before or as soon as possible after potential exposure to the virus lends promise to clinical application in the treatment of influenza in the horse. However successful, the use of antiviral drugs would not outweigh the benefits derived from prophylactic control of influenza through vaccination programs.

The most effective treatment for secondary complications resulting in myocarditis or myositis consists of complete "stall rest." The period of rest is contingent upon the severity of the complication. In most instances, one to two weeks are required for myositis complications, and four to six months are required for myocardial complications.

PREVENTION

Commercially prepared vaccines are available and contain antigens of the two subtypes. Most equine influenza vaccines consist of inactivated viruses, although isolated antigens (hemagglutinating and neuraminidase subunits) are sometimes utilized as vaccine preparations. The recommended vaccination program involves two primary injections four to six weeks apart followed by annual booster injections. Several studies indicate that adequate SN and HI titers result from vaccinations but fall to low levels within three to four months. If SN and HI titers are indicators of protection, vaccinated horses may need to be revaccinated every three to four months if continued protection is to be offered. Local secretory and cell-mediated responses to equine influenza have not been evaluated, particularly their roles in offering protection. It is likely that these immunologically mediated defense mechanisms also play important roles in immunity against influenza infections. The amount of exposure risk often determines the frequency of a vaccination program; i.e., horses with low exposure risk need not be vaccinated as frequently. Vaccination of asymptomatic horses during endemics or epidemics may be beneficial in controlling infections among susceptible populations.

The optimal period for initial vaccination of foals

*Banamine, Schering, Kenilworth, NJ
†Hi-Amine, Pitman-Moore, Washington Crossing, NJ
‡Robitussin, AH Robins Co, Richmond, VA

3

against influenza has not been determined. Most foals are vaccinated between the ages of two and six months.

Adverse reactions from immunizations are infrequent. Fever, malaise, and slight, localized swelling at the injection site may occur within 24 hours following vaccination. Reactions may persist for one to two days depending upon the vaccine product used and the sensitivity of the horse to the product. In all cases, horses should be rested for at least two days following vaccination. Normal activity can be resumed one week following vaccination.

References

1. Gabel, A. A., Heuschele, W. P., and Kohn, C. W. (eds.): Proceedings of 1980 Invitational Workshop on Equine Viral Respiratory Disease and Complications. Am. Assoc. Eq. Pract. Newsletter, 2:49, 1980.
2. Proceedings 4th International Conference Equine Infectious Diseases. J. Eq. Med. Surg. Suppl. 1. Vet. Publ., Inc., Princeton, NJ, 1978.

EQUINE HERPESVIRUS

Irwin K. M. Liu, DAVIS, CALIFORNIA

Three immunologically distinct types of herpesvirus are recognized in the horse and are designated as equine herpesvirus type 1 (EHV-1), type 2 (EHV-2), and type 3 (EHV-3).

EQUINE HERPESVIRUS TYPE 1
(Rhinopneumonitis)

EHV-1 is associated with three different clinical syndromes in the horse: respiratory, abortigenic, and neurologic.

RESPIRATORY FORM

This form is primarily associated with weanlings, yearlings, and two-year-olds. The disease is characterized by fever followed by a clear, yellow, mucoid discharge from the nostrils. Coughing and depression are rarely noticed; however, coughing becomes more apparent and productive when secondary complications occur. Secondary bacterial infections are inevitable with this viral infection with Streptococcus sp. being the most common bacteria involved. In older horses, although infection occurs and the virus multiplies, signs are usually not noted.

Treatment. In most instances, the respiratory difficulties caused by this form of EHV-1 will resolve in two weeks. In cases in which secondary bacterial complications produce a more chronic form of respiratory disease, antibacterial therapy is recommended based upon transtracheal aspiration and isolation of the bacterial agent(s).

Prevention. Two commercially available vaccines are currently being used to control the respiratory form of EHV-1 in young horses. The recommended protocol for use of the modified live virus preparation (Rhinomune)* begins with an initial immunization between three and four months, followed by a booster in four to eight weeks and semiannually until the horse reaches the age of two years or is no longer susceptible to a high risk of exposure. With the killed virus preparation (Pneumabort-K),* foals are immunized by the administration of two injections three to four weeks apart, with the second injection given about three weeks prior to weaning. Six months following the second dose, a booster injection is given followed by annual boosters thereafter.

ABORTIGENIC FORM

Following the infection of pregnant mares with EHV-1, clinical signs are not manifested for several weeks. Abortion of a virus-infected fetus (usually during the last trimester of pregnancy) or the birth of an EHV-1–infected foal that usually dies within hours after birth are the only signs of this form of EHV-1 infection. Although all susceptible pregnant mares in a herd may become infected with EHV-1, only a few will abort.

Treatment. There is no specific treatment for this form of EHV-1 infection.

Prevention. The killed virus preparation (Pneumabort-K) is the only available vaccine for the prevention of abortion in pregnant mares. For pregnant mares, vaccination at five, seven, and nine months of gestation is recommended. Revaccination annually during the same gestational periods is also recommended.

NEUROLOGIC FORM

This form of EHV-1 infection occurs in horses of various ages but primarily in horses over one year

---

*Rhinomune, Norden Labs, Lincoln, NB

*Pneumabort-K, Fort Dodge Labs, Fort Dodge, KS

of age. Posterior paresis, ataxia, and posterior paralysis may follow the respiratory and abortigenic forms of the disease or may occur spontaneously without any premonitory signs.

Treatment. Clinical evidence indicates that 10 mg of dexamethasone* or prednisolone at the rate of 400 to 500 mg per day orally or intramuscularly in an adult-sized horse for several weeks may be helpful if administered during the early stages of the disease. Since the effects of continuous administration of low-level corticosteroids on pregnant mares have not been determined, it is best to avoid their use in pregnant mares unless the mare's life is in jeopardy. For recumbent horses, a sling apparatus can be very useful if tolerated by the affected horse. It should be adjusted so that the horse can stand unassisted by the sling but should be supportive when needed. Good footing is imperative in all cases.

Prognosis for survival is favorable if the affected horse is able to stand and walk unassisted. Rarely is there complete recovery following treatment.

In conjunction with prophylactic immunization programs, every attempt should be made to isolate new arrivals and clinically ill horses from resident populations. In addition, every effort should be made to decrease stress in highly susceptible stock, particularly pregnant mares, weanlings, and yearlings.

EQUINE HERPESVIRUS TYPE 2

There is no known disease produced in horses by EHV-2 infections. Pharyngeal follicular hyperplasia and keratoconjunctivitis superficialis have been re-

*Azium, Schering, Kenilworth, NJ

ported to be associated with EHV-2; however, further investigations are needed to substantiate these findings.

EQUINE HERPESVIRUS TYPE 3 (Coital exanthema)

Equine coital exanthema is a venereally transmitted disease caused by EHV-3. It occurs in the mare and the stallion with lesions appearing initially as small (1 to 3 mm) vesicles on the epithelial surfaces of the vulva or the penis. The vesicles ulcerate and cause scabbed-over erosions and persist for about two weeks. EHV-3 infections do not appear to have any effects on fertility in the stallion or conception in the mare if copulation and ejaculation are complete. When the lesions are severe, copulation and ejaculation by the stallion may be inhibited.

Treatment. Antibacterial ointments, such as Furacin ointment, applied to the affected areas of the penis and vulva may be useful in preventing severe secondary bacterial infections and may also act as an emollient. Sexual rest is the most effective treatment, as continual irritation through copulation delays spontaneous recovery and enhances transmission of the virus to susceptible mares.

References

1. Gable, A. A., Heuschele, W. P., and Kohn, C. W. (eds.): Proceedings of the 1980 Invitational Workshop on Equine Viral Respiratory Disease and Complications. Am. Assoc. Eq. Pract. Newsletter, 2:49, 1980.
2. Proceedings of the 4th International Conference on Equine Infectious Diseases. J. Eq. Med. Surg. Suppl. 1., Vet. Publ., Inc., Princeton, NJ, 1978.

EQUINE ADENOVIRUS

Irwin K. M. Liu, DAVIS, CALIFORNIA

Equine adenovirus, although ubiquitously found in horses of all ages and all breeds, is not generally considered to be a disease-producing agent. In combined immune deficiency (CID) in Arabian foals, adenovirus occurs with bacteria and *Pneumocystis carinii* in the immunologically compromised host.

Diagnosis of equine adenovirus infection in the horse includes viral isolation, hemagglutination inhibition, serum neutralization, and fluorescent antibody technique on nasal and conjunctival smears.

No commercially prepared vaccines or reports of the treatment of adenovirus infection in the horse

are available. Prevention of secondary adenoviral complications in CID-affected foals with hyperimmune adenovirus antisera has been tried. Its effect has not been determined.

Reference

Gabel, A. A., Heuschele, W. P., and Kohn, C. W. (eds.): Proceedings of the 1980 Invitational Workshop on Equine Viral Respiratory Disease and Complications. Am. Assoc. Eq. Pract. Newsletter, 2:49, 1980.

EQUINE RHINOVIRUS

Irwin K. M. Liu, DAVIS, CALIFORNIA

Three antigenically distinct equine rhinoviruses (ERV) are recognized: ERV-1, ERV-2, and ERV-3.

Although rhinoviruses frequently infect horses without producing clinical signs, some investigators claim they cause severe pharyngitis and serous to mucopurulent nasal discharge with a fever lasting for one to two days, or a transient fever without any visible respiratory distress. A cause-and-effect relationship of equine rhinovirus and follicular hyperplasia has also been suggested. Evidence to support these claims is lacking.

Diagnosis of ERV infection in horses requires isolation of the virus and serum neutralization techniques.

There is no known treatment for ERV infections in the horse. Symptomatic treatment previously described for other viral diseases affecting the respiratory tract may be beneficial if secondary bacterial complications occur (p. 3). "Stall rest" for at least one week and isolation from other horses may prove helpful if ERV infection is suspected.

There are no commercial vaccines available for ERV infection.

Reference

Gabel, A. A., Heuschele, W. P., and Kohn, C. W. (eds.): Proceedings of the 1980 Invitational Workshop on Equine Viral Respiratory Disease and Complications. Am. Assoc. Eq. Pract. Newsletter, 2:49, 1980.

EQUINE VIRAL ARTERITIS

Leroy Coggins, RALEIGH, NORTH CAROLINA

Equine viral arteritis (EVA) is a contagious viral infection of horses that serologic studies reveal is much more common than the observed clinical disease. Certain equine populations have shown serologic reactivity as high as 75 to 80 per cent.

At least one strain of virus is highly fatal, but the majority of field viruses appear to be relatively avirulent and result in subclinical infections. Clinical disease is not commonly diagnosed but has occurred in epidemic form among horses at racetracks and in pregnant mares on farms, resulting in severe abortion storms. Recovery from infection stimulates a lifelong immunity. As yet, however, a commercial vaccine is not available, so control is accomplished through management of horses to reduce exposure to the virus.

CLINICAL SIGNS

Acute clinical disease is characterized by fever and serous nasal discharge, which in mild cases is not unlike equine influenza, rhinopneumonitis, and other respiratory infections. In more severe cases, there is conjunctivitis, palpebral edema, dyspnea, generalized weakness, depression, anorexia, colic, diarrhea, loss of weight, and dehydration. Affected animals may also exhibit keratitis, photophobia, and edema of the lower abdomen, legs, mammary gland, scrotum, and sheath. Clinical signs are extremely variable. Although some strains of the virus are highly fatal when injected experimentally, mortality is negligible in natural outbreaks. Abortion usually occurs during or shortly after the febrile period. Central nervous system disturbance is a less constant sign. Signs result from lesions caused by viral damage in the media of small arteries and venules, which leads to thrombus formation and necrosis of the surrounding areas.

DIAGNOSTIC AIDS

Diagnosis in individual cases may not be possible because of the mildness or absence of characteristic signs. In these instances, one may have to rely on confirmatory tests such as virus isolation or neutralization tests on several horses.

Nasal swabs and washings can be used in an attempt to isolate the virus in a tissue culture. For reasons that are not obvious, it appears that the virus can be isolated more readily by first transfusing blood from the suspect horse into a susceptible horse and then attempting virus isolation from the inoculated animal. The spleen is reported to be a reliable source of the virus. A fourfold increase in neutralizing antibody in convalescent serum is diagnostic of infection.

The history associated with the abortion may strongly suggest EVA. Abortion occurs during or shortly after the febrile illness, and the fetus shows no specific lesions or inclusions, as are usually found with equine rhinopneumonitis abortion. A panleukopenia occurs concurrently with fever; lymphocyte counts are more severely depressed than neutrophil counts.

THERAPY

There is no specific treatment; thus, each animal must be treated symptomatically. Recovered animals develop a long-standing immunity and have few or no aftereffects. Antibiotics and sulfonamides have no effect on the course of the viral infection but may be helpful in preventing secondary bacterial infection. Absolute rest for three to four weeks after clinical signs disappear is essential, and a gradual return to work with careful husbandry is essential for a favorable recovery.

PREVENTION

An experimental vaccine has been developed that promotes a solid immunity but as yet has not been produced commercially, apparently because of inadequate demand for the product. Preventive measures, therefore, are based on an interruption of the spread of the virus by good hygienic measures and isolation of infected horses during the infectious period (presumably the first four to six weeks after infection). New additions to a herd should be isolated for several weeks, and movement of horses on a farm involved in an epizootic should be avoided for four to six weeks after the last clinical case. It is thought that stallions may spread the virus via semen during the febrile and early convalescent periods. However, the most common means of spread is more likely to be by contact with respiratory secretions from recently infected horses.

The virus has characteristics of the RNA togavirus, which is enclosed by a lipid envelope and thus is susceptible to common disinfectants and detergents.

References

1. Burki, F.: Further properties of equine arteritis virus. Arch. Gesamte Virusforsch., *19*:123, 1966.
2. Crawford, T. B., and Henson, T. B.: Immunofluorescent, light-microscopic and immunologic studies of equine viral arteritis. Proceedings of the 3rd International Conference on Equine Infectious Disease, Karger, Basel, 1973, p. 282.
3. McCollum, W. H., Prickett, M. E., and Bryans, J. T.: Temporal distribution of equine arteritis virus in respiratory mucosa, tissues and body fluids of horses infected by inhalation. Res. Vet. Sci., *12*:459, 1971.
4. McCollum, W. H., and Bryans, J. T.: Serological identification of infection by equine arteritis virus in horses of several countries. Proceedings of the 3rd International Conference on Equine Infectious Disease, Karger, Basel, 1973, p. 256.

EQUINE INFECTIOUS ANEMIA

Leroy Coggins, RALEIGH, NORTH CAROLINA

Equine infectious anemia (EIA) is a retrovirus infection of horses and other Equidae. The disease is usually observed as an acute clinical infection but tends to become a subclinical infection with time and good care. The infected horse, however, has infectious leukocytes circulating in its bloodstream indefinitely.

DIAGNOSTIC AIDS

It is usually not difficult to make a diagnosis of acute EIA on the basis of recurrent febrile episodes that do not respond to antibiotic therapy and the presence of typical clinical signs of anemia, depression, loss of weight, and edema. A history of sudden death of a horse on pasture with other horses that then develop clinical disease is often an indication that an epizootic of EIA has occurred. Fever is usually the first sign of infection, and transmission takes place rapidly during the fly season.

Horses with subacute or chronic infections may have greatly enlarged spleens that are palpable by rectal examination. Such animals may also have extensive edema of the lower thorax and abdomen, sheath, and legs.

Animals in the subclinical phase of EIA may have a recrudescence of clinical signs following the administration of corticosteroids. A dosage of 5 mg per kg body weight of dexamethasone* given intra-

---

*Azium, Schering Co., Kenilworth, NJ

muscularly for five days will usually cause infected animals to become febrile and develop signs of EIA within seven days after initiation of the treatment.

A decrease in circulating platelets occurs commonly in EIA-infected horses and is closely associated with fever spikes. The number of platelets returns to normal rapidly as the fever recedes. The severity of anemia varies greatly, and the packed cell volume may become extremely low before the animal dies. There may be an increase in circulating monocytes, and some of these may contain hemosiderin. A hypergammaglobulinemia is primarily composed of class G immunoglobulins.

A biopsy examination of the liver may reveal its involvement in this infection. In acute cases, fatty degeneration, necrosis without cellular reaction, and incomplete focal necrosis of hepatic cells may be found. In cases of longer-standing involvement, infiltrations of histiocytic cells containing hemosiderin granules may be found in sinusoids. Sideroleukocytes and cells having phagocytized erythrocytes may be found in the central vein and/or sinusoids.

An examination of puncture fluids from a splenic biopsy may show the presence of basophilic round cells or small lymphoid cells.

The clinical diagnosis of EIA should be confirmed with the agar gel immunodiffusion (AGID) test. This test is capable of detecting all infected animals except those in the early incubation period, the first two to three weeks after infection. A horse suspected of being exposed should be retested after four to six weeks. Foals that have been nursed by infected mares may be temporarily positive in the AGID test but if not infected should be negative by six months of age.

Other serologic tests have not as yet been generally accepted for the diagnosis of EIA. The AGID is an accurate indicator of infection because of the large amount of precipitating antibody produced rapidly by infected horses. Unfortunately, the AGID test does not measure the degree of risk involved for the transmission of EIA from an individual horse.

Serologically positive horses remain infected indefinitely and are potential transmitters of the infection, but epidemiologic data suggest that the chance of transmission increases greatly when a horse is showing clinical signs and has a high titer of circulating infectious virus in its bloodstream. As yet, however, there is no satisfactory way quantitatively to measure the virus or its antigens in the blood of the infected horse.

THERAPY

No specific treatment is available, and one must rely on general supportive therapy and symptomatic treatment. Infected horses, especially those that are clinically ill, are ready sources of infection for other horses and therefore should be considered for immediate euthanasia or should be isolated in screened stalls.

Horses that recover rapidly and spontaneously may live relatively normal lives with little probability of spreading the infection to other horses, if they are isolated from other horses during the fly season and are not used for breeding purposes.

General supportive therapy should include resting the horse in a comfortable stable with no exposure to adverse environmental conditions and other infections. A good nutritious diet will help horses to return to normal weight. Mineral and vitamin preparations may aid in treatment of the anemia. Corticosteroids or other immunosuppressive treatments are contraindicated in this disease. Such drugs tend to result in a relapse of clinical illness and death of the infected animal. During the clinical phase, such an animal would more likely be a transmitter of the EIA infection.

PREVENTION

There is no safe and efficacious vaccine for EIA. The detection of numerous strains and the possibility of antigenic variation of the virus in the infected horse have diminished prospects of developing a satisfactory vaccine.

The control of horseflies, the principal mechanical vector of EIA virus, is extremely difficult because of their resistance to insecticides and their flight habits. These flies avoid enclosed barns in which insecticides would be most effective. Thus, screening of stables that house the infected horses is the only practical approach to this problem.

Since EIA may be spread by any transfer of blood, one must avoid contaminated equipment or disinfect it before using it on several horses. One should be especially careful with equipment that may cause skin or mucosal abrasions or absorb secretions or excretions, such as lip tatoos, dental floats, and stomach tubes. Disposable hypodermic needles or equipment cleansed with a detergent and sterilized by boiling in water or in an autoclave should be used. Multiple-dose vials of drugs and vaccines, if contaminated, may retain viable EIA virus in the refrigerator for months and perhaps years. Blood transfusions, which are a very effective means of transmitting EIA, should be made only after careful selection of donor blood.

The blood of an infected horse remains infectious throughout its lifetime, and such an animal should be considered a possible source of EIA infection. Serologically positive horses should be isolated from other horses, especially during the summer months to prevent transmission by blood-sucking insects. It is not recommended that infected horses be used for breeding, primarily because of the possibility of infection of the fetus or newborn foal and the risk that the foal may spread the infection to other foals or horses via horseflies. Clinically ill mares almost always infect their foals. Foals out of infected mares should be isolated from other horses until freedom of infection can be established by allowing for loss of maternal antibody, which may require as long as six months.

References

1. Coggins, L., Norcross, N. L., and Nusbaum, S. R.: Diagnosis of equine infectious anemia by immunodiffusion test. Am. J. Vet. Res., 33:11, 1972.
2. Ishii, S., and Ishitani, R.: Equine infectious anemia. Adv. Vet. Sci. Comp. Med., 19:195, 1975.
3. McGuire, T. C., and Crawford, T. B.: Immunology of a persistent retrovirus infection—equine infectious anemia. Adv. Vet. Sci. Comp. Med., 23:137, 1979.
4. Nakajima, H., Suguira, T., and Ushimi, C.: Immunodiffusion test for the diagnosis of equine infectious anemia. J. Eq. Med. Surg., Suppl. 1:339, 1978.

RABIES

Larry C. Booth, ST. PAUL, MINNESOTA

Rabies is a relatively rare disease in the horse. Since 1970, the Center for Disease Control in Atlanta, Georgia has reported from 18 to 52 confirmed cases in the United States annually. In Minnesota, the number of confirmed cases reported by the Minnesota Health Department averages approximately two per year. Even with the low prevalence in horses, the potential for human exposure makes it imperative to consider rabies in any peripheral or central nervous system disorder of the horse.

ETIOLOGY

Rabies is caused by a neurotropic rhabdovirus. The virus is readily killed by most detergents and disinfectants, including 40 to 70 per cent alcohol, povidone-iodine, tincture of iodine, and the quaternary ammonium compounds.

In the United States, rabies is primarily propagated by skunks, foxes, raccoons, insectivorous bats, and unimmunized domestic dogs. The skunk is an important vector in the Midwest and Southwest; fox rabies is prevalent in the Appalachian region from New England to the South Atlantic States and into Tennessee and Kentucky. Raccoon rabies is a growing problem in the Southeastern States, including Florida, Georgia, North Carolina, South Carolina, southeastern Alabama, and southern Virginia.

PATHOGENESIS

The virus is transmitted through saliva by the bite of an affected animal or contamination of an open skin wound with infective saliva. Following inoculation, the virus will remain for variable periods of time at the point of introduction before migrating centrally through the axoplasm of the peripheral nerves to the brain and spinal cord. Here the virus replicates almost exclusively in the gray matter. Dissemination of the rabies virus within the body then occurs through centrifugal migration by way of the cranial nerves and to a lesser extent the peripheral nerves. The extent and time course of the dissemination is variable. Concentration of the virus in saliva is the result of its ability to replicate within the secretory cells of the salivary gland.

The incubation period in the horse is believed to be similar to most other animal species, from three to six weeks, rarely as long as six months. The variability of the incubation period reportedly depends on the site of inoculation, with bites to the head and neck leading to a shorter incubation period than wounds more distally removed from the brain. Probably of greater significance is the anatomic nerve distribution. The head and neck has a relatively more dense plexus of nerve endings, which may aid the neurotropic virus in establishing itself.

CLINICAL SIGNS

Diagnosis of equine rabies can be difficult owing to the broad spectrum of clinical signs. The classical descriptions of furious and paralytic forms of the disease can be misleading. The most important guideline is to *think rabies first* when dealing with any unexplainable clinical syndrome.

Hyperesthesia is a strongly suggestive sign of the disease. It is present to some degree in a majority of cases. Skin mutilations are also prominent findings in animals with rabies and appear to be the result of a viral-induced neuritis. Hyperexcitability, ataxia, paresis, paralysis, and behavioral changes should all be viewed with the suspicion of rabies. Nonspecific symptoms such as depression, anorexia, and pyrexia may be present. Of paramount importance in the clinical recognition of rabies is the rapid progression of the disease, with most cases becoming terminal within five days.

Differential diagnoses to be considered include (1) tetanus, (2) equine herpesvirus 1 infection, (3) eastern, western, and Venezuelan equine encephalomyelitis, (4) botulism, (5) lead poisoning, (6) moldy corn poisoning, (7) cerebrospinal nematodiasis, (8) cervical spondylotic myelopathy, (9) equine degenerative myeloencephalopathy, (10) equine protozoal myeloencephalitis, and (11) certain plant poisonings such as yellow star thistle or Russian knapweed. The diagnosis of rabies can be confirmed by submitting the intact head or intact brain, under refrigeration, for examination by a laboratory designated by the local or state health department. Local health officials should be consulted regarding specific recommendations for the preparation and shipment of specimens. The person handling the carcass of a suspected rabid animal should use rubber gloves.

Laboratory procedures include the fluorescent antibody test performed on impression smears from the brain, as well as intracerebral inoculation of weaned mice with brain tissue. The presence of Negri bodies upon histologic search, although pathognomonic, is not a consistent finding.

PREVENTION OF RABIES AND MANAGEMENT OF THE EXPOSED HORSE

Immunization can be recommended for any valuable horse in an endemic area. The only vaccine currently approved for horses by the National Association of State Public Health Veterinarians in its 1981 Compendium is the Porcine Cell Line Origin, High Cell Passage, SAD strain.* Vaccination should begin at four months of age with a booster dose given annually.

---

*ERA Strain Rabies Vaccine, Jensen-Salsbery Laboratories, Kansas City, MO 64141

Management of potential exposure to rabies should begin with an epidemiologic investigation by the attending veterinarian in cooperation with local health officials to assess the potential risk to the horse(s) involved. The presence of a vector species, or confirmed rabid animal, on the premises accompanied by a recent wound to the horse constitutes sufficient evidence for exposure.

Managing the exposed horse depends on the circumstances and the reliability of the owner or handler. Not all exposed animals will develop rabies. There appears to be a definite quantitative threshold of virus necessary to establish infection. Therapy is directed at reducing the size of the inoculum through wound management. All such wounds should be treated by wide excision débridement followed by thorough cleansing and copious lavage with povidone-iodine. Wounds should not be sutured.

If the horse has been previously immunized against rabies, an immediate prophylactic booster dose with an approved vaccine may be justified. If the horse has not been previously immunized, postexposure immunization cannot be recommended because it may complicate the course of the disease by delaying the incubation period or modifying the clinical signs. In addition, there are no data to substantiate the safety or effectiveness of postexposure prophylactic immunization in the horse.

Strict quarantine and careful observation for six months are mandatory in all cases. If signs suggestive of rabies develop, the animal should be humanely destroyed and the intact head or intact brain submitted for diagnosis.

Supplemental Readings

1. Blood, D. C., Henderson, J. A. and Radostits, O. M.: Veterinary Medicine, 5th ed. Philadelphia, Lea & Febiger, 1979.
2. Gillespie, J. H., and Timoney, J. F.: Hagan and Bruner's Infectious Diseases of Domestic Animals, 7th ed. Ithaca, NY, Cornell University Press, 1981.
3. Joyce, J.R., and Russell, L. H.: Clinical signs of rabies in horses. The Compendium on Continuing Education for Practicing Veterinarians, 3:556, 1981.
4. Rabies prevention. Morbidity and Mortality Weekly Report, 29:265, 277, 1980.

ROTAVIRUS INFECTIONS

Bradford P. Smith, DAVIS, CALIFORNIA

Rotavirus infections have been recognized as a cause of diarrhea in 12 species of mammals, including horses. The virus typically causes neonatal diarrhea, which is clinically impossible to differentiate from that which is caused by other agents. Differentiation and definitive diagnosis of rotavirus diarrhea is based on either fluorescent antibody techniques, ELISA tests, electron microscopy, or isolation of the virus in cell culture. Because the virus is present in highest titer in the feces during the initial stages of the disease, it is important that samples be submitted to the diagnostic laboratory from foals that have had diarrhea for only a day or two.

Foals may be affected from a few days of age up to several months of age. The mortality rate in foals over two weeks of age is low (2 per cent in two outbreaks) but has been reported to be considerably higher in affected foals that are less than 14 days old. The disease may have a high morbidity rate in some outbreaks. Adult horses appear to act as one source of infection, and they may occasionally exhibit signs of diarrhea. The stool of affected foals is watery with a greenish-yellow to grayish-green color. Fever (up to 105° F) is present in most affected foals during the initial stages of disease. Once dehydration and other changes occur, fever may no longer be present. Depression is greatest in the foals with the highest rectal temperature.

Hematologic findings are not specific. In two reported outbreaks, none of the foals had a leukopenia or a lymphopenia, but several had a leukocytosis and neutrophilia. This may reflect secondary involvement with bacteria or bacterial toxins because of the damaged bowel. Concurrent infections with other pathogens such as Salmonella have been reported.

THERAPY

Therapy for diarrhea in foals is similar regardless of the cause. It is very likely that many outbreaks of diarrhea involve multiple etiologies. Therapy must often be initiated prior to receipt of laboratory results, but the clinician should always remember to take fecal and blood samples for diagnostic purposes prior to the initiation of treatment. It must also be kept in mind that most of what is recommended is either empirically derived or derived by interpolation from calves and other species in which rotavirus diarrhea has been more extensively studied.

Rotaviruses appear to attack mainly mucosal cells in the small intestines. The differentiated cells on the tips of villi are lost, resulting in stunting of the villi. These cells are responsible for digestion and absorption of lactose and other disaccharides, so that their destruction results in these sugars passing into the lower bowel. Bacterial fermentation of sugars in the lower bowel results in osmotic changes that prevent adequate water absorption in the colon and contribute further to the development of the diarrhea.

Therapy is aimed mainly at (1) preventing and correcting dehydration, electrolyte losses, and acid-base abnormalities, as in any neonatal diarrhea (p. 311); (2) decreasing the oral intake of disaccharides while attempting to supply some energy source; (3) preventing bacteremia and excessive growth of bacteria in the gut by administration of antimicrobial drugs. No specific therapeutic measures are currently in use against rotavirus infections.

Adequate volumes of fluids should be given intravenously to severely dehydrated foals, while oral fluids may be adequate in only slightly dehydrated foals. The fluids should contain glucose, bicarbonate, sodium, potassium, and chloride. There are commercial preparations available that possess the desired ingredients, or one can prepare fluids. Such fluids may also be beneficial orally, particularly if the foal is withheld from suckling the mare (in which case the mare must be milked out by hand). The rationale for not allowing the foal to suckle the mare for 36 to 48 hours is that lactose digestion is not occurring efficiently in the scouring animal, and the continued ingestion of milk may allow the diarrhea to continue or even to worsen. Antimicrobial drugs should be used with the recognition that repeated use in many animals on a farm may lead to the development of resistance, particularly if the antimicrobials are given orally. There is some indication that antimicrobial drugs may be of benefit in reducing the severity of viral diarrhea. Studies in calves have indicated that the disease syndrome produced by rotavirus is less severe in gnotobiotic calves than in calves with normal bacterial flora.

Intestinal protectants, adsorbants, antipyretics, antiprostaglandin drugs, mineral oil, and vitamins have been advocated by some as additional modes of therapy, but these have not proven beneficial in controlling neonatal foal diarrhea in the author's experience.

Some affected foals develop unformed stools that last from 2 to 18 months. Treatment does not alter the character of the feces in this chronic phase of the disease.

PREVENTION

Little research has been performed regarding prevention of rotavirus diarrhea in foals. There appears to be poor cross-protection in calves inoculated with foal or human rotaviruses and subsequently challenged with calf rotavirus, and a calf rotavirus vaccine was not effective in protecting colostrum-deprived piglets when they were challenged with swine rotavirus. Nevertheless, there are reports from uncontrolled field trials that vaccination of foals with an oral modified live calf rotavirus vaccine was effective in decreasing the occurrence of foal diarrhea on some farms.

In the face of an outbreak, all ill foals should be kept isolated from newborn animals. Moving mares for foaling to a part of the ranch not yet contaminated by sick foals may help to control the spread of the disease. Common-sense sanitation and disinfection with agents such as Clorox are also helpful. Vaccination of prepartum mares and newborn foals with calf rotavirus vaccines may be attempted, but the value of such a procedure has yet to be documented.

Supplemental Readings

1. Eugster, A. K., and Whitford, H. W.: Concurrent rotavirus and salmonella infections in foals. J. Am. Vet. Med. Assoc., *173*:857, 1978.
2. Flewett, T. H., Bryden, A. S., and Davies, H.: Virus diarrhea in foals and other animals. Vet. Rec., *96*:477, 1975.
3. Woode, G. N., Bew, M. E., and Dennis, M. J.: Studies on the cross protection induced in calves by rotaviruses of calves, children, and foals. Vet. Rec., *103*:32, 1979.
4. Scrutchfield, W. L., Eugster, A. K., Abel, H., and Ward, J. E.: Rotavirus infections in foals. Proceedings of the 25th Annual Convention of the American Association of Equine Practitioners, 1979, p. 217.

VESICULAR STOMATITIS

Irwin K. M. Liu, DAVIS, CALIFORNIA

Vesicular stomatitis virus (VSV) affects horses, cattle, and swine. Two distinct types of VSV have been reported in the United States: Indiana and New Jersey types. A third type antigenically related to the Indiana type has been isolated in Trinidad and Brazil and has been designated the Cocal type. All three types have been isolated from horses.

In horses, the disease is characterized by inflammation of the mucosa of the mouth and tongue with formation of vesicles 2 to 3 mm in diameter. Fever with depression and anorexia also occurs. On occasion, the vesicles may be present on the feet, the mammary glands of lactating mares, or on the prepuce of male horses. In severe cases the horse may be unable to eat, and in many instances the horse is presented with an edematous head with blood-tinged, frothy saliva.

The vesicular fluid is generally a clear or yellow serous fluid. Following rupture of the vesicles, denuded plaques appear. Recovery occurs in three to nine days unless the lesion present is complicated by secondary bacterial infection.

Transmission of VSV is believed to be via the Phlebotomus sandflies.

Diagnosis of VSV is based upon viral isolation or complement fixation and serum neutralization tests. Inoculation of experimental animals may also serve as a diagnostic tool.

TREATMENT AND CONTROL

Vesicular stomatitis in horses is a reportable disease. All affected horses must be quarantined, and strict isolation procedures should be enforced. Nitrofurazone (Furacin) ointment applied with a gloved hand to ruptured vesicles outside the mouth serves as an antibacterial agent and may also serve as an emollient. Soft feed and fresh water should be provided. No vaccines are commercially available.

Reference

Hanson, R. P.: Vesicular stomatitis. *In* Catcott, E. J., and Smithcors, J. F. (eds.): Equine Medicine and Surgery, 2nd ed. Wheaton, IL, American Veterinary Pub., 1972, pp. 57–63.

EQUINE EHRLICHIOSIS

John E. Madigan, UKIAH, CALIFORNIA

Equine ehrlichiosis (EE) is a seasonal rickettsial disease of horses observed chiefly in California. The organism was first identified in California in 1968. Since then EE has been observed in Colorado and Illinois. The disease was initially believed to be of low incidence, but it is not uncommon in northern California during the fall, winter, and early spring. Increased awareness of the disease and the method of diagnosis have accounted for the increase in the numbers of clinical cases.

CLINICAL SIGNS

The severity of the clinical signs of EE is a function of the age of the animal and the duration of illness. In horses less than one year old, the signs are quite mild and are limited to fever. Horses one to three years old develop a fever, depression, mild limb edema, and ataxia. Horses over three years of age show the characteristic signs of fever, partial anorexia, depression, limb edema, petechiation of the nasal septal mucosa, and reluctance to move. During the first one to two days of infection, fever is quite high and fluctuates from 103 to 107° F. The ataxia can be severe, with the horse assuming stances in which the elbows and hoofs touch the ground with the rear quarters elevated. Staggering is always seen, and the ability to place the feet out wide from the body leads one to suspect proprioceptive deficits. Heart rate is elevated to 50 to 60 per minute. A partial anorexia occurs with the horse eating some hay but preferring green grass.

As the disease continues for three to seven days, other signs develop, including icterus, petechiation, severe limb edema, reluctance to move, and severe depression. The limbs are often painful to the touch, and the horses can show reluctance and difficulty in lying down. Any concurrent infection such as a leg wound shows an exaggerated inflammatory response. Concurrent respiratory conditions that were mild or believed controlled are exacerbated at this time.

PATHOGENESIS

The mode of transmission and the incubation period are not known. In all cases, ticks have either been present or the horse has been exposed to ticks at the time of illness. The disease is not contagious. More than one case at a time has not been observed in groups of up to 50 horses in similar pasture conditions. Mortality in untreated animals given sup-

portive therapy is low. One fatality has occurred of 40 clinical cases treated. Death was due to concurrent bacterial pneumonia. Pregnant mares have not aborted because of the disease.

The hematologic changes are leukopenia, thrombocytopenia, elevated plasma icterus index, decreased packed cell volume, and inclusion bodies in the neutrophils. The leukopenia is only seen in the early stages of the disease, with a lymphopenia preceding the neutropenia. The increase in icterus corresponds to the decreasing packed cell volume. The thrombocytes decrease on about the third day of illness, and the decrease precedes the limb edema. Elevation of serum glutamic-oxaloacetic transaminase (SGOT), bilirubin, and sorbitol dehydrogenase (SDH) indicates a moderate degree of liver damage.

The exacerbation of minor infections during the disease leads one to suspect that the horse's immune system is compromised during an infection.

DIAGNOSIS

The diagnosis of equine ehrlichiosis is conclusively made only when the characteristic cytoplasmic inclusion bodies in neutrophils are seen in a standard blood smear. The organism is difficult to see except under oil immersion and is not readily seen in the early stages of the disease. Twenty to thirty minutes of scanning the blood smear are often required to observe a definitive inclusion body. Inclusions are pleomorphic, blue-gray to dark blue in color, and often have a spoke wheel–type appearance. More than one inclusion body in a cell is common. After 48 hours' duration of infection, inclusions are more readily seen in approximately 30 to 50 per cent of neutrophils.

Diagnosis requires an awareness of the sequential evolution of signs as well as changes in laboratory data. Differential diagnoses include viral encephalitis, primary liver disease, leptospirosis, equine infectious anemia, purpura hemorrhagica, and viral arteritis. When complicated by concurrent bacterial infection of the respiratory tract, EE must be differentiated from influenza or other primary respiratory disease.

TREATMENT

Horses definitively diagnosed as having EE should be treated with oxytetracycline* at a dose of

---

*Oxyvet Injection, Rachelle Laboratories, Inc., Long Beach, CA

7 mg per kg once daily intravenously. A prompt decrease in temperature occurs within 12 to 24 hours. Treatment is continued for a total of seven days by either daily oxytetracycline injections or oral oxytetracycline* following an initial 48 hours of intravenous treatment to lower the temperature and improve the appetite. A dose of 20 mg per kg of oxytetracycline is given twice daily for the oral treatment. No adverse effects due to tetracycline therapy have been noted in 40 cases.

A prompt improvement is noted in the degree of alertness within 12 hours of treatment. Ataxia persists for two to three days, and limb edema often persists for several days. Horses seen early in the disease and treated before edema is noted will still often develop swelling. Inclusion bodies are difficult to find after the first day of treatment and are no longer present within 48 to 72 hours of treatment.

Supportive measures include maintaining fluid and electrolyte balance, which can be done through oral therapy. Leg wraps are helpful to reduce the degree of limb edema. Confinement of severely ataxic horses may be necessary to prevent secondary physical injury. No antipyretics are needed owing to the rapid decrease in temperature provided by oxytetracycline. Corticosteroid therapy in the initial stages may help to lessen the degree of edema and possibly the ataxia. A dose of dexamethasone† (0.02

*Vetquamycin-324, Rachelle Laboratories, Inc., Long Beach, CA

†Azium, Schering Corp., Kenilworth, NJ

mg per kg per day) is adequate. Treatment with steroids beyond 48 hours is not needed. The possibility of concurrent infection should influence the decision to use steroids. The presence of a concurrent infection must be viewed as a serious complication, and appropriate therapy must be instituted for even a minor infection. Laminitis has not occurred in any cases and is not a feature of the untreated disease in experimental cases.

Horses identified as having EE early in the course of the disease and treated for less than seven days may relapse within one to two weeks. Penicillin, chloramphenicol (Chloromycetin), and streptomycin have no inhibitory effect on *Ehrlichia*. Sulfamethazine and cycloserine have some inhibitory effect but significantly less than oxytetracycline. Immunity to EE lasts at least two years.

The prognosis in EE is considered excellent in uncomplicated cases. This is in sharp contrast to the other diseases on the list of differential diagnoses, and it stresses the importance of an accurate diagnosis. A minimum of three weeks' rest is indicated after infection.

Supplemental Readings

Gribble, D. H.: Equine ehrlichiosis. *In* Catcott, E. J., and Smithcors, J. F. (eds.): Equine Medicine and Surgery, 2nd ed. Wheaton, IL, American Veterinary Pub., Inc., 1972, pp. 114–117.
Gribble, D. H.: Equine ehrlichiosis. J. Am. Vet. Med. Assoc., *155*:462, 1969.

ACTINOBACILLOSIS

Frederik J. Derksen, EAST LANSING, MICHIGAN

Actinobacillosis (shigellosis) is a highly fatal septicemic disease of newborn foals. The etiologic organism, *Actinobacillus equuli*, also occasionally causes abortion in mares and septicemia and peritonitis in mature horses.

EPIDEMIOLOGY

Actinobacillus equuli is a small, non–spore-forming, gram-negative rod. The organism is ubiquitous in the horse's environment and has been isolated from fecal material and pharyngeal cultures. In the past, actinobacillosis was a major cause of foal mortality, as up to 30 per cent of foal deaths occurring in the first week of life were attributed to *Actino-*

bacillus equuli septicemia. At present the disease in foals is sporadic and accounts for less than 2 per cent of foal mortality.[2] Since the organism is ubiquitous in the newborn foal's environment and since so few animals contract the disease, *Actinobacillus equuli* can be regarded as an opportunist, affecting stressed foals or foals with a compromised immunodefense system. Thus, prematurity, overcrowding, malnutrition of the dams, failure of passive transfer of immunoglobulins, and cold or wet environments may predispose a foal to Actinobacillus septicemia. Because some foals are born with clinical signs of septicemia and die shortly after birth, prenatal infection has been postulated. The source of this infection is obscure, as uterine cultures rarely yield the organism. Since enteritis is the most consistent early sign of the disease in newborn foals, the route of

TABLE 1. DIFFERENTIAL DIAGNOSIS OF THE WEAK NEONATE

Condition	Synonym	Predominant Clinical Signs	Pathogenesis	Therapy	Prognosis	See Page No.
Infectious Diseases						
Septicemia caused by *Escherichia coli*, Streptococcus sp, Staphylococcus sp, *Actinobacillus equuli*, Salmonella sp	Sleepy foal syndrome; joint ill	First week of life; fever and lethargy; reduced suck reflex; diarrhea; death in 24 hours	Organisms ubiquitous in environment; infection occurs in stressed foals, e.g., overcrowding, cold, prematurity, failure of immunoglobulin transfer or absorption	Broad-spectrum antimicrobial therapy *E. coli*—gentamicin, 2.0 mg/kg IM tid Streptococci—penicillin, 20,000 units/kg IM bid Staphylococci—kanamycin, 5 mg/kg IM tid Actinobacillus—gentamicin, 2.0 mg/kg IM tid Salmonella—gentamicin 2.0 mg/kg, IM tid Note: When using aminoglycosides in foals, renal function must be monitored.	Guarded	14, 22, 24, 36
Equine herpes virus 1		First week of life; respiratory distress; weakness; failure to nurse	Prenatal equine herpes virus 1 infection	None	Grave	4
Noninfectious Conditions						
Neonatal maladjustment syndrome	Barkers; convulsives; dummies	First 24 hours; respiratory distress; failure to nurse; aberrant behavior, e.g., chewing, blindness, aimless wandering, convulsions, opisthotonos	Birth hypoxia or trauma to CNS at birth; premature severance of the umbilical cord leads to brain injury	Symptomatic, including adequate restraint, force feeding, warm, safe environment, intravenous fluids	Guarded	
Prematurity, less than 325 days' gestation		Low birth weight (less than 45 kg for Thoroughbreds)	Fetal stress or endocrine disturbances	Provide a clean, warm, low-stress environment and supportive therapy	Favorable if gestation longer than 300 days	
Ruptured bladder		Frequent straining with passage of small amounts of urine; lethargy and failure to nurse; more common in colts	Incomplete closure of dorsal bladder wall; may also be caused by trauma	Surgical repair	Favorable	568
Neonatal isoerythrolysis	Isoimmune hemolytic anemia	First or second day; lethargy, frequent yawning; jaundice; red urine	Isoantibodies produced by the dam are passed to foal via the colostrum	Whole blood transfusion with cross-matched blood if erythrocyte count is less than $3 \times 10^6/\mu l$; prevent nursing and provide artificial milk	Favorable if detected early	321
Congenital cardiac defects		Dyspnea; heart murmurs; cyanosis; weakness	May be inherited	Surgical intervention could be attempted	Grave	146

infection is probably by ingestion, although entry via the umbilicus is also possible.

In older horses, *Actinobacillus equuli* infection is rare but has been reported to cause peritonitis, septicemia, and abortion. Usually these animals were stressed by malnutrition or parasitism.[3] The source and route of infection in older horses are unknown.

CLINICAL SIGNS

Actinobacillosis in foals is characterized by an acute fulminating and fatal septicemia within the first week of life. Affected foals may be weak, sleepy, or comatose at birth and die within 24 hours. These foals may never stand and do not nurse. Others are normal at birth but become ill within a week. Illness is characterized by depression, fever, anorexia, diarrhea, and hyperpnea. Signs of abdominal pain may also be observed. Terminally ill foals become comatose. In foals that survive the acute phase of the disease, arthritis with swollen joints and lameness is commonly observed.

Actinobacillosis in the adult horse is usually acute and is characterized by depression, fever, anorexia, difficulty in swallowing, and cardiovascular shock. Acute and chronic peritonitis have also been reported.[4]

PATHOLOGY

A severe enteritis is the most consistent lesion in foals that die within 24 hours after onset of clinical signs. Adrenal glands are often hemorrhagic. Foals succumbing two or three days after the onset of clinical signs have a characteristic purulent nephritis with small abscesses scattered throughout the renal cortex. When joints are affected, lesions range from a slight increase in synovial fluid to purulent arthritis involving the joint cavity and tendon sheaths. In rare cases, pleuropneumonia may also be present.[5]

DIAGNOSIS

Definitive diagnosis of neonatal foal diseases is difficult, as clinical signs of a variety of neonatal conditions are similar. Table 1 gives a list of differential diagnoses of the weak equine neonate and provides a basis for distinction between infectious and noninfectious conditions. This distinction needs to be made on the basis of clinical signs and will determine the course of therapy. Fever and diarrhea with leukocytosis or leukopenia suggest septicemia, while aberrant behavior, heart murmurs, or red-colored urine without fever or diarrhea and a normal

white blood cell count suggests a noninfectious etiology. There are practically no clues to differentiate between actinobacillosis and septicemia caused by *Escherichia coli*, Salmonella sp, Streptococcus sp, or Staphylococcus sp.

In the adult horse, diagnosis is based on culture of the organism from peritoneal fluid or blood cultures.

THERAPY

Since the course of the disease in foals is acute, there is usually no time for bacterial isolation and sensitivity testing. Therefore, the early administration of high levels of broad-spectrum antibiotics likely to be effective against the invading organism is essential for a favorable outcome. Gentamicin, 2.0 mg per kg intramuscularly three times a day, is usually effective against *Actinobacillus equuli*. However, aminoglycosides are nephrotoxic, and, therefore, renal function (blood urea nitrogen and serum creatinine) should be monitored in foals receiving gentamicin therapy. Since actinobacillosis cannot be distinguished from the more common streptococcal septicemia and since streptococci are often resistant to gentamicin, penicillin is used in combination. Initially, sodium penicillin, 80,000 IU per kg, should be administered intravenously every four hours to achieve high blood levels, followed by intramuscular procaine penicillin G, 20,000 IU per kg twice a day. If any doubt exists about the adequacy of colostrum intake by the newborn foal, 1 liter of compatible plasma should be transfused. Additional supportive measures include force feeding via a nasogastric tube, maintaining a quiet, clean, and dry environment, and fluid and electrolyte therapy. In the later stages of the disease when joints are affected, flushing with saline and antibiotic solutions may prevent chronic arthritis and lameness.

CONTROL

The incidence of septicemic conditions in foals may be reduced by careful management. Mares should deliver in the environment in which they have been residents for the month prior to foaling. Foals should be born in clean environments, and handlers should practice strict hygiene in all procedures in which infections could be introduced through the oral or umbilical routes. Although prophylactic antibiotics are commonly administered to the equine neonate, efficacy of this practice has not been substantiated. Instead, strict attention should be paid to adequate intake of good-quality colostrum, preferably within three hours of birth.

References

1. Dimak, W. W., Edwards, P. R., and Bruner, D. W.: Infections observed in equine fetuses and foals. Cornell Vet., 37:89, 1947.
2. DuPlessis, J. L.: The histopathology of Shigella viscosum equi infection in newborn foals. J. S. Afr. Vet. Med. Assoc., 34:25, 1963.
3. Gay, C. C., and Lording, P. M.: Peritonitis in horses associated with Actinobacillus Equuli. Aust. Vet. J., 56:296, 1980.
4. Vander Molen, E. J.: Een ondersoek naar de bacteriele oorsaken van de neonatale mortaliteit by het veulen. Tydschr. Diergeneesk., 104:165, 1979.
5. Zakapal, J., and Nesvadba, J.: Aktinobacillare Septikamie die Massenerkrankung in einer Zuchtstuten hede. Zbl. Vet. Med., 15A:41, 1968.

ANTHRAX

Mortimer Cohen, DAVIS, CALIFORNIA

Anthrax is an infectious disease caused by *Bacillus anthracis* and is characterized by septicemia and toxemia. The course in domestic animals is usually acute and rapidly fatal.

The infection is usually acquired by ingestion of spore-contaminated forage, especially tough, scratchy feed, which can abrade the oral mucosa. Confined grazing on heavily contaminated areas around water holes can also predispose animals to infection. There are also substantiated cases of mechanical transmission of anthrax by blood-sucking arthropods and by fomites.

Outbreaks in grazing animals occur primarily during the warmer seasons when the minimum daily temperature is above 16° C (60.8° F). Documented cases have occurred in midwinter, however. Epizootics tend to occur following periods of climatic change such as heavy rains following periods of drought. The organism is not normally found in soil with a pH of less than 6.

Upon ingestion of spores, infection may occur either through intact mucous membranes or through abraded mucosa. After entry, motile phagocytes carry the bacteria to local lymph nodes, where they proliferate and subsequently pass via the lymphatics to the bloodstream, resulting in a septicemia. The toxin produced by this bacteria causes edema and tissue damage. Death results from shock and acute renal failure.

CLINICAL SIGNS

Several syndromes are recognized in horses: acute, subacute, and chronic. The acute infection may be characterized by fever up to 107° F followed by a period of excitement that merges into depression, respiratory distress, stupor, staggering, convulsions, coma, and death within 48 hours. The subacute syndrome, which can persist up to eight days, frequently is manifested as a severe colic. The spleen is enlarged and can be palpated rectally, hemorrhages may be seen on mucous membranes, and there may be muscle rigidity. Hot, painful, rapidly progressing swelling may develop on the neck and lower abdominal region. Dyspnea, cyanosis, and coma ensue, and blood may exude from body openings. An infrequently encountered chronic form involves the tongue and pharynx. Local edema and bleeding from the mouth or nose may cause death due to suffocation. A few animals will recover, but the infection may persist in regional lymph nodes.

DIAGNOSIS

Diagnosis may be difficult in areas where the disease is not endemic. Anthrax certainly should be suspected when animals die suddenly in or near areas where the disease has appeared previously. Close questioning may be necessary, as stored spores have remained viable for as long as 60 years. The differential diagnoses should include sudden death due to lead poisoning, sunstroke, lightning stroke, malignant edema, purpura hemorrhagica, and colic.

In live animals, the organism may be detected in Wright- or Giemsa-stained smears of peripheral blood or edema fluid. Blood can be submitted as a dried specimen on a sterile swab, on a small piece of sterile cotton umbilical tape, or on slides. On examination of stained smears, *B. anthracis* will appear as single or short-chained bacilli with blunted ends. The important distinguishing feature is the presence of a capsule around the bacillus. In early cases, blood culture or injection of samples into guinea pigs is necessary for diagnosis. It is not advisable to open the carcass of suspicious cases, as the organisms present can then sporulate and become a focus of infection for years. Great care must be taken in handling of all samples from any suspect case, either living or dead. Blood or edema fluid samples from recently dead animals can be collected and submitted, carefully packed, to a laboratory. Tissue specimens other than dried blood should be shipped under refrigeration or frozen. Fluorescent antibody procedures can also be used diagnostically.

TREATMENT

Potassium or sodium penicillin G, administered intravenously at a dose of 50,000 to 100,000 units per pound (100,000 to 220,000 units per kg) divided into four daily doses may be effective in the earlier stages of the disease. This can be followed in three to four days by procaine penicillin G (30,000 units per pound, 65,000 units per kg intramuscularly, divided into two daily doses). Streptomycin (8 to 10 mg per lb, 20 to 25 mg per kg intramuscularly divided into two daily doses) has been reported to be highly effective in cattle. Oxytetracycline (3 to 5 mg per lb, 8 to 12 mg per kg intramuscularly or intravenously divided into two daily doses) has also been reported to be highly effective in cattle. The best choices are penicillin and streptomycin administered concurrently, or oxytetracycline. The simultaneous use of penicillin and oxytetracycline is contraindicated. Treatment should be continued for seven days. Although it is not commercially available in the United States, anthrax antiserum has been recommended at a daily dose of 100 to 250 ml intravenously for five days.

CONTROL

Hygiene is the single most important factor in preventing spread of the disease. Contaminated fomites, bedding, and manure should be destroyed or buried. Carcasses should be burned or buried at a depth of 2 meters and covered with quicklime (calcium oxide). A 3 per cent peracetic acid solution or a 10 per cent formaldehyde solution should effectively sterilize contaminated pasture. The former product appears not to be readily available in the United States. The area should be quarantined, and local regulatory and public health officials should be notified. Exposed animals should be isolated and closely observed, and antibiotic therapy should be instituted at the first sign of fever or any other suspicious findings. Contaminated clothing may be disinfected by soaking in a 10 per cent formaldehyde solution, and shoes may be sterilized using ethylene oxide.

PREVENTION

There are four commercially available vaccines on the market: Anthrax Vaccine,* Sternvac,† Anvax,‡ and Thraxol-Z.§ These Sterne-strain vaccines are administered subcutaneously. Directions on the manufacturer's label should be closely followed, as there is some variation in initial dose and boosters. Immunity is usually achieved about seven days after administration. Clients should be advised that these vaccines are not without side effects. Swelling is common, and some animals may become quite depressed and febrile. Analgesics such as phenylbutazone (1 gm intravenously every 12 hours) may be used, but antibiotics are contraindicated, as they will nullify the effects of the vaccine. Rest for 7 to 10 days after vaccination is recommended, and it is preferable not to vaccinate in hot weather.

References

1. Blood, D. C., Henderson, J. A., and Radostits, O. M.: Veterinary Medicine: A Textbook of the Diseases of Cattle, Sheep, Pigs and Horses, 5th ed. London, Bailliere Tindall, 1979, pp. 433–436.
2. Kaufmann, A. F., Fox, M. D., and Kolb, R. C.: Anthrax in Louisiana, 1971: An evaluation of the Sterne strain anthrax vaccine. J. Am. Vet. Med. Assoc., *163*:442, 1973.
3. Kaufmann, A. F.: Anthrax. *In* Howard, J. L. (ed.): Current Veterinary Therapy: Food Animal Practice. Philadelphia, W. B. Saunders Co., 1981, pp. 677–679.
4. Knight, H. D.: Anthrax. *In* Catcott, E. J., and Smithcors, J. F. (eds.): Equine Medicine and Surgery, 2nd ed. Wheaton, IL, American Veterinary Pub., Inc., 1972, pp. 101–103.

---

*Anthrax Vaccine, Colorado Serum Co., Denver, CO
†Sternvac, Haver-Lockhart, Shawnee, KS
‡Anvax, Jensen-Salsbery, Kansas City, MO
§Thraxol-Z, Bayvet-Cutter, Oakland, CA

BRUCELLOSIS

John E. Peel, DAVIS, CALIFORNIA

Brucella abortus has been recognized as a cause of disease in horses for many years. The prevalence of disease and the number of horses with high antibody titers to *Brucella abortus* is greater in rural horse populations than in urban ones. Eradication of brucellosis from cattle populations around the world has brought about a concurrent decrease in the incidence of equine brucellosis. These facts, together with reports of specific clinical cases having close contact with affected herds of cattle, lead to the belief that horses most commonly become infected from cattle.

Natural infection is most likely due to ingestion of infected material, though entry to the body could occur through skin wounds and abrasions. Many horses appear to have a latent infection manifested by the presence of positive brucella agglutination titers in the absence of clinical signs. Serologic surveys show numbers of horses varying from 2 to 15 per cent of populations to have positive agglutination titers; these are large numbers compared to those showing signs of active disease. The number of such horses varies depending upon the type and class of horse included in the survey and the criteria used to define a positive titer.

CLINICAL SIGNS

A generalized form of disease is recognized, with affected animals showing signs of depression, fever that fluctuates intermittently, muscle stiffness, and reluctance to move. These nonspecific signs must be coupled with rising antibody titers in order to make a diagnosis of brucellosis.

Equine brucellosis has also been associated with fistulous withers and poll evil. The organism has an apparent predilection for synovial structures, resulting in localized pain and swelling. The signs manifested in this type of infection are dependent on the structure involved. The most common sites affected are the supraspinous and atlantal bursae, giving rise to fistulous withers and poll evil, respectively. The reason for the frequent involvement of these sites is poorly understood, but an association with *Onchocerca cervicalis* infection has been made. *Actinomyces bovis* has frequently been cultured from these lesions along with *Brucella abortus.* Swelling of these bursae causes considerable pain and will result in reluctance to move the head and neck. These swellings ultimately fistulate, and the exudate that drains from them is typically copious and purulent. Once opened, these lesions are readily colonized by secondary bacteria, and so culture from lesions at this stage will yield a variety of organisms. If left untreated, such lesions commonly heal over but invariably recur, and the course of the disease is protracted and can lead to a situation in which there are multiple draining tracts at the affected sites.

Bursae and tendon sheaths in the limbs are sometimes infected with Brucella, and there are reports of joints being affected. The severity and nature of the resulting lameness is obviously dependent upon the site of the affected structure and the degree of inflammation present. The lameness typically is of an intermittent type, though even during periods of apparent remission the affected structure is still distended. Many diagnoses of this type of disease have been made on serologic grounds alone, but positive cultures from limb bursae, sheaths, and joints have also been made.

Brucella abortus has been isolated from an abscess in the vertebral column of a horse showing signs of weight loss, stiffness of the neck, and signs of involvement of local nerves.

There are reports of positive Brucella cultures from aborted fetuses, though this cannot be considered an important cause of abortion in horses.

There is one report of infertility in a stallion associated with *Brucella abortus.*

DIAGNOSIS

Diagnosis of brucellosis in horses is made tentatively on a history of association with cattle and the presence of clinical signs consistent with the disease. Confirmation of the diagnosis requires either the demonstration of rising antibody titers or a positive identification of the organism by culture.

Serologic surveys done on normal horses show low titers of antibodies to *Brucella abortus* to be common even in horses that have had no history of contact with the disease. Most authors agree that an agglutination titer greater than 1:40 is indicative of exposure to infection. However, the use of paired serum samples taken two weeks apart is the most accurate means by which to make a serologic diagnosis; fourfold or greater increases in titer indicate recent exposure.

Agglutination titers have been shown to be less reliable and less sensitive indicators of disease in the horse than complement fixation and Coombs' tests, so all three serologic tests should be performed in animals in which brucellosis is suspected.

TREATMENT

Brucella organisms are sensitive to a number of antibacterial agents in vitro, most notably to tetracyclines, chloramphenicol, streptomycin, and trimethoprim and sulfadoxine in combination. However, results of treatment of clinical cases with these preparations have been uniformly disappointing apart from the stallion mentioned earlier, which improved after treatment with 7 gm of chloramphenicol daily for 21 days. Semen quality improved, as did the conception rates in mares covered by the stallion, and the large numbers of leukocytes and Brucella organisms present in the semen prior to treatment disappeared.

The disappointing results of antibiotic therapy in other cases of equine brucellosis is probably due to the intracellular habitat favored by the organism, which renders it inaccessible to antibacterial agents. Antimicrobial drugs that achieve some intracellular levels, such as chloramphenicol and trimethoprim-sulphas, are recommended.

Many authors have treated horses with brucellosis with brucella vaccines, and good results have been claimed for this mode of therapy. Both killed vaccines and the live strain 19 vaccine have been used. A positive diagnosis must be made before vaccination is resorted to, and the dangers to public health should be considered if a draining wound is present. One author[2] advises the use of a single dose of strain 19 vaccine for the treatment of limb-associated bursal and sheath disease. The dose varies from 2 ml for a Thoroughbred yearling to 5 ml for an adult horse. This should be given subcutaneously in an aseptic manner; and the area should be massaged for several minutes after administration in an attempt to minimize the risk of abscess formation at the injection site. Vaccinated horses undergo a severe febrile reaction that begins within 12 hours and is associated with increased pulse and respiratory rates, injected mucous membranes, patchy sweating, and pawing with the forefeet. Complete loss of appetite is seen for 24 hours, and intense inflammation is present at the injection site between 24 and 48 hours. Local abscesses sometimes occur as a complication. Some improvement in horses treated by this method is expected in seven days, but complete resolution takes three weeks.

Another author[7] treated cases of fistulous withers by vaccination with three doses of strain 19 vaccine. The amount given varied from 5 ml in ponies to 8 ml in fully grown horses. The injections were made subcutaneously and were given at 10-day intervals. A similar reaction to that described previously was noted, and resolution of the problem occurred in the four cases described.

Use of the British Ministry of Agriculture equine Brucella vaccine has been reported.[4] This is prepared from strains of *Brucella abortus* isolated from cases of fistulous withers and poll evil and is a killed vaccine. Two or three doses are given at 10-day intervals. A local reaction is seen that increases in severity at each injection, and good claims are made for its efficacy.

It is interesting to note that in one case treated with this vaccine, the Brucella antibody titers fell rather than rose as might have been expected with such a treatment. Before use of Brucella vaccines, one should first be familiar with local regulations regarding its use in horses.

If these methods of treatment fail, then cases of fistulous withers and poll evil must be treated by surgical means[8] whereby the lesion is excised and all tracts are thoroughly curetted. In advanced cases, this can involve the removal of large quantities of tissue, and the difficulty in instituting ventral drainage leads to a prolonged recovery period.

It should be reemphasized that because of the danger of brucellosis to public health, adequate measures to protect personnel handling affected horses must be taken. This is particularly important where lesions are draining and discharges contain Brucella organisms.

PREVENTION

Minimizing contact between horses and affected cattle is the principal means of prevention.

References

1. Collins, J. D., Kelly, W. R., Twomey, T., Farrelly, B. T., and Whitty, B. T.: Brucella associated vertebral osteomyelitis in a Thoroughbred mare. Vet. Rec., 88:321, 1971.
2. Cosgrove, J. S. M.: Clinical aspects of equine brucellosis. Vet. Rec., 73:1377, 1961.
3. Dawson, F. L. M., and Durant, D. S.: Some serological reactions to Brucella antigen in the horse. Equine Vet. J., 7:137, 1975.
4. Denny, H. R.: Brucellosis in the horse. Vet. Rec., 90:86, 1972.
5. Denny, H. R.: A review of brucellosis in the horse. Vet. J., 5:121, 1973.
6. McCaughey, W. J., and Kerr, W. R.: Abortion due to brucellosis in a Thoroughbred mare. Vet. Rec., 80:186, 1967.
7. Millar, R.: Disease of the ligamentum nuchae associated with *Brucella abortus* infection in the horse, and its treatment with strain 19 vaccine. Br. Vet. J., 117:167, 1961.
8. Vaughn, J. T.: Physical restraint. *In* Catcott, E. J., and Smithcors, J. F. (eds.): Equine Medicine and Surgery, Wheaton, IL, American Veterinary Pub., 1972, pp. 690–709.

MALIGNANT EDEMA

Mortimer Cohen, DAVIS, CALIFORNIA

Malignant edema is an acute, frequently fatal disease caused primarily by *Clostridium septicum,* although *C. perfringens* and *chauvoei* have also been occasionally isolated. The usual mode of infection is through abrasions or lacerations of the skin. Iatrogenic introduction via injections with contaminated needles or poor surgical technique is known to occur. Castration is mentioned as a fairly frequent cause. Infection of the genitalia during parturition is also described.

Signs of infection appear within 12 to 48 hours after infection. The local site of involvement is marked by soft, doughy swelling, pain, and heat. Pitting edema is common. Subcutaneous emphysema and putrid odors are not necessarily present. The lesion spreads rapidly and is often marked with a gelatinous exudate. A blood-tinged fluid may ooze from the wound or may be aspirated. The animals are depressed, weak, lame, or stiff and generally have high fevers (104 to 107° F). Mucous membranes are often muddy, and capillary refill time is substantially prolonged.

Microscopic examination and cultural identification of organisms obtained from the wound can aid in diagnosis, but one should not wait for culture results before instituting therapy. A Gram stain of exudate should demonstrate chains of long, grampositive rods with rounded ends.

Diagnosis is based on history, physical examination, and microbiologic laboratory results.

THERAPY

Prompt treatment is essential in this potentially life-threatening disease. Wound care, systemic antibiotics, and supportive therapy are the main goals.

Wound Care. The wound should be opened, and all necrotic tissue and debris should be removed. Rigorous débridement is indicated, as necrotic tissue may allow continued elaboration of toxin. Following excision, intensive irrigation of the wound using large volumes of sterile saline or lactated Ringer's solution is recommended. The wounds are generally left open, although dressings are permissible if the wounds are in areas that are amenable to bandaging. Wounds that cannot be bandaged may be covered with topical antibiotics.

Systemic Antibiotics. Potassium or sodium penicillin G is the drug of choice. Intravenous therapy is recommended, as intramuscular injections appear not to be effective initially. The recommended dose is 25,000 to 200,000 units per lb (50,000 to 400,000 units per kg) divided into four daily doses. An av-

erage dose for a 1000 lb animal would be 15 million units every six hours for at least the first four days. Sodium ampicillin* at a rate of 20 to 100 mg per lb, (40 to 200 mg per kg)in four divided doses may also be used. After the first four days, if improvement is noted, therapy may be changed to 10,000 units per pound (20,000 units per kg) of procaine penicillin G intramuscularly every 12 hours. It is important to continue close monitoring of the patient, as some will start to regress following the switch to intramuscular antibiotics. Systemic antibiotics administered in massive amounts will be to no avail if proper wound management is not achieved.

Supportive Therapy. Careful monitoring of the animal's cardiovascular system is mandatory, as the toxins generally have a profound effect upon the body. Fluid sequestration and metabolic acidosis are not uncommon. Appropriate fluid therapy using a balanced lactated Ringer's solution and sodium bicarbonate in 5 per cent dextrose should be given as necessary. Secondary renal failure has occurred in patients without proper fluid replacement. Packed cell volume should be monitored, as toxin-induced hemolysis can occur. If possible, packed red cells or whole blood from compatible donors should be administered if a precipitous drop in the hematocrit indicates a life-threatening anemia.

Analgesics such as phenylbutazone (1 to 2 gm intravenously every 12 hours) or flunixin meglumine (500 mg intramuscularly or intravenously every 8 to 12 hours) are definitely indicated in this disease.

The use of steroids for treatment of shock in the face of toxemia is indicated. The dose should be 1 to 2 mg per kg of dexamethasone sodium phosphate intravenously. This may be repeated every three to six hours to effect.

The immunization status for tetanus should be ascertained in these animals. Tetanus antitoxin at a dose of 1500 units should be administered if the animal has not been previously vaccinated or if the animal has not been vaccinated within the past three to four years or if the history is unknown. If the vaccination status is current, a booster of tetanus toxoid is recommended. Although bacterins such as Clostri-Bac CSN† or C.C.S.N.S.‡ are available and effective, they are generally not used in horses because of the relative rarity of the disease. Prophylaxis is best achieved by aseptic surgical technique and the avoidance of contaminated needles.

---

*Penbritin, Beecham Labs, Bristol, TN
†Clostri-Bac CSN, Haver-Lockhart, Shawnee, KS
‡C.C.S.N.S., Dellen Labs, Omaha, NB

In conclusion, early and vigorous wound care and systemic antibiotics are the two most important components of successful treatment of malignant edema.

References

1. Blood, D. C., Henderson, J. A., and Radostits, O. M.: Veterinary Medicine: A Textbook of the Diseases of Cattle, Sheep, Pigs and Horses, 5th ed. Philadelphia, Lea & Febiger, 1979, pp. 445–447.
2. Knight, H. D.: Malignant edema. *In* Catcott, E. J., and Smithcors, J. F. (eds.): Equine Medicine and Surgery, 2nd ed. Wheaton, IL, American Veterinary Pub., 1972, p. 94.
3. Polk, H. C.: Gas gangrene and similar soft tissue anaerobic infections. *In* Conn, H. F. (ed.): Current Therapy. Philadelphia, W. B. Saunders Co., 1979, pp. 23–26.

SALMONELLOSIS

Bradford P. Smith, DAVIS, CALIFORNIA

Salmonella infections cause a variety of signs in the horse. Many veterinarians are most familiar with the acute diarrhea syndrome associated with enteric salmonellosis, which is discussed in detail in the gastrointestinal diseases section. In addition to the acute diarrhea syndrome, Salmonella also causes bacteremia and may localize in joints, resulting in septic arthritis (particularly in foals) or in localized sepsis in other body cavities or organs.

CLINICAL SIGNS AND DIAGNOSIS

The clinical signs associated with bacteremic salmonellosis vary greatly. Bacteremic foals are often febrile and have a rapid heart rate. Petechial hemorrhages may be present on the mucous membranes. The foal is usually weak, depressed, anorectic, and often in endotoxic shock. Peracute deaths may occur. Hematologic abnormalities include a neutropenia and sometimes a degenerative left shift. This change is not specific for salmonellosis and will occur with many gram-negative infections and other toxemias. Positive blood cultures using commercial trypticase soy broth blood culture bottles* inoculated with aseptically collected jugular blood are an aid in diagnosis. Three or more bottles should be inoculated over a period of time (approximately two to three hours apart) in order to increase the likelihood of finding a positive culture. These bottles are incubated at 37° C and are subcultured when visible growth (cloudiness) occurs or at 24 and 48 hours following inoculation. Initial bottle cultures and subcultures should be performed aerobically and anaerobically. Salmonella are relatively easy to isolate and can often be recovered by 24 hours either aerobically or anaerobically, but some other pathogens may be more fastidious. Isolation aids in

later treatment by allowing antimicrobial sensitivity testing to be performed.

Clinical signs in foals not dying acutely may include lameness and stiffness associated with septic arthritis in one or more joints. Infected joints usually have joint fluid that is watery, cloudy, and has poor mucin properties. Positive cultures from joints may occasionally be found, but blood or feces is more likely to yield Salmonella. Salmonella may also cause pneumonia, pleuritis, endocarditis, and septic nephritis. Occasionally it can be isolated in pure culture from localized abscesses.

In many foals, both enteric disease and bacteremia occur, so that death may occur very rapidly, and on postmortem exam typhlitis and colitis (involving mainly the proximal large colon) are the principal lesions found. Culture of organs and colonic and cecal contents will yield Salmonella if it is the causative organism. The organs most likely to yield a positive isolation are cecal and colonic lymph nodes and the cecal and colonic mucosa. In animals dying from bacteremia, most tissues are positive for Salmonella.

Horses may also act as asymptomatic carriers with or without fecal shedding of Salmonella. Fecal culture for Salmonella is relatively simple. An aliquot of fecal material should be placed in an enrichment medium such as selenite F or tetrathionate broth and incubated at 37° C. The size of the sample inoculated should be about 10 to 20 per cent of the volume of the enrichment medium. Subculture at 18 to 24 hours following inoculation onto an enteric medium such as brilliant green agar allows identification to proceed. Identification of a carrier horse through culture of the organism allows better disease control. Known shedders should be isolated. Treatment of carrier animals with antimicrobial drugs has been ineffective at eliminating the carrier state and thus is not recommended.

A clinical form of salmonellosis intermediate between the asymptomatic carrier and the acute diar-

---

*Trypticase soy broth with CO_2, Becton, Dickinson and Co., Rutherford, NJ

rhea and/or bacteremia forms also exists. In horses exposed to smaller doses or less pathogenic serotypes or in which other factors reduce disease severity, the clinical signs include fever, partial anorexia, and depression that last for a few days and then spontaneously improve. Some horses develop unformed cow-pat feces during the mild form of the disease.

THE ROLE OF STRESS

In addition to the virulence of the infecting serotype and the dose, the susceptibility of the individual horse plays a major role in determining whether or not a clinical disease state will ensue following exposure. Although it is possible to produce disease in healthy animals, under natural conditions salmonellosis usually strikes very young, debilitated, or stressed horses. Stresses such as prolonged shipping (particularly in hot weather), food deprivation, general anesthesia and surgery, or a major medical problem are most commonly associated with severe, usually enteric, salmonellosis. Stresses seem to act by altering the gut flora and thus reducing competitive inhibition and by suppressing immune functions.

TREATMENT

In formulating appropriate treatment for horses affected with salmonellosis, the clinician must consider the form of Salmonella infection present. Attempts to eliminate the asymptomatic shedding of Salmonella in feces by treatment with antimicrobial drugs have been largely unsuccessful. Therapy in horses with acute diarrhea is aimed in large measure at correction of fluid, electrolyte, and acid-base abnormalities through intravenous fluid therapy (p. 311). Large volumes of fluids are also a useful therapeutic mode in horses with Salmonella bacteremia and endotoxic shock. These individuals are suffering from poor peripheral circulation, lactic acidosis, and neutropenia (which makes them more susceptible to bacteremia). Thrombocytopenia, hypoglycemia, and many other metabolic aberrations also occur in some animals with endotoxemia (p. 57).

Antimicrobial drugs are of most benefit in treating or preventing bacteremic salmonellosis. Many pathogenic Salmonella strains are resistant to commonly used antimicrobial drugs. Based on antimicrobial sensitivity testing, it has been found that most of the equine Salmonella isolates are currently resistant to penicillin, streptomycin, neomycin, tetracycline, and sulfas. Some isolates have been resistant to ampicillin and the newer aminoglycosides, including kanamycin, and one recent Salmonella isolate was resistant to gentamicin and trimethoprim-sulfa and sensitive only to amikacin. Several chloramphenicol-resistant strains have also been documented. It is therefore imperative that culture and antimicrobial susceptibility testing be performed, so that the clinician may alter the original regimen if necessary.

The most appropriate antimicrobial drugs for initial treatment of suspected salmonellosis are either chloramphenicol or trimethoprim-sulfa. Chloramphenicol is given at a dose of 25 to 50 mg per kg every six hours. The initial dose should be given intravenously in order to establish blood levels. Follow-up doses are often given orally at the same dose level, but in the critically ill patient with a catheter in place, continued intravenous therapy is indicated. Trimethoprim-sulfa is given orally or intravenously at a dose of 4.0 mg per kg of the trimethoprim every 12 hours. The usual ratio of trimethoprim to sulfadiazine is 1 to 5. The third and fourth choice drugs would be gentamicin given intramuscularly at a dose of 1 to 2 mg per kg every six hours or ampicillin given intravenously at a dose of 25 mg per kg every six hours. The use of potentially nephrotoxic aminoglycoside such as gentamicin for prolonged periods in animals with compromised renal function should be carefully monitored. Chloramphenicol or trimethroprim-sulfa combinations are considered the drugs of choice because few resistant strains of Salmonella currently exist and because Salmonella are capable of living within macrophages and other cells where they are shielded from many antimicrobial drugs. Chloramphenicol and trimethoprim-sulfas probably achieve better intracellular levels than do drugs such as gentamicin.

Other forms of therapy are indicated in animals with evidence of endotoxemia. The nonsteroidal anti-inflammatory antiprostaglandin drugs (such as phenylbutazone and flunixin meglumine) are beneficial in experimental endotoxemia if given as a pretreatment. Their value in horses already suffering from endotoxic shock has not been documented. Corticosteroids in antishock doses are indicated if the horse is worsening or is in a serious condition that is not reversed promptly by plasma volume expansion with intravenous fluids. Corticosteroid therapy should not replace fluid therapy. The proper dosage for corticosteroids in treating endotoxic shock in the horse has not been determined, but based on interpolation from other species, a dose of 1 mg per kg or greater of dexamethasone or its equivalent is indicated. This may be repeated as needed every 12 hours, depending on the half-life of the steroid used. Antimicrobial therapy does not appear to markedly affect the course of diarrhea and intestinal disease caused by Salmonella, but it does treat or prevent bacteremia and aid in eliminating Salmonella localized in other areas of the body.

Local therapy, such as joint lavage with buffered saline or Ringer's solution and drainage of pleural effusions or other affected localized areas, is very important and should not be neglected. In young foals, the possibility that the foal did not absorb sufficient colostral immunoglobulin should be examined, and deficient individuals should be given intravenous plasma therapy.

CONTROL

The control of salmonellosis on a farm is based on (1) isolation of sick animals and shedding animals that have been identified by fecal culture, (2) elimination of stresses and crowding, especially in hot weather, (3) disinfection of the environment and boots of individuals moving about the farm or hospital, and (4) daily monitoring, via rectal temperatures and neutrophil counts, of animals coming down with disease so that they may be treated before severe illness develops.

Effective disinfectants include the phenolics,*† formaldehyde (2 per cent), nolvasan, and sodium hypochlorite (bleach at a ¹⁄₃₂ dilution). Phenolics

---

*Kerol Disinfectant, Jensen-Salisbery, Kansas City, MO
†One-Stroke-Environ, Vestal Labs, St. Louis, MO

may be the most effective for farm circumstances, but regardless of what disinfectant is used, a thorough cleaning to remove organic material before its use is mandatory.

The value of vaccination using killed bacterins is not proven, but in several uncontrolled clinical trials some benefit (decreased foal morbidity and mortality) has been attributed to bacterins given to the mare. Local swellings and sometimes adverse systemic reactions are often associated with Salmonella vaccines, and they should be used carefully. No commercial vaccines designed for use in horses are available. The clinician should rely for control principally on sanitation and the other aspects of control discussed before.

Supplemental Readings

1. Morse, E. V., Duncan, M. A., Page, E. A., and Fessler, J. F.: Salmonellosis in Equidae: A study of 23 cases. Cornell Vet., *66*:198, 1976.
2. Mahaffey, L. W.: *Salmonella typhimurium* in foals in western Australia. Aust. Vet. J., *28*:8, 1952.
3. Smith, B. P.: Atypical salmonellosis in horses: Fever and depression without diarrhea. J. Am. Vet. Med. Assoc., *175*:69, 1979.
4. Smith, B. P., Reina-Guerra, M., Hardy, A. J., and Habasha, F.: Equine salmonellosis: Experimental production of four syndromes. Am. J. Vet. Res., *40*:1072, 1979.
5. Smith, B. P.: Salmonella infections in horses. Compendium on Cont. Education, *3*(1):54, 1981.

STRANGLES

Gordon J. Baker, URBANA, ILLINOIS

Strangles is an acute upper respiratory disease of young horses characterized by inflammatory changes in the respiratory mucosa, mucopurulent nasal discharge, and abscess formation in the mandibular or retropharyngeal lymph nodes or both.

BACTERIOLOGY

The causal organism, *Streptococcus equi*, is well recognized but in many aspects is poorly understood. *S. zooepidemicus* is also commonly isolated from strangles abscess discharges. Both organisms give wide zones of hemolysis when cultured on blood agar, and serologic examination classifies them as members of Lancefield's group C. *S. equi* ferments salicin but not lactose, sorbitol, or trehalose. *S. zooepidemicus* ferments sorbitol and lactose but not trehalose.

S. zooepidemicus is readily isolated from the respiratory tract of normal horses, whereas the evidence for the existence of an *S. equi* carrier state is unclear. Woolcock[8] was unable to isolate the organism from the respiratory tract of wild horses and 28 yearlings from studs in Australia. He suggested that more intensive studies were needed to resolve the problem of *S. equi* carrier animals and pointed out epidemiologic similarities between strangles and group E streptococcal infections in pigs in which a discharging abscess is not requisite for transmission of the disease.

Bazeley[1] found that a 4.5 hour broth culture of *S. equi* was virulent for horses and mice and that the organisms were encapsulated and were capable of stimulating protective antibody. It was concluded that the capsular material reduced the rate of phagocytosis of the cocci and that protective antibodies acted directly on the capsule. Studies of the cell surface components of *S. equi* suggest, however, that the immune response is directed toward cell wall structures exclusively[4] and that mouse protection tests support the conclusion that a trypsin-labile antigen is responsible for the stimulation of protective antibody production. Young cultures of bacteria whose colony characteristics are compact rather than mucoid (i.e., have minimal capsule development) have yielded bacterins with satisfactory protective capacity.

CLINICAL SIGNS AND DIAGNOSIS

The infective organism is transmitted in the purulent discharges of affected horses. The disease may result from direct contact between animals or indirectly from fomites, such as buckets, feeders, fences, waterers, or from such sources as stomach tubes, balling guns, and endoscopes. Strangles epizootics show high morbidity (up to 100 per cent) and low mortality, and young animals are more frequently and severely affected.

Overcrowding, poor hygiene, and intercurrent diseases, such as parasitism and viral respiratory diseases, also influence the spread and severity of the contagion (see Prevention and Control).

The first clinical signs are seen two to six days after exposure. The horse or pony is depressed, anorectic, and pyrexic (39.5 to 41.1° C). A dry, "painful," throaty cough is frequently heard, and mandibular lymph node enlargement may be observed and palpated. The animal may stand with its head and chin held down and with its neck stretched. Because of the pharyngeal discomfort, it is reluctant to swallow. These signs are accompanied by serous ocular and nasal discharges that rapidly become mucopurulent.

Abscessation of one, some, or all of the mandibular, parotid, medial, and lateral retropharyngeal lymph nodes occurs from six days to three weeks after infection. Each abscess may drain and form a sinus or, when multiple and large, may cause other clinical signs. In gross abscessation, there may be respiratory obstruction and snoring dyspnea, and any dysphagia may result in inhalation pneumonia. Lymph nodes may drain into and cause empyema of the auditory tube diverticula (ATD, guttural pouches) and subsequent cranial nerve neuropathy, as witnessed either by laryngeal paralysis, facial nerve palsy, or Horner's syndrome.

Leukocytosis and increases in plasma fibrinogen were recorded by the sixth day in experimental S. equi infections. The changes reflected the clinical course of the disease and were paralleled by a significant decrease in the packed cell volume and in the hemoglobin levels.[6]

Laboratory confirmation of a clinical diagnosis of strangles should always be made because of the epizootic importance of the disease. Since S. zooepidemicus invades all such abscesses, attempts to isolate pure S. equi should be made from abscesses that have not drained spontaneously.

A milder form of the disease in mature horses is characterized by poor performance, anemia, low-grade fever, lymphadenopathy, and weight loss. In such cases the diagnosis is often uncertain unless the anamnesis reveals contact with strangles or unless cultures of one or more lymph nodes are made. Serologic testing is not of diagnostic value, but the detection of antibody to streptolysin O or antibody to streptococcal M protein may be of value in the future to assess the "immunodeficient" subject and so be of prognostic value.

COMPLICATIONS AND SEQUELAE

In most cases, the disease runs its clinical course and abscesses and sinuses resolve in three to six weeks. Persistent local lymphadenopathy and recurrent sinus formation occur in a few cases, probably because of either ineffective treatment or an impaired immune response. Such recurrent disease is a particular problem in burros.

"Bastard strangles" is a disseminated form of the disease with lymphadenopathy and abscess formation in visceral lymph nodes. Affected animals are virtually worthless and may have signs of alimentary obstruction, peritonitis, pneumonia, and pleuritis.

In young foals, S. equi bacteremia may result in septicemia, joint and vertebral infections, encephalitis, visceral abscessation, and death.

In epizootics, the incidence of complications is low. Knight et al.,[6] however, found that 9 of 20 yearling horses infected by intranasal inoculation developed ATD empyema. This perhaps indicates that complications are more frequent if the organism is inhaled and affects the retropharyngeal nodes rather than ingested where the primary lesion may be confined to the mandibular lymph nodes. Such lesions may take months to resolve, and surgical treatment may be necessary (see Treatment).

Anemia is a feature of strangles infections, even in mature horses. Anemic horses will not return to their earlier racing form for three months or more, and any attempt to accelerate this recovery time (such as by using antibiotics and glucocorticoids) may lead to irreversible or lethal complications. The pleuritis/pleural effusion syndrome of racehorses and traveling show horses may be such a sequela. It is important that only light work is given to the horse until packed cell volume and hemoglobin levels return to normal.

It has been suggested that horses may become sensitized to streptococcal antigens and that subsequent exposure may result in a hypersensitivity reaction. Purpura hemorrhagica is one such form of hypersensitivity reaction. Urticaria, dermatitis, obstructive respiratory disease, and various neuropathies have all been linked at some time with evidence of streptococcal hypersensitivity, but the evidence is far from solid.

TREATMENT

Horses with strangles must be isolated, rested, kept warm and dry, and their legs wrapped. Purulent discharges must be removed, and disinfection is necessary to reduce contamination of the environment. Extreme care must be taken to prevent direct and indirect contact with other horses on the premises. The owner or trainer must be aware that the use of antibiotic therapy is an adjunct to and not a replacement for strict and thorough nursing procedures. Abscesses will still need to be bathed, poulticed, and surgically drained to aid complete recovery.

S. equi is sensitive to penicillin, and penicillin G is the antibiotic of choice. It has been argued, on theoretical and rather specious clinical grounds, that the treatment of strangles with antibiotics, particularly penicillin, is contraindicated. It is argued that penicillin, by killing the organisms, indirectly affects the development of immunity and thereby increases the risk of bacteremia, septicemia, and metastatic abscessation.[3] It is far more likely that any "failures" of penicillin therapy in strangles are a result of local inhibitory factors, such as fibrosis, preventing minimum inhibitory concentrations (MIC) from reaching the locus of infection and the spontaneous formation of the L (i.e., noncapsulated) form of the Streptococcus. Consequently, I use penicillin in clinical cases, and in a series of eight cases of "bastard strangles" with alimentary (five), pelvic and perineal (two), and pleural (one) disease, no evidence was found to incriminate a failure of earlier antibiotic therapy.

Therapy is started with aqueous penicillin G given intravenously or intramuscularly (60,000 IU per kg) and is maintained with procaine penicillin G (5000 IU per kg). Such treatment for five days is the most effective form of therapy in clinical strangles. Mansmann[7] has recorded reduction in the size of intra-abdominal *S. equi* abscesses if 5000 IU per kg procaine penicillin G (PPG) is maintained for four weeks.

Contact animals should be treated with PPG (5000 IU per kg) at the earliest sign of pyrexia. Such treatment precludes serious clinical disease and is most effective in controlling any strangles epizootic in training yards or riding centers.

Severely affected horses may require surgical treatment. Large retropharyngeal abscesses or ATD empyema can cause obstructive dyspnea and dysphagia. A tracheostomy tube should be inserted to ensure an adequate airway and a cranial cervical esophagostomy used to feed the horse. Up to 10 kg of Andersen pellets or their equivalent mashed in 18 l of water in divided feeds can be used to maintain a 450 kg horse.

Drainage and irrigation of ATD empyema can be carried out via indwelling nasal catheters or by an incision into the distended structure through Viborg's triangle (p. 485). A warmed 3 to 5 per cent solution of povidine-iodine* or an equivalent antiseptic is used to flush any abscesses or the ATD cavities daily. Similarly, after incision, abscessed lymph nodes should be irrigated daily with the same solution.

Recovery from cranial nerve neuritis that results from streptococcal adenitis may be expected within six months. If after such a time there are no signs of recovery, surgical treatment, for example, of laryngeal paralysis, should be considered.

PREVENTION AND CONTROL

Epizootics can be controlled by a program of isolation of known contacts and diseased animals and by the use of procaine penicillin G. Since incubating carriers exist, strict quarantine measures are advised for all new arrivals whether or not they are known to come from contaminated premises.

A contaminated environment may provide a source of infective *S. equi* for up to one year, so the importance of hygiene measures to minimize contamination cannot be emphasized too strongly. Premises should be scrubbed and disinfected or steam sterilized.

Immunity to *Streptococcus equi* is strong after natural infection but wanes rapidly. A bacterin produced by the heat treatment of young, encapsulated organisms from rapidly growing cultures was shown to be effective when used in field trials of army horses in Australia.[2] In breeding stables, training yards, and remount camps that have an endemic strangles problem, the use of bacterin immunization is strongly advised. The vaccination should continue until two yearling crops have been reared free from disease.[2] In endemics, horses should be immunized by three 10 ml doses of bacterin injected intramuscularly at weekly intervals. Animals over 10 to 20 weeks of age are capable of mounting a protective antibody response. Booster doses are given annually or on contact with strangles cases. There may be local edema, soreness, and in some cases, induration at the site of injection of the bacterin.[3] There may also be a transient fever and a neutrophilia. Horses with a fever or nasal discharge should not be im-

---

*Betadine, Purdue-Frederick Co., Norwalk, CT

munized. Purpura hemorrhagica may follow immunization, and in development trials, four cases were observed among 3152 treated horses, although three of these were inadvertently given a second complete series of bacterin injections one year after the first.

Streptococcus equi bacterins are available in Australia and in North America* but not in the United Kingdom.

References

1. Bazeley, P. L.: Studies with equine streptococci. 2. Experimental immunity to *Streptococcus equi.* Aust. Vet. J., *16*:243, 1940.

2. Bazeley, P. L.: Studies with equine streptococci. 3. Vaccination against strangles. Aust. Vet. J., *18*:141, 1942.
3. Bryans, J. T.: Streptococcal diseases. *In* Catcott, E. J., and Smithcors, J. F. (eds.): Equine Medicine and Surgery. Wheaton, IL, American Veterinary Pub., 1972, pp. 79–82.
4. Erickson, E. D., and Norcross, N. L.: The cell surface antigens of *Streptococcus equi.* Can. J. Comp. Med., *39*:110, 1975.
5. Evers, W. D.: Effect of furaltadone on strangles in horses. J. Am. Vet. Med. Assoc., *152*:1394, 1968.
6. Knight, A. P., Voss, J. L., McChesney, A. E., and Bigbee, H. G.: Experimentally induced *Streptococcus equi* infections in horses with resultant guttural pouch empyema. V. M. S.A.C., *70*:1194, 1975.
7. Mansmann, R. A.: Antimicrobial therapy in horses. Vet. Clin. North Am., *5*(1):81, 1975.
8. Woolcock, J. B.: Epidemiology of equine streptococci. Res. Vet. Sci., *18*:113, 1975.

*Equibac II, Fort Dodge Labs, Fort Dodge, KS

TETANUS

Mortimer Cohen, DAVIS, CALIFORNIA

Tetanus is an infrequent, easily preventable, and often fatal disease characterized by local or generalized spasms of striated muscles. Tetanospasmin, the neurotoxin produced by the anaerobic spore-bearing gram-positive bacillus *Clostridium tetani,* acts on four areas of the nervous system: the motor end plate in skeletal muscle, the spinal cord, the brain, and the sympathetic nervous system.

The classical presentation of tetanus includes trismus, prolapsed nictitans, stiff, straddling gait, tail held out stiffly, erect carriage of ears, and an anxious, alert expression. The animal demonstrates an exaggerated response to normal stimuli. Inability to eat or drink and constipation and retention of urine are frequently observed. The disease can progress to a sawhorse stance and finally to lateral recumbency, opisthotonus, and respiratory failure. Overactivity of the sympathetic nervous system is clinically manifested by profuse sweating, tachycardia, cardiac dysrhythmias, hypertension, and tachypnea.

Fully developed tetanus is quite distinctive, allowing diagnosis to be made from clinical signs and a history of an inadequate immunization regimen. History of injury may not be present. Early in the course of the disease, however, tetanus may be confused with hypocalcemic tetany of lactating mares, hypomagnesemia, acute laminitis, and cerebrospinal meningitis. Hypocalcemic tetany and hypomagnesemia respond to administration of appropriate fluids. Acute laminitis does not demonstrate tetany or prolapse of the third eyelid. Cerebrospinal meningitis causes rigidity and hyperesthesia, but the presentation is one of depression and immobility. A markedly varying incubation period, ranging from three days to a month, and infrequently to three or four months, coupled with inapparent causative wounds may make initial diagnosis difficult.

TREATMENT

The principles of treatment are as follows: (1) prevention of further absorption of toxin by wound care and neutralization of free circulating toxin, (2) control of reflex spasms and tonic rigidity, (3) supportive therapy, and (4) prevention of complications.

PREVENTION OF FURTHER ABSORPTION AND NEUTRALIZATION OF TOXIN

Prompt and proper wound care is a critical part of the elimination of toxin production. It is not always possible to find the site of infection. Meticulous inspection, especially in and around the hoof, is mandatory. Removal of foreign bodies and débridement of any necrotic tissue followed by irrigation with 3 per cent hydrogen peroxide is the preferred regimen. It has been recommended that administration of antitoxin precede débridement to ensure neutralization of toxin in tissue close to the wound.

Tetanus antitoxin (TAT)* administered either intramuscularly or intravenously cannot penetrate

*Tetanus antitoxin, Haver-Lockhart, Shawnee, KS

nerve fibers to combine with toxin in transit to the central nervous system, nor can it effectively cross the blood-brain barrier. Nonetheless, its use is still recommended to bind any remaining toxin outside of the nervous system. Doses of 5000 units per 100 pounds (100 units per kg) body weight are probably adequate.

Intrathecal injection of antitoxin is controversial. Convulsions have been described in humans, horses, and other species. Apparently, the preservative phenol in a 0.25 to 0.50 per cent solution is the cause of convulsions. This author has had success with intrathecal therapy in three of four cases.

General anesthesia is accomplished using xylazine* (1 mg per kg) followed by thiopental† (8 to 12 mg per kg) or acepromazine‡ 0.09 mg per kg followed by glyceryl guaiacolate§ to effect (approximately 10 gm per 100 kg). The area between the occipital protuberance and the atlas is surgically prepped, and the cisterna magna is penetrated with an 18-gauge spinal needle.‖ Fifty ml of cerebrospinal fluid is withdrawn, and a similar volume of TAT (1000 units per ml) is injected slowly. In foals, 30 ml of TAT is used. One-hundred fifty mg of methyl prednisolone sodium succinate** may be mixed with the antitoxin to decrease irritation. The xylazine-ketamine combination is not recommended for general anesthesia because it is felt that the rigidity sometimes noted with this combination exacerbates the spasms of tetanus. Antitoxin thus introduced will not unbind toxin already attached to the neuroreceptor sites, but it can prevent further binding of toxin and may prevent development of further signs.

Penicillin therapy is also indicated for eradication of *Clostridium tetani*. Initial doses of 20,000 to 40,000 units per kg of potassium penicillin administered intravenously four times daily for the first three to four days can be followed by 20,000 units per kg twice daily of procaine penicillin G intramuscularly.

CONTROL OF REFLEX SPASMS AND TONIC RIGIDITY

Sedatives, hypnotics, general anaesthetics, neuromuscular blocking agents, and centrally acting muscle relaxants have all been suggested and have been used in humans for control of muscle spasms and tonic rigidity.

*Rompun, Haver-Lockhart, Shawnee, KS
†Biocentic, Parke Davis, Detroit, MI
‡Acepromazine, Ayerst Labs, New York, NY
§Glyceryl guaiacolate, Professional Veterinary Labs, Belle Plaine, MN
‖Monoject, Sherwood Medical Industries, Inc., St. Louis, MO
**Solumedrol, Upjohn Co., Kalamazoo, MI

The most frequently used drug in horses is acetylpromazine (0.5 mg per kg intramuscularly) every 6 to 12 hours. Many of the other drugs used in humans are either too expensive (such as diazepam) or are not logistically possible to administer in field situations. Neuromuscular blocking agents such as D-tubo-curare coupled with positive pressure ventilation could work but are impractical. Similarly, the use of barbiturates, while quite useful in smaller species, is not feasible in horses. Ventilation problems preclude long-term use of these drugs.

Centrally acting muscle relaxants such as methocarbamol* (10 cc intravenously every six to eight hours) or 5 per cent glyceryl guaiacolate in 5 per cent dextrose to effect may also be considered.

SUPPORTIVE THERAPY

Supportive therapy includes maintenance of proper environment, fluid and electrolyte balance, adequate nutrition, care of bowels and bladder, and relief of pain and pyrexia.

It is recommended that the patient be placed in a dark, isolated, and heavily bedded stall. If necessary, cotton can be placed in the animal's ears to reduce extraneous noise. Manipulation of the patient should be minimal. Body slings for support of the animal may be necessary in some situations.

Constant monitoring of fluid and electrolyte status is necessary, because fluid loss can be quite marked. Acidosis is not uncommon. Measurement of acid-base balance with the Harleco apparatus can be performed with ease and expediency. Appropriate fluid therapy using a balanced lactated Ringer's solution and sodium bicarbonate in 5 per cent dextrose should be given as necessary.

Soft foods should be available to the animal. Alfalfa meal is normally quite palatable and can provide adequate nutrition. If the patient is unable to eat, then alfalfa pellets soaked in water can be administered via a stomach tube and bilge pump. The daily ration should be divided into halves or thirds, and while some loss of muscle mass will occur, basal requirements can be met. The stomach tube should be secured in place to avoid the trauma of repeated passage.

When being handled, the animals should be tranquilized to reduce the likelihood of severe exaggeration of muscle spasms. A tracheostomy tube should be available in case of laryngospasm.

Enemas or manual evacuation of the rectum and catheterization of the bladder may be necessary. The stall should be checked daily for evidence of feces or urine. If none are seen, then appropriate therapy should be initiated.

*Robaxin, A. H. Robbins, Richmond, VA

Phenylbutazone* (1 gm intravenously twice a day) can be administered for control of pain and pyrexia.

Control of sympathetic nervous system overactivity is difficult and controversial in human medicine. Labetalol, which has both alpha- and beta-adrenergic blocking actions, may be effective. At this time, the drug is not commercially available. It is hoped that it will be both available and affordable in the near future.

PREVENTION OF COMPLICATIONS

Close observation of the respiratory system is essential, as respiratory complications, including pneumonia, buildup of excessive secretions in the bronchi and bronchioles, and laryngospasm are not uncommon. Aspiration of secretions via a polyethylene tube can be performed. The use of nebulization and broad-spectrum antibiotics for lung problems is in order if indicated.

Proper hydration is also important to prevent renal failure. Recent research has shown that the toxin also acts on the proximal tubules. The damage is reversible, provided hydration is adequate.

PREVENTION

Given the high mortality rate of the disease and the economic costs of nursing care, preventive measures are vitally important in the handling of a suspicious wound. Proper débridement of the wound is essential. Procaine penicillin G (20,000 units per kg twice daily) can be used. If the vaccination history is unsatisfactory or unknown, 1500 units of antitoxin should be administered. Indiscriminate use of tetanus antitoxin is inadvisable, as a serum-asso-

ciated hepatopathy has been observed in some animals 4 to 10 weeks following administration of this and other biologicals. The antitoxin vials carry a warning, so clients should be advised. One ml of tetanus toxoid* can be administered simultaneously as long as it is injected in a site different from that used for antitoxin. A second dose of toxoid should be administered three to four weeks following the initial vaccination. Yearly boosters are recommended thereafter. Some recent work has shown that immunity of up to 2½ years' duration can be achieved by using a toxoid in a water-in-oil emulsion. Actual duration of immunity from the standard aluminum hydroxide adjuvant is unknown. From a medicolegal viewpoint, however, yearly boosters should be given. It is important to note that the disease does not confer good immunity to the horse.

References

1. Beroza, G. F.: Tetanus in the horse. J. Am. Vet. Med. Assoc., *177*:1152, 1980.
2. Blood, D. C., Henderson, J. A., and Radostits, O. M.: Veterinary Medicine: A Textbook of the Diseases of Cattle, Sheep, Pigs and Horses, 5th ed. Philadelphia, Lea and Febiger, 1979, p. 438.
3. Jansen, B. C., and Knoetze, P. C.: The immune response of horses to tetanus toxoid. Onderstepoort J. Vet. Res., *46*:211, 1979.
4. Kerr, J. H.: Current topics in tetanus. Intens. Care Med., 5:105, 1979.
5. Knight, H. D.: Tetanus. *In* Catcott, E. J., and Smithcors, J. F. (eds.): Equine Medicine and Surgery, 2nd ed. Wheaton, IL, American Veterinary Pub., 1972, pp. 94–98.
6. Muylle, E., Oyaert, W., Ooms, L., and Decraemere, H.: Treatment of tetanus in the horse by injections of tetanus antitoxin into the subarachnoid space. J. Am. Vet. Med. Assoc., *167*:47, 1975.
7. Vakil, B. J.: Tetanus. *In* Kirk, R. W. (ed.): Current Veterinary Therapy. Philadelphia, W. B. Saunders Co., 1979, p. 67.

---

*Phenylbutazone, Med. Tech., Inc., Elwood, KS

*Tetoid, Beecham, Bristol, TN

TUBERCULOSIS

John E. Peel, DAVIS, CALIFORNIA

Tuberculosis has never assumed an importance in horses of the proportions that it has in other species. Even in areas and times when the disease is and was endemic in cattle and human populations, the incidence of clinical disease in the horse was low, on the order of 0.1 per cent, as evidenced by slaughterhouse surveys.

With control and eradication of tuberculosis from

cattle populations, there has been a parallel decrease in its occurrence in horses, and reports in the modern literature are scarce.

Horses seem to possess some natural resistance to tuberculosis organisms, and this is held to be responsible at least in part for the relative rarity of disease. Because of this rarity in modern populations, care must be taken to avoid overlooking the disease, particularly in parts of the world where it is still endemic in other species. Tuberculosis should be included in a list of differential diagnoses of progressive weight loss and debility.

ETIOLOGY AND NATURE OF DISEASE

Equine tuberculosis is caused by the acid-fast organism *Mycobacterium tuberculosis,* and of the three strains, bovine, avian, and human, disease is most commonly caused by the bovine type, occasionally by avian strains, and only very rarely by human strains. The nature of the disease caused by all strains is similar and will be discussed together, with differentiation being made by isolation of the organism and its behavior on inoculation in laboratory animals. Some strains isolated from horses appear to have reduced virulence for laboratory animals.

Infection is usually via ingestion, though primary respiratory infection does occur. After ingestion, the organism most commonly settles in the mesenteric lymph nodes and spleen, and these organs are the most usual sites in which lesions are found. It is not common to have visible intestinal lesions, but when present, these take the form of craterlike ulcers. A lesion similar to that seen in Johne's disease in cattle has been described in the bowel of horses affected by the avian strain of the tuberculosis organism. The infection is contained in the local lymph nodes or spleen or both where the lesion gradually enlarges or is spread via the bloodstream. The spread of tuberculosis can be miliary, where myriads of tiny nodules are found throughout the body, the lungs being the most severely affected. If fewer organisms are released into the bloodstream, then these settle in target organs, frequently the lungs, and lesions develop to a larger size. The clinical course of disease is longer than with miliary spread, since it takes longer for the function of the affected organ to become compromised.

The horse is different from other species in that the lesions do not assume the usual granulomatous nature with a caseous center and fibrous capsule but tend to have a tumorlike appearance with areas of liquefaction necrosis in the center and very little fibrous tissue present. On histologic section, the presence of epithelioid cells, Langhans' giant cells, and acid-fast organisms characterizes these lesions as tuberculosis.

Isolates have been made from lymph nodes, the spleen, liver, lungs, bowel, bony tissues, meninges, skin, mammary gland, and nasal mucosa. Only rarely have the kidneys been shown to be affected, and in contrast to other species, extensive involvement of the pleura and peritoneum is uncommon.

CLINICAL SIGNS

Clinical signs of tuberculosis can be extremely varied depending on the organs involved. The most common clinical picture seen is that of chronic progressive weight loss that occurs over a period of many months after a slow and insidious onset. This is followed eventually by depression, weakness, and sometimes anorexia and fever in terminal stages. Where miliary spread has occurred and is affecting the lungs, there will be a terminal phase of the disease in which raised body temperature and respiratory rate and coughing are prominent signs before death ensues.

There seems to be a predilection of the organism for cervical vertebrae, where it causes osteomyelitis, and pain and stiffness of the neck are very common signs reported in equine tuberculosis.

Polyuria is a sign frequently reported in terminal cases of tuberculosis, even in the absence of renal involvement.

DIAGNOSIS

The most effective and definitive means of diagnosing tuberculosis in the horse is to culture and demonstrate the presence of the causative organism. All discharges from animals showing signs suspicious of disease should be examined by direct smear for acid-fast organisms and by culture and inoculation in laboratory animals in order to characterize any bacteria seen. A positive isolation of *Mycobacterium tuberculosis* constitutes a definitive diagnosis.

Much has been written about the use of the intradermal tuberculin test in horses, and all authors agree that this is a very unreliable test in the horse, unlike in cattle, where it has been the basis of highly successful eradication programs throughout the world. Horses going to slaughter have been subjected to the intradermal test, and there has been absolutely no correlation between postmortem signs and positive skin tests.

TREATMENT

Treatment of equine tuberculosis is not generally a practical proposition. Firstly and most importantly, this should be precluded by the dangers to public health that would be inherent in such a course of action. Secondly, if embarked upon, a course of treatment would necessarily be prolonged, and so the cost would be prohibitive in most cases, especially in view of the likelihood that the disease is advanced to such a stage before a diagnosis is made that the prognosis for a cure would be poor.

It is possible that a very valuable stud animal might become infected and so, despite the problems listed above, make it worth an attempt to treat the disease. In such an exceptional situation, the protocol followed in treating the disease in humans should be used.

Streptomycin, isoniazid, rifampin, and ethambutol are the major agents used in human tuberculosis therapy, and these drugs are used in combination in order first to avoid toxicity associated with high levels of one particular drug and second to try and prevent the development of drug-resistant strains.

Regular culturing and sensitivity testing of infected discharges is performed throughout the treatment period in order to spot the development of resistant strains early and to tailor treatment accordingly. Isoniazid is the most useful therapeutic agent and is recommended in humans to be used in doses of 8 to 10 mg per kg daily. There are reports of the use of isoniazid in horses at doses varying between 3 and 20 mg per kg to treat conditions other than tuberculosis with no apparent side effects, and so this would appear to be a useful regimen to follow. Streptomycin could be given at a rate of 15 mg per kg daily for one month followed by this same dose twice weekly for three months. This is used only if there is no renal impairment. Ethambutol is used in humans at a rate of 25 mg per kg daily. The author has not found reports of its use in the horse. Therapy should be kept up for a minimum of two years before being withdrawn. It should be emphasized that treatment of equine tuberculosis has not been reported, and these principles are extrapolated from those used in treating human disease. As indicated earlier, only exceptional circumstances would warrant an attempt to treat the disease in the horse, and this would need to be sanctioned by the public health authority of the area in which the horse lived. If treatment is undertaken, then adequate precautions must be taken to protect persons in contact with the animal, and the prognosis for the animal would be poor.

References

1. Francis, J.: Tuberculosis in Animals and Man. London, Cassell and Co., 1958, pp. 193–203.
2. Goodman, L. S., and Gillman, A.: The Pharmacological Basis of Therapeutics, 5th ed. New York, Macmillan Pub. Co., 1975, pp. 1201–1216.
3. Jubb, K. V. F., and Kennedy, P. C.: Pathology of Domestic Animals, Vol. 1. New York, Academic Press, 1970, p. 247.
4. Luke, D.: Tuberculosis in the horse, pig, sheep, and goat. Vet. Rec., 70: 529, 1958.

ULCERATIVE LYMPHANGITIS

Mortimer Cohen, DAVIS, CALIFORNIA

Ulcerative lymphangitis is a chronic progressive inflammatory disease of the subcutaneous lymphatics, usually involving the lower hind limbs. The causative agent is *Corynebacterium pseudotuberculosis*, although similar lesions have been attributed to other pyogenic organisms, including streptococci, staphylococci, *C. equi*, and *Pseudomonas aeruginosa*. The disease was of considerable importance and was widely encountered during the height of the era when horses were used for transportation, but now is only infrequently encountered.

Infection occurs through abrasions of the lower limbs, especially around the fetlocks, and is more likely to occur when horses are crowded together in dirty stables. Generally, the disease is only mildly contagious; only sporadic cases occur in crowded situations.

Upon introduction of the organism through the skin, there is invasion of the lymphatic vessels. Diffuse swelling follows with subsequent development of dermal nodules. Animals are often markedly lame. These nodules abscess, ulcerate, and discharge a thick, creamy pus. The lesions may reach a size of 5 to 7 cm in diameter. The ulcers heal within 1 to 2 weeks but leave small areas of depilated, unpigmented skin. As the primary ulcers heal, new ones develop in the adjacent skin, and in this way progression occurs. As new nodules develop, the lymphatics between them cord. The lymphatics can be 1 to 2 cm thick. Fresh abscesses form along inflamed lymph vessels. Occasionally deep abscesses with extensive fibrosis are seen, as well as cellulitis with severe edema and exuberant fibrous tissue. The condition seldom extends beyond the hock, but there are reports of regional lymph node involvement and, rarely, widespread dissemination of lesions and death.

The disease must be differentiated from glanders, epizootic lymphangitis, and sporotrichosis. Glanders is no longer seen in the United States and generally involves the respiratory tract as well as the skin. Cutaneous lesions are most frequently encountered on the medial aspect of the hock. Epizootic lymphangitis, rarely encountered in the United States, also frequently is associated with pulmonary involvement as well as lesions on the nictitans or conjunctiva. Limb lesions are most often seen around the hock, although the distal extremities may also be involved, since entry is through abrasions. Cutaneous lesions are not restricted to the limbs. Sporotrichosis is quite similar to ulcerative lymphangitis in that the occurrence is sporadic in stables, distal hind limbs are usually involved, and ulcerating nodules around the fetlock are common. These nodules are purulent granulomas with a small core of creamy pus. These wounds heal more slowly than the Corynebacterium abscesses, are generally painless, and usually do not have the extensive swelling seen in ulcerative lymphangitis. Lymphangitis is usually not as marked either. Direct smear or culture of abscess material is diagnostic. Under microscopic examination, *C. pseudotuberculosis* appears as a small diphtheroid rod with a typical Chinese-letter configuration.

TREATMENT

The unfortunate aspect of this disease is that although it is rarely fatal, it is often debilitating and disfiguring. Once lymphatic fibrosis has occurred, there is virtually no chance for normalization of the affected limb. High doses of systemic penicillin (20,000 to 80,000 units per kg intramuscularly twice daily) for periods of one month or more may be effective in controlling the disease. Local treatment consists of incising the abscess and flushing with povidone-iodine solution. The limb may be wrapped with a Furacin or Furacin-glycerin sweat for five days or more. Hydrotherapy and exercise may also be helpful. Anti-inflammatory agents such as phenylbutazone (1 to 2 gm intravenously or orally twice a day) are also indicated. The use of an autogenous bacterin has been advocated in the early stage of the disease, but results are equivocal. Attempts to develop an efficient vaccine have not been successful.

CONTROL

Proper stable management and careful treatment of lower limb injuries usually afford adequate protection against the disease.

References

1. Blood, D. C., Henderson, J. A., and Radostits, O. M.: Veterinary Medicine: A Textbook of the Diseases of Cattle, Sheep, Pigs and Horses, 5th ed. London, Balliere Tindall, 1979, pp. 421–422, 712.
2. Jubb, K. V. F., and Kennedy, P. C.: Pathology of Domestic Animals, 2nd ed., Vol. 1. New York, Academic Press, 1970, pp. 141–144.
3. Knight, H. D.: Ulcerative lymphangitis. *In* Catcott, E. J., and Smithcors, J. F. (eds.): Equine Medicine and Surgery, 2nd ed. Wheaton IL, American Veterinary Pub., 1972, p. 90.

MYCOTIC DISEASES

Cheryl McCullough, DAVIS, CALIFORNIA

As a rule, deep mycotic diseases are insidious and fatal. Unfortunately, amphotericin B, the drug used in the therapy of these diseases, is not without its own serious side effects. A decision to treat an animal with antifungal agents should not be reached without the client being made fully aware of the poor prognosis, the experimental nature of therapy in horses, the toxic effects of amphotericin B, the prolonged duration of therapy, and the expense of both the drug and laboratory support necessary to monitor patients on treatment. The systemic mycoses are not considered to be contagious. However, since all of them affect humans, care should be exercised when handling tissues or other samples from horses suspected of having aspergillosis, cryptococcosis, coccidioidomycosis, histoplasmosis, blastomycosis, or rhinosporidiosis. Fortunately, these diseases are also relatively rare in horses. In the initial portion of this chapter, I will discuss signs of fungal disease and diagnostic criteria. Therapy of these diseases is discussed later.

ASPERGILLOSIS

Aspergillosis may be caused by one of several different species of Aspergillus, *Aspergillus fumigatus* being incriminated most frequently. Aspergillus species are widespread throughout the world, and they are readily propagated on damp feedstuffs.

Inhalation of spores is thought to be the source of infection. Severity of clinical disease is presumed to be directly proportional to the size of the inoculum inhaled. For this reason, horses kept in damp stables are at much greater risk than pastured horses. Also, those horses with a history of prolonged antibiotic therapy or of immunosuppressive therapy are at greater risk than other horses. As might be expected, pulmonary infections are most commonly observed, although meningeal and generalized infections have been reported. In the acute form of the disease, progression is quite rapid, with death occurring within two weeks. Severe diarrhea may be present. In its chronic form, aspergillosis is a wasting disease quite similar to tuberculosis. Respiratory difficulty and a moist cough are typical clinical signs. Hemoptysis may be noted. Findings on auscultation of the lung fields range from increased respiratory sounds to finding areas of decreased air flow and dullness. In acute cases, diffuse miliary nodules are present in the lung parenchyma. With time, the center of the nodule becomes necrotic and contains hyphae. The surrounding tissue becomes atelectic and may calcify.

An antemortem diagnosis of aspergillosis is difficult to establish, since Aspergillus organisms can be recovered from tracheal aspirates of normal horses. Aspergillosis should be suspected when the tracheal wash findings (large numbers of fungal hyphae plus a marked mononuclear inflammatory response) are supported by clinical and radiographic evidence of respiratory disease. History of exposure to large numbers of spores via stabling or being fed poor-quality hay should also be present. The hazards of therapy require that the diagnosis be based on evidence more substantial than finding a few Aspergillus organisms in a tracheal wash.

CRYPTOCOCCOSIS

Cryptococcosis is worldwide in its distribution and is caused by *Cryptococcus neoformans*. While the disease in dogs and humans is primarily meningeal in nature, in the horse, nasal and meningeal infections are reported with approximately equal frequency. Pulmonary and cutaneous manifestations are occasionally reported also.

The clinical signs vary with the location of the primary lesion. Rhinitis leads to a persistent nasal discharge. There may or may not be any other signs of disease. Cryptococcal meningitis causes central nervous system–related disturbances such as ataxia, blindness, and incoordination. Lesions that do not generate a tissue reaction are "slimy" or mucoid in appearance and are of a gelatinous consistency. Myxomatous neoplasms are similar in appearance and must be differentiated from cryptococcal lesions. When an infection does evoke a tissue response, the result is granuloma formation.

Diagnosis is based on the demonstration of the organism in tissue, discharges, or spinal fluid or by culture of the organism from these samples. The organism can often be detected by staining direct fluid or impression smears with a drop of India ink.

This provides a dark background against which the wide, transparent, gelatinous capsule that surrounds the organism is clearly demonstrated. The organism itself is round and thick-walled. Because the capsule is highly refractile, unstained preparations should be examined under low-intensity light.

The method of spread has not been determined. The organism has been closely associated with pigeon droppings; however, pigeons are not thought to be a source of infection; rather, the droppings are thought to serve as a selective growth medium.

COCCIDIOIDOMYCOSIS

Coccidioidomycosis is a disease of arid areas in North and South America and is caused by *Coccidioides immitis*. It is endemic in Texas, Arizona, New Mexico, California, and neighboring states, as well as northern Mexico, Venezuela, Honduras, and parts of Bolivia, Paraguay, and Argentina. *Coccidioides immitis* is dust-borne and may travel quite a distance from endemic areas via the dust on vehicles or in dust storms.

The usual form of the disease is a mild, self-limiting respiratory infection. In this form, the only indicators of Coccidioides infection are the positive skin test that can be elicited or a low titer positive complement fixation (CF) test. The chronic form of the disease is characterized by progressive weight loss. Low-grade fever or variable temperature, gradual abdominal distention, dry cough, and large quantities of abdominal or thoracic fluid may be observed. Decreasing packed cell volume (PCV) and increasing total white blood cell count may be noted in the hemogram. This form is generally fatal, and typically granulomatous lesions are found in the lungs, spleen, and kidney.

Diagnosis is based on observation of the organism in either lesions, body fluids, or discharges or by culture of the agent from these materials. High titer CF tests in association with illness or rising CF titers are also indicative of active illness.

HISTOPLASMOSIS

Histoplasmosis is caused by *Histoplasma capsulatum*. It is endemic in the Ohio and central Mississippi River Valleys and the Appalachian Mountains in the United States. Regions of Central and South America, Africa, Asia, and Europe have also been established as endemic areas. As with the cryptococcal organism, *H. capsulatum* has been associated with excreta and other products from several avian species (primarily chickens) and also with bat excrement.

Two forms of histoplasmosis exist, a mild or subclinical type and a general disseminated type. The mild form is the most common and can be detected by a positive histoplasmin skin test. Skin testing reveals that the incidence of infection is quite high in endemic areas. Although the incidence of infection is high, the number of cases of general disseminated histoplasmosis is very low. This is fortunate, since the disseminated form is often fatal. The disease is rarely reported in horses, and the clinical course of the disease has not been characterized. Marked hyperplasia of reticuloendothelial tissues is considered to be the hallmark of Histoplasma infection, although other tissues may be affected. In the equine cases described in the literature, lesions were found in various organs, including the fetal liver, bone marrow, lung, the colon (granulomatous colitis), the spleen, and fetal membranes.

In tissue sections, it is difficult to distinguish *H. capsulatum* from *H. farciminosus*, the causative agent of epizootic lymphangitis. Therefore, the definitive diagnosis is made by culturing the organism. *Histoplasma farciminosus* has been cited as the cause of granulomatous pneumonia in horses from the Sudan.

NORTH AMERICAN BLASTOMYCOSIS

North American blastomycosis is caused by *Blastomyces dermatitidis*. It occurs primarily in the Middle Atlantic, South Central, and Ohio-Mississippi River Valley states. It is also seen in Central America and Africa.

To date, only one case of systemic blastomycosis has been reported in the horse. In this animal, there was a 10-month history of recurrent abscesses in the perineal region. Abscesses eventually spread to the udder. During the last few weeks of life, there was a rapid loss of weight. The full extent of systemic involvement was not determined, as a full postmortem examination was not performed. Diagnosis was based on the histopathologic examination of the udder. Infection does occur, as evidenced by positive blastomycin skin tests. Unfortunately, this test is not specific (cross-reaction to histoplasmin occurs), and the true incidence of the disease is difficult to determine.

Positive diagnosis is made by culture of the organism or histopathologic examination of tissues. Like the other mycoses, blastomycosis is not thought to be contagious; however, human cases have been reported in which the source of infection was thought to be infected animals or tissue.

THERAPY

Although the majority of cases of systemic mycoses are diagnosed at necropsy or in their terminal stages, a therapy protocol is provided in the event that a practitioner or client may wish to attempt treatment of a particularly valuable animal. With the exceptions of cryptococcal meningitis and rhinosporidiosis, which will be discussed later, the current treatment of choice for the deep mycoses is parenteral amphotericin B (AMB). Reports of the use of AMB in the horse are sparse.[5, 8] No specific guidelines for the use of this drug in horses exist, and the following recommendations are adaptations of presently accepted practice in human medicine.

A 10 mg test dose is given initially. This amount is increased daily by 0.2 mg per kg until a maintenance dose of 0.5 to 1.0 mg per kg per day is being administered. After the critically ill patient is stabilized with daily AMB, the interval between doses is lengthened to 48 hours with no change in amount of drug per treatment. Human patients on this alternate day regimen feel and eat better on the nontreatment days, maintain effective blood levels of the drug over the 48-hour period, and require less of their physician's time.

The commercial AMB is hydrated with sterile water without preservatives to give a 5 mg per ml concentration. This is then suspended in 5 per cent dextrose in water to give a final concentration of 0.1 mg per ml. Heparin (20 units per kg) should be added to the infusion to help control the phlebitis generated by AMB. This preparation is infused intravenously over a period of one to two hours. Acidic solutions or those containing electrolytes should not be used as the final diluent, as they cause aggregation of the colloidal dispersion that AMB forms when hydrated.

Fever, chills, hypotension, and nausea are reported in humans during the infusion of AMB. Premedication with oral prednisolone (100 to 400 mg) is helpful in controlling these effects. Additional premedication with aspirin (40 mg per kg orally) and an antihistamine (20 to 25 mg per 100 lbs body weight of doxylamine succinate intramuscularly) can be used. In conjunction with intravenous therapy, intrathecal administration of AMB has been recommended for the treatment of coccidioidal meningitis.

AMB is not without drawbacks, the primary one being its nephrotoxicity. Pretreatment values for creatinine, blood urea nitrogen (BUN), PCV, serum K^+, and a urinalysis should be obtained. These parameters should be monitored twice weekly for the first four weeks of therapy and once weekly thereafter until cessation of treatment. The glomerular filtration rate (GFR) often stabilizes at 20 to 60 per cent of normal following several doses of AMB. If renal function continues to deteriorate, therapy should be discontinued for two to five days. It has been suggested that a sudden spike in urinary K^+ output can be used as a determinant of nephrotoxicity and that therapy should be stopped when this occurs. After renal function improves, therapy may be continued at the previous dosage. Five per cent or less of the daily dose is excreted in the urine; therefore, the dosage need not be adjusted for those patients with preexisting renal dysfunction. Other less common manifestations of AMB toxicity include hepatic dysfunction, allergic reactions, anemia, thrombocytopenia, and leukopenia. The duration of therapy has not been established; however, a course of 6 to 12 weeks is to be expected.

The recent development of 5-fluorocytosine, an antifungal agent with good activity against Cryptococcus and certain Aspergillus sp has altered the therapy of cryptococcal meningitis. 5-Fluorocytosine (flucytosine) is rapidly and almost completely absorbed following oral administration and achieves effective therapeutic levels in various body tissues and fluids, including the cerebrospinal fluid (CSF). For this reason, combined AMB and flucytosine therapy is recommended in cases of cryptococcal meningitis. An advantage of the combination of AMB with flucytosine is the markedly reduced dose of AMB that can be used. A daily dose of 0.2 to 0.3 mg per kg of AMB is used in conjuction with 150 mg per kg per day of flucytosine divided in four doses. Other advantages found in humans include more patients cured or improved, fewer failures or relapses, somewhat shorter duration of therapy, and more rapid sterilization of the CSF.

Although lower doses of AMB decrease its nephrotoxic effects, renal function must still be monitored because flucytosine is almost completely (80 to 90 per cent) excreted in the urine unchanged. Therefore, the dose must be adjusted to accommodate patients with renal impairment. The aim of therapy is to achieve peak serum levels of 50 to 75 μg per ml. Peak serum concentrations greater than or equal to 100 μg per ml seem to increase the incidence of toxic effects, particularly those associated with bone marrow depression. Indications of toxicity include hepatic dysfunction, diarrhea, and bone marrow depression. Primary resistance of organisms as well as the emergence of resistant organisms during treatment precludes the use of flucytosine alone in the treatment of crytococcal meningitis. For those cases in which resistance to the combined therapy occurs, intrathecal administration of AMB in conjunction with parenteral AMB and flucytosine is advocated.

Another class of drugs, the imidazole derivatives, is being explored for its antifungal properties. Miconazole is now available for parenteral administration. In spite of initial apparent success, miconazole is not thought to be as effective as AMB in the treatment of fungal diseases, and its use in human medicine has been restricted to those patients who respond poorly to or do not tolerate therapy with AMB. Ketoconazole is the newest imidazole derivative to be developed. Its advantages over miconazole include its good absorption following oral administration and the same spectrum of antifungal activity with fewer toxic effects.

RHINOSPORIDIOSIS

Rhinosporidiosis is caused by *Rhinosporidium seeberi* and occurs in India, South Africa, Uruguay, Venezuela, Argentina, and the United States.

It does not cause the granulomatous reaction that is typical of the other fungal diseases; instead, lesions are sessile or pedunculated and lobulated and soft. These growths are pink and dotted with small white areas that represent the sporangia. They bleed easily and are usually found unilaterally on the nasal mucosa. The disease can be life-threatening if the size and location of the polyps obstructs air movement. The diagnosis of the disease is based on the observation of sporangia in tissue sections of polyps or of spores in the nasal discharge. The organism is very difficult to culture. Although the source of infection and method of spread have not yet been determined, rhinosporidiosis is not thought to be contagious.

Surgical excision is the treatment of choice; however, recurrence is common. Recently rather impressive therapeutic results have been obtained in humans by combining surgical excision and cautery followed by oral dapsone therapy. Dapsone (diaminodiphenylsulfone) is used primarily in the treatment of leprosy. In the treatment of rhinosporidiosis, an empirical dose of 100 mg per day was given in addition to iron and vitamins. To the knowledge of this author, dapsone has not been used in the horse.

References

1. Ainsworth, G. C., and Austwick, P. K. C.: Fungal Diseases of Animals, 2nd ed. Commonwealth Agricultural Bureau, Farnham Royal, Slough, England, 1973.
2. Dade, A. W., Lickfeldt, W. E., and McAllister H. A.: Granulomatous colitis in a horse with histoplasmosis. VM SAC, 68:279, 1973.
3. Hall, A. D.: An equine abortion due to histoplasmosis. VM SAC, 74:200, 1979.
4. Krough, P., Basse, A., Hesselholt, M., and Bach, A.: Equine cryptococcosis: A case of rhinitis caused by Cryptococcus neoformans serotype A. Sabouraudia, 12(2):272, 1974.
5. McMullan, W. C., Joyce, J. R., Hanselka, D. V., and Heitmann, J. M.: Amphotericin B for the treatment of localized subcutaneous phycomycosis in the horse. J. Am. Vet. Med. Assoc., 170:1293, 1977.
6. Medoff, G., and Kobayashi, G. S.: Strategies in the treatment of systemic fungal infections. N. Engl. J. Med., 302:145, 1980.
7. Nair, K. K.: Clinical trial of diaminodiphenylsulfone (DDS) in nasal and nasopharyngeal rhinosporidiosis. Laryngoscope, 89:291, 1979.
8. Worthington, W. E.: Opportunistic fungus infections of horses. In Opportunistic Fungal Infections. Proceedings of the Second International Conference. Springfield, IL, Charles C Thomas, 1974.

BACTEREMIA

Corinne F. Raphel, KENNETT SQUARE, PENNSYLVANIA

In the horse, many infectious agents produce bacteremia, including Streptococcus, Staphylococcus, *Escherichia coli, Actinobacillus equuli, Corynebacterium equi,* and Salmonella organisms. Infections culminating in bacteremias account for a significant percentage of mortality in neonatal foals.

PATHOGENESIS AND PATHOLOGIC CHARACTERISTICS

In the neonatal foal, the most important predisposing factor for bacteremia is failure of passive transfer of antibody (that is, inadequate colostral absorption). Additionally, prematurity, weakness, stress, and patent urachus can also play a part in the pathogenesis of infection. Factors that reduce colostrum intake include deliberate deprivation (to prevent hemolytic disease), death of the dam, delayed or feeble suckling in weak or premature foals, or foals with "neonatal maladjustment syndrome" or other behavioral abnormalities soon after birth, as well as deformities that prevent rising, walking, suckling, or swallowing by the foal.

Except in the case of intravascular infection (such as bacterial endocarditis and suppurative thrombophlebitis), bacteria enter the circulation almost inevitably through the lymphatic system. Consequently, when bacteria multiply at a site of local infection in the tissues, the likelihood of septicemia is greatest in local conditions that favor drainage from the area to the thoracic duct and venous blood. Once bacteria enter the blood, they are removed rapidly by reticuloendothelial cells in the liver and spleen and by leukocytes in capillaries, especially those in the lungs. Transient bacteremia occurs in the early phase of many infections. If untreated, the septicemia/bacteremia can be responsible for "seeding" other previously uninfected organs.

Petechial hemorrhage or ecchymotic hemorrhage or both is a characteristic lesion of bacteremia. Localization of infection in the joints, peritoneum, kidney, liver, lungs, brain, and heart valves is common. Neonates frequently have multiple sites of abscessation owing to hematogenous spread to other organs following primary infection via the oral, nasal, or umbilical route of entry. The adult horse frequently has a single focus of infection (such as a lung abscess) that may periodically produce bacteremia.

CLINICAL SIGNS

Clinical signs depend on both the horse's age and the causative organisms but are remarkably similar for many etiologic agents.

In foals, bacteremia is characterized by fever, lethargy, and reduced strength of suckle. Other clinical signs include lameness, joint distention, uveitis, hypopyon, and depression, depending on localization of the infection in the joints, anterior chamber of the eye, peritoneum, gastrointestinal tract, brain, or other organs. Initial signs may be rapidly followed by prostration and death within a few hours.

Causes of bacteremias in the adult horse include Salmonella enteritis, pneumonia and/or lung abscessation, and, less commonly, suppurative thrombophlebitis and bacterial endocarditis. In the mature horse, bacteremias may have a more protracted course. Chronic bacteremias are usually characterized by persistent fever that may be intermittent or continuous, general disability, partial anorexia, depression, and usually progressive loss of condition. Submucosal petechial hemorrhage in the conjunctival, oral, or vulvar areas may be seen. Other clinical signs depend on the organ system that is the focus of infection. A cough, nasal discharge, and moist rales on auscultation of the thorax may be present in the horse that is bacteremic secondary to pneumonia, while a murmur might be heard in the horse with bacteremia associated with bacterial endocarditis.

DIAGNOSIS

Diagnosis is based on clinical signs, physical examination, and laboratory testing. The degree of inflammatory reaction may be reflected by leukocytosis or fibrinogenemia. To make a definitive diagnosis, a bacterial organism must be isolated. The bacterial organism may be isolated from blood or peritoneal, synovial, pleural, or cerebrospinal fluid.

Although blood cultures are not routinely done, they may be indicated for detection of bacteremia and determination of the causative organism and its antibiotic sensitivity. Bacteremia is usually intermittent and precedes the fever spike by approximately one hour so that by the time fever has appeared, the blood may be sterile. Because of this sequence of events, blood samples for culture must be taken a minimum of three times within a 24-hour period. The ability to obtain multiple samples is determined by clinical circumstances and the urgency to initiate antimicrobial therapy.

The simplest method of blood culture is to utilize a special vacutainer and blood culture tube. Blood collection must be performed aseptically. The area over the vein should be clipped and scrubbed with povidone-iodine solution and allowed to dry. Blood is removed with a sterile tube and needle, with care being taken to avoid contamination by the skin. Blood is drawn directly into the broth with a sterile disposable needle, and the tube is incubated and subcultured. Commercially available blood culture sets are manufactured, and sterile blood culturing needle sets are also available.

If bacteria grow from blood cultures, it is necessary to determine the significance by ruling out any contamination during sampling. The following criteria may be used in differentiating a positive blood culture from a contaminated specimen: (1) growth of the same type of organism in repeated cultures and (2) growth of a large number of a single type of organism. Growth of a small number of several different types of organisms and the isolation and identification of common skin flora suggest contamination. A pathogenic microorganism isolated from the blood is a significant diagnostic finding. If repeated culture examinations of the blood continue to reveal the presence of this microorganism, antibiotic sensitivity of the organism should be determined.

The success rate of isolation of organisms on blood cultures is low. Forty-three horses suspected of having bacteremia had a total of 107 blood cultures (average 2.5 cultures per horse). Some horses had only one culture, while several had up to six blood cultures. In only one horse was a causative organism (Pasteurella sp.) isolated from the blood cultures. Thus, the incidence of true positive cultures is approximately 2 per cent. Cultures of synovial, peritoneal, or pleural fluid will sometimes isolate the etiologic agent; in many cases no isolates will be found.

THERAPY

Antimicrobial therapy of bacteremias is almost always initiated on an empirical basis to cover the most likely etiologic agent. A broad-spectrum antibiotic such as penicillin with an aminoglycoside (such as kanamycin, neomycin, or gentamicin), sodium ampicillin, oxytetracycline, sulfamethazine, or chloramphenicol should be used initially. If a positive culture is obtained, the isolated organism and its sensitivity will dictate the choice of antibiotics. The suggested dosage rates and routes of administration of some recommended antimicrobical agents are given in Table 1.

Systemic administration of antibiotics is usually sufficient even if there is evidence of septic arthritis. Intra-articular administration of antibiotics, while ensuring at least temporary adequate concentrations locally, has the disadvantage of inducing chemical synovitis.

In the neonate that is suspected of being colos-

TABLE 1. SUGGESTED DAILY DOSAGE RATES AND ROUTES OF ADMINISTRATION OF SOME ANTIMICROBIAL AGENTS

Drug	Dose	Route	Times/Day
Procaine penicillin G	22×10^3 IU/kg	IM	2
K penicillin G	22×10^3 IU/kg	IV	4
Na penicillin G	22×10^3 IU/kg	IV	4
Ampicillin Na	11 mg/kg	IM, IV	4
Gentamicin	2.2 mg/kg	IM	4
Kanamycin	5.5 mg/kg	IM	2
Neomycin	5.5 mg/kg	IM	3
Oxytetracycline	5.5 mg/kg	IV	2
Sulfamethazine	200 mg/kg on day 1	IV	1
	100 mg/kg on day 2	IV	1
Trimethoprim	5.5 mg/kg	P.O. or IV	2
Chloramphenicol	25–50 mg/kg	P.O. or IV	4

trum deprived, 10 to 20 ounces of donor colostrum should be administered. Other supportive measures for the neonatal bacteremic foal include feeding and avoiding hypothermia.

In the absence of a suck reflex, mare's milk or reconstituted dry milk should be administered through a rubber stomach tube at a rate of 80 ml per kg body weight per day divided into a minimum of 10 equal feedings. Dry milk preparation should be reconstituted to provide 45 calories in 8 to 10 ml of water per kg body weight per day.

Hypothermia should be prevented by the use of woolen blankets, heat lamps, and an insulated stall.

Nonsteroidal anti-inflammatory drugs, including phenylbutazone* (4.4 to 8.8 mg per kg twice a day intravenously or orally), flunixin meglumine† (1 mg per kg once a day intravenously, intramuscularly, or orally) and meclofenamic acid‡ (2.2 mg per kg once a day orally) will be beneficial for both analgesic and antipyretic action in both the neonatal and mature horse. All anti-inflammatory drugs should be maintained at the lowest dose capable of producing the desired clinical response.

Steroids are contraindicated in horses with bacteremia unless the horse has signs of shock.

PREVENTIVE MEASURES

The incidence of bacteremic conditions in foals may be reduced by careful management procedures. It is beneficial to have mares foal in the en-

---

*Butazolidin, Jen-Sal Laboratories, Kansas City, MO
†Banamine, Schering Corp., Kenilworth, NJ
‡Arquel, Parke Davis and Co., Detroit, MI

vironment in which they have been residents for at least one month prior to parturition. The foal should be monitored to ensure that it receives adequate colostrum within two hours postpartum. The efficacy of routine prophylactic antibiotic injections in the foal during the first one to five days of life has never been substantiated.

In the mature horse, early detection and treatment of infections, such as pneumonia or enteritis, may decrease the incidence of bacteremia.

References

1. Knight, H. D., Sharon, K. H., and Jang, S.: Antibacterial treatment of abscesses. J. Am. Vet. Med. Assoc., *176*:1095, 1980.
2. Platt, H.: Septicemia in the foal. A review of 61 cases. Br. Vet. J., *129*:221, 1973.
3. Rossdale, P. D.: Neonatal problems in the horse. *In* Morrow, D. A. (ed.): Current Therapy in Theriogenology. Philadelphia, W. B. Saunders Co., 1980, pp. 755–767.
4. Washington, J. A.: Blood culture: Principles and techniques. Mayo Clin. Proc., *50*:91, 1975.

INTERNAL ABSCESSES

Gary E. Rumbaugh, DAVIS, CALIFORNIA

Chronic internal sepsis in the horse is an insidious, nonspecific, and often misleading diagnostic problem. Internal sepsis is usually characterized clinically by a persistent fever that may be intermittent or continuous, general debility, and progressive loss of condition. The clinicopathologic alteration will vary to some extent, depending on the location of the lesion, but may include leukocytosis with a left shift, increased sedimentation rate, increased plasma fibrinogen, normocytic anemia, hypergammaglobulinemia, hypoalbuminemia, vague abdominal pain or pleurodynia, partial intestinal obstruction, and cough. While an accurate diagnosis is a prerequisite to successful therapeutic intervention in these cases, their nonspecific presentation requires a skillful physical examination, prudent use of ancillary diagnostic aids, and a liberal endowment of empiricism.

There are reports in the veterinary literature outlining the clinical presentation of intrathoracic, intra-abdominal, and subcutaneous and/or lymphatic channel abscesses and their management. This chapter will concern itself primarily with those abscesses occurring in the intra-abdominal space and the subcutaneous lymphatic locations, leaving the lung and the pleural septic processes for discussion elsewhere (p. 523).

ABDOMINAL ABSCESSES

Horses with internal abdominal abscesses consistently present with one of two chief complaints. The first is a history of intermittent or prolonged colic. These animals are febrile with increased heart and respiratory rates, and most are depressed and anorectic. Constipation, decreased peristalsis, and dehydration are frequently noticed. Another consistent feature of these cases is a marked resistance by the animal to rectal examination. This is often shown as severe abdominal straining and rectal expulsive efforts.

The second form of presentation of abdominal abscesses is a chronic ongoing weight loss problem. These animals range from the emaciated horse to the thin "poor-doer." Inconsistent elevations in heart and respiratory rates and elevations in rectal temperatures are also presenting features in these cases. Depression is observed in all horses, but anorexia is not a consistent finding. Urination and defecation are usually normal. There does not appear to be any breed or sex predilection in this syndrome, but horses under five years of age are more commonly affected than older animals. While the previous medical history of these cases has no consistent pattern, most animals have a vague history of respiratory catarrh or superficial cutaneous abscessation.

Clinicopathologically, these cases present a fairly consistent pattern of abnormalities: (1) slight to moderate depression anemia with reduced numbers of red blood cells and a reduction in the hematocrit to 30 per cent or less, (2) leukocytosis with a relative and absolute neutrophilia, often with a left shift, (3) elevated plasma fibrinogen concentration, often greater then 1000 mg per dl (high normal is 400 mg per dl), and (4) elevated total plasma proteins due to hyperglobulinemia with below normal albumin levels. The albumin-to-globulin (A/G) ratio is well below normal, ranging from 0.17 to 0.63 (normal range is 0.65 to 1.46).

Analysis of peritoneal fluids is of diagnostic assistance in animals with abdominal abscesses (p. 224). All peritoneal fluid aspirates in these cases will be exudates, with varying amounts of fibrinogen, a large number of white blood cells, and increased protein content. In some cases, these samples will also contain bacteria if examined by the Gram staining method; however, attempts to culture this fluid are rarely successful, possibly owing to the bacteriostatic effect of peritoneal fluid.

Based on these clinical and laboratory findings, it is suggested that horses with prolonged colic or chronic weight loss with a more or less constant fever, with or without a rectally discernible mass, should be examined further by means of a complete blood count, plasma fibrinogen determination, serum protein fractionation, and cytologic examination of peritoneal fluid. Findings of depression anemia, leukocytosis, increased fibrinogen levels, and a decreased A/G ratio, as well as a peritoneal sample containing increased proteins and cells, should strongly suggest an intra-abdominal abscess.

The cause of internal abdominal abscesses in the horse has most often been attributed to unusual or metastatic infection with *Streptococcus equi, S. zooepidemicus,* and *Corynebacterium pseudotuberculosis.* The actual pathogenesis of internal abdominal abscesses has not been delineated, but it has been proposed that such internal infection is related to failure of the individual animal to develop adequate immunity to the organism, thereby allowing systemic spread of infection.[1] It has been further suggested that the formation of internal abscesses may be influenced by the therapy of active cases of strangles.[1] Treatment with penicillin prior to maturation and drainage of the typical strangles abscess are believed to lead to more frequent occurrence of metastatic abscesses. Other authors[2] have suggested that withholding treatment to allow for mature abscess formation does not aid in preventing septicemia and such hematogenous spread of the organisms.

It is possible to speculate that, rather than early therapy, inadequate penicillin therapy may have a role in the development of internal abscessation by failure to control the organisms already widely disseminated throughout the body. It is, therefore, suggested that once antimicrobial therapy is initiated in horses with respiratory catarrh and lymphoid abscessation, it should continue at appropriate levels for at least 10 days after cessation of all clinical signs. In humans, streptococcal infections are often treated for extended periods when dissemination of infection is suspected.

THERAPY

Medical management of these horses is based on the finding that the most common inciting organisms, *S. equi, S. zooepidemicus,* and *C. Pseudotuberculosis,* are all sensitive to concentrations of penicillin G that are attainable in the horse. Long duration penicillin therapy (40,000 to 100,000 units per kg of body weight divided into two doses daily)

is indicated and may be necessary for two to six months. Rectal palpation and repeated abdominal paracentesis examination, as well as repeated complete blood counts (CBC), can be utilized to measure the success of therapy. Analgesics, such as phenylbutazone dosed to effect (4 to 10 mg per kg), may be valuable in the more acute cases to reduce fever and to relieve pain and anxiety, allowing the horse to eat and drink normally.

Treatment of internal abdominal abscessation with or without concomitant peritonitis may be attempted surgically. Such treatment, however, is complicated by the need to drain the purulent material without further contaminating the peritoneal space. Many internal abdominal abscesses involve the mesentery or multiple organs, including the bowel, spleen, liver, or kidneys, and cannot be readily excised without damaging adjacent structures. Abscesses may be quite friable and may rupture when handled.

SUBCUTANEOUS ABSCESSES

Another abscess syndrome of the horse that is becoming more common is the subcutaneous or lymphatic channel abscess caused by *Corynebacterium pseudotuberculosis.* Classically, this bacterium has caused equine lymphangitis; however, a clinical entity recognized as lower pectoral or abdominal wall abscessation is becoming more frequent. There is no breed, sex, or age predisposition. One or more of these signs is generally observed: diffuse or localized swellings, ventral edema, lameness, depression, fever, and draining tracts. These abscesses are found in the pectoral area, ventral abdominal wall, prepuce, inguinal region, shoulder area, mammary gland, axilla, and internal abdominal organs.

The nature of the abscesses varies markedly. The involved area may range from 5 to 30 cm in diameter and may be accompanied by pitting edema of adjacent ventral tissue. Most abscesses are localized and come to the surface and rupture or are lanced without difficulty. However, some abscesses develop extensive capsules and require surgical exploration for resolution. The use of a sterile probe or needle or both to identify the site and the contents of the swelling is essential prior to therapy. Occasionally, needles of up to 15 cm long have been required to obtain a sample of swelling contents.

THERAPY

Most superficial abscesses resolve without extensive therapy, but medical and surgical treatment can expedite resolution. Hydrotherapy appears to increase the rate at which abscesses come to the surface; cataplasm ointments, however, seem to do little if any good. Whether antimicrobial therapy is beneficial is controversial. The use of antibiotics in this condition has been associated with chronic abscessation and when inadequately used may contribute to deeper, more chronic abscesses. The most commonly used antibiotic for the treatment of *C. pseudotuberculosis* abscesses is procaine penicillin G at a rate of 20,000 to 40,000 units per kg per day, divided and administered twice a day intramuscularly.

Certain types of deep abscess or abscess development associated with the elaboration of a thick fibrous capsule require more aggressive management. Surgical exploration of axillary, mammary, inguinal, and preputial abscess sites may be necessary to establish proper ventral drainage, following which recovery is usually rapid.

While the environmental reservoir and infective route of *C. pseudotuberculosis* are still speculative, it is prudent in periods when the disease is occurring to institute routine control methods. Such measures would include frequent removal of discharge from draining abscesses, environmental and local fly control, wound protection in cases of ventral midline dermatitis, and isolation of infected horses.

References

1. Bryans, J. T., and Moore, B. O.: Group C streptococcal infections of the horse. *In* Wannamaker, L. E., and Matsen, J. M. (eds.): Streptococci and Streptococcal Diseases: Recognition, Understanding, and Management. New York, Academic Press, 1972, p. 327.
2. Evers, W. D.: Effect of furaltadone on strangles in horses. J. Am. Vet. Med. Assoc., *152*:1394, 1968.
3. Knight, H. D., Heitala, S. K., and Jang, S.: Antibacterial treatment of abscesses. J. Am. Vet. Med. Assoc., *176*:1095, 1980.
4. Meirs, K. S., and Ley, W. B.: Corynebacterium pseudotuberculosis infection in the horse: Study of 117 clinical cases and consideration of etiopathogenesis. J. Am. Vet. Med. Assoc., *177*:250, 1980.
5. Rumbaugh, G. E., Smith, B. P., and Carlson, G. P.: Internal abdominal abscesses in the horse: A study of 25 cases. J. Am. Vet. Med. Assoc., *172*:304, 1978.

VACCINATION PROGRAMS

Gary E. Rumbaugh, DAVIS, CALIFORNIA

The organization of a program for the control and prevention of infectious diseases demands an accurate knowledge of disease etiology and the ecology of both the potential pathogen and the host animal. The horse is constantly exposed to a variety of organisms from endogenous and exogenous sources. Fortunately, for many of the commonly encountered infectious diseases, it is possible to predict with accuracy the offending organism and to use this organism or a part of it to induce a protective immune response in the horse.

An ideal vaccine should give prolonged strong immunity and should be free of adverse side effects. Unfortunately, these prerequisites tend to be mutually incompatible. Live organisms stimulate the best immune response but are liable to cause many side effects, including disease, while "killed" organisms are relatively poor immunogens but are less likely to cause adverse side effects. As a compromise, many of our currently available products are modified or attenuated in an attempt to reduce the virulence of the organism until, although living, it is not capable of causing disease. The most common method of attenuation is by prolonged tissue culturing, and most equine vaccines are now of this type. Current research in animal vaccination is attempting to isolate viral protein subunits that give rise to protective antibodies. Since these particles are not infectious, they would presumably be given in high doses and would produce high immunity. Possibly, in the near future these studies will produce more nearly ideal vaccines.

Many of the present commercially available equine vaccines are polyvalent, that is, containing several antigens, or mixed, containing different organisms. While the use of these vaccines has been shown to be safe, it is inadvisable to indiscriminately mix vaccines in the field. The possibility always exists of competition or even interference between the antigens when they react with sensitive cells.

A primary immune response to a vaccine depends upon vaccinating a healthy animal. For this reason, anthelmintic and vaccination programs should be combined in health programs, as severe parasitism and malnourishment impair the effectiveness of the response. Because the use of a vaccine or antiserum in an ill animal or in one incubating an infectious disease can give an unpredictable response varying from no immune response to a hypersensitivity reaction, vaccinating in the face of a disease outbreak is not recommended. In general, a vaccination program should include all horses on the farm or ranch, thus reducing the possibility of an unvaccinated nidus of infection for new additions. Animals added to the herd, including neonates, should be treated as individuals until their vaccinations bring them to the level of immunity in the herd.

A practical, well-maintained system of record keeping is essential in monitoring herd immunity. It should describe the immunizations performed, the product used, and the date of vaccinations, as well as other aspects of housing, management, and veterinary treatment that relate to disease prevention. Whenever possible, booster vaccinations should utilize the same product as the initial vaccination. It is mandatory not only from a medical standpoint but also from the possibility of legal actions that manufacturers' recommendations concerning storage, expiration dates, and routes and sites of administration be followed and recorded.

Based on these general recommendations concerning immunization in the horse, the following specific procedures are suggested.

TETANUS

Active immunization of horses against tetanus with tetanus toxoid should be a practice that would effectively eliminate the need for the use of tetanus antitoxin. However, under certain conditions, as in stables with heavy traffic of horses with unknown vaccination status or with new foals, this is not always possible. Tetanus toxoid should be used for active immunization of foals beginning at three to four months of age. A booster is administered in two to four weeks, approximately six to nine months later, and then annually. Although it has been suggested that tetanus toxoid "boosters" in adult animals may only be required every five years, the yearly booster program is generally recommended. Vaccinating pregnant mares each year during the last one to two months of gestation should provide adequate passive immunity in the newborn foal. Tetanus toxoid should also be given to any animal that sustains a tetanus-prone wound six months or more following its last booster. If an injury occurs and the toxoid immunization has not been completed or the vaccination status is unknown, it is safest to administer tetanus antitoxin at this time. While there are serious concerns about the relationship between the use of tetanus antitoxin and the development of serum hepatitis, the risk of tetanus is real, and tetanus antitoxin is effective in reducing the incidence of the disease when used early in the course of infection.

EASTERN AND WESTERN EQUINE ENCEPHALOMYELITIS

The immune response to the killed vaccines for eastern and western equine encephalomyelitis is generally not of long duration; thus, boosters are required frequently. The initial vaccination involves two injections two to four weeks apart administered before the biting insect season. In horses previously vaccinated, one booster injection should be given every five to six months unless colder weather intervenes. Concurrently with tetanus immunizations, the foal vaccination program is initiated at 8 to 10 weeks of age, and the vaccinations are continued for life.

VENEZUELAN EQUINE ENCEPHALOMYELITIS

Venezuelan equine encephalomyelitis vaccine produces immunity for at least three years and even perhaps for a lifetime. The vaccine produces better immune titers when given with eastern and western equine encephalomyelitis agents rather than after these agents. This occurs even though there is no cross-protection among the three agents. Vaccination for Venezuelan equine encephalomyelitis is not currently recommended in the United States, except for horses entering Texas and North Carolina.

INFLUENZA

The length of protective immunity derived from infection with clinical forms of either influenza A-1 or influenza A-2 virus is unclear. Serum antibody titers last only about six months but may not be correlated with protective immunity.

The vaccines currently available are designed to produce immunity against both the A-1 and the A-2 influenza viruses and are "killed" viral agents that give a short serologic response. Horses are given two vaccinations two to four weeks apart beginning when foals are 10 to 12 weeks of age. For maximal protection of horses at high risk, particularly young racing and show stock, booster vaccinations are given as frequently as every two to four months after an initial series of two injections. After the age of three years, boosters every six months or at yearly intervals may provide adequate protection. Injection of these vaccines produces little or no untoward reaction in the majority of animals. However, a few animals develop transient areas of induration at the site of injection and muscle stiffness.

EQUINE HERPESVIRUS

Respiratory disease and the associated complications of abortion and neurologic disease caused by equine herpesvirus 1 are problems that are even more difficult to control than that of equine influenza. As natural immunity to EHV-1 generated by clinical infection produces an immunity that lasts

TABLE 1. GUIDELINES FOR VACCINATION PROGRAMS

Vaccine	Age 2–4 Months	4–6 Months	1 Year	Booster	Note
Tetanus	Toxoid	Toxoid	Toxoid	Annual	Give toxoid if horse receives tetanus-prone wound 6 months after booster.
EEE/WEE	First injection	Second injection		Every 6 months of insect season	
VEE		First injection		Every 2 years	Not routinely recommended in United States
Equine influenza	First injection	Second injection		Every 4–6 months	
EHV-1	First injection	Second injection		Every 2–3 months	Only for upper respiratory infection; of questionable efficacy for prevention of abortion; use according to manufacturer's recommendations between conception and parturition
Strangles					Two injections 4 weeks apart only in areas of extremely high incidence
Rabies				Annual	Only in endemic areas
Anthrax				Annual	Only in endemic areas

EEE, WEE, and VEE = eastern, western, and Venezuelan equine encephalomyelitis, respectively
EHV = Equine herpesvirus

only three to four months, it is unlikely that protection provided by either of the two commercially available vaccines is of any longer duration. Because questions have been raised about the efficacy of the modified live virus vaccine in preventing abortions, no recommendations for its use for this purpose will be made in this article. For the possible prevention of respiratory disease, a result not conclusively proven, vaccination of young horses with modified live virus vaccine begins with an initial immunization between two and four months of age followed by booster injections every two to three months until the horse reaches the age of two years. Horses in training face constant reexposure, which usually results in a state of apparent immunity. Initial data suggest that a new killed EHV-1 vaccine provides protection against the acute respiratory form, abortion, and the neurologic form; however, it is still too early to judge its efficacy in large-scale field usage. For young horses, a vaccination program similar to that for the modified live vaccine is recommended, but for pregnant mares, it is recommended that the killed vaccine be administered at five, seven, and nine months of pregnancy.

STRANGLES (STREPTOCOCCUS EQUI)

There is presently only one bacterin available in the United States for this disease. Experimentally, the bacterin has been shown to prevent disease, but mass clinical use has not been successful. This has opened the question of antigenic change or modification in mass, commercially produced products of this type. While routine vaccination against strangles is not recommended, the vaccine, if given in two doses four weeks apart prior to an outbreak on an area-wide basis, has been shown to cause a reduction in new cases. At the present time, there is a cell-free strangles vaccine being produced in Australia that is apparently free of the common adverse side effects. If this vaccine becomes available in America, strangles preventive measures will be readjusted.

RABIES

In areas of high incidence of rabies in other animals, horses should be vaccinated. Active rabies in the horse always results in the death of the animal and, quite often, unnecessary exposure of humans and other animals. The porcine-kidney-tissue (ERA strain-fixed virus)* rabies vaccine is the only product available approved for use in the horse in America. In rabies endemic areas, yearly boosters are recommended.

---

*Jen-Sal Laboratories, Kansas City, MO

ANTHRAX

In endemic areas or with outbreaks occurring in cattle, an annual anthrax vaccination with Sterne-type nonencapsulated avirulent spore vaccine is recommended. This vaccine is not to be used in pregnant animals and must be used carefully, as it may produce severe inflammatory response (fever and myalgia) in the vaccinated animal.

CLOSTRIDIAL ORGANISMS

Horses appear to be susceptible to many of the clostridial infections other than tetanus. Clinical experience and experimental data on the use of clostridial vaccines in the horse are unavailable.

References

1. Verberne, L. R. M., and Mirck, M. H.: A practical health program for prevention of parasitic and infectious diseases in horses and ponies. Eq. Vet. J., 8:123, 1976.
2. Tyzick, I. R.: Veterinary Immunology. Philadelphia, W. B. Saunders Co., 1977.
3. Gibbs, E. P. J.: Equine viral encephalitis: Review article. Eq. Vet. J., 8:66, 1976.
4. Proceedings of the 1980 Invitational Workshop on Equine Viral Respiratory Diseases and Complications. Columbus, Ohio. Am. Assoc. Eq. Pract. Newsletter, May, 1980.
5. First, Second, Third, and Fourth International Conferences on Equine Infectious Diseases. *In* Bryans, J. T., and Gerber, H. (eds.): 1967, 1969, 1972, 1978.

ANTIBIOTICS

Waldir M. Pedersoli, AUBURN, ALABAMA

Antimicrobials constitute the most frequently used therapeutic drugs in equine practice. Notwithstanding their clinical availability in a variety of pharmaceutical forms over the last four decades, their mode of action, pharmacologic effects, and therapeutic uses are often misunderstood, resulting in improper use and a decrease in their clinical effectiveness.[9]

DEFINITION AND CHARACTERISTICS

Antibiotics, which are chemical agents produced by numerous species of microorganisms, are capable of inhibiting the growth of other microorganisms and, in many cases, destroying them. An increasing number of antibiotics are now partially or totally synthesized. The number of antibiotics identified extends into the hundreds, with the possibility of thousands or even millions becoming available through synthesis. Approximately 60 have been characterized enough to be of value in the treatment of infectious diseases (Table 1). In this paper, the words antibiotics and antimicrobial drugs are used synonymously for chemicals of natural, semisynthetic, or totally synthetic origin that are used clinically for their action against pathogenic microorganisms.

IS CHEMOTHERAPY REQUIRED?

This important question should always be answered before prescribing an antibiotic. The primary objective in using antibiotics is to kill and/or inhibit pathogenic microorganisms in affected animals and humans as quickly and efficiently as possible while causing minimal or no harm at all to the host. Antibiotics are used to treat infections, not diseases; therefore, there is no advantage in using antibiotics when the illness is not due to infection or when infection is present but results from microorganisms (such as viruses) known to be unaffected by antibiotic action.[23]

PHARMACOLOGIC CLASSIFICATION AND MECHANISMS OF ANTIMICROBIAL ACTION

Antibiotic agents are classified according to their chemical structure (Table 1); their spectrum of antibacterial activity (narrow, such as penicillins, erythromycin, and lincomycin, or broad, such as tetracycline, chloramphenicol, aminoglycosides, ampicillin, cephalosporins, sulfonamides, and nitrofurans); and their major direct effect on the microorganism (bactericidal or bacteriostatic). Some antibiotics have a killing (bactericidal) action at or close to the minimal inhibitory concentration (MIC), while others (bacteriostatic) only inhibit bacterial growth. The penicillins, cephalosporins, aminoglycosides, and polymyxins are considered bactericidal, while tetracyclines, chloramphenicol, macrolides, and lincomycin are generally bacteriostatic. Although the classic division of antibiotic activity into either bactericidal or bacteriostatic is often only of aca-

TABLE 1. CONDENSED CLASSIFICATION OF ANTIBIOTICS AND OTHER ANTIMICROBIAL AGENTS

A. Penicillins

Penicillin G benzathine	Amoxicillin	Hetacillin
Penicillin G potassium	Ampicillin	Methicillin
Penicillin G procaine	Carbenicillin	Nafcillin
Penicillin G sodium	Cloxacillin	Oxacillin
Penicillin V	Dicloxacillin	Teracillin

B. Cephalosporins

Cephazolin	Cephalothin
Cephalexin	Cephapirin
Cephaloglycin	Cepharadine
Cephaloridine	

C. Aminoglycosides

Amikacin	Paramomycin
Framycetin	Sisomycin
Gentamicin	Streptomycin
Kanamycin	Tobramycin
Neomycin	

D. Tetracyclines

Chlortetracycline	Minocycline
Demethylchlortetracycline	Oxytetracycline
Doxycycline	Tetracycline
Methacycline	

E. Chloramphenicol

F. Macrolides

Erythromycin
Oleandomycin and troleandomycin
Tylocin

G. Miscellaneous

Bacitracin	Polymyxin B
Clindamycin and lincomycin	Spectinomycin
Colistin	Vancomycin
Novobiocin	

H. Antifungals

Amphotericin
Griseofulvin
Nystatin

I. Antibacterials

Sulfonamides
Trimethoprim
Nitrofurans

J. Antituberculosis

Isoniazid
Para-aminosalicylic acid
Ethambutol
Rifampin

demic interest and not absolutely distinct, it may have important implications in the treatment of infections.[24] Bactericidal action is desirable in life-threatening situations in which a very rapid effect is required, when the physiologic antimicrobial defensive mechanisms are seriously impaired, or when trying to prevent a residue of dormant organisms that might lead to "carrier" states.[22] The use of bacteriostatic drugs implies that the normal antimicro-bial defense mechanisms of the animal participate effectively in order to rid the body of the infection; otherwise, relapse could ensue following cessation of chemotherapy.[24] In clinical practice, there is little need to select between bactericidal and bacteriostatic agents for treating mild to moderate infections in otherwise healthy individuals[22] as long as adequate amounts in high enough doses are used often enough.

MECHANISM AND SITE OF ACTION

The cellular and biochemical sites at which antimicrobial agents exert their primary action are presented in Table 2.

THE SELECTION OF ANTIMICROBIAL AGENTS

Choosing the proper antibacterial drug depends not only on the etiologic microorganism and the site of infection but also on the urgency of the therapy, probable duration of the disease, frequency and route of administration, estimated cost of the treatment, and the knowledge of possible adverse reactions resulting from the use of antimicrobial agents. The first decision the veterinarian must make is whether administration of an antimicrobial agent is really necessary. Ideally, initiation of antibiotic therapy necessitates the identification of the causative agent coupled with antibiotic sensitivity tests. However, because therapy often is required before microbiologic identification and sensitivity tests are completed, the veterinarian must use clinical experience and judgment in identifying the most likely microorganisms responsible for the infection, as well as the preferred drug and the route of administration; appropriate selection can also be helped by a Gram-stained smear of exudate or discharge. Antimicrobial sensitivity tests are most important when dealing with microorganisms that have considerable variation in sensitivity, such as coliforms, enterococci, Proteus sp, Pseudomonas sp, Salmonella sp, and staphylococci. Sensitivity tests are also usually necessary when body defense mechanisms are impaired and the most efficacious antimicrobial is required or when antibiotics (such as streptomycin) that permit the development of bacterial resistance are used. Sensitivity tests are usually not necessary with microorganisms with little or no susceptibility variation (streptococci), mixed infection when there is uncertainty concerning the etiologic microorganism, and when the number of organisms isolated by culturing is considered insignificant.[3]

Whenever the practitioner begins therapy on a presumptive bacteriologic diagnosis, cultures of blood and other body fluids should be taken before initiating chemotherapy. Bacterial identification and sensitivity tests are more useful in establishing which drugs are ineffective rather than those that are probably most efficacious.[17] Sensitivity tests are not infallible and are of little value or actually misleading if poor technique is used in securing specimens, growing cultures, or establishing results. No matter what technique is used by the practitioner for determining the proper antimicrobial therapy, constant clinical reevaluation and response to the treatment selected are still the best clues to suc-

TABLE 2. SITES OF ACTION OF ANTIMICROBIAL AGENTS[4, 22]

Antimicrobial	Site of Antibacterial Action
A. Bacitracin, cephalothin, cycloserine, novobiocin, penicillins, ristocetin, vancomycin	Cell wall
B. Amphotericin B, colistin, gentamicin, kanamycin, neomycin, novobiocin, nystatin, polymyxins, streptomycin	Cell membrane
C. 1. *Aminoglycosides*—amikacin, dihydrostreptomycin, gentamicin, kanamycin, neomycin, sisomycin, streptomycin, tobramycin 2. *Macrolides*—erythromycin, oleandomycin, tylosin 3. *Tetracyclines*—chlortetracycline, demethylchlortetracycline, doxycycline, methacycline, minocycline, oxytetracycline, tetracycline 4. *Miscellaneous*—chloramphenicol, clindamycin, lincomycin, spectinomycin	Protein synthesis
D. Griseofulvin, rifamycin, numerous others too toxic for clinical use	Nucleic acid synthesis
E. Sulfonamides, nitrofurans, isoniazid, para-aminosalicylic acid	Metabolites and enzyme systems

cessful treatment in an animal receiving an adequate supportive therapy regimen and maintained in a proper environment.

Although opinion seems to vary, initially a narrow-spectrum antimicrobial agent is preferred over one with a broad spectrum of activity. Penicillins are generally considered the drugs of choice because of the greater incidence of gram-positive infections in the horse. In mixed infections, the proven synergistic effect of penicillin and streptomycin and of trimethoprim and a sulfonamide should be considered, making sure that the full therapeutic dose of each drug is administered.[21] Antibiotics should always be used keeping in mind the patient's complete health picture and making sure that the basic principles of good surgical and medical practices are followed; antibiotics are not replacements for a thorough and complete physical examination and proper diagnosis. One must always bear in mind that accumulated pus under tension necessitates surgical drainage and that infection resulting from a foreign body, calculus, or blockage and obstruction of a body's passage requires correction of the causative condition before the infection becomes responsive to chemotherapy.

SOME REASONS FOR FAILURES WITH ANTIMICROBIAL THERAPY

The effectiveness of antimicrobial therapy is directly dependent on the microorganism(s) present, the patient, and the drug being used. In most situations, a five-day treatment will usually be sufficient to indicate if therapy is succeeding. If at the end of this period the animal's health condition has not improved substantially, the following possible reasons should be considered.

MICROORGANISM FACTORS[13, 19]

Drug Resistance. If the microorganism is naturally resistant or if it has acquired resistance during chemotherapy, then little or no antibacterial effect is achieved.[19] Acquired antimicrobial resistance can be induced by mutations, changes in the structure of chromosomal DNA, or transferable drug resistance, which is linked to extrachromosomal DNA. Plasmids are the extrachromosomal DNA molecules (R factors) that have the capacity to reproduce themselves. The R factors are present mainly in gram-negative enteric bacteria, including Enterobacter, *Escherichia coli,* Klebsiella, Proteus, Pseudomonas, Salmonella, Shigella, and Vibrio. A growing number of bacteriostatic antimicrobials (chloramphenicol, sulfonamides, and tetracyclines) are frequently associated with R factor resistance. In addition to drug-resistant microorganisms, there is a group of drug-destroying bacteria that are capable of inactivating the antibiotic agent through the action of specialized enzymes such as penicillinase.

Wrong Diagnosis. No microorganism is actually involved or responsible for the disease. This is a common reason for failure of chemotherapy; for example, antibiotics do not alter fever due to viral infections.

Mixed Infections. If two or more microorganisms are the causative agents of the infection, antimicrobial therapy against only one may not be fully effective.

FACTORS RELATED TO THE PATIENT

Associated Diseases. An infectious condition can change the in vivo distribution of a drug. It is known that penicillin G can cross the inflamed meninges more easily than the normal meninges. The homeostasis of the animal is also of vital concern. The pharmacokinetics of the antimicrobial agent (absorption, distribution, biotransformation, and excretion) may be significantly altered by the state of fluid and electrolyte (kidney function) balance and cardiovascular integrity. Most antibiotics have an optimal pH at which they perform best. The distribution of some antimicrobial agents can be altered by fibrinous, purulent, necrotic, and other materials linked with a bacterial infection.

FACTORS RELATED TO THE ANTIMICROBIAL AGENT[11, 12]

Wrong Dose. In order to be effective, the antimicrobial agent must reach its site of action at a high enough concentration and stay there for a time long enough to kill or inhibit the etiologic microorganism. In order to achieve those objectives, the antimicrobial agent must be given at the recommended dose, time intervals, route of administration, and proper pharmaceutical dosage form to ensure full bioavailability.

Mixing with Interfering Drugs.[2] Whenever two antimicrobial agents act simultaneously upon a homogenous bacterial population, the achieved effect can be of four types: indifference, additive, antagonism, or synergism. *Indifference* means that each drug acts totally independent of the other. The vast majority of antimicrobial combinations used clinically yield indifference type results. *Additive* effects may occur when both drugs are effective against a particular microorganism, causing an effect that theoretically is the algebraic sum of the effect of each individual drug. *Antagonism* occurs when the total effect is smaller than the algebraic sum produced by the effect of each single drug which constitutes the combination. *Synergism* is accomplished when two drugs acting simultaneously upon bacteria result in an effect greater than could be achieved by either one acting alone. The following rules are proposed as guidelines for antimicrobial therapy where combinations need to be used, so that antagonism may be avoided: (1) Avoid combining bacteriostatic and bactericidal drugs; (2) antagonism rarely, if ever, occurs between members of two bacteriostatic groups or between members of two bactericidal groups; (3) bactericidal antibiotics may be synergistic; (4) bacteriostatic antibiotics are never synergistic but may be additive; (5) if possible, combination therapy should be avoided when in vitro sensitivity testing has not been done.

In addition to improper drug combinations leading to an alteration of the expected antimicrobial effect, interactions of other kinds can also occur between antimicrobial drugs and other agents frequently used in therapy. Therefore, it is generally agreed that the practice of mixing antibacterial drugs with each other or with other drugs and vehicles in the same syringe (unless officially approved and recommended) is a poor if not dangerous practice. The chances of physical, chemical, and pharmacologic incompatibilities occurring are enormous.

Often physical and chemical incompatibilities are clearly visible upon mixing, but in many cases they are not evident; for example, with carbenicillin-gentamicin or kanamycin-methicillin; the formation of insoluble complexes when tetracyclines are mixed with high concentrations of aluminum, calcium, iron, or magnesium salts are well known. The concomitant use of chloramphenicol and other drugs that may be biotransformed in the liver may lead to a pharmacologic interaction due to the inhibitory effect of the antibiotic upon the hepatic microsomal enzyme system. A list of some incompatibilities related to antibiotics has recently become available and is presented in Table 3.

FIXED COMBINATIONS OF ANTIMICROBIAL DRUGS[12, 22]

Ever since a second antimicrobial agent became available, there has been a scientifically unjustified tendency to develop pharmaceutical preparations containing two or more antimicrobial agents on the assumption that the mixture is either more potent, less toxic, or has a broader spectrum of antibacterial activity than a single agent. Although the FDA and the National Academy of Sciences have long ago stated that use of combinations in the treatment of patients who can be cured by one drug "is irrational, illogical, unscientific and is a disservice to the patient," there are certain clinical situations in which the simultaneous use of two or more antimicrobial agents (preferably in nonfixed combinations) is not only desirable but necessary. The most important of these clinical situations are described next.

Overwhelming, Life-Threatening Infections. Septicemia induced by gram-negative bacteria, especially in immunodeficient patients, has been identified as the leading prerequisite for the use of combinations. Gentamicin is considered the drug of choice combined with ampicillin (for streptococci) and clindamycin (for anaerobes) to cover all the commonly pathogenic bacteria; other combinations being broadly advocated are carbenicillin plus gentamicin, polymyxin plus kanamycin, and kanamycin plus ampicillin.

Mixed Infections. Rarely, when no single antimicrobial agent is effective against each of two or more distinct bacteria causing a systemic infection, the use of two separate drugs may be justified. Mixed infections are often related to surface infections such as skin abrasions, wounds, and mucous membrane lesions. Antibiotics recommended for topical application only (bacitracin, neomycin, and polymyxin) are often used.

Prevention of Rapid Emergence of Resistance. In the treatment of some chronic infections, such as tuberculosis, the use of two antimicrobial agents (streptomycin plus para-aminosalicylic acid or isoniazid plus ethambutol) is extremely effective in preventing the rapid emergence of resistant mutants to a single drug. The use of gentamicin plus carbenicillin has also been recommended for Pseudomonas septicemia.

Synergistic and Additive Action. Occasionally, or maybe rarely, a true synergistic or additive action may take place when two antimicrobial agents are used simultaneously. Clinically useful synergism has been obtained in human patients with penicillin plus streptomycin (endocarditis), streptomycin plus para-aminosalicylic acid and isoniazid plus ethambutol (tuberculosis), streptomycin plus tetracycline (brucellosis), neomycin plus polymyxin (gut sterilization), carbenicillin plus gentamicin (Pseudomonas infections), and sulfamethoxazole plus trimethroprim (certain urinary tract infections).

PHARMACOLOGIC HAZARDS OF ANTIBIOTIC THERAPY

Although the penicillin group of antibiotics is exceptionally free from toxic effects even in dosages far in excess of those recommended for proper therapy, the general consensus is that there are no harmless antibiotics. Even the minimally toxic antibiotics such as erythromycin can cause liver pathology in some individuals. Diarrhea, collapse, and death following tetracycline and oxytetracycline administration to horses are well known. The undesirable effects may be direct or may be due to the antibiotic itself (ototoxicity by streptomycin), hypersensitivity reactions (penicillin), species with higher "susceptibility" (streptomycin, chloramphenicol in cats), or a drug interaction such as has been documented in humans (methoxyflurane plus tetracycline) and in dogs (chloramphenicol plus pentobarbital). A summary of some of the reported adverse effects of antimicrobial agents in animals and humans is presented in Table 4.

PATTERNS OF ANTIMICROBIAL SUSCEPTIBILITY IN HORSES

Antimicrobial susceptibility tests are used to determine the in vitro susceptibility and resistance of the microorganism to the agent being tested. Because the ultimate success of antimicrobial therapy is directly related to the sensitivity of the microorganism to the antimicrobial agent used, susceptibility tests are of utmost importance in helping the practitioner make the best possible selection of the antimicrobial agent to be used. The most comprehensive paper dealing with this subject in the horse was published recently,[15] from which most of the information presented here has been compiled.

TABLE 3. INCOMPATIBILITIES OF SOME ANTIBIOTICS[7]

Antibiotic	Incompatibility
Ampicillin	Do not mix with any drug.
Carbenicillin	Do not mix with: Chloramphenicol Erythromycin Gentamicin Lincomycin Tetracycline
Cephalothin	Do not mix with any drug.
Chloramphenicol	Do not mix with: Carbenicillin Erythromycin Nitrofurans Oxytetracycline Polymyxin B Sulfonamides Tetracyclines Vancomycin
Clindamycin	Compatible with most IV solutions.
Erythromycin	Do not mix with: Carbenicillin Chloramphenicol-lincomycin Oxytetracycline Iodides
Gentamicin	Do not mix with any drug. Compatible with IV solutions.
Kanamycin	Do not mix with any drug. Compatible with IV solutions.
Lincomycin	Do not mix with any drug. Compatible with IV solutions.
Methicillin	Do not mix with: Oxytetracycline Tetracycline
Oxacillin	Do not mix with any drug.
Oxytetracycline	Do not mix with: Ampicillin Calcium salts Chloramphenicol Erythromycin Methicillin Nitrofurans Oxacillin Penicillin Polymyxin B Ringer's lactate Sodium bicarbonate
Penicillin G	Do not mix with: Chlortetracycline Oxytetracycline Tetracycline Sodium bicarbonate
Tetracycline	Do not mix with: Calcium salts Carbenicillin Cephalosporins Chloramphenicol Erythromycin Nitrofurans Penicillin G Polymyxin B Sodium bicarbonate Sulfonamides

(From Davis; L. E., and Abbitt, B.: Clinical pharmacology of antibacterial drugs in the uterus of the mare. J. Am. Vet. Med. Assoc., *170*:205, 1977. With permission.)

TABLE 4. SOME POSSIBLE ADVERSE EFFECTS OF ANTIMICROBIAL DRUGS IN HUMANS AND ANIMALS[1, 5, 6, 10, 18, 21, 26]

Antimicrobial Drug	Adverse Effect	Animal
A. *Penicillins*		
1. Penicillin G benzathine	Hypersensitivity, colitis X syndrome	Humans, horse, cattle
	Anaphylaxis, CNS stimulation	Horse
2. Penicillin G potassium	Cardiac arrest	Foal
3. Ampicillin, lincomycin, clindamycin	"Pseudomembranous colitis" with bloody diarrhea, death	Humans, horse
4. Ampicillin	Anaphylactoid reaction	Cattle
B. *Aminoglycosides*	Cardiovascular depression, ototoxicity, peripheral neuromuscular blockade	Man, horse, cat, dog
	Renal damage	Dog
Gentamicin	Partial blindness	Cattle
C. *Tetracyclines*		
1. Tetracycline	Diarrhea, colitis X, anaphylaxis	Horse
	Teeth staining, liver damage	Humans
	Malignant hyperthermia	Cat
2. Oxytetracycline	Colitis X, collapse, death	Horse
	Anaphylaxis	Horse, cattle
D. *Cephalosporins*		
1. Cephaloridine	Tubular necrosis	Monkeys, rabbits
E. *Miscellaneous*		
1. Chloramphenicol	Depression of hepatic microsomal enzyme system	Humans, cat, dog
	Aplastic anemia	Infants, cat
	Anorexia, depression, leucopenia	Cat
	Anaphylaxis	Cat
2. Trimethoprim	Anaphylactoid reaction	Horse
3. Erythromycin lactobionate	Intense local reaction	Horse

The term *minimal inhibitory concentration* (MIC), usually reported in micrograms (μg) or international units (IU) per ml, represents the lowest concentration of the antimicrobial agent inhibiting bacterial growth. Generally speaking, a microorganism is considered susceptible if it is inhibited by a value of at least one half the mean blood concentration or one fourth the average peak blood concentration; it is declared resistant if the MIC is greater than the peak blood concentration. If the MIC is situated above one half the mean blood concentration or one fourth the mean peak blood concentration but below the peak blood concentration, the strains are declared intermediate in susceptibility. The percentage sensitivity of the 11 most common bacteria isolated from all animals by a veterinary diagnostic laboratory in Illinois (1972 to 1977) is presented in Table 5. Also shown are data indicating the total number of isolates of bacteria generally considered pathogenic to horses and their percent-

age by site of isolation (Table 6). The total number of bacterial isolates from horses, the percentages that are sensitive or intermediately sensitive and resistant to 17 frequently administered antimicrobial agents are indicated in Table 7. The blood serum MIC of seven antibiotics tested against 12 bacteria considered pathogenic and often isolated from equine specimens is shown in Table 8.

CLINICAL PHARMACOLOGY OF ANTIMICROBIAL AGENTS IN HORSES

Several authors who have reviewed the literature pertaining to the clinical use of antibiotics in the horse from 1969 to 1975 have expressed surprise that relatively little information was available. More recently, other investigators have agreed that the basic principles of antimicrobial therapy as well as some therapeutic regimens for specific equine dis-

TABLE 5. PERCENTAGE OF BACTERIA SENSITIVE TO 16 ANTIMICROBIAL DRUGS

Microorganism	Total Isolates Tested	AMP	BAC	CLI	CHL	ERY	GEN	KAN	NEO	NOV	PEN	POL	STR	TET	NIT	SUL	TRI
Bordetella bronchiseptica	143	27	11	4	97	88	99	92	94	38	7	98	4	90	13	28	34
Corynebacterium pyogenes	280	96	95	82	99	86	97	89	65	98	94	23	48	77	89	13	9
Escherichia coli	2658	59	1	1	89	32	99	60	57	10	2	97	19	28	96	79	28
Klebsiella pneumoniae	210	18	1	1	80	10	94	72	70	8	1	97	33	50	81	78	56
Pasteurella hemolytica	247	58	42	2	99	86	94	83	59	20	52	94	29	59	99	88	42
Pasteurella multocida	514	96	35	5	99	88	94	83	67	54	89	92	40	88	96	66	17
Proteus mirabilis	246	80	1	2	88	6	99	91	87	48	44	4	68	5	63	76	61
Pseudomonas aeruginosa	425	4	2	19	27	9	90	13	40	4	3	96	17	13	8	35	56
Salmonella sp	242	83	2	2	99	12	99	74	71	4	14	96	23	63	92	60	17
Staphylococcus aureus	1003	65	97	87	96	94	99	95	96	95	50	83	70	71	99	41	34
Streptococcus (beta)	564	99	93	73	97	92	74	13	12	34	96	12	8	28	86	8	7

AMP = ampicillin, BAC = bacitracin, CLI = clindamycin, CHL = chloramphenicol, ERY = erythromycin, GEN = gentamicin, KAN = kanamycin, NEO = neomycin, NOV = novobiocin, PEN = penicillin, POL = polymyxin B, STR = streptomycin, TET = tetracycline, NIT = nitrofurazone, SUL = sulfachloropyridazine, TRI = triple sulfa. (Modified from Rhoades, H. E.: Sensitivity of bacteria to 16 antibiotic agents. VM SAC, 74:976, 1979). (With permission.)

TABLE 6. SITE OF ISOLATION OF BACTERIA GENERALLY CONSIDERED PATHOGENIC TO HORSES[15]

		Percentage of Total Isolates											
Microorganism	Total No. of Isolates	Abscesses, Wounds	Bone	Blood	Ear, Eye	Endo-trach. Tubes	Feces	Joint	Perito-neal Fluid	Pleu-ral Fluid	Repro-ductive Tract	Respira-tory Tract	Urine
Actinobacillus suis and *equuli*	31	14	3	3	—	—	—	—	3	—	—	77	—
Bordetella	20	—	—	—	—	5	—	—	—	—	—	95	—
Corynebacterium equi	13	—	—	—	—	—	—	8	—	—	—	92	—
Enterobacter	10	30	—	—	—	—	—	10	—	—	40	20	—
Escherichia coli	12	17	4	—	—	—	1	5	6	8	31	16	12
Klebsiella pneumoniae and *oxytoca*	16	6	—	6	—	—	—	—	6	6	57	13	6
Nonhemolytic streptococci	19	42	11	—	—	—	—	5	—	—	16	26	—
Pasteurella sp	40	22	3	—	—	—	—	—	3	8	5	59	—
Pasteurella ureae	22	18	—	—	—	—	—	—	—	5	—	77	—
Proteus mirabilis	9	56	—	—	—	—	—	11	—	—	11	11	11
Pseudomonas	35	9	2	—	11	—	—	—	—	—	50	11	17
aeruginosa	12	8	—	—	—	—	67	—	—	17	—	8	—
Salmonella	63	57	3	2	4	—	—	13	—	—	3	16	2
Staphylococcus aureus													
Streptococcus	10	20	10	—	10	—	—	—	—	—	—	60	—
zooepidemicus	39	32	8	—	8	—	—	—	—	—	11	36	5
*Miscellaneous													

*Miscellaneous bacteria include Actinobacter, Aeromonas, Alcaligenes, Citrobacter, Enterococcus, Eubacteria, Erwinia, Flavobacterium, Hemophilus, Micrococcus, Moraxella, Peptostreptococcus, Proteus, Pseudomonas, Serratia, and *Staphylococcus epidermides.*

TABLE 7. BACTERIA ISOLATED FROM HORSES AND PERCENTAGE SENSITIVE, INTERMEDIATELY SENSITIVE, AND RESISTANT TO COMMONLY ADMINISTERED ANTIMICROBIAL AGENTS[15]

Microorganism	No. of Isolates		Percentage Sensitive (S), Intermediately Sensitive (I), and Resistant (R) to Antibiotics Tested																
			AMP	CEP	CHL	ERY	GEN	KAN	LIN	MET	NEO	OXA	PEN	POL	STR	TET	SUL	FUR	CAR
Actinobacillus suis and *equuli*	31	(S)	71	97	100	83	100	68	—	—	42	—	65	94	42	87	81	100	—
		(I)	3	3	0	8	0	23	—	—	42	—	6	6	19	6	0	0	—
		(R)	26	0	0	9	0	9	—	—	16	—	29	0	39	7	19	0	—
Bordetella	20	(S)	0	61	100	33	100	90	—	—	90	0	0	100	0	100	68	0	—
		(I)	0	22	0	50	0	5	—	—	5	0	0	0	0	0	0	0	—
		(R)	100	17	0	17	0	5	—	—	5	100	100	0	100	0	32	100	—
Corynebacterium equi	13	(S)	—	54	92	100	100	90	8	13	100	0	23	—	92	77	—	58	—
		(I)	—	0	8	0	0	0	0	0	0	0	31	—	8	0	—	17	—
		(R)	—	46	0	0	0	10	92	87	0	100	46	—	0	23	—	25	—
Enterobacter	10	(S)	20	30	80	0	100	90	—	—	80	0	0	83	56	70	100	83	—
		(I)	10	20	20	0	0	0	—	—	10	0	0	0	33	20	0	17	—
		(R)	70	50	0	100	0	10	—	—	10	100	100	17	11	10	0	0	—
Escherichia coli	12	(S)	59	62	84	3	99	68	—	—	0	0	2	99	28	45	28	99	—
		(I)	4	19	3	0	1	7	—	—	4	4	1	1	10	8	10	1	—
		(R)	37	19	13	97	0	25	—	—	96	96	97	0	62	47	62	0	—
Klebsiella pneumoniae and *oxytoca*	16	(S)	13	94	81	0	100	94	—	—	81	0	0	100	63	56	79	67	—
		(I)	0	0	0	0	0	0	—	—	6	0	0	0	6	13	0	0	—
		(R)	87	6	19	100	0	6	—	—	13	100	100	0	31	31	21	33	—
Nonhemolytic streptococci	19	(S)	73	65	90	79	70	15	64	—	20	45	70	100	28	63	0	64	57
		(I)	0	0	5	11	10	23	0	—	10	0	10	0	22	11	0	0	0
		(R)	27	35	5	10	20	62	36	—	70	55	20	0	50	26	100	36	43
Pasteurella sp	40	(S)	92	97	100	89	100	89	—	—	67	17	75	86	68	100	70	95	—
		(I)	3	0	0	3	0	3	—	—	18	0	15	5	15	0	3	0	—
		(R)	5	3	0	8	0	8	—	—	15	83	10	9	17	0	27	5	—
Pasteurella ureae	22	(S)	91	100	100	90	100	65	—	—	59	0	77	100	45	95	95	100	—
		(I)	0	0	0	10	0	35	—	—	36	10	9	0	9	0	0	0	—
		(R)	9	0	0	0	0	0	—	—	5	90	14	0	46	5	5	0	—
Proteus mirabilis	9	(S)	22	56	63	0	100	67	—	—	71	0	0	25	22	33	50	38	—
		(I)	0	0	0	0	0	0	—	—	0	0	22	0	22	0	0	13	—
		(R)	88	44	37	100	0	37	—	—	29	100	88	75	56	67	50	49	—
Pseudomonas aeruginosa	35	(S)	0	0	6	0	89	3	—	—	24	0	0	100	14	14	16	0	—
		(I)	0	0	6	0	3	9	—	—	29	0	0	0	3	6	6	0	—
		(R)	100	100	88	100	8	88	—	—	47	100	100	0	83	80	78	100	—
Salmonella	12	(S)	42	50	92	100	100	33	—	—	33	0	0	100	25	33	67	100	—
		(I)	0	17	0	0	0	0	—	—	0	0	0	0	0	0	0	0	—
		(R)	58	33	8	0	0	67	—	—	67	100	100	0	75	67	33	0	—
Staphylococcus aureus	63	(S)	42	100	100	95	100	96	98	100	95	91	27	100	47	87	83	100	—
		(I)	0	0	0	0	0	0	0	0	0	3	2	0	0	0	0	0	—
		(R)	58	0	0	5	0	4	2	0	5	6	71	0	53	13	17	0	—
*Streptococcus equi	1	(S)	—	—	—	—	—	—	—	—	—	—	—	—	—	—	—	—	—
		(I)	—	—	—	—	—	—	—	—	—	—	—	—	—	—	—	—	—
		(R)	—	—	—	—	—	—	—	—	—	—	—	—	—	—	—	—	—
Streptococcus zooepidemicus	10	(S)	100	100	100	100	100	66	100	100	50	75	100	—	71	57	—	100	—
		(I)	0	0	0	0	0	17	0	0	13	0	0	—	0	14	—	0	—
		(R)	0	0	0	0	0	17	0	0	37	25	0	—	29	29	—	0	—
Miscellaneous bacteria	39	(S)	45	61	82	79	94	79	50	8	81	27	29	79	47	73	77	63	—
		(I)	3	5	5	5	0	12	10	0	8	0	16	5	11	11	0	7	—
		(R)	52	34	13	16	6	9	40	92	11	73	55	16	42	16	23	30	—

AMP = ampicillin, CEP = cephalothin, CHL = chloramphenicol, ERY = erythromycin, GEN = gentamicin, KAN = kanamycin, LIN = lincomycin, MET = methicillin, NEO = neomycin, OXA = oxacillin, PEN = penicillin, POL = polymyxin B, STR = streptomycin, TET = tetracycline, SUL = sulfanilamide, FUR = nitrofurantoin (Furadantin), CAR = carbenicillin

eases are well established. What seems to be still inadequate are data obtained from properly conducted clinical trials and information related to pharmacokinetic studies of antimicrobial agents in the horse. A compilation of the biologic half-life (β) (Table 9) determined by different authors for various antimicrobials in the horse as well as suggested guidelines for dosage, route of administration, and mean blood serum concentrations are presented in Table 10. Also presented are data concerning the in vitro MIC of several antimicrobials to bacteria generally considered pathogenic to horses (Table 11) and a summary of the mean blood plasma concentrations of various antibiotics and sulfonamides after a single administration to adult horses (Table 12).

DRUG THERAPY IN THE NEONATAL FOAL

Many problems related to drug therapy in the neonate can be due to incomplete development of the biologic mechanisms involved in the pharmacokinetics (absorption, distribution, biotransformation, excretion, etc.) of the drug being used. A newborn animal has a deficient drug-biotransforming hepatic enzyme system until it is approximately 30 days old. Thus, owing to the augmented risks of drug therapy in the neonate, special care should be taken to properly identify the microorganism responsible for the infection and its antimicrobial susceptibility so that the benefit: risk ratio is maximized.[8] Since identification of the microorganism is not always possible, microscopic examination of ex-

udates, aspirates, and urine coupled with the knowledge of the pathogenic microorganisms most likely to be found in horses (see Table 6) is of tremendous help in selecting the most appropriate antibiotic (Table 13).

SUGGESTED GUIDELINES FOR ANTIMICROBIAL THERAPY IN HORSES

1. It is impractical to base antimicrobial therapy solely on the basis of bacterial culture and susceptibility. Appropriate choice can be made by examining a Gram-stained smear of exudate or discharge.
2. An immediate decision can usually be made based on the clinician's evaluation of the disorder, which will guide him or her to the probable etiologic agent, first choice drug, and route of administration.
3. Initially a narrow-spectrum antibiotic such as penicillin is preferred owing to the high incidence of gram-positive infections. In mixed infections, consider the use of penicillin and streptomycin.
4. Be alert for the possibility of drug-induced adverse reactions. Document and report every case to the FDA's Bureau of Veterinary Medicine.
5. If no significant clinical improvement occurs within 48 hours of initial therapy, be prepared to change therapy.
6. Do not use suboptimal dosage regimens or prophylactic therapy.
7. Avoid combining bactericidal and bacteriostatic drugs.
8. Continue therapy for at least three days after clinical recovery has occurred.

TABLE 8. BLOOD SERUM MINIMUM INHIBITORY CONCENTRATIONS (μg/ml) OF SOME ANTIBIOTICS TESTED AGAINST BACTERIA CONSIDERED PATHOGENIC AND FREQUENTLY ISOLATED FROM EQUINE SPECIMENS[13]

Microorganism	AMP	CHL	ERY	GEN	KAN	OXY	PEN
Actinobacillus equuli	16	8	ND	16	64	1	ND
Bordetella bronchiseptica	≥16	16	ND	8	32	4	ND
Corynebacterium equi	2–4	4.9	1.25	0.25	ND	2	4
Corynebacterium pseudotuberculosis	0.12	ND	<0.25	0.05	ND	0.25	0.06
Escherichia coli	5	3	ND	1	2	3.1	64
Klebsiella sp	ND	0.5	ND	0.06	0.12	6.3	ND
Pasteurella hemolytica	0.5	1	4	2	8	0.1	0.5
Salmonella sp	1.5	0.5	ND	0.25	1	4.2	>9
Staphylococcus aureus	0.05	1	0.5	0.12	0.5	1.6	0.03
Streptococcus fecalis	1	ND	1.5	8	8	6.3	2
Streptococcus equi	0.5	ND	0.25	ND	ND	4.2	0.002
Streptococcus zooepidemicus	ND	ND	ND	ND	ND	4.2	0.002

ND = not determined, AMP = ampicillin, CHL = chloramphenicol, ERY = erythromycin, GEN = gentamicin, KAN = kanamycin, OXY = oxytetracycline, PEN = penicillin G

TABLE 9. BIOLOGIC HALF-LIVES (T1/2 β) OF
ANTIMICROBIAL DRUGS IN THE HORSE[9]

Antimicrobial	Dosage (mg/kg)	Half-life (hours)
Ampicillin sodium	40	1.55
Chloramphenicol	9–26	0.98
Chloramphenicol	22	0.9
Chloramphenicol	20–40	1.0
Gentamicin	5	2.54
Kanamycin	10	1.41
Penicillin G sodium	21–36*	0.88
Oxytetracycline	2.5	10.5
Oxytetracycline	4	15.7
Sulfadimethoxine	60	11.3
Sulfadimidine	60	9.8
Sulfamethyldiazine	60	11.9
Sulfamethylphenazole	60	11.4
Sulfaphenazole	60	8.8
Trimethoprim	5.5	4.1

*1 mg = approximately 1667 IU (From English, P. B., and
Roberts, M. C.: Antimicrobial chemotherapy in the horse. I.
Pharmacological considerations. J. Eq. Med. Surg., 3:259, 1979.
With permission.)

TABLE 10. DAILY DOSAGES, ROUTES OF ADMINISTRATION, AND MEAN BLOOD SERUM
CONCENTRATIONS OF SOME ANTIMICROBIALS ADMINISTERED TO HORSES[13, 15, 21]

Antimicrobial	Total Dosage mg/kg or IU/kg	Dose Divided	Route of Administration	Serum Concentration µg/ml
Ampicillin	80–200	q.i.d.	Im, IV	0.6–1.24
Chloramphenicol	100–200	q.i.d.	PO	ND
Chloramphenicol	100–200	q.i.d.	IV	23
Erythromycin	10	t.i.d. or q.i.d.	IV	ND
Erythromycin	4	t.i.d.	IV	0.8
Gentamicin	2–2.5 gm	s.i.d.	IU in 250 ml saline	ND
Gentamicin	1.3–3	t.i.d.	IM	2.4–7.64
Gentamicin	6–18	t.i.d.	IM	ND
Isoniazid	10–30	s.i.d.	PO	ND
Kanamycin	15	t.i.d.	IM	19
Neomycin	50–100	t.i.d. or q.i.d.	PO	ND
Oxacillin	50–100	b.i.d. or t.i.d.	IM, IV	ND
Penicillin G benzathine	40,000	at 5-day intervals	IM	ND
Penicillin G potassium	50,000–200,000	q.i.d.	IM	0.4–2.2
Penicillin G potassium	50,000–400,000	q.i.d.	IV	3.4–19.2
Penicillin G procaine	40,000–100,000	b.i.d.	IM	0.45–3.62
Penicillin G sodium	120,000	q.i.d.	IM	6.1
Oxytetracycline	4.4–10	s.i.d. or b.i.d.	IV	7
Streptomycin	15–20	b.i.d., t.i.d.	IM	ND
Sulfamethazine	60–150	s.i.d.	IV, SC, PO	ND
Sulfamethylphenazole	110	s.i.d.	PO, IV	ND
Amphotericin B	100	every other day	IV in 250 ml saline	
Griseofulvin	10	s.i.d.	PO	ND
Nystatin	2.4–10^6 units	s.i.d.	IV in 250 ml saline	ND

ND = not determined, IM = intramuscular, IV = intravenous, PO = per os, SC = subcutaneous, IU = international units.

TABLE 11. MINIMUM IN VITRO INHIBITORY CONCENTRATION (µg/ml) OF ANTIBIOTIC NECESSARY TO CAUSE 100% GROWTH INHIBITION OF SOME BACTERIA COMMONLY PATHOGENIC TO HORSES [15]

Microorganism	AMP	CAR	CEP	CLI	CHL	ERY	GEN	KAN	LIN	MET	OXA	PEN	POL	STR	TET	TOB	FUR	SUL
Actinobacillus	—	8–16	—	0.5–2	—	0.25–0.5	0.25–1	1–4	64	1–2	4	0.12–0.5	—	1	0.25–1	—	—	64
Bordetella bronchiseptica	—	8–16	0.25–2	—	0.5–4	—	1–8	—	0.5–1	—	—	—	—	—	—	0.5–2	0.25–16	—
Corynebacterium equi	—	—	—	—	—	0.25	0.25	—	—	16	—	4	—	—	—	0.25	—	—
Enterobacter	—	—	—	—	—	—	—	—	—	—	64	—	—	—	—	—	—	—
Escherichia coli	16	—	—	2	—	4	0.25–4	64	64	16	64	—	—	—	—	0.25–5	—	—
Klebsiella	—	64	—	—	—	—	—	—	64	—	64	4–512	—	64	—	—	—	—
Nonhemolytic streptococci	—	—	—	—	—	0.25–2	—	0.5	—	16	—	—	—	—	—	—	0.5	—
Pasteurella sp	—	—	—	—	0.5–4	—	0.25–1	1–4	—	—	—	—	—	—	0.25–2	0.25–2	0.25–2	—
Pasteurella ureae	—	—	1–2	—	0.5–6.5	—	0.25–0.5	—	—	16	—	0.25	—	0.5	—	—	—	0.5
Proteus mirabilis	4–8	128–512	2–8	—	—	—	0.5–1	—	64	16	—	2	—	4–8	16	0.5–1	—	16
Pseudomonas aeruginosa	—	8–64	—	—	16–32	—	—	—	64	16	—	—	1	32–64	—	—	16	16
Salmonella	—	—	—	—	4	—	—	—	—	—	—	—	—	—	—	1–4	64	—
Staphylococcus aureus	—	—	—	—	0.5–8	—	—	—	—	—	0.5	—	—	—	—	—	—	—
Streptococcus zooepidemicus	0.12	—	1	—	0.25–5	—	1–2	—	—	0.25–1	—	0.06	—	—	—	—	8	—

— = MIC not determined or percentage growth inhibition below 100%

AMP = ampicillin, CAR = carbenicillin, CEP = cephalothin, CLI = clindamycin, CHL = chloramphenicol, ERY = erythromycin, GEN = gentamicin, KAN = kanamycin, LIN = lincomycin, MET = methicillin, OXA = oxacillin, PEN = penicillin, POL = polymyxin B, STR = streptomycin, TET = tetracycline, TOB = tobramycin, FUR = nitrofurantoin (Furadantin), SUL = sulfonamide

TABLE 12.   MEAN BLOOD PLASMA CONCENTRATION (µg/ml) OF VARIOUS ANTIBIOTICS AND SULFONAMIDES (mg/dl) AFTER SINGLE PARENTERAL OR ORAL ADMINISTRATION TO ADULT HORSES[9]

Antimicrobial	Number of Animals	Dose mg/kg or IU/kg	Route of Administration	0.5	1	2	3	4	6	8	9	12	24	36	48	72	120
Penicillins																	
Ampicillin sodium	3	8.8	IM	—	7.9	4.55	—	1.56	0.49	0.18							
Ampicillin sodium	4	13.5	IV	—	14.3	15.8	—	3.3	—	1.2							
Penicillin G potassium	18	1100	IM	—	0.47	0.23	—	0.01	0.00	—							
Penicillin G potassium	5	4400	IM	—	3.68	2.77	—	0.25	0.00	—							
Penicillin G sodium	12(<2 yrs)	1100	IM	—	0.43	0.19	—	0.01	0.00	—							
Penicillin G sodium	10	1100	IV	—	0.05	0.00	—	—	—	—							
Penicillin G sodium	5(foals)	2200	IM	—	0.52	0.11	—	0.00	—	—							
Penicillin G sodium	4	26,000	IM	—	52.0	39.4	—	13.7	—	1.4							
Penicillin G sodium	4	30,000	IV	—	16.2	9.0	—	4.0	—	1.5							
Penicillin G procaine	4	4000	IM	—	0.02	—	—	—	—	—	—	0.05	0.00	—	—	—	—
Penicillin G procaine	6	5000	IM	—	0.26	—	—	—	—	—	—	0.08	0.06	—	0.01	0.00	—
Penicillin G procaine	5	8200	IM	—	0.02	—	—	—	—	—	—	0.07	0.05	—	0.01	0.00	—
Penicillin G procaine	3	13,000	IM	—	0.11	—	—	—	—	—	—	0.08	0.07	—	0.01	0.00	—
Penicillin G procaine	5(foals)	24,000	IM	—	0.31	—	—	—	—	—	—	0.15	0.05	—	0.04	0.03	—
Penicillin G benzathine	12	25,000	IM	—	1.3	—	—	—	—	—	—	—	0.09	—	0.07	0.05	0.02
Penicillin G benzathine	12	50,000	IM	—	1.0	—	—	—	—	—	—	—	0.10	—	0.06	0.05	0.02
Aminoglycosides																	
*Dihydrostreptomycin	6	5.5	IM	—	9	11	—	12	7	—	—	2	—	—	—	—	—
*Dihydrostreptomycin	6	5.5	IM	—	11	11	—	10	6	—	—	1	—	—	—	—	—
*Dihydrostreptomycin	6	7.3	IM	—	46	—	—	11	—	—	4	—	—	—	—	—	—
Gentamicin	4	1.7	IM	—	10.2	7.2	—	3	1.2	—	0.7	—	—	—	—	—	—
Gentamicin	4	4.4	IM	—	15.1	10.4	—	6	2.7	—	1.4	—	—	—	—	—	—
Gentamicin	6	5	IV														
Streptomycin HCl	4(<2 yrs)	4.4†	IM	—	8	2	—	10	7	—	8	8	—	—	—	—	—
Streptomycin HCl	2	4.4†	IM	—	12	12	—	24	12	—	16	16	—	—	—	—	—
Streptomycin HCL	4(foals)	8.8†	IM	—	14	12	—	20	12	—	12	16	—	—	—	—	—
Chloramphenicol (CHL)																	
CHL aqueous suspension	4	30	IM	—	2.6	2.9	—	2.6	—	1.7	—	—	—	—	—	—	—
CHL aqueous suspension	4	50	IM	—	3.0	35	—	3.6	—	2.5	—	—	—	—	—	—	—
CHL micronized powder suspension	10	20	Oral	3.7	2.5	1.4	—	0.2	—	—	—	—	—	—	—	—	—
CHL micronized powder suspension	2	20	IV	12.5	5.4	3.3	—	0.6	—	—	—	—	—	—	—	—	—
CHL micronized powder	9	30	IM	0.6	1.0	1.2	—	0.5	—	—	—	—	—	—	—	—	—
CHL sodium succinate	4	30	IM	—	17.8	9.3	—	3.9	—	1.1	—	—	—	—	—	—	—
CHL sodium succinate	4	50	IM	31.9	32.9	24.3	—	13.3	—	16.5	—	—	—	—	—	—	—
Tetracyclines																	
Chlortetracycline	6	11	IV	—	5	—	—	1.3	—	—	—	0.2	0	—	—	—	—
Chlortetracycline	6	22	IV	—	30	—	—	10	—	—	—	1.3	0.1	—	—	—	—
Oxytetracycline	6	4.4	IV	5.6	—	—	—	4.2	—	—	—	2.3	1.5	—	—	—	—
Oxytetracycline	6	4.4	IV	0.5	0.8	—	—	1.3	—	—	—	1.5	0.7	—	—	—	—
Oxytetracycline	8	4.4	IV	23.8	8.0	—	—	1.8	—	—	—	1.2	0.4	0.1	—	—	—
Oxytetracycline	8	4.4	IM	0.7	0.8	—	—	1.2	—	—	—	1.3	1.0	0.5	—	—	—
Oxytetracycline	6	10	IV	—	32	—	—	4	—	—	—	4	1	0	—	—	—
Oxytetracycline	6	10	IM	—	1	—	—	4	—	—	—	4	2	2	—	—	—
Sulfonamides																	
Rapidly excreted:																	
Sulfadimidine	4	150	Oral	—	—	—	6	—	10	—	—	9	5	—	—	—	—
Sulfadimidine	4	75	IV	—	—	—	11	—	12	—	—	11	6	—	—	—	—
Sulfadimidine	4	150	SC	—	—	—	11	—	10	—	—	9	6	—	—	—	—
Sulfanilamide	14	220	Oral	—	15	—	16	—	13	—	—	—	3	—	—	—	—
Sulfamethazine	5	60	IV	—	16	—	13	—	10	—	—	7	4	1	—	—	—
Slowly excreted:																	
Sulfadimethoxine	5	60	IV	—	—	—	16	—	14	—	—	6	3	1	—	—	—
Sulfadimethoxine	3	100	Oral	—	—	—	—	—	6	—	—	6	5	3	—	—	—
Sulfamethoxypyridazine	4	110	Oral	—	11	—	13	—	12	—	—	8	6	2	—	—	—
Sulfamethylphenazole	4	220	Oral	—	18	—	21	—	19	—	—	17	13	61	—	—	—
Sulfamethylphenazole	4	110	IV	—	19	—	15	—	11	—	—	8	5	3	—	—	—
Sulfamonomethoxine	3	20	IM	—	—	—	—	—	—	—	—	16	—	—	—	—	—
Sulfaphenazole	5	60	IV	—	—	—	32	—	19	—	—	17	4	1	—	—	—

*Each one is a different commercial preparation
†Dose repeated at 3, 6, 9, and 12 hours

TABLE 13. RECOMMENDED FIRST AND ALTERNATE SELECTION OF ANTIMICROBIAL AGENTS BASED ON THE MICROORGANISMS IDENTIFIED OR MOST LIKELY TO BE ISOLATED[14, 16]

Microorganism	Antimicrobial Choice	
	First	*Alternate(s)*
Gram-Positive		
B-hemolytic streptococci	Penicillin	Cephalothin, erythromycin
Non-hemolytic streptococci	Penicillin + kanamycin	Gentamicin, ampicillin
Corynebacterium equi	Erythromycin	Gentamicin, chloramphenicol
Clostridium sp	Penicillin	Metronidazole, chloramphenicol
Corynebacterium pseudotuberculosis	Erythromycin	Penicillin
Corynebacterium pyogenes	Penicillin	Cephalothin, erythromycin
Staphylococcus aureus Penicillinase producer	Penicillinase resistant Penicillins	Cephalothin, erythromycin Vancomycin
Staphylococcus aureus Non–penicillinase producer	Penicillin	Cephalothin, erythromycin Vancomycin
Anaerobic cocci	Penicillin	Clindamycin, erythromycin
Gram-Negative		
Actinobacillus sp	Gentamicin, ampicillin	Kanamycin, chloramphenicol, tetracycline
Bacteroides fragilis	Metronidazole	Clindamycin, chloramphenicol
Bacteroides melaninogenicus	Penicillin	Metronidazole, chloramphenicol
Bordetella bronchiseptica	Gentamicin, kanamycin	Tetracycline, chloramphenicol, trimethoprim, sulfonamide
Enterobacter sp	Gentamicin, kanamycin	Chloramphenicol sulfonamides
Escherichia coli	Gentamicin	Kanamycin, ampicillin, cephalothin
Fusobacterium sp	Penicillin	Metronidazole
Klebsiella sp	Cephalothin, gentamicin, kanamycin	Chloramphenicol
Pasteurella sp	Cephalothin, ampicillin, gentamicin	Kanamycin, chloramphenicol, tetracycline
Proteus sp other than *Proteus mirabilis*	Kanamycin, carbenicillin	Gentamicin
Proteus mirabilis	Penicillins	Cephalothin
Pseudomonas aeruginosa	Gentamicin or gentamicin + carbenicillin	Polymyxin B
Salmonella sp	Chloramphenicol	Ampicillin

References

1. Anderson, G., Ekman, L., Månsson, I., Persson, S., Rubarth, S., and Tufvesson, G.: Lethal complications following administration of oxytetracycline in the horse. Nord. Vet. Med., 23:9, 1971.
2. Aronson, A. L.: The use, misuse, and abuse of antibacterial agents. Mod. Vet. Pract., 56:383, 1975.
3. Aronson, A. L., and Kirk, R. W.: Rational use of antimicrobial drugs. Proc. Am. An. Hosp. Assoc., 36:234, 1969.
4. Aronson, A. L.: Some considerations in the rational use of antibacterial drugs. Proc. Am. An. Hosp. Assoc., 44:331, 1975.
5. Baker, J. R., and Leyland, A.: Diarrhea in the horse associated with stress and tetracycline therapy. Vet. Rec., 93:583, 1973.
6. Baker, J. R.: Diarrhea in horses associated with tetracycline therapy. Vet. Ann., 15:178, 1975.
7. Davis, L. E., and Abbitt, B.: Clinical pharmacology of antibacterial drugs in the uterus of the mare. J. Am. Vet. Med. Assoc., 170:205, 1977.
8. Davis, L. E.: Drug therapy in the neonatal foal. J. Eq. Med. Surg., 3:175, 1979.
9. English, P. B., and Roberts, M. C.: Antimicrobial chemotherapy in the horse. I. Pharmacological considerations. J. Eq. Med. Surg., 3:259, 1979.
10. Farmer, C. G.: Penicillin: Adverse reaction in horses. Vet. Rec., 106:298, 1980.
11. Hamilton-Miller, J. M. T.: The logical use of antibiotics. J. Sm. An. Pract., 16:679, 1975.
12. Jawetz, E.: Actions of antimicrobial drugs in combination. Vet Clin. North Am., 5:35, 1975.
13. Knight, H. D.: Antimicrobial agents used in the horse. Proceedings of the 21st Annual Meeting of the American Association of Equine Practitioners, 131–144, 1975.
14. Knight, H. D.: Infectious diseases of the newborn foal. Proceedings of the 24th Annual Meeting of the American Association of Equine Practitioners, 433–447, 1978.
15. Knight, H. D., and Heitala, S.: Antimicrobic susceptibility patterns in horses. Proceedings of the Second Equine Pharmacology Symposium; 63–88, 1978.
16. Knight, H. D., Sharon, K. H., and Jang, S.: Antibacterial treatment of abscesses. J. Am. Vet. Med. Assoc., 176:1095, 1980.
17. Larson, V. L.: Antimicrobial therapy in ruminants. Vet. Clin. North Am., 5(1):101, 1975.
18. Potter, W. L.: Collapse following intravenous administration of oxytetracycline in two horses. Aust. Vet. J., 49:547, 1973.
19. Powers, T. E.: Antimicrobial agents: Pharmacology. Proceedings of the 9th Annual Convention of the American Association of Bovine Practitioners, 94–95, 1976.

20. Rhoades, H. E.: Sensitivity of bacteria to 16 antibiotic agents. VM SAC 74:976, 1979.
21. Roberts, M. C., and English, P. B.: Antimicrobial chemotherapy in the horse. II. The application of antimicrobial therapy. J. Eq. Med. Surg., 3:308, 1979.
22. Sanford, J.: The selection of antibiotics. Vet. Rec., 99:61, 1976.
23. Smith, H.: Antibiotics in Clinical Practice, 3rd ed. Baltimore, University Park Press, 1977.
24. Watson, A. D. J.: Antimicrobial Therapy. *In* Kirk, R. W. (ed.): Current Veterinary Therapy VI. Philadelphia, W. B. Saunders Co., 1977, pp. 15–26.
25. Witter, R. S., and Hayes, M. E.: Equine antimicrobial therapy. Proc. Am. An. Hosp. Assoc., 42:22, 1975.
26. Yeary, R. A.: Systemic toxic effects of chemotherapeutic agents in domestic animals. Vet. Clin. North Am., 5(1):51, 1975.

ENDOTOXEMIA

Dolores J. Kunze, RALEIGH, NORTH CAROLINA

The severest manifestation of endotoxemia is endotoxin shock, which is a form of septic shock. Septic shock results from both gram-positive bacterial toxins and gram-negative bacterial endotoxins, the clinical signs being the same regardless of the Gram staining characteristics of the instigating bacteria. Since gram-negative bacteria are the predominant source of septic shock in horses, this discussion will be limited to endotoxin shock and endotoxemia.

Endotoxin, which is a lipopolysaccharide with amino acid side chains, originates from the outer part of the cell wall of enteric bacteria. It is continuously released during the normal turnover of the intestinal microflora. Endotoxin is not "released" from intact gram-negative bacteria but rather is freed upon bacteriolysis. Endotoxin causes a clinical problem when an imbalance among various enteric bacterial populations allows the rapid growth of one or more of those populations. As increased numbers of gram-negative bacteria die, larger amounts of endotoxin are presented to the host organism. A very small amount of free endotoxin, as is the case under normal conditions, is readily tolerated. This small amount of enteric endotoxin is absorbed by the intestinal mucosa, enters the portal blood, and is detoxified by the liver. Endotoxin coming from other sites in the body is also handled in this manner. However, when this detoxifying capacity is overcome, as it is when a large amount of endotoxin is present or when liver function is severely compromised, clinical signs of endotoxemia develop.

CLINICAL SIGNS

Endotoxemia is a frequent component of several diseases of horses, including gastroenteritis, abdominal visceral displacement, ileus, aspiration pneumonia, wounds with gram-negative sepsis, and gram-negative urogenital infections. Endotoxin provokes an intense stimulation of host defense systems (Fig. 1), which results in the clinical manifestation of endotoxemia. While the exact mechanism of action remains unknown, it is felt that when endotoxin attaches to a susceptible cell, it somehow alters membrane stability and thereby exerts its pathobiologic effects.

The horse is extremely sensitive to endotoxin. The clinical signs observed vary depending on the amount of endotoxin present and the amount of time elapsed (Table 1). The earliest indications may be fever, mild depression, and anorexia, or at the other extreme, the affected horse may be in shock.

Endotoxin shock varies from the other forms of shock in several ways. Early in the course, pyrexia is a common finding, the extremities are warm, the mucous membranes may be bright pink, and capillary refill time may be decreased, in contrast to other forms of shock, in which the mucous membranes are pale or cyanotic and capillary refill time is prolonged. Later in endotoxin shock, the mucous membranes become "muddy" as cyanosis is superimposed on the already hyperemic mucous membranes. In advanced cases as the patient sweats, the fever subsides and the body temperature decreases. At this time, the patient's extremities become clammy and cool. As in other forms of shock, hyperpnea occurs, and a horse in severe endotoxin shock may be dyspneic. An occasional cough may be noted, and in a terminal case, bloody foam may appear at the nose and mouth. If improperly treated, the inevitable outcome of endotoxin shock is death.

PATHOPHYSIOLOGY

The hemogram is a very sensitive indicator of the presence of endotoxin. Initially a severe leukopenia (primarily neutropenia) develops, and the platelet numbers may decrease because neutrophils and platelets facilitate the handling of endotoxin by the

TABLE 1. CLINICAL SIGNS OF ENDOTOXEMIA AND ENDOTOXIN SHOCK

Depression
Anorexia
Altered body temperature regulation
 —Fever initially: Shivering, sweating, warm extremities
 —Decreased body temperature later: Cold, "clammy" extremities
Tachycardia
 —Hypertension initially: Hyperemic mucous membranes with rapid capillary refill time
 —Hypotension later: Superimposed cyanosis—"muddy" mucous membranes with prolonged capillary refill time
Hyperpnea
 —In severe cases, dyspnea, occasional cough
 —In terminal cases, bloody foam at nose and mouth
Prolonged or decreased bleeding times
 —Disseminated intravascular coagulation
Progressive cardiovascular decline
Prostration and death if shock is left untreated

lymphoreticular system. Endotoxin-platelet interactions result in (1) the release of vasoactive amines (serotonin and histamine), (2) the formation of intravascular occlusive aggregates, and (3) the induction of disseminated intravascular coagulation (DIC) (Fig. 1).

With the development of DIC, microthrombi form in various organs, particularly the kidneys and lungs. An endotoxemic patient may with adequate medical support survive the initial insult and sub-

sequent shock only to develop renal failure, pneumonitis, or laminitis as a result of microthrombi.

Within neutrophils, endotoxin adheres to lysosomal membranes, disrupts membrane transport, and causes enzyme leakage. Eventually, neutrophil chemotaxis is inhibited or overcome by humoral factors released from other cells under endotoxin influence, but the major neutrophil functional defect stems from alterations in adhesiveness. These changes in adherence are complement-dependent and support the histologic evidence of sequestration of platelets and neutrophils in pulmonary capillary beds and other small vessels.

If the patient survives an initial endotoxemic episode, granulocytosis will be observed (Fig. 2). As a result of an increase in circulating segmented and nonsegmented neutrophil numbers, not only do the previously marginated mature neutrophils return to the circulating pool but also immature granulocytes appear in greater numbers. Bone marrow endothelium is destroyed following endotoxin exposure, and mature and immature cells are released at an accelerated rate. Thus, the granulocytosis is the sum of the return of sequestered cells and the early release of cells from the bone marrow.

The effect of endotoxin on the lymphoreticular system is not well understood, but lymphopenia follows the early neutropenia after a few hours. This lymphopenia may be an indirect effect as a result of increased serum cortisol.

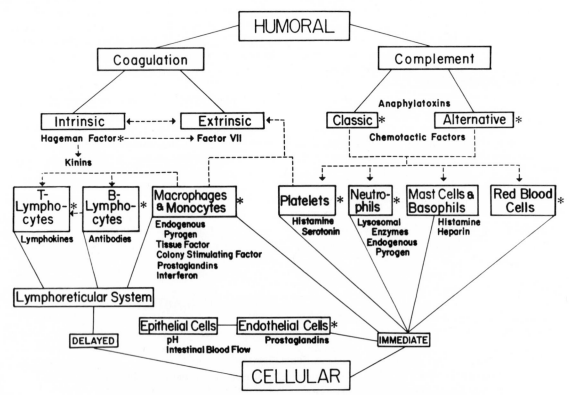

Figure 1. Humoral and cellular defense mechanisms invoked by endotoxin.

Red blood cells also are affected by endotoxin. Direct red blood cell damage has not been reported in the horse; however, a marked elevation in packed cell volume (PCV) is observed following endotoxin infusion. The arterial hypotension of advanced endotoxin shock increases sympathoadrenal activity, which results in splenic contraction and ejection of erythrocytes into the general circulation.

Following slow intravenous infusion of a shock dose of endotoxin in a horse, there is an immediate increase in pulmonary arterial pressure, a marked decrease in systemic arterial pressure, and sometimes a mild increase in central venous pressure. There is a striking early rise in pulmonary vascular resistance, producing central venous pooling. Shortly thereafter, the systemic arterial pressure returns to normal levels and remains there for several hours. Still later, hypotension becomes severe, total peripheral resistance is low, and generalized venous pooling occurs.

The hemodynamic and hematologic events are interrelated; white blood cell and platelet numbers decrease simultaneously with the early pressure changes. Platelets are essential for the hemodynamic pathophysiology; as platelet numbers decrease, serum concentrations of several vasoactive substances increase and cause the changes in hemodynamics. Plasma serotonin reaches a maximal level 15 seconds after endotoxin injection but then rapidly disappears. An increase in bradykinin occurs and may contribute to the hypotension. Also, following endotoxin administration, histamine and catecholamine levels are measured at higher than normal levels.

DIAGNOSTIC PROCEDURES

If untreated, progressive endotoxemia leads to shock. Since any form of shock is an emergency state, the attending veterinarian initiates treatment without the benefit of extensive diagnostic support.

TABLE 2. DIAGNOSTIC PLAN

Physical examination
Packed cell volume determination
Total serum solids determination
Blood gas analysis and determination of acid-base status
Serum electrolyte determination
Central venous pressure measurement
Complete blood count and white blood cell differential
Serum protein determination
Determinations of blood chemistries
Clotting profile if coagulopathy is suspected
Bacterial culture and antibiotic sensitivity determination

The first and most important diagnostic step is a thorough physical examination, which forms the basis of a therapeutic plan. When the condition of the patient permits and when the technology is available, a series of diagnostic procedures will allow the attending veterinarian to appropriately alter or augment the initial treatment (Table 2).

The hematocrit and total plasma solids measurements further define the patient's hydration. The splenic capsule contraction early in the course of an endotoxemic episode greatly increases the PCV without altering the total plasma solids, and the horse is not dehydrated at this time. Conversely, in some gastroenteritis or peritonitis cases, the PCV may be high owing to dehydration but the total plasma solids might be quite low owing to the alimentary or exudative loss of protein. In general, the dehydrated horse will have an increased PCV and increased total solids.

The blood pH, $PaCO_2$ and HCO_3^- values provide information on the functional state of the cardiovascular system and allow some estimation of the level of tissue hypoxia and injury. With this data, the base excess or deficit can readily be determined and used to calculate HCO_3^- replacement (p. 200). In advanced shock, the patient will be acidotic.

Recently, blood lactate levels have been employed to arrive at a prognosis. An elevated blood lactate value indicates that the rate of anaerobic gly-

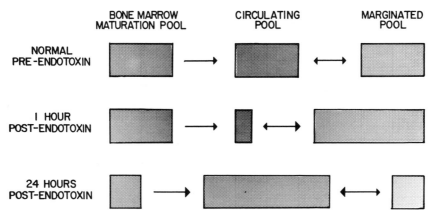

Figure 2. Schematic representation of the changes in leukocyte numbers during endotoxin shock.

colysis has increased because cellular oxygen tension is reduced following decreased tissue perfusion. The prognosis for an animal in shock can be derived using serial lactic acid determinations, since the mortality rate increases with rising lactic acid levels.

Depending on the shock-initiating event, serum electrolyte levels may be altered. Generally, an electrolyte imbalance is of more concern in protracted shock or the recovery phase of shock than it is in acute shock. With decreased perfusion and cellular hypoxia, potassium leaks out of cells, which initially increases serum potassium levels. Overall, however, there is a decrease in total body potassium.

The monitoring of central venous pressure (CVP) can be useful as a diagnostic aid and as a means of determining the efficacy of fluid therapy. The normal range of CVP in the standing adult horse is approximately 5 to 10 cm H_2O. The evaluation of the CVP may assist in the decision to administer vasoactive drugs if the CVP is low or could provide warning of possible fluid volume overload if the CVP increases too rapidly. It is very difficult to overfill the adult equine cardiovascular system by intravenous fluids given by gravity alone. However, in ponies or foals or if fluid administration is mechanically assisted, overhydration is possible and should be avoided.

In chronic endotoxemia or recovery from shock, the data from complete blood counts and white blood cell differentials, blood chemistries, serum protein values, and bacterial cultures and sensitivities will assist in the treatment plan. This information may also assist in identifying the original problem if it has not been previously determined. Very early in the course of an endotoxemic episode, the sudden neutropenia (less than 1000 neutrophils) is very good evidence of the presence of endotoxin, and a decrease in lymphocyte numbers is also a common finding. Later, especially in recovery, there is a pronounced granulocytosis. Generally, serum globulins rise in the face of an infection, but serum albumin may decrease in the patient with gastroenteritis or widespread sepsis. While bacterial culture and sensitivity determinations will greatly influence the therapeutic plan, antimicrobial therapy will usually have been initiated earlier. The treatment plan should be regularly reevaluated and updated as new data are collected.

TREATMENT

Mild or low-grade endotoxemia encountered as a feature of another disorder may not be identified as a problem requiring specific therapy. An aspiration pneumonia or a wound infected with gram-negative bacteria should be treated with the appropriate an-

TABLE 3. TREATMENT PLAN

Maintain adequate ventilation
Restore circulating blood volume
Correct base deficit or base excess
Correct electrolyte imbalances
Administer corticosteroids (with judgment)
Administer antimicrobial agents (with judgment)
Maintain oncotic pressure
Administer vasodilators (with judgment)
Administer analgesics (with judgment)
Administer sedatives or tranquilizers (with judgment)
If coagulopathy is present, administer heparin while monitoring coagulation profiles

timicrobial agent or agents. It should be remembered, however, that some bactericidal drugs may potentiate the endotoxemia. Severe endotoxemia, and specifically endotoxin shock, can be more of a therapeutic challenge (Table 3). The maintenance of ventilation should be a primary consideration; oxygen therapy is indicated whenever hypoxemia is present or is suspected. Oxygen can be administered via a face mask, through a nasogastric tube passed into the trachea, or through an intratracheal catheter (p. 478). If the upper airway is compromised, a tracheostomy may be required. Some excitable horses may not tolerate the necessary equipment required to administer oxygen and will require additional restraint.

The restoration and maintenance of adequate circulating blood volume is paramount. Large intravenous volumes of balanced electrolyte solutions are necessary and require the use of a large indwelling catheter or needle. Any of several isotonic electrolyte solutions can be used, but lactated Ringer's solution is used most frequently with physiologic saline as another common choice. The volume of fluid required can be very large, particularly if the fluid loss is ongoing. In a severe case of shock, up to 150 ml per kg of body weight of solution may be required over a 24-hour period. The volume required will vary with each case, but a very general rule of thumb is to administer the fluids as rapidly as possible until the horse urinates. Once the vascular volume is high enough to thus adequately perfuse the kidneys, the rate of flow should be decreased to minimize the excessive urinary loss of fluid and electrolytes. Oral fluid replacement can and should be used as well, as long as the horse tolerates it and has no contraindication for it, such as gastrointestinal obstruction or ileus.

Acid-base or electrolyte imbalances should be corrected over several hours. If exact deficits cannot be determined, 50 to 100 gm of bicarbonate can be given to the equine patient with suspected acidosis, taking care not to combine bicarbonate with calcium-containing solutions. It is dangerous to attempt to replace potassium empirically, but administration of 10 mEq per l is safe up to a total of 1600 mEq over a 24-hour period. If a sodium or chloride deficit develops, physiologic saline is the solution of choice. The shock patient will also benefit from a 5 per cent dextrose solution or a half-strength solution of lactated Ringer's or saline plus 2.5 per cent dextrose, particularly later in the course of therapy. The choice of solution is important, but adequate volume replacement is the more immediate concern.

The horse with peritonitis or prolonged diarrhea may lose large amounts of serum protein, which could lead to a loss of plasma oncotic pressure. Large volumes of plasma can be used for replacement of this protein, but securing this much plasma is difficult and expensive. High molecular weight solutions (dextran) can also be used, but again large amounts will be needed, and the cost is high. Also, the protein loss is often ongoing, and the course of the disease may be long; these factors increase the expense and risk of untoward effects.

Once the circulating blood volume has been restored, a vasodilator can be used to improve tissue perfusion and decrease tissue hypoxia. It should not be used before adequate fluid replacement is accomplished because it will exacerbate the hypotension. Isoproterenol hydrochloride,* a beta stimulator, can be diluted (0.2 mg in 1 liter of saline) and given to effect as a slow infusion to increase myocardial contractility and to produce vasodilatation. It can also induce arrhythmias; therefore, careful cardiac monitoring is required. Acetylpromazine† can also be used as a vasodilator because it is an alpha-adrenergic blocker. Its sedative properties may also be useful once the patient's condition is stable.

The use of pharmacologic doses of corticosteroids in endotoxin shock is a generally accepted practice. An intravenous dose of 1 to 4 mg per kg of prednisolone sodium succinate‡ or 2 to 4 mg per kg of dexamethasone§ every four to six hours has been recommended for use in horses. A dose of 30 mg per kg of prednisolone sodium succinate has been used in experimental endotoxemia in ponies. People and horses appear to have a similar sensitivity to the effects of endotoxin, yet the intravenous dose of dexamethasone that is recommended for use in people with septic shock is 15 mg per kg every four to six hours. This is judged less effective than the recommended dose of hydrocortisone sodium succinate of 150 mg per kg every four to six hours. Only at such high levels have physicians detected a statistical increase in the survival rate. These dosages would be prohibitively expensive for use in equine practice. It is possible that larger doses of corticosteroids could be used in horses with increasing degrees of success; however, the economic constraints of veterinary practice may preclude the widespread use of such large amounts. If they are to be used, corticosteroids should be given very early in the course of treatment to be of maximal benefit. The prostaglandin synthetase inhibitors (phenylbutazone and flunixin meglumine) are also indicated in endotoxic shock and may prevent coagulopathies.

The use of antimicrobial agents in endotoxin shock is also an accepted practice. If a bacterial infection is present or pending, antimicrobial therapy is justifiable, but bactericidal drugs can potentially worsen the severity of shock as bacteria are destroyed and further endotoxin is released. Many drugs, including chloramphenicol, dihydrostreptomycin, neomycin, kanamycin, and gentamicin, are effective against many gram-negative bacteria. However, high levels of the aminoglycosides should be used with caution because of the possibility of producing neuromuscular blockade (particularly in very sick horses). Penicillin is useful against most anaerobes and is especially effective in conjunction with one of the aminoglycosides. The tetracyclines are also effective against gram-negative bacteria, but they can cause enteritis in stressed horses and are therefore not recommended for use in the endotoxemic patient. The only antimicrobial agent that directly interferes with the bioactivity of endotoxin is polymixin B sulfate. This drug was used by the author in ameliorating some of the pathophysiology of low-level experimental endotoxemia. However, the toxicity of polymixin B greatly limits its clinical use.

Since many of the conditions that precipitate endotoxin shock are painful, analgesics are often required. If possible, their use should be delayed until the patient has been carefully evaluated. Xylazine* has analgesic as well as sedative properties, but its use should be delayed until blood volume is restored because it may cause bradycardia and hypotension. Some other commonly used analgesics include dipyrone,† pentazocine,‡ and meperidine hydrochloride.§

Tranquilization or sedation may also be necessary. The risks of using acetylpromazine and xylazine in a hypotensive horse have been discussed. Smaller than usual doses may prove effective when used following the administration of pentazocine or meperidine hydrochloride.

The treatment of coagulopathies in horses has been very frustrating. One reason for this may be that the disease process is quite advanced by the time that it is discovered. Various doses of heparin have been suggested, including 20 to 30 units per

---

*Isuprel, Sterling Drug, Inc., New York, NY
†Acepromazine, Ayerst Laboratories, New York, NY
‡SoluDelta Cortef, The Upjohn Company, Kalamazoo, MI
§Azium, Shering Corp., Kenilworth, NJ

*Rompun, Haver Lockhart Laboratories, Shawnee, KS
†Novin, Haver Lockhart Laboratories, Shawnee, KS
‡Talwin-V, Winthrop Laboratories, New York, NY
§Demerol, Winthrop Laboratories, New York, NY

kg body weight given at six-hour intervals. Monitoring the anticoagulation effect is a major problem, but the basic goal is to double the normal partial thromboplastin time.

Supplemental Readings

Kohn, C. W.: Preparative management of the equine patient with an abdominal crisis. Vet. Clin. North Am. (Large Anim. Pract.), *1*:289, 1979.

Moore, J. N., Garner, H. E., Shapland, J. E., and Schaub, R. G.: Equine endotoxemia: An insight into cause and treatment. J. Am. Vet. Med. Assoc., *179*:473, 1981.

Morrison, D. C., and Ulevitch, R. J.: A review: The effects of bacterial endotoxins in host mediation systems. Am. J. Pathol., *93*:527, 1978.

Stashak, T. S.: Clinical evaluation of the equine colic patient. Vet. Clin. North Am. (Large Anim. Pract.), *1*:275, 1979.

Weil, M. H., Shubin, H., and Biddle, M.: Shock caused by gram-negative microorganisms: Analysis of 169 cases. Ann. Intern. Med., *60*:384, 1964.

Section 2
NUTRITION
Edited by H. F. Hintz

ENERGY AND PROTEIN 65

MINERALS 71

VITAMINS 84

FEEDING PROGRAMS 91

SAMPLE RATIONS AND COMMERCIAL FEEDS 97

HOOF GROWTH AND NUTRITION 100

EXERTIONAL MYOPATHY 101

FOUNDER 104

HYPERLIPEMIA 107

HEAT BUMPS, SWEET FEED BUMPS, SWEET ITCH 110

ECLAMPSIA 111

NUTRITION OF THE SICK HORSE 111

BILIRUBINEMIA 116

ENERGY AND PROTEIN

H. F. Hintz, ITHACA, NEW YORK

H. F. Schryver, ITHACA, NEW YORK

Energy

Providing an incorrect amount of energy is one of the most common mistakes in the feeding of horses. Acute overfeeding can cause a variety of problems, such as enterotoxemia, colic, and founder. Chronic overfeeding can result in obesity, impaired performance, needless expense, and perhaps skeletal problems. The treatment of overfeeding is simple. The energy intake must be decreased, but the decrease should not be too drastic and abrupt, as metabolic disorders may result (see Hyperlipemia). Unfortunately, some clients do not appreciate the difference in energy concentration among feedstuffs, nor will they accept the fact that under some conditions horses do not need any grain. Furthermore, overfeeding frequently occurs in the preparation of animals for shows and sales. Even though trainers know excess fat is of no value and perhaps harmful, the excess fat makes the animals look better in the eyes of many people and increases sales prices.

Underfeeding can result in loss of weight or reduced weight gain, delay in onset of sexual maturity in young animals, reduced resistance to disease, impaired performance, rough hair coats, and unthrifty appearance.

Inadequate energy can result from several problems other than simply underfeeding. Parasites, dental problems, and malabsorption can all cause decreased utilization of feed. In group feeding situations, some horses may not obtain reasonable access to the feed. Feed intake may be decreased if the water supply is not adequate. Furthermore, many owners fail to recognize chronic weight loss until the situation is severe. They may see the animals every day, but the change is so gradual that they do not realize that the animals are in trouble. For example, a pony was brought to the clinic at Cornell University because the owner thought the pony had a broken leg. The pony had been housed in a run-in shed with a larger pony. It was winter and the pony had a long hair coat. Upon examination, it was found that the pony did not have a broken leg; rather, it was emaciated and could not walk simply because it was starved. The ponies had been fed together, and apparently the larger pony got most of the feed, and the situation was aggravated because the cold weather increased the energy requirement. The long hair coat masked the weight loss. Thus, it is recommended that owners weigh their horses regularly. If scales are not available, measuring tapes placed around the heart girth can be used. Several feed companies supply such tapes, and they are reasonably accurate.

Estimates of energy requirements for various classes of horses are shown in Table 1, but these are only guidelines. If the horse is not in the desired condition and factors such as parasites (p. 267) and dental problems (p. 186) have been corrected, then the amount of grain should be adjusted accordingly.

SOURCES OF ENERGY

Horse owners often feel that energy of one type may be good for certain activities but not for others. That is, they want a source of energy that allows the horse to run fast but will not fatten the horse or a source of energy for weight gain but they do not want the horse to get "high." Unfortunately, methods to fraction energy in such divisions have not been developed, and energy must be considered as energy.

GRAINS

The energy content of some grains is shown in Table 2. Horse owners prefer to feed oats to their horses. Oats are an excellent feed but are often more expensive than other grains. They have the lowest digestible energy (DE) concentration and the lowest weight per volume of most common grains (Table 3). Thus, oats are the safest grain, since owners are much less likely to overfeed oats than other grains. For example, there may be twice as much energy in a quart of shelled corn as there is in a quart of oats. Oats also have a higher protein content than corn, and the protein quality is slightly better than that of corn.

Unfortunately, the quality of oats varies more than the quality of the other grains. The digestible energy content is negatively correlated with the fiber content, and the greater the fiber content the less weight per bushel. The weight may vary from 25 to 40 lb or more per bushel. The energy content may vary from 2.4 to 3.0 megacalories (Mcal) of DE per kg.

Oats are also frequently dusty and may also contain other excess foreign material unless they are properly cleaned. Thus, care should be taken when purchasing oats.

TABLE 1. ENERGY AND PROTEIN REQUIREMENTS OF VARIOUS CLASSES OF HORSES*

| | Expected Mature Weight (kg) | | | | | |
| | 400 | | 500 | | 600 | |
	DE† Mcal/day	Protein kg/day	DE Mcal/day	Protein kg/day	DE Mcal/day	Protein kg/day
Maintenance, mature	13.86	0.54	16.39	0.63	18.79	0.73
Mares, last 90 days of gestation	15.52	0.64	18.36	0.75	21.04	0.87
Lactating mare, first 3 months	23.36	1.12	28.27	1.36	33.05	1.60
Lactating mare, 3 months to weaning	20.20	0.91	24.31	1.10	28.29	1.29
Weanling	13.03	0.66	15.60	0.79	16.92	0.86
Yearling	13.80	0.60	16.81	0.76	18.85	0.90
Two-year-old	13.89	0.52	16.45	0.63	19.26	0.74

*(From the National Research Council. Nutrient Requirements of the Horse. NAS-NRC Publication, Washington, DC, 1978.)
†Digestible energy

In parts of the United States, corn is the most economical grain for feeding many horses. However, it has a high DE concentration and, therefore, requires better feeding management than oats.

Although many horse owners feel that corn is a "hot" food and that horses do not perform at their best when fed corn, many experiments have demonstrated that these complaints are incorrect when reasonable feeding care is taken. For example, polo ponies at Cornell performed as well when fed alfalfa and corn as when fed timothy and oats, but the feed intakes were adjusted so that DE intakes were similar. Arabian horses ridden 50 miles in five hours performed satisfactorily when fed alfalfa and corn. As mentioned earlier, corn is much easier to overfeed and, if overfed, produces more heat; when corn and oats are fed to provide the same intake of DE, oats actually provide more heat because of the greater fiber content. Oats or corn can be fed whole, although crimping of oats may improve energy utilization by 7 to 10 per cent.

Barley is also excellent for horses and has been used as a horse feed for many years. Barley has a DE content somewhere between that of oats and corn, but the energy concentration is still such that it is relatively easily overfed. Barley may be less palatable than oats or corn. The protein content is similar to that of oats. Some horse owners also consider barley to be a "hot" feed. One owner claimed that barley was a "hot" feed unless you cooked the heat out of it by steaming it. As with corn, it is a matter of feeding the correct amount of DE. Barley should be processed by crimping or rolling. No studies have been conducted on the value of steam-flaking barley for horses, but early studies indicated that cooking provided no benefits above those of crimping or rolling.

Milo has a digestible energy content similar to that of corn. It is an economical grain in the southwestern United States and is a satisfactory grain for horses when properly processed and supplemented. As with corn, if management is not careful, over-eating can result in enterotoxemia, colic, or founder.

Rye is seldom fed to horses because of the relatively high price and because horses do not like it. A grain mixture should contain no more than one third rye to avoid decreases in feed intake.

Wheat can sometimes be an economical source of energy. It has a high DE content and must be fed with caution. Milo, rye, and wheat should be pro-

TABLE 2. AVERAGE COMPOSITION OF SOME COMMON ENERGY SOURCES*

Grain	DE Mcal/kg	Protein (%)	Fiber (%)	Calcium (%)	Phosphorus (%)
Barley	3.2	11	6	0.08	0.40
Brewers' grains	2.6	27	15	0.27	0.48
Corn (yellow)	3.5	9	2	0.02	0.31
Distillers' grains (corn)	3.2	27	12	0.09	0.37
Oats (high quality)	3.0	13	10	0.10	0.35
Oats (low quality)	2.4	11	13	0.09	0.30
Rye	3.2	12	2	0.06	0.34
Sorghum (milo)	3.4	11	2	0.04	0.29
Wheat	3.5	13	3	0.05	0.36
Molasses, beet	2.6	7	0	0.16	0.01
Molasses, cane	2.4	3	0	0.89	0.04

*(From the National Research Council. Nutrient Requirements of the Horse. NAS-NRC Publication, Washington, DC, 1978.)

TABLE 3. RELATIVE WEIGHTS OF SOME COMMON FEEDS*

Feed	Weight of 1 Quart (lbs)	Volume of 1 lb (qts)
Alfalfa meal	0.6	1.7
Barley	1.5	0.7
Beet pulp	0.6	1.7
Corn	1.7	0.6
Cottonseed meal	1.5	0.7
Linseed meal	0.9	1.1
Molasses, cane	3.0	0.3
Oats	1.0	1.0
Rye	1.7	0.6
Soybean	1.8	0.6
Wheat	1.9	0.5
Wheat bran	0.5	2.0

*(From Morrison, F. B.: Feeds and Feeding. Ithaca, NY, Morrison Publishing Co., 1957.)

cessed (cracked, rolled, or steam-rolled) for efficient utilization.

HAYS

Hays contain a lower concentration of energy than grains. Legume hays, such as alfalfa, clover, birdsfoot trefoil, and lespedeza, usually contain a higher amount of digestible energy, calcium, protein, and vitamins than grass hays such as Bermuda, bluegrass, fescue, orchardgrass, reed canary, or timothy (Table 4). The most important criterion to consider when buying hay is not species but rather nutritive value in relation to cost. The primary factor that influences nutritive value is stage of maturity at harvesting.

Young plants contain a greater concentration of DE and nutrients than do old plants. As the plant matures, the amount of lignin and structural components increases. These fractions are not utilized efficiently by horses. The effect of stage of maturity on value is demonstrated in Table 5, and the recommended stage of maturity for harvesting is summarized in Table 6. If the plant is too young when harvested, the nutrient concentration is greatest, but the yield per acre is greatly decreased.

Good quality hay should be harvested at the proper stage of maturity, should be free from mold, dust, and weeds, and should not be excessively weathered. Weathering can cause loss of leaves and decreased vitamin content. Unless proper harvesting methods are used, legume hay is more likely to be moldy or dusty than grass hay because it has more leaves and drying is more difficult.

Some owners feel that the excess protein in alfalfa causes kidney damage. Other owners feel that alfalfa causes horses to sweat more. Neither of these opinions is supported by scientific evidence. Horses fed legumes may urinate more, and there may be a stronger smell of ammonia in the barn because of

TABLE 4. ENERGY CONTENT OF HAY AND OTHER NONCONCENTRATE FEEDS*

	Dry Matter (%)	Digestible Energy Mcal/kg	
		1†	2‡
Alfalfa, grazed prebloom	21	0.52	2.51
grazed fullbloom	25	0.57	2.29
hay, earlybloom	90	2.18	2.42
hay, midbloom	89	2.04	2.29
hay, fullbloom	89	1.92	2.16
meal, dehydrated, 17 per cent protein	92	2.26	2.46
Bahiagrass, grazed	30	0.63	2.11
hay	91	1.72	1.89
Barley hay	89	1.68	1.89
straw	90	1.47	1.63
Beet pulp	91	2.60	2.86
Bluegrass, grazed early	31	0.76	2.46
grazed, posthead	35	0.77	2.20
Citrus pulp	90	2.69	2.99
Clover (red), grazed, earlybloom	20	0.50	2.51
hay, late	89	1.92	2.16
Corn cobs	90	1.22	1.36
Cottonseed hulls	91	1.32	1.45
Fescue, hay	88	1.78	2.02
Lespedeza hay	91	1.88	2.07
Timothy, hay, prehead	89	1.96	2.20
head	88	1.74	1.98

*(From the National Research Council. Nutrient Requirements of the Horse. NAS-NRC Publication, Washington, DC, 1978.)
†As is
‡Dry matter basis

TABLE 5. PROTEIN CONTENT OF ALFALFA AND TIMOTHY AT DIFFERENT STAGES OF MATURITY*

Date	Alfalfa		Timothy	
	Stage	*Protein*	*Stage*	*Protein*
May 25	Vegetative	19%	Vegetative	15%
June 5	Bud	16	Boot	12
June 15	Early flower	14	Early head	10
June 20	Flower	11	Heading	9
July 5	Late flower	8	Flower	6
July 25	Green seed	5	Early seed	3

*Dates under New York conditions

TABLE 6. STAGE OF GROWTH FOR HARVESTING HAY CROPS TO OBTAIN GREATEST AMOUNTS OF DIGESTIBLE NUTRIENTS

Crop	Stage to Harvest
Perennial grasses:	
Coastal Bermudagrass	14–16 in height (maximum 4 weeks' growth)
Common Bermudagrass	Early bloom
Bluestem, introduced and native	Boot—early bloom
Johnsongrass	Boot
Lovegrass	Boot
Timothy	Early head
Smooth bromegrass	Early to medium head
Orchardgrass	Boot to early head
Annual grasses:	
Millet, pearl or cattail	Boot
Sorghum, forage	Bloom-soft dough
Sudan varieties and sudan hybrids	Boot
Oats	Early bloom
Ryegrass	Early bloom
Legumes:	
Alfalfa	Full bud
Clover (crimson, hop, red, white, Persian, and arrowleaf)	¼ to ½ bloom
Birdsfoot trefoil	¼ bloom
Peanut	Harvest to retain maximum leaves
Vetch	Early bloom

the higher nitrogen content of alfalfa hay. It is true that alfalfa will usually contain more protein and DE than needed by mature horses. In fact, mature horses fed good quality legume hay free choice may become overweight.

Alfalfa is used to greatest advantage when fed to growing horses or lactating mares, as these animals have high protein and calcium requirements. Swerczek[5] suggested that the incidence of "shaker foal syndrome" could be reduced by not feeding an excessively nutritious diet such as alfalfa to mares nursing foals. He further suggested that the alfalfa caused an increase in the corticosteroid content of the mare's milk, which in turn made the foal more susceptible to toxicoinfectious botulism and hence shaker foal syndrome. Further studies are needed to establish such relationships.

OTHER ENERGY SOURCES

Molasses is an excellent source of energy and is often added to horse rations to reduce dust and increase palatability. However, some horses prefer feeds without molasses; that is, some horses will select the feed without molasses if given a choice. Furthermore, molasses may be an expensive source of energy.

The use of pelleted rations has enabled the use of many feeds that would not normally be consumed by horses. Apple skins, corn cobs, peanut hulls, sunflower hulls, almond hulls, ryegrass straw, corrugated paper boxes, and ammonia-treated straw are examples of unconventional feeds that have been used in horse rations. Many of these feeds provide little nutrition other than DE and fiber, but they are well utilized when properly supplemented. Many of these feeds are not economical at present but are likely to be used in increasing amounts in the future as the prices of primary feedstuffs increase.

Protein

In the evaluation or formulation of rations, protein is usually the next nutrient considered after energy status has been examined. Theoretically the best measure of protein value for nonruminants is the amount and balance of available essential amino acids. Unfortunately, little information is available on the amino acid requirements of the horse. It has been estimated that weanlings require rations containing about 0.7 per cent lysine, but no values are available for the other amino acids. Generally, therefore, the crude protein content is used to evaluate the ration. Crude protein is estimated by determining the nitrogen content of the feed and multiplying by 6.25 because most proteins contain about 16 per cent nitrogen. This method (Kjeldahl) may overevaluate certain feedstuffs such as silage that contain significant amounts of nonprotein nitrogen, but it is widely used because it is a relatively easy and inexpensive procedure and results in reasonable values for most common feedstuffs.

Knowledge of the digestibility of the feedstuffs would be beneficial. Again data are limited, but fortunately most protein supplements appear to be digested efficiently.

PROTEIN DEFICIENCY

Protein is too ubiquitous a part of the animal to show a specific set of deficiency signs. Deficiency depresses metabolic activities, food intake is decreased, growth is impaired, and reproduction and lactation are suboptimal. Anemia and hypoproteinemia may develop. The animal appears unthrifty, is not alert, and the hair coat is dull. In other species, brain development and learning ability in young animals can be impaired by protein deficiency.

PROTEIN REQUIREMENTS

Requirements can be expressed as daily intakes of protein or as a percentage of the diet. The latter method is probably the one used most commonly. Estimates of the daily crude protein requirements are shown in Table 1. Requirements as a percentage of the diet are shown in Table 7. The daily intake of protein (grams per day) required is constant for a given horse. The percentage of crude protein required in the diet, however, depends on several factors, such as concentration of DE. That is, when significant amounts of grain are fed, the concentration of the DE is greater, and the crude protein content of the total ration should be higher than when only hay is fed, since the horse will need fewer pounds of feed to meet its energy needs. Therefore, the protein concentration must be higher to provide the required protein intake when grain intake is great.

The protein content of the grain mixture needed when feeding grass or legume hay is shown in Table 8. As mentioned earlier, the diet of young growing horses should contain 0.7 per cent lysine, but further studies are needed to determine the requirements for other amino acids.

Although protein requirements are listed for several classes of horses, it is obviously not practical to have numerous grain mixtures on the farm. A protein supplement could be added to a basic grain mixture at feeding time according to the horse's needs, but such a practice is often confusing when several horses are involved or when more than one person is doing the feeding. A more practical solution might be to have only four grain mixtures. One mixture would be for creep feed, one for weanlings, one for yearlings and producing mares, and one for mature horses. Of course, if only a few horses are involved, it might be more economical to have only one or two grain mixtures.

SOURCES OF PROTEIN

The composition of some protein sources is shown in Table 9. Legume hay harvested at the proper stage of maturity provides a significant amount of protein. Alfalfa meal is used in many horse rations, particularly the complete pelleted rations, and in addition to protein provides minerals and vitamins.

Good quality pasture also provides protein. For example, legume pasture such as clover may contain 18 to 20 per cent protein on a dry matter basis. Even grasses such as bluegrass and timothy may contain as much as 15 per cent protein during the early growth stages, but the moisture content of pas-

TABLE 7. ESTIMATES OF PROTEIN REQUIREMENTS EXPRESSED AS PERCENTAGE OF DIET ON 90% DRY MATTER BASIS*

Class	Crude Protein (%)
Mature horse, maintenance	7.7
Mares, last 90 days of gestation	10.0
Lactating mare, first 3 months	12.5
Lactating mare, 3 months to weaning	11.0
Creep feed	16.0
Weanling (6 mos)	14.5
Yearling	12.0
Two-year-old	9.0
Mature working horse	7.7

*(From the National Research Council. Nutrient Requirements of the Horse. NAS-NRC Publication, Washington, DC, 1978.)

TABLE 8. MINIMUM PROTEIN CONTENT NEEDED IN GRAIN MIXTURES WHEN FEEDING LEGUME HAY OR GRASS HAY*

Class of Horse	Legume Hay† (%)	Grass Hay† (%)
Creep feed	16	18
Weanlings	14.5	18
Yearlings; pregnant mares (last 90 days); lactating mares	10–11	15–16
Mature horses	‡	8

*When using hay:grain ratios shown in Table 6
†Values will depend on protein content of hay. In this example, it was assumed that the legume hay contained 14.5% crude protein and the grass hay contained 8% crude protein.
‡In most cases, the legume hay could provide nearly all of the protein needed.

TABLE 9. COMPOSITION OF SOME PROTEIN SOURCES*

	Protein (%)	Lysine (%)	Lysine: Protein (%)	Calcium (%)	Phosphorus (%)
Alfalfa hay—early bloom	16	0.85	5.5	1.58	0.23
—mid bloom	14	0.81	5.6	1.35	0.22
—full bloom	13	0.62	4.6	1.16	0.21
Alfalfa meal—15%	15	0.68	4.5	1.32	0.22
—17%	18	0.88	5.0	1.60	0.23
—20%	21	0.95	4.6	1.70	0.24
Brewers' grains	27	0.90	3.3	0.27	0.48
Cottonseed meal	41	1.76	4.2	0.23	0.90
Distillers' grains, dried	27	0.60	2.2	0.09	0.37
Fish meal (herring)	72	5.70	7.9	2.08	1.55
Linseed meal	33	1.20	3.6	0.39	0.81
Meal and bone meal	50	3.20	6.4	9.42	5.09
Peanut meal	45	1.60	3.6	0.20	0.65
Skim meal (dried)	33	2.60	7.8	1.32	1.05
Soybean meal	45	3.00	6.7	0.25	0.60
Soybean meal, dehulled	48	3.20	6.7	0.25	0.60
Sunflower meal, dehulled	47	1.82	3.9	0.36	0.90

*90% dry matter basis

ture is high and may limit intake. The level of protein in the pasture depends greatly on the stage of maturity, fertilizing practices, and weather conditions.

Animal protein supplements such as dried skim milk, fish meal, and meat and bone meal are efficiently utilized, contain a relatively high amount of lysine, and are usually a high quality protein source. Such sources also provide significant amounts of calcium and phosphorus. However, animal protein supplements are usually much more expensive per unit of protein than vegetable proteins.

Most vegetable protein sources, such as cottonseed meal, have a relatively low content of lysine and a higher content of phosphorus (P) than calcium (Ca) (Table 9). Fortunately, soybean meal has a higher lysine content than most other oil meals. Soybean meal is an excellent protein source for horses, and in most parts of the United States is usually the most economical source. Linseed meal, peanut meal, cottonseed meal, sunflower meal, and brewers' or distillers' grains should not be used as the primary protein source for young horses unless they are fed at higher levels (which is usually uneconomical) or combined with additional lysine sources. The value of the protein sources can be greatly influenced by the method of processing. Untreated legume seeds such as soybeans, raw soybean meal, or kidney beans should not be fed to horses because these feeds contain many factors, such as trypsin inhibitors, that decrease utilization of the feed and decrease feed intake. Heat destroys the deleterious factors, but excess heat decreases the value of the protein because high temperatures cause the protein to bind with carbohydrate fractions. Excessive heat during processing has been reported to decrease the value of soybean meal, alfalfa meal, and brewers' or distillers' grains.

PROTEIN TOXICITY

No studies have demonstrated protein toxicity in horses. Excess protein is broken down, the carbon chain is used for energy, and nitrogen is excreted in the urine. Of course, feeding excess protein is costly because the protein supplement is usually an expensive component of the ration. Furthermore, energy is required to excrete nitrogen.

It has been stated that feeding high levels of protein causes crooked legs and other skeletal deformities in young, fast-growing horses, but it is probably not protein per se that causes the problems. Feeding an unbalanced diet containing high levels of protein results in problems. For example, if protein is added to increase rate of growth without ensuring that necessary amounts of other nutrients such as Ca and P needed for bone formation are present, problems will develop. Studies with rats and humans indicate that high levels of protein cause hypercalciuria, but further studies are needed to determine the effect of protein on calcium metabolism in horses.

NONPROTEIN NITROGEN UTILIZATION

Nonprotein nitrogen compounds such as urea are often added to rations for ruminants. The microflora of the rumen use the nitrogen to synthesize protein, which then can be digested and utilized by the host animal. The principal advantages of using nonprotein nitrogen in ruminant rations are reduction of feed costs and utilization of materials that could not be used directly by nonruminants such as humans.

The horse, however, does not appear to be an efficient utilizer of nonprotein nitrogen. Much of the dietary nonprotein nitrogen is absorbed from the small intestine. If the nonprotein nitrogen is urea, most of the absorbed nitrogen is excreted in the urine because mammalian systems do not contain the enzyme urease, which is needed to break down urea into ammonia and carbon dioxide. Some absorbed urea can be secreted into the large intestine, where bacteria can utilize it, and some of the urea reaches the large intestine directly. Unfortunately, quantitative measurements of the amounts of amino acids produced by bacteria and subsequently utilized by the horse are not available. Some studies indicate that amino acids of bacterial origin make significant contributions to the nutritional status of the horse, whereas other studies suggest they do not. However, it appears that the economic advantage of feeding urea to horses is not nearly as great as that of feeding urea to cattle because the horse does not utilize urea as efficiently as cattle. Furthermore, in the classes of horses that require high dietary levels of protein, such as young horses, protein quality of the diet is important.

NONPROTEIN NITROGEN TOXICITY

Ammonia is toxic, but urea per se is not toxic. As mentioned earlier, mammals do not have enzymes to form ammonia from urea. Excessive feeding of urea to cattle can result in ammonia toxicosis because of rapid ammonia release from the rumen by the bacteria. Horses are more tolerant of urea ingestion than cattle because much of the urea is absorbed before it reaches the site of bacterial activity. Ammonia toxicosis was produced in ponies by feeding one pound of urea. Clinical signs were characteristic of severe central nervous system derangement. The earliest signs were aimless wandering and incoordination, followed by head-pressing against fixed objects. Death followed shortly after head-pressing began. Convulsions occasionally occurred as a terminal episode. One pound of urea is much greater than the amount needed to produce ammonia toxicosis in ruminants, and it is highly unlikely that horses will obtain that level of intake under field conditions.

In summary, horse owners should not be concerned about ammonia toxicosis if their horse happens to eat a cattle ration containing urea. If the feed is safe for cattle, it will be safe for horses.

References

1. Cunha, T. J.: Horse Feeding and Nutrition. New York, Academic Press, 1980.
2. Evans, J. W., Borton, A., Hintz, H. F., and Van Vleck, L. D.: The Horse. San Francisco, Freeman, 1977.
3. National Research Council: Nutrient Requirements of the Horse. NAS-NRC Publication, Washington, DC, 1978.
4. Roberts, S. J.: Veterinary Obstetrics and Genital Diseases, 2nd ed. Ithaca, NY. Published by author, 1971.
5. Swerczek, T. W.: Experimentally induced toxicoinfectious botulism in horses and foals. Am. J. Vet. Res., *41*:348, 1980.

MINERALS

H. F. Schryver, ITHACA, NEW YORK
H. F. Hintz, ITHACA, NEW YORK

Minerals comprise about 4 per cent of the weight of the animal body. Among the minerals of concern in equine nutrition are calcium, phosphorus, potassium, sodium, chlorine, magnesium, sulfur, iron, zinc, copper, manganese, iodine, and selenium. These elements are known to perform many vital functions in the structure and metabolism of the body.

Plants, and ultimately the soil in which the plants are grown, are the sources of minerals in the nutrition of the horse. A large number and variety of factors influence the pathway of minerals from soil to plant to animal. The soil may contain too little or too much of essential elements, or alternatively, factors in the soil may reduce the ability of plants to obtain essential elements. These and related factors often result in regional mineral problems in animal agriculture. Some examples of regional problems are the large areas of iodine-deficient soils or regions in which the soil contains an excess or deficiency of selenium. Such areas are often well known and have been mapped (Figs. 1 and 2). Information about regional mineral problems is often available from the local extension service, state college of agriculture, or regional United States Department of Agriculture office.

The soil-plant-animal pathway of minerals is one of changing relationships. The content and avail-

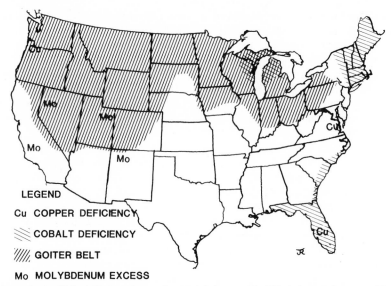

Figure 1. Areas in the United States where mineral deficiency or toxicity is known to occur. (Courtesy of the Plant, Soil, and Nutrition Laboratory of the United States Department of Agriculture, Ithaca, NY.)

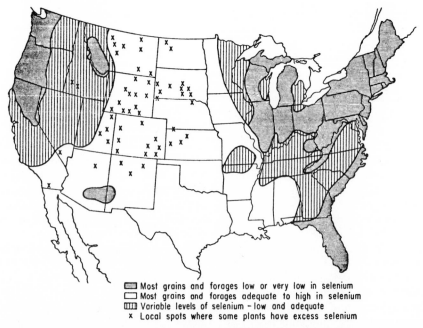

Figure 2. Areas of selenium deficiency and toxicity in the United States. (Courtesy of A. H. Allaway, Plant, Soil, and Nutrition Laboratory of the United States Department of Agriculture, Ithaca, NY.)

ability of minerals in soils and plants may be altered by agricultural techniques, such as fertilizing, spraying, and harvesting. The mineral content and distribution in soils and plants may also be altered by air- or water-borne deposition of elements from industrial pollution and other sources. Changing relationships also develop from plant breeding, which introduces new species and varieties that differ in their ability to extract minerals from soils. Animal breeders and husbandmen exert increased pressure on the soil-plant-animal system by demanding more rapid rates of growth from their animals. These and other factors have altered the soil-plant-animal pathway of minerals in the recent past and will continue to do so in the future. Mineral problems that were considered unlikely to occur 25 years ago are now observed frequently in some species of livestock. Similar problems may be expected in horse husbandry in the future.

There are complex interrelationships that exist among minerals themselves. For example, dietary calcium influences phosphorus, magnesium, zinc, copper, and other minerals in the diet, while calcium is itself influenced by phosphorus, magnesium, or iron in the diet. The organic composition of a diet also influences mineral nutrition. Calcium absorption is enhanced or inhibited by dietary protein, certain amino acids, some carbohydrates, lipids, and by specific organic substances such as oxalate, phytate, and vitamin D. These relationships determine the availability of minerals in the diet. The presence of natural or synthetic chelating agents also influences the availability of minerals. To be beneficial in nutrition, the chelation or binding of minerals to the chelator must be weaker than the binding capacity of the tissue for the same element. The chelating agent must be able to "deliver" the mineral element to the tissues. Unfortunately, some natural and synthetic chelating agents bind some minerals very strongly and do not release the minerals to the tissues. On the other hand, some chelating agents exchange one mineral for another at the tissue level. Thus, a chelating agent may increase the availability of one mineral but at the expense of creating a deficiency of another. There is no evidence that chelated trace minerals are more effective sources than simple inorganic forms of trace minerals for horses.

Determination of the mineral status of animals suspected of having deficiency, excess, or imbalance of minerals is done most directly and accurately by considering the nutritional history of the animals in question. The nutritional history should include the age and function of the animal and the types and amounts of feeds that have been fed. Soil analysis may provide useful information if home-grown feeds are used. Mineral analysis of feeds is also potentially useful, provided that proper sampling techniques

are followed. The feeds sampled must represent feeds that were used during the period of development of the suspected nutritional problem. In agricultural regions, personnel of the extension service or dairy herd improvement services are often equipped with the proper tools and techniques for obtaining useful soil, feed, and water samples.

Determination of the concentration of minerals in blood serum or plasma may be helpful in some cases. However, homeostatic controls and the body stores of minerals may minimize or prevent significant changes in the concentration of some minerals in blood. For example, neither a very low nor a very high calcium diet alters the plasma calcium concentration in horses. A high phosphorus diet may cause plasma calcium to fall, but only to the low normal range. Quite large dietary increases in zinc or copper in horses produce only small increases of the plasma concentration of these elements. On the other hand, severe, prolonged, experimental deficiency of zinc and magnesium causes a marked decrease in concentration of these elements in blood plasma. Blood selenium analysis may be useful in determining selenium status. However, blood analysis should not be the sole criterion for diagnosis of mineral problems even when blood concentration tends to reflect mineral status. The investigator should seek additional evidence.

Blood samples taken for trace element analysis are easily contaminated. Syringes, needles, and evacuated blood sample tubes are common sources of contamination. For example, spuriously high zinc values occur when blood contacts the rubber stoppers of some evacuated blood sample tubes for only a brief period. Special blood sampling tubes are available for obtaining samples for trace element analysis.

Analysis of hair is sometimes suggested as a means of determining the mineral status of horses. A great variety of factors affect the mineral content of hair. These include hair color, rate of hair growth, site on the body, and season of the year. For example, colored hair has three to four times as much calcium, magnesium, and manganese as white hair. The calcium, magnesium, iron, and manganese concentration of hair can vary twofold in different seasons. Contamination of hair by urine, feces, feed, soil, and other environmental sources is a serious and unsolved problem in obtaining hair samples for analysis. The few scientific studies that have been reported indicate that hair analysis is valueless for determining the calcium, phosphorus, copper, or molybdenum status of horses.

CALCIUM AND PHOSPHORUS

Calcium and phosphorus are the most abundant elements in the body, comprising more than 70 per cent of the "ash" of the body. The minerals are commonly considered together because they occur together in bone and because they strongly influence each other in nutrition and metabolism. A deficiency or an excess of one affects the metabolism of the other nutrient.

Greater than 99 per cent of calcium and 80 per cent of the phosphorus of the body occurs in crystalline form in bone as hydroxyapatite, which has the empirical formula $Ca_{10}(PO_4)_6(OH)_2$. The bone crystal, which has a Ca:P ratio of about 2:1, is intimately associated with collagen. Bone also contains carbonate, citrate, and the elements sodium, potassium, fluorine, magnesium, and many other elements. The relationship of these components in the inorganic phase of bone can be influenced in part by diet.

Calcium and phosphorus have a large number of functions in addition to constituting bone crystal. Calcium is necessary in the blood clotting mechanism for the conversion of prothrombin to thrombin. Calcium is involved in transmission of nerve impulses, muscle contraction, and the secretion of many hormones and is necessary for the activation of a number of enzymes. Phosphorus is part of many structural and functional compounds in the body, such as phosphoproteins, phospholipids, and nucleoproteins. Phosphate is an active part of a large number and wide variety of enzyme systems.

Bone acts not only as a structural element in the body but also as a store of calcium and phosphorus that can be mobilized and transported by blood to other sites to serve some of the metabolic functions mentioned before. The concentration of calcium in blood plasma is closely regulated by the activities of parathormone, secreted by the parathyroid gland (p. 160), calcitonin, secreted by the C cells of the thyroid gland, and by metabolites of vitamin D. These substances, alone or in combination, influence the intestinal absorption and renal excretion of calcium as well as the mobilization and deposition of calcium in bone. Mobilization of calcium from bone under the influence of parathormone occurs when dietary sources are inadequate for body needs. During mobilization of calcium, both mineral and organic phases are usually removed from bone. Thus, a net loss of bone substance occurs, which may be severe after prolonged calcium mobilization due to dietary deficiency.

Calcium deficiency may be due to simple lack in the diet or may be due to factors that limit calcium utilization in diets in which the calcium level is adequate. Factors that limit dietary calcium utilization include excess dietary phosphate as inorganic phosphate or as phytate phosphate and oxalic acid. Phytate phosphate is a hexaphosphoric acid ester of inositol that occurs in many seed grains and protein supplements. Oxalic acid is found in many species of grasses, particularly those grown in tropical areas. Both of these substances bind dietary calcium (and other divalent cations) and make it less available for absorption from the intestinal tract. Both phytate and oxalate are probably digested in the large intestine of the horse, causing release of the chelated calcium. However, this is of little value to the individual because calcium is poorly absorbed from the large intestine of the horse.

CLINICAL SIGNS OF CALCIUM AND PHOSPHORUS DEFICIENCY

Signs of calcium deficiency are generally seen in the skeletal system. Calcium is mobilized from skeletal stores to maintain other metabolic functions that are calcium-dependent. Thus, deficiency signs relating to calcium-dependent metabolic functions are rare. Skeletal signs depend on the severity and duration of calcium deficiency, on the age, and on the phosphorus or vitamin D status of the affected animals. The net result of calcium deficiency is the formation of too little bone. The cortices of the long bones may be thin-walled, porous, and fragile. The trabeculae of cancellous bone of the axial and appendicular skeleton become thin and sparse. In rickets and ricketslike disorders in which calcium and vitamin D deficiency is combined, mineralization of the organic phase of bone does not take place normally. In nutritional secondary hyperparathyroidism (NSH), a low or marginal intake of calcium is combined with an excessive phosphorus intake. The entire skeleton is affected, but the enlarged facial bones of affected horses have given the name "bighead disease" to the condition.

Calcium deficiency may be undetected for many weeks or months. The skeleton of mature animals contains a very large reserve of calcium that can be called upon to meet other metabolic needs. More than half of the skeletal mineral may be removed before clinical signs appear. Young animals may grow in stature at a normal or only slightly reduced rate while fed a calcium-deficient diet. Bone elongation continues during deficiency because bone is constantly remodeled during growth. Bone mineral removed during remodeling may be deposited at sites of new bone formation. For example, bone mineral removed from an endosteal surface may be reutilized at periosteal surfaces or at the growth plate. The result is that skeletal mass does not keep pace with increasing body size, and the skeleton is more injury-prone.

Phosphorus deficiency affects the skeleton in similar ways. However, young animals fail to grow, probably because they eat poorly and because phosphorus-deficient forage crops are frequently deficient in protein as well. Phosphorus-deficient animals are often lame and walk with a stiff, painful gait. Deficient animals often have a depraved appetite and eat wood, bones, stones, and other objects. Behavioral studies have shown that phosphorus-deficient sheep with depraved appetites do not clearly prefer phosphorus-containing supplements. This indicates that the depravity or pica of phosphorus deficiency is not an example of "nutritional wisdom" or "phosphorus appetite" as commonly thought.

Reproductive inefficiency is a frequent sign of phosphorus deficiency. Affected animals show anestrus or irregular estrus and reduced rate of conception.

Hypophosphatemia is a frequent finding in phosphorus deficiency. In well-documented field cases of phosphorus deficiency in cattle, serum phosphorus may decrease to less than one third of normal levels.

CALCIUM AND PHOSPHORUS REQUIREMENTS

The calcium and phosphorus requirement of horses depends on the age and function of the individual. Young, growing horses have high requirements to meet the needs of skeletal development. The requirement of the mare is increased during late pregnancy for bone formation in the developing fetus and during lactation for secretion of calcium and phosphorus in milk. Table 1 shows the estimated dietary requirements of calcium and phosphorus for different classes of horses. Amounts of calcium greatly in excess of the requirement should be avoided. Excess calcium intake appears to inhibit the turnover or remodeling process in bone and interferes with the utilization of phosphorus and other essential minerals. Phosphorus greatly in excess of the requirement and in excess of the calcium intake should also be avoided. Excess phosphorus intake inhibits absorption of calcium and other elements and may alter calcium homeostatic mechanisms and the rate of bone turnover.

The calcium and phosphorus content of some common feeds is shown in Table 2. Cereal grains are poor sources of calcium but moderately good sources of phosphorus. Byproducts of the oil seeds, such as soybean oil meal, contain more calcium and phosphorus than the cereal grains. Hays generally contain considerably more calcium than cereal grains or oil seed products. Legume hays are rich sources of calcium. However, the mineral content of roughage can be very variable depending on the type of roughage, type of soil on which the hay was grown, stage of maturity when hay was cut, handling after harvest, and other factors. The calcium and phosphorus of roughage is highly available to horses. That of cereal grains and oil seed meals is slightly

TABLE 1. APPROXIMATE CALCIUM AND PHOSPHORUS REQUIREMENTS FOR HORSES*

	Percentage in the Diet		Daily Nutrients (gm)	
	Ca	P	Ca	P
Foals, to 6 months	0.80	0.55	33	20
Weanlings	0.60	0.45	34	25
Yearlings	0.50	0.35	31	22
Two-year-olds	0.40	0.30	25	17
Mare, late pregnancy	0.45	0.30	34	23
Mare, lactation	0.45	0.30	50	34
Mature horses, maintenance	0.30	0.20	23	14

*Assuming 500 kg mature weight

less available, possibly owing to the phytate content of these products (Table 3).

CALCIUM AND PHOSPHORUS SUPPLEMENTS

The calcium and phosphorus content of some common mineral sources is shown in Table 4. The minerals in those sources are readily assimilated by horses. The ratio of the minerals in the sources varies so that it is possible to choose a supplement to correct a deficiency or imbalance in a particular diet. Thus, a diet deficient only in calcium can be most easily corrected with limestone, while a diet equally deficient in calcium and phosphorus can be corrected with dicalcium phosphate.

The available experimental evidence indicates that horses, like ruminants, do not have a nutritional sense or nutritional wisdom to select the amount of calcium and/or phosphorus needed from free choice supplements. The horse is not able to balance a ration or to make up a deficit in a ration if offered calcium and phosphorus free choice. This applies even when the free choice minerals contain salt. Free choice calcium and phosphorus give a false sense of security to the horse manager but do little for the horse.

DIAGNOSIS OF CALCIUM AND PHOSPHORUS DEFICIENCY

Diagnosis of suspected calcium and/or phosphorus deficiency may be difficult. Skeletal changes are generally not clinically evident until the disease is well advanced. Conventional radiographic procedures usually are unable to detect loss of skeletal mineral until the losses exceed about 30 per cent. Plasma or serum phosphorus concentration may be decreased in phosphorus deficiency.

Plasma calcium concentration is usually found to be normal in calcium deficiency because the ho-

TABLE 2. APPROXIMATE MINERAL COMPOSITION OF SOME COMMON FEEDS FOR HORSES

	Ca	P	Mg	K	Zn	Fe	Cu	Mn
	Percentage				*Ppm*			
Roughages:								
Alfalfa	1.3	.25	.29	1.9	17	180	13	30
Bluegrass	.30	.29	.16	1.7	—	260	9	93
Brome grass	.32	.22	.13	2.0	—	100	7	100
Oat hay	.30	.26	.75	1.2	—	400	4	120
Orchard grass	.35	.31	.20	3.0	18	110	14	40
Timothy	.41	.20	.16	1.6	—	140	5	46
Grains:								
Barley	.05	.37	.15	.45	17	90	9	19
Corn	.05	.60	.03	.35	21	30	4	6
Oats	.07	.37	.19	.44	33	80	7	43
Wheat	.05	.45	.11	.41	30	40	7	40
Protein Supplements:								
Cottonseed meal	.16	1.20	.60	1.50	80	300	20	23
Linseed meal	.43	.90	.67	1.53	—	360	28	42
Skim milk	1.30	1.09	.13	1.66	68	10	1	2
Soybean meal	.31	.70	.30	2.19	48	130	30	48
Miscellaneous:								
Beet pulp	.75	.10	.30	.20	10	330	14	38
Molasses, cane	1.05	.15	.47	3.80	30	250	80	57
Wheat bran	.12	1.43	.59	1.60	120	190	14	138

The compositions shown in the table are expressed on a dry matter basis and are average compositions for each type of feed. Composition will vary depending on the origin of the feed, stage of maturity at harvest, processing techniques, and many other factors. (Adapted from National Academy of Sciences: Nutrient Requirement of Horses, 4th ed. Washington, DC, National Academy of Sciences–National Research Council, 1978.)

meostatic mechanisms are effective in maintaining plasma calcium at normal levels. Maintenance of plasma calcium concentration is at the expense of the skeleton. Serum alkaline phosphatase may be intermittently elevated in severe and rapidly developing calcium or phosphorus deficiency. Hair analysis has been suggested as a diagnostic procedure;

TABLE 3. AVAILABILITY OF CALCIUM AND PHOSPHORUS IN SOME COMMON HORSE FEEDS AND SUPPLEMENTS

	Ca (Percentage)	P (Percentage)
Corn	—	38
Timothy hay	70	42
Alfalfa hay	77	38
Linseed meal	68	45
Milk products	77	57
Wheat bran	—	34
Limestone	67	—
Dicalcium phosphate	73	44
Bone meal	71	46
Monosodium phosphate	—	47

Availability was determined as the percentage of calcium or phosphorus absorbed by experimental horses when the ingredient listed was the primary source of either calcium or phosphorus in the diet.

(From Feeding the foal. Stud Managers' Handbook, Vol. 9. Clovis, CA, Agriservices Foundation, 1973, p. 66.)

however, hair does not reflect the calcium or phosphorus status of horses.

Comparison of the urinary clearance ratio of phosphorus to creatinine has been suggested as a useful diagnostic procedure. In practice, the concentration of phosphorus and creatinine in a single urine sample is measured, and the ratio of the concentration of phosphorus to the concentration of creatinine $\left(\frac{[PO_4]}{[Creatinine]} \times 100 \right)$ is calculated. The rationale behind the test is that a relatively constant amount of creatinine is generally excreted by the kidney. The ratio decreases in phosphorus deficiency owing to decreased urinary phosphorus excretion. The ratio increases in calcium deficiency or phosphorus excess owing to increased renal excretion of phosphorus. Unfortunately, there are few reported applications of this procedure. Those wishing to use this procedure should compare results obtained from suspect animals to results obtained from control horses of similar age, sex, and breed that have been fed adequate levels of calcium and phosphorus.

The most direct and most effective diagnostic procedure is a thorough review of the dietary history of animals suspected of deficiency. If possible, the review should include visual inspection of the feeds used on the farm and should include chemical anal-

TABLE 4. APPROXIMATE CALCIUM AND PHOSPHORUS CONTENT OF SOME COMMON MINERAL SUPPLEMENTS

	Ca (Percentage)	P (Percentage)	Gm of Element in 30 Gm of Supplement	
			Ca	*P*
Calcium carbonate	34	0	10	0
Defluorinated phosphate	32	15	10	5
Bone meal	30	14	9	4
Dicalcium phosphate	27	21	8	6
Monocalcium phosphate	17	21	5	6
Monosodium phosphate	0	22	0	7

These are approximate or average values. The calcium content of bone meal, for example, may vary from 27 to 32 per cent.

30 Gm is approximately one tablespoon. Thus, one tablespoon of calcium carbonate provides 10 gm of Ca or about one third of the daily requirement of a yearling of 500 kg mature weight (see Table 1).

Limestone or oyster shells are common calcium carbonate sources that are used for mineral supplements for livestock.

ysis of the feeds for calcium and phosphorus content.

THERAPY

Calcium or phosphorus deficiency is treated by supplying the deficient nutrients in the diet. This may be done by using feeds that are rich in these nutrients (Table 2) or by using mineral supplements. Table 4 shows the composition of some commonly used calcium and phosphorus supplements and the grams of element supplied by one tablespoon (about 30 gm) of supplement.

MAGNESIUM

Magnesium is involved with calcium and phosphorus metabolism and is an activator or cofactor of numerous enzymes. Magnesium is particularly important in cellular energy metabolism.

Deficiency of magnesium has been produced experimentally in foals fed purified diets containing only 7 to 8 ppm of magnesium. Some of the deficient foals developed severe signs of central nervous system irritability, including nervousness, muscular tremors, and ataxia. Handling or loud noise caused the foals to develop convulsive seizures with paddling of the legs, hyperpnea, and sweating. Serum magnesium values of deficient foals were less than 1 mg per 100 ml. Serum phosphorus and calcium levels were normal. At postmortem examination of the magnesium-deficient foals, the elastic fibers of the aorta, the pulmonary artery, and other large arteries were found to be mineralized. Mineral deposits were also observed in elastic tissues of the lung and spleen and in the Purkinje fibers in the heart. Degeneration of cardiac and skeletal muscle was observed.

TRANSIT TETANY

Naturally occurring magnesium deficiency has not been described in horses. However, a tetany associated with hypomagnesemia and hypocalcemia has been reported in the midwestern United States and in England. The signs of "equine transit tetany" include sweating, hyperpnea, muscular fibrillation, difficult or uncertain locomotion, incoordination, and collapse with muscular twitching. Death may occur during convulsions. Affected animals respond to intravenous administration of magnesium and calcium salts. The syndrome appears to be brought on by a stressful situation such as shipping. The condition does not appear to be a simple magnesium deficiency, but tetany-prone animals may be helped by providing additional magnesium in the diet.

Horses require about 0.1 per cent magnesium in the diet or about 4 to 6.5 gm per day for a 1000-pound horse. The magnesium in common feeds and supplements appears to be readily available to horses.

SODIUM AND CHLORIDE

The major functions of sodium and chloride are the regulation of tissue osmotic pressure and acid-base balance. Sodium is important in maintenance of cell membrane potentials and the transmission of nerve impulses. The two elements are usually considered together as sodium chloride and have related functions in tissues.

Horses have a clear salt drive. The needs of the horse can easily be met by providing salt "free choice" either as salt blocks or as loose salt. Salt consumption varies greatly among individual horses. Measurements at Cornell University's Equine Research Park over a 12-month period show consistent daily intakes of salt that vary from 15 gm

TABLE 5. MICRONUTRIENT MINERAL ALLOWANCES FOR HORSES

	Mg Element/Kg Diet
Iron	50.0
Zinc	40.0
Manganese	50.0
Copper	9.0
Iodine	0.1
Selenium	0.1
Cobalt	0.1

The amounts given in this table are considered to be adequate for growth and maintenance (National Research Council, 1978).

for one horse to over 200 gm for others. Most of the horses in the survey consumed 50 to 75 gm of salt per day.

Iodized, trace mineral salt is highly recommended for horses. It provides a simple, safe, dependable means of meeting the requirements for salt and part of the need for iodine and other trace minerals (Table 5). Table 6 shows the contribution of a commercially available trace mineral salt mixture to the estimated trace mineral requirements of a mature horse, assuming that the horse consumed about 50 gm of salt per day. This is well within the range of salt intake of most horses.

The sodium content of urine and feces has been used in determining sodium status. Sodium levels below 10 mg per dl in urine and 1 to 1.5 gm per kg of dry feces generally indicates an insufficient supply of sodium in the diet.

Salt poisoning can occur in salt-starved horses that are given access to salt without adequate water. Signs of salt poisoning include colic, diarrhea, frequent urination, weakness, staggering, and paralysis of the hind limbs.

TABLE 6. CONTRIBUTION OF A TRACE MINERAL SALT MIXTURE TO THE REQUIREMENTS OF A MATURE HORSE FOR TRACE MINERALS

Composition of the Salt Mixture	Mg of Mineral in 50 gm Salt	Multiple of the Requirement
	%		
Cobalt	0.010	5.0	10.0
Copper	0.023	11.5	.2
Iodine	0.007	3.5	7.0
Manganese	0.225	112.5	.6
Zinc	0.200	100.0	.5
Magnesium	0.100	50.0	.002
Iron	0.232	116.0	.6

The salt mixture is typical of an iodized, trace mineralized salt that is commercially available as loose salt or salt blocks. A typical daily consumption by a 1000 lb horse from free choice feeders would be about 50 gm. A daily intake of 50 gm would supply the multiple of the NRC estimated requirements for trace elements as shown.

POTASSIUM

Potassium, like sodium and chloride, is important in maintaining tissue osmotic pressure and acid-base equilibrium. It is intimately involved in regulating the passage of nutrients into cells and in water metabolism. Potassium plays an important role in muscle contraction. Most of the body potassium is intracellular.

Potassium deficiency has been studied experimentally in a number of species. Signs in affected animals include decreased rate of growth, loss of appetite, and decreased serum potassium levels. Naturally occurring or experimental potassium deficiency has not been reported in the horse.

The potassium requirement of the horse is estimated to be about 0.4 to 0.5 per cent of the diet. Most forage crops contain about 1.5 per cent potassium. Thus, dietary potassium deficiency seems unlikely in horses that receive forage as 35 per cent or more of their ration. On the other hand, grains generally contain 0.4 per cent or less of potassium. Thus, rations very high in grains may cause problems as a result of low potassium intake. Increased potassium loss may occur as a result of prolonged hard work as in endurance rides or as a result of diarrhea, acute intestinal obstruction, adrenal cortical dysfunction, and in other pathologic states.

IRON

Iron is an integral part of hemoglobin, the oxygen-carrying protein in red blood cells, of myoglobin in muscle, and of respiratory enzymes such as cytochrome C, peroxidase, and catalase.

Deficiency of iron results in anemia. The red blood cells may be reduced in size, number, and hemoglobin content (p. 303). Anemic animals have pale mucous membranes and are often weak, inactive, and tire easily. The greatest need for iron occurs in the newborn, which has a rapidly expanding red blood cell mass and small iron stores. At the same time, dam's milk is generally a poor source of iron. Thus, iron stores and intake may be insufficient to meet the needs of the newborn, and anemia results. Access to soil and to feeds other than dam's milk provide a source of iron to the newborn and can help prevent anemia.

Under normal circumstances, the body excretes very little iron. The iron stores are reused in hemoglobin synthesis. However, repeated hemorrhage increases iron loss, may deplete iron stores, and may result in anemia. This may occur in certain parasite infestations.

The mature horse is estimated to require about 40 ppm of iron and rapidly growing foals about 50 ppm of iron in the diet. Good quality feeds easily supply this level of iron.

Simple iron deficiency anemia is probably a very rare occurrence in the horse. Anemic horses should be examined carefully, and causes of anemia other than iron deficiency should be sought.

Ferrous salts (Fe^{++}) are more efficiently absorbed and are more effective iron supplements than ferric salts (Fe^{+++}). Chelated iron salts do not appear to be more efficiently utilized by horses than simple inorganic iron salts or the iron that is contained in feeds. Injectable iron supplements provide iron immediately to the body, but this is probably of doubtful utility. Some injectable iron dextran supplements that are meant for treating baby pig anemia have produced a severe, shocklike syndrome in horses and should be avoided.

Iron supplements given to normal horses or to horses that do not have simple or induced iron deficiency are of little value. Iron does not stimulate hemoglobin synthesis. Prolonged high iron consumption interferes with phosphorus utilization in ruminants and may do so in horses as well.

COPPER

Copper is important for the utilization of iron in hemoglobin synthesis and in the maturation of red blood cells. Copper is also involved in the function of many enzymes associated with amino acid metabolism and with cellular respiration. Copper is part of the enzyme tyrosinase, which is needed for conversion of tyrosine to melanin in skin. Normal collagen and elastin formation and osteoblast activity are dependent on copper. Copper is an integral part of lysyl oxidase, an enzyme that is responsible for the cross-linking of collagen molecules in the maturation of collagen.

Copper deficiency may be due to simple lack of copper in the diet, or deficiency may be induced by excess molybdenum intake. Horses seem more tolerant of dietary molybdenum than ruminants. Several reports indicate that high molybdenum pastures that have resulted in severe disease in cattle have not affected horses that have also grazed the pastures. Nevertheless, short-term experiments in the horse show that when molybdenum intake exceeds copper intake by several times, copper metabolism may be influenced without producing signs of copper deficiency. The complex interaction of sulfate with molybdenum and copper that has been observed in ruminants has not been studied in horses. Dietary supplements containing copper have been used to counteract excess molybdenum intake in ruminants and presumably would do so in horses.

CLINICAL SIGNS OF COPPER DEFICIENCY

The signs of copper deficiency are often directly referable to the various functions of copper in the body. Thus, deficient animals may be anemic. The anemia of copper deficiency resembles iron deficiency anemia because iron is poorly utilized in copper deficiency. Copper-deficient anemic animals do not respond to iron supplements. The hair of deficient animals may become gray owing to the defect in melanin synthesis in the skin.

Affected animals may have bone abnormalities due to defects in collagen maturation and altered osteoblast activity. In dogs and swine, copper deficiency causes a bone disease that resembles rickets. The joints of affected animals are swollen, and the limbs may be deformed. The cortex of the long bones is thin, the trabeculae are few and small, and the growth plates of the bones are widened.

Horses appear to tolerate diets that produce copper deficiency in ruminants. Uncomplicated cases of copper deficiency have not been reported in the horse, but copper deficiency has been implicated in skeletal disease in young horses in copper-deficient areas of Western Australia. In Ireland, copper-responsive osteodystrophies have been described in foals, and a molybdenum-induced copper deficiency has been suggested as a cause of a ricketslike disease. In each of these instances, bone cortices of affected horses have been thin and the joints enlarged, and in some cases there have been limb deformities.

COPPER REQUIREMENTS

The copper requirement for maintenance of mature ponies has been estimated to be 3.5 ppm of the diet. Young horses probably require 10 ppm in the diet.

Ponies appear to be resistant to chronic copper toxicity and have tolerated up to 80 ppm in the diet for long periods.

ZINC

Zinc plays an essential role in the function of a large number of enzyme systems that are involved in digestion and metabolism.

CLINICAL SIGNS OF ZINC DEFICIENCY

Naturally occurring zinc deficiency has not been reported in horses, but experimental zinc deficiency has been produced in foals. The deficiency inhibited growth of the foals and caused skin lesions similar to those seen in zinc-deficient pigs. The lesions, called parakeratosis, began on the lower limbs and then extended upward on the body as the deficiency progressed. The first signs were hair loss, followed by scaling of the dried, outer layers of the skin.

Subsequently the affected skin was encrusted by a rough layer of serous exudate and desquamated epithelium. Skin wounds in the affected foals healed poorly. Serum alkaline phosphatase levels were below normal, as were tissue and blood concentrations of zinc. Skeletal abnormalities were not reported in the experimentally deficient foals, but zinc deficiency has resulted in short, thick bones in chickens and in bone deformities in calves. Reproductive and behavioral abnormalities have been observed in zinc-deficient rats, but such findings were not described in experimental zinc deficiency in horses.

ZINC TOXICITY

Excess zinc intake can be toxic. Growing horses fed diets containing 5000 ppm (0.50 per cent) of zinc developed anemia, swelling of the epiphyses of the long bones, stiffness, and lameness. Such a high intake level of zinc may result from contamination of soil and feeds by metal smelters.

ZINC REQUIREMENTS

Young horses fed practical rations containing 40 ppm of zinc grew well and maintained their tissue concentrations of zinc, suggesting that this level of zinc is adequate for growth. However, other factors in the diet may affect zinc utilization. For example, high levels of calcium or copper increase the requirement of the pig for zinc. Phytin, a phosphorus-containing chelating agent found in cereal grains and byproducts and in protein supplements such as soybean meal, combines with zinc to decrease its absorption from the digestive tract. Diets high in calcium enhance the detrimental effect of phytin on zinc absorption in pigs. The presence of these factors in horse rations causes some nutritionists to recommend that the horse be given diets containing at least 100 ppm of zinc.

The requirements of the horse for zinc can generally be met from good quality roughage and from trace mineralized salt. Oral zinc supplements such as zinc oxide, carbonate, and sulfate are effectively utilized.

COBALT

Cobalt occurs in the molecule of vitamin B_{12}. Cobalt may have other functions in the body, but these are not yet well studied. Horses are able to graze pastures that contain levels of cobalt that are deficient for sheep and cattle without ill effects. Cobalt deficiency or toxicity has not been described for horses.

Rations that contain 0.1 ppm of cobalt should be adequate for horses.

IODINE

Much of the body content of iodine is found in the thyroid gland, where the element is incorporated into the thyroid hormone thyroxine. Soils and plants in large areas of the world, including the northern tier of the United States, are iodine-deficient.

Iodine deficiency results in goiter, or enlargement of the thyroid gland. Goiter is also caused by goitrogenic substances found in plants of the cabbage genus Brassica. These include cabbage, Brussels sprouts, kale, and rape. Goitrogens are also found in linseed, peanuts, soybeans, and other legumes. Generally, goiter caused by these goitrogenic plants can be prevented by feeding additional iodine to animals at risk.

Iodine deficiency or the activity of goitrogenic substances results in decreased production of thyroxine. This in turn stimulates production of thyrotropic hormone by the pituitary gland, which causes hyperplasia and enlargement of the thyroid gland. Young animals are most subject to iodine deficiency and goiter. Young born of iodine-deficient dams are often stillborn. Others are weak and unable to nurse. Affected foals have been born with forelimb contracture.

Iodine deficiency affects reproduction in mature animals. Affected mares may exhibit irregular estrus cycles and prolonged gestation.

Thyroid function can be estimated by a competitive protein binding assay for serum levels of thyroxine (T_4 test). The T_4 test has been shown to be more reliable as a test of thyroid function than the protein-bound iodine (PBI) test in thyroidectomized ponies.

IODINE REQUIREMENTS

The horse probably requires about 0.1 ppm of iodine per day. Iodine deficiency is a well-recognized problem, and the use of iodized salt is so widespread and common that iodine deficiency is not encountered often. On the other hand, cases of goiter in foals due to excess iodine intake have been reported several times in Maryland, Virginia, Kentucky, New York, Great Britain, and Japan. The goitrous foals have been born of mares given excess amounts of iodine supplements during pregnancy. Excessive iodine intake has come about through the enthusiastic use of iodine supplements or through the use of several iodine supplements simultaneously. Kelp, which is a rich source of iodine, has been an ingredient in each of the cases of iodine-induced goiter.

SULFUR

There appears to be little need for elemental or inorganic forms of sulfur by the animal body. Sulfur is required as organic compounds, such as the sulfur-containing amino acids and vitamins. Excess intake of inorganic forms of sulfur influences the toxicity of molybdenum in ruminants, but its effect in horses is not known.

MANGANESE

Manganese is required in enzymes that are involved in protein metabolism and fatty acid and cholesterol synthesis. Manganese plays a central role in the synthesis of glycosaminoglycans and glycoproteins, which are important constituents of cartilage and bone.

A condition thought to be manganese deficiency has been described in horses in a ranching community where the soils have been heavily limed to combat acidity produced by a nearby zinc smelter. The area soils tend to be marginal or low in manganese, and availability to plants is reduced by soil alkalinity. Samples of alfalfa hay contained as little as 13 ppm of manganese. Mares suffered from reproductive dysfunction that was manifested as delayed estrus, reduced fertility, and spontaneous abortion. Foals were often born with skeletal deformities and muscle contractures. Lesions included asymmetry of the skull, curvature of the vertebral column, shortened limb bones, and enlarged joints. Contracture of neck muscles resulted in a peculiar positioning of the head. Affected foals were often unable to flex their limbs.

The manganese requirements of the horse have not been determined, but estimates place the requirement at about 40 ppm. Some grains such as corn are poor sources of manganese, but roughage tends to be a good source.

SELENIUM

Selenium is a component of glutathione peroxidase, an antioxidant enzyme that catalyzes the conversion of peroxides to alcohols in tissues. Vitamin E and the sulfur-containing amino acids also have antioxidant properties and are able partly to replace one another and selenium in the diet.

Selenium-deficient areas occur in most of the Northeastern United States, the eastern seaboard, the Pacific Northwest, and adjacent areas of Canada (Fig. 2). Grains and forages grown in these areas tend to be low in selenium. Selenium deficiency results where animals are fed solely on home-grown feeds or on feeds grown in the adjacent selenium-deficient areas. Animals are often protected against deficiency when part of their ration contains feeds shipped from selenium-adequate areas.

SELENIUM DEFICIENCY (WHITE MUSCLE DISEASE)

Selenium deficiency leads to muscular dystrophy. The severe dystrophy that occurs in young foals is called white muscle disease. This disease has been recognized with increasing frequency in recent years in the eastern United States and Canada. Affected foals are weak, reluctant to move, tremble when standing, and walk with a stiff gait. The muscles are often bilaterally affected and are swollen and hard or rubbery. Inability to eat leads to rapid inanition. There may be fever and increased heart and respiratory rates. Blood serum selenium and glutathione peroxidase concentrations may be low, and serum glutamic-oxaloacetic transaminase (SGOT) levels may be elevated in affected foals. Low serum selenium and glutathione peroxidase levels may be observed in other animals on the premises. There is some uncertainty about the normal concentration of selenium in blood, but horses at selenium-deficient farms where foals or horses have died with lesions of muscular dystrophy have generally had less than 4 μg Se per dl of serum or blood. Glutathione peroxidase activity and blood selenium concentrations are highly correlated in horses. The foal may have myoglobinuria, which colors the urine brown. Foals may die acutely as a result of cardiac myopathy. Affected muscles are white or gray and may look like fish flesh. Fat deposits are often discolored yellowish brown.

White muscle disease may respond to oral or intramuscular treatment with selenium–vitamin E. Success depends in large part on the extent of lesions at the time of treatment. Commercial injectable preparations of selenium (as sodium selenite) and vitamin E (alpha-tocopherol) are available.*

Rations that meet the estimated selenium requirement of 0.1 ppm should prevent selenium deficiency and white muscle disease on the farm. Pregnant and lactating mares may also be supplemented with selenium at a rate of about 1 mg of selenium per day. However, only small amounts of selenium cross the placenta. Thus, supplementing the pregnant mare may not benefit the foal. Breeders in selenium-deficient areas should try to employ some

---

*E-SE, Burns Biotec, Omaha NB

TABLE 7. SUMMARY OF MINERAL FUNCTIONS, DEFICIENCY SIGNS, AND FEED SOURCES

Mineral	Some Functions	Some Deficiency Signs	Good Feed Sources	Poor Feed Sources
Calcium	Constituent of bone mineral; blood clotting; transmission of nerve impulses; muscle contraction; secretion of hormones; activation of some enzymes	Impaired mineralization of bone and skeletal development: rickets; osteomalacia; nutritional secondary hyperparathyroidism; osteoporosis; possible bone deformities and/or fracture	Good quality hay, especially legumes; limestone; oyster shells; bone meal; dicalcium phosphate	Most grains; poor quality grass hay
Phosphorus	Constituent of bone mineral; constituent of some structural and functional proteins such as phosphoproteins, phospholipids, nucleoproteins; involved in fat, carbohydrate, and energy metabolism	Impaired mineralization of bone; decreased growth rate; reproductive problems; low blood phosphorus concentration	Most grains; soybean meal; linseed meal; brewers' yeast; bone meal; dicalcium phosphate; monosodium phosphate	Grain straws; beet pulp; citrus pulp; molasses
Magnesium	Constituent of bone mineral; activator or cofactor of numerous enzymes involved in cellular energy metabolism; alkaline and acid phosphatases	Central nervous irritability: nervousness, muscle tremors, ataxia, convulsive seizures; mineralization of elastic tissues of aorta, pulmonary artery, lung, and spleen; serum magnesium less than 1 mg/dl	Good quality hay, especially legumes; protein supplements	Most grains; poor quality grass hay
Sodium, potassium, and chloride	Maintenance of tissue osmotic pressure and acid-base equilibrium; control of water balance and passage of nutrients into cells; involved in transmission of nerve impulses and muscle contraction	Craving for salt; hyperexcitability; decreased growth rate; loss of appetite; decreased serum potassium	Salt is a good source of sodium and chloride; most roughages are good sources of potassium.	Most feeds are inadequate sources of sodium and chloride; grains are generally inadequate sources of potassium.
Iodine	Component of thyroxine; needed for thyroid functions	Goiter; reduced rate of growth, low body temperature; impaired development of hair and skin; foals weak at birth	Iodized salt.	Most animal feeds in iodine deficient regions.
Manganese	Involved in protein, fatty acid, and cholesterol synthesis; synthesis of glycoproteins and glycosaminoglycans necessary in chondrogenesis and osteogenesis	Reproductive dysfunction: delayed estrus, reduced fertility, spontaneous abortion in mares; foals born with skeletal deformities, shortened limb bones, enlarged joints, and contractures	Roughage is generally a good source except on heavily limed soils.	Grains; some roughage grown on heavily limed soils; milk and milk products
Selenium	Constituent of glutathione peroxidase, which catalyzes the removal of peroxides from tissues	Muscular dystrophy: white muscle disease; low serum selenium and serum glutathione peroxidase concentration; elevated serum glutamic-oxaloacetic transaminase concentration	Depends on soil content	All feeds grown in regions with selenium-deficient soils
Molybdenum	Constituent of xanthine oxidase			

Table continued on opposite page

TABLE 7. SUMMARY OF MINERAL FUNCTIONS, DEFICIENCY SIGNS, AND FEED SOURCES *(Continued)*

Mineral	Some Functions	Some Deficiency Signs	Good Feed Sources	Poor Feed Sources
Iron	Constituent of hemoglobin, myoglobin, cytochrome C, peroxidase, catalase; involved in oxygen transport	Anemia: pallor, low endurance; depressed growth	All roughage	Milk and milk products; wheat; corn; sorghum
Copper	Involved in iron absorption and hemoglobin synthesis; involved in melanin synthesis in skin; synthesis and cross-linking of collagen	Anemia; pigment loss in hair; ricketslike disease of bone: swollen joints, deformed long bones with thin cortices	Legume hay; molasses; linseed meal; soybean meal	Milk and milk products
Zinc	Cofactor or activator of large number of enzymes in digestion and metabolism	Parakeratosis: hair loss, scaling of skin, serous exudation and desquamation of skin; poor wound healing; low serum alkaline phosphatase; reproductive, behavioral, and skeletal abnormalities in some species	Insufficient data available	Beet pulp

feeds imported from the selenium-adequate areas of the midwestern United States, between the Mississippi River and the Rocky Mountains. Soybean meal, linseed meal, and alfalfa are generally good sources of readily available selenium.

"Tying-up" disease is an exercise-related myopathy and associated myoglobinuria. Affected horses appear to be "myopathy-prone" rather than selenium-deficient. Nevertheless, "myopathy-prone" horses often appear to respond to selenium–vitamin E administration (p. 101).

SELENIUM TOXICITY

Selenium is toxic. Supplements should be given and recommended with caution. The use of multiple selenium supplements for the same animal or animals should be avoided. Toxicosis also results when animals in areas where the selenium content of the soil is high are supplemented. Soils that contain greater than 0.5 ppm of selenium are considered potentially dangerous. Seleniferous soils are located in the northern Great Plains, parts of Colorado and Eastern Kansas, and northern New Mexico (Figs. 1 and 2). Horses suffering from selenium toxicosis, also called blind staggers or alkali disease, lose the hair from the mane and tail, the hooves may slough, and the affected horse may become blind and paralyzed.

MOLYBDENUM

Molybdenum is a constituent of the enzyme xanthine oxidase and is an essential element in nutri-

tion. The molybdenum requirement for most animals is not known, and molybdenum deficiency disease has not been described. Horses appear to absorb molybdenum readily from the intestinal tract and to excrete excess molybdenum in the urine. Balance studies suggest that horses fed up to 100 ppm of molybdenum in the diet do not store appreciable amounts of the element in their tissues.

Excess molybdenum intake increases the need for dietary copper and can result in a syndrome identical to copper deficiency. Horses appear to be more tolerant of high molybdenum intake than cattle and have successfully grazed pastures that cause overt molybdenum toxicosis in cattle.

FLUORINE

Fluorine is often classified as an essential element because it appears to reduce the incidence of tooth decay and possibly of osteoporosis in humans. There is no direct evidence to indicate that fluorine is essential or beneficial to horses.

FLUORINE TOXICITY

Fluorine is better known in animal nutrition for the harmful effect of chronic excess intake. The resulting toxicosis, known as fluorosis, may result from long-term ingestion of pasture, hay, water, or mineral supplements that have been contaminated by certain industrial operations. Fluorosis may also occur from consumption of water or mineral supplements that contain naturally high levels of fluorine. For example, certain rock phosphates contain excessive fluoride and require special treatment before they may safely be used as mineral supplements.

Horses seem less susceptible to fluorosis than sheep or cattle. Excess fluoride accumulates in bones and teeth and damages both structures. Dental lesions occur only when horses ingest excess fluorine during tooth development. Tooth enamel becomes mottled, chalky, and brittle. The defective enamel may chip, exposing the softer, underlying sensitive tooth structures, which wear more readily. Horses with severely affected teeth eat less and slobber poorly masticated food. Affected horses are frequently stiff and lame. The bones of the limbs, skull, mandible, and ribs show periosteal hyperostosis, particularly at tendon and ligament insertions.

The amount of fluoride considered safe for consumption by horses is controversial. The National Research Council Subcommittee on Horse Nutrition (1978) recommends that horse rations contain no more than 50 ppm. Others consider this level to be far in excess of a safe amount.

References

1. National Academy of Sciences: Nutrient Requirement of Horses, 4th ed. Washington, DC, National Academy of Sciences-National Research Council, 1978.
2. Maynard, L. A., Loosli, J. K., Hintz, H. F., and Warner, R. G.: Animal Nutrition, 7th ed. New York, McGraw-Hill Book Co., 1979.
3. Cunha, T. J.: Horse Feeding and Nutrition. New York, Academic Press, 1980.
4. Underwood, E. J.: Trace Elements in Human and Animal Nutrition, 4th ed. New York, Academic Press, 1977.
5. Swenson, M. J. (ed.): Dukes' Physiology of Domestic Animals, 9th ed. Ithaca, NY, Comstock Publishing Associates of Cornell University Press, 1977.

VITAMINS

H. F. Schryver, ITHACA, NEW YORK

H. F. Hintz, ITHACA, NEW YORK

Vitamins are a group of unrelated organic compounds that are required in very small amounts in metabolism. Not all vitamins are dietary essentials for the horse. Some vitamins are synthesized in the tissues of the horse or by microorganisms in the large intestine. For example, under normal conditions, enough ascorbic acid is produced by the liver of the horse to meet metabolic needs even in the absence of a dietary source of the vitamin. Microorganisms in the cecum and colon of the horse are known to synthesize an abundance of B vitamins. It is not known how efficiently these substances are absorbed and utilized by the horse. The factors that modify the rates of synthesis by microorganisms and of absorption by the horse are also not known.

Vitamins are commonly classified into two groups: the fat-soluble vitamins, A, D, E, and K, and the water-soluble B vitamins and vitamin C. The classification also distinguishes some aspects of the source and metabolism of the vitamins.

Vitamins are frequently used as therapeutic agents for a variety of conditions. The conditions that are treated sometimes bear a superficial clinical or metabolic resemblance to specific signs of vitamin deficiency that have been observed in one or more species. For example, hemorrhage as a deficiency sign of vitamin C or vitamin K would be treated by very high doses of either or both vitamins C and K. There is little clear-cut experimental evidence that indicates conclusively that vitamins or other nutrients are effective therapeutic agents. Provision of vitamins and other nutrients at the required level or slightly in excess will correct or prevent specific deficiency signs. However, "megadose" therapy is without value at best, and since some vitamins and other nutrients are toxic at very high levels, the practice may be dangerous.

VITAMIN A

Vitamin A is important in vision, in development and maintenance of epithelial cells, in bone development, and in reproduction. Many of the functions of vitamin A are related to the stabilizing effect of the vitamin on the membranes of lysosomes—the subcellular particles that contain degradative enzymes. Controlled release of enzymes from lysosomes is necessary for the removal of cells and intercellular substances during the turnover and remodeling of tissues. For example, failure of release of lysosomal enzymes due to vitamin A deficiency results in failure of maturation and removal of epiphyseal cartilage cells and intercellular matrix. As a consequence, endochondral bone growth is affected.

Vitamin A is involved in the formation, development, and differentiation of epithelial cells. In vitamin A deficiency, differentiated epithelial cells are replaced by relatively undifferentiated stratified squamous, keratin-producing cells. These changes are most prominent in the respiratory, reproductive, urinary, and digestive tracts. The replacement of one cell type by another alters the function and the resistance to infection of the affected epithelial surfaces.

Bone growth and remodeling are markedly influenced by vitamin A. The vitamin is essential for the normal sequence of growth, maturation, and degeneration of epiphyseal cartilage cells and for normal functioning of osteoblasts and osteoclasts. Deficiency of vitamin A results in decreased rate of endochondral bone growth and a decreased rate of bone resorption at endosteal and other resorption surfaces. Failure of resorption results in relative diminution of the internal dimension of certain bones and foramina. In severe cases of vitamin A deficiency in young animals, bony orifices do not enlarge sufficiently to accommodate important structures such as the spinal cord or optic nerve, resulting in severe nervous signs.

CLINICAL SIGNS OF VITAMIN A DEFICIENCY

Marginal vitamin A deficiency has been produced in young ponies by diets low in carotene. Growth in height, weight, and heart girth of the ponies was impaired. The deficient ponies had decreased serum concentration of iron, albumin, cholesterol, and vitamin A.

Conditions resembling vitamin A deficiency have been reported in horses that have been fed poor quality feeds for long periods. In the past, military horses on long campaigns have often been affected owing to the difficulties in obtaining green feeds.

Signs of experimental vitamin A deficiency took as long as one to one and a half years to develop. The first signs were night blindness followed by corneal cloudiness and keratinization. Reproductive problems developed in some of the horses when the deficiency disease was far advanced. Problems in mares included inability to conceive and abortion. Stallions experienced loss of libido. The testes of affected stallions were soft and flabby with a decreased number of seminiferous tubules and an increase in interstitial cells. Foals born of vitamin A-deficient mares were weak and unable to nurse. Signs of experimental vitamin A deficiency developed more rapidly in young horses fed semipurified diets that contained very little vitamin A. Signs included anorexia, lacrimation, polyuria, and convulsive seizures. The seizures were initiated by excitement. The horses in seizure fell and made paddling movements with the legs. Cerebrospinal fluid pressure in affected horses was elevated to 550 mm of saline.

CLINICAL SIGNS OF VITAMIN A TOXICOSIS

Excess dietary vitamin A is stored in the liver, and the accumulated excess can be toxic. Prolonged excess intake may cause bone resorption with subsequent bony deformities, fragility, and fractures. Naturally occurring cases of excess vitamin A intake have not been reported in the horse. Experimental vitamin A intoxication has been produced in young ponies by feeding about 1000 times the level of vitamin A that is suggested as the requirement by the National Research Council (NRC). Vitamin A intoxication impaired the growth of the ponies in terms of gains in body weight, height at the withers, and heart girth. Plasma vitamin A was elevated in affected ponies.

SOURCES OF VITAMIN A

Vitamin A occurs in feeds as precursors called provitamin A. The common provitamin A in horse feeds is carotene. Some carotene is metabolized to vitamin A in the wall of the intestine of the horse, but much of the dietary carotene is absorbed and stored in the liver and adipose tissues. The NRC assumes that the horse converts 1 mg of carotene to about 400 IU of vitamin A.[1]

Carotene is most abundant in green feeds. However, the compound is highly unstable and easily oxidized. Large losses of carotene occur during the curing and storage of hay. For example, losses of carotene in field-cured alfalfa hay may be 90 per cent or greater. Half to three quarters of the carotene remaining in the cured hay may be lost during six months' storage of the hay. Thus, field-cured hay stored for six months or longer may contain less than 5 per cent of the carotene content of the original, uncut, fresh green plant. Hay that has been artificially cured in a hay drier has a much higher carotene content than field- or sun-cured hay. Generally, the degree of greenness of stored hay is a fair index of its carotene content. The carotene of alfalfa hay is more available to horses than that of grass hay. Among the grains, only corn contains carotene, but the amounts in corn are only about one tenth that of good roughage.

VITAMIN A REQUIREMENTS

Horses require about 25 IU of vitamin A per kg of body weight for maintenance, 40 IU per kg for growth, and 50 IU per kg for pregnancy and lacta-

TABLE 1. VITAMIN CONTENT OF SOME COMMON HORSE FEEDS

	Carotene	Thiamine	Riboflavin	Vitamin E
		Mg/kg		
Alfalfa hay	26	3	11	90
Alfalfa meal	131	4	14	135
Barley	1	5	2	18
Red clover hay	20	2	18	60
Corn	3	2	2	26
Linseed meal	0	9	3	18
Oats	0	7	2	18
Oat hay	15	3	5	12
Rye	1	3	2	17
Skimmed milk, dry	0	4	20	10
Soybean meal	0	6	3	2
Timothy hay	9	2	12	63
Wheat bran	3	7	5	13
Brewers yeast	0	100	40	2

These are approximate and average values. Many factors alter the vitamin content of feeds. The hays listed are sun cured. (Adapted from National Academy of Sciences: Nutrient Requirement of Horses, 4th ed. Washington, DC, National Academy of Sciences–National Research Council, 1978.)

tion. This translates to about 4 to 5 mg of carotene per kg of feed. The carotene content of some feeds is shown in Table 1.

DIAGNOSIS OF VITAMIN A DEFICIENCY

Determination of vitamin A status is commonly done by measuring the vitamin A content of blood serum or plasma. A range of 20 to 175 μg of carotene per dl of plasma or serum has been considered normal for horses. Young ponies fed approximately adequate amounts of vitamin A (12 μg per kg of body weight per day) had 27 ± 2 μg of total vitamin A per dl of plasma. Serum vitamin A levels of 8 μg per dl or less have been observed in experimental vitamin A deficiency in young horses. Hepatic stores of vitamin A may sometimes maintain serum levels until deficiency is far advanced. Thus, serum vitamin A levels may be less reliable than is commonly thought for diagnosis of deficiency. Response of experimentally deficient animals to parenteral vitamin A administration is often prompt. The response may be used as an indication of vitamin A status.

VITAMIN A SUPPLEMENTATION

Horses that have not had access to green feeds for four to six months and that have been fed poorly cured or poorly stored hay may benefit from a vitamin A supplement. Feed sources of carotene include almost any green feed such as pasture or alfalfa meal. Supplemental, oral sources of vitamin A include fish liver oils such as shark, halibut, swordfish, and cod liver oils. Unfortunately, these sources vary greatly in stability, quality, and in vitamin A activity. Long-term oral vitamin A supplementation that exceeds the NRC recommendation of 25 IU of vitamin A per kg of body weight for maintenance, 40 IU per kg for growth, and 50 IU per kg for pregnancy and lactation should be avoided. A variety of commercially available parenteral vitamin A preparations are available.

VITAMIN D

Vitamin D facilitates the absorption and utilization of calcium and phosphorus for bone formation. Metabolites of vitamin D have complex interrelationships with parathormone (p. 160) and calcitonin to regulate the concentration of blood calcium by means of intestinal absorption of calcium, resorption of calcium from bone, and urinary calcium excretion. Vitamin D is converted to 25-hydroxycholecalciferol in the liver. This substance is modified to 1,25-dihydrocholecalciferol—$1,25(OH)_2D_3$—in the kidney under the influence of parathyroid hormone. $1,25(OH)_2D_3$ is the most physiologically active form of vitamin D and acts to facilitate calcium absorption by stimulating the synthesis of intestinal calcium-binding protein (CaBP). CaBP actively transports calcium across the mucosal cells of the intestinal tract.

CLINICAL SIGNS OF VITAMIN D DEFICIENCY

Deficiency of vitamin D results in rickets in young animals. The disease is basically a defect in the mineralization of newly formed bone. Bone so formed is weak, soft, and easily deformed. The ends of the long bones tend to enlarge, and the shafts of the bones tend to bend, resulting in the characteristically bowed limbs of rickets. Affected animals may have hypocalcemia, hypophosphatemia, and elevated alkaline phosphatase levels in serum. Well-documented cases of rickets in foals under natural conditions have not been described.

CLINICAL SIGNS OF VITAMIN D TOXICOSIS

Excess intake of vitamin D is toxic. Horses fed 100 times the NRC recommended level of vitamin D became anorexic, developed lameness and hypercalcemia, and died as a result of mineralization in the heart, great vessels, lungs, upper digestive tract, and costal musculature. Horses fed 50 times the NRC recommended level of vitamin D did not show clinical signs but absorbed more calcium from the intestine than did control horses. Levels of vitamin D fed to pigs at 50 times the NRC recommended level produced detrimental effects on bone cells. The calcium content of the diet, the potency of the vitamin D preparations, age of the animals, and other factors may modify the toxicity of vitamin D.

A condition resembling vitamin D intoxication in horses results from ingestion of plants that contain compounds with potent vitamin D activity. These include *Trisetum flavescens* (yellow oat grass), a plant of the European Alps; *Solanum malocoxylon*, a South American relative of the potato; and *Cestrum diurnum* (day blooming jessamine), an ornamental plant grown in the West Indies and recently introduced into the Southern United States. Horses intoxicated by ingestion of these plants lose weight, are lame, and have hypercalcemia. Widespread calcinosis is observed at postmortem examination.

SOURCES OF VITAMIN D

There are two forms and sources of vitamin D. Ergosterol is found in plants and forms ergocalciferol or vitamin D_2 when the plant is cut and subjected to ultraviolet irradiation, as in the sun curing of hay. Growing plants, grains, and grain byproducts do not contain significant amounts of D_2, but sun-cured hay may contain 150 to 3000 IU per kg. Cholecalciferol or vitamin D_3 is found in animals and results from the ultraviolet irradiation of 7-dehydrocholesterol in the skin. Both vitamin D_2 and D_3 have equal value for many mammals and probably do so for the horse as well.

VITAMIN D REQUIREMENTS

The current estimate of the dietary vitamin D requirement for horses is 6.6 IU per kg of body weight

TABLE 2. VITAMIN ALLOWANCES FOR HORSES

	Units/kg of Body Weight	Units/kg of Feed
Vitamin A (IU)		
Growth	40	1800
Pregnancy and lactation	50	2500
Maintenance	25	1500
Vitamin D (IU)	6	275
Vitamin E (mg)	0.4	15
Thiamine (mg)	0.04	3
Riboflavin (mg)	0.07	2

These are approximate amounts of vitamins that are thought to be adequate for growth of young horses or maintenance of mature horses. (Adapted from National Academy of Sciences: Nutrient Requirement of Horses, 4th ed. Washington, DC, National Academy of Sciences–National Research Council, 1978.)

or about 3000 IU for a 1000-pound horse. Horses normally obtain adequate amounts of vitamin D from exposure to sunlight and from sun-cured forages. Under most circumstances, there is little need for vitamin D supplements for horses. Vitamin D supplements that provide more than 6.6 IU of vitamin D per kg of body weight should be recommended with caution because of the danger of toxicosis. There is no evidence that supplemental vitamin D is of benefit to horses when the level of calcium and phosphorus in the diet is low or the ratio between them is not correct. Fish oils and fish meals are good sources of vitamin D_3. Irradiated yeast is a common and inexpensive source of vitamin D_2.

VITAMIN E

Vitamin E is an antioxidant. It prevents peroxidation of the lipids of cell membranes and thus preserves the structural integrity of cells.

Signs of vitamin E deficiency vary greatly among species, but reproductive problems and muscular dystrophy are commonly seen. However, not all reproductive problems and muscular dystrophies are vitamin E–responsive. For example, white muscle disease of foals often responds to selenium but does not respond to vitamin E (alpha-tocopherol). There is only contradictory evidence of a relationship between vitamin E and some reproductive problems in the horse.

CLINICAL SIGNS OF VITAMIN E DEFICIENCY

Experimental vitamin E deficiency has been produced in young horses fed a semipurified diet. Serum tocopherol levels in the deficient foals were about 120 μgm per dl. Other signs included increased erythrocyte fragility, elevated serum glutamic-oxaloacetic transaminase (SGOT), intermittent leukocytosis, and hemoglobinuria. Postmortem examination of deficient foals showed acute glomerular nephritis and dystrophic changes in the muscles of the right ventricle, the intercostal and other skeletal muscles, and muscles of the tongue. Deficient foals required 27 µgm per kg of body weight of parenteral alpha-tocopherol or 233 µgm per kg of body weight of oral tocopherol to maintain the stability of erythrocytes.

SOURCES OF VITAMIN E

Animal feeds are generally rich in vitamin E. Cereal grains, grain byproducts, green forage, and hay are excellent sources of vitamin E. On the other hand, the oil meals such as linseed or soybean oil meals often have very little vitamin E because the modern oil extraction process removes the vitamin. Because the vitamin is readily oxidized, rancidity, heating, grinding, pelletting, and long storage of feeds decrease the vitamin E content. Among the natural feedstuffs, alfalfa meal is a particularly rich source of vitamin E.

Alpha-tocopherol, which is the most potent form of vitamin E, is readily available as a synthetic product. One mg of alpha-tocopherol equals 1 IU of the vitamin.

Large doses of vitamin E have been used in attempts to treat barren mares, to improve racing performance, and to improve performance in endurance horses in uncontrolled studies. There is no evidence to indicate that large doses of vitamin E have value. Fortunately, vitamin E appears to be relatively nontoxic.

VITAMIN K

Vitamin K is involved in synthesis of prothrombin in the liver and thus is important in blood coagulation.

Deficiency of vitamin K occurs in birds and results in hemorrhagic disease. Vitamin K deficiency may result in mammals in cases of biliary dysfunction because bile is necessary for the intestinal absorption of vitamin K and other fat-soluble vitamins. However, vitamin K is synthesized in large amounts by the intestinal microflora of many species. It is assumed that this is so in horses as well. Deficiency has not been reported in the horse.

All green, leafy feeds such as hay or pasture are rich sources of vitamin K.

VITAMIN C

Ascorbic acid or vitamin C is the antiscorbutic factor. All species appear to require vitamin C in

metabolism, but only humans, guinea pigs, subhuman primates, and some bats, birds, and fish have a dietary requirement for vitamin C. These species lack the enzyme necessary for the synthesis of vitamin C from simple sugars. The horse is among the species that are able to synthesize ascorbic acid in the liver.

Vitamin C is important in the hydroxylation of proline and lysine to hydroxyproline and hydroxylysine during collagen synthesis. Deficiency of the vitamin impairs the synthesis of collagen. Many of the signs of scurvy are related to this metabolic defect. In humans these include altered capillary integrity, sore, spongy gums, loosening of the teeth, subcutaneous hemorrhages, edema, joint pain, and anorexia. Plasma ascorbic acid values in human scurvy may fall to 0.05 mg per dl from a normal level of 0.5 to 1.2 mg per dl. Horses fed diets that were free of ascorbic acid for up to six months maintained their whole blood and plasma ascorbic acid levels at the same levels as horses fed normal diets. The horses also excreted as much ascorbic acid in urine as horses fed diets containing ascorbic acid. These findings indicate that the horse is able to synthesize ascorbic acid in the dietary absence of the vitamin. The excess that is synthesized in the tissues is excreted in urine. Whole blood ascorbic acid in horses ranged from 0.35 to 0.48 mg per dl and plasma levels from 0.32 to 0.40 mg per dl.

Large doses of vitamin C have been used in treatment of reproductive problems in the horse. This application needs controlled study.

THIAMINE

Thiamine serves as a coenzyme in the oxidative decarboxylation of pyruvate to acetate in cellular metabolism. A deficiency of thiamine results in accumulation of pyruvic and lactic acids in tissues. Thiamine deficiency has characteristic signs in certain species and has been given special names such as beriberi in humans, Chastek paralysis in foxes, and polyneuritis in birds. Deficiency results in a wide range of signs, including loss of appetite, weight loss, reduced growth rate, peripheral and central nervous system signs, bradycardia, muscular weakness, and twitching.

CLINICAL SIGNS OF THIAMINE DEFICIENCY

Thiamine deficiency has been studied experimentally in horses by feeding diets containing little or no thiamine or by inducing the deficiency by means of thiamine antimetabolites. Biochemical changes that can be observed before clinical signs develop include hypoglycemia and elevated blood pyruvic acid concentration. As the deficiency progressed,

TABLE 3. SUMMARY OF VITAMIN FUNCTIONS, DEFICIENCY SIGNS, AND FEED SOURCES

Vitamin	Some Functions	Some Deficiency Signs	Good Feed Sources	Poor Feed Sources
Vitamin A	Stability of lysosomal and other cell membranes; growth and development of epithelial cells; growth, development, and remodeling of bone; vision; dark adaptation; maintenance of visual purple	Night blindness; corneal cloudiness, keratinization; impaired growth; reproductive problems: inability to conceive; abortion, loss of libido in the male; testicular degeneration; convulsions; elevated cerebrospinal fluid pressure; decreased tissue and serum vitamin A concentration	Provitamin A is abundant in all green feeds; good quality, well-cured hay, especially alfalfa	All grains; poorly cured hays and those subjected to long storage in poor conditions
Vitamin D	Synthesis of intestinal calcium binding protein (CaBP); absorption of dietary calcium and phosphorus; resorption of calcium from bone; control of urinary calcium excretion	Skeletal disease: defective mineralization of newly formed bone, bone deformities; impaired growth; hypocalcemia; hypophosphatemia; elevated serum alkaline phosphatase	Sun-cured hay; vitamin D_3 formed in the skin of animals exposed to sunlight; fish oils; fish meal; irradiated yeast	Grains and grain byproducts
Vitamin E	Antioxidant in tissues: prevents peroxidation of lipids of cell membranes; cofactor in synthesis of ascorbic acid	Decreased serum tocopherol concentration; increased red blood cell fragility; elevated serum glutamic-oxaloacetic transaminase (SGOT) levels; muscular dystrophy	Grains; grain byproducts; green forages; hay	Solvent-extracted oil meals
Vitamin K	Synthesis of blood clotting factors	Hemorrhagic disease in species that require the vitamin	All green feeds	
Thiamine	Serves as the coenzyme cocarboxylase for the enzymatic decarboxylation of α-ketoacids in energy metabolism	Accumulation of pyruvic and lactic acids in tissues; loss of appetite; weight loss; impaired growth; bradycardia; peripheral and central nervous system disturbances; incoordination, weakness in hindquarters, muscular weakness and twitching; hypoglycemia; elevated blood pyruvate; increased thiamine pyrophosphate effect; elevated sorbitol dehydrogenase and creatine in serum	Most horse feeds, especially grains and grain byproducts; brewers' yeast	Poorly cured hay
Riboflavin	Serves as a coenzyme (flavin mononucleotide—FMN—and flavin adenine dinucleotide—FAD) in many enzyme systems	Impaired growth and feed efficiency; photophobia; corneal vascularization; conjunctivitis; lacrimation	Leafy feeds, especially alfalfa, yeasts	Cereal grains and byproducts
B_{12}	Coenzyme in several enzyme systems; involved in metabolism of propionic acid in ruminants	Deficiency signs have not been described in horses.	The vitamin is probably synthesized in adequate amounts in the tissues of the horse.	
Ascorbic acid	Important in collagen synthesis in the hydroxylation of proline and lysine to hydroxyproline and hydroxylysine	Deficiency of vitamin C has not been described in the horse.	The vitamin is synthesized in the tissues of the horse.	

affected experimental horses showed bradycardia, dropped heart beats, ataxia, muscular fasciculations, and periodic hypothermia of the hooves, ears, and muzzle. Some horses lost weight, developed diarrhea, or became blind. Gait changes were among the most prominent clinical signs of induced thiamine deficiency. Weakness in the hindquarters caused swaying. A slow, shuffling gait was necessary to maintain balance. The forelegs often crossed when the horse walked in a circle. Backing was difficult and often ended in a dog-sitting position.

Thiamine deficiency results in many changes in clinical biochemistry. Among the more specific changes are increased blood concentration of pyruvate and an increased thiamine pyrophosphate (TPP) effect. Sorbitol dehydrogenase (SDH) and creatine phosphokinase (CPK) are elevated in serum. In addition to these biochemical changes, blood thiamine levels may be useful in estimating thiamine status.

ANTITHIAMINE FACTORS AND THIAMINE SUPPLEMENTATION

There are many antimetabolites of thiamine. These include thiaminase, which occurs in bracken fern (*Pteridium aquilinum*) and horsetail (*Equisetum arvense*). Other antithiamine factors include amprolium, which is a coccidiostat, caffeic acid, and substances in cotton seed. Increased intake of dietary thiamine can often be used to offset the effects of these antithiamine substances. The thiamine requirement of the horse has been estimated to be 3 mg per kg of diet or about 15 to 20 mg for the maintenance of a mature horse. Horses working vigorously may require additional thiamine. Most horse feeds contain liberal amounts of thiamine. Grains and grain byproducts are very good sources. Thiamine tends to be lost during the sun curing of hay. Among the natural feedstuffs, brewers' yeast is an exceptionally good source of thiamine.

RIBOFLAVIN

Riboflavin serves as part of many enzyme systems. Some of the prominent and important signs of human riboflavin deficiency include photophobia, corneal vascularization, conjunctivitis, and lacrimation. These signs bear some resemblance to periodic ophthalmia of horses. However, attempts to treat horses affected with periodic ophthalmia with riboflavin supplementation have not been successful.

The riboflavin requirement of horses is estimated to be about 2.2 mg per kg of feed. Leafy feeds such as hay are good sources. Alfalfa is a very good source. Yeast is a very rich source that can be used as a natural supplement. Cereal grains and byproducts are not good sources of riboflavin.

VITAMIN B$_{12}$

Vitamin B$_{12}$ is a generic term used for a group of compounds that have similar functions. The vitamin is a metabolic essential in all species that have been studied. Some species, such as humans, require a dietary source, while others, such as ruminants and probably horses, synthesize sufficient vitamin B$_{12}$ in the digestive tract. The large intestine of the horse contains microorganisms that synthesize B$_{12}$, and the concentration of B$_{12}$ increases as digesta moves down the intestinal tract. Cobalt is the limiting factor for vitamin B$_{12}$ synthesis by ruminal microflora. This is probably true for the large intestinal microflora in the horse as well. Vitamin B$_{12}$ is necessary for the metabolism of propionic acid, an important product of large intestinal fermentation in the horse. Experimental attempts to produce vitamin B$_{12}$ deficiency in the horse have not been successful. Excretion of large amounts of B$_{12}$ in feces and urine has suggested that the horse does not have a dietary requirement for the vitamin under normal circumstances. Excretion of B$_{12}$ in feces has been found to be 0.5 mg per day and in urine to be 0.007 mg per day. This is several thousand times greater than the urinary excretion in humans and the fecal excretion of the vitamin in cattle. Serum vitamin B$_{12}$ values have been found to be 6 to 7 μgm per ml in the horse.

OTHER B VITAMINS

Other B vitamins and related compounds are known to be dietary essentials for one or more species. Among these are niacin, pantothenic acid, pyridoxine, biotin, choline, folic acid, and inositol. It is assumed that these substances are required by the horse as metabolic essentials, but it is not known if they are required in the diet of the horse. Feeds that are commonly fed to horses tend to be good sources of these compounds, and many of these and other B vitamins are synthesized in the lower bowel of the horse. Nevertheless, these and other substances are frequently added to vitamin premixes and to vitamin supplements for horses. The value of such supplements is not known.

References

1. National Academy of Sciences: Nutrient Requirement of Horses, 4th ed. Washington, DC, National Academy of Sciences–National Research Council, 1978.
2. Maynard, L. A., Loosli, J. K., Hintz, H. F., and Warner, R. G.: Animal Nutrition, 7th ed. New York, McGraw-Hill Book Co., 1979.
3. Cunha, T. J.: Horse Feeding and Nutrition. New York, Academic Press, 1980.
4. Underwood, E. J.: Trace Elements in Human and Animal Nutrition, 4th ed. New York, Academic Press, 1977.
5. Swenson, M. J. (ed.): Dukes' Physiology of Domestic Animals, 9th ed. Ithaca, NY, Comstock Publishing Associates of Cornell University Press, 1977.

FEEDING PROGRAMS

H. F. Hintz, ITHACA, NEW YORK

The following section outlines feeding programs for the mature horse at maintenance, the working horse, the brood mare, the stallion, and growing horses. Sample rations are presented here and in the next section, but many different combinations of feedstuffs can be fed satisfactorily to horses, and of course there are differences of opinion as to the best methods of providing the nutrients. The sample rations were selected to reflect regional differences in relative availability of feedstuffs and to reflect differences in opinions of various authorities.

HOW MUCH HAY?

Most feeding programs are based on hay or pasture. How much hay *must* a horse be fed? The answer of course, is none. Hay is not essential. Fiber is essential, but many feedstuffs, for example, beet pulp, peanut hulls, or citrus pulp, can provide fiber. Nevertheless, when horses do not have access to pasture, the feeding of good quality hay greatly simplifies ration formulation and is usually one of the easiest methods of providing needed nutrients. Hay intake is usually equivalent to 1 to 2 per cent of body weight.

MATURE HORSES

The feeding program for maintenance of the average mature horse can be very simple. Good quality hay consumed at a rate of $1\frac{1}{2}$ to $1\frac{2}{3}$ kg of hay per 100 kg of body weight, water, and trace mineralized salt fed free choice should supply all the needed nutrients. Additional mineral supplements may be needed if the hay was grown on soil lacking in minerals such as selenium, copper, or phosphorus. If the climate is harsh, energy requirements should be increased, and some grain will be needed. The preceding recommendation also assumes reasonable parasite control and no dental problems. Some highly nervous horses may require additional energy.

Merits of legume and grass hays were discussed earlier (p. 67). Average grass hay will provide the 8 per cent protein, 0.30 per cent calcium, and 0.20 per cent phosphorus needed by the mature horse. Legume hay will provide much more protein and calcium than needed. The excess is not likely to be harmful but could be expensive.

WORKING HORSES

One of the primary concerns in the development of working horse rations is energy intake, and of course energy need depends on the amount and type of energy expenditure. Horses used in equitation classes may be ridden several hours per day yet may not require a great deal of energy because the work is not intensive. Equitation horses at Cornell working two to three hours per day maintained weight when fed 8 kg of hay and 3 kg of oats. On the other hand, racehorses at the track work fewer hours but may require 7 to 10 kg of hay and 8 to 10 kg of grain daily.

Thus, it is difficult to provide simple guidelines on the energy intake of working horses. The values in Table 1 provide some information that can be used as starting points in the feeding of working horses, but the body condition of the horse is the best guide, and energy should be regulated accordingly (p. 65).

The protein requirement of the horse is not greatly increased by work. The nitrogen lost in sweat is easily compensated for by the increased intake of the total ration. High levels of protein (24 per cent) were neither beneficial nor harmful to horses ridden 50 miles per day at a rate of 9 miles per hour. However, the excess protein may increase the water requirement and thus may be detrimental if water availability is limited. Excess protein is also expensive.

Although amino acids are often ingredients of supplements or injections given to performance horses, we are not aware of any controlled studies on their benefits, assuming the horse is fed a balanced diet.

Working increases the mineral requirements because of the losses in sweat, but, as with protein, if the diet contains a percentage of minerals adequate for maintenance, the horse will in most cases obtain additional minerals when eating to meet energy needs. There are exceptions, however. Electrolyte losses may be of particular concern in horses that sweat profusely, such as endurance horses or three-day event horses (p. 318). Synchronous diaphragmatic flutter (thumps) has been related to low serum Ca and K levels in endurance horses. The British Horse Society recommends that 1 oz of salt be added per gallon of water provided to such horses. Several commercially packaged electrolyte supplements are available. They can be added to the water or dosed if the horse does not drink. The amount of sweat loss influences the response to electrolytes.

TABLE 1. EXAMPLES OF FEED INTAKE OF HORSES AT WORK

Description of Work	Hay (Kg/Day)	Grain (Kg/Day)
Equitation classes	8–10	2–3
Standardbreds at the track	9–10	7–9
Thoroughbreds at the track	7–9	6–8
Polo ponies (indoor)	8–10	3–6
Draft horses—light work	7–8	2–3
(600 kg) —medium work	6–7	5–6
—heavy work	6–7	7–9

We found no electrolyte problems in horses going 50 miles per day at nine miles per hour even at temperatures of 90° F.

As energy intake increases, the requirement for B vitamins increases because the vitamins are cofactors necessary for energy utilization. Reports have suggested that some racehorses have marginal intakes of thiamine, one of the first signs of which is anorexia. Two tablespoons of brewers' yeast daily should supply the requirement for thiamine.

BROOD MARES

Brood mares can be divided into three categories: open mares, pregnant mares, and lactating mares. Energy intake is often suggested to influence breeding performance. While underfeeding of the filly could delay the onset of first heat, for most mares overfeeding is perhaps of greater concern than underfeeding. Several studies have suggested that the mares gaining weight (flushed) during breeding season have increased chances of conception. If the mare is excessively overweight at the start of the breeding season, flushing cannot be used. Therefore, it is recommended that barren mares be kept in reasonable condition and their feed intake be increased during breeding season.

Obesity cannot be blamed for all cases of barren mares. As Roberts[10] pointed out, it is difficult to determine if some mares are barren because they are fat or fat because they are barren. If they do not have foals, their energy requirements are greatly reduced, and they are much more likely to gain weight.

The nutrient requirements of mares are summarized in Table 2. In the following text, the requirements of the 450 kg mare (open, pregnant, or lactating) will be used to illustrate the effect of physiologic condition on nutrient requirements.

An open mare weighing 450 kg needs 15 Mcal digestible energy. If the hay contains 2.15 Mcal per kg, the mare would need to eat 7 kg of hay daily or approximately 1.5 kg of hay per 100 kg of body weight. Of course, more than 7 kg of hay would need to be fed because some hay is usually wasted.

TABLE 2. NUTRIENT CONCENTRATION IN DIETS FOR MARES (EXPRESSED ON 90% DRY MATTER BASIS)

Mare	Digestible Energy (Mcal/kg diet)	Crude Protein (%)	Ca (%)	P (%)
Open	2.0	7.7	0.30	0.20
Pregnant (last 90 days)	2.3	10.0	0.45	0.30
Lactating (early)	2.6	12.5	0.45	0.30
Lactating (late)	2.3	11.0	0.40	0.25

The National Research Council recommends that the ration of the open mare contain at least 7.7 per cent protein. Most hays and grains of average or greater quality contain at least 8 per cent protein. Thus, protein supplements are not usually needed by the open mare.

The ration of the open mare should contain at least 0.3 per cent calcium and 0.2 per cent phosphorus. As discussed earlier (p. 76), the mineral content of hay varies according to many factors, such as species, soil type, and age of the plant at harvest. Good quality grass hay could be expected to contain at least 0.35 per cent calcium and 0.2 per cent phosphorus; legumes such as alfalfa may contain 1 to 1.5 per cent calcium and 0.2 to 0.25 per cent phosphorus. Thus, calcium and phosphorus problems would not be expected when the open mare is fed hay of reasonable quality.

Crops grown in many parts of the United States, such as the Northeast, eastern coast, and Northwest, contain low levels of selenium. It has been suggested that feeding rations with low levels of selenium may cause decreased fertility. The requirement for selenium has been estimated to be 0.1 ppm (p. 81).

One study suggested that high levels of vitamins A and E may improve reproductive performance of mares, but in another study no benefit of vitamin supplementation was found. Of course, the basic ration must contain concentrations of protein, minerals, and vitamins that are adequate for maintenance.

The pregnant mare early in the gestation period does not have nutrient requirements greatly different from those of the open mare. During the last 90 days of gestation, the fetus is developing rapidly, and the mare's needs are increased. The National Research Council suggests that the energy requirement of the mare during the period of rapid fetal growth is about 12 per cent greater than for maintenance.

During the last 90 days of gestation, about 17 Mcal of digestible energy would be needed by the 450 kg mare. That amount of energy could be supplied by 5.5 kg of hay and 1.5 kg of grain daily.

The pregnant mare's need of protein, as for energy, is increased significantly over that of maintenance only during the last 90 days of gestation. The National Research Council estimates that at least 10 per cent protein is needed then. Even though the increase is 20 per cent above maintenance, the actual amount needed is not really high. Mares fed legume hays such as alfalfa or clover (usually 11 to 15 per cent protein) and grain such as oats (12 per cent protein) or corn (9 per cent protein) would not need a protein supplement. When a grass hay such as late-cut timothy hay is fed, a protein supplement may be needed. For example, if grass hay contains only 8 per cent protein and 5.5 kg of the hay and 1.5 kg of grain are fed, the grain mixture should contain about 16 per cent protein. Grain mixtures calculated to contain 16 per cent protein are shown in Table 3.

The calcium and phosphorus requirements, when expressed as a percentage of the diet, are similar for pregnant and lactating mares. Of course, total intake is much greater for the lactating mare because she eats more feed.

The pregnant or lactating mare needs 0.45 per cent calcium and 0.30 per cent phosphorus in the ration. Thus, the pregnant or lactating mare fed grass hay and grain would need a mineral supplement. When grass hay is fed, the grain mixture should contain at least 0.55 per cent calcium. The addition of 1 per cent dicalcium phosphate and 1 per cent limestone to the grain mixture usually supplies adequate levels of calcium and phosphorus. When legume hay is fed, a calcium supplement is usually not needed.

The energy needs of the lactating mare are a function of the level of milk production. The amount of milk produced varies greatly among mares, but the National Research Council states that some mares will produce amounts of milk equivalent to 2 to 3 per cent of their body weight during early lactation (1 to 12 weeks) and late lactation (13 to 24 weeks), respectively. A 450 kg mare milking at these levels would require about 70 per cent more energy during early lactation than for maintenance and about 48 per cent more energy during late lactation than for maintenance. A 450 kg mare producing 13.5 kg of milk would need almost 26 Mcal of digestible energy (about 6 kg of hay and 4.5 kg of grain daily). A mare producing 9 kg of milk would need about 22 Mcal of digestible energy (4.5 kg of hay and 3.5 kg grain).

The lactating mare needs about 12.5 per cent protein in her ration. If 6 kg of alfalfa hay containing 14 per cent protein was fed, the 4.5 kg of grain mixture would need to contain about 11 per cent protein. When feeding oats containing 12 per cent protein and alfalfa hay, no protein supplement is needed, but if corn containing 9 per cent protein is fed, a

TABLE 3. EXAMPLES OF GRAIN MIXTURES (A, B, and C) CALCULATED TO CONTAIN 12 OR 16% PROTEIN*

Ingredient	12%			16%		
	A	B	C	A	B	C
Corn	28	46	—	26	39	—
Oats	60	40	45	50	35	39
Barley	—	—	45	—	—	39
Soybean meal	6	8	4	18	20	16
Molasses	6	6	6	6	6	6

*Based on National Research Council (1978) reports of feed analysis

protein supplement may be necessary. A grain ration containing 12 per cent protein would be reasonable to ensure adequate protein intake. Grain mixtures containing 12 per cent protein are shown in Table 3.

If the lactating mare is fed a hay containing 9 per cent protein, the grain mixture should contain 16 per cent protein (see Table 3).

Note that soybean meal is used as the protein in all the mixtures shown in Table 3. Soybean meal is recommended because it is of higher protein quality (better array of essential amino acids) than other vegetable proteins such as cottonseed meal.

Many horse owners give brood mares a supplement containing milk products or milk substitutes. Such products are usually excellent sources of amino acids and often of vitamins and minerals. Little benefit should be expected from the addition of such products to the mare's ration when the ration is adequately balanced.

The calcium and phosphorus requirements were discussed with those of the pregnant mare.

Estimates of hay and grain needed for various classes of mares are summarized in Table 4. Re-

TABLE 4. ESTIMATES OF DAILY FEED REQUIREMENTS OF MARES*

Mare	Feed†	Weight of Mare (Kg)				
		400	450	500	550	600
Open	Hay (kg)	6.4	6.9	7.4	8.0	8.6
Pregnant	Hay (kg)	5.0	5.4	5.9	6.3	6.6
	Grain (kg)	1.6	1.7	1.8	1.9	2.0
Lactating (early)	Hay (kg)	4.5	5.0	5.4	5.8	6.1
	Grain (kg)	4.0	4.5	5.0	5.5	5.9
Lactating (late)	Hay (kg)	4.0	4.5	5.0	5.5	5.9
	Grain (kg)	3.4	3.6	4.0	4.6	4.9

*Based on National Research Council (1978) report
†Values for hay and grain are based on representative analyses. Actual intake that is needed will depend on several factors such as quality of feed, environment, and individual status of the mare.

member that many factors influence the energy requirement. Cold environment, parasites, or dental problems are examples of factors that can increase the energy needs. The total digestible nutrient (TDN) content of feeds varies. For example, the TDN content of some hays is different from that of others, but the estimates in Table 4 can be used as starting points. If the mare is too fat, the amount of feed, particularly that of grain, should be decreased.

STALLIONS

Little research has been conducted on the effect of nutrition on stallion performance. Some stallion managers claim excess protein is detrimental to the proper production of sperm. However, there is no evidence to support such a theory, nor is there any evidence to suggest that the protein requirement of the stallion is significantly greater than for maintenance.

Ration formulation for the stallion is simple. Feed the same grain the mare receives plus good-quality hay, water, and trace mineralized salt free choice. A problem on many farms may be the amount of feed given. Stallions that are slightly to moderately overweight probably do not have greatly impaired function, but it would seem prudent to attempt to keep stallions in good, trim condition—not too lean or too fat. Excessive fat has been shown to impair reproduction in other species. Furthermore, stallions that receive limited exercise and are chronically overfed are prime candidates for founder. In fact, several outstanding stallions have had their careers shortened because of founder.

GROWING ANIMALS

Newborn Foals

Mare colostrum contains about five times the protein concentration and twice the energy concentration of mare milk. Furthermore, colostrum is an excellent source of vitamin A. Recent studies have demonstrated that foals deprived of colostrum have lower vitamin A stores. For example, when antibodies were provided by serum, the vitamin A intake was lower than when foals received colostrum. Therefore, it is recommended that supplemental vitamin A be given to foals deprived of colostrum. The requirement for foals is estimated to be about 4000 IU of vitamin A daily.

Foals that are much smaller at birth than normal foals may require additional care and may have difficulty nursing. Mares fed rations lacking in energy or protein or obese mares may have smaller foals

than mares in good nutritional state. Although the heritability of birth weight is only 0.15 to 0.25, the size of the mare can greatly influence birth weight, presumably because of the environment and nutrition afforded to the fetus by the mare. That is, a large mare bred to a small stallion will probably have a larger foal than a small mare bred to a large stallion.

Dams younger than 8 years of age or older than 12 years of age are likely to have lighter, shorter foals than mares 8 to 12 years of age. The average colt is bigger than the average filly at birth. Foals born in May, June, or July are bigger at birth than foals born in January, February, or March.

Orphan Foals

Orphans can be reared on nurse mares or even nurse goats. Cow's milk contains more fat and less sugar than mare's milk and should be modified if fed to foals. Many old-time recipes are available. For example, Morrison[8] suggested one fourth pint of limewater and one teaspoonful of sugar be added to one pint of cow's milk and that the foal be fed about one half pint of the mixture every two hours for the first few days after birth. Fortunately, several commercial products such as Borden's Foal-Lac are now available, and they have been used successfully.

Creep Feeding

Creep feeding is often recommended because some mares do not produce adequate amounts of milk and because it is more efficient to feed the foal directly than feeding the mare to produce milk. It is also suggested that creep feeding allows the foals to grow faster and helps prevent setbacks at weaning. On the other hand, some authorities suggest that creep feeding may induce such rapid growth that the foals are predisposed to skeletal problems such as epiphysitis. Although there has been much speculation about the advantages and disadvantages of creep feeding and discussion of the pros and cons of rapid growth, few controlled studies have been conducted. In particular, much more research is needed to determine the effects of rate of growth on performance of the horse as a two-year-old and as a mature animal. Growth rate will be discussed in more detail in the section on the feeding of weanling foals.

The National Research Council recommends that creep rations contain 16 per cent protein, 0.8 per cent calcium, and 0.55 per cent phosphorus. The grain should be cracked, crimped, or rolled.

Weanlings

The weanling is much more susceptible than older horses to nutritional problems. The protein requirement, expressed as a percentage of the diet, is almost twice that of the mature horse at maintenance. The National Research Council estimates of the energy, protein, calcium, phosphorus, and vitamin A requirements of growing horses are shown in Table 5.

Of course, the requirements are dependent upon the desired rate of growth. The expected rate of growth (weight gain) is higher now than during the 1950s and before. For example, a 1978 NRC bulletin suggests that a six-month-old foal with an expected mature weight of 500 kg should gain about 0.8 kg per day. The 1949 bulletin suggests 0.6 kg per day. The 1978 bulletin indicates that a light horse should reach about 46 per cent of its mature weight at six months of age and 75 per cent of its mature weight at 12 months of age. The comparable values in the 1949 bulletin were 40 per cent and 56 per cent at six and 12 months, respectively.

The increased rate of gain requires careful nutritional considerations. For example, in 1951 Morrison suggested that good legume hay and oats would be satisfactory for weanlings. Such a diet might be expected to contain 13 per cent protein or less, which would not support the rate of gain expected by some owners. When protein is added to produce more rapid growth, the requirements for other nutrients are increased. When rapid growth is obtained but essential minerals are lacking, skeletal problems are likely to develop.

Problems Associated with Improper Nutrition of Growing Horses

The optimal growth rate of young horses varies with the type and use of the animal and the objectives of the owner. Several studies with other species have clearly demonstrated that longevity can be increased by feeding a balanced diet but at a level lower than that required for maximal growth rate. Studies with dogs and pigs indicate that young animals fed a highly palatable diet at high levels of intake may grow rapidly but develop a higher incidence of skeletal diseases such as osteochondrosis dissecans, hypertrophic osteodystrophy, enostosis, elbow dysplasia, and hip dysplasia. The conditions developed even though the diets were balanced according to present knowledge.

Overfeeding has long been claimed to cause problems in horses. Henry[2] wrote that "liberal feeding must be counterbalanced by an abundance of outdoor exercise. In no other way can colts be ruined so surely and so permanently as by liberal feeding

TABLE 5. SUMMARY OF NUTRIENT CONCENTRATION NEEDED IN RATIONS OF GROWING HORSES*

	Digestible Energy (Mcal/kg diet)	Crude Protein (%)	Ca (%)	P (%)
Weanling (3 mos)	2.9	16	0.8	0.55
Weanling (6 mos)	2.8	14.5	0.6	0.45
Yearling (12 mos)	2.6	12	0.5	0.35
Long yearling (18 mos)	2.3	10	0.4	0.30

*90% dry matter basis

and close confinement." Henry recommended that colts 6 to 12 months of age be fed 1 to 1.4 kg of grain daily, which is considerably below most feeding standards of today. In 1968, Miller,[7] a prominent breeder, trainer, and driver of Standardbreds, wrote: "Horsemen have preached for years that stock farms should market ready-to-race yearlings that are not 'hot-housed' and not stuffed with feed during the last few months before the sale. But it is also a fact that more owners and trainers, despite what their natural inclination might be, seem to prefer slick, stout yearlings that actually have been overfed. Apparently this is an occupational hazard of the yearling selection business and it is doubtful that it will ever change."

Stromberg[12] reported an increasing incidence of osteochondrosis in young fast-growing horses. He postulated that a genetic predisposition is associated with rapid growth and excessively high energy feeding. Overfeeding also appears to be involved in the etiology of certain types of wobbles.[6] Kronfeld[5] suggested that overfeeding of genetically predisposed animals but not overfeeding per se might be responsible for skeletal disorders.

Epiphysitis. Epiphysitis has been claimed to be induced by overfeeding. This problem, characterized by abnormalities in the epiphyses of the long bones (particularly the distal epiphysis of the radius, metacarpus, tibia, and metatarsus) consists of enlargement and lipping of the physes, premature closure, and, frequently, metaphyseal osteosclerosis or osteomalacia.

Epiphysitis is perhaps most often seen when young animals are fed rations high in protein and energy and low in calcium, such as heavy concentrate feeding with grass hay as the main forage. However, even when calcium supplements are provided in these circumstances, the problem may still occur. Further studies are needed to define the relationship of diet to epiphysitis, but decreasing grain intake frequently seems to be of therapeutic value.

Contracted Tendons. The condition of "contracted tendons," generally affecting foals 4 to 12 months old, involving the superficial and/or the deep flexor tendons, can also be associated with overfeeding.[10] "Contracted tendons" is a misnomer because it is unlikely that the tendons contract. The pathogenesis of the condition may involve overfeeding of protein and energy, causing the long bones to grow at a more rapid rate than the tendons, thus producing an unnatural length of the tendons relative to bone length, or perhaps the muscles do not develop properly. However, further studies are needed to substantiate the role of nutrition in the development of contracted tendons. Evidence to support the hypothesis that the condition may be associated with undernutrition followed by overnutrition has been reported by Hintz et al.[3] In this study, four of six foals weaned at four months of age and subsequently fed limited amounts of high-energy feed for four months developed a condition similar to "contracted tendons" within one to three months of being fed the diet free choice. None of the six control foals fed the same diet free choice from weaning developed the condition. Weight gains during the first four months for restricted and control foals were 0.23 kg per day and 0.85 kg per day, respectively, and during the second period 0.81 kg per day and 0.56 kg per day, respectively. Foals with restricted growth rates in their early months may require special consideration when growth-inhibiting factors are removed. If flexure abnormalities appear, measures to restrict growth rate may be helpful.

Enterotoxemia. Enterotoxemia may be caused by acute overfeeding, and although Diekie et al.[1] claimed that "enterotoxemia in the foal occurs infrequently," Swerczek[13] reported that the condition is one of the most important causes of mortality of young horses, accounting for the death of 28 of 935 foals necropsied at University of Kentucky from 1973 to 1975. The largest and most aggressive foals in group feeding situations are the most affected.[15] The foals appeared healthy at feeding but were found dead shortly thereafter, often with no clinical signs, although flatulent colic and acute dyspnea were sometimes observed. Posterior ventral subcutaneous edema and emphysema were found at necropsy, and the gastrointestinal tract was filled with grain and was dilated from gas formation. The cortex of the kidneys was degenerative. It was concluded that the enterotoxemia was due to *Clostridium perfringens* Type D. As mentioned earlier, careful management is necessary to prevent acute overeating.

In summary, the optimal growth rate for young horses is not known, but the average light horse might be expected to obtain about 47 per cent, 67 per cent, and 80 per cent of mature weight by 6, 12, and 18 months, respectively.[4] The average light horse obtained about 83 per cent, 91 per cent, and 95 per cent of mature height at the withers by 6,

TABLE 6. ESTIMATES OF BODY WEIGHT AT VARIOUS AGES FOR HORSES OF VARIOUS MATURE BODY WEIGHTS

Age (Months)	Mature Weight (Kg)					
	200	400	500	600	800	1000
2	60	105	130	155	150	210
4	85	150	180	220	250	315
6	110	185	230	275	340	420
8	125	220	275	320	400	500
10	140	245	310	360	450	565
12	150	270	335	400	500	630
14	160	290	360	435	540	670
16	165	305	380	460	580	730
18	170	320	400	480	620	780

12, and 18 months, respectively.[4] Estimates of body weight at various ages for horses of various mature body weights are shown in Table 6.

EARLY WEANING

The average foal is now weaned at a younger age than in the past. Traditionally, many farm managers weaned at six months of age or later. Weaning at four months or even two months is now common. Earlier weaning allows the mare to be returned to use sooner, makes more efficient use of feed, appears to cause less setback at weaning time, and may increase the growth rate of the foal. However, earlier weaning requires greater attention to the diet of the foal. A four-month-old foal given only oats

TABLE 7. ESTIMATES OF DAILY FEED REQUIREMENTS OF GROWING HORSES

Age of Foal (Mos)	Type of Feed	Expected Mature Weight (kg)		
		400	500	600
		Weight of feed (kg)*		
4	Hay	1.4	1.5	1.8
	Grain	3.0	3.5	4.2
6	Hay	1.6	1.8	1.9
	Grain	3.2	3.8	4.3
8	Hay	1.9	2.2	2.5
	Grain	3.4	4.1	4.7
12	Hay	2.7	3.2	3.7
	Grain	2.8	3.4	3.9
14	Hay	3.2	3.7	4.3
	Grain	2.7	3.3	3.7
18	Hay	3.7	4.3	4.9
	Grain	2.4	2.9	3.3

*Values may be used as initial guidelines. Amount of feed will vary according to desired rate of gain, quality of feed, individual status of the foal, and environmental conditions.

and grass hay cannot be expected to grow and develop properly. The requirements for foals are shown in Table 5. Complete feeds, either pelleted or a mixture of chopped hay and grain, are useful for growing foals. Once the foals are adjusted to the ration, the feed can be in front of the foals at all times without danger of overfeeding. The ratio of hay to grain in the mixture can be increased as the foal matures, thus preventing the animal from getting too much energy or becoming overweight. The complete feed makes the balancing of rations easier because the foals cannot sort the feed, and all foals in a group are eating the same percentage of hay. The complete feed may also save labor costs and works well with three-sided run-in shed arrangements. However, some long hay should be fed with complete feeds. Foals fed complete rations free choice may be expected to eat amounts equivalent to 3 to 3.5 per cent of their body weight. Some foals will consume even greater amounts. Estimates of daily feed requirements are shown in Table 7.

References

1. Diekie, C. W., Klinkerman, D. L., and Petrie, R. J.: Enterotoxemia in two foals. J. Am. Vet. Med. Assoc., *173*:858, 1978.
2. Henry, W. A.: Feeds and Feeding. Madison, WI, published by author, 1901.
3. Hintz, H. F., Schryver, H. F., and Lowe, J. E.: Delayed growth response and limb conformation in young horses. Proc. Cornell Nutr. Conf., 94, 1976.
4. Hintz, H. F., Hintz, R. L., and Van Vleck, L. D.: Growth rate of Thoroughbreds. Effects of age of dam, year and month of birth and sex of foal. J. Anim. Sci., *48*:480, 1979.
5. Kronfeld, D.: Feeding practices on horse breeding farms. Proc. 24th Annu. Conv. Am. Assoc. Eq. Pract., 461, 1978.
6. Mayhew, I.: Spinal cord disease in the horse. Cornell Vet., *68*, Suppl. 6:205, 1978.
7. Miller, D.: Feeding. *In* Harrison, J. C. (ed.): Care and Training of the Trotter and Pacer. Columbus, OH, United States Trotting Association, 1968.
8. Morrison, F. B.: Feeds and Feeding. Ithaca, NY, Morrison Pub. Co., 1951.
9. National Research Council. Nutrient Requirement of Horses. Washington, DC, National Academy of Sciences–National Research Council, 1978.
10. Owen, J. M.: Abnormal flexion of the corono-pedal joint or "contracted tendons" in unweaned foals. Eq. Vet. J., 7:40, 1975.
11. Roberts, S. J.: Veterinary Obstetrics and Genital Disease. Ithaca, NY, published by author, 1971.
12. Stromberg, B.: A review of the salient features of osteochondrosis in horses. Eq. Vet. J., *11*:211, 1979.
13. Swerczek, T. W.: The etiology, pathology and pathogenesis of diseases of foals and weanlings. Proc. Soc. Theriogenol., 19, 1976.
14. Swerczek, T. W.: Experimentally induced toxicoinfectious botulism in horses and foals. Am. J. Vet. Res., *41*:348, 1980.
15. Swerczek, T. W., and Crowe, C. W.: Enterotoxemia in young horses due to *Clostridium perfringens* Type D. Chicago, Proc. 54th Conf. Res. Workers Anim. Dis., 1978.

SAMPLE RATIONS AND COMMERCIAL FEEDS

H. F. Hintz, ITHACA, NEW YORK

SAMPLE RATIONS

As stated earlier (p. 65), many different combinations of feedstuffs can be fed satisfactorily to horses, and of course there are differences of opinion as to the best methods of providing the nutrients. Furthermore, local conditions such as availability and price of feedstuffs should influence formulation. Many companies also manufacture feeds specifically designed for various classes of horses.

It must be stressed, however, that the success of any feeding program depends on good management. Horses should be observed closely and frequently. Routine weighing (or estimating weight with tapes placed around the heart girth) is an excellent management aid, as even experienced horsemen can sometimes be fooled as to the extent of weight changes.

On many farms, a considerable amount of feed is wasted because of inadequate or poorly designed feeding equipment or because of carelessness. Also, many injuries to horses result because of feeding equipment that is not used properly or designed properly.

The results of surveys of feeding practices at four racetracks are shown in Table 1. In addition to hay and grains, almost all the trainers fed or injected vitamin and mineral supplements.

Rations for breeding animals are shown in Table

TABLE 1. SURVEY OF FEEDING PRACTICES AT FOUR RACETRACKS

Track	Type	Average Weight of Horse (kg)	Hay* (kg)	Oats (kg)	Corn (kg)	Sweetfeed (kg)	Wheat Bran† (kg)
Roosevelt‡	Standardbred	475	8.8	4.4	0.5	1.8	0.2
Vernon Downs	Standardbred	452	8.3	4.5	0.5	1.6	0.2
Finger Lakes	Thoroughbred	489	6.6	6.2	—	1.0	0.5
Belmont	Thoroughbred	486	7.3	5.8	—	1.3	0.5

*Most trainers fed grass or grass-legume mixed hay. Ten percent fed alfalfa or clover hay or alfalfa cubes.
†Average of those trainers feeding wheat bran. Approximately 50 per cent of the trainers used wheat bran.
‡At least 10 trainers were surveyed at each track.

TABLE 2. EXAMPLES OF RATIONS SUGGESTED BY VARIOUS AUTHORITIES

Mares*	Gestation Per Cent by Weight	Lactation Per Cent by Weight
Oats	30	15
Corn or milo	10	10
Barley	12¼	26
Wheat bran	10	7
Soybean meal	11	13
Linseed meal	4	4
Alfalfa meal	10	7
Molasses	7	7
Dicalcium phosphate	2	1¼
Limestone	¾	¾
Salt	1	1
Vitamins	2	1

Lactating Mares (550 kg)†

1. Alfalfa hay (7.3 kg) and corn (2.7 kg)
2. Red clover hay (7.3 kg) and barley (1.3 kg), corn (1.3 kg)
3. Timothy hay (7.3 kg) and oats (1.3 kg), wheat bran (1.3 kg), soybean meal (0.45 kg) plus mineral supplement

Pregnant Mares‡

1. Grass-legume hay plus grain mixture containing 80 per cent oats and 20 per cent wheat bran; mineral mixture fed free choice
2. Grass-legume hay plus grain mixture containing 45 per cent barley, 45 per cent oats, and 10 per cent wheat bran; mineral mixture fed free choice

Pregnant or Lactating Mares§	Fed with Legume Hay (Per Cent)	Fed with Grass Hay (Per Cent)
Corn	43.0	38.0
Oats	40.5	35.5
Soybean meal	5.0	14.0
Molasses	6.0	6.0
Wheat bran	5.0	5.0
Dicalcium phosphate	0.5	0.5
Limestone	—	1.0

Fed with good-quality hay

*Cunha, T. J.: Horse Feeding and Nutrition. New York, Academic Press, 1980.
†Morrison, F. B.: Feeds and Feeding. Ithaca, NY, Morrison Pub. Co., 1951.
‡Ensminger, E.: Horses and Horsemanship, 5th ed. Davisville, IL, Interstate Pub. Co., 1977.
§Hintz, H. F.: Cornell University, unpublished information.

2. The rations vary from simple to complex. Unfortunately, the rations have not been compared with each other to determine which is best.

Rations for growing animals are shown in Tables 3 and 4. Amounts of feed were discussed in the article on feeding programs.

COMMERCIAL FEEDS

The sales of commercial horse feeds have increased greatly since the 1960s. It has been suggested that most modern horse owners have little experience in formulating rations and are not interested in mixing their own feed. Many suburban horse owners are much more comfortable buying a complete feed for their horses, just as they would buy one for their cats or dogs. Consequently, the sales of complete pelleted feeds have greatly increased.

Pellets have several advantages: decreased feed waste, economy of space in storage and transportation, more attractive horses because of loss of hay belly, more opportunities for mechanization of feeding, less labor, prevention of sorting of feed by the horse, and reduced dust. Complete pelleted diets also permit the use of properly supplemented by-products, feeds, or ingredients that might not normally be accepted by horses.

The disadvantages of pellets include the cost of pelleting and increased incidence of vices such as wood chewing, tail chewing, and cribbing. The vices are probably due to boredom or perhaps simply a desire to chew. If complete pelleted rations are fed, some hay should be provided as a source of roughage. Some veterinarians have also reported that the feeding of pellets increases the incidence of choke. We have not observed this problem in our horses and ponies fed complete rations.

Many companies manufacture horse feeds, and most companies have different formulations for various classes of horses to give the horse owner a wide variety from which to select. Factors to consider when selecting feed include cost, nutrient content, quality control, reliability of the manufacturer, and services provided by the manufacturer. The feed tag

TABLE 3. EXAMPLES OF CREEP RATIONS

I*	Fed with Alfalfa Hay (Per Cent by Weight)	II†	Fed with Mixed Hay (Per Cent by Weight)
Cracked corn	38	Cracked corn	53
Crushed oats	38	Soybean meal	33
Molasses	6	Molasses	10
Soybean meal	17	Trace mineral salt	1
Dicalcium phosphate	1	Limestone	1
		Dicalcium phosphate	1
		Brewers' yeast	0.5
		Vitamin supplement	0.5

*Cornell University
†William Tyznik, Ohio State University

TABLE 4. EXAMPLES OF RATIONS FOR WEANLINGS

I*	Fed with Alfalfa Hay (Per Cent by Weight)	Fed with Grass Hay (Per Cent by Weight)	II†	Per Cent
Corn	45	39	Oats	25.0
Oats	36	27	Corn or barley	30.8
Soybean meal	12	25	Milo or corn	15.0
Molasses	6	6	Soybean meal	15.0
Limestone	—	2	Dehydrated alfalfa meal	5.0
Dicalcium phosphate	1	1	Molasses	5.0
			Vitamin supplement	0.7
			Dicalcium phosphate	2.0
			Limestone	0.5
			Salt	1.0

Barley can replace corn and oats; steamed bone meal or a similar Ca-P supplement can replace dicalcium phosphate. Trace mineralized salt is given free choice. If hay is of poor quality, a vitamin supplement should also be fed.
*Hintz, H. F.: Cornell University, unpublished information.
†Cunha, T. J.: Horse Feeding and Nutrition. New York, Academic Press, 1980.

TABLE 5. ESTIMATES OF MINIMUM NUTRIENT CONTENT NEEDED IN COMMERCIAL FEEDS IN ORDER TO MEET NUTRIENT REQUIREMENTS FOR VARIOUS CLASSES OF HORSES

Class of Horse	Nutrient (Per Cent by Weight)	Type of Forage Feed			
		Legume Hay	Mixed Hay	Grass Hay	None*
Weanlings	Crude protein†	14.5	16	18	14.5
	Calcium	0.4‡	0.6	0.9	0.70
	Phosphorus	0.6	0.6	0.6	0.45
Yearlings	Crude protein	10	12	14	12
Mares Late gestation and lactation	Calcium	0.1‡	0.3‡	0.7	0.50
	Phosphorus	0.5	0.5	0.5	0.35
Mature horses	Crude protein	8	8	10	10
	Calcium	—§	—§	0.2‡	0.30
	Phosphorus	0.3	0.3	0.3	0.25

*Feeding small amounts of hay even when using complete feeds will help alleviate such vices as wood chewing.
†The protein should be of good quality; that is, it should supply the essential amino acids. Soybean meal, milk proteins, and meat meal are examples of reasonable protein sources.
‡Many mixtures will contain calcium levels greater than 0.4 per cent, but the extra calcium is not harmful when an adequate level of phosphorus is provided.
§The forage will normally provide all the calcium needed.

should list the minimal amount of crude protein and crude fat and the maximal amount of fiber. Some companies also list the Ca and P content. Even if not listed, the latter information should be available from the dealer. Estimates of the amount of nutrients required in commercial feeds for various situations are shown in Table 5. The feed tag may also list ingredients, but most tags now list ingredients according to groups of feeds and not individual feeds. The tag may say cereal grain instead of corn or plant protein instead of soybean meal. The wording is more general so that companies can take advantage of low-cost formulas and thereby minimize feed cost. Sometimes the basic ingredients in any given brand of feed may vary greatly among shipments. Drastic changes in ingredient quality may influence the feed intake of horses.

References

1. Cunha, T. J.: Horse Feeding and Nutrition. New York, Academic Press, 1980.
2. Ensminger, E.: Horses and Horsemanship, 5th ed. Davisville, IL, Interstate Pub. Co., 1977.
3. Morrison, F. B.: Feeds and Feeding. Ithaca, NY, Morrison Pub. Co., 1951.

HOOF GROWTH AND NUTRITION

H. F. Hintz, ITHACA, NEW YORK

What can I feed my horse to make his hooves grow faster and tougher? This question is frequently asked by horse owners whenever nutrition is discussed. Of course, fast growth is not necessarily highly correlated with high-quality hooves, but it may be desired to grow out a hoof with a problem such as a quarter crack or for horses such as endurance or racehorses that must have their shoes replaced frequently. Unfortunately, it is not easy to give an answer that satisfies the horse owner. Many factors other than nutrition are known to influence hoof growth, and it may not be possible to increase growth by nutritional changes.

Although I could not find any studies on the genetics of hoof growth in horses, I suspect that the heritability of hoof growth and quality is quite high. Many horsemen claim that certain horses' families have superior hooves. Studies with other species support the importance of genetics. For example, Brinks and coworkers[1] concluded that the heritability of hoof growth in cattle was quite high and that selection for hoof growth or for normal hooves should be effective in cattle. They were considering selecting for slow growth because cattlemen prefer slow hoof growth in order to decrease the time and effort required to trim feet. Other studies indicated that heritabilities for hoof characteristics such as heel depth in dairy cattle were significant and that genetic variation in hooves could be recognized even if trimming were practiced.

Foals under one year of age have a much faster rate of hoof growth than older animals. Foals may have a growth rate of 0.5 mm per day, whereas a rate of 0.2 to 0.3 mm per day might be expected in older animals. Differences in rates of hoof growth have also been found between animals seven years or older and animals three years or younger.

Several studies have shown that hoof growth varies with the time of year, although moisture and temperature appear to affect growth more than season per se. Hoof growth is faster during periods with warmer temperatures and greater rainfall. Studies in Texas indicate that the most rapid growth is in October and the slowest in December. Studies in New York indicate that hooves grow faster in September and October than during January and February.

Most studies indicate that hind hoofs grow faster than front ones, but it appears that use, age, and weight distribution may influence the difference.

It is commonly thought that increasing the blood supply to the hoof increases rate of growth. Thus, irritants, blisters, or other circulation-stimulating agents are sometimes applied to the coronet. Daily massage of the coronet to stimulate circulation has also been reported to increase hoof growth. Further studies are needed to evaluate these practices. Some practitioners feel that the more rapid hoof growth produced by the use of irritants results in hoof tissue of poor quality.

Several nutrients are known to influence hoof growth. A reduced energy intake can result in decreased rate of hoof growth in growing animals. A complete pelleted ration was fed in limited amounts or ad libitum to two groups of Shetland pony foals for 117 days. The limited group was fed an amount to allow a weight gain of about 0.2 lb per day. The ad libitum group gained 1 lb per day. The hoof growth in the limited group was 0.25 mm per day, compared to 0.38 mm per day in the ad libitum group. Of course it might be possible that any factor that decreases body weight gain will decrease rate of hoof growth. Several studies have shown a high correlation between rate of hoof growth and rate of weight gain.

Protein deficiency can also result in decreased hoof growth. The hoof growth of weanlings fed 10 per cent protein was only two thirds that of weanlings fed 14.5 per cent protein. Several studies have been conducted to determine if additional protein or amino acids, that is, supplements in excess of the requirements, will enhance hoof growth. Butler and Hintz[3] found no benefit from the addition of gelatin to a commercial complete pelleted feed. The hoof growth was 0.33 mm per day for those weanling ponies fed the pellets and 0.31 mm per day for those ponies fed the pelleted diet plus 90 gm of gelatin per 100 kg of body weight.

Studies with amino acid supplementation also failed to demonstrate special effects on hoof growth. However, if the amino acid supplementation of a deficient horse stimulates weight gain, it is likely to stimulate hoof growth.

Vitamins and minerals can also influence hoof growth. Good-quality hay would normally be expected to provide adequate levels of vitamins, but poor-quality hay could be deficient in vitamin A.

Zinc is essential for a normal epidermis, and in a recent symposium it was suggested that zinc deficiency could be a cause of foot problems in cattle. Although zinc deficiency has not been reported under field conditions in horses, such a possibility cannot be ignored because it was previously thought that zinc deficiency was not a problem in ruminants.

Selenium toxicity in horses can result in hair loss from the mane and tail, degeneration of hoof quality, and eventually complete loss of the hoof.

In summary, a complete, balanced diet is essential for proper hoof growth. There is no evidence to suggest that the addition of extra nutrients to balanced diets promotes hoof growth.

References

1. Brinks, J. S., Davis, M. E., Mangus, W. L., and Denham, A. H.: Genetic aspects of hoof growth in beef cattle. *In* Colorado Feeder Day Report, Colorado State University, Fort Collins, 1980, pp. 12–14.
2. Butler, D.: The Principles of Horseshoeing. Ithaca, NY, published by author, 1974.
3. Butler, K. D., and Hintz, H. F.: Effect of level of feed intake and gelatin supplementation on growth and quality of hoofs of ponies. J. Anim. Sci., *44*:257, 1977.

EXERTIONAL MYOPATHY

Karl K. White, ITHACA, NEW YORK

Exertional myopathy is a clinical problem familiar to most equine veterinarians. The syndrome has been called azoturia, Monday morning disease, paralytic myoglobinuria, exertional rhabdomyolysis, tying-up syndrome, and myositis. Some authors consider the tying-up syndrome to be distinct from the azoturia complex; however, most evidence points to a common origin with somewhat different clinical manifestations.

Rhabdomyolysis is an apt descriptive term for the pathology of exertional myopathy and has been well described by Lindholm et al.[3] At the cellular level, hyalin degeneration is followed by necrosis of muscle with little initial inflammatory response.

The pathophysiology of exertional myopathy is poorly understood. Historically, excessive storage of glycogen within the muscles during periods of rest, resulting in release of destructive amounts of lactic acid during subsequent exercise, has been blamed. Results of more recent work suggest that, although the preceding mechanism may play a role in the syndrome, it is not the primary etiology. Poor perfusion of the affected musculature, resulting in decreased cellular oxygenation and increased local levels of metabolic byproducts including lactic acid, appear to be important. Likewise, an intracellular energy deficit resulting from poor perfusion, aberrant metabolic pathways, as in the malignant hyperthermia-myopathy syndrome in humans and swine, and other ill-defined mechanisms have been suggested.

Exertional myopathy often occurs in muscularly fit horses maintained on a high plane of nutrition that are rested for one or more days with no decrease in nutritional intake. Resumption of work triggers the onset of acute azoturia, or Monday morning disease. Unfit, overweight animals maintained at relatively high nutritional levels that are suddenly put to work are likewise predisposed to the disease.

Younger horses, particularly fillies, in the early stages of training appear to suffer a higher incidence of myopathy, especially the milder form described as tying-up. Horses with massive development of the croup, loin, and thigh musculature like the working Quarterhorse and draft breeds are at risk for the severe azoturic form of myopathy. A possible association has been made between the occurrence of exertional myopathy and nervous animals or animals exercised in a cold, damp environment.

CLINICAL SIGNS

Clinical signs usually relate to pain and stiffness of the croup, loin, and thigh musculature with associated abnormalities of gait. The forelimb muscle masses are only occasionally involved. In mild cases, a stiff, somewhat stilted rear limb gait is apparent. As severity increases, the animal may appear to have muscle cramps and may be reluctant to move or refuse to move at all. A very severe episode of exertional myopathy may result in recumbency with inability to rise or in assumption of what has been described as the "dog-sitting" position.

Other clinical signs show a similar gradation. Characteristically, croup, loin, and thigh musculature is firm and painful to palpation. Sweating may be apparent only over the affected muscle masses or may be generalized. The horse may appear to be anxious and may present with elevated pulse and respiratory rates and occasionally fever. Myoglobinuria is observed with moderate to severe myopathy.

Laboratory data are helpful in the diagnosis of mild cases of exertional myopathy but are most useful in monitoring response to treatment in severe cases. Elevations of serum glutamic oxaloacetic transaminase (SGOT), lactate dehydrogenase (LDH), and creatine phosphokinase (CPK) levels provide evidence of muscular damage. CPK, the most sensitive indicator, peaks about six hours subsequent to muscle damage and clears within a few days if damage does not continue. SGOT and LDH peak in approximately 24 and 12 hours, respectively, and clear in one to two weeks. It is important to note that heavy exercise alone may increase these enzyme levels severalfold in the normal horse. In severe cases, blood urea nitrogen and serum creatinine levels should be monitored to assess the effects of myoglobin clearance on renal function.

DIAGNOSIS

Clinically, exertional myopathy must be differentiated from abdominal pain or colic and hypoxic myopathy of the rear limbs associated with iliac thrombosis. Differentiation is usually not difficult if the history and physical findings are considered.

The clinician should be aware, however, that colic and myopathy may occur simultaneously from a common stress or the one condition from the other. The combination is most commonly observed in animals worked over long distances, such as endurance or timber racers and occasionally three-day event animals. Recognition of the combined syndrome is critical, since forced walking of the moderately affected myopathy case may exacerbate the condition severely.

Residual effects of an episode of exertional myopathy on the musculoskeletal system vary from no clinically significant abnormalities in mild cases to fibrosis and loss of muscle mass in severe cases, which result in obvious gait and aesthetic abnormalities. Renal dysfunction may be an important sequela of severe or repetitive attacks. Individuals that have experienced myopathy episodes appear to be predisposed to additional bouts, although increasing age tends to reverse this trend.

THERAPY

Treatment must address not only the myopathy syndrome but also associated electrolyte disturbances resulting from colic or exhaustion (p. 311). Serum calcium, phosphorus, potassium, and sodium levels may be abnormal in such cases and contribute to the development or exacerbation of the muscular pathology.

In mild cases of myopathy in which stiffness becomes apparent near or at the conclusion of an exercise period, the horse should be kept warm, by blanketing if necessary, and should be walked slowly until additional treatment is available. If acute, severe muscular pain begins shortly after exercise begins, walking is contraindicated, as it may result in refusal to move or recumbency. Even walking the animal to a more convenient treatment location may be disastrous. The animal should be blanketed and kept as quiet as possible until specific treatment is available.

In all cases, use of nonsteroidal anti-inflammatory agents such as phenylbutazone is indicated. Considerable pain relief is usually achieved at a dosage level of 4 to 8 mg per kg intravenously. Severe pain may warrant the use of narcotics such as meperidine, especially if the animal is recumbent and continuously struggles unsuccessfully to rise. Seemingly, relief of pain and associated anxiety allows most animals to relax and break the vicious circle of pain and muscular tenseness. Tranquilization may prove beneficial in the extremely nervous animal by providing additional relief from anxiety. The phenothiazine class of tranquilizers provides such an effect and may be used. Caution is advisable, as this class of drug also acts as an alpha blocking agent for the sympathetic nervous system. Alpha blockade may be useful in increasing perfusion of the muscle masses, thus allowing increased oxygenation and waste removal. However, if significant dehydration is present, relative hypovolemia with possible shock may ensue. Thus, general circulatory status must be assessed and volume deficits corrected prior to use of phenothiazine derivatives. If deficit correction is not immediately possible, xylazine at a dose of 0.5 to 1 mg per kg may be used intravenously for its tranquilizing and mild analgesic properties.

In moderate or severe cases of exertional myopathy, corticosteroid therapy is useful. Dexamethasone at a dose of 0.1 to 0.2 mg per kg intravenously or prednisolone sodium succinate at 1.0 to 2.0 mg per kg is recommended. The muscle relaxant methocarbamol* has been recommended at a dosage of 15 to 25 mg per kg given slowly intravenously. We have not thought this to be particularly helpful, but it is certainly rational therapy and should be utilized in recumbent patients or those in danger of becoming so. Methocarbamol may be repeated at six-hour intervals if desired.

Fluid and electrolyte management of severely affected recumbent individuals is critical. Evaluation of acid-base and electrolyte status on at least a daily basis is necessary for reasonably specific management of imbalances; however, some general concepts are applicable. Affected animals are usually acidotic, making bicarbonate therapy desirable. When myoglobinuria is present, maintenance of adequate renal perfusion and alkalinization of the urine is absolutely critical to minimize pigment damage to the kidneys. Intravenous administration of sodium bicarbonate until myoglobin begins to clear from the urine is suggested. The bicarbonate should be administered with a volume of balanced electrolyte solution adequate to maintain urine production. The balanced solution may likewise be "spiked" with appropriate amounts of electrolytes, such as potassium, as deficits become apparent. Lactated Ringer's solution is probably the most reasonable choice as the carrier fluid owing to its ready availability and reasonable cost, although some would argue against inclusion of lactate because of its role as a possible causative agent of myopathy. Clinically, this concern does not seem to be an important consideration, since the destructive action of lactic acid is localized and apparently secondary to poor perfusion. In addition, most myopathy patients have liver function adequate to metabolize the modest lactate levels introduced by fluid therapy.

Diuretics have been recommended but should be used cautiously if at all in moderate or severe cases of myopathy pending evaluation of electrolyte sta-

tus. Diuresis induced by fluid therapy is the much safer and more desirable course. If stranguria or urinary retention appear to be significant problems, the animal may be catheterized. Urine quantity and quality is then easily monitored. As mentioned previously, significant pigmenturia necessitates daily BUN and serum creatinine determination.

Physical management of the affected animal entails common sense and good nursing practices. If able to stand, the animal should be kept warm and in a quiet environment. Feed should be restricted to hay with water freely available. After all signs have disappeared, rest should continue for several days to several weeks, depending on the severity of the attack. During the recuperative period, feed may be increased slightly and hand-walking may be begun. Training should resume slowly, with nutritional increases lagging somewhat behind those calculated for the amount of daily exercise. A preventive program should be initiated (see Prevention section).

MANAGEMENT OF THE RECUMBENT PATIENT

Management of the recumbent patient is a difficult undertaking. In addition to the recommendations made for the standing patient, deep, soft bedding and frequent turning of the animal are desirable to prevent decubitus ulcers. The nutritional plane should be decreased further, since gastrointestinal upset in the recumbent horse is a constant concern and is a potentially disastrous complication in the myopathy patient. The most important quality for the clinician managing a recumbent myopathy case is patience. Intuitively, we all dislike seeing a downed horse and thus have a great tendency to rush the standing process. Premature or frequent attempts to get the horse to its feet often result in further attacks of myopathy, which may preclude the horse from ever standing. Patience, adequate symptomatic and replacement therapy, and judicious assistance in standing when the animal is sufficiently strong provide the most favorable results.

PREVENTION

As with most medical problems, prevention of exertional myopathy is the most desirable treatment. Parenterally administered vitamin E and selenium have been used widely to prevent recurrence of exertional myopathy. Evaluation of this treatment is difficult, since it is usually initiated in conjunction with the administration of other drugs and the institution of appropriate changes in dietary

---

*Robaxin, A. H. Robins Co., Richmond, VA

and exercise management. The product E-Se* is used intramuscularly at a dose of 10 ml per 500 kg weekly for one month. Injections are then given biweekly or monthly as desired. A variety of other agents such as B vitamins, oral sodium bicarbonate, corticosteroids, and dipyrone have been suggested to prevent the syndrome, but none appear to have gained wide acceptance.

The clinician should be aware that dantrolene sodium is presently being evaluated for the treatment of postanesthetic myopathy and for prophylaxis of the tying-up syndrome in racehorses. Results to date are promising. The drug appears to work intracellularly as a calcium binder. It is used successfully in humans and swine to prevent the malignant hyperthermia syndrome. Unfortunately, the manufacturer has decided not to pursue marketing approval for use in the horse. The drug is rather insoluble and usually is given orally; however, successful intravenous administration in the horse has been reported. A significant drawback to the chronic prophylactic treatment of performance animals may be the hepatotoxic potential of dantrolene.

Management of dietary and exercise regimens is the most important factor in prevention of exertional myopathy, especially in its most severe forms. The key is establishment of a routine for feeding and exercise that varies little from day to day. A well-balanced feeding program designed to maintain the horse slightly on the lean side is desirable. If daily exercise must vary, then daily nutritional intake must do likewise. For the average horse owner, a balanced, commercially prepared grain mix may be advisable, since it varies less from batch to batch

---

*E-Se, Burns-Biotec, Omaha, NB

than home-formulated "eyeball" mixtures. A combination of grass or oats and alfalfa hay has been recommended rather than alfalfa alone. However, in a recent three-year experiment at Cornell University comparing the effects of dietary fat and protein levels on the performance of endurance horses, exertional myopathy was not observed in any animal despite the exclusive use of alfalfa as the hay source and performance distances of 50 to 75 miles.

The most difficult recommendation to implement is an exercise regimen that is constant from day to day. The vast majority of owners today are weekend riders. If such is the case and a satisfactory nutrition-exercise program cannot be achieved, it may be better for the owner to acquire a horse less sensitive to these variations. Likewise, if an owner requires a slick, show ring–fit horse rather than a lean one, perhaps a different horse is the answer.

In summary, the plane of nutrition must correlate on a daily basis with the exercise level. Ideally, neither should vary as to amount or even timing from day to day. Vitamin E and selenium and in the future possibly dantrolene may be beneficial prophylactically, but the veterinarian must impress on the owner that the daily management of the horse is paramount in prevention of exertional myopathy.

References

1. Adams, O. R.: Lameness in Horses, 3rd ed. Philadelphia, Lea and Febiger, 1974.
2. Hammel, E. P., and Raker, C. W.: Myopathies. *In* Catcott, E. J., and Smithcors, J. F. (eds.), Equine Medicine and Surgery, 2nd ed. Wheaton, IL, American Veterinary Pub., 1972.
3. Lindholm, A., Johansson, H. E., and Kjaersgaard, P.: Acute rhabdomyolysis in Standardbred horses. A morphological and biochemical survey. Acta Vet. Scand. 15:325, 1974.

FOUNDER

J. E. Lowe, ITHACA, NEW YORK

Founder is a metabolic derangement resulting in ischemia, inflammation, and often necrosis and separation of the sensitive from the insensitive laminae of the hoof. The disease first appears at the distal end of the toe and may involve any percentage of the laminae extending from the toe. The disease is complicated by the mechanical effects that result from separation of laminae and subsequent rotation of the third phalanx (P3) toward the sole, coupled with recurrence of the metabolic derangement and/or inflammation resulting from the weakening and mechanical tearing of the remaining healthy laminae.

Founder can be acute or chronic. Although the terms are generally understood by veterinarians and horsemen, it can be argued that laminitis can be caused by concussion, infection, and acute trauma of the foot, which in some cases lead to chronic laminitis of that foot or at least a disease process that cannot be clinically distinguished from chronic laminitis.

In spite of considerable investigation, acute founder is a poorly understood disease process. It occurs in all breeds, but ponies have the reputation of being likely candidates. The etiologic agent or agents are multiple. They include carbohydrate engorgement, massive tissue destruction and infection, lush grass ingestion, induced founder, especially from corticosteroid hormones, and unidentified agents contained in black walnut shavings used for bedding. Carbohydrate overload is the only inducing method that has been used as a repeatable model for study of the pathogenesis.

CLINICAL SIGNS

The signs of acute founder are a characteristic reluctance to move forward, a pronounced heel-toe landing when forced to move, a so-called walking-on-eggs attitude when placing the front feet on the ground, a warm or hot foot, a pounding digital pulse, a reluctance to have one foot held up for examination, and, if willing to allow one foot to be held up, a definite tenderness to the use of hoof testers on the sole ahead of the apex of the frog.

The front feet are most often affected, but all four may be affected. In severe cases, the animal may be unable to rise or stand, and P3 may rotate sufficiently to protrude through the sole. The etiologic agent may be responsible for fever and other systemic signs; however, the pain associated with acute founder can cause elevation of temperature, pulse, and respiration plus anorexia and weight loss.

THERAPY

Acute founder is an emergency situation. Therapy is aimed at controlling or eliminating the inciting disease or agent and returning the circulation within the hoof to normal or tolerable levels before separation and rotation takes place. If therapy is successful and rotation does not occur, then the possibility of a chronic condition is eliminated. Unfortunately, therapy is not uniformly successful. Refractory laminitis may appear with some drug-associated founder and in spontaneous founder of unknown etiology.

Therapy for metritis, retained placenta, pneumonia, digestive dysfunction, and other conditions is of foremost importance in the face of acute founder. Removal of inciting agents such as access to lush grass and fresh walnut bedding is also essential. When applicable, removal of corticosteroid hormone administration is indicated. When diagnosed within the first 24 hours after signs appear, the judicious use of palmar digital nerve block using 2 per cent mepivacaine or 2 per cent lidocaine is beneficial. The horse is also walked for five minutes every hour until the block has worn off. The block may be repeated once or twice during the first 24 hours of the disease. Apparently the nerve block helps restore circulation by allaying pain, allowing normal walking, and probably by relieving vasospasm

within the foot. The danger with this treatment is that if rotation or necrosis has already taken place, the block is likely to promote separation of hoof and bone by allowing the horse to walk on a mechanically incompetent foot.

Phenylbutazone is the nonsteroidal anti-inflammatory agent of choice. It is also the least expensive. Administer 8 to 10 mg per kg intravenously followed by 4 to 5 mg per kg every 24 hours for as long as needed. It is best to use the intravenous route until recovery is evident, whereupon the oral route can be used. Corticosteroids such as dexamethasone and flumethasone are contraindicated.

Investigations have shown a decrease in sulfur-containing amino acids at weakened or ruptured laminae. Therefore, supplementation of the diet with methionine (10 gm per day) for as long as recovery takes is sometimes recommended. No studies have demonstrated that extra methionine will ensure buildup of the hoof, but the rationale seems reasonable, and 10 gm of methionine per 1000 lbs should not be harmful. Higher levels could lead to amino acid imbalances and other problems.

Mechanical support for the soles to help prevent rotation is indicated. A stall filled with moist sand provides gentle support and allows the horse to lie down comfortably. Standing the patient in mud or in a running sand-bottom stream has also been used successfully; however, it does not allow the animal to lie down if it wishes. Absolutely rigid support by plaster of Paris casts to fill the sole has not been successful in our hands.

The use of hot or cold running water or packs on the feet is under debate. Cold water is nearly always available. Because the foot is hot and throbbing, the natural reaction of humans is to use cold water applications. Maintaining continual hot applications is impractical. Recent findings of ischemia at the laminar junction have led to the debate over hot and cold packs. We still apply unheated tap water. A foot dressing in the form of an elastic gauze bandage or similar cotton and gauze covered by porous adhesive tape stays on for many days and allows the foot to be kept moist and cool. These dressings are used even when the animal stands in sand.

Remove the shoe unless it is too painful for the patient to hold one foot up. Even then the nails can sometimes be cut with a sharp chisel. If a nerve block is used, removal of the shoes is made easier.

Antihistamine injections may help recovery from the inciting disease, but their direct effect on founder is questionable.

CHRONIC FOUNDER

If rotation of P3 has occurred, the front of the hoof wall may be concave in appearance; the sole may be flat or even convex. If P3 has rotated sufficiently so that it protrudes through the sole, secondary infection of the sole and the diseased laminae is likely. Infection also occurs with flat thin soles that crack or become too soft from prolonged soaking. Infection adds another complication to an already major problem. The prognosis has to remain guarded to poor as long as infection is present. Whenever rotation is sufficient for protrusion of the tip of P3 through the sole, the prognosis is poor. Drainage, antiseptics, and local and/or systemic antibiotics are used to overcome the infection. Do not shoe with pads until the infection is completely under control.

In most cases of chronic founder, infection is not present. Therapy is aimed at protection of the weakened foot through trimming, shoeing, body weight control, and pain control. A lateral radiograph of the foot shows clearly how much the leading edge of P3 diverges from the leading edge of the hoof wall, giving one a good indication of the degree of rotation. The greater the rotation, the greater the weakening, the poorer the prognosis, and the more difficult the treatment. Corrective trimming can to some extent make the rotation appear less pronounced on radiographs.

Control of body weight by restricting the diet is essential in treatment of chronic founder. Many chronically foundered ponies are obese, but unfortunately some owners are reluctant to restrict feed. Pain control is achieved through the results of diet restriction (if necessary), administration of phenylbutazone, and the results of therapeutic shoeing. The skills of the farrier are essential. Trimming the heels lower and "dubbing" the toe help the patient to place the foot flat and level for more even weight-bearing when landing. A wide-web shoe that is concave on the inner edge next to the sole is used to help prevent sole pressure. Leather pads provide protection, and an additional leather rim pad may be necessary to help prevent ground contact by the tender sole.

The type of packing that provides the most protection is being debated. We have no preference as long as the packing is not hard and does not ball up under the sole. A soft formula acrylic plastic for the sole and a hard formula to replace diseased hoof wall are useful in some cases. We prefer the less expensive methods described earlier.

The prognosis for founder depends on severity and duration. Many chronically foundered animals that are well cared for continue to be serviceably sound. On the other hand, if P3 protrudes through the sole or the coronary bands begin to ooze serum and you have visions of the hoof falling off, it is usually best to refrain from attempting to be a hero but rather recommend euthanasia.

References

1. Ackerman, N., Garner, H. E., Coffman, J. R., and Clement, J. W.: Angiographic appearance of the normal equine foot and alterations in chronic laminitis. J. Am. Vet. Med. Assoc., *166*:58, 1975.
2. Amoss, M. S., Hood, D. M., Miller, W. G., Hightower, D., McGrath, J. P., McMullan, W. C., and Scrutchfield, W. L.: Equine laminitis. II. Elevation in serum testosterone associated with induced and naturally occurring laminitis. J. Eq. Med. Surg., 3:171, 1979.
3. Coffman, J. R., Johnson, J. H., Guffy, M. M., and Finocchio, E. J.: Hoof circulation in equine laminitis. J. Am. Vet. Med. Assoc., *156*:76, 1970.
4. Dorn, C. R., Garner, H. E., Coffman, J. R., Hahn, A. W., and Tritschler, J. G.: Castration and other factors affecting the risk of equine laminitis. Cornell Vet., 65:57, 1975.
5. Garner, H. E., Coffman, J. R., Hahn, A. W., Hutcheson, D. P., and Tumbleson, M. E.: Equine laminitis of alimentary origin: An experimental model. Am. J. Vet. Res., 36:441, 1975.
6. Hood, D. M., Amoss, M. S., Hightower, D., McDonald, D. R., McGrath, J. P., McMullen, W. C., and Scrutchfield, W. L.: Equine laminitis. I. Radioisotopic analysis of the hemodynamics of the foot during the acute disease. J. Eq. Med. Surg., 2:439, 1978.
7. Hood, D. M., Gremmel, S. M., Amoss, M. S., Button, C., and Hightower, D.: Equine laminitis. III. Coagulation dysfunction in the developmental and acute disease. J. Eq. Med. Surg., 3:355, 1979.
8. Obel, N.: Studies on the histopathology of acute laminitis. Almqvist and Wiksells Bocktryckeri ab Uppsala, 1948.
9. Robinson, N. E., Scott, J. B., Dabney, J. M., and Jones, G. A.: Digital vascular responses and permeability in equine alimentary laminitis. Am. J. Vet. Res., 37:1171, 1976.
10. True, R. G., Lowe, J. E., Heissen, J., and Bradley, W.: Black walnut shavings as a cause of acute laminitis. Proceedings of the Annual Meeting of the American Association of Equine Practitioners, 511–516, 1978.

HYPERLIPEMIA

Jonathan M. Naylor, SASKATOON, SASKATCHEWAN, CANADA

Hyperlipemia syndrome has been used traditionally to describe a severe disease in ponies characterized by cloudy plasma and severe fatty infiltration of the liver. The advent of modern laboratory screening tests, which include serum triglyceride, cholesterol, and total lipid measurements, has led to the detection of both horses and ponies with mild lipemia. The condition is subclinical, and there is no evidence of associated fat-induced liver damage. There is a problem in terminology in that although these animals are by definition hyperlipemic, they do not fit into the traditional usage of this term in equine medicine as used by Wensing[12] and Schotman.[8, 9] In order to differentiate these two entities, the term *hyperlipemia syndrome* will be reserved for members of the Equidae family with gross lipemia, fatty livers, and a severe clinical syndrome, whereas the term *hyperlipidemia* will be used to describe mild lipemias.[3, 5] Equidae members with serum triglycerides less than 500 mg per dl and no evidence of liver dysfunction should be classified initially in the hyperlipidemia category.

LIPID METABOLISM

Most cases of hyperlipemia and hyperlipidemia are seen in underfed ponies.[9] During fasting, triglycerides in adipose tissue are broken down into free fatty acids and glycerol, which are released into the blood.[1, 5, 15] Some free fatty acids are used directly by peripheral tissues such as muscle; the rest are taken up by the liver. Fatty acids may be oxidized in the liver completely to provide energy or partially to yield ketone bodies, or they may be re-esterified to triglycerides and phospholipids (Fig. 1). In the fasting horse, serum concentrations of triglycerides and to a lesser extent phospholipids rise,[1, 5, 15] but ketonemia is not marked.[5] One difference between disorders of lipid metabolism in ruminants and Equidae is that hypertriglyceridemia is seen in fasting Equidae. In contrast, fasting milk cows show only a mild elevation in serum triglycerides,[7] and there is a net hepatic uptake of triglycerides in fasting cows.[7] Equidae with the hyperlipemia syndrome may be mildly ketotic; in contrast, ketonemia is marked in ketotic cattle and sheep with pregnancy toxemia. Thus, hepatic metabolism of fatty acids favors triglyceridemia in Equidae and ketonemia in ruminants.

HYPERLIPIDEMIA

Many sick, anorectic horses have mild elevations of serum lipids. There is no visible opacity to the plasma, and laboratory tests record serum triglyceride values of less than 500 mg per dl.[5] In the absence of clinicopathologic evidence of liver damage, this mild lipemia signals the need for nutritional supportive therapy rather than the diagnosis of the hyperlipemia syndrome.

THE HYPERLIPEMIA SYNDROME

PATHOPHYSIOLOGY

The severe lipemia of the hyperlipemia syndrome is characterized by a serum cloudy with the presence of fat. Triglyceride values are in the 500 to 9000 mg per dl range,[5, 12] and fat has begun to accumulate in the liver. Mild ketonemia is present in some cases.[2] Severe fatty infiltration of the liver with resultant hepatic dysfunction may be responsible for some of the signs of hyperlipemic disease.

Although fasting alone can produce severe lipemia and clinical disease in ponies,[15] fasting horses usually only develop hyperlipidemia. Horses are usually both aphagic and azotemic before hyperlipemia develops.[5] This combination of events is probably effective in producing hyperlipemia because lipid utilization during fasting is disrupted by an inhibition of peripheral removal of triglycerides during azotemia,[4] resulting in the accumulation of lipids within the blood. This effect may be due to an inhibitory effect of azotemia on lipoprotein lipase, an enzyme that plays a crucial role in the removal of triglycerides from blood by peripheral tissues. In a recent case series of horses with hyperlipemia, all were azotemic, usually because of renal lesions.[5] Renal lesions have also been reported in ponies and may contribute to the development of hyperlipemia in these breeds.[3]

Fatty infiltration of the kidney occurs in the late stages of starvation-induced hyperlipemia in ponies, and the intriguing possibility exists that this may in turn give rise to a secondary azotemia. If this is the case, then removal of lipids from the blood could be further inhibited and the hyperlipemia exacerbated.

CLINICAL FINDINGS

There are no clinical findings specific for the hyperlipemia syndrome. Affected Equidae are depressed, and in some cases this depression is very marked.[3, 9] Diarrhea has been reported in some affected ponies, but it is unclear to what extent this reflects intercurrent parasitism. A percentage of healthy horses denied food develop diarrhea after more than three to five days of food deprivation.[5, 10]

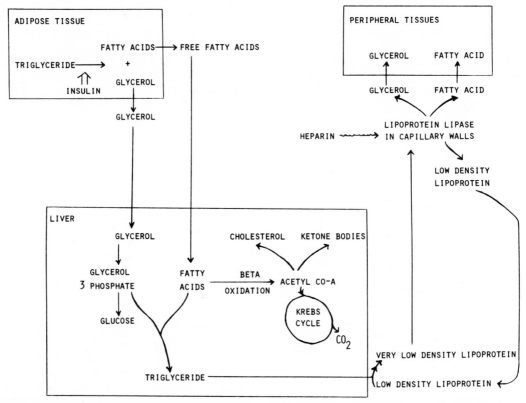

Figure 1. A simplified diagram of lipid metabolism in the horse. Inhibitors are indicated by ⟹, activators by ⌢.

This suggests that imbalances in gut function brought on by lack of food may produce diarrhea in horses, and this may account for some instances of diarrhea in hyperlipemic Equidae. Jaundice is also seen in some cases of hyperlipemia,[9] presumably as a result of the combined effects of food deprivation and liver dysfunction.

The hyperlipemia syndrome is most common in ponies[9] but has also been reported in donkeys and horses.[5] Affected ponies are often fat, but this is not an invariable finding.[9] Affected horses are in good to thin bodily condition. Pregnant and lactating ponies are particularly susceptible,[2, 3] and because of this, most cases are seen in the spring in the Northern Hemisphere.[9] Transport can also predispose to the development of the condition.[2]

Affected ponies are in negative energy balance, usually because a primary disease process depresses food intake. Heavy parasite burdens are a common inciting cause;[9] parasites can both depress food intake and compete for available nutrients. The condition is also seen as a sequela to underfeeding, usually in out-wintered ponies. In horses, negative energy balance does not result in the hyperlipemic disease unless the affected horse is also azotemic.[5]

An unusual presentation of hyperlipemia in ponies is in association with pituitary tumor. These animals often eat readily, and the hyperlipemia is thought to be secondary to prolonged fat mobilization in response to hormonal imbalances.[5]

DIAGNOSIS

Diagnosis is based on examination of the blood. Lipemic blood tends to have a blue tinge, and serum or plasma is opaque and varies in color from white to yellow, depending on the relative degrees of hyperlipemia and hyperbilirubinemia. Early cases of hyperlipemia are characterized by a faint cloudiness to serum or plasma; this is easier to see in a test tube than in a microhematocrit tube. Sometimes normal plasma can appear slightly hazy and may be confused with hyperlipemia; repeated centrifugation at high speed will clear the opacity, which is probably due to the residual platelets. Hyperbilirubinemia is common in anorectic horses and imparts a yellow color to plasma or serum, which are nevertheless clear—opacity indicates hyperlipemia. Clot tubes can sometimes appear cloudy if the red cells sediment out before the blood clots; if clot retraction is poor, the upper phase will be gelatinized by fibrin and will appear opaque. Inverting the tube or stirring it with an applicator stick allows the identification of fibrin by its gel-like consistency.

When the hyperlipemia syndrome is diagnosed on the basis of clinical signs and the appearance of the blood, serum should be submitted for triglyceride assay to quantify the degree of lipemia. It is also important to conduct liver function tests, particularly the BSP clearance test, to determine the degree of liver dysfunction. Serum enzyme activities, such as sorbitol dehydrogenase and alkaline phosphatase, help quantify the degree of active liver destruction. The blood glucose concentration can be low and should be measured. Serum creatinine should be determined because azotemia can contribute to the pathogenesis of the condition. Some commercially available laboratory screening tests offer an inexpensive method of measuring triglyceride, glucose, creatinine, and enzyme activities in serum.

Metabolic acidosis may develop in severe cases of the syndrome, and attempts should be made to quantify this; base deficits have been reported as large as 24 mEq per l.[12]

TREATMENT

The first priority is to treat the inciting cause of hyperlipemia and to attempt to improve feed intake. Ponies that are febrile or in pain may benefit from the administration of antipyretics or analgesics. Feed intake may also be improved by offering a variety of feeds and allowing the patient to choose. Patients that eat bedding may prefer poor-quality hay to better hays. Fresh grass is often the last food to be refused by a sick horse; allowing ponies to graze has been used as part of some successful therapeutic regimens.[11] Patients that refuse all food should be tube-fed. Gruels of dried grass or a complete feed can be fed by stomach tube (p. 114). Supportive therapy should include maintenance of the patient's hydration in order to avoid prerenal azotemia.

There are a number of therapeutic regimens aimed at speeding the removal of lipids from the blood. On a long-term basis, these treatments may also decrease lipid accumulation in the liver. The treatments fall into two categories: those that inhibit mobilization of lipids into blood from adipose tissue stores and those that speed the removal of triglycerides from blood. Insulin and glucose decrease mobilization of adipose tissue lipids, whereas heparin speeds the removal of triglycerides from the circulation. At present, no treatment for hyperlipemia has been approved by the FDA.

Only limited information is available on the dosage of heparin. One recommendation is that ponies be given from 100 to 250 IU per kg body weight twice daily.[8] We have used somewhat lower dosages (40 USP units per kg) and have observed a temporary beneficial effect on the severity of the hyperlipemia. Heparin inhibits blood clotting in vivo, and this danger should not be overlooked.

Insulin therapy is usually combined with carbohydrate administration. Combinations of glucose and insulin alone are reported to produce a severe lactic acidosis and a poor recovery rate. A treatment in which insulin administration is combined with glucose and galactose administration on alternate days is reported to give better results than either glucose and insulin or heparin treatments.[11, 14] Using this regimen, a 200 kg pony would be given 30 IU protamine zinc insulin intramuscularly twice daily with 100 gm of glucose orally twice daily on the first and succeeding odd days. On even days, 15 IU protamine zinc insulin is given intramuscularly twice daily with 100 gm of galactose orally once daily.[11, 13, 14] Treatment is administered until the serum is no longer grossly lipemic, although insulin can be administered in decreasing doses for an additional three days if required.

Acidosis may be corrected with a replacement solution fortified with sodium bicarbonate as necessary. Acid-base status, blood glucose concentration, and the degree of lipemia should be monitored during therapy. If heparin therapy is used, blood clotting studies should be performed during therapy, and the patient should be monitored for bleeding problems.

The success rate in treatment of hyperlipemia is usually low. Cases in which the inciting disease process is responsive to therapy and in which the hyperlipemia is less than 2 gm total lipids per dl have the best prognosis (Table 1). Foaling or abortion during treatment may also improve the prognosis.[8] The prognosis for horses with hyperlipemia is very poor unless the associated azotemia can be corrected.

TABLE 1. RELATIONSHIP BETWEEN TOTAL BLOOD LIPIDS AND RECOVERY IN PONIES TREATED FOR HYPERLIPEMIA

Total Lipids, gm/dl	Total Number of Ponies	Percentage Recovered
1–2	8	75
2–3	14	50
3–4	7	14
4–7	35	26

(Modified from Schotman, A. M., and Wagenaar, G.: Hyperlipemia in ponies. Zbl. Vet. Med., *16*:1, 1968.)

PREVENTION

Most cases of hyperlipemia in ponies can be avoided by maintaining feed intake. Adequate food should be available, and supplemental feeding is necessary for animals outwintered at pasture. Ponies that are being trucked long distances should be rested periodically and allowed to eat. The development of hyperlipemia secondary to disease-induced aphagia can be prevented by tube feeding. These precautions are particularly important if the pony is pregnant or lactating. Prolonged restriction of feed intake for therapeutic purposes, such as in overweight laminitic ponies, should be done with care. The risk of hyperlipemia may be reduced by feeding a half-maintenance ration rather than complete feed withdrawal.

References

1. Baetz, A. L., and Pearson, J. E.: Blood constituent changes in fasted ponies. Am. J. Vet. Res., 33:1941, 1972.
2. Eriksen, L., and Simesen, M. G.: Hyperlipemia in ponies. Nord. Vet. Med., 22:273, 1970.
3. Gay, C. C., Sullivan, N. D., Wilkinson, J. S., McLean, J. D., and Blood, D. C.: Hyperlipemia in ponies. Aust. Vet. J., 54:459, 1978.
4. Gregg, R. C., Diamond, A., Mondon, C. E., and Reaven, G. M.: The effects of chronic uremia and dexamethasone on triglyceride kinetics in the rat. Metabolism, 26:875, 1977.
5. Naylor, J. M., Kronfeld, D. S., and Acland, H.: Hyperlipemia in horses: Effects of undernutrition and disease. Am. J. Vet. Res., 41:899, 1980.
6. Reid, I. M., Stark, A. J., and Isenor, R. N.: Fasting and refeeding in the lactating dairy cow. I. The recovery of milk yield and blood chemistry following a six day fast. J. Comp. Pathol., 87:241, 1977.
7. Reid, I. M., Collins, R. A., Roberts, C. J., Symonds, H. W., and Baird, G. D.: Pathogenesis of fatty livers in fasted cows. Proc. Nutr. Soc., 36:41A, 1977.
8. Schotman, A. J. H., and Wagenaar, G.: Hyperlipemia in ponies. Zbl. Vet. Med., 16:1, 1968.
9. Schotman, A. J. H., and Kroneman, J.: Hyperlipemia in ponies. Neth. J. Vet. Sci., 2:60, 1969.
10. Tasker, J. B.: Fluid and electrolyte studies in the horse. IV. The effects of fasting and thirsting. Cornell Vet., 57:658, 1967.
11. Wensing, T. H.: Hyperlipemia in ponies. Vet. Rec., 91:209, 1972.
12. Wensing, T. H., Schotman, A. J. H., and Kroneman, J.: Various new clinical chemical data in the blood of normal ponies and ponies affected with hyperlipemia (hyperlipoproteinaemia). Tijdschr. Diergeneeskd., 98:673, 1973.
13. Wensing, T. H., Schotman, A. J. H., and Kroneman, J.: A new method in the treatment of hyperlipemia (hyperlipoproteinaemia) in ponies. Neth. J. Vet. Sci., 5:145, 1973.
14. Wensing, T. H., Schotman, A. J. H., and Kroneman, J.: Effect of treatment with glucose, galactose and insulin on hyperlipemia (hyperlipoproteinaemia) in ponies. Tijdschr. Diergeneeskd., 99:919, 1974.
15. Wensing, T. H., Schotman, A. J. H., Remmen, J. L. A. M., and Kroneman, J.: Inducing hyperlipemia (hyperlipoproteinaemia) in ponies by fasting or transfusion of lipaemic blood. Tijdschr. Diergeneeskd., 99:855, 1974.

HEAT BUMPS, SWEET FEED BUMPS, SWEET ITCH

J. E. Lowe, ITHACA, NEW YORK

Heat bumps are a noninfectious, noncontagious dermatitis seen in the warmer months. The bumps are 0.5-mm diameter swellings in the skin; they may be unilateral, or they may be confined to the saddle and girth area. The bumps are most common on horses that are bathed or hosed daily.

The etiology is unclear. The bumps are seen more often on horses fed on a high plane of nutrition. Some reports suggest that the bumps are an allergenic response to certain feedstuffs; hence, the name "sweet feed bumps." Allergy to grass has also been suggested as a cause. Baker[1] listed other possible causes such as photosensitization, onchocerciasis, and allergy to biting insects, particularly *Culicoides pulicaris* and *C. robertsi*. He concluded, however, that evidence was not conclusive and that further research was required.

The bumps seldom get better and seldom get worse in spite of treatment, and therapy for uninfected bumps is discouraging unless they are treated in the fall. When cold weather comes, the bumps usually disappear spontaneously, leading to the conclusion that insects are more involved with the dermatitis than is sweet feed. Steroids systemically or topically help suppress the bumps, but when therapy is discontinued, the bumps may return. McCaig[2] suggested that regular antihistamine injections (every 6 to 12 hours) together with creams such as diphenhydramine* help relieve the condition but that such regular injections are almost impossible for the average owner. Fly repellents may be of some use.

*Caladryl, Parke-Davis, Morris Plains, NJ

Occasionally the "bumps" are rubbed bare of hair or rubbed raw. Secondary bacterial infection can occur with subsequent tenderness, swelling, weeping, and heat in the area involved. Secondary infection is treated topically with iodine surgical soap scrubs and broad-spectrum antibiotic ointment application. Systemic treatment with penicillin or ampicillin for three days is also indicated if cellulitis develops.

In conclusion, the bumps are a nuisance. Once horsemen realize that no one can treat bumps successfully and consistently, they usually resign themselves to the fact that the bumps have to be tolerated. Manipulating the diet by trial and error may help some horses, but the percentage of successes is so small that most horsemen give up in frustration just as the veterinarian does.

References

1. Baker, K. P.: The rational approach to the management of sweet itch. Vet. Ann., *18*:163, 1978.
2. McCaig, J.: Recent thoughts on sweet itch. Vet. Ann., *15*:204, 1975.

ECLAMPSIA

H. F. Hintz, ITHACA, NEW YORK

Equine eclampsia or hypocalcemia is generally considered to be less of a problem now than when draft horses were the prevalent type of horses, but occasionally cases are reported.

Traditionally the hypocalcemia has been thought to occur most commonly around the tenth day postpartum or one to two days after weaning, but recent case reports included mares in midgestation and midlactation, and males.

The serum calcium level of affected horses is usually 4 to 6 mg per 100 ml. Clinical signs are variable but can include increased muscular tension and tremors, anxiety, rear limb ataxia, dilation of the nostrils, salivation, grinding of the teeth, and synchronous diaphragmatic flutter. Hypomagnesemia may also be present. However, hypermagnesemia, hyperphosphatemia, and hypophosphatemia have also been reported.

Treatment with an intravenous injection of a 500 ml solution containing 8.42 gm Ca, 1.88 gm Mg, and 4.8 gm PO_4 has been effective. In some cases, two injections may be required.

We are not aware of any studies in which the effect of diet on the incidence of eclampsia was examined. A high calcium intake prior to the onset of lactation predisposes cows to milk fever. Perhaps a similar effect could predispose mares or horses ridden in endurance rides to hypocalcemia, but further studies are needed.

Supplemental Readings

1. Arnbjerg, J.: Hypocalcemia in the horse. Nord. Vet. Med., *32*:207, 1980.
2. McAllister, E. S.: Hypocalcemia in the horse. J. Eq. Med. Surg., *1*:230, 1977.
3. Rach, D. J., Moore, D. W., and Sturn, R.: Equine eclampsia. Can. Vet. J., *13*:78, 1972.

NUTRITION OF THE SICK HORSE

Jonathan M. Naylor, SASKATOON, SASKATCHEWAN, CANADA

D. E. Freeman, KENNETT SQUARE, PENNSYLVANIA

Nutrition as supportive therapy is often neglected in the treatment of sick horses. Energy or protein deprivation has adverse effects on the immune response and on wound healing.[4, 14, 20, 22] Nutritional support can also prevent death from cachexia, which occurs when the animal has lost 20 to 30 per cent of its body weight. The following sections describe some of the techniques and uses of nutritional support in clinical situations. The simplest regimens can be readily applied in the field with cooperation between stablehand and veterinarian. The more complex regimens are often best carried out under close supervision in a veterinary hospital.

ASSESSMENT OF NUTRITIONAL STATUS

Body shape is used by clinicians to gauge nutritional status. Mature animals lose fat and muscle tissue but maintain skeletal elements during periods of negative energy balance. Thus, flesh falls away from the bones. Loss of body tissue is first apparent over the lumbar vertebrae and rump; the ribs become prominent later. Growing animals in negative energy balance show a similar pattern of weight loss. Studies with cattle and sheep suggest that moderate restrictions of energy intake in growing ruminants result in slower growth, but body proportions are similar to those seen in normal animals of the same weight.[1] Therefore, nutritional status in the growing horse is best judged using expected weight for age growth curves.

Food intake is the other commonly used index of nutritional status (p. 65). Assessment of food intake and bodily condition should be a routine part of physical examination. In the examination of a thin horse, it is particularly important to establish whether cachexia is due to poor feed intake or some other problem before proceeding with more specialized tests of digestive or metabolic function. In people, prolonged starvation from any cause can itself cause a malabsorption syndrome.[23] Decreased food intake has recently been advanced as a cause of malabsorption in a horse.[16]

Blood chemistry offers some guidance as to a horse's nutritional status. The best indices of food deprivation are plasma-free fatty acid and glycerol concentrations, but these are not routinely available at present. Some laboratories measure serum triglycerides and give a normal range of 6 to 78 mg per dl; mild elevations in the 100 to 500 mg per dl range are usually consistent with a period of poor food intake.[21] Normal serum triglycerides do not rule out poor food intake, since there is much variation in the triglyceridemic response to food deprivation. Also, a lag of more than 40 hours between the removal of food and an elevation in serum triglycerides is common (p. 107).

Low serum albumin values usually reflect protein-losing enteropathy or renal or liver disease rather than long-term protein deprivation.

DIETS FOR SICK HORSES

The ideal diet for the sick horse should be palatable and digestible and should have a high protein content. Protein content is important because disease increases both protein and energy requirements. Depot lipid is available to meet some of the energy demands, but there is no comparable store to replace lost protein, so positive nitrogen balance should be maintained to inhibit breakdown of muscle and visceral protein. In general, alfalfa hay meets these requirements more closely than orchard grass or timothy hay because of its better palatability and protein content.

SPECIAL DIETS

Chronic Pulmonary Disease. Horses with chronic pulmonary disease usually do best at pasture but, if kept indoors, often improve if they are taken off hay, fed pelleted feeds, and placed in a well-ventilated stall. When hay has to be fed, it should be thoroughly soaked with water either with a hose or preferably placed in a net and completely immersed in a tub of water for at least five minutes.[6] Soaked feed should be replaced frequently because it can easily mold. There will be less dust if hay cubes are fed in place of loose hay, but these again should be soaked. This dietary program and environmental management are the cornerstones of the successful treatment of many horses with chronic pulmonary disease (p. 505).

Diarrhea. Diarrhea is another circumstance in which special diets may be indicated. Some horses, particularly those on high grain diets and in good physical condition, will respond to decreasing the grain content of the ration and feeding more grass hay. In contrast, horses that have primarily large intestinal lesions (such as chronic salmonellosis), which impair fiber digestion may maintain condition better on grain diets. In the latter case, the improvement in bodily condition is presumably due to increased absorption of nutrients from grain in the small intestine even though fecal quality is not improved.

Colonic Impaction. In horses prone to recurrent colonic impactions, we restrict hay intake and provide pellets because hay diets are associated with more large intestinal filling than are grain diets.[11] Pelleted feeds may be beneficial not only because gut fill is limited but also because resistance to flow through the gut may be decreased. Resistance to flow of ingesta through the gut is proportional to particle size,[2] and feeds that are processed into pellets are ground up before compaction into pellets. Horses fed pellets also have soft feces, which presumably helps minimize the chance of further impactions.

Choke. Horses prone to esophageal obstruction should not be fed pellets. A soft food such as grass or a sloppy mash is preferable. If the horse is a greedy eater, large round stones placed in the grain will slow down the rate of eating and decrease the probability of further episodes of choke.

IMPROVING VOLUNTARY FOOD INTAKE

Palatable feeds are usually the first line of attack in improving voluntary feed intake in the horse or pony that eats poorly. Young leafy grass has a high palatability and digestibility and may be preferred by horses that refuse other foods. In general, alfalfa hay is more palatable than grass hays, and grains are more palatable than bran. "Sweet feeds"—usually mixtures of molasses and rolled grains—can often increase palatability when added to whole grain feeds. However, some sick horses will reject a good alfalfa hay and grain and will eat poor hay or their bedding. For this reason, it is important to offer the sick horse a variety of foods and to let it have its own preference. There may be an initial preference for a novel food such as apples or carrots, but this can soon diminish, and the person who feeds the horse should be constantly searching for foods preferred by the horse.

Bran mashes are a popular food for sick horses, although they can be low in palatability. Palatability can be improved by mixing a quart of oats with a quart of bran. The mixture is steeped with boiling water and served warm but not hot. Molasses (up to 250 ml) can be added as flavoring, as can up to 20 gm of salt. Steamed oats, barley, and well-boiled linseed meal may be particularly palatable to some horses and can be substituted for part of the oats in the mash.

The site at which food is offered can be important, as some horses prefer to eat from the ground rather than a manger or hay rack.

It is important to guard against overfeeding and sudden dietary changes. A sudden change to alfalfa hay can cause diarrhea; alfalfa should be gradually introduced over a five-day period as the amount of grass hay is reduced. Increases in the grain fraction of the diet should not exceed 0.5 kg a day for a 450 kg horse. Fresh feed should be offered in small amounts and should be replenished as necessary, and feed should be discarded as it gets stale. Partially eaten feeds contaminated by saliva mold quickly and will be refused by the horse.

Fever and pain depress feed intake. Antipyretics can improve intake.[3] Analgesics can be particularly effective in improving feed intake in horses with chronic laminitis or crippling orthopedic problems. In cases in which systemic derangements accompany pain, analgesics have a much less pronounced effect on food intake.

Feed stimulants such as diazepam that have a direct effect on feeding centers in the brain can improve feed intake in horses.[5] We do not recommend diazepam for feed intake modification in sick horses because in our experience it produces tranquilization and ataxia with little benefit on feed intake. Anabolic steroids increase feed intake, but because the effect may take up to 10 days, they are unlikely to be of use in the immediate treatment of the sick horse. However, they can be useful in building up horses in the convalescent period.

Vitamin supplementation may be beneficial to some horses. Normally the diet and synthesis of vitamins by the gut flora provide plenty of B vitamins, and the average horse has adequate stores of vitamins for short-term food deprivation. Horses that have been off feed for a number of days and horses that have disturbed gut function because of diarrhea or oral antibiotic therapy may benefit from vitamin B complex administration.

FORCE FEEDING

There are two approaches to nutritional supplementation in sick horses unable or unwilling to eat. The first approach is only to supplement part of the horse's requirements; the other is to provide all nutrients.

Partial supplementation, which involves dosing with a high-protein food, is used with patients that are in fairly good bodily condition and still have some voluntary food intake. The rationale behind high-protein supplements is that improving the balance between protein requirements and protein intake will minimize catabolism of muscle and visceral protein. The horse is still in negative energy balance, and depot lipid is broken down to meet the energy deficit. One type of therapy involves the use of 50 gm of dehydrated cottage cheese made into a slurry and administered by a dose syringe three times a day. This provides only a third to a quarter of maintenance protein requirements but may convert a patient with marginal food intake into positive protein balance. Dehydrated cottage cheese is used as a supplement because it contains a high proportion of casein and is 90 per cent digestible to the horse.[19] Its amino acid spectrum is particularly good, and the protein is likely to have a high biologic value for the horse.[12]

Complete nutritional support is indicated in patients that are either severely cachectic or are expected to be unable to eat for more than five days. Complete nutritional support may also be given early in the therapeutic regimen if it is thought that any further loss of body condition is undesirable, such as a horse that is recumbent and is losing body weight so that it cannot regain sufficient strength to stand. We tend to reserve complete nutritional support for horses wanting to eat but unable to ingest food because of painful, neurologic, or intestinal obstructive diseases.

Complete nutritional support can be given orally or intravenously. Intravenous therapy is both costly and time-consuming. Solutions and infusion sets must be sterile. Contamination of solutions occurs readily when making additions to the intravenous fluid bottles,[7] and bacterial contaminants multiply in the medium of the intravenous solutions. This is a special problem with intravenous feeding, since the bottle of nutrient solution can hang for long periods before being exhausted. Particular care must also be taken with catheter placement. Solutions are hypertonic, and the catheter should be in a large vessel to minimize the risk of thrombosis. The tubing and catheter should be changed regularly to decrease the risk of contamination.[7]

Another problem with intravenous nutrition is that large loads of glucose are given by a route that bypasses many of the normal homeostatic mechanisms. In contrast, during oral feeding, gut hormones are released that aid insulin release;[15] this potentiation of insulin release is decreased when glucose is administered intravenously. Furthermore, portal blood from the gut passes through the liver before entering the general circulation. These mechanisms are bypassed in intravenous feeding, and hyperglycemia may develop, particularly in septic patients. Fat would be particularly useful as an alternative energy source, and Intralipid,* a preparation used successfully in Europe,[10] is now available for this purpose in the United States.

Intravenous feeding may be indicated in the treatment of foals with diarrhea. Their small size reduces some of the costs of intravenous feeding, and Hoffsis's formulation for calves[13] can be used (Table 1).

Sick animals are more prone to derangements of glucose metabolism than healthy animals, and blood glucose should probably not be allowed to rise above 200 to 300 mg per dl. Hyperglycemia will result in urinary loss of glucose and osmotic diuresis; very high blood glucose concentrations may induce convulsions.[9]

When feeding intravenously, the flow of nutrients should be kept as even as possible. Nutrient intake should slowly be built up from half maintenance to maintenance over the course of two days. Additions to the fluid bottles should be minimized and should be made using a closed technique, preferably under a laminar flow hood. Making additions to intrave-

*Intralipid, Cutter Labs, Inc., Berkeley, CA

TABLE 1. FORMULATION OF INTRAVENOUS FEEDING SOLUTION FOR FOALS

Amount	Item
750 ml	5% fibrin hydrolysate with 5% dextrose*
400 ml	50% dextrose
30 mEq	Sodium bicarbonate
30 mEq	Potassium chloride
	Injectable multivitamins

These items are mixed aseptically to yield a solution with a final volume of 1200 ml and an osmolality of 1629 mOsm/kg. The solution is administered at the rate of 2.5 l to a 45 kg foal. Based on recommendations for calves. (From Hoffsis, G. F., Gingerich, D. A., Sherman, D. M., and Bruner, R. R.: Total intravenous feeding of calves. J. Am. Vet. Med. Assoc., *171*:67, 1977.)
*Aminosol 5% in D5-W, Abbott Labs, North Chicago, IL

nous solution bottles in a laboratory resulted in a 25 per cent contamination rate.[7] Adding a broad-spectrum antibiotic to the intravenous fluid may limit bacterial growth. When mixing intravenous fluids, beware of drug interactions and always inspect the bottles for precipitates before infusing. Also remember that incompatibilities may not be physically evident. Addition of vitamin complexes and tetracycline can produce precipitates. Antibiotics are best given through a separate catheter.

Oral alimentation is the alternative to intravenous feeding and is used more frequently because it is inexpensive and sterile solutions are not needed. Foals can be fed a commercial foal milk replacer,* and this can be given through a nasogastric tube if necessary.

Adult horses can be fed a liquid diet of electrolytes, dextrose, dehydrated cottage cheese, and dehydrated alfalfa meal (Table 2).[18] The electrolyte mixture is shown in Table 3. The mixture is low in sodium and rich in potassium, like many natural horse feeds. These proportions of electrolytes are suitable for maintenance purposes but not for replacement purposes. Horses with fluid losses as a result of diarrhea or sweating require additional sodium-rich replacement electrolyte solutions (p. 318). Horses have been successfully maintained on this electrolyte mixture for up to four weeks. Occasionally a mild hyponatremia may develop, and in these cases, 15 gm of sodium chloride can be added daily to the electrolyte mixture. Routine supplementation of additional sodium salts is not recommended. The diet is introduced gradually and slowly is increased to maintenance amounts (Table 3). The diet is rich in highly digestible protein and should induce positive balance. Figures for digestible energy contents in Table 3 are estimates, but the diet gives close to the maintenance energy requirement of the normal horse. Water intake is more than sufficient for maintenance purposes, and the urine is often dilute. Sometimes an improvement in hydration is noted following the use of this regimen even though the horse had previously been receiving intravenous fluids.

This diet can be difficult to pass through a stomach tube because it is viscous. The limiting factor is the amount of dehydrated alfalfa meal added. Alfalfa swells up in contact with water and should only be added immediately before the mix is poured into the stomach tube. A large-diameter stomach tube facilitates passage of the mix, and if persistent difficulties occur, the alfalfa meal can be cut back to 600 gm per feeding.

Two problems in horses that are tube-fed this diet are diarrhea and laminitis. The risk of laminitis can be minimized by avoiding the diet in horses that are

*Foal-Lac, Borden International, New York, NY

TABLE 2. RECOMMENDED TUBE FEEDING SCHEDULE FOR A 450 KG HORSE

	Day						
	1	2	3	4	5	6	7
Electrolyte mixture, grams	210	210	210	210	210	210	210
Water, liters	21	21	21	21	21	21	21
Dextrose, grams	300	400	500	600	800	800	900
Dehydrated cottage cheese,† grams	300	450	600	750	900	900	900
Dehydrated alfalfa meal, grams	2000	2000	2000	2000	2000	2000	2000
Megacalories/day, DE*	7.4	8.4	9.4	10.4	11.8	11.8	12.2

The above allowances should be divided and fed in three feedings daily. Maintenance requirements for a 450 kg horse are 15 Mcal of DE and 580 gm of crude protein.

*Digestible energy

†Dehydrated cottage cheese, 82% crude protein, less than 2% lactose. American Nutritional Labs, Burlington, NJ

foundering, that have chronic laminitis, or that have rotation of the pedal bones. Diarrhea associated with tube feeding is not accompanied by fever or changes in the hemogram and responds to withdrawal of tube feeding and intravenous electrolyte solutions to maintain hydration. The incidence of diarrhea can be greatly reduced by making sure that alfalfa meal is not left out of the oral alimentation mix.

ESOPHAGOSTOMY

Oral alimentation diets are fed through a stomach tube. There are two methods of placing this tube. Frequently, tube feeding is accomplished using a nasogastric tube. Alternatively, protracted feeding of a horse through an indwelling esophagostomy tube may be indicated following surgical procedures on the nasal passages, oral and pharyngeal tissues, and upper esophagus in order to spare healing surfaces from the friction and abrasion of an indwelling nasogastric tube. The tube is inserted through an esophagostomy at the junction of the middle and lower third of the neck, where the esophagus is readily accessible and has little contact with any major structures.[8] The surgery is performed on the sedated horse following infiltration of the area with a local anesthetic.[8]

Feeding through an esophagostomy tube can be performed cleanly and efficiently by one person with minimal restraint of the patient. When a small-bore stomach tube is used in the esophagostomy, the horse can be allowed access to normal food material without risk of esophageal obstruction. This is advantageous if it is desired to put the horse on a period of trial feeding, as the esophagostomy tube is still in place should it become necessary to resume extraoral feeding. When it is decided to discontinue feeding through the esophagostomy tube, it can be removed and the esophagostoma allowed to heal spontaneously.

Healing is usually rapid and should be complete within two weeks. Complications following this procedure are rare and usually mild. Some cellulitis and edema may develop during the first three days after surgery, but this regresses rapidly and is usually localized to the surgical site. The most common complication is the development of a fistulous tract along the route that was occupied by the esophagostomy tube. As with any procedure performed on the cervical esophagus, damage to the left recurrent laryngeal nerve is also a possible sequela.

Cases should always be carefully selected so that the possible development of complications can be justified on the basis that failure to perform the surgery could jeopardize the animal's life or well-being. The procedure should only be used when other methods are not feasible or practical.

Care must be taken when feeding a pony through an esophagostomy tube because the capacity of its stomach is small. If a large amount is given at each feeding, the combination of food and the influx of gastric secretions will cause distention, colic, and reflux of stomach contents around the tube. If reflux is of sufficient volume, some gastric fluid can be lost through the esophagostomy incision with subsequent metabolic consequences.

TABLE 3. MAINTENANCE ORAL ELECTROLYTE MIXTURE (One Day's Requirement for a 450 kg Horse)

Sodium chloride, NaCl	10 gm
Sodium bicarbonate, NaHCO₃	15 gm
Potassium chloride, KCl	75 gm
Potassium phosphate (dibasic anhydrous), K₂HPO₄	60 gm
Calcium chloride, CaCl₂ · 2H₂O	45 gm
Magnesium oxide, MgO	24 gm

References

1. Allden, W. G.: The effects of nutritional deprivation on the subsequent productivity of sheep and cattle. Nutr. Abstr. Rev., *40*:1167, 1970.

2. Argenzio, R. A., Lowe, J. E., Pickard, D. W., and Stevens, C. E.: Digest passage and water exchange in the equine large intestine. Am. J. Physiol., *226*:1035, 1974.

3. Baile, C. A., Naylor, J. M., McLaughlin, C. L., and Catanzaro, C. A.: Endotoxin-elicited fevers and anorexia and elfazepam-stimulated feeding. Physiol. Behav., *27*:271, 1981.

4. Blackburn, G. L., Bristrain, B. R., Maini, B. S., Schlamm, H. T., and Smith, M. F.: Nutritional and metabolic assessment of the hospitalized patient. J. Parent. Enter. Nutr., *1*:11, 1977.

5. Brown, R. F., Houpt, K. A., and Schryver, H. F.: Stimulation of food intake in horses by diazepam and promazine. Pharmacol. Biochem. Behav., *5*:495, 1976.

6. Cook, W. R.: Chronic bronchitis and alveolar emphysema in the horse. Vet. Rec., *99*:448, 1976.

7. Flack, H. L., Gans, J. A., Serlick, S. E., and Dudrick, S. J.: The current status of parenteral hyperalimentation. Am. J. Hosp. Pharmacol., *28*:326, 1971.

8. Freeman, D. E., and Naylor, J. M.: Cervical esophagostomy to permit extraoral feeding of the horse. J. Am. Vet. Med. Assoc., *172*:314, 1978.

9. Goldberger, E.: A Primer of Water, Electrolyte and Acid-Base Syndromes, 5th ed. Philadelphia, Lea and Febiger, 1975.

10. Greatorex, J. C.: Intravenous nutrition in the treatment of tetanus in the horse. Vet. Rec., *97*:498, 1975.

11. Hintz, H. F., Hogue, D. E., Walker, E. F., Lowe, J. E., and Schryver, H. F.: Apparent digestion in various segments of the digestive tract of ponies fed diets with varying roughage-grain ratios. J. Anim. Sci., *32*:245, 1971.

12. Hintz, H. F., Schryver, H. F., and Lowe, J. E.: Comparison of a blend of milk products and linseed meal as protein supplements for growing horses. J. Anim. Sci., *33*:1274, 1971.

13. Hoffsis, G. F., Gingerich, D. A., Sherman, D. M., and Bruner, R. R.: Total intravenous feeding of calves. J. Am. Vet. Med. Assoc., *171*:67, 1977.

14. Irvin, T. T.: Effects of malnutrition and hyperalimentation on wound healing. Surg. Gynecol. Obstet., *146*:33, 1978.

15. Kraegen, E. W., Chisholm, D. J., Young, J. D., and Lazarus, L.: The gastrointestinal stimulus to insulin release. II. A dual action of secretin. J. Clin. Invest., *49*:524, 1970.

16. Mackay, R. J., Iverson, W. O., and Merritt, A. M.: Exuberant granulation tissue in the stomach of a horse. Eq. Vet. J., *13*:119, 1981.

17. Morrison, F. B.: Feeds and Feeding. Ithaca, NY, Morrison Publishing Co., 1944.

18. Naylor, J. M.: The nutrition of the sick horse. J. Eq. Med. Surg., *1*:64, 1977.

19. Naylor, J. M.: Studies on an all-liquid, zero fiber, elemental diet in the horse. Dig. Dis. Sci., *22*:50, 1977 (abstract).

20. Naylor, J. M., and Kenyon, S. J.: Nutrition and neutrophil function in the horse: Implications for supportive therapy of sick horses. Proc. Am. Assoc. Eq. Prac., *24*:505, 1978.

21. Naylor, J. M., Kronfeld, D. S., and Acland, H.: Hyperlipemia in horses: Effects of undernutrition and disease. Am. J. Vet. Res., *41*:899, 1980.

22. Skinsnes, O. F., and Woolridge, R. L.: The relationship of biological defense mechanisms to the antibiotic activity of penicillin. 1. The modifying influence of penicillin on the pattern of pneumococcic infection and the immune response in the protein-depleted rat. J. Infect. Dis., *83*:78, 1948.

23. Viteri, F. E., Flores, J. M., Alvarado, J., and Behar, M.: Intestinal malabsorption in malnourished children before and during recovery. Relation between severity of protein deficiency and the malabsorption process. Am. J. Dig. Dis., *18*:201, 1973.

BILIRUBINEMIA

Jonathan M. Naylor, SASKATOON, SASKATCHEWAN, CANADA

Most cases of icterus in sick horses represent a physiologic response to poor food intake and are not indicative of hepatic damage or hemolytic anemia. For example, horses with colic may become icteric, and this is thought to be a response to anorexia. Fasting hyperbilirubinemia has been documented in many species, including cows,[4] but only in the horse is fasting bilirubinemia severe enough to cause icterus and to be confused with pathologic bilirubinemias (Table 1).

Icterus is the clinical manifestation of bilirubinemia. It imparts a yellow hue to the oral and vaginal mucosa and, most visibly, to the sclera. Dim or artificial lighting makes icterus less easy to see. The development of icterus lags behind bilirubinemia. In one study, serum bilirubin values had to be elevated above 5 mg per dl for at least 24 hours before an obvious icterus developed, and icterus persisted after the bilirubinemia returned to normal.[3]

During food deprivation, there is a progressive increase in serum bilirubin for the first three days before its concentration reaches a plateau. Serum bilirubin concentrations average a fourfold increase in fasting horses (Fig. 1), but there is much variation among individuals, and values range from 1 to 9 mg per dl.[3, 5] Breed also affects bilirubinemia. Ponies have lower resting serum bilirubin concentrations than horses and exhibit a less pronounced bilirubinemic response to fasting.[5]

The increase in total bilirubin during fasting is almost entirely due to an increase in the "indirect" or unconjugated fraction. Abnormally elevated conjugated or "direct reading" values for bilirubin indicate hepatic dysfunction or biliary obstruction. Bilirubinemia during fasting is the result of decreased hepatic clearance of bilirubin.[2] The mechanism is unknown, but there is a close correlation between the development of bilirubinemia and the

TABLE 1. CAUSES OF ICTERUS

Hemolytic
    Isoimmune hemolytic anemia
    Equine infectious anemia
    Autoimmune hemolytic anemia
    Transfusion reactions
    Babesiosis
    Phenothiazine poisoning
    Red maple poisoning
    Onion poisoning

Hepatic
    Reduced food intake
    Pyrrolizidine alkaloid poisoning
    Theiler's disease—serum hepatitis
    Tyzzer's disease
    Mycotoxicosis
    Equine infectious anemia
    Lupinosis

Cholestasis
    Usually secondary to hepatocellular damage
    Ascarids
    Cholangitis
    (Bile stone)

rise in free fatty acid concentrations (Fig. 2). It has been suggested that there may be some interference between hepatic metabolism of free fatty acids and bilirubin in fasting, possibly because of competition for transport and storage by the hepatocyte binding protein ligandin.[3]

The diagnosis of liver disease in horses rests on the detection of abnormally elevated "liver-specific" serum enzyme values (p. 251). Liver function tests such as the BSP clearance test (prolonged) and determination of prothrombin time (prolonged) and serum albumin are valuable in the diagnosis of chronic liver damage and in judging the severity of liver dysfunction. Serum urea nitrogen may also be low in some cases of severe liver disease. Abnormally elevated conjugated bilirubin values are a reliable reflection of liver dysfunction in horses. Conjugated bilirubin is water-soluble; elevated urine bilirubin indicates conjugated bilirubinemia. Interestingly, in experimental total hepatic obstruction, conjugated bilirubin is only about 50 per cent of the total.[1] The associated unconjugated bilirubinemia

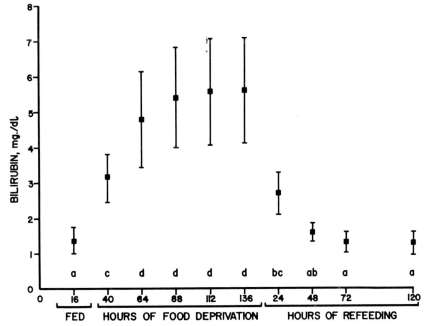

Figure 1. Effects of caloric deprivation on total serum bilirubin in six horses. Values are means ± 1 standard deviation. Letters denote significant differences at the $p < 0.05$ level using Duncan's multiple range test. (Reproduced with permission from Naylor, I. M., Kronfeld, D. S., and Johnson, K.: Fasting hyperbilirubinemia and its relationship to free fatty acids and triglycerides in the horse. Proc. Soc. Exp. Biol. Med., *165*:86, 1980.)

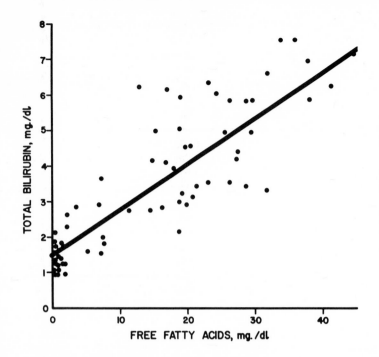

Figure 2. Graph of total bilirubin against free fatty acids. Data were gathered from eight horses during feeding and total caloric deprivation. (Reproduced with permission from Naylor, J. M., Kronfeld, D. S., and Johnson, K.: Fasting hyperbilirubinemia and its relationship to free fatty acids and triglycerides in the horse. Proc. Soc. Exp. Biol. Med., *165*:86, 1980.)

may reflect effects of secondary hepatocellular damage and anorexia.

Icterus without liver disease may indicate hemolytic anemia (p. 299). The bilirubinemia is due to elevations of the unconjugated fraction. Tests for conjugated bilirubin may give slightly elevated values (up to 0.4 gm per dl), probably because of cross-reaction with unconjugated bilirubin.

References

1. Ford, E. J. H., and Gopinath, C.: The excretion of phyllo-erythrin and bilirubin by the horse. Res. Vet. Sci., *16*:186, 1974.
2. Gronwall, R., and Mia, A. S.: Fasting hyperbilirubinemia in horses. Am. J. Dig. Dis., *17*:473, 1972.
3. Naylor, J. M., Kronfeld, D. S., and Johnson, K.: Fasting hyperbilirubinemia and its relationship to free fatty acids and triglycerides in the horse. Proc. Soc. Exp. Biol. Med., *165*:86, 1980.
4. Reid, I. M., Harrison, R. D., and Collins, R. A.: Fasting and refeeding in the lactating dairy cow. 2. The recovery of liver cell structure and function following a six-day fast. J. Comp. Pathol., *87*:253, 1977.
5. Tennant, B., Baldwin, B., Evans, C. D., and Kaneko, J. J.: Disease of the equine liver. Proc. 21st Annu. Conv. Am. Assoc. Eq. Pract., 410, 1975.

Section 3

CARDIOVASCULAR DISEASES

Edited by Christopher M. Brown

EXAMINATION OF THE CARDIOVASCULAR SYSTEM 121

LIMITATIONS OF ELECTROCARDIOGRAPHY 125

INDIRECT BLOOD PRESSURE MEASUREMENT 128

CARDIAC ARRHYTHMIAS 131

CARDIAC MURMURS 141

CONGENITAL CARDIAC LESIONS 146

BACTERIAL ENDOCARDITIS 147

THE ECG AND PERFORMANCE PREDICTION: HEART SCORE 148

PERICARDITIS 149

THROMBOPHLEBITIS 151

DISEASES OF THE GREAT VESSELS 152

AORTOILIOFEMORAL ARTERIOSCLEROSIS 153

EXAMINATION OF THE CARDIOVASCULAR SYSTEM

Christopher M. Brown, EAST LANSING, MICHIGAN

A basic evaluation of the cardiovascular system is part of any routine physical examination of a horse. A more detailed examination is often indicated in situations in which a specific problem has been previously identified or if there is reason to believe that a reduction in performance is related to cardiac disease. Often only minor abnormalities may be detected, and the problem then is to decide if such an abnormality is significant. Defining normality is often very difficult, and a familiarity with the normal equine cardiovascular system can only be obtained by careful examination of a large number of animals.

A variety of different techniques are available for the examination and evaluation of the equine cardiovascular system, and these will be considered separately. The use and usefulness of the electrocardiogram (ECG) is an important and at times controversial topic and will also be discussed separately (pp. 125 and 131).

HISTORY

As with any clinical evaluation, a detailed and accurate history can often uncover valuable information and reduce the time needed for an investigation. Frequently, horses with reduced performance are suspected of having cardiovascular problems, whereas the cause is more often related to respiratory or musculoskeletal disease. It is important to establish the duration of the problem. Horses that have never performed to expectation may well have significant cardiovascular problems, but equally it is often difficult to convince owners and trainers that an individual horse has no significant lesions and just does not have the expected potential.

OBSERVATION

Observation of the horse from a reasonable distance can be very informative. The general disposition (alert or dull, nervous or quiet, and so forth) should be noted. These behavioral and psychological factors will influence the heart and will affect the findings on auscultation and ECG. General observation will also give an opportunity to check for edema, ascites, and venous engorgement, although these are uncommon signs of heart disease in the horse. Some degree of jugular pulsation is not unusual in the normal horse. With the head in the normal position, the lower quarter of the jugular may fill and empty with each cardiac cycle. If the horse has its head down, as when grazing, both jugulars may be distended, and pulsations may pass along their whole length. This should not be misinterpreted as a clinically significant finding, as the filling is passive; the head is below the level of the right atrium.

PALPATION

Manual examination of the horse gives useful information on the functioning of the cardiovascular system. The contracting heart strikes the chest wall during systole, and this can often be felt by placing the hand on the left side of the chest in the cardiac area. The maximal impulse will usually be felt at the fifth intercostal space. The ease with which it can be felt is influenced by the conformation of the chest and the amount of subcutaneous fat. It is more easily felt in lean, narrow-chested, fit racehorses than in obese, barrel-chested ponies. The impulse is less frequently palpated on the right. The diagnostic value of the impulse beat in the horse is limited. Graphic recording of the beat is used in human apex cardiography and has been utilized in the dog. It has, however, proved difficult to record in the horse. If the impulse is palpable over a greater area than normal, it may be suggestive of cardiac enlargement; however, as conformation can influence the detection of the impulse beat, even this finding is difficult to evaluate unless the apparent change is large.

If there are severe flow disorders present in the heart or great vessels, then the low-frequency components of the murmurs they generate may be detected by palpation as a thrill. The presence of a thrill is usually indicative of a severe abnormality.

The state of the peripheral circulation can also be evaluated by palpation. The temperature of the limbs, the strength and quality of the pulse, and the capillary refill time of the mucous membranes are all helpful in evaluating the cardiovascular system. The pulse can be taken at a variety of sites, and each has its advantages and disadvantages. One most commonly used site is the facial artery where it passes from the medial to the lateral aspect of the mandible at the rostroventral border of the masseter muscle. This is a convenient site, as it can be readily palpated while holding the horse's head. However, if the horse is head-shy or has a bit in its mouth, then the constant movement will make it difficult to palpate the pulse for an adequate period of time. Another less frequently used site is the transverse facial artery, situated caudal to the lateral canthus of the eye and ventral to the zygomatic arch. This is a smaller vessel than the facial artery, and similar advantages and disadvantages apply to it. Another useful vessel is the brachial artery high on the medial aspect of the forelimb. This site allows simultaneous auscultation of the chest and palpation of the pulse. This facilitates the detection of pulse deficits and also the timing of murmurs. Rectal palpation of the terminal aorta and the cranial mesenteric and internal iliac arteries can also be helpful in assessing the state of the peripheral vasculature.

PERCUSSION

This technique for the evaluation of the equine thorax is particularly useful for conditions affecting the lungs and pleurae. It is much less useful, however, for determining cardiac enlargement and will give a convincing positive result only if the heart is markedly enlarged. The area of cardiac dullness is more readily identified on the left than on the right. Increased dullness in the cardiac area will also occur with pericardial effusion, pleural effusion, and consolidation of the ventral part of the lung. The exact cause requires additional investigation.

AUSCULTATION

Auscultation is the most valuable of all the available techniques for cardiovascular examination and, with practice, can yield a large amount of useful data concerning equine cardiac function and malfunction. The technique is simple; however, it requires patience and practice to obtain the maximal amount of information. It is advisable to always use the same stethoscope and to become very familiar with sounds of the normal horse's heart. The relationships of the equine heart to the chest wall are shown in Figure 1. Although these valve areas can be identified, they are only approximations, and the rest of the cardiac area should not be ignored during auscultation.

In many normal horses, it is possible to hear all four heart sounds. The first and second sounds are easily identified, and at heart rates below about 45, the atrial or fourth sound is audible, preceding the first. The third sound may be heard in some horses as a soft sound following the second. The relationship of the heart sounds to hemodynamic events is shown in Figure 2. Thus, on auscultation of a slowly

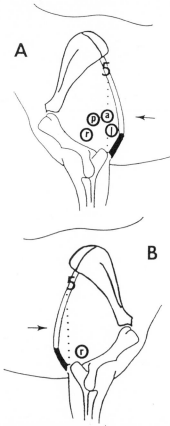

Figure 1. Approximate relationships of the heart valves to the left (*A*) and right (*B*) chest wall. The vertical broken line represents the caudal edge of the triceps muscle. The arrow is at about the level of the shoulder joint. a, aortic valve; p, pulmonic valve; r, right atrioventricular valve (tricuspid); l, left atrioventricular valve (mitral). The position of the fifth rib is also indicated.

beating horse's heart the heart sounds will be heard as

$$\begin{array}{ccccc}
\text{"Lu}-\text{lup} & \text{(pause)} & \text{dup}-\text{bup"} \\
\rightarrow \text{diastole} \quad 4 & 1 & \text{systole} \quad 2 & 3 & \text{diastole} \rightarrow
\end{array}$$

The close association of the atrial sound with the first and that of the third sound with the second may lead to the impression that the first and second sounds are split in the horse. This is not usually the case, and it is therefore very important to become familiar with the normal sounds. Equally important is the fact that sounds may vary in intensity at different sites in the cardiac area. A thorough auscultatory examination should therefore include the entire cardiac area on both sides of the chest. Just as the impulse beat is influenced by the conformation of the horse, so is the audibility of heart sounds and murmurs. Their intensity at the chest surface will also be influenced by the presence of fluid in the pericardial sac or within the pleural space.

Murmurs are often graded on their intensity at the chest surface, and an arbitrary grading system

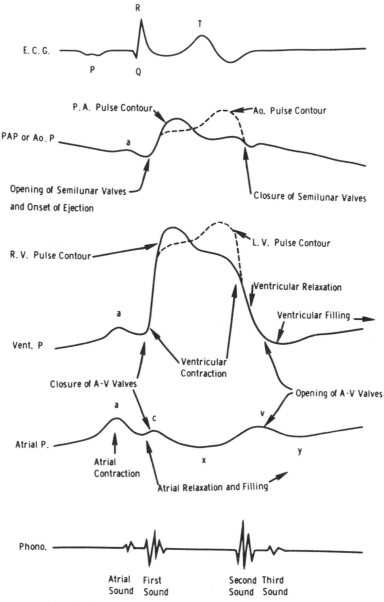

Figure 2. Schematic representation for the pressure wave forms of the right and left chambers and vessels. The illustration depicts relative shapes and timing only and bears no relationship to actual pressure values, which differ markedly between the two sides of the heart. E.C.G., bipolar electrocardiogram; PAP, pulmonary artery pressure; AOP, aortic pressure; L or RVP, left or right ventricular pressure; L or RAP, left or right atrial pressure. Phono, phonocardiogram. (From Brown C. M., and Holmes J. R.: Hemodynamics in the horse. 1. Pressure pulse contours. Equine Vet. J., *10*:188, 1978. With permission.)

has been devised to document this. The grades are one through five; Grade 1 is barely audible and very localized; Grade 2 is of low intensity, audible after careful auscultation; Grade 3 is immediately audible over a fairly wide area; Grade 4 is very loud but inaudible when the stethoscope is removed from the chest, and a thrill may also be present; Grade 5 is the loudest, widely radiating and audible with the stethoscope about 1 cm from the chest wall, and has a prominent thrill. Although numerical, this classification is qualitative and as such is very subjective.

Direct comparisons between one observer's findings and those of another cannot be too stringent. Such subdivisions as grade 2½ should be avoided. Grading a murmur is merely one individual's understanding of what is heard. It is valid only for that particular observer and that particular horse.

Disorders in flow are the usual cause of audible murmurs, but it should be remembered that not all obvious murmurs arise from significant lesions and not all significant lesions give rise to loud murmurs (p. 141). The same lesion in two horses of very different conformation may give rise to a similar murmur at the site of the lesion, which, by the time it has radiated to the chest surface, may sound very different in the two animals. Thus, comparison of Grade 2 murmur in one horse with that in another is not justified. It is possibly more useful to determine the area over which a murmur can be heard. A widely radiating murmur usually arises from a more significant lesion than one that is very localized.

The preceding paragraphs are not meant to discourage attempts to describe auscultatory findings but are presented merely to point out their limitations. It is very valuable to adopt a method for describing and recording cardiologic findings. This is particularly so if the animal is to be reevaluated at a later date. Various methods can be used, but the simplest is to have diagrams of left and right cardiac areas and then to map out the site of maximal intensity of a murmur and its area of radiation. A diagrammatic or phonetic description of the murmur can then be made alongside the diagram to show its timing, shape, duration, and quality.

PHONOCARDIOGRAPHY

Phonocardiography is the graphic recording of heart sounds and murmurs using a chest surface microphone and recording device. The technique can be useful in certain cases when timing and typing of a murmur have proved difficult by auscultation alone. It can also provide a permanent record for comparison if the animal is to be reevaluated later. Intracardiac phonocardiography has also been developed in the horse. These techniques are usually beyond the scope and needs of most practitioners.

ECHOCARDIOGRAPHY

This technique allows direct recordings of the movements and thickness of various parts of the beating heart. The initial results from the horse are extremely promising, but as yet it is still not in wide use. It will remain a technique predominantly for the specialist.

CARDIAC CATHETERIZATION

Cardiac catheterization can be very helpful, particularly in the diagnosis of suspected congenital lesions. Pressures within the cardiac chambers and great vessels can be measured, and blood can be withdrawn for gas analysis. Right heart catheterization via the jugular vein is fairly straightforward, but access to the left side via a peripheral artery is more difficult and involves greater risk. Cardiac catheterization with suitable equipment also allows cardiac output measurements to be made. However, the indications for cardiac output measurements in equine clinical cases are rare. These techniques are essentially limited to specialized practices.

RADIOGRAPHY

Thoracic radiography of adult horses yields only limited information for the cardiologist. Only lateral radiographs can be taken, and detail is often poor. Cardiac enlargement or pericardial effusion has to be great in order to make a convincing diagnosis. Intravascular contrast studies are not feasible in adult horses. However, both plain and contrast studies can be very useful in foals, particularly for the evaluation of congenital lesions.

PROTOCOL FOR EXAMINING THE EQUINE HEART

It is a good idea to develop a consistent routine for examining the cardiovascular system. The dangers of overlooking a significant problem will then be reduced. The following are personal ideas and may well not suit everyone.

After a history has been taken, the horse should be examined in a quiet, well-lit area. Preferably, someone familiar with the animal should handle it, and a miminal amount of restraint should be used. Bridles with bits are a nuisance, as the horse often mouths on the bit, making auscultation difficult. The animal should be observed at a distance and then examined manually. Any abnormality should be noted. The heart should be auscultated, usually starting on the left. This is the most important part of the examination, and it is worth spending five or more minutes on it, covering all areas on both sides. It is often difficult to examine the cranial parts of the cardiac area in heavily muscled horses. The stethoscope has to be pushed cranially on the chest wall under the caudal edge of the triceps muscle mass. This area can be better exposed if the forelimb is drawn forward, but this may be resisted by some horses.

The following are two initial questions to be asked when auscultating the heart: (1) Is the rhythm regular? (2) Are the sounds normal? If any irregularity is present, then careful auscultation may determine its cause. The presence of an audible atrial sound in most horses may be very helpful, as it indicates that the atria have contracted. Its absence in an arrhythmia suggests an absence of atrial activity. If the arrhythmia cannot be typed with confidence by auscultation, then it is wise to record an ECG at this time (p. 131). This is important, as further investigations, including exercise, may alter or abolish the arrhythmia. If the rhythm is regular but a murmur is present, then a careful determination of its type and radiation should be made before exercise, as again this may alter the findings.

After a full examination has been made at rest, it may then be necessary to exercise the horse in order to further evaluate cardiac function. This will be true if a definitive diagnosis of a serious disorder has not been made in the initial examination or if an abnormality has been detected and the influence of exercise upon it has to be determined. The amount and type of exercise to be given will vary with each case and will be determined by the age, breed, degree of fitness, and current use of the horse. There is little to be gained from working a broodmare to the point of exhaustion but equally little value in a 100-yard trot for a three-year-old in full training. Wherever the limit of exercise is set, it is often valuable to reach that level by a series of exercise periods, gradually increasing the intensity until the maximal level is obtained. The heart should be evaluated immediately after each period and alterations in rhythm and sounds noted. It may be necessary to perform additional ECG examinations, either by conventional methods or radiotelemetry, to determine the nature of an arrhythmia at high heart rates.

Either before the exercise tests or after the animal has recovered, a full ECG examination using a variety of lead systems may be considered necessary. The reasons for this and its limitations will be considered in the next section.

LIMITATIONS OF ELECTROCARDIOGRAPHY

P. W. Physick-Sheard, GUELPH, ONTARIO, CANADA

The first electrocardiographic work on the horse was published by Norr in 1913.[6] Since that time, numerous papers have been published on the equine electrocardiogram (ECG), but these data have been of limited value, in part because of a lack of standardization of recording methods and use of inappropriate lead systems.

In clinical medicine, the ECG is used in two ways: (1) a single ECG lead used to monitor cardiac rhythm and (2) multiple electrocardiographic leads used to assess changes in chamber size, to monitor intracardiac conduction defects, and, more recently, as a means of assessing cardiac size and predicting performance (p. 148). To appreciate the limitations of the ECG in the horse, a brief review of the origin and nature of the electrical activity of the heart is presented.

ORIGIN AND NATURE OF THE ECG

Each contraction of the heart is preceded by a wave of electrical activity originating in the myocardium, which is composed of a large number of individual muscle cells, each retaining a negative internal charge at rest. Depolarization results in a flow of positively charged ions into the cell, reversing the polarity. The change in charge is measured in volts, while the flow of particles or ions is electrical current.

Depolarization originates in the sinoatrial node, traverses the atria and the atrioventricular node, and is passed to the ventricular myocardium via the Purkinje system. From here the signal is passed from muscle cell to muscle cell. The resultant depolarization of sheets or "fronts" of myocardial cells generates a wave of electrical activity that sweeps through the heart. Although the signal to depolarize is almost simultaneously delivered to most areas of the myocardium, depolarization does not commence at the same time or spread in the same direction in all areas. A large number of distinct fronts are therefore generated simultaneously.

Considering only the ventricular muscle mass, at any single instant during depolarization, there is a complex three-dimensional distribution of electrical activity within and around the heart, with contributions being made by the various fronts. These areas of activity interact, some being additive, some canceling one another. Thus, at the surface of the heart, the three-dimensional or spatial pattern of electrical activity represents the algebraic sum of what is happening within the myocardium.

The various forces distributed in and around the heart at any single instant can be resolved into a single force with magnitude (volts) and direction referred to as a vector. The justification for this treatment lies in the assumption that the heart generates electrical activity as though it were a single, fixed dipole.

Just as the pattern and strength of fronts of depolarization are changing constantly during the cardiac cycle, so is the pattern that the distribution of this electrical activity describes in space around the heart. If the duration of the ventricular depolarization (QRS) were divided into an infinite number of discrete instances and if the instantaneous spatial vector were calculated at each instant, then this vector would change constantly in magnitude and direction. If these vectors were each constructed in a three-dimensional model, then their tips could be joined, and the result would be a vector loop described in space. This loop would represent an approximation of the result of all the electrical forces being generated within the heart during depolarization of the ventricles.

SINGLE-LEAD TRACINGS—CARDIAC RHYTHM

Since the electrical activity of the heart is distributed "in space," it can be viewed from any direction. By electrical convention, if from the viewpoint selected, the current flow is toward the electrode, then an upward deflection is recorded on the ECG. If the flow is away from the electrode, a negative deflection is recorded. Flow occurring at right angles to the observer results in no deflection.

Because rhythm tracings are being used to indicate the time sequence of electrical activity, it is of little consequence where the electrodes are attached, as long as the position gives a signal of large amplitude that is easy to read. The popularity of a base-apex lead results from the large deflection provided in the QRS (see section on arrhythmias).

MULTIPLE-LEAD TRACINGS—HEART AND CHAMBER SIZE

The ECG is also used to monitor the spatial distribution of cardiac electrical forces (the three-dimensional pattern referred to before). Multiple electrodes are used to view the heart from several different directions in an attempt to determine the myocardial mass. Before considering the use of the ECG, the limitations of the technique should be appreciated:

1. An ECG, recorded at the surface of the heart or at the surface of the body, represents the result of all the component electrical forces acting within the heart during the cardiac cycle. While the single resultant dipole theory holds that these components are not of individual significance, information of diagnostic value may lie only in these components and not in the results. This consideration is particularly important in the horse, in which the Purkinje system ramifies deeply into the myocardium, resulting in simultaneous depolarization of much of the ventricular mass. As a result of this, it has been suggested that most of the ventricular depolarization in the horse is electrically silent on the body surface ECG and that only the apical portion of the ventricular septum may contribute to the QRS. The body surface ECG may, therefore, contain very little information and, in the absence of any means of detecting the local component forces, may be of limited diagnostic value.

2. The ECG recorded at the body surface is modified by the electrical resistance of the tissues around the heart. This resistance is affected by breathing, changes in posture, and also by pathologic processes such as pericardial effusion.

3. While the healthy heart may approximate a dipole generator, the diseased heart may not. Since most methods of attaching the electrodes to the body (lead systems) are based upon the dipole theory, such systems may not detect significant changes occurring in equine cardiac electrical activity in the disease state.

4. Since the body surface ECG has distinct limitations as a diagnostic tool, further limitations must not be introduced by the recording method. The lead system must record the true distribution of body surface potentials with reasonable accuracy.

Einthoven's system of limb leads or modifications thereof are the methods most commonly applied to studies of the equine cardiac electrical field. The system was developed for humans and has been applied directly to the horse, in which it has severe limitations because it does not adequately sample the cardiac electrical field. Results obtained in the horse show a very wide range of normal values, and studies have shown that the conventional lead systems do not reflect the true distribution of body surface potentials. Recordings are subject to wide variations if limb position is not carefully maintained. More accurate results are obtained using a semiorthogonal system developed by Holmes.[3]

Ideally, the interpretation of the body surface ECG would be based upon a thorough understanding of the relationship between the ECG pattern and the sequence and pattern of depolarization of the different parts of the myocardium. This would allow ECG changes to be correlated with specific functional and structural abnormalities within the heart. Unfortunately, very little is known of depolarization patterns, especially in the horse, and at this time it is not possible to confidently relate the pattern of the body surface ECG to internal changes.

Further problems are encountered as a result of limited opportunity to correlate ECG changes with confirmed diagnoses. The horse possesses tremendous cardiovascular reserve and shows a low incidence of cardiovascular disease. In those cases in which dysfunction is clinically detectable, the size and value of the animal often precludes the use of such supportive studies as radiography and postmortem examination.

Using a semiorthogonal lead system to examine a series of 190 horses referred specifically for examination of the cardiovascular system, Holmes noted some association between ECG pattern and clinical findings, though the sensitivity and specificity of these changes was not determined.[3] A large number of confirmed diagnoses, preferably with detailed cardiovascular data and heart chamber weights, will be required before the correlative approach to ECG interpretation can yield results that can be applied on a routine basis.

In summary, the use of the single-lead ECG in the monitoring of cardiac function and in the definition and diagnosis of cardiac arrhythmias is well established and is of value equal to that in all other domestic species and humans. The use of multiple-lead systems to monitor changes in cardiac chamber size and conduction defects is currently a research tool. The semiorthogonal system, while showing promise, is experimental and of little immediate value for routine clinical application. The clinician is thus advised not to depend upon the multiple-lead ECG to determine changes in cardiac chamber size, to detect generalized cardiac hypertrophy, or to localize ventricular myocardial disease processes in the horse.

ATRIAL DEPOLARIZATION

Spontaneous changes in P wave occur frequently in the horse. While such changes almost certainly indicate variation in the pathway of depolarization, the large size of the sinoatrial (SA) node makes it difficult to determine whether the changes represent the activity of ectopic foci or variations in SA nodal activity, even when they are associated with arrhythmias.

The sequence of depolarization of the atria in the horse is understood to some degree, as is the relationship this bears to P wave conformation. However, the literature contains little objective information on the relationship between changes in atrial size and changes in atrial electrical activity. The multiple-lead ECG for investigating atrial function is of no more use at present than it is in investigating disease of the ventricles. The technique may, however, be of value in the definition of arrhythmias.

VENTRICULAR REPOLARIZATION

The T wave in the horse is a notoriously labile waveform. While it shows a fairly consistent pattern in the resting, fully relaxed animal, it changes progressively with rate and can change spontaneously in response to changes in autonomic tone, release of adrenal medullary hormones, exercise, and any factor modifying the load placed on the myocardium. Virtually no work has been done on the significance of changes in the spatial distribution of electrical forces during the T wave in the horse.

Before even attempting to interpret the T wave, it is essential to ascertain that the animal was fully relaxed during the recording. If this condition is met and the waveform deviates from what is normally expected in the lead recorded, then it may be in order to register the change as abnormal. The changes, however, are generally nonspecific and are of little help in arriving at a definitive diagnosis. They may be used with great caution as an indicator that there may be some primary or secondary abnormality of the ventricular myocardium. Conversely, failure of the T wave to achieve the contour usually seen under circumstances of increased load may also imply myocardial dysfunction. While loss of amplitude of the T wave is seen in hypokalemia, the actual waveform will depend very much upon heart rate and upon the type of arrhythmia precipitated by the electrolyte imbalance. Similar observations can be made with regard to the ST segment. Identification of abnormality depends very much upon thorough familiarity with the normal range of variation under defined conditions. Ideally, the clinician should avoid placing too much significance on changes in the T wave in the equine electrocardiogram.

References

1. Getty, R.: Sisson and Grossman's The Anatomy of the Domestic Animals, 5th Ed. Philadelphia, W. B. Saunders Co., 1975, p. 556.
2. Hamlin, R. L., Smetzer, D. L., and Smith, C. R.: Analysis of QRS complex recorded through a semiorthogonal lead system in the horse. Am. J. Physiol., 207:325, 1964.
3. Holmes, J. R.: Spatial vector changes during ventricular depolarization using a semiorthogonal lead system—a study of 190 cases. Equine Vet. J., 8:1, 1976.
4. Holmes, J. R., and Darke, P. G. G.: Studies on the development of a new lead system for equine electrocardiography. Equine Vet. J., 2:12, 1970.
5. Muylle, E., and Oyaert, W.: Equine electrocardiography. The genesis of the different configurations of the "QRS" complex. Zbl. Vet. Med., 24:762, 1977.
6. Norr, J.: Das Elektrokardiogram des Pferdes seine Aufnahine und Form. A. Biol., 61:197, 1913.

INDIRECT BLOOD PRESSURE MEASUREMENT

B. W. Parry, WERRIBEE, VICTORIA, AUSTRALIA

The values obtained by indirect blood pressure (BP) measurement are an approximation of actual arterial pressures, which can only be truly measured by arterial puncture. Indirect methods are atraumatic, noninvasive, and therefore readily repeatable.

Recently, ultrasonic probes that detect blood flow[*, †] and arterial wall motion[‡] and an electronically modified oscillometric technique[§] have been verified, by comparison with directly measured arterial pressure, to be reasonably accurate methods for BP measurement in the horse. The ultrasonic probes utilize Doppler frequency shifts to produce audible sounds that correlate with the arterial events of systolic pressure (SP) and diastolic pressure (DP). The new oscillometric technique measures SP, mean arterial pressure (MAP), and DP by electronic observation of pressure fluctuations in the occlusive bladder.

TECHNIQUE

The middle coccygeal artery is the most common site for indirect BP measurement in the horse, as it is readily accessible, reasonably immobile, surrounded by little perivascular tissue or muscle, backed by bone, and maintained under high pressure, despite its small size, owing to its proximity to the aorta.

To measure BP, a pneumatic rubber bladder is centered squarely over the middle coccygeal artery, at the base of the tail, and secured snugly in place by its outer inelastic self-adhesive cloth sleeve. If the cuff is applied very tightly, the artery may be partially or totally occluded, resulting in spuriously low BP readings. Conversely, BP may be overestimated by a loosely applied cuff. In general, snug application of the cuff is easily achieved, and errors due to incorrect cuff tension would be unusual. Little practice is required to ensure that cuff application is standardized between measurements.

The bladder is connected to an inflation/deflation device and manometer calibrated in millimeters of mercury (mm Hg). With the oscillometric method, no further steps are necessary; however, the Doppler probes must be aligned over the artery so that good pulse sounds are audible. To facilitate acoustic contact, an ultrasonic coupling gel is interfaced between the probe and skin. The occlusive bladder is inflated to at least 20 mm Hg above the anticipated SP (at least 20 mm Hg after sounds are abolished) and then deflated slowly at a rate not exceeding 2 to 3 mm Hg per heartbeat to ensure that BP is not underestimated.

SP and DP criteria vary with the instrument used. The first audible sound is taken as SP with both types of ultrasonic probe. Diastolic pressure is recorded as the entry of a distinct second sound when using a blood flow detector. Occasionally DP readings are not possible owing to poor or absent DP sounds. However, with probes that sense arterial wall motion, DP is read at the point at which there is an audible change in volume or pitch or both, or the point at which two distinct sounds disappear or a constant rumble begins. The new oscillometric technique uses electronic circuitry to note the point at which bladder pressure fluctuations begin to increase in amplitude, taken as SP, then the point of maximum bladder pressure oscillations, taken as MAP, and finally the point at which bladder pressure fluctuations cease to decrease in amplitude, taken as DP. With all techniques, the bladder should be fully deflated between readings to allow the return of trapped venous blood.

Accurate indirect BP measurement requires that the correct occlusive bladder width (BW) be used. The appropriate size is proportional to the tail girth (TG), measured at the base of the tail. Recommendations vary with the technique employed. Thus, with the ultrasonic blood flow detector, a BW:TG ratio of 0.48 underestimates SP and overestimates DP by about 9 per cent, while for the oscillometric technique a BW:TG ratio of 0.20 to 0.25 has been recommended for measurement of MAP. Use of a bladder that is too narrow results in overestimation of BP, while one that is too wide underestimates BP. The former effect is more pronounced than the latter, and, therefore, it is generally better to use a BW larger than recommended if the correct one is unavailable.

To date, little work using the electronic oscillometric technique on horses has been published, and all further comments will be restricted to studies utilizing Doppler probes.

Bladder widths of 9, 10, and 11 cm have been advocated for equine BP measurement with Doppler probes. As the TG of mature horses is about 21

---

*Ultrasonic Stethoscope, BF4A, Medasonics, Inc., Mountainview, CA
†Parks Electronics Laboratory, Beaverton, OR
‡Arteriosonde, Hoffman-La Roche, Inc., Cranbury, NJ
§Dinamap, Applied Medical Research, Tampa, FL

128

to 23 cm, SP and DP would be respectively underestimated and overestimated by about 5 to 12 per cent with these bladders when using an ultrasonic blood flow detector. A few ponies and young horses (TG about 18 cm) require narrower bladders, while mature draught horses (TG often 25 cm) usually need wider ones. Provided a BW:TG ratio of about 0.5 is employed, BP values may be recorded as read.

Blood pressure readings may be corrected to heart level or may be quoted unchanged as coccygeal, uncorrected values (CUCV). Two external landmarks have been used as reference points for correction to heart level: the notch on the lateral tuberosity of the humerus (correction to shoulder level) and the olecranon (correction to elbow level). A 1 cm column of blood exerts the same pressure as 0.77 mm Hg. In mature horses, where the notch on the lateral tuberosity of the humerus is about 35 cm below the level of the tail, approximately 27 mm Hg must be added to the coccygeal BP value to correct it to shoulder level. Similarly, to correct to elbow level, on average about 54 cm below the level of the tail, approximately 42 mm Hg must be added. The former landmark is a good external reference point for the position of the cranial vena cava in standing horses and consequently a better site than the olecranon for correction to heart level. Corrected readings should be quoted as coccygeal, shoulder-corrected values (CCV_{Sh}) or coccygeal, elbow corrected values (CCV_E).

Correction to heart level is generally unnecessary, as the middle coccygeal artery has become the standard site for indirect BP measurement in horses. However, most direct BP studies correct their readings to either the shoulder or the elbow, and comparison of coccygeal BP values would require appropriate corrections.

When measuring resting BP, it is advisable to have an attendant restrain the horse in a normal, relaxed, standing posture. Gentle halter restraint facilitates acceptance of the BP measurement routine by the subject and helps to limit changes in head height. Coccygeal BP may decrease by 25 mm Hg if the horse lowers its head about 120 cm. Some horses initially resist cuff application or bladder inflation and must be allowed a few minutes to become accustomed to the procedure. The importance of gentle, patient handling to prevent excitement cannot be overemphasized. Environmental disturbances should be minimal; resting values may not be obtained if the horse has been recently exercised, is being fed, or is distracted by noises. Occasionally animals will persistently fidget, making BP measurement difficult and the recording of true resting values doubtful. In all cases, at least three consecutive BP readings should be made to ensure that the values recorded are representative of the horse's

cardiovascular status at that time. If marked variations in both SP and DP occur between consecutive readings, the animal should be reassured and further readings made after a brief pause. Such horses may or may not be overtly nervous but usually settle down after a few minutes, and consistent values may then be recorded. Sometimes DP is steady but SP fluctuates between observations. Such subjects often fail to settle down, and they are noted to have labile SP. The significance of this finding has not been established, but these horses are often fractious in nature. In quiet, resting horses, BP values do not usually change by more than 6 mm Hg between consecutive readings; frequently this variation is only 2 to 3 mm Hg.

NORMAL VALUES

Normal resting BP (all values are reported as systolic pressure ± SD/diastolic pressure ± SD) for 456 Thoroughbreds in the United States were reported as $111.8 ± 13.3/69.7 ± 13.8$ mm Hg CUCV. A similar study of 97 Thoroughbreds in Australia quoted resting pressures of $117.8 ± 17.1/84.4 ± 13.4$ mm Hg CUCV. The latter survey included 97 Standardbreds and 102 nonracing horses with resting values of $107.5 ± 15.1/72.1 ± 13.9$ mm Hg CUCV and $111.1 ± 15.9/75.4 ± 13.0$ mm Hg CUCV, respectively. The overall average for 296 horses was $112.1 ± 16.5/77.3 ± 14.3$ mm Hg CUCV. Both surveys showed no significant age or sex effect on BP, and the Australian study demonstrated no significant effect of heart rate on BP; however, there was a significant effect of class on BP.

Although three or more consecutive readings are suggested to record a horse's resting BP, a single, normal BP value for an individual is a concept, not a reality. Blood pressure varies from moment to moment, depending on physiologic demands, environmental stimuli, and so forth; hence, for any animal there will be a range of normal BP values, with changes of up to about 15 mm Hg possible between observations. Thus, measurements of resting BP attempt to determine a value within the individual's range of normal pressures.

Similarly, it is difficult to define limits for normal BP. Hypertension and hypotension are valuable concepts, but the points at which they are deemed to occur are arbitrarily defined, and unless pathologic processes can be consistently ascribed to "abnormally" high or low readings, their merit is dubious. From the survey of American Thoroughbreds it was suggested that normal equine BP might be defined as ± 1SD from the mean value. Such a narrow range would define approximately one sixth of horses surveyed as hypertensive. Wider limits on normality (for human BP) have been advocated by some workers, with normal defined as ±40 per cent from the mean, borderline hypertensive and borderline hypotensive as the following 7.5 per cent above and below these limits, and abnormally hypertensive and abnormally hypotensive as the remaining 2.5 per cent beyond the borderline limits. At present, limits for normal equine BP are fairly subjective. Until more work is reported, it is probably wise when quoting an animal as hypertensive or hypotensive to state the BP value recorded and possibly the range of values considered normal.

USE IN ANESTHESIA

Preanesthetic BP measurement should be encouraged as part of the routine case work-up, to help define good and poor anesthetic risk cases and thus permit the anesthetist to tailor premedication and anesthetic regimens to suit the individual horse.

No correction of BP readings to heart level is needed in the recumbent horse because the tail and the heart are at nearly the same height. Blood pressure measurement is an extremely useful anesthetic monitor. It is a reliable guide to the depth of anesthesia, decreasing with increasing blood concentration of inhalation anesthetic agent. Further, it is generally a more sensitive indicator of cardiovascular status during surgery than are cardiac auscultation, arterial palpation, or electrocardiography. Blood pressure will vary according to the anesthetic regimen used. In the stable, surgically anesthetized horse, SP will usually be in the range of 75 to 100 mm Hg, and unless the plane of anesthesia or the status of the cardiovascular system is changing, it will usually vary by less than 5 mm Hg between readings. When monitoring anesthetic cases, the BP cuff is usually left in place between readings. Doppler probes may be connected to or may have a built-in loudspeaker so that continuous audible information on the character of the middle coccygeal arterial pulse, namely its rate, rhythm, and amplitude, are broadcast between BP readings.

USE IN CASES OF ACUTE ABDOMINAL DISEASE

Blood pressure measurement is an important aid in the routine clinical evaluation of equine abdominal crises. When used in conjunction with heart rate, oral mucosal membrane color, hydration and capillary refill rate, jugular filling rate, and hematocrit, an accurate assessment of the horse's cardiovascular status can be made and appropriate therapy initiated and monitored.

Hypertension, normotension, and hypotension have all been described in equine colic cases and may all occur at some stage in each case. Visceral pain frequently results in arterial hypertension (BP about 145/105 or higher) and moderate tachycardia. Treatment of the inciting cause of pain, for example, gastric distention relieved by passing a stomach tube or palliative analgesic therapy or both, is often successful in controlling overt signs of pain and consequently lowering heart rate and BP. Acetylpromazine and other phenothiazine derivatives are ill-advised in colic cases, especially without prior BP measurement, as their hypotensive side effects may exacerbate mild, clinically inapparent shock.

Shock is a common complication of equine abdominal accidents, colitis X, and severe salmonellosis. It may be due to a number of factors, including hypovolemia, endotoxemia, and bacteremia. Blood pressure measurement helps to define the degree of cardiovascular collapse and the urgency for supportive therapy. It does not preclude a thorough physical and clinicopathologic investigation of the case but does provide valuable ancillary information. Colic cases with a SP of less than 80 mm Hg CUCV generally have a poor prognosis; however, aggressive fluid therapy, possibly coupled with large doses of short-acting corticosteroids, may help to bolster circulating blood volume, thus restoring venous return and consequently arterial BP. Systolic pressures of approximately 40 mm Hg CUCV have been recorded in some cases of shock. Severely hypotensive horses may often have no detectable arterial sounds and therefore indeterminable BP. Prolonged hypotension (generally less than 70 mm Hg CUCV for several hours) usually causes irreparable tissue damage due to ischemia, and even if BP can be restored to normal levels, the prognosis is usually grave.

When measuring BP in colic cases, it is important to make certain that the animal is standing in a normal relaxed posture (p. 129). Mentally depressed horses tend to hang the head, consequently lowering systemic arterial pressure. If an attendant physically raises the animal's head, coccygeal BP usually rises, often by about 10 to 15 mm Hg. Obviously when BP is being used as a prognostic guide, this may alter the assessment of the case.

The efficacy of fluid therapy is best monitored by arterial BP measurements. Indwelling jugular catheters to measure central venous pressure are probably unnecessary in the horse, especially if arterial pressure is measured, as overhydration is very unlikely, and it is not possible to distinguish an increase in central venous pressure due to improved venous return (associated with effective fluid administration) from venous congestion due to cardiac failure. On the other hand, when monitoring arterial BP, improved circulatory function is readily demonstrated by an increase in systemic pressure.

In summary, arterial BP can now be simply and reliably measured in horses. Currently, hypertension and hypotension have been observed in a few diseases, and some therapeutic implications have resulted. However, clinical equine BP measurement is in its infancy, and much work has yet to be done. The present noninvasive techniques will allow veterinarians the opportunity to investigate the role of BP abnormalities in equine medicine.

Supplemental Readings

Garner, H. E.: Update on equine laminitis. Vet. Clin. North Am. Large Anim. Pract., 2:25, 1980.

Gay, C. C., Carter, J., McCarthy, M., Mason, T. A., Christie, B. A., Reynolds, W. T. and Smyth, B.: The value of arterial blood pressure measurement in assessing the prognosis in equine colic. Eq. Vet. J., 9:202, 1977.

Geddes, L. A.: The Direct and Indirect Measurement of Blood Pressure. Chicago, Year Book Medical Pub., 1970.

Hood, D. M.: Current concepts of the physiopathology of laminitis. Proc. 25th Annual Meeting, Am. Assoc. Equine Pract., December 1979, pp. 13–20.

Meagher, D. M.: Clinical evaluation and management of shock in the equine patient. Vet. Clin. North Am., 6:245, 1976.

Soma, L. R.: Textbook of Veterinary Anesthesia. Baltimore, The Williams and Wilkins Co., 1971.

CARDIAC ARRHYTHMIAS

Ronald W. Hilwig, TUCSON, ARIZONA

The most important consideration in the treatment of cardiac arrhythmias in horses is an accurate diagnosis of the arrhythmia coupled with an assessment of its significance. Corrective therapy should not be attempted without first determining the probable cause of the arrhythmia. The horse has a higher incidence of cardiac arrhythmias at rest than any other domestic livestock species, the autonomic nervous system being responsible for most of these resting arrhythmias. Arrhythmias in a resting horse should not be looked upon as abnormal in an otherwise healthy animal, since autonomic-induced arrhythmias almost invariably disappear when the heart rate is elevated by exercise, excitement, or administration of anticholinergic drugs. Numerous organic diseases and underlying physiologic imbalances as well as myocardial disease may precipitate resting cardiac arrhythmias. Frequently, treatment of the primary disease or correction of imbalances corrects the arrhythmia.

Postexercise or excitement alterations in cardiac rhythm, excluding simple increased heart rate, should be viewed with suspicion, especially if accompanied by reduced performance, weakness, or dyspnea. Many changes occur in normal electrocardiogram (ECG) waveforms at increased heart rates, and these must not be confused with abnormalities. A thorough ECG examination must include tracings obtained at rest, immediately after exercise, and during the cool-down period, since some arrhythmias may be evident only transiently or during one of these periods.

The majority of arrhythmias are initially detected by careful auscultation of the patient, and some can be adequately diagnosed by this means alone. Signs and symptoms that may accompany an abnormal cardiac arrhythmia include lack of exercise tolerance and poor performance, labored breathing, pulmonary edema, ascites and dependent edema, abnormal arterial pulses, and jugular vein pulsations. A thorough physical examination should be performed on the animal suspected of having an abnormal heart rhythm.

The most reliable means of diagnosing normal and abnormal cardiac arrhythmias is with the ECG. Treatment, if any, should be deferred until the ECG examination is completed. A simple single-channel recorder is adequate for routine diagnosis. Chart speeds of 25 mm per sec and 50 mm per sec are preferable, but a single speed of 25 mm per sec will suffice for most cases.

If the limb leads are used, then muscle tremor and subtle shifting movements to maintain body position often result in ECG recordings that are of little value. Various "monitor" leads have come into use for evaluation of cardiac electrical activity. These have the advantages of minimizing movement artifacts and allowing the generation of relatively larger waveforms. One such lead system found satisfactory by the author places the right forelimb electrode on the right side of the neck along the jugular groove about one third of the way up the neck from the torso. The left forelimb electrode is placed on the ventral midline under the apex of the heart. Alligator clips, preferably copper, are used with suitable electrode paste to attach the electrodes to the skin. The ground electrode (right hindlimb) is usually placed on the left forelimb, but any site remote from the heart may be used for placement of this electrode. Lead I is selected on the recorder. This monitor lead has the advantages of being relatively indifferent to limb position and positional changes and provides large amplitude waveforms that allow the sensitivity of the recorder to be reduced, thereby reducing muscle tremor artifacts. Figure 1 illustrates a typical ECG tracing recorded with this lead system.

The duration of ECG waveforms and time inter-

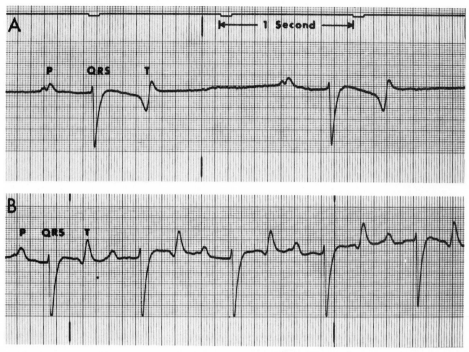

Figure 1. Recording from a normal horse at a resting heart rate of 33 BPM (*A*) and the same horse after light exercise at a rate of 80 BPM (*B*). At increased heart rates, all time intervals and waveforms are abbreviated, and the two positive components of the P wave are less evident. The T wave has lost much of its negative component and is of higher positive amplitude. Paper speed 50 mm per sec.

vals for normal adult horses and ponies is shown in Table 1.

All time durations are shortened at higher heart rates. Resting ECG durations should be determined at heart rates greater than 22 but less than 50 beats per min. Resting rates outside these limits should be considered as bradycardia and tachycardia, respectively, except in ponies, which may have resting rates exceeding 50.

Postexercise or excitement alterations in the ECG include increased amplitude and peaking of the P and T waves, shifting of T wave polarity, and deviation of the S–T segment. Figure 1 shows the normal resting ECG and the changes following exercise. The S–T segment usually slopes toward the initial limb of the T wave. S–T segment deviations greater

TABLE 1. DURATION IN MILLISECONDS OF ECG WAVEFORMS AND INTERVALS FROM NORMAL ADULT HORSES AND PONIES

	P Wave	P–R Interval	QRS Complex	Q–T Interval
Horses				
Range	80–200	220–560	80–170	320–640
Mean	140	330	130	510
Ponies				
Range	85–106	209–226	66–86	420–483
Mean	100	217	78	462

than 0.2 mv above or below baseline in the resting ECG are considered abnormal.

DETECTION AND SIGNIFICANCE

SUPRAVENTRICULAR ARRHYTHMIAS

Sinus Arrhythmia (Fig. 2). This normal resting arrhythmia appears on the ECG tracing as a varying P–P or R–R interval and missed beats. This condition is normal at resting heart rates and is attributed to waxing and waning of vagal tone. The arrhythmia is eliminated by increased heart rates or by administration of anticholinergic drugs such as belladonna alkaloids (e. g., atropine).

Wandering or Shifting Atrial Pacemaker (Fig. 2). This condition appears as a progressive or abrupt alteration in P wave contour and may, but not always, be accompanied by changes in the P–R interval. Sinus arrhythmia or missed beats or both accompany this condition. The wandering pacemaker cannot be detected by auscultation, but the missed beats are diagnosed as a silent period during the time a beat is expected. Occasionally the fourth (atrial) heart sound alone can be heard during a missed beat. While some authors consider this condition abnormal, others feel that it is a normal shifting of the pacemaker within the sinoatrial node. Approximately 30 per cent of normal resting horses

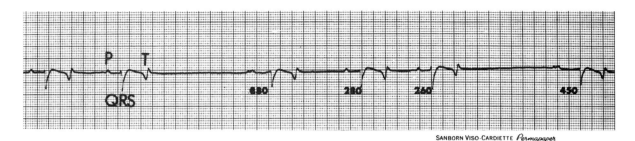

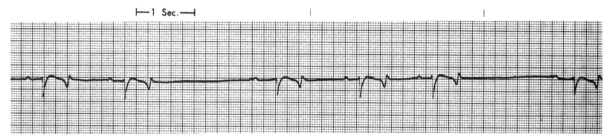

Figure 2. Continuous recording from a normal horse showing sinus arrhythmia and wandering atrial pacemaker. This rhythm was correlated with respiratory activity. The long pauses between sets of three beats occurred during expiration. The P–R (P–Q) interval, shown in milliseconds, is longest on the beat following the pause, and the P wave configuration is much different for that beat. One might argue that SA block had occurred during the long pause, since another beat would almost fit perfectly into the rhythm during this period. The simple surface ECG recording could not detect this condition if it occurred. Paper speed 25 mm per sec.

exhibit this wandering pacemaker, but during excitement or exercise when vagal tone is overridden, it is abolished. No treatment is indicated with either sinus arrhythmia or wandering atrial pacemaker.

Supraventricular Premature Beats (Figs. 3 and 9). Spontaneous discharge of a pacemaker located within the SA node, the atria, or the AV junction before the normal pacemaker discharges may elicit a supraventricular premature beat. The P wave may or may not appear and be different from normal, but the QRS complexes are similar to those of the basic rhythm. The P wave may be superimposed on the trailing edge of the preceding T wave, thereby distorting its configuration. SA node and atrial premature beats are not usually followed by a compensatory pause, although AV junction premature beats may occasionally be followed by a compensatory pause. Most authors view this condition as being indicative of cardiac disease.

Careful auscultation can detect the presence of premature beats, but the focus of origin cannot be determined without use of the ECG machine. Most premature beats of supraventricular origin result in first and second heart sounds of less than normal intensity that may or may not be followed by a compensatory pause. The arterial pulse for the premature beat is weaker than normal, and the beat following the premature beat produces a pulse of normal or increased amplitude.

Tachycardias (Fig. 3). Short bursts of supraventricular premature beats are termed paroxysmal nodal, atrial, or junctional tachycardia. If the tachycardia persists, the term paroxysmal is dropped.

These conditions can be detected by auscultation as an abrupt change in heart rate accompanied by rapid and weak arterial pulsations. The differentiation between supraventricular and ventricular origin cannot be made by auscultation alone. The supraventricular tachycardias should be considered to indicate myocardial disease predisposing to atrial fibrillation and should be treated to prevent its onset.

Atrial Fibrillation (Fig. 4). Atrial fibrillation is characterized by an absence of discrete P waves preceding each QRS complex. The P waves are replaced by fine, coarse, or variable atrial waves known as F waves or fibrillation waves. The frequency of occurrence of these waves may be as high as 500 per minute. The ventricles are not able to respond this frequently, and the QRS complex occurs irregularly at 50 to 120 beats per minute at rest. Occasionally a relatively slow but irregular QRS frequency of 25 to 35 beats per minute may appear with this arrhythmia. At higher ventricular rates, S–T segment deviation from baseline and T wave peaking may be observed on the ECG. A variable intensity of heart sounds, absence of the fourth (atrial) heart sound, a very irregular heart rate, and arterial pulsus alternans and pulse deficit are invariably observed with this condition. Some horses at rest have no outward signs of the arrhythmia, whereas others exhibit dyspnea, dependent edema, ascites, and jugular pulsations. Invariably animals with atrial fibrillation have reduced exercise or work performance, and this is sometimes the only complaint that initiates the cardiac examination.

An unfavorable prognosis should be given if a

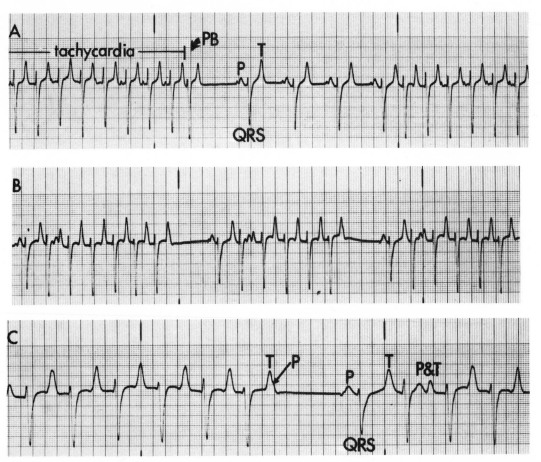

Figure 3. Supraventricular tachycardia. Tracing *A* (paper speed 25 mm per sec) shows paroxysmal atrial tachycardia with a heart rate of 180 BPM, followed again by the tachycardia. A supraventricular premature beat (PB) interrupts the tachycardia and is followed by a compensatory pause, which allows the sinus node pacemaker to capture the rhythm for four beats before another supraventricular premature beat precipitates a bout of tachycardia. Tracing *B* shows atrial tachycardia with a heart rate of 160 BPM interrupted by an occasional sinus beat. Tracing C was recorded at twice the speed (50 mm per sec) as *B* to show the P wave superimposed upon the T wave preceding the sinus beat. The P wave blocked the tachycardia pacemaker and allowed the sinus node to capture the ventricle for a beat before the atrial pacemaker assumed control again. Note the P wave between the QRS complex and T wave of the first postsinus beat.

murmur or AV valve insufficiency is auscultated in the presence of this arrhythmia. Occasionally, atrial fibrillation develops for no apparent reason or is secondary to organic disease or electrolyte imbalance. Most horses with this type of fibrillation can be converted to sinus rhythm, and many will return to equal or better than prearrhythmia performance. Those with valvular disease–caused fibrillation usually do not have a favorable outcome.

Cases of paroxysmal atrial fibrillation have been reported in young racehorses. They performed poorly in a race and were found to be fibrillating immediately afterward. They reverted to sinus rhythm within 24 hours. Some then returned to normal performance. The incidence of this condition in racehorses is unknown.

Atrioventricular (AV) Block (Fig. 5 and 6). This arrhythmia takes three major forms: (1) first degree, which is seen as a prolonged P–R interval; (2) second degree, in which some P waves are not followed by a QRS complex; and (3) third degree, in which P waves and QRS complexes occur independently from each other. First-degree AV block is due to waxing and waning of vagal tone. Second-degree block is of two types, type 1 or Wenckebach phenomenon and type 2. The type 2 block is uncommon and appears as a missed QRS complex without impending ECG signs. The type 1 block is characterized by progressive lengthening of the P–R interval until a P wave is not followed by a QRS complex. Minor variations of this progressive-type block have also been reported. The first postblock beat is characterized by a decreased Q–T interval and diminished T wave amplitude and high-amplitude arterial pulse. The missed beats are detected on auscultation as described before. If missed beats appear infrequently, no treatment is indicated, since this is thought to be vagally induced. First- and second-

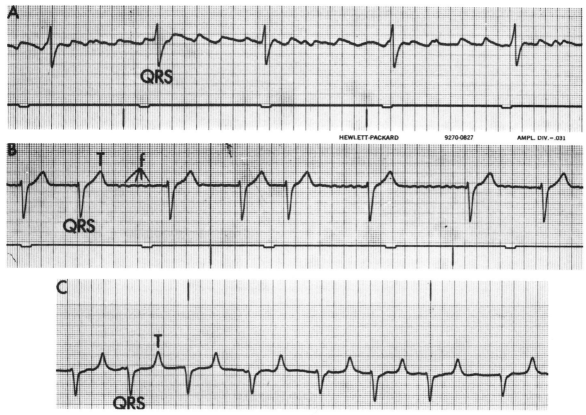

Figure 4. Tracings of atrial fibrillation from three different horses showing the variability of this arrhythmia. Tracing *A* shows coarse undulations of the baseline, which represent the electrical activity of the atria. QRS complexes occur at quite regular intervals at 60 BPM. T waves cannot be distinguished from the atrial waves. Tracing *B* shows fine undulations of atrial activity and a relatively fast, irregular heart rate of approximately 98 BPM. Both QRS complexes and T waves are readily observed. Tracing *C* shows atrial fibrillation with almost no baseline undulations of atrial origin and a rapid, quite regular heart rate of 120 BPM. QRS complexes and T waves are well defined. Paper speed in all tracings was 50 mm per sec.

degree blocks normally disappear at elevated heart rates.

Third-degree AV block is a pathologic condition characterized by a relatively slow heart rate that may not be altered by excitement or exercise. Pauses of 40 to 50 seconds between beats have been observed, and fainting or staggering bouts may occur especially upon exertion. The QRS complexes may appear quite normal or may be bizarre, depending upon the site of origin of the pacemaker. First and second heart sounds are altered only minimally, if at all. In some cases, discrete fourth (atrial) sounds are audible but are not correlated with the first and second sounds. Cardiac diseases cannot always be demonstrated in animals with this arrhythmia, and treatment is usually unsuccessful.

VENTRICULAR ARRHYTHMIAS

Ventricular Premature Beats (Fig. 7). Spontaneous discharge of a latent pacemaker located in the specialized conduction tissue of the interventric-ular septum or ventricular myocardium may result in a bizarre-appearing ventricular ECG waveform. Premature ventricular beats appear earlier than expected and are characterized by prolonged and large QRS and T waves. The beat may be either interpolated, wherein it falls between two normal beats (a true extrasystole), or noninterpolated, wherein the abnormal beat is followed by a compensatory pause with little or no change in heart rate. The origin of the premature beat may be determined by the polarity of the QRS complex. Using the monitor lead system described before, a beat originating from the right ventricle will have a positive QRS complex, and one originating from the left ventricle will have a negative QRS complex. Presence of ventricular premature beats at rest is indicative of myocardial disease or cellular electrolyte imbalances. This arrhythmia is frequently noted during inhalation anesthesia, especially if surgery is being performed on the gut for obstruction or torsion.

Auscultation alone is not sufficient to differentiate this arrhythmia from supraventricular premature beats, although several circumstances may suggest

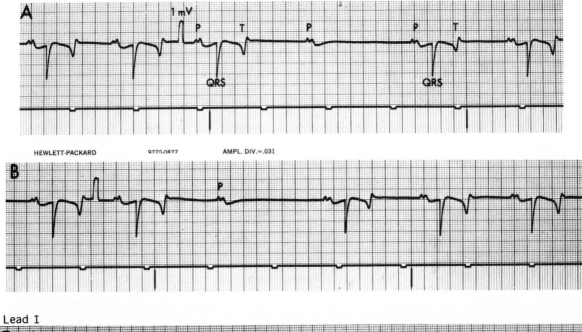

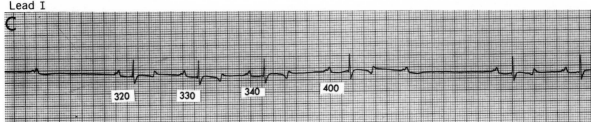

Figure 5. Tracings *A* and *B* are continuous and show type 2 second-degree atrioventricular block wherein the electrical signal from the atria is not conducted to the ventricle. This type of block has no pattern and appears as a random P wave that is not followed by a QRS complex. Tracing *C* shows type 1 second-degree atrioventricular block, which is characterized by an increasing P–R (P–Q) interval (shown in milliseconds) until a P wave is not followed by the QRS complex. Paper speed 25 mm per sec.

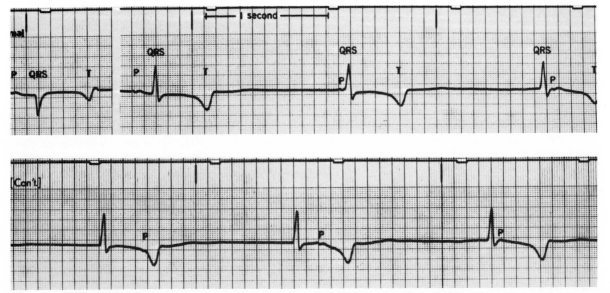

Figure 6. Continuous recording showing complete or third-degree atrioventricular block. A normal waveform is shown as a reference on the upper left. P waves occur at regular intervals but are not conducted to the ventricle. A right ventricular focus has assumed pacemaker function at a relatively fixed rate of 40 BPM. Paper speed 50 mm per sec.

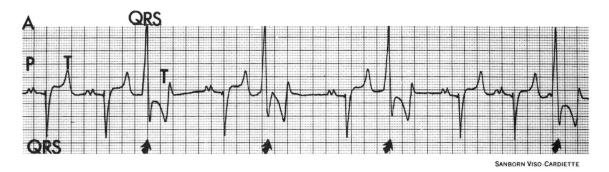

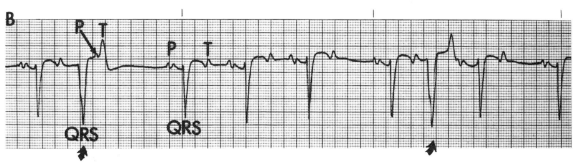

Figure 7. Tracing *A* shows ventricular premature beats or extrasystoles (arrows) originating from the right ventricle. The QRS complexes of these ectopic beats are large and wide and are followed by a large, opposite-polarity T wave. Tracing *B* shows ventricular premature beats (arrows) originating from the left ventricle. The QRS complexes of the ectopic beats are large and wide and are followed by a large, opposite-polarity T wave. The ectopic beat on the left of this tracing is noninterpolated, since it is followed by a compensatory pause, whereas the ectopic beat on the right of this tracing is interpolated and does not disrupt the basic rhythm. Paper speed 25 mm per sec.

a ventricular origin. In many cases, the extra ventricular beat results in louder than normal first, second, or first and second heart sounds, and the arterial pulse is weak or absent. Compensatory pauses more frequently accompany ventricular premature beats than atrial premature beats. The first postpremature ventricular beat produces louder than normal heart sounds and a stronger than normal arterial pulse. Premature supraventricular beats frequently produce less than normal intensity first and second heart sounds and only a slight change in arterial pulse amplitude on the first postpremature beat. These circumstances are only presumptive, and ECG diagnosis must be established prior to treatment if any is to be undertaken.

Ventricular Tachycardia (Fig. 8). Short or long bursts of ectopic ventricular depolarizations may periodically appear on the ECG tracing. This condition is known as paroxysmal ventricular tachycardia and may be accompanied by premature ventricular beats. If long-standing over several seconds or minutes, the term paroxysmal is dropped. Paroxysmal ventricular tachycardia and ventricular tachycardia are ominous signs of cardiac disease and predispose to ventricular fibrillation, a terminal event. During a bout of tachycardia, the ECG may show occasional P waves, normal QRS complexes, and fusion beats (a normal beat superimposed upon an ectopic beat) that are inscribed during a relatively quiet period of electrical activity. The ectopic focus of activity may be unifocal or multifocal, giving either one or more types of ventricular waveforms, respectively. Multifocal ventricular tachycardia is highly suggestive of myocardial disease but also appears as a result of a combination of inhalation anesthetic administration and electrolyte imbalance. This arrhythmia must be treated vigorously to prevent its progression to ventricular fibrillation. Auscultation alone cannot differentiate this condition from paroxysmal supraventricular tachycardias, since they both are heard as abrupt changes in heart rate. More frequently in a ventricular-induced tachycardia, the first and second heart sounds become much louder and the heart rate much higher than in supraventricular-induced tachycardias. Exceptions to this generality, of course, exist.

Ventricular Fibrillation (Fig. 8). This arrhythmia is terminal, and all organized electrical and contractile activity of the heart ceases. The ECG shows irregular oscillations of varying amplitudes and frequencies. No heart sounds are heard, and arterial pulsations are absent. Treatment is universally unsuccessful.

Complex arrhythmias with several ECG abnormalities are also seen occasionally (Fig. 9). Multiple pacemaker sites can be demonstrated by the varia-

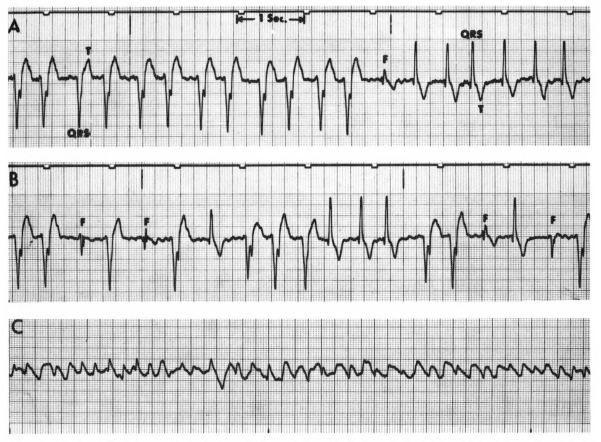

Figure 8. Tracing *A* illustrates ventricular tachycardia from a left ventricular focus in the left two thirds of the tracing. A fusion beat (F) is seen at the end of this section of the recording wherein two pacemakers discharged at the same time, giving rise to two different ventricular waveforms that summated in the fusion beat. Immediately following this beat, a right ventricular pacemaker assumed control, resulting in tachycardia. Tracing *B* shows multifocal ventricular tachycardia with fusion beats interspersed. A suggestion of P waves or other atrial electrical activity can also be observed on the baseline and T waves in both tracings. Tracing *C* shows ventricular fibrillation in which no organized activity occurs. Paper speed 25 mm per sec.

tions in waveforms. These types of arrhythmias pose a problem to simple, therapeutic regimens, since it is sometimes difficult to determine which particular arrhythmia is most significant and what agent should be employed without making the condition worse. Caution in administration of drugs and careful ECG and clinical monitoring must be undertaken in all antiarrhythmia therapy but especially in complex arrhythmias.

TREATMENT

Treatment of abnormal cardiac arrhythmias is not always successful and may be only temporary. Arrhythmias occasionally arise secondarily to another disease state that, when corrected, will result in spontaneous disappearance of the arrhythmia. The potential hazards of treatment must be weighed against those of not treating, and the subsequent

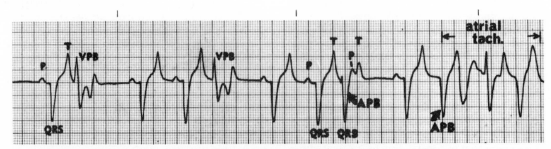

Figure 9. This tracing shows a variety of abnormalities, including ventricular premature beats (VPB), atrial premature beats (APB), and atrial tachycardia as well as some normal sinus beats. Paper speed 25 mm per sec. (From Hilwig, R. W.: Cardiac arrhythmias in the horse. J. Am. Vet. Med. Assoc., *170*:153, 1977.)

decision should be a joint one between the owner and attending veterinarian. After initiation of therapy, the arrhythmia sometimes appears worse for a period before it gets better and therefore requires good judgment and confidence in diagnosis and choice of therapeutic agents. Frequent ECG evaluation and clinical monitoring must accompany the antiarrhythmic therapy to guard against undesired outcomes.

It is assumed in this section on therapy that most conditions that could have precipitated cardiac arrhythmias, such as electrolyte imbalances, have been corrected or ruled out by careful clinical examinations or assessment of what was being done to the animal at the time. Unless otherwise stated, dosages have been calculated for the adult 450 kg horse and should be adjusted as necessary based upon the weight of the animal being treated.

QUINIDINE

Quinidine sulfate has been used to treat supraventricular arrhythmias, including frequent premature beats, especially if they are multiple or multifocal, paroxysmal atrial tachycardia, atrial tachycardia, and atrial fibrillation. Frequent ventricular premature beats or extrasystoles, paroxysmal ventricular tachycardia, and ventricular tachycardia may also be controlled with quinidine. Possible undesirable side effects from the administration of quinidine include swelling of the nasal mucosa, which may become extensive enough to close off the nasal passages, development of urticarial wheals, laminitis, gastrointestinal upset, cardiovascular collapse, atrioventricular block or other arrhythmias, and sudden death. For these reasons, a small test dose of 5 gm orally is administered to observe adverse reactions, if any, before treatment is undertaken. Quinidine should not be given to animals that are showing signs of congestive heart failure or those having atrioventricular block on the ECG. The negative inotropic effects on the myocardium and the slowed atrioventricular conduction time resulting from quinidine therapy may accentuate both of these conditions. Digitalis glycosides have been used prior to or simultaneously with quinidine in congestive states, since the glycosides have a positive inotropic action upon the myocardium, but they should not be used in the presence of atrioventricular block.

Limited experience indicates that intravenous dihydroquinidine gluconate or quinidine gluconate can be used successfully to abolish arrhythmias, but because of their greater toxicity hazard, they should not be used for long-term therapy.

Several therapeutic regimens using quinidine have been employed to abolish arrhythmias, and the choice depends upon the circumstances. Several methods are presented here as starting points only.

ORAL ADMINISTRATION OF QUINIDINE SULFATE (BY STOMACH TUBE OR IN LARGE GELATIN CAPSULES)

Method 1

Day 1: 5 gm test dose
Days 2 and 3: 10 gm twice a day
Days 4 and 5: 10 gm three times a day
Days 6 and 7: 10 gm four times a day
Days 8 and 9: 10 gm every five hours
Day 10 and thereafter: 15 gm four times a day

Method 2

Day 1: 5 gm test dose
Day 2: 10 gm every two hours until a total dose of 80 gm or less has been given.

Once the arrhythmia is abolished the total dose can be reduced by one half every two days until a maintenance dose that prevents reestablishment of the arrhythmia is reached. In cases of atrial fibrillation, quinidine administration can usually be discontinued one or two days after reversion to sinus rhythm. Oral doses of quinidine exceeding 40 gm per day predispose to undesirable side effects.

INTRAVENOUS ADMINISTRATION OF QUINIDINE SULFATE OR DIHYDROQUINIDINE GLUCONATE

These preparations are about 10 times more soluble in water than the sulfate form and should be diluted to a 1 per cent solution in glucose or physiologic saline solution for administration via slow drip at a rate not exceeding 40 to 50 ml per minute. Continuous ECG monitoring is required, and administration should be stopped if the P–R interval or QRS complex elongates beyond 125 per cent of the pretreatment values. Atrial fibrillation has been reported to revert to sinus rhythms after a total of 5 to 20 gm of quinidine has been given intravenously. If a maintenance dose is required, the animal should receive oral quinidine sulfate.

Some arrhythmias, particularly paroxysmal atrial tachycardia, may transiently appear to get worse before they get better, but for the confident and courageous, continued administration of quinidine often results in beneficial effects on cardiac rhythm.

PROPRANOLOL

Some investigators have employed propranolol for controlling tachyarrhythmias. Its quinidine-like action and beta-adrenergic blockade properties may result in slowed atrioventricular conduction time and reduced myocardial contractility. For these reasons, it should not be used in the presence of atrioventricular block or congestive heart failure. Digitalis glycosides have been used in conjunction with propranolol in congestive states to overcome negative inotropic effects. The efficacy of propranolol therapy is dependent upon the intrinsic adrenergic activity at the time of administration, and the beneficial results are thus not predictable. Propranolol has not received the high acclaim of quinidine in reverting atrial fibrillation to sinus rhythm. Beneficial results are obtained using propranolol for controlling ventricular extrasystoles and tachycardias, and it is quite effective in slowing ventricular rate even in the presence of atrial fibrillation.

ORAL ADMINISTRATION OF PROPRANOLOL

Days 1 and 2: 175 mg three times a day
Days 3 and 4: 275 mg three times a day
Days 5 and 6: 350 mg three times a day

INTRAVENOUS ADMINISTRATION OF PROPRANOLOL

Days 1 and 2: 25 mg twice a day
Days 3 and 4: 50 mg twice a day
Days 5 and 6: 75 mg twice a day

Atropine (0.045 mg per kg) should be available for intravenous administration in the event of excessive ventricular slowing or atrioventricular block.

LIDOCAINE

The local anesthetic lidocaine may be employed as an antiarrhythmic agent for short-term control of some arrhythmias and as a relatively simple presumptive diagnostic aid in differentiating a supraventricular tachyarrhythmia from a ventricular tachyarrhythmia. Do not use preparations of lidocaine that contain epinephrine. An intravenous bolus of 1 to 1.5 mg per kg of lidocaine is usually temporarily effective in slowing ventricular rate during a bout of ventricular tachyarrhythmia but has no such effect on a supraventricular tachyarrhythmia. This fact allows it to be used in the differential diagnosis of these conditions. The antiarrhythmic effects are lost within a few minutes. A slow intravenous drip of lidocaine is useful in controlling ventricular arrhythmias that may develop during some surgical procedures involving the gastrointestinal tract or extensive muscle trauma. Convulsions have been reported to occur after administration of a bolus of lidocaine.

DIGITALIS GLYCOSIDES

Digitalis glycosides have been used successfully for the treatment of congestive heart failure and for certain cardiac arrhythmias. The best antiarrhythmic responses occur with supraventricular tachyarrhythmias, since the glycosides slow atrioventricular conduction and thus effect ventricular slowing. Atrial fibrillation does not revert to sinus rhythm with these drugs; in fact, atrial activity may increase, but the reduced ventricular rate and increased contractility of the myocardium often result in remission of signs of congestive heart failure. Signs of digitalis intoxication include increased P–R interval and atrioventricular block, prolongation of the QRS complex, and additional cardiac arrhythmias, particularly ventricular extrasystoles. Mental depression, lack of appetite, and diarrhea may also indicate intoxication.

ORAL ADMINISTRATION OF DIGITALIS GLYCOSIDES

Digitalization is accomplished by five to six doses at eight-hour intervals. The dose is dependent upon the product used. Powdered digitalis or digitoxin is given at 0.03 to 0.06 mg per kg, digoxin at 0.06 to 0.08 mg per kg, or digitalis tincture at 0.3 to 0.6 ml per kg. These dosages may be increased by one fourth to one half every two days until the arrhythmia is abolished or signs of intoxication develop. The daily maintenance dose after digitalization usually consists of one eighth to one fourth of the digitalizing dose.

INTRAVENOUS ADMINISTRATION OF DIGITALIS GLYCOSIDES

Rapid digitalization may be effected by intravenous administration of 2.5 to 3.0 mg of ouabain every 1½ to 2 hours until heart rate slows, a total dose of 10 mg has been given, or signs of intoxication develop. Frequent ECG monitoring is required during this interval. When digitalization has been achieved, a maintenance dose not to exceed one fifth of the digitalizing dose may be used. Usually oral administration of another digitalis glycoside is used for maintenance. Daily doses of digitalis should be adjusted as dictated by clinical and ECG signs.

ATROPINE

This drug is usually employed as a diagnostic or short-term palliative agent to remove parasympathetic influences on the heart to effect increased heart rate. It will usually abolish first- and second-degree atrioventricular blocks and bradycardias that are vagally induced but is not effective in increasing the rate of idioventricular rhythm in the event of third-degree atrioventricular block. Long-term administration is not done because of the undesirable side effects, which include drying of mucous membranes and alterations in gastrointestinal motility and secretory activity. The parenteral dose is 0.045 mg per kg.

Supplemental Readings

1. Proceedings Academy of Veterinary Cardiology: Standards for Equine Electrocardiography. Boston, 1977.
2. Amada, A., and Kurita, H.: Five cases of paroxysmal atrial fibrillation in the racehorse. Exp. Rep. Equine Health Lab., No. 12, 89–100, 1975.
3. Buss, D. D., Rawlings, C. A., and Bisgard, G. E.: The normal electrocardiogram of the domestic pony. J. Electrocardiog., 2(3):229, 1969.
4. Hilwig, R. W.: Cardiac arrhythmias in the horse. J. Am. Vet. Med. Assoc., 170:153, 1977.
5. Senta, T., Smetzer, D. L., and Smith, C. R.: Effects of exercise on certain electrocardiographic parameters and cardiac arrhythmias in the horse. A radiotelemetric study. Cornell Vet., 60:552, 1970.

CARDIAC MURMURS

P. W. Physick-Sheard, GUELPH, ONTARIO, CANADA

Routine auscultation of the heart in the horse may reveal a murmur in an animal whose condition and performance have given no cause for concern. The clinician must interpret the significance of the sound and must provide accurate advice to the client. While many variations in cardiac sound in the horse are unassociated with organic heart disease, there is a significant incidence of valvular lesions. However, the association between the murmurs and lesions is complex and incomplete. Difficulties in interpretation are complicated by the tendency of murmurs to vary, particularly those occurring in the absence of valvular abnormality.

While the clinician must always be concerned that a cardiac murmur does not constitute a hazard to the rider or driver, serious risk is far more likely to be posed by an arrhythmia, particularly if this is the result of a valvular lesion. For the majority of cardiac murmurs in the horse that are unassociated with any other signs of cardiovascular dysfunction, the principal questions are to what extent will the findings affect the animal's exercise performance, and what are the chances of the problem progressing?

ACQUIRED VALVULAR DISEASE

While murmurs in the horse can occur in the absence of valvular abnormality, the majority are probably associated with some degree of change. In a study of 1557 horses[4, 5] examined pre- and postmortem, acquired, structural abnormalities of the valves were found in 23 per cent of the animals, with better than 50 per cent of these exhibiting a murmur. In contrast, murmurs in the absence of valve changes were noted in only 2 per cent of horses.

In the majority of cases of valvular abnormality in the horse, lesions are mild and consist of subendothelial proliferation of fibrous tissue, usually on the outflow surface of the valve. Fibrous thickening may be diffuse but is more often in nodules or bands, which predispose to flow disturbance. Distortion of the valve cusps or leaflets is rare and restricted to cases in which the inner, fibrous skeleton of the valve is involved in the pathologic process. Such a change is associated with severe valve dysfunction. Microscopic villi on the atrial surface of the mitral valves are common but not associated with abnormal sound. Rarely, areas of fibrous thickening may ulcerate, but the majority of these lesions are benign with minimal infiltration of inflammatory cells.

Additional acquired lesions include endocarditis (p. 147) and rupture or fibrosis of the chordae tendineae. Fibrosis of the chordae may result in shortening and failure of the valve to close. Alternatively, they may stretch or even rupture, resulting in prolapse of the atrioventricular (AV) valve into the atrium during ventricular systole. Such findings are surprisingly rare in the horse despite the incidence of valve change in general and the vigorous work performed by the equine heart.

The pathogenesis of valve changes in the horse is unclear. Valve trauma during function and natural aging changes, possibly predisposed by the poor vascular supply to the free margin of the valve, are generally considered to be the most important factors. This hypothesis is supported by the greater incidence of such lesions in the left heart, principally of the aortic valve. The greater pressures generated on the left could be expected to produce a greater load on the aortic and mitral valves. In addition, the lesions appear more frequently on the valve margins, the areas that come into contact during valve closure. Histologically, the changes appear to be degenerative rather than inflammatory. The very low incidence of endocarditis in the horse would make healed septic lesions an unlikely cause of valve distortion, and there are no recognized viral diseases that affect the equine endocardium. There is on the other hand experimental evidence that chronically increased workload, as in systemic arterial hypertension or chronic arteriovenous shunt, will predispose toward valve change and endocarditis. In the studies of Else and Holmes,[4, 5, 6] there was a significantly higher incidence of valvular abnormality in Thoroughbreds and hunters, while the author has noted significant outflow tract murmurs in a greater percentage of Standardbred racehorses than grade animals. Vigorous exercise may be a factor in their development.

Only occasionally, fenestrations of a valve margin may be found. While this is unlikely to produce a murmur in the case of the AV valve, as it has a wide area of apposition during closure, such an abnormality of the aortic or pulmonic valves can result in a very distinct and high-pitched musical murmur, either diastolic or systolic, though such sounds are rarely of clinical significance.

Migration of the larvae of *Strongylus vulgaris* has been said to cause valve lesions, and caseous and calcified endocardial nodules in the apex of the left ventricle have also been ascribed to this parasite. It would appear from the studies of Else and Holmes[4, 5, 6] that *S. vulgaris* may only rarely be responsible for lesions beyond the bulb of the aorta and that valve lesions are of another etiology.

While it may be expected that the incidence of valve lesions would increase with the age of the population in view of the proposed pathogenesis, there does not appear to be any obvious correlation between the age of the patient and the likelihood of a clinically significant valve lesion. Bearing in mind the fact that younger horses tend to be examined more closely more often, especially in the case of the racehorse, there is as good a chance of coming across a significant valve change in a two-year-old as in a ten-year-old.

CLASSIFICATION OF CARDIAC MURMURS[2]

SYSTOLIC MURMURS

The majority of murmurs are systolic and can be subdivided as follows.

Systolic Murmurs Associated with the Ventricular Outflow Tracts (Pulmonary Artery and Aorta)

Murmurs originating in the outflow tracts are the most common type of systolic murmur and may be benign or may be the result of obstruction to flow.

BENIGN OR FUNCTIONAL MURMURS

These murmurs occur in the absence of organic heart disease. The sound is typically of high frequency and low intensity, rarely exceeding grade II at rest. It occurs early in systole, starting after the first heart sound (S1) and ending well before the second sound (S2). It is crescendo-decrescendo in shape and is usually loudest over the pulmonic valve on the left. It is thus necessary to auscultate well forward and high up to locate the sound. It can rarely be heard on the right and does not radiate widely. The murmur may become louder (grade III) and may be heard over a wider area in states of elevated cardiac output, such as anemia, exercise, excitement, and pregnancy. Our clinical impression is that this murmur is common in young horses.

The predisposing causes appear to be (1) increases in cardiac output, (2) increases in the velocity of blood flow, and (3) the presence of minor obstructions or structural characteristics of the outflow tracts that predispose to vortex shedding but that may not cause sufficient disturbance of flow in the normal, fully relaxed animal to produce an audible murmur.

Very loud murmurs are sometimes heard in horses with colic or in very excited animals that have just been shipped. Reexamination of the same animal after treatment or rest reveals no murmur at all. These sounds have the characteristics described before except that they appear to be associated with the aortic rather than the pulmonic valve. In cases of aortic systolic murmur, the clinician should examine the animal at a later date. If the murmur has subsided, there should be no cause for further concern. The significance of this murmur in exercise is unknown.

OBSTRUCTIONS OF THE OUTFLOW TRACT

Although murmurs in this category are associated with abnormalities of the outflow tract, their clinical significance varies. Compared with benign murmurs, they are louder, longer in duration, of lower pitch, and radiate more widely. Outflow tract murmurs that are always louder on the left than the right may start right after S1 and run into S2, being distinctly crescendo-decrescendo with the peak of intensity occurring in midsystole. In severe stenosis of a semilunar valve, the peak may occur later. The coarse, harsh, or noisy character and the shape and intensity together with the area of maximal intensity combine to produce a typical sound referred to as an ejection murmur. While the murmurs of both pulmonic and aortic stenosis tend to radiate dorsally along the outflow tracts (aorta and pulmonary artery), the distribution of the sounds differs toward the apex, each being most easily heard over the respective ventricle. Aortic murmurs, however, are generally louder than pulmonic murmurs.

In the study of valvular disease referred to before,[4, 5, 6] 87 per cent of affected horses had lesions on the aortic valves. In contrast, only 37 per cent of affected horses had pulmonic valve changes. Because lesions of the aortic valve are generally the more severe and more common, murmurs of outflow tract obstruction are most likely to be of aortic origin.

While in general the intensity of the murmur can be related to the severity of the valve change and to the degree of obstruction, the majority of obstructive semilunar valve lesions in the horse are mild in degree.

It is unlikely in the majority of cases of outflow tract obstruction that the increased cardiac load will result in a clinically apparent ventricular hypertrophy, although during vigorous exercise the size of the outflow tract could conceivably become limiting, resulting in both a sudden increase in myocardial work load at that level of work and a tendency to tire rapidly. As a rough guide, an ejection-type murmur is likely to be of clinical significance if it is grade III or louder, especially if it can be heard on both sides of the chest. Evidence of cardiomegaly is a further indication of a functionally significant lesion. In horses not asked to perform vigorously, mild to moderate outflow tract stenosis may be of little or no significance.

Systolic Murmurs Associated with the Atrioventricular Valves

The atrioventricular (AV) valves are open throughout ventricular diastole and closed during ventricular contraction. Failure of the valve to seal effectively results in retrograde flow into the atria, a situation referred to as regurgitation, insufficiency, or incompetence. The murmur produced tends to be of low frequency and has a blowing or rumbling character. It lasts throughout systole and is described as pansystolic, starting with rather than after S1 and often continuing through S2. The murmur is of uniform intensity (band-shaped) and rarely exceeds grade III. Because of its low frequency and blowing character, a quiet murmur is easily missed. In some cases, a mid to late systolic murmur of low frequency and intensity may be noted. Though uncommon, this sound may indicate mitral valve prolapse.

Mitral insufficiency is more common than tricuspid insufficiency and produces a more intense murmur. Else and Holmes[4, 5, 6] reported lesions on the mitral valve in 23 per cent of 356 animals with valve changes; frequently, mitral lesions were associated with lesions of the aortic valve. Tricuspid lesions were found in only 10 per cent of the affected horses. It is likely that the majority of AV valve lesions do not give rise to murmurs, since the valve cusps are in contact over a wide area during ventricular systole and do not easily become incompe-

tent. A murmur indicative of AV insufficiency, especially one of grade III or better, therefore suggests the presence of moderate to severe valve damage.

Differentiation of tricuspid and mitral insufficiency is simple. Mitral insufficiency results in a murmur best heard on the left side toward the posterior limit of the area of auscultation and loudest just behind and approximately 1 to 2 inches above the point of the elbow. Unless the sound is of grade III intensity or better on the left, it is unlikely to be heard on the right. Regurgitation of large volumes of blood through the mitral valve causes pulmonary venous hypertension and a tendency to pulmonary congestion and edema. This results in clinical signs initially indistinguishable from chronic obstructive airway disease, with coughing and an expiratory effort. Mild cases may show a predisposition to pulmonary hemorrhage during vigorous exercise.

Insufficiency of the tricuspid valve is occasionally seen in the horse, either in association with cardiac dilatation or endocarditis, though neither is a common event. The regurgitation results in a jugular pulse. When the jugular vein is manually emptied after distal obstruction with the thumb, it will refill rapidly in a pulsatile manner. Occasionally, a tricuspid insufficiency will not produce this sign either because there is a small regurgitant stream or because the stream is directed into the posterior vena cava. Tricuspid insufficiency is always of clinical significance and is likely to be progressive or associated with complications, particularly in an animal undergoing vigorous exercise. Ultimately, the elevation of central venous pressure and chronic passive venous congestion resulting from regurgitation produce organ dysfunction and classical signs of congestive heart failure. Murmurs of AV insufficiency should therefore be treated with greater caution than those of outflow tract obstruction of equivalent intensity.

DIASTOLIC MURMURS

Diastolic murmurs of either the outflow tract or the AV valves are of greater clinical significance than a systolic murmur of equal intensity. With the possible exception of aortic insufficiency, diastolic murmurs are not common, and because the murmurs are usually of low frequency, they are easily missed.

Diastolic Murmurs Associated with the Outflow Tract

The aortic outflow tract is the most likely source of a diastolic murmur in the horse. In Else and Holmes'[4, 5, 6] study, of 1557 horses examined, 32 had lesions of the aortic valve associated with a diastolic murmur, while another 17 had a diastolic murmur with lesions on both the aortic and mitral valves. It is unlikely that a diastolic murmur occurs in the absence of valvular abnormality.

The murmur of aortic insufficiency starts immediately upon closure of the aortic valve (S2), increasing in intensity transiently, then slowly falling to end with or just before the next S1. The murmur is thus crescendo-decrescendo with a very early peak. The sound produced is characteristically soft and blowing, occasionally even whistling, though harsh, noisy, diastolic murmurs of aortic insufficiency may occur and are associated with severe valvular damage. The sound is best heard over the left ventricle, with the area of maximal intensity being just below the aortic valve and the murmur radiating toward the apex. Occasionally, the murmur will also be heard on the right side. The hemodynamic conditions created by the valvular insufficiency will often result in an associated systolic murmur in the left ventricular outflow tract of the benign or functional type. This sound may on occasion exceed the original diastolic sound in intensity.

Abnormality of the pulmonic valve is rare. Were this valve to become incompetent, the low pressure gradient between the pulmonary artery and the right ventricle would result in a very low intensity murmur of limited duration, heard well forward and high up on the left. A murmur of pulmonic insufficiency of sufficient intensity to be detected easily would probably be accompanied by a systolic flow murmur with detectable ventricular hypertrophy and would indicate severe valve damage. As disease of the pulmonic valve is rare, a diastolic murmur of this origin is uncommon.

Insufficiency of the semilunar valves results in reduced foward flow of blood and an increased volume of blood in the ventricle at the end of the diastole. Response is an eccentric hypertrophy of the ventricle. In the case of the aortic valve, insufficiency is also associated with a hard, short, and very distinct pulse wave that falls away rapidly.

Diastolic Murmurs Associated with AV Valves

Early in diastole when the AV valves open, the early rapid phase of ventricular filling commences and blood rushes into the ventricular chambers. The end of rapid filling is marked by the third heart sound (S3) (p. 122), a distinct sound clearly separated from S2, being short in duration and low in frequency. Although S3 may be heard in many horses, it should be regarded as abnormal if it is particularly evident at resting heart rates, especially if it rivals S1 and S2 in intensity. This may occur in cases of excessive myocardial tone, as in moderate to severe hypertrophy of the ventricles, and also in

the case of a relatively flaccid, failing myocardium. Although in such cases the sound is usually short and distinct, it may be quite prolonged and complex and may be interpreted as a murmur. If this occurs, differentiation from the murmur of mitral stenosis may be difficult, though generally the murmur will commence very soon after S2, the abnormal S3 sound occurring later. The clinician should note that an accentuated third heart sound is a normal finding in the horse during cardiac acceleration and deceleration and is most pronounced at heart rates of 60 to 120 beats per minute.

Various so-called "flow" or "functional" diastolic sounds have been described, usually occurring very late in diastole (immediately before S1) or very early in diastole (between S2 and S3). They are usually low in intensity and frequency and not easily heard, though they may be accentuated in any condition increasing flow across the atrioventricular valves. The sounds occur at the peaks of blood flow across the AV valve and likely reflect this flow rather than any structural abnormality. In young horses, a high-pitched diastolic squeak may occur just before S3. Though quite distinct, this sound tends to be transient and is not associated with any cardiac pathology. Its origin is unknown.

True diastolic murmurs associated with the AV valves are indicative of AV stenosis, a condition that is rare in the horse. The sound is most likely to be heard during rapid ventricular filling early in diastole and at the end of diastole, periods when blood is moving rapidly across the AV valve. The murmur may last throughout diastole, but it is likely to be quieter in the middle of diastole in the horse where the heart rate is slow and the diastolic interval quite long. A murmur of AV stenosis extending throughout diastole would indicate a severe obstruction sufficient to hold back the blood during early diastole and thus would interfere with rapid ventricular filling.

The murmur of AV stenosis is typically low frequency and of slightly noisy or rumbling character and is best heard immediately beneath the valve of origin and over the ventricle. It is unlikely to radiate widely, though it may be heard on both sides of the chest. In most cases, it is of grade II intensity or less. The higher incidence and greater severity of lesions of the mitral valve make mitral stenosis a more common entity than tricuspid stenosis. However, in the studies of Else and Holmes,[4, 5, 6] no clinical cases of isolated AV stenosis were recorded, most cases of diastolic murmurs in the left heart being associated with aortic valve lesions, which could also have contributed to the sound. The findings in this series would suggest that AV stenosis may be an uncommon primary finding and more likely associated with generalized valvular disease. Because of the nature of the murmur of AV stenosis, it is likely that a severe degree of narrowing would have to be present for the murmur to be clearly audible.

In cases of severe mitral stenosis, with the murmur lasting throughout diastole, there is likely to be pulmonary venous hypertension interfering with normal lung function and predisposing the animal to exercise-related pulmonary hemorrhage, though this is probably a very uncommon cause of epistaxis. While there could be a secondary effect on right heart function, the horse is likely to show respiratory signs and a significant fall in exercise performance long before this point.

CLINICAL SIGNIFICANCE OF MURMURS

MYOCARDIAL HYPERTROPHY AND PERFORMANCE

Valvular abnormality may place either a pressure load (such as in aortic stenosis) or a volume load (such as in aortic insufficiency) on the heart. The heart's response is some combination of myocardial hypertrophy and dilation. The response depends upon the severity of the valvular defect and also upon the nutritional status of the myocardium (for example, blood supply), the speed of onset of the valve lesion, and the presence of additional factors also placing a load on the heart. An equivalent degree of valvular stenosis in two different animals, therefore, may produce very different responses. With currently available techniques, quantification of ventricular enlargement is difficult and is further complicated by the wide range of individual variation in heart size. If cardiomegaly is clinically detectable by percussion or ECG, then it can safely be assumed that the valve lesion is significant and will affect performance.

In the horse with valvular lesions, the prognosis for survival is good, since the cardiovascular reserve of the species makes decompensation unlikely with any but the most severe lesion. Valve lesions of a progressive type are uncommon.

The vast majority of valve lesions are unlikely to stop a horse from working. Whether performance will deteriorate with the development of a valve lesion or whether poor performance can be blamed upon a previously existing valvular abnormality is almost impossible to determine unless very extensive assessment of cardiovascular functional capacity has been carried out on the animal at the onset of the problem. The significance of the lesion will depend upon the animal's reserve capacity, the amount of that reserve capacity being used to overcome the effects of the lesion and the type of work the animal is being asked to perform. Severe changes are likely to have a detectable effect upon both maximal speed and stamina. Since such animals are unlikely to perform satisfactorily, there would appear to be little justification for maintaining them in vigorous work. Prognosis for the use of such animals in occupations requiring a low rate of work is likely to be good, however. The degree of dysfunction caused by mild valve changes is unlikely to be clinically detectable and may have no measurable effect upon performance.

Repeated episodes of maximal performance in an animal with cardiac hypertrophy and limited reserve may accelerate degenerative changes in the myocardium and increase the likelihood of serious cardiac arrhythmia and myocardial failure. The clinician is therefore well advised to carry out periodic reexamination of animals with significant cardiac lesions.

In general, murmurs of outflow tract stenosis are of less significance than an equivalent murmur associated with the AV valves, and they are also far more common. In either case, if the animal is brought in to work gradually, maintained in good condition, and not required to undertake sudden episodes of strenuous exercise, the condition may remain stable for long periods.

MURMURS ASSOCIATED WITH ARRHYTHMIAS

A hypertrophied myocardium is by definition abnormal and under severe stress is predisposed to arrhythmias. The tendency toward arrhythmias increases with the severity of valvular lesions but is disproportionately large with AV valvular insufficiency. In this case, the atrial myocardium is exposed to excessive pressures. Stretching and dilatation lead to atrial tachyarrhythmia. In a case in which an arrhythmia is secondary to valvular abnormality, the onset of the arrhythmia is a poor prognostic sign and initiates a downward spiral of events by placing a further load on an already abnormal myocardium. In this situation, serious arrhythmias may develop during vigorous exercise. Fortunately this is a relatively uncommon sequela to valvular abnormality in the horse. The majority of equine cardiac arrhythmias arise spontaneously and are not associated with valvular disease. The presence of a cardiac arrhythmia poses a far more significant risk to the rider or driver than the murmur and valvular abnormality.

While they are extremely uncommon sequelae, rupture of the atrium secondary to AV insufficiency and rupture of the aorta in cases of severe aortic stenosis are possibilities. Such an event would be caused by unaccustomed episodes of vigorous exercise.

References

1. Bruns, D. L.: A general theory of the cause of murmurs in the cardiovascular system. Am. J. Med., 27:360, 1959.
2. Criscitiello, M. G.: Pathophysiology of heart sounds and murmurs. *In* Levine, J. H. (ed.): Clinical Cardiovascular Physiology. New York, Grune & Stratton, 1976, p. 259.
3. Detweiler, D. K., and Patterson, D. F.: The cardiovascular system. *In* Catcott, E. J., and Smithcors, J. F. (eds.): Equine Medicine and Surgery, 2nd ed. Wheaton, IL, American Veterinary Pub., 1972, p. 227.
4. Else, R. W., and Holmes, J. R.: Cardiac pathology in the horse. 1. Gross pathology. Equine Vet. J., 4:9, 1972.
5. Else, R.W., and Holmes, J. R.: Cardiac pathology in the horse. 2. Microscopic pathology. Equine Vet. J., 4:57, 1972.
6. Holmes, J. R., and Else, R. W.: Cardiac pathology in the horse. 3. Clinical correlations. Equine Vet. J., 4:195, 1972.

CONGENITAL CARDIAC LESIONS

Christopher M. Brown, EAST LANSING, MICHIGAN

All the common mammalian congenital cardiac defects, as well as many of the more bizarre ones, have been described in the horse. The list includes interventricular septal defects, patent ductus arteriosus, patent foramen ovale, tetralogy and pentalogy of Fallot, persistent right aortic arch, persistent common truncus, dextraposition of the aorta, atresia of the tricuspid valve, three-chambered heart, and congenital aortic valvular insufficiency. It is also possible for various combinations of these defects to occur. Of these defects, the commonest is interventricular septal defect, followed in frequency by various valvular defects.

Clinical signs vary depending upon the severity of the hemodynamic derangement. In some cases, the problem may go undetected until the animal is presented for veterinary examination as a yearling or older. It may not become apparent until the horse is put into training and shows reduced stamina. On the other hand, the defect may be so severe that the animal may live only a few minutes or hours. Many are associated with poor growth and development, cyanosis, weakness, and eventually heart failure.

On auscultation, the majority of these lesions are associated with obvious murmurs. It is not uncommon to detect a cardiac murmur in a foal up to four days old. This probably arises from patency of the ductus arteriosus. This is usually functionally closed by the fifth day. If an apparent "machinery" murmur is detected beyond this date, then it may be abnormal, and the foal should be rechecked at 10 to 14 days of age. With other defects the murmurs vary but are essentially the same as those described for congenital defects in other species. Careful auscultation with mapping of the site and extent of the murmur may be very helpful. A thrill may also be present.

If a congenital lesion is suspected, then confirmation can be obtained by a more detailed examination. This may include plain and contrast cardiac radiographs, cardiac catheterization for pressure measurement, blood sampling for gas analysis, and in some cases echocardiography. These are obviously techniques for the specialty practice.

Once diagnosed, treatment of many of these lesions is unrealistic. Surgical closure of patent ductus arteriosus can be attempted, and foals have been successfully placed on cardiac bypass so open heart surgery is possible. However, the possible genetic factors involved in congenital cardiac disease in the horse are unknown, and therefore one must consider the ethical factors in raising breeding animals with corrected congenital cardiac defects.

In most cases, severe congenital cardiac defects can be diagnosed on the basis of examination and clinical signs. Once diagnosed, the owner can be fairly certainly informed that the animal is unlikely to be a useful athlete, and treatment in most cases is unrealistic.

Supplemental Readings

1. Button, C., Gross, D. R., Allert, J. A., and Kitzman, J. V.: Tricuspid atresia in a foal. J. Am. Vet. Med. Assoc., 172:825, 1978.
2. Glazier, D. B., Farrelly, B. T., and O'Connor, J.: Ventricular septal defect in a 7-year old gelding. J. Am. Vet. Med. Assoc., 167:49, 1975.
3. Rooney, J. R., and Franks, W. C.: Congenital cardiac anomalies in horses. Pathol. Vet., 1:454, 1964.

BACTERIAL ENDOCARDITIS

P. W. Physick-Sheard, GUELPH, ONTARIO, CANADA

Bacterial endocarditis is the only commonly encountered inflammatory lesion of the endocardium in domestic animals, being found with some frequency in the pig and cow. However, the condition is not common in the horse, despite the impression created by the literature. The rarity of the lesion and the significance empirically attached to cardiac lesions in the horse in general have resulted in inappropriate attention being paid to this infrequent though none-the-less serious condition.

PATHOGENESIS AND ETIOLOGY

Though reference to an allergic factor in the pathogenesis of endocarditis in the horse has been made, there appears to be little evidence to support this hypothesis, the theory being largely extrapolated from the occurrence of rheumatic heart disease in humans. The occurrence of bacterial endocarditis in the horse appears to be a sporadic, perhaps chance event. The principal predisposing factor is probably recurrent episodes of bacteremia, though theoretically a single episode involving a highly pathogenic organism may cause the lesion. The infection could localize in any tissue, but under as yet undefined circumstances, it localizes on the heart valves. The literature states that most lesions are found in the left heart, usually involving the aortic valve, though this author has seen principally right-sided lesions involving the triscupid valve.

While in cattle and the pig the origin of the infection is often either current or identifiable in the animal's history, the majority of equine cases cannot be easily explained. It is not known for how long the condition may remain subclinical, and the primary source of infection may thus have been forgotten. Alternatively, the source may be the minor, transient bacteremia that probably occurs frequently as a result of minor disruptions of the skin and mucous membranes.

The organisms commonly involved in the horse are Streptococcus sp, principally *Streptococcus zooepidemicus*, and Actinobacillus sp, both groups of organisms that can be found as commensals. This would tend to support the suggestion that bacterial endocarditis in the horse may be largely a chance event. Cases of endocarditis caused by distinct pathogens such as *Streptococcus equi* are occasionally encountered under circumstances of recent infection or contact with cases of strangles.

CLINICAL AND LABORATORY FINDINGS

Affected animals usually present with a history of lethargy and depression. Pyrexia may have been noted during episodes of depression, and in protracted cases, weight loss may be apparent. History of pyrexia responsive to antibiotics is common, with relapses occurring when therapy is withdrawn.

Clinical findings usually include mild tachypnea and tachycardia, depression, and possibly pyrexia. Auscultation may reveal a murmur, though often none is found, especially if the lesion is located on the tricuspid valve. In these cases, a degree of jugular pulsation may help in identifying the location of the lesion. Though uncommon, the possibility of more than one valve being involved should be considered.

A soft, intermittent cough may also be noted in cases of tricuspid endocarditis as a result of embolic showering of the lungs, whereas the detachment of pieces of a vegetative mass in the left heart can result in embolic infarction in any organ. Commonly the kidney is affected, though there may be no clinical signs. Emboli entering the coronary arteries will cause myocardial infarction, with arrhythmias becoming apparent, principally ventricular ectopic beats.

Laboratory studies reveal mild to moderate anemia, mature neutrophilia, and usually an elevated fibrinogen level. Fractionation of serum proteins reveals elevated serum globulins, principally gamma globulin, in all but the most recent cases, and total serum protein may reach greater than 10 gm per dl. In the majority of uncomplicated cases, the remaining laboratory findings are normal.

DIAGNOSIS

Most of the clinical signs and laboratory data are nonspecific and in the absence of a murmur could be consistent with any deep inflammatory or bacterial process, for example abscessation. In all cases of recurrent pyrexia responsive to antibiotics, a blood culture should be taken. Blood should be drawn with asepsis from the jugular vein on three occasions at four- to six-hour intervals. The test should only be carried out during a pyrexic episode, preferably greater than 24 hours after the withdrawal of antibiotics, to increase the chances of obtaining a positive culture. Antibiotic sensitivity tests should be conducted. Blood cultures are often negative. However, a positive result together with the clinical picture justifies a diagnosis of bacterial endocarditis. Cases of fungal and possibly chlamydial endocarditis may occur but are exceedingly rare.

THERAPY

A tentative diagnosis may be followed by treatment with penicillin, since most of the commonly encountered organisms in bacterial endocarditis in the horse are sensitive to this antibiotic. The results of blood culture and sensitivity tests may subsequently indicate a change in therapy. Antibiotics should be administered at high levels for three to six weeks and *should not* be discontinued when pyrexia subsides. There is no advantage to constantly changing the antibiotic once appropriate therapy has been identified, assuming that effective serum levels are maintained. In most cases, crystalline penicillin will be as effective as the more expensive members of this group, and in view of the need for prolonged therapy, considerably cheaper. In applying antibiotic therapy, the dosage regimens recommended by Knight should be employed.[2] Some advantage may be gained by utilizing synergy for the first two weeks of therapy, though this should not

result in reduction in the levels of the primary antibiotic administered.

Despite vigorous therapy, the prognosis remains poor. Relapse at variable intervals is the rule, and in the very small number of cases that do respond to treatment, severe valve distortion and dysfunction are highly likely. The clinical course of the condition involves embolic sequelae to the detachment of pieces of the vegetative mass. Endocarditis in the right heart results in pulmonary embolism, which in the case of a large thrombus may cause acute respiratory distress and even death. Embolic showering from the left heart may cause renal damage and myocardial infarction. A very guarded prognosis should thus be given in all cases. Successful therapy is likely to depend upon early diagnosis.

References

1. Kay, M. D.: Infective Endocarditis. Baltimore, University Park Press, 1976.
2. Knight, H. D.: Antimicrobial agents used in the horse. Proc. 21st Annu. Conv. Am. Assoc. Eq. Pract., p. 131, 1975.
3. Lillehei, C. W., Bobb, J. R. R., and Bisscheu, M. G.: Occurrence of endocarditis with valvular deformities in dogs with arteriovenous fistulae. Proc. Soc. Exp. Biol. NY, 75:9, 1950.
4. Wagenaar, G.: Endocarditis in the horse. Blue Book for the Vet. Prof., *12*:38, 1967.

THE ECG AND PERFORMANCE PREDICTION: HEART SCORES

P. W. Physick-Sheard, GUELPH, ONTARIO, CANADA

Many attempts have been made to use easily measurable physiologic parameters to predict performance. Electrocardiography is no exception. Specifically, attempts have been made to correlate performance with QRS duration (QRS interval), performance being defined as total stakes monies won, earnings per start, and kilometer times (time in seconds to run one kilometer). The QRS interval is calculated as the mean of the duration in each of the three limb leads in seconds and is referred to as the heart score.

Steel[3] gives a correlation coefficient of $+0.44$ (P < 0.01) for the relationship between QRS interval and total stakes monies won, while Nielsen and Vibe-Petersen[2] show QRS interval to be negatively correlated with kilometer time. Both workers have shown the relationship to be closer in the stallion than the mare and have also found an increase in

heart score with age up to four to five years, the closest association being seen in two-year-old horses and animals over four years of age. As a result of such studies, the measurement of heart score has been widely used to screen two-year-olds entering training.

Heart score is based on the assumption that QRS duration reflects the time taken for depolarization to traverse the ventricular muscle mass and thus relates directly to the volume of muscle or heart size. This is supported by data indicating the heart score to be directly related to heart weight.[3]

The QRS duration represents the period of time during which electrical forces generated during depolarization of the ventricles produce a measurable resultant potential at the body surface. As noted before (p. 126), the waveform probably only represents the depolarization of a portion of the interventricular septum,[1] and variations in the configuration of the QRS are indicative of variations in the sequence of depolarization in this area. It may be, therefore, that heart score is dependent upon the pattern or sequence of ventricular depolarization and that this pattern is itself dependent upon heart mass. Alternatively, the results may imply some relationship between heart mass and the distribution of the conducting system in the interventricular septum.

In terms of the practical application of heart score, it should be noted that QRS duration may be affected by pathologic processes. Ectopic ventricular contractions, ventricular conduction system defects, myocardial infarcts, cardiomegaly, and aberrant conduction pathways may all prolong QRS. The ECG should thus be examined carefully to detect deviations from normal before QRS duration is measured. Since the limb leads have very limited sensitivity in this context, these tracings should be interpreted with great caution.

As performance and thus winnings are dependent upon so many factors, heart score has a surprisingly strong correlation with performance. The more athletic members of the more athletic breeds generally have a large heart weight:body weight ratio. Preliminary studies by the author indicate that QRS duration is positively correlated with body weight. Applying this to the two-year-old, animals with high heart scores may in fact be the better developed, more mature individuals that could be expected to have some advantage in competitive situations.

Since the male of a species often shows greater growth rate and earlier maturity than the female, it could be expected that males would have a competitive advantage correlated with higher heart score. Once an animal has shown ability, management is generally to optimize performance, thus maintaining the correlation between heart score and performance.

Thus, while there appears to be a significant relationship between heart weight and QRS duration and while there can be little doubt that a physiologically large heart confers a competitive advantage, the correlation between heart score and performance may in part result from the effect on performance of other factors that have an incidental relationship to heart weight. Such factors would be body weight and maturity together with secondary environmental factors such as nutrition and management.

References

1. Muylle, E., and Oyaert, W.: Equine electrocardiography: The genesis of the different configurations of the QRS complex. Zentralbl. Veterinaermed. [A], *24*:762, 1977.
2. Nielsen, K., and Vibe-Petersen, G.: Relationship between QRS-duration (heart score) and racing performance in trotters. Equine Vet. J., *12*:81, 1980.
3. Steel, J. D.: Studies on the Electrocardiogram of the Horse. Sydney, N.S.W. Australasian Medical Publishing Co., 1963.

PERICARDITIS

Pamela C. Wagner, PULLMAN, WASHINGTON

Pericarditis refers to inflammation of the parietal and visceral surfaces of the pericardial sac. The inflammation is usually accompanied by pericardial effusion that in turn gives rise to signs of right heart failure, i.e., peritoneal effusion, increased venous pressure, and decreased arterial blood pressure. Ascites and peripheral edema are indications of more chronic pericardial disease.

Several types of pericarditis have been described. *Effusive pericarditis* results in accumulation of large volumes of fluid in the pericardial sac. The effusion may be blood due to trauma, vessel rupture, or neoplasia. It may be a transudate, usually secondary to congestive heart failure, or it may be an exudate due to infection of the pericardium or an idiopathic effusion. *Constrictive pericarditis* is usually more chronic in nature and is manifested by extreme thickening of the pericardium resulting in constriction of the chambers of the heart.[8]

The occurrence of pericarditis in the horse is rare. In most cases, it is secondary to bacterial infections or pleuritis[4, 5] and has been observed following respiratory diseases such as equine influenza and equine viral arteritis.[1] In one report, three cases were idiopathic with no causative agent isolated, while a fourth case was due to external trauma and infection with Pseudomonas sp.[8]

DIAGNOSIS

Physical signs of pericarditis are absent if there is no impairment of cardiac function. As the condition progresses and fluid accumulates in the pericardial sac, clinical signs appear. These include depression, anorexia, dyspnea, reluctance to lie down, and muffled heart sounds. Most cases also show jugular pulse, abnormal wide-based stance, and some edema, usually on the ventral midline.

Hemograms of the horse with pericarditis may reflect the chronicity of the condition and the type of pericarditis present. Most cases have a low hematocrit (23 to 32 per cent), elevated white blood cell counts (13,000 to 30,000 per μl), and elevated fibrinogen levels (700 to 1200 mg per dl). As the condition becomes more chronic, blood urea nitrogen levels increase, indicating prerenal or renal failure. Electrolyte imbalances noted in terminal cases include severe hyponatremia and hyperkalemia and in humans are indicative of a poor prognosis.[7]

Electrocardiograms (ECG) show a decreased amplitude of the QRS complex in all leads. This decrease in amplitude can also be seen in chronic pleuritis and chronic wasting diseases with anemia and must be carefully interpreted in light of the hemogram findings.[8] As the heart becomes more compromised by fluid accumulation or constriction by fibrosis of the pericardium, the peripheral arterial pressure decreases and the central venous pressure increases. Cardiac tamponade can occur if pericardial fluid increases enough to hamper cardiac filling. Accumulation of fluid outside the pericardium in the thorax, cardiac arrhythmias, and ventricular tachycardia are terminal events.[2, 8]

Diagnostic tools for confirmation of pericarditis include radiology and pericardiocentesis. Lateral radiographs of the chest may show increased size of the pericardium; however, this is difficult to evaluate if the radiograph is suboptimal or if extensive knowledge of normal variations is lacking. The lung field is usually unaffected until advanced disease causes heart failure. Radiographs are not useful in determining the origin of the pericarditis.

PERICARDIOCENTESIS

Pericardiocentesis is helpful in determining whether there is fluid in the pericardial sac and in assessing the etiology of the effusion.[2] A pleuritis may accompany pericarditis in the horse, and prior to pericardiocentesis, the fluid from the thorax should be removed. Pericardiocentesis should only be performed if fluid still surrounds the heart after the thorax has been drained and if all clinical and ancillary examinations confirm pericardial disease. An area 10 cm × 10 cm is clipped over the left fifth, sixth, and seventh intercostal spaces at the level of the costochondral junctions. An ECG may be recorded in the usual manner during sampling but is not essential. The horse is restrained by physical methods or with small amounts of a tranquilizer.

Local infiltration of the skin at the fifth intercostal space is accomplished using lidocaine. The area is surgically prepared with alternating scrubs of alcohol and povidone-iodine (Betadine). A small skin incision is made using a No. 15 blade. A 60 cc syringe is attached to a 3 to 5 in 18 gauge needle, which is passed through the skin incision and the chest wall. Negative pressure is maintained by withdrawing the barrel of the syringe while advancing the needle. When the pericardium is encountered, a thrust may be needed to enter, especially if the condition is chronic and the pericardium is thickened. If the ECG is being monitored, there will be no abnormalities seen until the needle touches the epicardium. A premature ventricular contraction will indicate that this has occurred, and the needle can be withdrawn slightly to withdraw fluid from the pericardial sac. If no fluid can be withdrawn, the pericarditis may be of a constrictive rather than an effusive type, or the fluid may be too viscous to withdraw through an 18 gauge needle.

When bloody fluid is obtained, it is observed for clotting time. If it clots immediately, it is fresh hemorrhage, and the procedure should be abandoned immediately. If it has some appearance other than bloody, a small sample should be submitted for analysis and the remainder drained if possible. The most common exudates in the horse are infectious or benign idiopathic ones. In both cases, the protein is elevated above normal (72.5 mg per dl), and the white cell count is increased. In infectious pericarditis, the fluid may have very high numbers of white blood cells (greater than 20,000 per μl), and an organism may be identified by culturing the fluid. Idiopathic pericardial effusions are usually serosanguineous and will not clot. The white cell count may be elevated, but infectious organisms cannot be demonstrated by cultures or stains of the fluid.

TREATMENT

The prognosis for recovery in any case of pericarditis in the horse is poor. There are no recorded cases of successful therapy once the horse shows severe clinical signs. Medical management in humans has been described for infectious pericarditis, and systemic antibiotic therapy has been found to be efficacious.[7] If fluid can be obtained from the pericardial sac and an organism identified, antibiotic therapy in the horse is indicated. Pericardial antibiotic levels equal those of the blood, so therapeutic, not massive, doses are indicated. Supportive treatment should include fluid and electrolyte therapy to correct imbalances. The use of corticosteroids in idiopathic benign pericarditis has been advocated in the dog.

Surgical treatment of constrictive pericarditis in

the cow has been described.[3] A left lateral pericardectomy was performed, adhesions were broken down, and a strip of pericardium was resected and left open. Complete recovery was achieved. There are no reports of surgical therapy of pericarditis in the horse.

References

1. Detweiler, D. K., and Patterson, D. F.: The cardiovascular system. *In* Catcott, E. J., and Smithcors, J. F. (eds.): Equine Medicine and Surgery. Wheaton, IL, American Veterinary Pub., 1972, pp. 334–335.
2. Ettinger, S. J., and Suter, P. F.: Canine Cardiology. Philadelphia, W. B. Saunders Co., 1970, pp. 403–420.
3. Nigam, J. M., and Manohar, M.: Pericardectomy as a treatment for constrictive pericarditis in a cow. Vet. Rec., *92*:202, 1973.
4. Rainey, J. W.: A specific arthritis with pericarditis affecting young horses in Tasmania. Aust. Vet. J., *20*:204, 1944.
5. Ryan, A. F., and Rainey, J. W.: A specific arthritis with pericarditis affecting horses in Tasmania. Aust. Vet. J., *21*:146, 1945.
6. Scribner, B. H.: University of Washington Teaching Syllabus for the Course on Fluid and Electrolyte Balance, 7th revision. Seattle, Bookstore of the University of Washington, 1979, pp. 34–37.
7. Tan, J. S., Holmes, J. C., Fowler, N. O., Manitasas, G. T., and Phair J. P.: Antibiotic levels in pericardial fluid. J. Clin. Invest., *53*:7, 1974.
8. Wagner, P. C., Miller, R. A., Merritt, F., Pickering L. A., and Grant B. D.: Constrictive pericarditis in the horse. J. Equine Med. Surg., *1*:242, 1977.
9. White, N. A., and Rhode, E. A.: Correlation of electrocardiographic findings to clinical disease in the horse. J. Am. Vet. Med. Assoc., *164*:46, 1974.

THROMBOPHLEBITIS

Christopher M. Brown, EAST LANSING, MICHIGAN

Jugular phlebitis, often with thrombosis, is a not uncommon complication of intravenous injection in the horse, particularly if the agents are irritants (such as phenylbutazone and thiobarbiturates). Similar problems can arise with long-term indwelling intravenous catheters. Such problems can be avoided if intravenous medication is given with care and if aseptic technique is followed for catheter placement. Fewer problems will be encountered if catheters long enough to reach the thoracic inlet are used. Problems will be further reduced if the catheter does not pass through the skin directly over the vessel. A subcutaneous tunnel can be made from the jugular vein to a site 10 to 15 cm dorsal to the vein and the catheter passed down from there to the vein and then into the vein. The risk of "pumping" organisms directly from the skin surface to the vein is reduced. Again it must be emphasized that these catheters should be placed using a stringent aseptic technique. If not being used for continuous infusions, then the catheters should be flushed regularly with heparinized saline. If any resistance to flushing is encountered, this can indicate either a kink in the catheter or a blockage of the tip with a clot. If the latter is suspected, then the catheter should be replaced.

Problems will arise if a catheter is left in place for too long. Many catheters are made of thrombogenic materials, and also their tips tend to continually traumatize the endothelium. This is particularly true of short, rigid catheters. Generally speaking, correctly placed jugular catheters should not be left in place for more than four to five days, and in foals three days is a more acceptable maximum.

CLINICAL SIGNS

Clinical signs depend upon the site of venous obstruction and upon the presence of tissue necrosis or sepsis or both. In cases in which the problem arises owing to perivascular injection of irritant substances, the area will be swollen, hot, and painful. Patency of the vein may be difficult to determine owing to swelling. Without treatment, extensive necrosis of muscle and skin may occur, and a large area may slough. The vagosympathetic trunk or the recurrent laryngeal nerve or both may be damaged, giving rise to a variety of clinical signs, including laryngeal hemiplegia and Horner's syndrome. The tissue defect can be very large and may take many months to heal.

If the lesion is entirely intravascular, then the only localized sign may be cording of the vessel that has filled with a thrombus. Initially the site will be swollen and painful, and there may be local infection, particularly if the thrombophlebitis arose at a site of catheterization. Over time the thrombus will organize and contract to a fibrous cord much narrower than the original vessel. Septic or nonseptic thromboembolism may also occur if fragments of the thrombus detach. They will usually be trapped in the lungs, and if septic, may give rise to pulmonary abscesses.

Loss of one jugular vein does not usually cause serious permanent problems. Initially there may be some prominence of the facial veins, and the contralateral jugular will be filled. However, adequate adaptation rapidly develops, and no permanent engorgement results. If the problem is bilateral and develops rapidly, then venous engorgement of the head may occur. This leads to swelling and edema, which may cause upper airway obstruction and difficulty in eating. However, collateral vessels, such as the vertebral veins, often expand to handle the load, and the swelling reduces.

THERAPY

Initial therapy in cases of perivascular injections with irritant solutions should include local irrigation with physiologic saline to dilute the irritant. Concurrent injection of local anesthetic solution (without epinephrine) has also been advocated to reduce spasm of blood vessels and also to reduce pain. Frequent "hot packing" of the affected site may also be beneficial. If sepsis or extensive tissue necrosis occurs, then it may be necessary to surgically establish drainage.

In cases in which there is a high risk of venous thrombosis, prophylactic anticoagulant therapy has been advocated. In a study by Scott et al. (1980), crystalline sodium warfarin given orally was the main agent used, although injectable warfarin and also heparin were given concurrently in certain cases. Of four cases with thrombophlebitis, two had a favorable outcome and two did not. Complications included subcutaneous hemorrhages on the ventral abdomen and limbs. Throughout the course of therapy, coagulation parameters were monitored frequently and the dosage was adjusted to keep prothrombin times 1.5 to 2.5 times greater than normal. Dosages varied from 30 to 75 mg per day for full-sized horses. If the animals were considered to be in danger from overtreatment, then they were given 40 to 150 mg of vitamin K_1.

Anticoagulation therapy of this type should be undertaken cautiously and only if the coagulation system can be evaluated on a regular basis. The risks of precipitating warfarin poisoning are such that empirical therapy should be avoided.

Supplemental Readings

1. Gulick, B. A., and Meagher, D. M.: Evaluation of an intravenous catheter for use in the horse. J. Am. Vet. Med. Assoc., *178*:272, 1981.
2. Scott, E. A., Byars, T. D., and Lamar, A. M.: Warfarin anticoagulation in the horse. J. Am. Vet. Med. Assoc., *177*:1146, 1980.

DISEASES OF THE GREAT VESSELS

Christopher M. Brown, EAST LANSING, MICHIGAN

Lesions affecting the pulmonary artery or the aortic root or both have been reported to cause clinical problems in horses. Those affecting the aorta have been described more frequently. Rupture of the aorta just above the valve has been well documented, resulting in sudden death from cardiac tamponade. Similar aortic ruptures, but through the fibrous aortic ring, have been described in stallions. A typical history is that the stallion bred a mare, often early in the season, then collapsed and died. Death may not be so sudden, and the animal may live a few hours. Occasionally the horse does not die and shows progressive signs of heart failure with jugular pulsations, edema, and various murmurs. Histopathology of these cases, either those rupturing the aortic ring or rupturing through the ring, shows medionecrosis of the aortic wall. The role of these changes in the etiology of the condition is unknown. A sudden and marked elevation in blood pressure may be the precipitating cause, particularly in the breeding stallion.

Dissecting aortic aneurysm that ruptured into the pulmonary artery has been described. Clinically the animal showed signs of congestive heart failure. Fatal rupture of the pulmonary trunk has also been described in an adult horse with a patent ductus arteriosus.

Thoracic aortic strongylosis was reported in 9.4 per cent of horses at a British slaughterhouse. This was associated with ischemic myocardial fibrotic lesions. It was suggested that larval activity in the aortic root produced thromboemboli, which then seeded into the coronary vasculature. These occluded small vessels and caused small areas of ischemia. The clinical significance of these findings is unknown. However, the possibility that these small ischemic areas could be the cause of some of the equine arrhythmias is intriguing.

Supplemental Readings

1. Cranley, J. J., and McCullogh, K. G.: Ischemic myocardial fibrosis and aortic strongylosis in the horse. Equine Vet. J., *13*:35, 1981.
2. Rooney, J. R., Prickett, M. E., and Crowe, M. W.: Aortic ring rupture in stallions. Pathol. Vet., *4*:268, 1967.

AORTOILIOFEMORAL ARTERIOSCLEROSIS

P. W. Physick-Sheard, GUELPH, ONTARIO, CANADA

M. G. Maxie, GUELPH, ONTARIO, CANADA

Aortoiliofemoral arteriosclerosis (AIFA) is an acquired, progressive vascular disease of the horse involving the terminal aorta, aortic bifurcation, internal and external iliac arteries, and their major divisions, notably the femoral arteries and their main branches. Clinical signs are those of exercise-associated vascular insufficiency (intermittent claudication) in the hindlimbs. The condition occurs almost exclusively in young (three years old or less) male racehorses, usually animals whose performance shows great promise; it is occasionally seen in geldings, though such animals have often been castrated since the onset of prodromal signs, and it has been recorded in mares. AIFA is distinguished from acute thromboembolism or saddle thrombus by the absence of the typical acute history, by the absence of postmortem evidence of a primary site of thrombus formation, and by the histology of the lesion. The condition has previously been referred to as aortic-iliac thrombosis, aortoiliac thrombosis, and aortic-iliac-femoral thrombosis.

CLINICAL SIGNS

Animals usually present with a prodromal history of vague hind end lameness or poor performance of several weeks' to months' duration, with treatment having been applied empirically for "loose" stifles, trochanteric bursitis, bone spavin, or shoeing problems. Despite failure to achieve expected standards, performance is often adequate during the prodromal period as long as the animal is kept in work. A tendency for the horse to move roughly after a race is frequently referred to by trainers. In cases examined by the authors, acute signs have invariably been preceded by a period of rest, usually undertaken because of a deterioration in race performance, without a definitive diagnosis having been made. Affected animals return from this rest period with significant lameness becoming evident at work. The rate of working that produces lameness varies from case to case and may be as little as light jogging or trotting in severe cases. The horse shows a progressive stiffness of usually one hindleg initially, occasionally both, the stiffness resulting in a tendency to go on the toe, to knuckle or to trip, and to circumduct behind. Disability is progressive with work until, in many cases, the animal is unable to go on and may even fall. One or both limbs are carried stiffly, the back is arched, and the gait is very stilted.

The animal is often very anxious and may sweat profusely from the barrel, head, and neck but not over the affected limbs. The extent to which these acute signs are shown will depend upon the extent of the horse's vascular impediment and the rate of working, mildly affected cases showing only very transient signs.

Palpation of the hindlimbs reveals them to be cold, particularly from the lower thigh distally, and no arterial pulse can be palpated in the affected limb. The saphenous vein, normally full immediately after light exercise and within 10 seconds of completing heavy exercise, may in affected cases remain collapsed for a minute or more. The animal may tread with the hindlimbs and in mild cases may kick out. Clinical signs subside rapidly so that by 30 to 45 minutes postexercise, the animal appears clinically normal and ready to return to work.

Hematologic and biochemical studies both at rest and postexercise have shown only those changes normally associated with vigorous exercise in the horse; there is no abnormal elevation of serum muscle enzymes in association with this condition. Clinical examination of affected horses at rest reveals a typical collateral pulse contour in affected limbs. Coolness is inconsistent. In severe cases, the pulse may not be detectable. Rectal examination reveals a loss or weakening of the pulse and asymmetry and unusual firmness of the iliac vessels, though careful palpation may be necessary to detect the thrombus at the aortic bifurcation. In advanced cases, there may be muscle wasting over the hind end, although this is not often a prominent feature. Affected stallions are usually infertile, occasionally by virtue of the thrombosis of testicular arteries but more likely because blood is shunted away from the testes as a result of development of collateral blood supply to the hindlimbs.

Though the clinical signs in severe cases are quite distinct, difficulty may be encountered in confirming a diagnosis in cases of partial obstruction. While arteriography is the technique of choice, the introduction of a sufficiently large bore catheter to allow opacification of the proximal vascular tree of the hindlimbs may present problems, especially since the femoral and saphenous arteries are usually involved in the disease process. Such techniques as the measurement of blood velocity using ultrasound probes or definition of pulse contour may provide supportive evidence, but definitive diagnosis would rest upon demonstration of the actual obstruction.

These difficulties may in part explain the somewhat confused picture with regard to treatment.

PATHOLOGY

Postmortem examination reveals partial to total occlusion of the external and internal iliac arteries and their major divisions. Evidence points to simultaneous development of the primary lesions at several sites in the affected vessel, with the femoral arteries showing primary involvement as low as the level of division into the posterior femoral and popliteal arteries. Invariably a large, locally formed thrombus has been found in the aorta at the bifurcation. The thrombus shows moderate to firm fibrous attachment to the vessel wall over a wide area dorsally but is not always continuous with the thrombi lying in the iliac arteries. There may or may not be some asymmetry in the degree of involvement of the two sides. Unilateral involvement of the femoral artery and its major branches has been diagnosed in one horse.

In all cases, the primary lesion appears to be an intimal proliferation consisting mainly of fibrous tissue with moderate vascularity. Thrombus formation appears to occur subsequently, with this secondary lesion ranging from fresh local thrombus formation through areas of partial organization to a mature, firm, organized fibrous mass. Attempts at recanalization are seen at some sites, while in areas of partial occlusion, the thrombus may have a smooth endothelial covering. At sites of primary involvement, the internal elastic lamina frequently shows discontinuity and fragmentation.

The histologic findings in cases examined by the authors justify a diagnosis of primary arteriosclerosis. In most cases, the vascular occlusion is enough to totally preclude vascular supply via either the internal or external iliac vessels. Thorough postmortem examination has revealed diffusely distributed though mild vascular lesions at other sites in the body. No evidence has been found of parasitism within the aortoiliac lesion or of primary thromboembolism. Cardiac disease has not been recorded in cases of AIFA with the exception of one horse that had in addition a ventricular septal defect.

ETIOLOGY

The etiology and pathogenesis of AIFA are not understood. No attempt has been made in the literature to differentiate between aortic thromboembolism and AIFA, and analogies have been drawn with saddle thrombus or aortic thromboembolism in the cat, though the evidence indicates that AIFA in the horse is a primary degenerative vascular disease possibly predisposed to in part by vigorous exercise.

True thromboembolism is occasionally seen in the horse; the onset is acute. Predisposing causes of such episodes may include abdominal abscessation, extensive parasite damage to the aorta, and atrial fibrillation. Cases surviving the acute stage of thromboembolism may show clinical signs similar to AIFA. Conversely, the horse suffering from AIFA and subsequently rested may show an apparent sudden onset of clinical signs upon returning to work.

Observations made by the authors suggest that the hemodynamics of blood flow in the affected vessels may be a primary factor in the development of the AIFA lesion. In the horse, predisposition to nonlaminar, possibly turbulent flow may be the result of several factors, notably the anatomy of the aortic bifurcation and the large diameter of these vessels, the unique and marked fibrous union of the terminal aorta and aortic bifurcation to the deep lumbosacral fascia, the external stresses to which the vessel is subjected during locomotion, and the very heavy blood flow to the muscles of the hindlimb during exercise. Damage to the vascular endothelium that may result from turbulent flow and stress on the blood vessel wall may predispose to intimal proliferation and to local adhesion of platelets and fibrin. Progressive development of the intimal plaque and mural thrombi results in eventual occlusion of the vessel. Developing lesions will further contribute to local turbulence. Reduction in flow at rest is not likely to result in clinical signs until the size of the vessel lumen approaches 20 per cent of normal. However, much less marked reduction in lumen size is likely to result in clinical signs during exercise. Individual variations, such as congenital narrowness of the aorta and iliac vessels with hemodynamically unfavorable angles of bifurcation and unfavorable area ratios, will predispose to turbulent flow and stress-related vascular injury. Individual variations in the efficiency of vascular repair and fibrinolysis may also predispose toward the growth of thrombus. While the higher incidence of the condition in the male is unexplained, the situation parallels that in men, where the aortoiliac bifurcation is a predilection site for degenerative vascular disease and occlusive thrombogenesis. However, while a hemodynamic theory may help to explain the pathogenesis of the lesions, the factors that mediate individual predisposition and those that moderate the clinical picture remain unclear.

TREATMENT

The recommended therapy for obstructive vascular disease in the hind end of the horse has been to administer sodium gluconate by slow intravenous infusion (90 to 250 min) at the dose of 450 mg per kg body weight. It has been suggested that the administration of 100 mg prednisolone sodium succinate intravenously 30 min prior to the sodium gluconate will eliminate the frequent systemic reactions associated with the drug. Using this regimen, cures have been claimed.[1, 3]

This therapy is based upon a report that was published in 1966[3] suggesting that sodium gluconate together with a dialyzable constituent of recalcified human plasma clots was capable of stimulating in vivo fibrinolysis in cats and dogs. The clots that were dissolved were fresh and were formed by the injection of partially clotted homologous blood into a segment of evacuated clamped jugular vein. Clot breakdown in response to treatment was partial and localized to areas of the clot in direct contact with the vascular endothelium. The experiment did not appear to have been controlled, and there have been no studies to suggest that sodium gluconate has any effect on a mature thrombus.

In those cases cited in the literature[2] in which a clinical response to the use of sodium gluconate was seen, the diagnosis was not confirmed prior to treatment, and no objective studies were reported to have been carried out to quantify the nature and extent of response to treatment. Several of the cases appear to have been acute in onset and may have been cases of true thromboembolism. Only two cases of true thromboembolism of the aortic bifurcation have been seen in the horse in this clinic in the last 10 years, both occurring in pleasure horses. The onsets were typically acute in contrast to the progressive picture seen in AIFA, and severe systemic response to the infarctive sequelae was apparent. In diseased arteries in humans, evidence of predisposition to spasm has been found, while the presence of a fresh thrombus as opposed to simple vascular occlusion has been shown to interfere with the development of collateral circulation in the cat. In those cases cited as having responded to treatment,[2] therefore, the sodium gluconate may have had some modifying influence on these factors, in addition to possibly assisting in the lysis of a relatively fresh blood clot.

The use of the recommended therapeutic regimen by the authors in nine horses showing typical clinical signs of AIFA has had no clinical effect, either beneficial or deleterious. Five of these cases were confirmed by postmortem examination. In view of the nature of the lesions found, a response would not have been expected.

While affected animals may show a very significant exercise intolerance, their ability to perform can be improved by progressive increase in exercise so as to stimulate the development of a collateral blood supply. It is likely that this collateral supply is responsible for the animal's ability to perform adequately during the prodromal period and prior to the period of rest. During rest the collateral circulation regresses rapidly in the absence of constant exercise demand, resulting in a marked exacerbation of clinical signs on return to work.

Collateral supply is most likely to be provided by the posterior mesenteric artery via the anterior hemorrhoidal artery and by the caudal epigastric arteries. Additional supply will occur via the lumbar arteries and circumflex iliac vessels and via numerous smaller collaterals. This circulation will be very inefficient because of the small diameter and length of the vessels involved. In the mare, the ovarian (anterior uterine) artery is capable of making a very significant contribution to vascular supply and may be part of the reason for the low incidence of the clinical condition in the female.

References

1. Azzie, M. A. J.: Aortic/iliac thrombosis of Thoroughbred horses. Equine Vet. J., *1*(3):113, 1969.
2. Branscomb, B.L.: Treatment of arterial thrombosis in a horse with sodium gluconate. J. Am. Vet. Med. Assoc., *152*:1643, 1968.
3. Kopper, P. H.: In vivo fibrinolysis with a dialysable constituent of recalcified human plasma clots and gluconate. Nature, *211*:43, 1966.
4. Moffett, F. S., and Vaden, P.: Diagnosis and treatment of thrombosis of the posterior aorta or iliac arteries in the horse. Vet. Med. Sm. Anim. Clinician, 73:184, 1978.
5. Stehbens, W. E.: Haemodynamics and the Blood Vessel Wall. Springfield, IL, C. C Thomas, 1979, p. 294.

Section 4
ENDOCRINE DISEASES
Edited by V. K. Ganjam

THYROID DISEASES 159

NUTRITIONAL SECONDARY HYPERPARATHYROIDISM 160

TUMORS OF THE PITUITARY GLAND (PARS INTERMEDIA) 164

DIABETES MELLITUS 169

ANHIDROSIS 170

THYROID DISEASES

John E. Lowe, ITHACA, NEW YORK

Thyroid disease with disturbed thyroxine secretion or release appears to be an uncommon problem in the horse. Clinical states of hypothyroidism or hyperthyroidism are rarely recognized and confirmed by thyroid function tests. As reliance on function tests becomes more widespread and perhaps with improvements in function test sensitivity, we may be able to recognize borderline thyroid disturbance. For all that has been blamed on thyroid dysfunction in the horse, the evidence is still not available to substantiate its importance.

The thyroid gland produces thyroxine from thyroid cells and calcitonin from C cells within the gland. Thyroxine has profound effects on growth, maintenance, and function of all tissues, especially in the young, growing animal. Calcitonin is a regulator of calcium homeostasis at the upper end of the narrow normal range.[9] It is not the only regulator and may not be the primary one.

HYPERCALCITONINISM

Hypercalcitoninism induced by experimental diets rich in calcium has been implicated as a cause of osteopetrosis and in the pathogenesis of osteochondritis dissecans and vertebral malformation leading to spinal cord trauma.[8] However, since no clinical entity of calcitonin dysfunction is recognized, no rational therapy can be recommended.

HYPOTHYROIDISM

A dietary source of iodine is essential for normal production and release of thyroxine, which is stored in the follicles of the thyroid gland. Retention of thyroxine with gross enlargement of the thyroid lobes (goiter) occurs in conditions of too little and too much dietary iodine. These conditions are widely recognized. The excess iodine problem is seen most frequently as a result of feeding excess vitamin-mineral supplements that contain seaweed (kelp), a rich iodine source.[1] Correction is simply removal of the source of excess iodine. Goiter from lack of iodine has been seen in the past in all domestic animals, particularly sheep. This type of goiter is rare today because iodized salt is fed or provided free choice to most horses.

The extent to which goiter has to exist before functional effects of a lack of circulating thyroxine are seen is difficult to define. Protein-bound iodine, resin sponge uptake of labeled tri-iodothyronine (T_3), and total serum thyroxine (T_4) have all been used to evaluate the function of the thyroid gland.

At present, T_4 is the only reliable indicator of thyroid function in the horse. Normal values (1 to 3 μg per cent) are lower than in other species, and for reasons that are unknown, the fit horse has particularly low values.[4] A value of 0.5 μg per cent should be found before a state of hypothyroidism is diagnosed.[5, 6, 7] The newborn has excessively high T_4 values for a few days.

Some weak foals with goiter are born to mares receiving excessive dietary intake of iodine during gestation. The functional significance of goiter in these foals is unknown. Some do recover, and the goiter regresses in three to six weeks. Others may die of complications or of other causes only to have the goiter implicated as the primary cause because it is so easily observed.[1] Experimentally, thyroidectomy in young foals severely curtails growth and may cause death within one to two months.[5]

Hypothyroidism has been diagnosed in obese mares that are subject to recurring laminitis and erratic reproductive function, but thyroid function tests either have not been used or have not confirmed hypothyroidism. A cheap, readily available thyroxine source, iodinated casein,* has been used in these animals. Weight loss ensues but may be the result of creating a hyperthyroid state. There is no clear-cut prescription for success in treatment of these cases. Iodinated casein contains approximately 1 per cent thyroxine. In totally thyroidectomized horses, 5 gm of iodinated casein per day are necessary to maintain normal T_4 levels.

Surgical thyroidectomy without concurrent parathyroidectomy is possible in the horse and has shown that totally hypothyroid horses have subnormal body temperature, reduced appetite, lethargy, dry, scaly coats that shed later in the spring than in normal horses, slowed growth with delayed eruption of teeth, delayed closure of epiphyseal growth plates, edema of pendant parts, especially the rear limbs from the hock distally, elevated serum cholesterol, depressed serum phosphorus, and a low-grade anemia. These animals can reproduce, although libido is depressed, total sperm cell production is decreased, and cycling of mares is inconsistent.[7] Thus, total thyroidectomy except in the neonate is not life-threatening. Thyroxine supplementation results in correction of signs associated with the hypothyroid condition. Five gm of iodinated casein per day added to the ration brings T_4 levels up to 1 to 3 μg per cent. If iodinated casein is used as an added source of thyroxine, adjustment of the dose should be based on clinical response and T_4 levels.[6]

---

*Protonome, Agri Tech, Kansas City, MO

HYPERTHYROIDISM

Documented cases of hyperthyroidism have not been found in the literature by the author. We have performed or recommended total thyroidectomy on three fractious uncontrollable hunters. One result was excellent, one fair to good, and one poor. The one in the excellent category went on to win championships while on a regulated low level of thyroxine supplementation; one became capable of being trained and ridden in a ring but not the hunt field, and one was totally unmanageable. These animals were not confirmed hyperthyroid by thyroid function tests. The ethics of this procedure are subject to legitimate debate; however, it is unlikely to ever become a procedure of widespread use.[6]

Pituitary tumors of the pars intermedia occasionally occur in old horses (p. 164). They sometimes cause a secondary hypothyroidism through suppression of thyroid stimulation hormone (TSH) because of pressure on the anterior pituitary gland. Because of interference with the pituitary gland, a mixture of signs is noted, including polyuria, polydipsia, hirsutism, poor shedding, dull dry hair coat, lethargy, and sometimes blindness because of pressure on the optic chiasm. In these cases, a TSH response test is useful. A blood sample is drawn for T_4 determination, then 20 IU TSH is given intramuscularly, and blood is drawn again for T_4 after 12 hours. A rise of greater than two times baseline indicates normal function of the gland and thus confirmation of suspected secondary hypothyroidism.

THYROID ADENOMA

Thyroid adenomas are seen in old horses as a nonpainful swelling, usually of one lobe of the thyroid. They may become quite large (up to 10 cm diameter). To our knowledge none have been reported to be functional. If indicated because of space-occupying problems or aesthetics, the involved lobe can be removed surgically.

References

1. Baker, H. J., and Lindsey, J. R.: Equine goiter due to excess dietary iodide. J. Am. Vet. Med. Assoc., *153*:1618, 1968.
2. Hightower, D., Miller, L., and Kyzar, J.: Comparison of serum and plasma thyroxine determinations in horses. J. Am. Vet. Med. Assoc., *159*:449, 1971.
3. Kallfelz, F. A.: Thyroid function in the dog. Vet. Clin. North Am., 7(3):497, 1977.
4. Kallfelz, F. A., and Lowe, J. E.: Some normal values of thyroid function in horses. J. Am. Vet. Med. Assoc., *156*:1888, 1970.
5. Lowe, J. E., and Kallfelz, F. A.: Thyroidectomy and the T-4 test to assess thyroid dysfunction in the horse and pony. Proc. 16th Annu. Conv. Am. Assoc. Eq. Pract. 1970, pp. 135–154.
6. Lowe, J. E., Baldwin, B. H., Foote, R. H., Hillman, R. B., and Kallfelz, F. A.: Equine hypothyroidism: The long term effects of thyroidectomy on metabolism and growth in mares and stallions. Cornell Vet., *64*:276, 1974.
7. Lowe, J. E., Baldwin, B. H., Foote, R. H., Hillman, R. B., and Kallfelz, F. A.: Semen characteristics in thyroidectomized stallions. J. Reprod. Fertil., Suppl., 23:81, 1975.
8. Mayhew, I. G., deLahunta, A., Whitlock, R. H., Krook, L., and Tasker, J. B.: Spinal cord disease in the horse. Cornell Vet., *68*, Suppl. 6:1, 1978.
9. Whitlock, R. H.: The effects of high dietary calcium in horses: A metabolic, radiological, morphological, and biophysical study. Thesis, Cornell University, 1970.

NUTRITIONAL SECONDARY HYPERPARATHYROIDISM

Charles C. Capen, COLUMBUS, OHIO

Calcium plays a key role in many fundamental biologic processes, including neuromuscular excitability, membrane permeability, muscle contraction, enzyme activity, hormone release, and blood coagulation, in addition to being an essential structural component of the skeleton. The precise control of calcium in extracellular fluids is vital to the health of animals and humans. To maintain a constant concentration of calcium despite marked variations in intake and excretion, endocrine control mechanisms have evolved that primarily consist of the interaction of three major hormones. Although the direct roles of parathyroid hormone (PTH), calcitonin, and cholecalciferol (vitamin D) are frequently emphasized

in the control of blood calcium, other hormones such as adrenal corticosteroids, estrogens, thyroxine, somatotropin, and glucagon may contribute to the maintenance of calcium metabolism and skeletal homeostasis under certain conditions.

Parathyroids in horses consist of two pairs of glands. The larger pair of parathyroids is situated in the ventral cervical region near the level of the first rib at the bifurcation of the bicarotid trunk.[8] The upper pair of parathyroid glands is present along the thyroid artery, dorsocranially to each thyroid lobe, and outside of the thyroid capsule.

Parathyroid glands are composed of a single type of secretory cell, termed a chief cell, that is responsible for the synthesis and secretion of parathyroid hormone.[3] Recent evidence suggests that a larger biosynthetic precursor ("proparathyroid hormone") is first synthesized on the rough endoplasmic reticulum from which active PTH is cleaved enzymatically during transport through the Golgi apparatus prior to storage in secretion granules and secretion from chief cells (Fig. 1).

In contrast to most endocrine organs, which are under complex controls involving both long and short feedback loops, the parathyroids have a unique feedback control by the concentration of calcium (and to a lesser degree, magnesium) ions in serum. Parathyroid hormone is the principal hormone involved in the minute-to-minute fine regulation of blood calcium in mammals. It exerts its biologic actions by directly influencing the function of target cells, primarily in bone and kidney.[4]

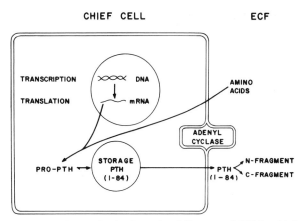

Figure 1. Biosynthesis of parathyroid hormone (PTH) by chief cells. Parathyroid hormone is synthesized as part of a larger biosynthetic precursor molecule (pro-PTH) that is converted to active PTH prior to storage and secretion from the cell.

PATHOPHYSIOLOGIC MECHANISMS

The increased secretion of PTH in this metabolic disorder is a compensatory mechanism directed against a disturbance in mineral homeostasis induced by nutritional imbalances. The disease occurs particularly in young horses, as well as in other animals, such as pigs, cattle, cats, dogs, laboratory animals, and certain nonhuman primates.

Dietary mineral imbalances of etiologic importance in the pathogenesis of nutritional secondary hyperparathyroidism are (1) excessive phosphorus with normal or low calcium, (2) a low content of calcium, and (3) inadequate amounts of vitamin D_3. The significant end result is hypocalcemia, which results in the parathyroid stimulation.

In horses, the most frequent nutritional imbalance involves the ingestion of excessive phosphorus. This results in an increased intestinal absorption of phosphorus and elevation of blood phosphorus concentration (Fig. 2). Hyperphosphatemia does not stimulate the parathyroid gland directly but does so indirectly by virtue of its ability to lower blood calcium. Horses that develop the disease usually have been fed high-grain diets with below-average quality roughage. Evidence of high phosphorus intake may be difficult to establish inasmuch as the excess phosphorus may be fed by the owner in the form of a bran supplement added to a grain diet in order to improve the health of the horse. The diet usually is palatable and nutritious except for the imbalanced phosphorus (excessive amounts) and calcium (marginal or deficient) content. A diet deficient in calcium fails to supply the daily requirement even though a greater proportion of ingested calcium is absorbed, and hypocalcemia develops. Occasionally, horses may develop nutritional hyperparathyroidism after pasturing on grasses with a high oxalate

content. This results in intestinal malabsorption of calcium.[9]

In response to the nutritionally induced hypocalcemia, all parathyroid glands undergo cellular hypertrophy and hyperplasia with ultrastructural evidence of increased secretory activity.[5] Since kidney function is normal, the increased levels of PTH result in diminished renal tubular reabsorption of phosphate and increased reabsorption of calcium, returning blood levels toward normal (Fig. 2). In addition, bone resorption is accelerated, and release of calcium elevates blood calcium levels to the low normal range. Continued ingestion of the unbalanced diet sustains the state of compensatory hyperparathyroidism, leading to the progressive development of metabolic bone disease.

CLINICAL SIGNS

Initial clinical signs in horses with nutritional secondary hyperparathyroidism usually include a transitory shifting lameness in one or more limbs, generalized tenderness of joints, and a stilted gait.[8] Although skeletal involvement is generalized with hyperparathyroidism, it does not affect all parts uniformly. Skeletal lesions become apparent earlier and reach a more advanced stage in certain areas. The lameness develops as a result of increased osteoclastic resorption of outer circumferential lamellae with disruption of tendinous insertions and bone trabeculae supporting the articular cartilage, resulting in disruption of joint cartilage on weight-bearing. Resorption of alveolar socket bone and loss of lamina dura dentes occur early and may result in loose teeth.

Later in the course of the disease, severe lesions develop in bones of the skull, especially the maxilla

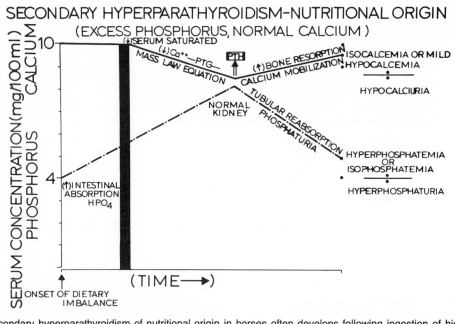

Figure 2. Secondary hyperparathyroidism of nutritional origin in horses often develops following ingestion of high phosphorus diets with normal or deficient amounts of calcium. Parathyroid glands are stimulated by the hypocalcemia that develops reciprocally as the blood phosphorus is elevated. Parathyroid hyperactivity returns the blood calcium and phosphorus to near normal levels and results in the development of fibrous osteodystrophy.

and mandible, resulting in bilateral firm enlargements of the facial bones immediately above and anterior to the facial crests. The horizontal rami of the mandibles are irregularly thickened by a progressive hyperostotic fibrous osteodystrophy ("big head") that develops in horses with nutritional secondary hyperparathyroidism.

The hyperostosis of skull bones results from osteoid and fibrous connective tissue deposition in excess of the volume of bone resorbed. The chronic excess intake of phosphorus and increased secretion of PTH result in stimulation of osteoblasts to form osteoid in excess of the amount of bone resorbed by osteoclasts and progressive enlargement of skeletal bones. The hyperostotic fibrous osteodystrophy may impinge upon the nasal cavity, resulting in dyspnea, especially after exertion.

CLINICAL PATHOLOGY

Analysis of the serum for calcium, phosphorus, and alkaline phosphatase should be undertaken with an appreciation that one determination may be of limited diagnostic value. Since the body's compensatory mechanisms with nutritional secondary hyperparathyroidism are complex and usually operational when the horse is seen clinically for the first time, serum calcium and phosphorus levels usually are in the low normal range (Fig. 2) (Table 1). Serum alkaline phosphatase levels often are in the high nor-

mal range or elevated in horses with overt bone disease, reflecting the increased osteoblastic and osteoclastic activity in hyperparathyroidism. Under experimental conditions, horses fed a high phosphorus diet (phosphorus, 1.4 per cent; calcium, 0.7 per cent) are able to more rapidly normalize their blood calcium following an ethylenediaminetetra-acetic acid (EDTA)-induced hypocalcemia than controls fed a balanced diet (phosphorus, 0.6 per cent; calcium, 0.7 per cent) owing to the increased parathyroid activity.[2]

Changes in urine calcium and phosphorus are more consistent and useful in the clinical diagnosis of nutritional secondary hyperparathyroidism in

TABLE 1. SERUM AND URINE CALCIUM AND PHOSPHORUS AND SERUM ALKALINE PHOSPHATASE IN HORSES WITH NUTRITIONAL SECONDARY HYPERPARATHYROIDISM (NSH)

Laboratory Parameter	NSH	Normal Range
Serum calcium (mg/dl)	10.5	10.5–12.5
Serum phosphorus (mg/dl)	4.8	2–5
Serum alkaline phosphatase (sigma units/ml)	6.7	2–6
Urine calcium (mg/dl)	7.9	20
Urine phosphorus (mg/dl)	160.8	4–18

(Modified from Joyce, J. R., Pierce, K. R., Romane, W. M., and Baker, J. M.: Clinical study of nutritional secondary hyperparathyroidism in horses. J. Am. Vet. Med. Assoc., *158*:2033, 1971.)

horses. The increased secretion of PTH acts on the normal kidneys to markedly increase urinary phosphorus excretion but decrease calcium loss in the urine compared to normal horses.[7] Blood urea nitrogen, serum creatinine, and other parameters used to assess renal function are within normal limits in horses with nutritional hyperparathyroidism.

The diet should be carefully analyzed in horses suspected of having clinical evidence of nutritional secondary hyperparathyroidism. Often wheat bran (calcium:phosphorus 1:10.9) or rice bran (calcium:phosphorus 1:30) are major ingredients of the ration in horses with the disease.[7, 8] The onset of clinical signs and development of bone lesions occur more rapidly in young horses fed diets both low in calcium and containing excessive phosphorus. Horses fed diets containing large amounts of phosphorus initially have hyperphosphatemia (Fig. 2), resulting in intense osteoblastic stimulation and excessive deposition of osteoid, leading to the development of the hyperostotic form of fibrous osteodystrophy.

Nutritional secondary hyperparathyroidism may be encountered occasionally in horses on pasture with a normal phosphorus and calcium content but containing large amounts of oxalates.[9] The oxalates appear to form insoluble complexes with calcium in the intestine, resulting in an elevated fecal calcium:phosphorus ratio (2.35:1) compared with horses on a similar calcium and phosphorus intake but without the oxalate-rich plants (fecal calcium:phosphorus ratio 1.2:1). The interference in intestinal calcium absorption results in the development of progressive hypocalcemia that leads to parathyroid stimulation and development of the metabolic bone disease. The facial hyperostosis that may develop in horses without an increase of blood phosphorus appears to be due to the anabolic effects of the long-term moderate elevation in PTH levels on osteoblastic activity and deposition of osteoid.

THERAPY

The aim of treatment is to decrease PTH secretion by correcting the dietary mineral imbalance or deficiency. Diet supplementation with grain products containing phosphorus-rich bran should be stopped immediately. Since analysis of the diet often reveals a marginal or deficient content of calcium, supplementation with a calcium-rich low phosphorus source is indicated, particularly in young horses. Good-quality alfalfa hay is a useful dietary supplement for horses with severe nutritional secondary hyperparathyroidism due to a high content of calcium and a favorable calcium:phosphorus ratio (approximately 6:1).[7]

The dietary calcium intake should be calculated to provide for amounts in excess of the National Research Council's (1978)[1] daily requirement for either yearling horses (35 gm per day), two-year-old horses (31 gm per day), or mature horses (27 gm per day). Clinical evidence of lameness usually disappears within one to two months of feeding the corrected ration with supplementation, but the facial swellings only slowly, if ever, regress to normal.

Calcium has been fed to horses at five times the required levels without detrimental effects, provided the level of dietary phosphorus is adequate to compensate for the decreased efficiency of intestinal calcium absorption.[6] However, increased calcium intake may result in greater bone density and decreased bone remodeling with a greater proportion of lamellar than osteonic bone, which could influence bone strength unfavorably if continued for an unnecessarily long interval after bone healing has occurred in young horses.[10]

Horses that develop nutritional secondary hyperparathyroidism on pasture of grasses with a balanced calcium:phosphorus ratio that have a high oxalate content should be removed from the pasture and fed a high-calcium diet as described previously.

References

1. Anonymous: Nutritional requirements of horses, 4th revised ed. Washington, DC, National Academy of Sciences, 1978.
2. Argenzio, R. A., Lowe, J. E., Hintz, H. F., and Schryver, H. F.: Calcium and phosphorus homeostasis in horses. J. Nutr., *104*:18, 1974.
3. Capen, C. C.: Functional and fine structural relationships of parathyroid glands. *In* Brandly, C. A., and Cornelius, C. E. (eds.): Advances in Veterinary Science and Comparative Medicine. New York, Academic Press, *19*:249–286, 1975.
4. Capen, C. C.: The calcium regulating hormones: Parathyroid hormone, calcitonin, and cholecalciferol. *In* McDonald, L. E. (ed.): Veterinary Endocrinology and Reproduction, 3rd ed. Philadelphia, Lea & Febiger, 1980, pp. 60–130.
5. Fujimoto, Y., Matsukawa, K., Inubushi, H., Nakamatsu, M., Satoh, H., and Yamagiwa, S.: Electron microscopic observations of the equine parathyroid glands with particular reference to those of equine osteodystrophia fibrosa. Jap. J. Vet. Res., *15*:37, 1967.
6. Jordan, R. M., Myers, V. S., Yoho, B., and Spurrell, F. A.: Effect of calcium and phosphorus levels on growth, reproduction and bone development of ponies. J. Anim. Sci., *40*:78, 1975.
7. Joyce, J. R., Pierce, K. R., Romane, W. M., and Baker, J. M.: Clinical study of nutritional secondary hyperparathyroidism in horses. J. Am. Vet. Med. Assoc., *158*:2033, 1971.
8. Krook, L., and Lowe, J. E.: Nutritional secondary hyperparathyroidism in the horse. Pathol. Vet., Suppl. 1:1, 1964.
9. Walthall, J. C., and McKenzie, R. A.: Osteodystrophia fibrosa in horses at pasture in Queensland: Field and laboratory observations. Aust. Vet. J., *52*:11, 1976.
10. Whitlock, R. H., Schryver, H. F., Krook, L., Hintz, H. F., and Craig, P. H.: The effects of high dietary calcium in horses. Proc. 25th Annu. Conv. Am. Assoc. Eq. Pract., pp. 127–134, 1979.

TUMORS OF THE PITUITARY GLAND (PARS INTERMEDIA)

Jill Beech, KENNETT SQUARE, PENNSYLVANIA

Adenomas of the pars intermedia of the pituitary gland have been described as occurring primarily in aged horses.[9, 10, 15, 21, 23, 24, 28, 29] The youngest recorded in the literature is seven years, and usually horses are much older. There is no breed predilection, but females are said to be more frequently affected than males.[15] The tumor may be an incidental necropsy finding but also can cause clinical signs.

PHYSIOLOGY

In the horse, the pars intermedia is a source of melanocyte stimulating hormone (alpha-MSH, beta-MSH, gamma$_3$-MSH), beta endorphins (BEND), corticotropin-like intermediate lobe peptide (CLIP), and ACTH.[27] All these molecules come from a common precursor molecule, pro-opiomelanocortin (POMC) or pro-opiolipomelanocortin (POLMC), which is present in both the pars intermedia and pars distalis. Initial studies in horses with Cushing's disease show that the pattern of secretion of POLMC peptides is similar to that in normal horses. Unlike in humans, the hypersecretion is from the pars intermedia, not the pars distalis, and is insensitive to glucocorticoid negative feedback; dexamethasone does not have the suppressive effect seen in humans with Cushing's disease.[27] It has also been shown in rats that the secretion of ACTH in response to feedback-mediated changes is different in the pars intermedia than in the pars distalis.[22] Nicholson and colleagues[27] found that certain POLMC peptides were found only in tumor tissue and not in normal pars intermedia. The tumor POLMC concentrations were also higher than those in normal pars intermedia, and plasma levels were much higher. They found that in contrast to the lack of response to high doses of dexamethasone, the dopaminergic agonist pergolide* decreased both POLMC peptides and cortisol levels to high normal ranges. It is probable that these horses also have some secretion from the pars distalis, as dexamethasone combined with pergolide caused an even further decrease in plasma cortisol.[27]

CLINICAL SIGNS

Afflicted horses are usually presented to the veterinarian mainly because of polyuria and polydipsia (PUPD) and also because of hirsutism and failure to shed (Table 1). Horses may drink enormous quantities of water. More than 80 liters a day may be imbibed compared to the normal intake of 20 to 30 liters for a resting horse. Urine volumes are increased accordingly. Appetite may be normal or ravenous. If secondary complications such as infections intervene, anorexia may occur. The hair coat is often coarse and brittle and long and shaggy. It may become wavy or curly. The skin may be dry and scaly or greasy. The long hair may be diffuse or limited to the limbs, withers, and over the thoracic and croup regions. The mane and tail are normal. Animals frequently appear "sway-backed" and "potbellied" with loss of muscle, especially the dorsal epaxial and gluteal muscles; the tuber coxae and tuber sacrale appear prominent. These horses lose condition despite a normal or increased appetite. They also appear more susceptible to infections. It is common to see skin infections, such as streptothricosis; respiratory diseases, such as bronchitis and sinusitis; periodontal disease; and even infections of tendon sheaths or joints. Intramuscular and intravenous injection sites seem to be abnormally prone to infections, and wound healing is delayed. Several of our patients have had ulcers on the buccal mucosa. Laminitis may occur. Although other authors have not observed neurologic signs, Brandt described two of five cases that staggered and seemed tired.[4] Long-standing cases may become blind owing to optic nerve compression by the tumor. Bulging supraorbital fat pads and/or a "bug eyed" expression may be present. Animals may also suffer bouts of sweating, and the long curly hair becomes sticky and matted. Episodes of tachypnea have also been seen. When horses are turned out, it is possible for many of these signs to be missed. It is interesting that most of our cases were presented in late spring or summer; the long hair coat had not been noted to be abnormal until the horses had not shed in the spring. PUPD is often not noticed until horses are stabled for long periods.

When a horse is presented with the preceding history, careful physical examination and clinical laboratory testing are necessary for diagnosis. Chronic debilitation due to poor management and nutrition, ill-kept teeth, parasitism, and other systemic diseases must be eliminated from consideration. PUPD of unknown etiology may occasionally be seen in otherwise healthy horses (possibly psychogenic polydipsia), and it may also accompany chronic renal failure. Pheochromocytomas may cause bouts of hyperhidrosis, hyperthermia, and

---

*Pergolide mesylate, Eli Lilly and Co., Indianapolis, IN

TABLE 1. SUMMARY OF COMMON CLINICAL SIGNS

Signs	Suggested Pathogenesis
Polyuria	Increase in GFR by cortisol Osmotic diuresis due to glucosuria Cortisol may block ADH release or its renal action
	Compression of posterior pituitary and/or hypothalamus causing lack of ADH
Polydipsia	Secondary to polyuria to maintain hydration; hypothalamic dysfunction
Long shaggy coat and hyperhidrosis	Hypothalamic dysfunction possible; idiopathic
Muscle wasting and weight loss	Deranged carbohydrate metabolism due to increased cortisol secretion and peripheral insulin resistance resulting in protein catabolism and gluconeogenesis
Infection Poor wound healing	Elevated cortisol levels

GFR—glomerular filtration rate
ADH—antidiuretic hormone

tachypnea as well as weight loss; PUPD could occur if the hyperglycemia and glucosuria were sufficient to result in osmotic diuresis.

CLINICAL LABORATORY TESTS

Laboratory testing initially should include a complete blood count, chemistry screen (including glucose, creatinine, and electrolytes), and a urinalysis (Table 2). Always observe the plasma for any gray or bluish hue, which indicates gross lipemia, which may occur in affected ponies. Unless there is an infection causing leukocytosis, the white blood cell count will be normal or even low; however, typically there is an absolute or relative neutrophilia and a lymphopenia and eosinopenia. The packed cell volume (PCV) and red blood cell count are often normal, but a mild normocytic normochromic anemia may exist in some cases. Where infection has supervened, an anemia of chronic disease may be found. Affected horses are usually hyperglycemic, with values exceeding 150 mg per dl and even greater than 300 mg per dl. The test should be repeated to assess its consistency; affected untreated horses usually maintain a high blood glucose. Electrolyte values and creatinine are usually normal unless there are complicating factors. For example, anorexia or diarrhea may result in low potassium levels, or superimposed renal disease may cause an elevation in creatinine. Urinalysis reveals a variable specific gravity that may be low or within normal limits. There is glucosuria and sometimes ketonuria when the animal is in a negative energy balance.

Usually the preceding findings are sufficient to warrant the following additional tests: IV insulin tolerance test, plasma hydrocortisone (cortisol) or total corticoid levels, and ACTH stimulation and dexamethasone suppression tests (Table 3). All plasma samples to be assayed for hydrocortisone (cortisol) should be kept cool and centrifuged as soon as possible to allow immediate freezing of the plasma. Plasma hydrocortisone levels vary somewhat among the different laboratories. As competitive protein binding assay techniques are less expensive then radioimmunoassay, many laboratories measure total corticoids and not specifically hydrocortisone. The latter comprises the major portion of total corticoids; its value is usually the total corticoid level less 0.5 μg per 100 ml.[12] Therefore, total corticoids are adequate for assessing the adrenal function. If no normal values are available from your laboratory, control samples should be submitted. Preferably the samples should be sent to a laboratory specializing in hormonal assays. In addition to hormonal analysis, further chemistry screen analyses may reveal increased triglycerides, a high cholesterol level, and sometimes evidence of impaired hepatic function if there has been sufficient hepatocellular change.

TABLE 2. SUMMARY OF LABORATORY RESULTS WHICH MAY BE OBTAINED IN HORSES WITH TUMOR OF THE PARS INTERMEDIA OF THE PITUITARY

Results of Clinical Laboratory Tests	Suggested Pathogenesis
Neutrophilia Lymphopenia and eosinopenia	Increased cortisol
Anemia (mild)	Chronic infections suppress bone marrow
Insulin-resistant hyperglycemia Ketosis Hyperlipidemia Increased triglycerides Hypercholesterolemia	Increased cortisol secretion and possible pancreatic B cell exhaustion. Deranged carbohydrate metabolism
Increased plasma cortisol Exaggerated response to ACTH	Adrenal cortex hypertrophy
Lack of response to dexamethasone	Autonomous secretion of ACTH or an ACTH-like compound not affected by negative feedback
Low T_3 and T_4	Possible decrease in TSH release due to elevated cortisol or change in secretion secondary to tumor

TABLE 3. SUMMARY OF ENDOCRINE FUNCTION TESTS USED IN DIAGNOSIS OF TUMORS OF THE PARS INTERMEDIA OF THE PITUITARY GLAND

Hormone Test	Normal Value	Reference
Hydrocortisone (cortisol)	6–0 μg/100 ml	Garcia, 1981
	≤13 μg/100 ml	James et al., 1970
	2.67 μg/100 ml	Bottoms et al., 1972
	8.6 and 11 μg/100 ml	Eiler et al., 1979
	7 μg/100 ml	Gribble, 1972
Total corticoids (resting horse)	5.1 μg/100 ml	Hoffsis et al., 1970
(Standardbred)	8.2 μg/100 ml	Hoffsis et al., 1970
ACTH stimulation (rise in cortisol)		
1 unit/kg ACTH gel IM	2–3 times increased by 8 hours	James et al., 1970
Pre and 8-hour sample		Hoffsis et al., 1970
		Gribble, 1972
200 IU corticotropin gel* IM	100% increased by 1 hour and persisting at least 4 hours	Eiler et al., 1979
100 IU cosyntropin† IV	80% increased by 2 hours	Eiler et al., 1979
Pre and 2-hour sample		
1 unit/kg ACTH IV	2–3 times increased by 2 hours	Gribble, 1972
Combined test with dexamethasone (DXM)		Eiler et al., 1979
10 mg DXM IM; pre and 3-hour sample; then 100 IU cosyntropin† IV and sample 2 hours later	Decrease to ⅓ baseline and then approximately 2 times increase of baseline by cosyntropin†	
Dexamethasone suppression (decrease in cortisol)		
40 μg/kg IM	66% decrease by 12 hours	Gribble, 1972
20 mg IM	50% decrease at 2 hours	Eiler, 1979
	70% decrease by 4 hours	
	80% decrease at 6 hours	
	Still decreased at 31% baseline value at 24 hours	
Insulin tolerance (decrease in glucose)		
0.4 units/kg insulin BP	76% decrease at 2 hours	James et al., 1970
0.8 units/kg insulin PP	120 mg% decreased at 30 minutes to 20 mg% and then decreased at 2 hours to 9 mg%	
ACTH level	0800 hours—35 ± 11.8 pg/ml	Orth, 1981
	2200 hours—21.4 ± 9.6 pg/ml	
T₃	.09 ± .02 μg/100 ml	Garcia, 1981
T₄	1.8 ± .8 μg/100 ml	Garcia, 1981
TSH‡ response		
15 units TSH SQ	4 times increase in T₄; normal in 3 days	Lowe, 1971
5 units TSH SQ	2 times increase in T₃ and T₄ at 2 hours. Peak remains high at 6 and 12 hours. Normal by 24 hours	Purohit, 1980
pre, 2- 6- 8- and 24-hour samples		

*Adrenomone, Burns Biotec Laboratory, Oakland, CA
†Cortrosyn, Organon, Inc., West Orange, NJ
‡Dermathycin, Jen Sal Laboratories, Kansas City, MO

Response to IV insulin is abnormal, as these horses are resistant and do not show the normal decrease in blood glucose. When performing the test on horses with only mild hyperglycemia, intravenous glucose solution should be readily available for use should the horse show signs of hypoglycemia (such as restlessness, sweating, weakness, and staggering). We have used 0.8 units per pound (1.76 units per kg) crystalline insulin subcutaneously in affected horses without response. Other authors have found horses to be resistant to insulin at doses ranging from 40 units of crystalline insulin to 200 units of protamine zinc insulin.[23] Even doses as high as 3 units per lb of protamine zinc insulin failed to decrease the glucose in one horse.[21] James et al. gave 0.2 units per lb (0.4 units per kg) insulin BP to two normal ponies and found a 76 per cent decrease in blood glucose. By 30 minutes the level was low, and this decrease was maximal at two hours.[20]

Intravenous glucose tolerance tests in normal horses have been highly variable and depend on the type of diet as well as the fasting status; therefore, their use is not of particular value in working up suspected cases of pituitary tumors.[15] Gribble and Dybdal found that insulin levels were high normal or increased.[16] However, even control values have been very variable.[14]

Plasma corticoid levels are variable, and values differ slightly among different laboratories. Levels may vary from 5.12 μg per ml in a resting horse to 8.2 μg per ml in Standardbred racehorses.[18] Mean values for hydrocortisone found by Eiler et al. range from 8.6 to 11 μg per dl.[7] Evening levels (6 to 10 P.M.) are said to be two thirds of the morning values (6 to 10 A.M.).[3, 20, 33] However, levels fluctuate, and secretion appears to be episodic and not diurnal.[11] In affected horses, plasma cortisol or corticoid levels are variable.

Affected horses often have an exaggerated response to ACTH owing to adrenal hyperplasia. Whereas normal horses respond with a twofold to threefold increase in cortisol between four and eight hours after 1 unit per kg of ACTH gel, horses with pituitary tumors may have fourfold rises.[15, 18, 20] Eiler in 1979 reported that the level reached at two hours was the least variable and that intravenous cosyntropin* gives more consistent results than intramuscular corticotropin.†,[7]

Dexamethasone suppresses plasma cortisol in normal horses because of negative feedback on ACTH. Horses with pars intermedia pituitary tumors are nonresponsive. This could occur because pars intermedia ACTH and POLMC peptide production is regulated differently and not under normal glucocorticoid negative feedback (unlike pars distalis secretion). Gribble and Dybdal state that affected horses show less suppression than normals (whose cortisols are suppressed to less than 1 μg per 100 ml) or that their levels return to pretest levels by 12 hours, unlike normal horses, in which levels are still low at 24 hours.[16] Use of the combined dexamethasone suppression–ACTH stimulation test prevents assessment of this delayed effect, and, therefore, separate tests may be preferable. Neither the dexamethasone suppression test nor ACTH stimulation test is specific for diagnosing pituitary tumors, as responses may be inconsistent; however, an exaggerated response to ACTH and decreased response to dexamethasone in a horse with clinical signs would be highly suggestive of the diagnosis. If autonomous hypersecretion from an adrenocortical neoplasm was causing signs of Cushing's syndrome, one would not expect to see a response to either ACTH or to dexamethasone. Ectopic ACTH secretion has not been described in horses, although it is recognized in certain neoplastic conditions in humans. In humans, some ACTH-secreting pituitary tumors are resistant to dexamethasone and may appear to secrete autonomously; these may also occur in horses.[26] Two of our horses in which T_3 and T_4 were measured had low levels; this could be caused by changes in TSH release.[17]

Assays for equine ACTH, MSH, and other POLMC peptides would provide the diagnosis, as the tumors have been shown to produce and secrete high levels of these hormones. In two mares with pituitary tumors, immunoreactive levels of the POLMC peptides were markedly elevated. Because one of the horses' cortisol level was only slightly elevated yet markedly responsive to ACTH, it was suggested that the circulating ACTH may have been relatively biologically inactive.[26] Gribble[15] reported that plasma levels of MSH were consistently elevated in five of six affected horses. In people, MSH levels may also be elevated in Cushing's syndrome and in cases of ectopic tumors producing ACTH.[32] At the time of this writing, none of these assays are readily or cheaply available to practitioners.

Lysine vasopressin tests are used in people and may have some application in horses. Lysine vasopressin increases the release of hypothalamic ACTH releasing factor or mimics the action of the latter on the pituitary. Its administration, therefore, increases ACTH release and increases plasma 17 hydroxycorticosterone to a much greater extent in Cushing's disease than in Cushing's syndrome, where the adrenal glands are not under ACTH pituitary control.[5]

PATHOLOGY

Necropsy examination of these horses usually reveals a tumor of the pars intermedia of varying size. The size of the tumor does not necessarily correlate with clinical signs. Tumors are nonencapsulated but sharply delineated. There is prominent vascularization, minimal necrosis, and a low mitotic rate. The neoplastic spindle-shaped cells have well-developed rough endoplasmic reticulum and secretory granules and small Golgi apparatus. The tumor usually expands dorsally and causes pressure on the posterior lobe of the pituitary and the hypothalamus. The posterior lobe and infundibular stalk may be infiltrated peripherally, but there is no metastasis. The tumor may cause pressure on the optic chiasm. The adrenal cortex is usually hypertrophied, and multiple sites of infection are frequently found.

*Cortrosin, Organon, Inc., West Orange, NJ
†Adrenamone, Burns Biotec Laboratory, Oakland, CA

TREATMENT

Few of these horses have been treated because of the nature of the disease and general severity of clinical signs when the horses are presented. More mild cases, however, may merit treatment. Several horses have been treated with oral OP[1]-DDD. In one pony, daily oral administration of 30 mg per kg did appear to decrease the plasma cortisol levels and cause a temporary improvement in signs, but the pony's course was not significantly altered, and when it was necropsied, adrenocortical hyperplasia was quite marked.[2] Gribble and Dybdal found that OP[1]-DDD, even in massive doses, did not have any effect when it was given to five normal mares; there was no decrease in cortisol or decrease in size of the adrenal glands on postmortem examination.[16] Treatment of one horse with a pituitary tumor had no effect.[16] The drug is expensive, and if it is used the animal should be carefully monitored.

Recently Gribble and Dybdal have used cyproheptadine* to treat horses with tumors of the pars intermedia.[16] One was terminal and was treated only for a short time and showed no change, but three horses showed remarkable improvement clinically and biochemically. Their blood glucose levels, cortisol levels, and dexamethasone suppression tests returned to normal after one to two months. One horse was on medication for almost a year and two for about six months. There are owners' anecdotal reports of clinical improvement in several others. No untoward effects were seen. Postmortem examination of the three horses revealed that they had large pituitary tumors, but their adrenal glands were only slightly larger than normal compared to untreated horses that had extremely large adrenal glands.[15] The usual treatment regimen has been initiation at a dose of 0.6 mg per $kg^{3/4}$ (58 mg for a 450 kg horse) with an increase over several weeks to 1.2 mg per $kg^{3/4}$ (117 mg for a 450 kg horse) given orally in the morning. (For reference, 200 $kg^{3/4}$ = 53.2 kg; 300 $kg^{3/4}$ = 72.1 kg; 500 $kg^{3/4}$ = 105.7 kg.) Gribble reports responsive horses usually improve in six to eight weeks. One of the treated horses remained improved on alternate-day dosing after the initial three-month treatment period, and one horse was still improved about four months following total cessation of therapy.[16] The drug is usually given two to three times a day in people. Doses used in dogs have varied from 0.3 to 3.0 mg per kg daily, and it has sometimes been combined with bromocriptine; both drugs can induce remission, but their use is limited by frequent relapses and infrequent success.[6] The drug has anticholinergic, antihistaminic, and antiserotonin activity. It competes with serotonin for receptor sites and therefore may prevent

---

*Periactin, Merck, Sharp & Dohme, West Point, PA

serotonin from regulating ACTH release. As the physiology of equine pars intermedia tumors still remains largely unknown, the exact role of cyproheptadine remains somewhat speculative. Its effect on reproduction in the horse is unknown. In humans, its use is contraindicated in nursing mothers. It would seem that the drug deserves further use and evaluation.

Recently pergolide, a dopaminergic agonist, has been reported to be effective in decreasing cortisol and POLMC peptide levels in two mares.[27] The drug could have some clinical application and warrants further investigation. It is an ergot alkaloid; side effects are due to intense vasoconstriction, damage to vascular endothelium of small peripheral blood vessels, and smooth muscle contraction. Toxic effects may be seen acutely and with chronic dosing. Nicholson et al.[27] and Orth[28] have treated two affected horses for three months with 2 to 5 mg orally once daily. Their clinical signs improved in six weeks, and their hormonal and biochemical abnormalities also improved. No undesirable side effects were seen. (There could be concern of laminitis because of the drug's effect on blood vessels; this could not be fully evaluated in the two treated horses, as both had preexisting laminitis; however, there was no exacerbation of their signs.) It may be possible and perhaps preferable to attempt use of a lower dose.[28] I have used pergolide (1.0 mg per day) in an aged pony unresponsive to cyproheptadine. There was clinical improvement, and blood glucose was normal within two weeks, but the dexamethasone suppression of cortisol was still abnormal after six weeks. No undesirable side effects were observed during two months of observation. Medication is continuing.

If the owner elects to maintain a horse with a pituitary tumor for a period of time, a high plane of nutrition, adequate nursing, and attempts to minimize infections are necessary. Any infections should be treated, and one should keep in mind that wounds will be slow to heal and that these animals are probably more prone to stresses than are normal animals. Use of cyproheptadine or pergolide deserves further investigation.

References

1. Backstrom, G.: Hirsutism associated with pituitary tumors in horses. Nord. Vet. Med., *15*:778, 1963.
2. Beech, J., and Ganjam, V.: Unpublished data, 1978.
3. Bottoms, G. D., Roesel, O. F., Rausch, F. D., and Akins, E. L.: Circadian variation in plasma cortisol and corticosterone in pigs and mares. Am. J. Vet. Res., *33*:785, 1972.
4. Brandt, A. J.: Uber Hypophysenadenome bei Hund und Pferd. Skand. Vet. Tidskrift, *30*:875, 1940.
5. Coslovsky, R., Wajchinbery, B. L., and Nogueira, O.: Hyperresponsiveness to lysine-vasopressin in Cushing's disease. Acta Endocrinol., *74*:125, 1974.
6. Drucker, W. D., and Peterson, M. E.: Pharmacologic treat-

ment of pituitary dependent canine Cushing's disease. Abstr. 62nd Annu. Meet. Endocr. Soc., *60*:89, 1981.

7. Eiler, H., Goble, D., and Oliver, J.: Adrenal gland function in the horse: Effects of cosyntropin (synthetic) and corticotropin (natural) stimulation. Am. J. Vet. Res., *40*:724, 1979.

8. Eiler, H., Oliver, J., and Goble, D.: Adrenal gland function in the horse: Effect of dexamethasone on hydrocortisone secretion and blood cellularity and plasma electrolyte concentrations. Am. J. Vet. Res., *40*:727, 1979.

9. Ericksson, K., Dyrendahl, S., and Grimfelt, D.: A case of hirsutism in connection with hypophyseal tumor in a horse. Nord. Vet. Med., 8:807, 1956.

10. Evans, D. R.: The recognition and diagnosis of a pituitary tumor in the horse. Am. Assoc. Eq. Pract. Newsletter, *18*:417, 1972.

11. Ganjam, V.: Episodic nature of the -ENE and -ENE steroidogenic pathways and their relationship to the adrenogonadal axis in stallions. J. Reprod. Fertil., Suppl., *27*:67, 1979.

12. Ganjam, V.: Personal communication, 1981.

13. Garcia, H. O.: Personal communication, 1981.

14. Goeldner, D.: Equine Cushing's syndrome due to hyperpituitarism and its treatment with cyproheptadine. Second Annual House Officer Seminar, VMTH, University of California, Davis, March, 1980.

15. Gribble, D. H.: The endocrine system. *In* Catcott, E. J. and Smithcors, J. F. (eds.): Equine Medicine and Surgery, 2nd ed. Wheaton, IL, American Veterinary Pub. Inc., 1972, pp. 433–457.

16. Gribble, D. H., and Dybdal, N.: Personal communication, 1981.

17. Hershman, J. M., and Pittman, J. A.: Control of thyrotropin secretion in man. N. Engl. J. Med., *285*:997, 1971.

18. Hoffsis, G. F., Murdick, P. W., Tharp, V. L., et al.: Plasma concentration of cortisol and corticosterone in the normal horse. Am. J. Vet. Res., *31*:1379, 1970.

19. Holscher, M. A., Linnabary, R. L., Netsky, M. G., and Owen, H. O.: Adenoma of the pars intermedia and hirsutism in a pony. VM SAC, 1197, Sept., 1978.

20. James, V. H. T., Horner, M. W., Moss, M. S., and Rippon, A. E.: Adrenocortical function in the horse. J. Endocrinol., *48*:319, 1970.

21. King, J. M., Kavanaugh, J. F., and Bentinck-Smith, J.: Diabetes mellitus with pituitary neoplasms in a horse and a dog. Cornell Vet., *52*:133, 1962.

22. Kraicer, J., Gosbee, J. L., and Bencosme, S. A.: Pars intermedia and pars distalis: Two sites of ACTH production in the rat hypophysis. Neuroendocrinol., *11*:156, 1973.

23. Loeb, W. F., Capen, C. C., and Johnson, L. E.: Adenoma of the pars intermedia associated with hyperglycemia and glycosuria in two horses. Cornell Vet., *56*:623, 1966.

24. Lombard, L. S., Lawrence, A. M., and Phillips, T. N.: Multiple primary endocrine tumors in American horses with Cushing-like disease. Proc. 5th Perugia Quad. Internat. Conf., Excerpta Medica, Amsterdam, 1973, p. 435.

25. Lowe, J. E.: Thyroidectomy and the T_4 test to assess thyroid dysfunction in the horse and pony. Proc. 16th Annu. Conv. Am. Assoc. Eq. Pract., 1970, pp. 135–174.

26. Moore, J., Steiss, J., Nicholson, W. E., and Orth, D. N.: A case of pituitary adrenocorticotropin-dependent Cushing's syndrome in the horse. Endocrinology, *104*:576, 1979.

27. Nicholson, W. E., Wilson, M. G., Holscher, M. A., Sherrell, J., Mount, C. D., and Orth, D. N.: Tissue and plasma levels of proopiolipomelanocortin (POLMC) peptides in the normal and Cushing's horse. Abstr. 62nd Annu. Meet. Endocr. Soc., *403*:183, 1981.

28. Orth, D. N.: Personal communication, 1981.

29. Pauli, B. U., Rossi, G. L., and Straub, R.: Swischenzelladenom der Hypophyse mit "Cushing-ähnlicher:" Symptomatologie beim Pferd. Vet. Pathol., *11*:417, 1974.

30. Purohit, R. C., Ganjam, V. K., Slone, D. E., Woodham, D. B., and McLeod, C.: Effect of age, breed, and sex on the circulating levels of thyroxine and triiodothyronine and development of a simple thyroid function test in the horse. Proc. Am. Coll. of Vet. Intern. Med., 1980, Washington, D.C.

31. Tasker, J. B., Whiteman, C. E., and Martin, B. R.: Diabetes mellitus in the horse. J. Am. Vet. Med. Assoc., *149*:393, 1966.

32. Williams, R. H.: Textbook of Endocrinology, 5th ed. Philadelphia, W. B. Saunders Co., 1974.

33. Zokolovick, A., Upson, D. W., and Eleftheriou, B. E.: Diurnal variation in plasma glucocorticosteroid levels in the horse (Equus caballus). J. Endocrinol., *35*:249, 1966.

DIABETES MELLITUS

A. M. Merritt, GAINESVILLE, FLORIDA

Practically every published case of "diabetes mellitus" in the horse has been the result of a pituitary tumor.[2, 3] Thus, by strict definition, these horses do not have diabetes mellitus, which is glucosuria due to hyperglycemia caused by pancreatic islet beta cell deficiency. Instead, their hyperglycemia is due most probably to excess endogenous ACTH or growth hormone (GH) release. It appears that true diabetes mellitus in the horse is an extremely rare condition; this author can find only one published case that seems to qualify.[1] The animal described was a seven-year-old pony that was underweight, polydipsic, and emitted "a strange urine odor." Clinical laboratory analysis revealed a persistent hyperglycemia, with daily values ranging between 300 and 500 mg per dl, 4+ glucosuria, and 2+ ketonuria. The hyperglycemia was insulin-responsive, although a very large dose of 8 units per kg of regular insulin intravenously still would not drop the blood sugar concentration into the normal range. Protamine zinc insulin, at doses of 0.5 and 1.0 units per kg, was much more effective in combatting the hyperglycemia. In contrast, horses with hyperglycemia secondary to pituitary tumor seem to be totally insulin-resistant.

Pathologically, the pony with the apparent true diabetes mellitus had a chronic pancreatitis, with islets present but surrounded by fibrosis instead of

TABLE 1. PERTINENT CLINICAL FEATURES OF TRUE DIABETES MELLITUS VS. TUMOR OF THE PARS INTERMEDIA OF THE PITUITARY GLAND IN HORSES

Clinical Features	Diabetes Mellitus	Pituitary Tumor
Hirsutism	No	Yes
Hyperhydrosis	No	Yes
Polydipsia/polyuria	Yes	Usually
Hypothalamic dysfunction*	No	Often
Glucosuria	Yes	Yes
Ketonuria	Yes	No
Fasting hyperglycemia (mg/dl)	300–500	150–300
Insulin-responsive hyperglycemia	Yes	No

*Includes wildly fluctuating appetite and body temperature. Occasionally seizures are seen.

healthy acinar tissue. The pancreas of a horse with a pituitary tumor is grossly and histologically normal.

Table 1 lists the most important clinical features that differentiate hyperglycemia due to insulin deficiency (diabetes mellitus) from hyperglycemia due to pituitary tumor (p. 164).

References

1. Jeffrey, J. R.: Diabetes mellitus secondary to chronic pancreatitis in a pony. J. Am. Vet. Med. Assoc., *153*:1168, 1968.
2. King, J. M., Kavanaugh, J. F., and Bentink-Smith, J.: Diabetes mellitus with pituitary neoplasms in a horse and dog. Cornell Vet., *52*:133, 1962.
3. Tasker, J. B., Whiteman, C. E., and Martin, B. R.: Diabetes mellitus in the horse. J. Am. Vet. Med. Assoc., *149*:393, 1966.

ANHIDROSIS

Angeline Warner, KENNETT SQUARE, PENNSYLVANIA

Anhidrosis, the inability to sweat in response to an adequate stimulus, is a problem affecting many horses in the Gulf Coast states today. It is seen most often in hot, humid climates. Historically, the disorder crippled the athletic performance of many English Thoroughbreds taken to the tropical colonies. Sweating is the major heat dissipation mechanism of the horse, and affected horses are unable to thermoregulate in extreme heat. Rectal temperature may reach 107 to 108° F, resulting in collapse if exertion is continued. Thus, competition performance is often severely compromised.

A survey of contemporary cases in Florida[1] shows that anhidrosis affects horses of all ages, breeds, colors, and horses native to hot, humid climates as well as those undergoing acclimatization. Horses in rigorous training for racing, polo, or showing and those on a high concentrate diet have been reported as more commonly affected, but these recent data show that brood mares and idle pleasure horses are affected with equal frequency. No particular diet, vitamin or mineral supplement, or lack thereof can be incriminated in the etiology. Hereditary predisposition appears unlikely considering evidence to date. Etiology is as yet uncertain, and no consistently effective therapy has emerged.

CLINICAL SIGNS

Signs commonly noted at the onset are tachypnea, poor exercise tolerance, and alopecia, especially of the face. Profuse sweating prior to onset of anhidrosis is part of the classical description in the unacclimatized horse but is not seen frequently in contemporary cases. Decreased appetite, changes in water consumption, and loss of body condition are occasionally seen. Onset is usually during the spring or summer and may be abrupt or gradual. Cessation of sweating may be partial or complete. Many horses will maintain residual sweat production under the mane and over the brisket and perineum, but sweat is scant with little or no lather production. Partial anhidrosis frequently remits (i.e., more normal sweating occurs) during winter.

The diagnosis is made on the basis of inadequate sweat production after appropriate stimulation. Affected horses uniformly display blowing rapid respiration during hot weather in their attempt to thermoregulate. Rectal temparature may be markedly elevated. Laboratory values for hematology, electrolytes, and serum enzymes are frequently unremarkable in the anhidrotic horse. Skin biopsies are not diagnostic. Inadequate gland response may be confirmed by intradermal epinephrine challenge.[4] The equine sweat gland is apocrine and responds to postganglionic adrenergic stimulation and circulating catecholamines. Intradermal injection of 0.5 cc of 1:1000 epinephrine will lead within an hour or less to sweating over the bleb and in tracks radiating outward in normal skin. The response will be decreased or absent and may be delayed up to 4 to 5 hours in affected horses. The area under the mane (if that skin has been observed to sweat) or a normal horse should be used as a positive control. Total lack of sweat production at the site of epinephrine injection in the affected skin is considered a poor prognostic sign, as the concentration of transmitter is locally very high. Intravenous challenge should be avoided, since although the whole body sweating pattern may be demonstrated, a prolonged refractory period may follow.

POSSIBLE PATHOGENESIS OF ANHIDROSIS

Onset of anhidrosis may not be secondary to poor acclimatization, as once thought, but it does appear to be precipitated by heat stress in a humid environment whether or not the individual has previously experienced such conditions. Equine anhidrosis could be accounted for by changes in sweat gland stimulation, gland function, or impaired extrusion of sweat onto the skin surface. Accommodation of sweat glands to higher than normal concentrations of circulating epinephrine secondary to heat stress has been the most widely accepted explanation for tropical anhidrosis. It is also feasible that the process of sweat gland secretion could be fatigued after prolonged demand, and there is evidence of degenerative changes in normal equine sweat glands after repeated epinephrine injection. Obstruction of the sweat duct can occur in people owing to hydration and swelling of keratin after prolonged sweating, and anhidrosis may persist until the obstructing keratin layer undergoes normal sloughing with epidermal turnover. The equine apocrine duct empties into the hair follicle above the sebaceous gland duct, and interference with delivery of sebaceous secretion might contribute to the poor coat condition and alopecia seen in many cases.

The dry skin, alopecia, and decreased exercise tolerance in hot weather seen with anhidrosis have led to the suggestion of hypothyroidism as a contributing factor. Serum T_3 and T_4 are reported to be low in some anhidrotic horses, but there are no data available on changes in thyroid secretion in normal horses during heat stress, and experimentally thyroidectomized horses have been seen to sweat normally. Empirically, some nonsweating horses have been reported to improve after administration of NaI, KI, iodinated casein, or thyroid hormone replacement, but presently no experimental evidence exists suggesting hypothyroidism as an etiology.

Horses can lose up to 45 l per day of fluid via sweat during strenuous exercise, and the major electrolytes lost in equine sweat are chloride and potassium.[1] Inappropriate aldosterone secretion initiated by sweat electrolyte and fluid losses in a hot humid environment can facilitate continued potassium loss through the urine. Chronic minor metabolic imbalance could thus occur after prolonged heat stress and may account for secondary signs associated with anhidrosis.

THERAPY

A variety of empirical approaches have been tried to induce sweating in affected horses with variable to poor success. These include intravenous and oral electrolytes, oral vitamin E and iodinated casein supplements, dietary change to minimize concentrates, and ACTH injection. Oral supplementation of electrolytes is the most common therapy used today, and some horses do appear to improve. A number of commercial electrolyte supplements have been used,* and there appears to be no difference among them. There is to date no consistently effective therapy to induce sweating. Symptomatic efforts should be aimed at providing a cooler environment via fans or shade, clipping the body, and wetting the horse down with water to provide for evaporative cooling. Many anhidrotic horses are maintained using such measures and judicious exercise during cooler hours of the day. Moving the horse to a temperate climate or providing air conditioned quarters during the summer will obviously make the animal more comfortable, and frequently the decreased heat stress is associated with more normal sweating.

References

1. Carlson, G., and Ocen, P.: Composition of equine sweat following exercise in high environmental temperatures and in response to intravenous epinephrine administration. J. Eq. Med. Surg., *3*:27, 1979.
2. Correa, J., and Calderin, G.: Anhidrosis, dry-coat syndrome in the Thoroughbred. J. Am. Vet. Med. Assoc., *149*:1556, 1966.
3. Currie, A., and Seager, S.: Anhidrosis. Proc. 22nd Annu. Conv. Am. Assoc. Eq. Pract., 1976, pp. 249–251.
4. Evans, C., Smith, D., Ross, K., et al.: Physiologic factors on the condition of "dry-coat" in horses. Vet. Rec., *69*:1, 1957.
5. Warner, A., and Mayhew, I.: Equine anhidrosis: A survey of affected horses in Florida. J. Am. Vet. Med. Assoc., *180*:627, 1982.

---

*Electrofin, Haver Lockhart Laboratories, Shawnee, KS

Section 5

GASTROINTESTINAL DISEASES

Edited by Robert H. Whitlock

CLINICAL SIGNS OF SOME DISORDERS OF THE GASTROINTESTINAL TRACT 175

CLEFT PALATE 177

CRIBBING 181

SALIVARY GLAND DISEASE 183

GLOSSITIS 185

CARE OF THE TEETH 186

ESOPHAGEAL OBSTRUCTION 192

GASTRIC DISEASES 196

COLITIS-X 200

ENTERIC SALMONELLOSIS 207

INTESTINAL CLOSTRIDIOSIS 210

FOAL HEAT DIARRHEA 213

ANTERIOR ENTERITIS 214

CHRONIC DIARRHEA 216

MEDICAL MANAGEMENT OF COLIC 220

SMALL BOWEL OBSTRUCTION 224

LARGE BOWEL OBSTRUCTION 231

FLATULENT COLIC 236

THROMBOEMBOLIC COLIC 238

PERITONITIS 241

GRASS SICKNESS 244

MALABSORPTION SYNDROMES 245

ACUTE HEPATITIS 249

CHRONIC LIVER DISEASE 251

CHRONIC PANCREATITIS 253

RECTAL PROLAPSE 254

RECTAL TEARS 256

GASTROINTESTINAL NEOPLASIA 259

RETAINED MECONIUM 260

ASCARIASIS 262

STRONGYLOSIS 267

STRONGYLOIDOSIS 281

BOTS 283

CESTODE INFECTION 287

OXYURIS INFECTION 288

CLINICAL SIGNS OF SOME DISORDERS OF THE GASTROINTESTINAL TRACT

Robert H. Whitlock, KENNETT SQUARE, PENNSYLVANIA

Recognition of the clinical signs of equine gastrointestinal disease may seem simple when one considers diarrhea, colic, melena, salivation, and dysphagia but is more complex when anorexia and weight loss are added to the list.

Anorexia, the animal's refusal to readily ingest available, palatable food, may be due to a local lesion in the mouth or pharynx or more commonly is due to a centrally mediated inhibition of the normal desire to eat and drink. This latter mechanism is easily understood when one considers that fever, acute or chronic pain, localized abscesses, generalized infection, metabolic or endocrine disturbances, and central nervous system disorders are all frequently accompanied by anorexia. Several therapeutic approaches may be utilized to treat centrally mediated anorexia. Correction of the underlying disease problem is most important in the therapeutic approach to anorexia. Additionally, antibiotics for infectious processes and analgesics such as phenylbutazone to minimize pain and to decrease the fever are very important in this regard. Recently a new class of chemical compounds has been recognized that can stimulate increased feed consumption during disease states. Elfazepam and its close relative, diazepam, have been found to increase feed intake in sick horses.[1] Diazepam and several sister compounds are available, but elfazepam is not. Diazepam (5 to 10 mg per kg per animal) may be utilized as an initial test dose.[2]

Excessive salivation or *sialosis* rarely occurs in any species, including the horse. Apparent sialosis is most often due to a decrease in the swallowing of saliva, as occurs in choke with complete esophageal obstruction. Organophosphate toxicosis or extensive oral lesions, such as those that occur with blister beetle poisoning, may induce sialosis.

Recently a new syndrome has been recognized in young foals between one and five months of age. Salivation and foam at the mouth are characteristic clinical signs along with prominent odontoprisis, mild dullness, depression, and anorexia. The foamy saliva on the muzzle would suggest choke, but in all cases the esophagus is patent. The nasogastric tube should be passed into the stomach to ascertain the possibility of gastric distention. Gastric fluid often flows out of the tube spontaneously. These foals nurse the mare but not adequately; thus, they lose weight. Diarrhea is not a characteristic of the disease. The apparent excessive salivation, grinding the teeth, and gastric reflux all strongly implicate a subacute to chronic duodenal ulcer that effectively causes a duodenal stricture. The partial duodenal obstruction appears to be responsible for all the clinical signs.

Acute duodenal ulcers lead to vastly different clinical signs, which include profound dullness, depression, shock, loose stool, possible respiratory distress, and cessation of nursing. The clinical signs are more abrupt, and the foal is more severely affected than with duodenal strictures; however, the clinical signs are much less specific. Peritoneocentesis will give valuable information, confirming the peritonitis with degenerate leukocytes and bacteria in macrophages. Most affected foals with acute duodenal perforating ulcers are between 30 and 45 days of age. The etiology and pathogenesis of this very unusual disease is completely unknown.

Therapy for acute perforating duodenal ulcers must include systemic antibiotics, fluids, and gastric decompression. Most affected foals die. Occasionally the local peritonitis can be walled off and controlled by medical therapy. Surgical extirpation of the lesion is virtually impossible. The primary lesion, be it an acute perforating ulcer or chronic cicatrix (duodenal stricture), is usually located within 3 cm of the common bile duct. Foals with the syndrome of duodenal cicatrix have been successfully treated using a gastroduodenostomy or gastrojejunostomy; however, the surgical procedure is difficult and requires considerable expertise.

Dysphagia occurs occasionally in horses, associated with a variety of diseases, including rabies, botulism, moldy corn poisoning (encephalomalacia), severe pharyngitis, fractures of the mandible or maxilla or hyoid bones, guttural pouch tympanites, guttural pouch mycosis, and other neurologic diseases. The oral cavity should be explored carefully and extensively for any possible lesion. Treatment then must be directed at the primary cause. An indwelling nasogastric tube or periodic tubing of the horse with a highly nutritious feed will often provide the caloric and protein requirements better than intravenous hyperalimentation. An example of a nutritious mixture would contain electrolytes, dextrose, dehydrated cottage cheese, and alfalfa meal.[4] The mixture should be divided equally and added to 6 to 7 l of water and given by tube three times

TABLE 1. RECOMMENDED TUBE FEEDING SCHEDULE FOR A 450 KG HORSE*

	1	2	3	4	5	6	7
Electrolyte mixture,† gm	210	210	210	210	210	210	210
Water, l	21	21	21	21	.21	21	21
Dextrose, gm	300	400	500	600	800	800	900
Dehydrated cottage cheese, gm	300	450	600	750	900	900	900
Glycerine, ml	300	400	500	600	800	800	900
Alfalfa meal, lbs	½–1‡	1–2	1–2	1–2	1–2	1–2	1–2

Continue feeding day 7 diet until horse can eat or until diarrhea develops.

*To be divided into three equal feedings per 24 hrs

†Electrolyte mixture—1 day:

NaCl	10 gm
$NaHCO_3$	15 gm
KCl	75 gm
K_2HPO_4	60 gm
$CaCl_2 \cdot 2H_2O$	45 gm
MgO	24 gm

‡Add only enough alfalfa meal so that the mixture will easily flow through the stomach tube. The addition of alfalfa meal tends to lengthen the period for which the mixture can be fed before diarrhea begins.

per day (Table 1). When horses are maintained on this diet for longer than 10 days, they may develop a self-limiting diarrhea.

Weight loss as a clinical sign is not specific for gastrointestinal disease but does characterize many abdominal disorders including protein-losing enteropathy and subacute to chronic peritonitis (p. 241). Additional gastrointestinal disorders causing weight loss include parasitism, especially strongylosis; dental problems, such as malocclusion and sharp teeth; mesenteric abscesses; gastrointestinal neoplasia, such as gastric squamous cell carcinoma or lymphosarcoma; and chronic liver disease. The reader is referred to the articles on the specific diseases for a more complete discussion of these disorders.

Abdominal or mesenteric abscesses warrant further comment because of their incidence. Weight loss leading to emaciation and chronic intermittent colic are the most common complaints associated with mesenteric abscesses, which occur most commonly in younger horses. Additional findings are often vague but include moderate pyrexia, a palpable mass on deep rectal examination located in or about the mesenteric artery, moderate leukocytosis, hypergammaglobulinemia, and abnormal peritoneal fluid compatible with an abscess.[5] Most equine abdominal abscesses are due to metastatic streptococcal infections and should be responsive to penicillin. Inadequate penicillin therapy may predispose to internal abscessation; therefore, when penicillin is given in horses with strangles or respiratory catarrh, it should be continued at appropriate levels: 40,000 to 100,000 U per kg body weight divided in two doses daily for at least 10 days after cessation of all clinical signs in order to minimize the danger of internal abscess formation. Once the presence of an abscess is confirmed, long-term penicillin therapy is recommended and may be necessary for two to

six months. The duration of therapy will be determined by repeated close monitoring of the horse by rectal palpation, abdominal peritoneocentesis, and complete blood counts. Horses that are unresponsive to antibiotics, especially those with concurrent colic, may require surgical intervention. Several techniques have been utilized successfully, including marsupialization and intestinal anastomosis, to bypass the lesion.[6] The injection of antibiotics into the lesion and iodines have seemed to be of value. Although isoniazid has been utilized to treat abscesses for many years, there is no evidence to suggest that it is effective.[3]

Colic and diarrhea are common signs of abdominal disease in horses. For more complete discussions of these problems, the reader is referred to other articles in this book. Melena is an uncommon sign of abdominal disease in horses but often occurs with gastric carcinomas and less commonly with massive colonic ulceration. Blood loss rarely occurs in association with gastric ulcer disease in horses.

Abdominal distention, a common sign of gastrointestinal disease, can be due to a variety of disorders, but a simple guideline listing possible causes exists: fat, fetus, fluid, flatus, and feces. A complete physical examination, rectal examination, peritoneocentesis, and gastric intubation are often necessary to more completely define the nature of the distention. Therapy should be aimed at eliminating the underlying cause and not the sign.

References

1. Baile, C. A., and McLaughlin, C. L.: A review of the behavioral and physiological responses to elfazepam, a chemical feed intake stimulant. J. Anim. Sci., 5:1371, 1979.
2. Brown, R. F., Houpt, K. A., and Schryver, H. F.: Stimulation

of food intake in horses by diazepam and promazine. Pharmacol. Biochem. Behav., 5:495, 1976.
3. Hietala, S., and Knight, H. D.: Ineffectiveness of isoniazid against three equine pathogens. J. Am. Vet. Med. Assoc., 179:806, 1980.
4. Naylor, J. M.: The nutrition of the sick horse. J. Eq. Med. Surg., 1:64, 1977.

5. Rumbaugh, G. E., Smith, B. P., and Carlson, G. P.: Internal abdominal abscesses in the horse: A study of 25 cases. J. Am. Vet. Med. Assoc., 172:304, 1978.
6. Taylor, T. S., Martin, M. T., and McMullan, W. C.: Bypass surgery for intestinal occluding abscesses in the equine: A report of two cases. Vet. Surg., 10:136, 1981.

CLEFT PALATE

A. W. Nelson, FORT COLLINS, COLORADO

T. S. Stashak, FORT COLLINS, COLORADO

Cleft palates can be divided into clefts of the primary palate (external nares and lip) and secondary palate (hard and soft palate).[3] The most common area involved is the caudal half or three quarters of the soft palate. This defect occurs in approximately 0.1 to 0.2 percent of horses.[1] Defects in the palate are thought to result from a failure of the lateral palatine processes to unite on the midline.[4] They are considered heritable in approximately 10 per cent of the cases. However, other factors, such as vitamin deficiencies, irradiation, toxic chemicals, hormonal deficiencies, infective agents, and immunologic disease, are thought to be responsible for the majority of cases.[3] Whether the cleft develops in the lips or hard or soft palate depends on the stage of embyrologic development affected.

CLINICAL SIGNS

Clefts in the lips are disfiguring and can cause difficulty in suckling, whereas milk coming out of the nostrils is the most common clinical sign seen in foals with cleft of the soft or hard palate.[2] A definitive diagnosis can be made with oral examination or endoscopic examination or both. If untreated, aspiration pneumonia usually develops and generally leads to death of the foal in a few weeks to months.

TREATMENT

Surgical correction is more successful if it is performed by the time the foal is six weeks old.[2] The foal is still nursing, boluses of hard feed are not driven into the surgical area, and the depth of the surgical field is less. Even at this young age, instruments used are normally the longest available without being especially made. The approach to this area is made through a mandibular symphysiotomy with

the foal placed in dorsal recumbency.[5, 6] A temporary tracheotomy is made so that the endotracheal tube may be placed at this site while the surgical procedure is being performed.

Preoperative preparation includes thorough flushing of the oral cavity with water to clear any feed, followed by repeated flushings with a 10 per cent iodophor antiseptic.* A full-strength coating of iodophor antiseptic is then flushed deep into the oral cavity and not rinsed out. A complete surgical preparation of the ventral intermandibular space follows.

The surgical approach is illustrated in Figure 1. A skin incision is made on the ventral midline extending from the level of the mandibular angles anteriorly through the lower lip. The labial incision is extended down through the musculature of the chin to expose the ventral edge of the mandibular symphysis, the labial mucosa, and gingiva. The labial gingiva is then incised on its midline to the space between the central incisor teeth. Mandibular lymph nodes are now divided along their normal midline cleavage plane in order to give clear access to the mylohyoideus muscle, which is incised along its midline insertion from the level of the lingual process of the hyoid bone to the mandibular symphysis in order to expose the underlying paired bellies of the genioglossus and geniohyoideus msucles.

Prior to mandibular symphysiotomy, two ASIF drill holes are preplaced in the mandible just posterior to the incisor teeth. These holes are preplaced at this time because the mandible is stable and in good anatomic alignment. The mandibular symphysis is then separated by using a scalpel in the young foal and an osteotome in older horses. The lingual gingiva of the oral mucosa and submucosal fascia are incised at the midline of the frenulum linguae. This allows partial separation of the mandibular rami, which in turn provides good exposure of

---

*Betadine, Purdue Fredrick Co., Norwalk, CT

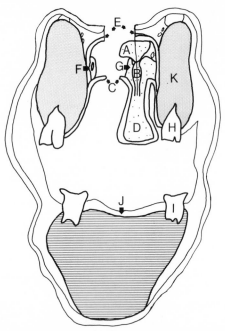

Figure 1. Drawing of a transverse section through the head of a horse at the level of the fourth cheek tooth, showing the plane of surgical approach to the oral cavity. Geniohyoideus muscle (A), genioglossus muscle (B), oral mucosa (C), tongue (D), mylohyoideus muscle (E), sublingual salivary gland with duct of mandibular salivary gland (F), styloglossus muscle (G), fourth lower cheek tooth (H), fourth upper cheek tooth (I), hard palate (J), and ramus of the mandible (K). (From Nelson, A. W., Curley, B. M., and Kainer, R. A.: Mandibular symphysiotomy to provide adequate exposure for intraoral surgery in the horse. J. Am. Vet. Med. Assoc., *159*:1025, 1971.)

the origin of the genioglossus and geniohyoideus muscles. Approximately 1 to 2 cm from their mandibular origin, these muscles are severed and reflected on the approach side of the tongue. Care is taken to avoid the anterior polystomatic openings of the sublingual salivary gland and duct of the mandibular salivary gland. These structures lie in the origin of the muscles previously mentioned, and their stomas exit in the mucosa of the floor of the mouth.

The incision is deepened by blunt dissection along the lateral edge of the geniohyoideus and styloglossus muscles (Fig. 1). This natural tissue plane lies medial to the anterior portion of the sublingual salivary gland, the ducts of the mandibular salivary gland, and the vertical portion of the mylohyoideus muscle. By spreading apart the mandibular rami, the mucous membranes of the floor of the mouth can be visualized reflecting from the lingual gingiva onto the tongue. The mucous membrane is cut with scissors, working caudad to the level of the anterior pillars of the soft palate. The mandibular rami are gradually separated, and once the mucous membrane is cut, they are retained in position without retractors by hooking the lower teeth over the

lateral edge of the upper teeth. The tongue is reflected laterally out of the field, and the hard and soft palates of the oropharynx are readily visualized. This plane of dissection has the advantage of avoiding vital structures. Major vital structures medial to the dissection plane are the hypoglossal and lingual nerves. Lateral to the dissection are the sublingual salivary glands and mandibular salivary duct (Fig. 1). Occasionally the location of the lingual nerve will be such that it is necessary to transect it to get adequate exposure. This does not appear to affect the motor function of the tongue, as no postoperative complications have been noted.

The distal border of the cleft palate must be identified and secured with traction sutures at the caudal end of the proposed site of anastomosis (Fig. 2). These sutures are best placed with the aid of 14- to 18-in needle holders. After suture placement, medial traction is put on them to assess the ability to bring the edges of the cleft together. If these edges can be approximated even under slight tension, the surgery progresses in a relatively simple manner. The free edge of the cleft palate is now placed under longitudinal tension by these traction sutures. An incision is made with a No. 11 Bard Parker blade from anterior to posterior along the free edge of the palate (Fig. 3). This splits the palate mucosa into two layers, the oral and nasal sides. This incision is now carried deeper with either a scalpel blade or Metsenbaum scissors until the palate musculature

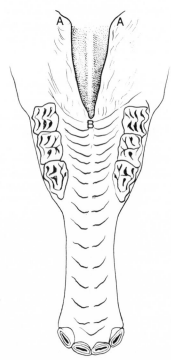

Figure 2. Ventral surface of the hard and soft palate demonstrating a cleft in the soft palate between points A and B.

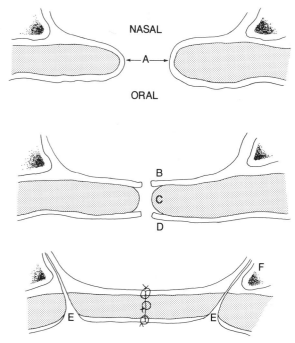

Figure 3. A diagram of the cross-section through the soft palate in the region of the cleft. The location of the incision (A) in the free edge of the cleft is indicated. This provides three tissue layers to suture: nasal mucosa (B), muscularis (C), and oral mucosa (D). Relaxing incisions (E) are made in the oral mucosa and muscularis of the soft palate, which are extended dorsal along the medial sides of the pterygoid bones (F) to the level of the dorsum of the nasal passage.

of suppleness left in these tissues. Any tension will result in failure. The soft palate should be able to be depressed dorsally until it touches the dorsal border of the nasopharynx. Any resistance at all, even the slightest, to this procedure will indicate the need for lateral relaxing incisions. In the authors' experience, these incisions are usually necessary. The lateral relaxing incisions extend from the region of the posterolateral border of the soft palate anteriorly along the medial border of the molar teeth to the level of the hard palate (Figs. 3 and 4). The incision is bluntly and sharply dissected deeper into the soft tissues until the medial border of the pterygoid bone can be palpated. Blunt dissection with the fingertips usually can carry the incision deep along the medial border of the pterygoid bone until the base of these bones is reached. These relaxing incisions remain open during the healing process of the palate and gradually close by ingrowth of granulation tissue.

Since the soft palate tissues are very delicate in the young foal, all surgical manipulation, including suturing, must be done as atraumatically as possible. Sutures should be 3–0 to 4–0 size and placed approximately 5 mm apart. Any bleeding vessels should be handled as delicately as possible, leaving minimal devitalized tissue.

After the cleft palate surgery has been completed,

is exposed. A similar incision is carried out on the opposite side of the cleft. This dissection provides an opportunity for a three-layer suture closure of the palate (Fig. 3).

The nasal side of the palate is sutured first. Simple interrupted 4–0 absorbable sutures on a cutting edge needle are used. The sutures are placed so that knots will be on the nasal side. The placement of the suture line is facilitated by maintaining traction on tension sutures with a long instrument, keeping the palate stress slightly in a caudal direction. Stay sutures can also be placed in the oral mucosa on each side of the incision, and the edges of the oral mucosa can be retracted laterally. This gives good exposure to the incision on the nasal side and keeps the edges of the palate properly aligned. Nasal-mucosal sutures are placed along the entire length of the incision. Similar sutures are placed in the muscular portion of the soft palate. These sutures include the muscular tissue and a little connective tissue left on the palate musculature during dissection. This suture line provides considerable strength to the closure. The oral mucosa is then closed in a similar manner (Figs. 3 and 4).

After the palate suturing procedure has been completed, the surgeon must ascertain the degree

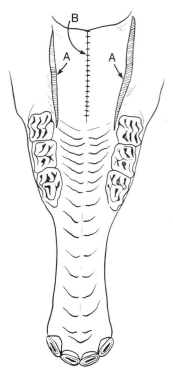

Figure 4. Same projection as Figure 2 demonstrating the length of the relaxing incisions (A) and the sutured cleft (B) in the soft palate.

the mouth, oropharynx, and nasopharynx are cleared of any blood clots and other debris that could be inhaled during the recovery process. The rami of the mandible are relaxed by unhooking the teeth from the dorsal molars. This allows the mandible to come together as the mucosal incision is sutured. Owing to the depth of surgical incision in this area, the tissues must be closed simultaneously from the deep to more superficial levels. This is done because the closure of the superficial tissues requires the approximation of the mandibular symphysis, which obstructs exposure of the deeper tissues.

After thorough lavage and application of iodophor antiseptic, a simple continuous 2–0 medium chromic gut suture is begun in the oral mucosa at the deepest portion of the incision. Approximately 10 to 20 per cent of the length of the mucosal incision is closed with this suture pattern before interrupted sutures are placed in the deep loose connective tissues. At the same time, a Penrose drain is inserted so that its deepest end will lie in the deepest part of the dissection. The loose areolar tissue is closed as the suture line in the oral mucosa is continued. The oral mucosal suture is continued until the rami of the mandible become too close to allow further suture placement. At this point, the suture material is passed through the mucosa into the oral cavity and is left there until the remaining part of the incision is closed, at which time the mouth is opened and the suture is continued on the oral side. While suturing the mucosa, care must be taken to avoid the mandibular salivary gland ducts as they course in the frenulum of the tongue. The mandibular symphysis is now stabilized by placing two ASIF cortical bone screws in the predrilled holes. The process of interfragmental compression is utilized.

Owing to the midline and ventral locations of the incision between the mandibles, the Penrose drain is brought out through the primary incision. This appears to be the best way to handle drainage of the area. The drain is removed in a stepwise fashion (4 to 8 cm at a time) during the ensuing 72 hours. Contamination that occurs during the surgical procedure is reduced by flushing of the surgical site several times during the suturing procedures with full-strength iodophor antiseptic solution.

The origins of the geniohyoideus and genioglossus muscles are rejoined to their mandibular attachments using an interrupted horizontal mattress suture (3–0 medium chromic surgical gut). The mylohyoideus muscle and subcutaneous tissues are sutured simultaneously with simple interrupted sutures (3–0 medium chromic surgical gut).

Skin of the ventral mandibular area is closed with simple interrupted sutures of the surgeon's choice. Owing to the prehensile nature of the lower lip of the horse, considerable movement may occur in the postoperative period in these tissues. This tends to cause dehiscence of the suture line in the lip. This can be avoided by placing quill tension sutures, supported by rubber tubing, through the mentalis muscle of the lip. Also, undermining of the cutaneous tissues off the mentalis muscle to a depth of 2 cm will further help to stabilize the primary incision line. Both these procedures decrease the motion of the tissues at this level. After the tension sutures are placed, the mucosa of the lip is sutured with simple interrupted absorbable 2–0 suture material. The ventral intermandibular suture line is continued around the rostral side of the lip, approximating the skin in a routine manner. Particular attention is paid to good alignment of the mucocutaneous junction because this is where dehiscence most frequently begins. The tendency for dehiscence of this suture line is much decreased in the suckling foal as opposed to those eating grass or hay.

POSTOPERATIVE CARE

Postoperatively, the foal is maintained on systemic antibiotics for approximately five days, and the oral cavity is checked daily for the accumulation of feed materials in and around the oral side of the mandibular symphysiotomy incision. This usually occurs between the lower lip and teeth. It is desirable to maintain the neonatal foal on milk during the first 14 days postoperatively. For the weanling, there are two approaches to postoperative feeding. The preferred approach is providing a softened gruel of one of the complete horse feed pellets. The gruel is made by adding sufficient water to make a moist slurry. If this is not eaten, a small soft stomach tube can be passed to force feed the weanling.

The mandibular symphysiotomy approach has few complications, and in most cases foals and weanlings do not demonstrate much reluctance or difficulty in eating immediately after surgery. However, there is usually a moderate amount of swelling associated with the surgical site with increased salivation noted for three to four days postoperatively. Tension sutures are removed at approximately 10 days, and skin sutures are removed approximately 14 days after surgery. Any accumulation of milk in the external nares after the surgical procedure may be due to paralysis of the soft palate rather than a failure of suture closure. Three to four weeks should be allowed to pass before the decision is made to examine the palate for fistula formation. Generally during this period of time, the passage of milk into the nasal cavity decreases or stops if the suture line remains intact. Small fistulas are no problem as long as the major portion of the repair holds.

References

1. Batstone, J. H. F.: Cleft palate in the horse. Br. J. Plast. Surg., *19*:327, 1966.
2. Frank, E. R.: Veterinary Surgery, 7th ed. Minneapolis, Burgess Pub. Co., 1964, p. 145.
3. Hammer D. L., and Sacks, M.: The palate. *In* Bojrab, M. J. (ed.): Current Techniques in Small Animal Surgery. Philadelphia, Lea and Febiger, 1975, pp. 75–84.
4. Jones, R. S., Maisels, D. O., DeGeus, J. J., and Lovius, B. B. J.: Surgical repair of cleft palate in the horse. Eq. Vet. J., *7*(2):86, 1975.
5. Nelson, A. W., Curley, B. M., and Kainer, R. A.: Mandibular symphysiotomy to provide adequate exposure for intraoral surgery in the horse. J. Am. Vet. Med. Assoc., *159*:1025, 1971.
6. Stickle, R. L., Gobel, D. O., and Braden, T. D.: Surgical repair of cleft soft palate in a foal. [VM SAC], Feb., 1973, pp. 159–162.

CRIBBING

Stephen B. Adams, LAFAYETTE, INDIANA

Cribbing or crib-biting is a common acquired vice in which horses grasp an object with the incisor teeth, flex the neck, and pull backward. Horses that swallow air during this procedure are called wind suckers. The vice appears to be a displacement activity most frequently noted in horses that are bored by confinement, isolation, or lack of a suitable roughage to eat. It has not been reported in feral horses. Confined horses may learn cribbing from stable mates, and foals have been noted to learn the vice from their dams.

Cribbing causes excessive wear of the incisor teeth and may cause enlargement of the ventral neck muscles. The habit usually does not seriously impair the horse's health. A horse that wind sucks may exhibit weight loss, unthriftiness, poor performance, digestive disturbances, and flatulence. Wind sucking is considered an unsoundness. Horses that crib or wind suck should be distinguished from horses that chew wood. The latter vice is generally less objectionable to most horse owners.

CONSERVATIVE MANAGEMENT

Removing fixed objects that the horse grasps while cribbing may deter the horse that has just learned the vice. Some horses that crib in a stall will not crib when placed in a pasture. However, management changes rarely deter established cribbers, some of which may be capable of swallowing air without grasping a fixed object.

A cribbing strap will help control cribbing and wind sucking in many horses. This strap is placed snugly around the throatlatch of the horse to prevent contraction of the ventral neck muscles and flexion of the neck and head. The strap may contain metal prongs that pierce the skin when the neck is flexed or a rigid metal piece that conforms to the relaxed neck muscles. The cribbing strap should be adjusted to allow the horse to eat and breathe normally (Fig. 1). It is worn at all times except during exercise.

SURGICAL MANAGEMENT

Myectomy of the ventral neck muscles was described in 1926 by Forssell.[2] The muscles partially excised are the sternocephalicus, omohyoid, and sternothyrohyoid. The action of the sternocephalicus muscles is to flex the head and neck when acting in unison and to turn the head sideways when acting singly. The action of the omohyoid and sternothyrohyoid muscles is to retract and depress the hyoid bone, the base of the tongue, and the larynx during deglutition.[5]

Following induction of general anesthesia, the horse is placed in dorsal recumbency with the head and neck extended. A 40 cm midline incision is made through the skin, fascia, and ventral neck muscles starting at the level of the hyoid bone and extending caudally. The skin edges are elevated and retracted laterally. The omohyoid muscle on one side is isolated in the caudal aspect of the incision by blunt dissection before it passes beneath the sternocephalicus muscle and is transected. The ipsilateral sternothyrohyoid muscle is likewise isolated and transected at the caudal aspect of the incision. These muscles are reflected cranially and removed from their attachments on the thyroid cartilage, basihyoid bone, and lingual process of the hyoid bone. The sternocephalicus muscle is severed obliquely in a craniodorsal direction at the caudal aspect of the incision, and the section of muscle is removed after transection of the tendon of insertion. Hemorrhage is generally profuse during surgery and should be controlled with ligation or electrocoagulation. The same procedure is then repeated on the muscles of the opposite side of the neck. Prior to skin closure

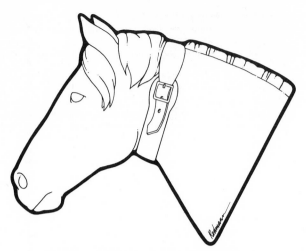

Figure 1. Proper position of a cribbing strap.

with interrupted sutures of a nonabsorbable material, wound drainage should be established. This is best accomplished with a drain placed in the wound and exiting caudal to the skin incision to provide gravity drainage. However, the caudal 4 cm of the skin incision may be left open for drainage. The neck should be bandaged and the skin sutures removed in 10 to 14 days. A review of the records of 73 horses undergoing Forssell's procedure revealed that 53 per cent of the horses had complete remission, 19 per cent improved, and 27 per cent showed no improvement.[3]

Forssell's myectomy may cause considerable postoperative disfigurement of the neck due to loss of ventral neck muscle mass. This disfigurement is especially objectionable in show horses. A modification of this technique has been developed that results in less disfigurement.[1] A skin incision is made over each sternocephalicus muscle starting where the linguofacial vein crosses the muscle and extending 10 cm caudally. A section of each sternocephalicus muscle is excised, and the ventral branch of the accessory nerve is severed. A third skin incision 15 cm long is made on the ventral midline. This incision extends caudally from the region of the hyoid bone. After isolation of the left and right omohyoid and sternothyrohyoid muscles, a 10 cm length of each is removed. The skin wounds are closed with a nonabsorbable suture material.

Neurectomy of the ventral branches of the spinal accessory nerves is another surgical technique useful for controlling cribbing.[4] The ventral branches provide motor innervation to the sternocephalicus muscles, which are the major muscles used by the horse to flex the neck. The nerves originate in the atlantal fossae and pass caudoventral under the parotid glands to enter the sternocephalicus muscles at the junction of the muscle belly and tendon of insertion.

Surgery may be performed on the tranquilized standing horse using local anesthesia or with the horse in lateral recumbency under general anesthesia. The neck should be slightly extended to facilitate location of the surgical landmarks. A skin incision is made just ventral to the jugular vein starting at the point where the linguofacial vein crosses the sternocephalicus muscle and extending 8 cm caudally. The sternocephalicus muscle is separated from the jugular vein with combined blunt and sharp dissection using Metzenbaum scissors. This exposes the dorsal surface of the sternocephalicus muscle where the ventral branch of the spinal accessory nerve passes a short distance through a groove on the surface of the muscle prior to entering it (Fig. 2). The nerve is isolated from the fascia on the surface of the muscle and elevated with a pair of curved hemostats. Identification of the nerve is confirmed by pinching it with hemostats. This will produce contraction of the sternocephalicus muscle unless local anesthetic has been infiltrated directly around the nerve. A 2 to 3 cm section of nerve is excised with a sharp scalpel blade. The subcutaneous fascia is closed with several interrupted absorbable sutures, and the skin is closed with vertical mattress sutures of a nonabsorbable material. The procedure is repeated on the opposite side of the neck, and the incision sites are bandaged. The skin sutures can be removed in seven days and training resumed. Horses normally confined to stalls should be housed in a paddock for three weeks.

The spinal accessory neurectomy is a simpler operation than Forssell's myectomy or the modification and results in less disfigurement of the neck. The success rate following this procedure is similar to the success rate of the myectomy. Failure of the neurectomy to eliminate cribbing does not preclude a successful result from a myectomy done secon-

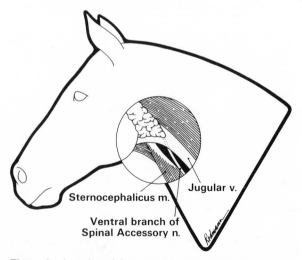

Sternocephalicus m.

Jugular v.

Ventral branch of
Spinal Accessory n.

Figure 2. Location of the ventral branch of the spinal accessory nerve.

darily. The neurectomy should be the surgical procedure of choice for most cribbers. Horses that exhibit severe and long-standing cribbing or horses that crib following a neurectomy are candidates for the more radical myectomy.

References

1. Berge, E. and Westhues, L. (eds.): Veterinary Operative Surgery. Copenhagen, Medical Book Co., 1965, p. 179.
2. Forssell, G.: The new surgical treatment against crib-biting. Vet. J., 82:538, 1926.
3. Hermans, W. A.: Kribbebijten-Luchtzuigen. Tijdschr. Diergeneeskd, 98:1132, 1973.
4. Hamm, D.: A new surgical procedure to control crib-biting. Proc. 23rd Annu. Meet. Am. Assoc. Eq. Pract., 23:301, 1977.
5. Sisson, S., and Grossman, J. D.: The Anatomy of Domestic Animals, 4th ed. Philadelphia, W. B. Saunders Co., 1975, pp. 389–391.

SALIVARY GLAND DISEASE

Debra Deem Morris, KENNETT SQUARE, PENNSYLVANIA

PTYALISM

The most common affection of the salivary glands is functional. Ptyalism, increased secretion of saliva, is identified by an abnormal accumulation of saliva in the mouth and must be differentiated from the more common problem, failure to swallow. Possible causes of ptyalism include heavy metal poisoning, parasympathomimetic (e.g., pilocarpine) toxicosis, encephalitis, and most commonly stomatitis. Toxicosis and encephalitis are usually attended by other signs referable to the gastrointestinal and central nervous systems.

When an animal has saliva draining from the mouth without other clinical signs, choke or dysphagia must be ruled out by passing a stomach tube and observing the animal swallow water or feed without nasal reflux. A thorough oral examination with the aid of a speculum should be performed in search of foreign bodies in the tongue, cheeks, or gums, tooth disease, oral ulceration, or other lesions within the mouth. If due to oral disease, the excessive salivation decreases once the source of irritation has been removed.

Ptyalism may be observed in horses that have grazed or consumed legumes parasitized by the fungus *Rhizoctonia leguminicola*. This fungus produces a mycotoxin, slaframine, that causes salivation when ingested. Animals seem to suffer no other ill effects, and the ptyalism ceases when the toxin is no longer being consumed. *Rhizoctonia leguminicola* has a wide geographic distribution, and the mycelial growth is usually not grossly visible because it is the color and texture of well-cured legume hay.

SIALOADENITIS

Sialoadenitis is uncommon in animals, as there is no specific infection that has a predilection for salivary tissue.[2] Salivary glands may be involved in any inflammatory process. In the region of the salivary glands, trauma is the frequent cause of inflammation. It is unusual but possible for infection to ascend the parotid or other salivary gland ducts, or the gland may become inflamed by hematogenous as well as local spread of infection. Strangles (*Streptococcus equi* infection) is rarely associated with sialoadenitis.

Inflammation results in duct obstruction by exudate, desquamated cells, and mucus. Obstruction with continued secretion produces dilation of the ducts, and acini swell and rupture from retained secretion. Leukocytes infiltrate the gland, and clinically it becomes enlarged, hot, and painful. A course of appropriate antimicrobial therapy may be indicated after isolation and identification of the organism have been attempted. Once the initial inflammation has subsided, the gland frequently atrophies and is replaced by extensive fibrous connective tissue. Since an inflammatory condition is very unlikely to affect all salivary glands, aptyalism does not occur.

Kernels of grain, plant awns, and other foreign bodies sometimes become lodged in the parotid or submandibular ducts (which lie opposite the third upper cheek teeth and canine teeth, respectively),[4] causing inflammation, obstruction and dilatation of the duct. Treatment consists of retrieval of the foreign body and appropriate antimicrobial therapy.

SIALOLITHS

Chronic inflammation in the salivary duct or gland may provide desquamated cells or consolidated exudate to act as a nidus for precipitation of calcium salts and the formation of salivary calculi. They are more common in horses than any other species, are composed largely of calcium carbonate, and are whitish, hard, and laminated.[2] Parotid calculi sometimes reach several centimeters diameter in the horse. Most calculi lodge at the duct orifice and cause some degree of salivary retention and a predisposition to infection and further inflammation. When identified, they should be surgically removed. Depending on the degree of damage to the duct or gland or both, total excision may be advisable to prevent salivary cysts or fistulae (see next section).

SALIVARY CYSTS

When a salivary duct is occluded by a sialolith, foreign body, or inflammation, the imprisoned secretion dilates the duct proximally to form a cyst. Ranula is a term applied to a cystic distention of a sublingual salivary duct in the floor of the mouth and presents as a smooth, rounded, fluctuating prominence with a bluish tinge. The contents may be serous or thick, tenacious mucus. Accumulation of salivary secretions in single or multiloculated cavities adjacent to ruptured ducts (mandibular, parotid, or sublingual) are referred to as salivary mucoceles or sialoceles. Unlike ranulae, these do not have an epithelial lining and can occur anywhere from the mandibular symphysis to the middle of the neck. Most are subcutaneous and vary up to 10 cm diameter. The contents are brown and mucinous and progressively become inspissated and tenacious.

Although quite common in dogs, sialoceles are rarely observed in horses. The treatment of choice in dogs has been removal of the gland whose duct has been traumatized. Simple excision or drainage of the cyst is unsuccessful because until the source of secretion is removed, the cyst usually recurs or an external fistula develops. The same procedure is required in horses.[1] Owing to the extensive and complicated nature of the parotid and mandibular salivary glands, nests of salivary tissue are easily left in place, which continue their secretory activity and create fistulae, which drain to the exterior. Successful ablation of all glandular tissue and cessation of secretion have been reported.[1] Ranulae are only very rarely seen and seem to respond to simple drainage. The polystomatic sublingual gland is situated between the body of the tongue and the incisive part of the mandible and is not easily accessible for removal.

SALIVARY GLAND NEOPLASIA

Primary salivary gland neoplasia are rare in horses and all species of domestic animals, but adenocarcinomas, benign mixed tumors, and acinic cell tumors arising within salivary glands have been reported.[3, 5, 6] The parotid and mandibular salivary glands are the most common sites of origin. Local invasion by tumors originating in adjacent tissue probably occurs more frequently than primary neoplasia.

The affected gland is enlarged by infiltration of neoplastic cells and becomes apparent as a mass occupying the space below the external ear, behind the mandibular ramus. Sometimes the intermandibular space and ventral cervical area become edematous. Abscesses and cysts must be clinically distinguished from salivary gland tumors. Needle aspiration is sometimes helpful, but nonspecific inflammation may be misleading if the neoplastic cells are not retrieved in the aspirate. A wedge biopsy is usually diagnostic when the mass is neoplastic.

Metastasis of salivary tumors is variable, depending upon the type of tumor. Adenocarcinomas usually spread to involve the deep cervical and mediastinal lymph nodes and are not amenable to therapy. Benign mixed tumors do not metastasize, but their peculiar growth results in marginal projections along the channels of peripheral vessels. Surgical excision is imperative to prevent recurrence because projections left in situ are a source of additional tumor growth. Acinic cell tumors are locally invasive but do not usually metastasize.

References

1. Bracegirdle, J. R.: Removal of the parotid and mandibular salivary glands from a pony mare. Vet. Rec., 98:507, 1956.
2. Jubb, K. V. F., and Kennedy, P. C.: Pathology of Domestic Animals, Vol. 2. New York, Academic Press, 1970, pp. 44–45.
3. Koestner, A., and Buerger, L.: Primary neoplasms of the salivary glands in animals compared to similar tumors in man. Pathol. Vet., 2:201, 1965.
4. Sisson, S.: Equine digestive system. *In* Getty, R. (ed.): Sisson and Grossman's Anatomy of the Domestic Animals, 5th ed. Philadelphia, W. B. Saunders Co., 1975, pp. 454–497.
5. Stackhouse, L. L., Moore, J. J., and Hylton, W. E.: Salivary gland adenocarcinoma in a mare. J. Am. Vet. Med. Assoc., 172:271, 1978.
6. Sundberg, J. P., Burnstein, T., Page, E. H., Kirkham, W. W., and Robinson, F. R.: Neoplasms of equidae. J. Am. Vet. Med. Assoc., 170:150, 1977.

GLOSSITIS

Virginia Reef, KENNETT SQUARE, PENNSYLVANIA

Glossitis, inflammation of the tongue, can be primary as a result of trauma or contact with irritant chemicals or secondary to some neurologic diseases and poisoning. Iatrogenic lingual lacerations and torn frenulum can be consequences of floating teeth, overzealous oral examination, or unconventional training practices. Maloccluded teeth, stemmy feedstuffs, or foreign bodies can also cause lacerations and can result in lingual abscessation.

CLINICAL SIGNS

Partial or complete dysphagia accompanied by lingual swelling and salivation is the most prominent clinical sign associated with glossitis. The breath has a fetid odor if there is bacterial invasion of the lesion or retention of decomposing food between the cheeks and molar arcades. Pain may be exhibited in association with mastication or oral examination.

TRAUMATIC GLOSSITIS

Traumatic lesions of the tongue have a good prognosis, and rapid healing can be expected owing to the good vascular supply. Foreign bodies should be removed coupled with drainage of the associated abscesses. If a suspected foreign body cannot be localized upon oral examination of the tongue, radiographs may be of value to visualize radiopaque foreign bodies such as wires. Radiolucent foreign bodies such as wood should be suspected with intermittent swelling of the tongue, dysphagia, draining fistulous tracts, and no foreign bodies visible on radiographs. Dental malocclusions or points can be corrected with proper dental care and periodic floating (p. 188). Tongue lacerations should be allowed to heal by secondary intention. Anti-inflammatory drugs, such as phenylbutazone and flunixin meglumine, supportive feeding, and frequent rinsing of the mouth are the preferred treatments. A solution of 1 per cent potassium permanganate can be used as an effective disinfectant mouthwash, or the mouth can be frequently rinsed with water. Supportive feeding with an alfalfa slurry, moistened pellets, bran mash, or a tube-fed diet are important until normal mastication can resume. The high-protein, low-residue diet with the addition of alfalfa meal is successful in maintaining horses via a nasogastric or esophagostomy tube (p. 111).

CONTACT GLOSSITIS

A contact glossitis occurs in horses secondary to the exposure of the lingual and buccal mucosa to counterirritants, especially mercury blisters. Proper protective measures to prevent the horse from licking or chewing the blistered limb were either not followed or were circumvented by the horse. Affected horses present with profound swelling and ulceration or vesiculation of the muzzle, lingual and buccal mucosa, pharynx, and larynx. These horses have severe dysphagia, with both water and feed being regurgitated through the nose. Salivation is profuse, and the horse resists oral examination. Dorsal displacement of the soft palate may be seen in association with a chemical glossitis. If the pharyngeal and laryngeal swelling is severe, respiratory distress may require a tracheotomy tube. Aspiration pneumonia is a complicating factor if the dysphagia is severe, and thus the horse should be muzzled and only allowed controlled access to food and water. If total supportive feeding is required, a nasogastric tube should be passed three times daily or an esophagostomy tube left in place for feeding three times a day. Anti-inflammatory drugs, potassium permanganate, and antimicrobials are indicated. The antimicrobial should be based on the likelihood or existence of aspiration pneumonia. The blistered limbs should be bandaged and the horse muzzled, cradled, or prevented from further exposure to the offensive chemical. Prognosis is guarded, as aspiration is a common and significant secondary complication.

SECONDARY GLOSSITIS

Glossitis occurs secondary to a wide variety of primary disease processes. A variety of neurologic conditions can result in dysphagia and a secondary lingual inflammation. Paralysis of the hypoglossal and glossopharyngeal nerves results in lingual inflammation owing to the horse's inability to retract the tongue into the mouth. Dysphagia is a classical sign of botulism and is occasionally a presenting sign with equine protozoal myeloencephalitis, tetanus, chronic lead poisoning, mandibular or maxillary fractures, or temporomandibular dislocations and guttural pouch mycoses. Vesiculation of the lingual and buccal mucosa can be seen in association with herpesvirus infection and the vesicular diseases.

Treatment and prognosis of the preceding conditions depend upon diagnosis of the underlying disease. Supportive treatment for secondary glossitis is the same as described previously for primary glossitis.

References

1. Blood, D. C., Henderson, J. A., and Radostits, O. M.: Veterinary Medicine, 5th ed. Philadelphia, Lea & Febiger, 1979, pp. 107–108.
2. Cook, W. R.: Observations of the aetiology of epistaxis and cranial nerve paralysis in the horse. Vet. Rec., 78:396, 1966.
3. deLahunta, A.: Veterinary Neuroanatomy and Clinical Neurology. Philadelphia, W. B. Saunders Co., 1977, pp. 107–108, 370.
4. Freeman, D. E., and Naylor, J. M.: Cervical esophagostomy to permit extraoral feeding of the horse. J. Am. Vet. Med. Assoc., 172:314, 1978.
5. Naylor, J. M.: The nutrition of the sick horse. J. Eq. Med. Surg., 1:64, 1977.
6. Swerczek, T. W.: Toxicoinfectious botulism in foals and adult horses. J. Am. Vet. Med. Assoc., 176:217, 1980.

CARE OF THE TEETH

G. Marvin Beeman, LITTLETON, COLORADO

Dental problems that interfere with mastication or contribute to systemic infection should always be considered as a cause of chronic weight loss. Dental problems will often also affect performance when the horse is being directed by a bit in the mouth.

When a horse is presented with a history that suggests a dental problem, age, sex, use, diet, and eating habits should be considered in arriving at a diagnosis. Age is important because of the eruption of the various teeth and the shedding of the deciduous teeth, both of which are often accompanied by dental disease. Also, there are many dental problems that occur much more frequently in older horses. Sex is a consideration because the mare has fewer teeth than the stallion, which may dictate the type of problem encountered (such as presence of rudimentary lower canine teeth in the mare, which often do not erupt and may cause gingival irritation). Use is considered because a bit will often cause severe lacerations to the cheeks if forced against sharp enamel points of the premolars. Abnormal eating habits such as dropping of grain, excessive salivation, "quidding" of hay or grass, or tilting of the head are indications of painful dental problems. Because age and sex are significant factors when evaluating a dental condition, the formulas for deciduous and permanent teeth (Table 1), along with the eruption table (Table 2), should be known.

The canine teeth of the mare are very small or do not erupt, while those of the male are almost always present, are longer than the wolf teeth (P1), and are located in the rostral half of the interdental space. The lower canine teeth are more rostral than the upper ones. Canines should not be confused with the wolf teeth (P1), which are commonly found only in the upper arcade and vary from small, round (5 mm in diameter) needlelike structures just erupting from the gum to rather large (10 to 15 mm wide)

concave teeth with the concavity on the lingual side. Even larger round wolf teeth have been encountered. Wolf teeth in the upper arcade may be located several millimeters rostral to or touching the second premolar. When the lower P1 is present, it is quite small and needlelike and is adjacent to the lower P2.

Several anatomic factors influence dental wear and thereby the incidence of dental disease. The upper (maxillary) arcades of molars and premolars are more widely separated than the lower (mandibular) arcades, the distance between the mandibulae being least at the fourth premolar and first molar. The upper teeth, therefore, overlap the lower teeth on the buccal surface, and the lower teeth overlap the upper teeth on the lingual suface. The occlusal surfaces of the upper cheek teeth viewed from in front slope outward and downward, while those of the lower teeth angle inward and upward. This angulation of the occlusal surfaces, coupled with the overlapping of teeth described before and the side-to-side pattern of mastication, causes the development of sharp enamel points on the buccal surface (outside) of upper teeth and the lingual surface (inside) of lower teeth.

Prominent points occur on rostral and middle portions of the upper teeth. On lower teeth, points are evenly distributed. Upper points are more angled, while lower points are more vertical. These differences in points in upper and lower arcades determine the angle at which the float blade is applied to the points. Because of the anatomy and method of mastication, the upper fourth cheek tooth (first molar) is subject to most wear and is the commonest site of serious dental disease.

Parrot mouth (brachygnathia of the lower jaw) or undershoot (prognathia of the lower jaw) cause long points on the rostral border of the upper second

TABLE 1. FORMULAS FOR DECIDUOUS AND PERMANENT TEETH

Deciduous Teeth
$2 \left(\text{Di} \dfrac{3}{3} \ \text{DC} \dfrac{0}{0} \ \text{Dp} \dfrac{3}{3} \right) = 24$

Permanent Teeth
$2 \left(\text{I} \dfrac{3}{3} \ \text{C} \dfrac{1}{1} \ \text{p} \dfrac{3 \text{ or } 4}{3} \ \text{M} \dfrac{3}{3} \right) = 40 \text{ or } 42$

premolar and the caudal border of the lower third molar, respectively. This is especially true in horses older than seven years.

EXAMINATION OF TEETH

By correlating the history, particularly the age of the horse, with a thorough understanding of anatomy of the head and teeth, the examination routine is established. Before the oral cavity is examined, the exterior of the head should be examined for (1) any abnormal swellings and/or draining tracts over the maxilla or mandibles, (2) abnormal head tilt, and (3) unilateral, purulent, flaky nasal discharge with a fetid odor of necrotic bone. The exterior of the

TABLE 2. ERUPTION TIMES FOR THE TEETH

Deciduous	
Tooth	*Eruption*
1st incisor	Birth or first week
2nd incisor	4–6 weeks
3rd incisor	6–9 months
No deciduous canine	
No deciduous wolf teeth	
2nd premolar	
3rd premolar	Birth–first 2 weeks
4th premolar	

Permanent			
Tooth			*Eruption*
1st incisor	I1		$2\frac{1}{2}$ years
2nd incisor	I2		$3\frac{1}{2}$ years
3rd incisor	I3		$4\frac{1}{2}$ years
Canine	C		4–5 years
1st premolar (wolf tooth)	PM1		5–6 months
2nd premolar	PM2		$2\frac{1}{2}$ years
3rd premolar	PM3	3 years	Lowers may erupt about 6 months earlier
4th premolar	PM4	4 years	
1st molar	M1		9–12 months
2nd molar	M2		2 years
3rd molar	M3		$3\frac{1}{2}$–4 years

cheeks should be palpated over the upper cheek teeth for painful sites.

The majority of horses object to having the oral cavity examined and must be restrained. The degree of restraint should be determined by the horse's response. The examination should be done with the least amount of discomfort and restraint possible; however, if the dental lesions are quite painful, the examination may not be possible without the use of chemical restraining agents. Various agents such as xylazine* alone or in combination with acepromazine maleate† and/or pentazocine lactate injection‡ are very useful for this examination and certainly should be used before the horse is upset or abused.

The first step in the examination is to position the horse in optimal light so it cannot back away from the examiner. This is best done in a corner of a stall or in stocks with a darkened background. An assistant should be instructed in the way to hold the horse. Be certain the halter is large enough to allow the mouth to be opened to the maximal amount and without discomfort to the horse.

Rinse the mouth free of debris, preferably with cold water. In a fractious horse, warm water will be more readily tolerated. Note if pain is evidenced or if there is halitosis.

The incisor teeth are visually examined first for abnormalities and the determination of age. The interdental space, gums, and the cheek opposite the upper premolars are palpated and observed for injuries. Examination of the cheek teeth is most often accomplished without a dental speculum. However, if a speculum is necessary, care must be taken to prevent injury to the horse and/or the examiner. The left side of the dental arcade can be visually examined by inserting the fingers of the left hand through the right interdental space and grasping the tongue and withdrawing it out of the right side of the mouth. This will force the horse to open its mouth and to pull back. To avoid injury to the tongue if the horse should react violently, the little finger of the hand grasping the tongue should also grasp the halter. The mouth can be forced open further by applying pressure to the hard palate with a finger of the right hand. Visual examination is facilitated by a head lamp or pocket penlight. Palpation of the left arcade can be accomplished with the tongue held in the same manner and the right hand introduced into the left interdental space, forcing the tongue between the right cheek teeth with the

*Rompun, Haver-Lockhart, Bayvet Division, Cutter Laboratories, Shawnee, KS

†Acepromazine Maleate-Injectible, Fort Dodge Laboratories, Inc., Fort Dodge, IA

‡Talwin-V, Veterinary Products Division, Winthrop Laboratories, Division of Sterling Drug, Inc., New York, NY

back of the hand while palpating those of the left arcade. The examination of the right cheek teeth is done in the same manner by reversing all procedures.

If additional examinations are needed, further narcosis may be necessary and a dental speculum may be applied. Use of a short-acting general anesthetic is reasonable to facilitate a complete examination. A laryngoscope will facilitate close visual evaluation of an involved tooth. Extreme care must be taken to avoid damage to the scope. A dental pick is helpful in determining if an infundibulum is defective. Injection of a colored fluid into a draining tract will determine if the lesion opens into the oral cavity (periodontal disease). Radiographs are quite helpful in determining the extent to which dental disease involves the periodontal tissue.

Since the age of the horse dictates to a large extent what might be the cause of dental disease, the diagnosis and therapy are categorized by age groups.

AGE 10–18 MONTHS

History. Not masticating well.

Examination. Reveals lacerations of cheeks from sharp points on upper premolars. This is not a common problem but may cause poor mastication in this age group.

Therapy. Float down the enamel points. The deciduous teeth are soft and will not require much rasping (see next section).

AGE 18–24 MONTHS

History. Poor mastication and bleeding from the mouth after riding with snaffle bit, objecting to bridle training, throwing head.

Examination. Ulcerated area of cheeks is present opposite the second upper premolar, tongue lacerations, small, very sharp points on all premolars, particularly the upper second premolar. Wolf teeth present.

Therapy

1. Remove wolf teeth. This should be done before the floating because they will likely be broken off or rasped down, thus making their removal difficult. In my opinion, this is the optimal time to remove these teeth because they are not as firmly embedded as they will be at an older age. Often the only restraint necessary to remove these teeth is a nose twitch; however, tranquilization and narcosis with or without local anesthesia may be necessary. The twitch and head must be held in a manner so that the wolf tooth can be seen. To do this, the twitch must be pushed toward the side being operated on while the head is held firmly. One method of removing the wolf teeth is to elevate the gingiva from the lateral, rostral, and caudal surface with an instrument specifically designed for this purpose or an orthopedic gouge (5 to 8 mm in width). The medial surface is left alone because of the danger of injuring the palatine artery. If the wolf tooth is quite close to the second premolar, forcing the instrument between the two teeth will loosen the wolf tooth sufficiently so that it can be pried out using the second premolar for support. If this is not possible, the tooth can then be pulled with a pair of wolf tooth extraction forceps. It is advisable to remove the teeth intact, but if they are broken off well above the gum line, it is best to leave the fragment in place because it seldom will create a problem and unnecessary damage will be done to the alveolus trying to remove it. Note should be made that the fragment may appear within a year's time and may be mistaken for another wolf tooth. Normally the fragment is easily removed when it appears. Removal of the wolf tooth without breaking it off is facilitated by grasping the tooth with forceps as deep into the gum and alveolus as possible. Apply traction straight down while rotating the tooth back and forth on its long axis rather than rocking the tooth medially and laterally. Also avoid the horse's mandibular movement, which will put lateral pressure on the forceps, causing the tooth to break off. When lower wolf teeth are present, they are removed in the same manner. They are usually small and easy to extract.

2. The sharp enamel points are rasped off. The floating procedure should be started with a minimal amount of restraint. Many horses can be floated completely with simple restraint; however, as objection increases, the level of restraint must be increased. A twitch is useful, but most horses will not tolerate a twitch for the length of time necessary to complete the floating. In some horses, a lip chain applied to the upper incisor gingiva will provide better restraint than a twitch. It is much more desirable to use chemical restraint than it is to fight the horse (the same products or combinations thereof as mentioned previously are very helpful). Even the short-acting general anesthetics (such as xylazine and ketamine hydrochloride injection NF*) are preferred over excessive physical restraint to float or carry out a simple surgical procedure involving the teeth.

The noseband of the halter should be sufficiently large so that the horse's mouth can be opened to its maximum. The halter and assistant's arm should not put pressure on the horse's face, as this will cause the float to injure the cheeks. To enable the pro-

---

*Vetalar, Parke-Davis & Co., Detroit, MI

cedure to be carried out without excessive restraint, the teeth causing the most trouble should be floated first because most horses will tolerate some floating before objecting. Therefore, the upper cheek teeth are most often floated first (the premolars in young horses and molars in older horses). The lower cheek teeth are floated last because horses seem to object to this portion of the procedure more than any other and because horses are much more prone to chewing the float when doing the lower arcade. This can be prevented by holding the tongue out of the side of the mouth opposite the side being worked on. However, as soon as the process is started, many horses will set their lower jaw and will actually stand quieter if the tongue is released.

In the actual floating process, the float (dental rasp) should be started on the teeth with relatively easy strokes until the rasps have established grooves. Then more pressure can be applied. Changing direction of the floats causes the most work; therefore, the longer the stroke, the better for the patient and the operator. Care needs to be taken to avoid injuring the mouth. One of the most vulnerable sites is beyond the last molar in both the upper and lower arcade. The rasp should be placed at approximately a 90° angle to the enamel points on the buccal surface of the upper cheek teeth and the lingual surface of the lower cheek teeth.

Because of the buccal ulcerations that are often caused by pressure from a snaffle bit against the sharp enamel points of the upper second premolar (either deciduous or permanent), this condition is often a problem when a gag snaffle is used (as in polo ponies). In order to tolerate the bit, the upper and lower second premolars should have the rostral aspect rounded from the table surface to the gum line and from the lingual surface to the buccal surface. For the buccal surface of the uppers, a short-handled 30° float is inserted from the opposite side of the mouth through the interdental space. (Some operators prefer a file blade rather than a rasp.) A short straight float is used for the lingual side of the uppers and lowers from the same side of the mouth through the interdental space. Caution is necessary to avoid injuring the roof of the mouth. Occasionally the buccal side of the lowers is most easily reached with the same instrument from the opposite side.

There are many different types of floats and blades available today. The choice should be the one that best fits the operation. The blades should be sharp because the fewer strokes needed to remove the sharp points, the better it is for the horse and the operator. In my opinion, the blades that have carborundum pieces fixed to them* are the best be-

*Jorgensen float blades, Jorgensen Laboratories, Inc., Loveland, CO

cause they are extremely sharp and stay that way with considerable use.

AGE 2½ YEARS THROUGH 4 YEARS

History. Same as in the preceding section. Often more obvious signs of painful mastication with a sudden onset and halitosis.

Examination. Same as in the preceding section, and the presence of retained deciduous premolars (commonly called dental caps). These horses present many different signs. Deciduous premolars (DcPm) should be considered retained when the permanent tooth has grown beyond the gum line and a definite demarcation between the cap and the permanent tooth can be seen. Often the infundibulae of DcPm are shallow or absent (this is a good identifying and differentiating feature of the DcPm). Occasionally the examination will reveal an upper cap that has split transversely or longitudinally with a portion missing or displaced laterally, causing buccal lacerations and facial swellings. One case was observed in which buccal penetration from a cap fragment was complete, causing an oral fistula. Caps of the lower arcade occasionally split transversely but rarely displace medially or laterally. Retained caps commonly occur in pairs. The lower third and fourth premolars may erupt six months earlier than the corresponding uppers.

Chronic ossifying alveolar periostitis observed as swelling of the maxilla or more commonly the mandible over the roots of the cheek teeth is caused by impacted, overcrowded DcPms. The swelling may be accompanied by draining tracts. This condition is a common finding in three-year-olds of breeds with relatively small heads (such as Arabians).

Caps that are attached to gingiva entirely around their circumferences should be removed *only* if there is a definite indication that they are causing a problem. Not only will removal be difficult and result in excessive damage to the gum, but also it will be some time before the permanent tooth will erupt sufficiently to allow for proper mastication.

Therapy. Often buccal and/or lingual lacerations will be from the retained DcPms, which should be removed before any floating is done. Caps should also be removed if chronic ossifying alveolar periostitis is present to the extent that considerable irritation or a draining tract is evident. Mild alveolar periostitis will often recover with the normal loosening and loss of the caps. Therefore, a conservative approach to this condition is warranted. Caps should be removed before the permanent tooth is removed to treat the draining tract. The exterior swelling will be slow to disappear.

Removal of caps can be accomplished with a combination of a screwdriver (with a shaft 10 to 14 in long and the tip rounded and bluntly wedged) and small dental equine forceps. The forceps are most useful for the lower caps and occasionally the upper second DcPm, while the screwdriver is the most efficient instrument for the upper three and four DcPms. The tongue is held out the contralateral side of the mouth. For the upper caps, the blade of the screwdriver is inserted between the permanent tooth and the cap at the rostrolingual quarter by directing the shaft from the opposite interdental space. The instrument can often be forced between the cap and permanent tooth with little pressure, then rotated to cause the cap to be freed. Occasionally tapping the screwdriver with a solid object will be necessary to force the blade between the DcPm and the premolar to separate the two. Care must be taken to be certain the instrument is directed properly to avoid injury to the mouth. The lower DcPms three and four can often be removed with forceps, but the screwdriver will work quite well also. The site of insertion between the lower cap and the permanent premolar is more rostral than for the upper teeth. Sometimes it is necessary to direct the shaft of the instrument along the table surface of the teeth to loosen the lower DcPms three and four.

Retained deciduous incisors often cause displacement of the permanent incisors toward the lingual side. When retained, they are embedded in the buccal gingiva, and most often they can be removed with dental forceps. Occasionally they will have to be loosened as described for the wolf teeth. Fragments need to be removed unless excessive damage will result, and then they should be left for a time to allow the permanent teeth to further displace the fragments.

Following any interruption to the gingiva, the oral cavity should be rinsed two to three times daily with strong salt water for three to five days.

After removing those caps that are creating problems, floating of the remaining teeth may be necessary.

FIVE YEARS AND OLDER

History. Most commonly will be painful mastication and weight loss.

Examination. The examination may reveal a single entity or any combination of the following.

1. Sharp enamel points on upper cheek teeth (most commonly the molars) causing buccal lacerations; points on the lower cheek teeth (most commonly the third and fourth) causing lingual lacerations.

2. Canine teeth that are long and sharp (occasionally those that do not erupt cause a gingival cyst).

3. Brachygnathia of the lower jaw (parrot mouth) creates a long point on the rostral border of the upper second premolar and the caudal border of the lower third molar. If the lower jaw protrudes, points occur on the rostral border of the second lower premolar and the caudal border of the upper third molar.

4. Abnormally long cheek teeth (usually opposite the defect left by the loss of the corresponding tooth in the opposing arcade).

5. When dental pain is observed, periodontal disease is most likely to be the cause. Dental pain will be manifested by (a) slow and careful mastication that is exaggerated with pelleted feed and occasionally with grain (the affected horse will often leave grain but eat hay), (b) exaggerated tongue movements, (c) holding the head rotated with the affected side up (especially when eating pellets), (d) excessive drooling of saliva and grain, (e) dropping of feed boli (quidding), (f) avoiding cold water or showing pain when the mouth is washed with cold water, or (g) pain exhibited when the teeth are floated. Halitosis is further evidence of periodontal disease. The source can be identified by palpating the suspected tooth and getting the odor of necrotic bone from the palpating finger. The gum will recede from the affected tooth. A unilateral flaky purulent nasal discharge with a fetid odor is most commonly caused by advanced disease of the upper cheek teeth causing maxillary sinusitis. The roots of the third and fourth cheek teeth are usually located within the anterior maxillary sinus, and those of the fifth and sixth cheek teeth are within the posterior maxillary sinus. If the diseased alveolus ruptures to the exterior of the maxilla or mandible, a fistula results.

Therapy. A combination of the following may be necessary.

1. Rasping of enamel points may be necessary. In older horses, the upper molars will cause the most damage to the cheeks, so they should be floated first. There is a tendency to over-rasp the cheek teeth. The only rasping that is necessary is to remove the sharp enamel points. This is especially true in very old horses because their teeth can be inadvertently extracted by the rasp.

2. The canine teeth that are long, sharp, and perhaps are interfering with the bridle should be rasped down rather than removed. By grasping the horse's mandible at the level of the interdental space with the thumb on one side and the index and middle fingers on the other, the lower labia can be held down and away from the lower canines. The upper canines are done in the same manner by elevating the upper labia with the thumb of the free hand. They can be rasped or filed down by placing the instrument of choice directly over the tooth and at right angles to it. Most often this procedure is nec-

essary to satisfy the owner rather than improve the horse's condition.

3. Elongation of the second upper premolar caused by parrot mouth can usually be corrected with a dental float, but often the elongation on the lower third molar will have to be cut off with molar cutters.

4. Excessively long cheek teeth that cause a masticating problem can be shortened by rasping at three- to six-month intervals. All the occlusal surfaces of the affected tooth must be rasped down. Sedation and a dental speculum will greatly enhance this procedure. Many times these cases are presented only after the affected tooth is quite long, and the only practical method of correction is cutting the tooth off with molar cutters or a similar instrument. Wire saws can also be used. There are various types of cutters. The compound molar cutter is the most effective, especially for large teeth. Extreme care must be taken in the proper placement of the instrument, and the pressure must be applied at 90° to the tooth with no rotational torque because the tooth can be fractured down into the alveolus. After the excess has been cut off, the buccal and lingual surfaces must be rasped smooth. This procedure can be done in the standing horse under sedation and local anesthesia. Even so, most horses will object to the pressure and excessive manipulation, which enhances the possibility of fracturing the tooth. Therefore, one of the short-acting general anesthetic regimens is indicated (an acepromazine, Rompun, and ketamine combination is very effective). A good dental speculum is also necessary. Care must be taken to prevent tooth fragments from being aspirated into the trachea in anesthetized horses.

5. The most common conditions causing dental pain are periodontal disease, defects of infundibulae, alveolar periostitis, and the resulting dental fistulas and/or sinus infections. These conditions are often seen in combination rather than as single entities. In my experience, they most commonly affect the fourth upper cheek tooth (first molar). Necrosis of the infundibulum is the commonest condition seen in our horse population. In many cases, the condition does not progress to the point that more serious sequelae develop. The affected tooth can be left in place and the entire arcade given regular examinations and conservative (floating) treatment at two- to four-month intervals to maintain normal mastication.

The lesion may progress to the point that the tooth splits, alveolar periostitis develops, and a sinus empyema occurs. When an upper cheek tooth splits, the fragment on the buccal side is displaced laterally, causing considerable cheek irritation. These fragments must be removed. Most often this

can be accomplished with a small tooth extractor and dental speculum on the standing, sedated animal. That portion of the tooth left in place (usually on the lingual surface) is often quite stable, and the tooth will stay viable and will not require extraction. This has been successful in enough cases to warrant conservative treatment before removal of the entire tooth. If sinus empyema or a fistula does develop, removal of the tooth is necessary either by extraction or repulsion. Though less common, mandibular teeth can be affected with infundibular defects and can develop all of the previously mentioned sequelae. If a lower cheek tooth splits, the fragment on the lingual side most often will be displaced toward the tongue, causing considerable irritation and interference in mastication.

When periodontal disease causes empyema or fistulae, it is necessary to remove the tooth and establish drainage. However, it is possible to prevent the advancement of the disease if the initial lesions of gingivitis (hyperemia, edema, and open defects) are treated. Systemic antimicrobial and nonsteroidal anti-inflammatory medication in conjunction with frequent astringent mouthwashes and floating to maintain normal dental tables and mastication will correct the disease. Occasionally an early fistula will dry up if vigorously flushed with hydrogen peroxide and one of the tamed iodine products. Unfortunately, the early signs of the disease are often undetected.

The extraction or repulsion of the cheek teeth is adequately explained in the literature. In our hands, repulsion is the most efficient and satisfactory method of tooth removal. Extraction is very difficult, and sufficient drainage is difficult to establish for proper postoperative treatment and recovery. The very old horse is the most amenable patient for tooth extraction. A case can be approached by first attempting extraction, but if not successful, repulsion should be the final procedure. Inhalation general anesthesia is preferred because adequate ventilation is maintained while working in the mouth, and the head can be manipulated without interference with the airway.

References

1. Baker, G. J.: Some aspects of equine dental disease. Eq. Vet. J., 2:105, 1970.
2. Baker, G. J.: Some aspects of equine dental radiology. Eq. Vet. J., 3:46, 1971.
3. Baker, G. J.: Surgery of the head and neck. *In* Catcott, E. J., and Smithcors, F. J. (eds.): Equine Medicine and Surgery, 2nd ed. Wheaton, IL, American Veterinary Pub., 1972, pp. 752–779.
4. Baker, G. J.: Some aspects of equine dental decay. Eq. Vet. J., 6:127, 1974.
5. Beeman, G. M.: Equine dentistry. Proc. 8th Annu. Meet. Am. Assoc. Eq. Pract., pp. 235–240, 1962.

6. Frank, E. R.: Affections of the teeth. *In* Frank, E. R. (ed.): Veterinary Surgery, revised ed. Minneapolis, Burgess Pub. Co., 1973, pp. 131–140.
7. Hofmeyr, C. F. B.: The digestive system. *In* Oehme, F. W., and Prier, J. E. (eds.): Textbook of Large Animal Surgery. Baltimore, Williams & Wilkins Co., 1974, pp. 364–382.

8. St. Clair, L. E.: Equine digestive system. *In* Getty, R. (ed.): Sisson & Grossman's Anatomy of the Domestic Animals, Vol. 1, 5th ed. Philadelphia, W. B. Saunders Co., 1975, pp. 460–470.
9. Vail, C. D.: Tips on equine dentistry. Lincoln, NB, Norden Laboratories, Norden News, 55(22):15, 1980.

ESOPHAGEAL OBSTRUCTION

Edward A. Scott, EAST LANSING, MICHIGAN

The esophagus connects the oropharynx with the lesser curvature of the stomach, originating dorsal to the larynx and passing left lateral of the median plane in the cervical region. As it approaches the thoracic inlet, the esophagus courses ventral to the trachea, then ascends dorsally within the chest and passes over the aortic arch. Its termination is at the gastric cardiac orifice, just caudal to the esophageal hiatus of the diaphragm. Over 50 per cent of its length is made up of the cervical segment.

There are four layers to the esophageal wall: (1) a fibrous layer termed the *tunica adventitia;* (2) muscular layers (*tunica muscularis*); (3) a submucosal layer (*tela submucosa*); and (4) mucous membrane (*tunica mucosa*). Muscle is striated from the pharynx to the base of the heart, where it becomes smooth muscle. Approaching the stomach, esophageal wall thickness increases as the lumen diminishes. Except at the cranial and caudal sphincters, muscular layers are spirally and elliptically arranged.

Vascular supply to the esophagus originates from carotid, bronchoesophageal, and gastric arteries. Innervation is supplied by the ninth and tenth cranial nerves and sympathetic nerves, with ganglia within muscular layers.

ETIOLOGY OF ESOPHAGEAL DISORDERS

Equine esophageal disorders that result in dysphagia and regurgitation "the flowing backwards or expulsion of swallowed contents in small amounts" can be classified as anatomic and/or physiologic (Table 1). Anatomic disorders, particularly food choke, are the most common and mechanically impede the passage of food. Physiologic disorders are less common and are caused by motor dysfunction of the esophagus or its sphincters.

Congenital abnormalities of the aortic arch or esophagus or both may cause esophageal obstruction in horses up to a year or more of age.[1, 2, 7] A foal weak at birth with septicemia or generalized myopathy may also have signs of dysphagia and regur-

gitation. Defects of the hard and soft palate in the newborn, while not resulting in esophageal obstruction, can cause dysphagia or regurgitation of food through the nasal cavity of neonates. While mural tumors of the esophagus are typically congenital, they may not produce clinical signs until the tumor is sufficiently large to prevent passage of food.

Stricture and diverticuli of the esophagus occur secondary to foreign bodies, swallowing of caustic agents, or esophageal surgery.[3–6] Excessively rough use of the nasogastric tube in the diagnosis or treatment of food choke can also cause esophagitis and promote stricture.

CLINICAL SIGNS

Esophageal obstructions in the horse are characterized by ptyalism, dysphagia, coughing, pneumonia, and regurgitation. "Choked" horses may repeatedly swallow or retch as if attempting to vomit. Extension of the head and neck with constant chewing movements is occasionally seen. In some instances, intermittent esophageal obstruction is self-corrected, and clinical signs vary according to duration and location of the lesion.

Any horse that regurgitates with dysphagia or ptyalism or both should be considered "choked" until diagnostic findings prove otherwise. It is imperative to remember that ptyalism and dysphagia are clinical signs that accompany central nervous system disorders (such as rabies). Integration of history, clinical signs, physical examination, and other diagnostic findings places a differential diagnosis list in proper prospective.

History may reveal one of the following: (1) prior choke episodes of unknown cause apparently responsive to passage of a nasogastric tube, (2) administration of medicinal boluses, (3) cellulitis or trauma in the cervical area associated with cuts, strangles, or perivascular injections, (4) fast eating and "bolting down" of concentrates, or (5) an appetite for foreign materials, such as wood, tree bark, plastic, or cloth materials.

TABLE 1. CAUSES OF REGURGITATION

Anatomic	Physiologic
Cleft palate	Sphincter disorders
Foreign body	Achalasia
Food choke	Cranial nerve injury
Stricture	Encephalopathy (e.g., moldy corn,
Diverticulum	lead, or toxic plants)
Tumors	Nutritional myopathy (e.g., vitamin
Esophagitis	E or selenium deficiency)
Congenital anomalies of	Infectious disease (e.g., rabies and
the esophagus	other encephalitides)
Congenital anomalies of	
the aortic arch	

Oropharyngeal diseases, such as foreign bodies, dental disease, glossitis, and oropharyngeal tumors that cause ptyalism, should be identified by a thorough oral examination. Manual examination may define the soft and hard palate and pharyngeal and epiglottic abnormalities. In foals, intractable horses, or those with possible neurologic dysfunction, endoscopy is essential to examine the nasal cavity, pharynx, and esophagus.

Observation of the horse and palpation of the esophageal area may reveal distention of the cervical esophagus in a choked horse. Early in the course of this disease, external palpation may reveal the point of obstruction if it is located in the pharyngeal or cervical area. Thereafter, esophageal spasm, inflammation, and enlargement of intraluminal contents produce a more diffuse area of firmness. Cellulitis and crepitation of the head and neck area are suggestive of a perforating pharyngeal, tracheal, or esophageal injury or clostridiosis. If oral, visual, or manual examination is inconclusive, nasogastric tube passage will confirm partial or complete esophageal obstruction and the approximate site of involvement.

Thoracic radiographs are indicated when esophageal disease may be complicated by aspiration pneumonia, a serious sequela.

ESOPHAGOSCOPY

Esophagoscopy is an aid to the evaluation of all patients with esophageal disease. Rigid endoscopes are of little value and are dangerous and, therefore, should not be used in the horse. With the emergence of flexible fiberoptic endoscopes, equine esophagoscopy has become a safe, quick, and definitive diagnostic tool. If the endoscope length is sufficient (150 cm or greater), all of the esophagus may be viewed in a normal horse. If food is withheld from the horse for 36 to 48 hours, gastroscopy is possible. When any type of endoscope is used on an animal with acute or necrotizing esophagitis, care must be exercised to prevent perforation. Endo-scopic examination is typically performed on the restrained standing animal, and the flexible endoscope is passed like a nasogastric tube. Most fiberoptic endoscopes allow irrigation and insufflation of the esophagus, which improve visibility and allow the clinician to observe changes in luminal size and character.

Normally, the folds of mucosa that line the lumen are arranged longitudinally and appear white when the esophagus is viewed in a relaxed position. As air is forced into the esophagus via the endoscope, these folds flatten and become pinker as the esophagus distends. The outline of the dorsal arch of the tracheal rings may then be seen in the ventral cervical esophagus. Transverse folds can be produced iatrogenically by caudal, then rostral movement of the endoscope. Transverse mucosal folds, when not artifactual, are pathognomonic of mural (wall) lesions of the esophagus. Swallowing results in peristaltic waves that obscure the view and produce alternate constrictions and diverticuli, all of which may appear abnormal to the untrained viewer. Angry-red localized or diffuse lesions indicate esophagitis as a result of loss of mucosa and exposure of submucosal or muscular layers.

An inability to distend the esophagus with air indicates a mucosal, mural, or extraesophageal lesion. If mucosal integrity is altered, localized mural reactions will promote a decrease in the lumen. When the mucosa is intact but transverse bridging folds are seen, rather than the normal longitudinal folds, a mural lesion should be suspected. Contrast radiography is necessary to separate mural from extraesophageal lesions in most instances.

Food material and foreign objects can be viewed through an esophagoscope. To aid visualization, secretions should be removed by suction using the endoscope or a stomach tube.

ESOPHAGEAL RADIOGRAPHY

Contrast radiography in conjunction with survey films and esophagoscopy are necessary for accurate evaluation of esophageal obstruction. Because of the horse's size, thoracic esophageal evaluation may be limited by the capacity of radiographic equipment. In the author's experience, the majority of choke cases are cervical and are within the capabilities of x-ray units used by practitioners.

Survey films establish technique and can demonstrate pathologic alterations visible without contrast media. Contrast radiography is a simple technique that yields valuable information. A nasogastric tube or small endotracheal tube with an inflatable cuff at its tip is introduced into the esophagus. Cuff inflation prevents the reflux of contrast media into the pharynx and airways. Liquid barium (6 to 12 oz) is administered under manual pressure. Esophageal obstructions, fistulas, and mural lesions are easily visualized with this technique. Following a barium injection, approximately 500 ml of air can be introduced to produce a double contrast study. The air-barium interface differentiates mural lesions from intraluminal obstructions.

Interruption of the normal linear pattern of mucosal folds is the principal change observed in esophageal strictures, esophagitis, and diverticulae. A normal esophagus distended with contrast media will lack longitudinal folds, but folds will return when the esophagus is relaxed. Normal peristaltic waves during contrast studies will produce "false strictures."

Correlation of physical examination, esophagoscopy and esophageal radiography should lead the examiner to a definitive diagnosis of esophageal disease. Successful medical or surgical management is dependent to a great degree on the accuracy of the initial diagnosis.

THERAPY

FOOD CHOKE

A nasogastric tube is passed to confirm the site of obstruction and as a first line of therapy. Certain drugs such as xylazine may make it difficult for the horse to swallow the tube and also may increase upper airway resistance, making breathing difficult. With a nasogastric tube in place and the animal slightly sedated, water is lavaged under pressure with a stomach pump. A combination of external massage, to and fro tube movements, and water infusion under pressure will dislodge the majority of food chokes. Infused water with food material will be regurgitated, and the head must be kept down during this maneuver. Refractory cases should be muzzled to prevent food or water intake and should be left alone for 8 to 12 hours, and then treatment should be repeated. Hydration and electrolyte needs are met by intravenous fluid administration (p. 311).

Reflux can be prevented by use of an endotracheal tube with an inflatable cuff. This tube is introduced via the nasal passages into the esophagus, and the cuff is inflated. Water can then be infused, and a small stomach tube passed through the endotracheal tube lumen permits lavage and mechanical breakup of the obstruction. Typically, a rubber endotracheal tube* (22 F) is used. This is placed in hot water to soften, providing easier movement through the na-

---

*Murphy Eye Endotracheal Tube (Order #30V-22), Bivona Surgical, Inc., Hammond, IN

sal passages. A 500 kg horse has sufficient room for a 22 to 26 F tube under these conditions.

Intractable horses increase the risk of esophageal trauma from mechanical action of a nasogastric tube. General anesthesia alleviates this and affords some esophageal muscular relaxation. If possible, a nasogastric tube should be introduced into the esophagus prior to general anesthesia. When the horse is anesthetized, the head can be inclined downward to prevent aspiration, or a cuffed endotracheal tube can be used as previously described. Additional care must be exercised with the anesthetized horse to prevent esophageal perforation and separation of the layers of the esophageal wall.

SURGICAL TREATMENT

If the site of choke is amenable to surgical intervention, an esophagotomy can be used to relieve refractory choke. The author emphasizes the use of surgery as an alternative to the repetitive esophageal trauma that results from over-rigorous use of the nasogastric tube. Surgical intervention may be necessary to remove foreign bodies, to correct strictures, congenital abnormalities, and diverticula, or to repair perforation and remove tumors.

Surgical removal of foreign bodies or food material is possible when the obstruction is in the cervical portion of the esophagus. Thoracic esophageal obstructions are theoretically amenable to removal; however, thoracic surgical approaches to the esophagus can have a favorable outcome only if wounds heal by first intention. In contrast, esophagotomy in the cervical area can heal adequately by second intention. Surgical complications of esophagotomy (wound dehiscence, fistulas, strictures, and diverticula) can be partially or completely circumvented when they occur in the cervical esophagus but not in the thoracic portion. In this author's opinion, thoracic esophageal surgery will not become a reality until technical expertise is developed in (1) closure of esophageal incisions, (2) equine thoracic surgery, (3) parenteral alimentation that prevents postsurgical catabolism, (4) improved diagnostic methods, and (5) a team approach to postsurgical care.

Cervical esophagotomies can be performed under general or local anesthesia.[8] Choice of anesthetic technique is based upon the nature of the obstructing object, the tractability of the animal, the cost, and the surgeon's preference. When a foreign body or food material is to be removed, esophageal incisions are located adjacent but caudal to the obstruction, if surgically possible. This position allows food and water to be administered irrespective of the time necessary for removal of the obstructing material. Incisions should be located ventrally or ventrolaterally to promote drainage of exudate or secretions. Some esophageal incisions are left to heal by secondary intention. In others, dehiscence may occur following primary wound closure. In both instances, exudate and secretions are present and must be allowed to drain.

The surgical approach to the esophagus is through a 7 to 10 cm midline skin incision. The paired sternothyrohyoideus muscles are separated, and the trachea is reflected to the right of the midline. The esophagus is recognized by its tubular structure or the presence of the firm, obstructing intraluminal material. If a stomach tube is passed, it can aid in recognition of the esophagus. A 2 to 3 cm longitudinal incision is made through the esophageal muscular layer and the mucosa is grasped with forceps and is transversely or longitudinally incised. Blunt forceps such as sponge forceps are introduced into the esophagus, and the food material is broken down and removed. Foreign objects are grasped and gently removed with the aid of lubricants. A stomach tube introduced toward the stomach allows irrigation of the esophagus and fluid and food administration. If food material or water is forced toward the pharynx, aspiration must be prevented by lowering the horse's head or by introduction of an endotracheal tube.

Following removal of the obstruction, a stomach tube is passed through the esophagotomy site and is secured to the neck. A complete pelleted horse feed and water are mixed and fed as a gruel until esophagitis recedes. Removal of the tube is followed by return to normal feeding with the esophagotomy site cleansed daily until healing is complete.

If a decision is made to suture the esophagus, the incision may be closed as follows: (1) a simple continuous pattern in the mucosa using monofilament 2–0 nylon, (2) apposition of esophageal muscular layers with interrupted absorbable sutures, and (3) placement of a chain of sutures in the dead space ventral to the esophagus. An indwelling stomach tube for five to seven days postoperatively prevents excessive stress on the internal esophageal layers. Removal of the tube is followed by a gradual return to normal feeding. The principal complication of esophageal closure is dehiscence with fistula formation. Fistulas normally heal with routine wound management. Traction diverticula may form but should not adversely affect food passage.

OTHER MODES OF THERAPY

The use of various specially designed instruments for dilation of the esophagus (bougienage) and removal of foreign bodies is an art practiced by few. Extensive experience and good judgment are essential prerequisites. Foreign bodies in the proximal cervical esophagus can be removed using long forceps introduced through the mouth with the horse under general anesthesia. Forceps may also be used

to break up and extract some food material; the remainder is then gently forced into the stomach. These maneuvers can also be performed through an esophagotomy as previously described.

SUPPORTIVE THERAPY

Following relief of an esophageal obstruction, a nasogastric tube can be left in place for food and water administration, or the animal can be withheld from food for 48 to 72 hours. Inflammation and spasm at the choke site persist for days, and balanced electrolyte solutions are administered intravenously until the horse is returned to voluntary food intake. Before returning to voluntary food intake, the patency of the esophagus is tested by allowing access to a small amount of food and water. The horse that drinks water without regurgitation can be maintained on a slurry of pelleted feed and water. This diet enhances healing of most esophageal wounds.

COMPLICATIONS

The major complication of esophageal surgery is stricture. If a choked horse has been surgically treated and thereafter begins to regurgitate through both nostrils, stricture should be suspected. Passage of the nasogastric tube may be difficult or impossible. Stricture is confirmed by esophagoscopy or contrast radiography. The primary means of correcting esophageal stricture are surgical resection and anastomosis.

Aspiration pneumonia is a serious complication of esophageal obstruction. Broad-spectrum antibiotics and prevention of further regurgitation are essential, but even so the prognosis is guarded for life and unfavorable for return to athletic performance.

Complications are best prevented by treating choke as an emergency. Horse owners should be advised that the horse is its own worst enemy, as it may continue to eat while choked. Food, water, and bedding must be removed immediately when choke is suspected. If a choked horse responds to conservative therapy, an attempt should be made to ascertain the contributory causes. Prevention of recurrence may require slowing of eating by placement of rocks in the manger. Regular dental care will improve mastication, and regular treatment for bots will reduce esophageal inflammation due to Gasterophilus migration (p. 283).

References

1. Bartels, J. E., and Vaughan, J. T.: Persistent right aortic arch in the horse. J. Am. Vet. Med. Assoc., *154*:406, 1969.
2. Bowman, K. F., Vaughan, J. T., Quick, C. B., Hankes, G. E., Redding, R. W., Purohit, R. C., Rumph, P. F., Pow-

ers, R. D., and Harper, N. K.: Megaesophagus in a colt. J. Am Vet. Med. Assoc., *172*:334, 1978.

3. Fretz, P. B.: Repair of esophageal stricture in a horse. Mod. Vet. Pract., 53:31, 1972.
4. Hoffer, R. E., Barber, S. M., Kallfelz, F. A., and Petro, S. P.: Esophageal patch grafting as a treatment for esophageal stricture in a horse. J. Am. Vet. Med. Assoc., *171*:350, 1977.
5. Lowe, J. E.: Esophageal anastomosis in a horse. A case report. Cornell Vet., *54*:636, 1964.
6. Raker, C. W., and Sayers, A.: Esophageal rupture in a Standardbred mare. J. Am. Vet. Med. Assoc., *133*:371, 1958.
7. Scott, E. A., Snoy, P., Prasse, K. W., Hoffman, P. E., and Thrall, D. E.: Intramural esophageal cyst in a horse. J. Am. Vet. Med. Assoc., *171*:652, 1977.
8. Stick, J. A., Krehbiel, J. D., Kunze, D. J., and Wortman, J. A.: Esophageal healing in the pony: Comparison of sutured vs. nonsutured esophagotomy. Am. J. Vet. Res., *42*:1506, 1981.

GASTRIC DISEASES

James L. Becht, KENNETT SQUARE, PENNSYLVANIA

PARASITISM

Gastric parasites of the horse include *Habronema muscae*, *H. microstoma*, *Draschia megastoma*, *Trichostrongylus axei*, *Gasterophilus intestinalis*, and *G. nasalis*. Infestation by these parasites is relatively common but rarely results in clinical gastric disease, although conjunctivitis or pulmonary abscessation may result from invasion of the eye or lungs by Habronema and Draschia sp. *Draschia megastoma* is more pathogenic than *Habronema muscae* or *H. microstoma* and frequently causes abscessation and granulomatous lesions in the glandular gastric wall, where the worms live in colonies. The major clinical significance of these parasites is the contamination of wounds or skin abrasions with larvae, producing lesions known as "summer sores." These lesions are usually characterized by exuberant granulation tissue and delayed healing. *Trichostrongylus axei*, the minute stomach worm, also infects cattle, sheep, and goats. Chronic infestations in horses may cause catarrhal or proliferative gastritis.

Gasterophilus nasalis and *G. intestinalis* are the most common "bots" that parasitize the equine stomach. *G. intestinalis* larvae characteristically attach to the nonglandular gastric mucosa in clusters, whereas *G. nasalis* larvae attach to the mucosa near the pylorus. Attachment of the larvae is deep in the wall and has occasionally been incriminated as a cause of gastric perforation.

Diagnosis of gastric parasitism is often presumptive. The eggs of Habronema sp. and *Draschia megastoma* are not recovered by conventional fecal flotation methods. Occurrence of cutaneous habronemiasis or "summer sores" should raise suspicion of gastric infestation by these parasites. Upon fecal flotation, eggs passed by adult *Trichostrongylus axei* worms resemble Strongylus eggs but have a char-acteristic flattened side and a pointed end and are usually more developed when they appear in the feces. Unless Gasterophilus sp. larvae are passed in the feces, definitive diagnosis of infestation by these parasites is difficult. Eggs attached to the body hair are usually sufficient evidence to incriminate internal infection. Gasterophilus larvae and mural abscesses caused by *Draschia megastoma* can be visualized with a flexible fiberoptic endoscope, but this method of diagnosis is not practical in most instances.

Most available anthelmintics have poor efficacy against *Habronema muscae*, *H. microstoma*, and *Draschia megastoma*. Carbon disulfide continues to be useful in the control of habronemiasis. Its effectiveness is enhanced by 4 l of 2 per cent sodium bicarbonate solution administered just prior to its use. Sodium bicarbonate solution removes excess gastric mucus to enhance exposure of the parasite to the anthelmintic. The recommended dose of carbon disulfide is 2.5 ml per 45 kg (100 lbs) body weight. Cambendazole* at 20 mg per kg body weight appears to have some activity against *Habronema muscae*, but it is ineffective against the other stomach worms. It can be administered as a paste or pellet or as a suspension given by stomach tube. Pyrantel†‡ at 6.6 mg (base) per kg body weight is slightly active against *Habronema muscae*, *Draschia megastoma*, and *Trichostrongylus axei*. It can be administered by a dose syringe, stomach tube, or mixed with feed. Thiabendazole§ at 44 mg per kg or 2 gm per 100 lbs body weight has greater than 90 per cent effectiveness against *Trichostron-*

---

*Camvet, Merck & Co., Rahway, NJ
†Imathal, Beecham, Bristol, TN
‡Strongid-T, Pfizer, New York, NY
§Equizole, Merck & Co., Rahway, NJ

gylus axei. This anthelmintic is available as a suspension for administration by stomach tube, a paste, or as a wettable powder.

Anthelmintics effective against Gasterophilus sp. include carbon disulfide, dichlorvos* at 3.2 gm per 200 lbs body weight, and trichlorfon.†‡ The recommended dosages of trichlorfon in these preparations are 16 gm per 1000 lbs body weight (Combot) and 9.1 gm per 500 lbs body weight (Dyrex TF). Dyrex TF also contains phenothiazine and piperazine and is administered in suspension via stomach tube. Anthelmintics for Gasterophilus control should be administered approximately two weeks after bot fly eggs are first deposited on the hair coat and again in late summer (p. 283).

Ivermectin (22, 23-dihydroavermectin B$_1$), an anthelmintic presently undergoing many experimental trials, is effective against Gasterophilus sp., Habronema sp., *Draschia megastoma*, and *Trichostrongylus axei*.

GASTRIC DILATATION

Dilatation of the stomach due to excessive ingesta, water, or gas usually causes sudden, intense abdominal pain. Gastric dilatation may be primary or secondary. Primary dilatation results from overeating of concentrates or fermentable grains (especially wheat), excessive consumption of water following deprivation or a period of exercise, or following excessive swallowing of air (cribbing). Secondary gastric dilatation, which occurs more frequently than primary dilatation, usually results from intestinal reflux into the stomach during intestinal ileus or following intestinal obstruction. All cases of intestinal obstruction are prone to develop secondary gastric dilatation (p. 224, 231).

CLINICAL SIGNS

The primary clinical sign in a horse with gastric dilatation is the sudden onset of continuous, moderate to severe abdominal pain. The degree of pain is proportional to the severity of gastric distension. Distention compromises the blood flow to the stomach wall and, by increasing intra-abdominal pressure, may make breathing more difficult. To relieve anterior abdominal pressure and assist diaphragmatic movement, the horse may lean back on the rear limbs or assume a "dog sitting" position. The "dog sitting" posture is rarely observed. Primary

---
*Equigard, Shell Chemical Co., San Ramon, CA
†Combot, Haver-Lockhart, Shawnee, KS
‡Dyrex-TF, Fort Dodge, KS

gastric dilatation (overeating) is further complicated by an increased osmotic pressure within the stomach. The fluid drawn into the lumen of the stomach to dilute the hypertonic fluid causes further distention, increased pressure, and more severe pain. Integrity of the stomach wall is then compromised, and toxin absorption can occur, resulting in toxemia and often laminitis. Hypovolemic shock may result if massive volumes of fluid are drawn into the stomach and gastric rupture follows. With gastric dilatation, ingesta may be present at the external nares. This should alert the veterinarian to the possibility of significant gastric distention. Ingesta at the nares in such cases does not mean the stomach has ruptured. Temperature, pulse rate, and respiratory frequency are usually elevated secondary to anxiety and abdominal pain. Retching or vomiting may occur secondary to gastric dilatation, but these are rare in the horse. Exaggerated digital pulses and lameness will be present if laminitis accompanies primary gastric dilatation.

Most horses with gastric dilatation have variable degrees of hemoconcentration (packed cell volume [PCV] 50 to 70 per cent), hypokalemia (serum K$^+$ less than 3 mEq per l), hyponatremia (serum Na$^+$ less than 130 mEq per l), and hypochloremia (serum Cl$^-$ less than 98 mEq per l). In contrast to most horses exhibiting abdominal pain due to other causes, horses with gastric dilatation may be alkalotic (venous blood pH greater than 7.45 and plasma bicarbonate greater than 28 mEq per l) owing to the intraluminal sequestration of hydrogen and chloride ions in the stomach. Metabolic acidosis can occur if gastric dilatation follows intestinal obstruction.

DIAGNOSIS

Diagnosis of gastric dilatation is best confirmed by passage of a nasogastric tube, which is followed by the escape of fluid (usually greater than 2 l) and gas from the stomach. It then becomes important to determine if the gastric dilatation is primary or secondary. A history of free access to grain or other highly fermentable feedstuff suggests that primary gastric dilatation is the etiology. If the duration of abdominal pain is greater than three to four hours and the vital signs, capillary refill time, and mucous membrane color have not changed appreciably, primary gastric dilatation is less likely, and secondary dilatation from intestinal fluid reflux must be considered. Palpation of abdominal structures per rectum may also be an important diagnostic tool to differentiate primary and secondary gastric dilatation. Detection of distended loops of small intestine (smooth cylindrical structures that lack teniae or longitudinal bands) strongly suggests gastric dilatation secondary to intestinal obstruction. The spleen may be displaced caudally by the distended stomach and palpated in the posterior abdomen or even in the pelvic inlet. This finding is not specific for gastric dilatation, since the spleen can be palpated in most horses and its location within the abdomen varies.

If the dilatation is secondary to small intestinal obstruction, decompression of the stomach will only partially ameliorate the abdominal pain and signs of systemic disease, whereas gastric decompression in primary dilatation should render the horse clinically normal if other more serious complications (laminitis, hypovolemic shock, or gastric rupture) have not occurred. Intestinal sounds, which are normally minimal during both types of dilatation, often return following gastric decompression if the dilatation is primary. The pH of the fluid removed during decompression may be of some diagnostic value; that is, a pH of 4 to 5 suggests gastric fluid, whereas a pH of 7 to 8 suggests small intestinal reflux. However, this parameter can be misleading, and the entire animal must be closely evaluated to determine the origin of the fluid and the type of dilatation present.

THERAPY

Initial therapy for primary or secondary gastric dilatation should be decompression via nasogastric tube. A tube with a large diameter is preferable, but since many horses exhibit severe abdominal pain, a standard equine nasogastric tube may be easiest to pass. If resistance at the cardia is encountered, administration of 5 to 10 ml of 2 per cent lidocaine through the tube will relax the cardia and may facilitate passage of the tube. Aspiration of the stomach with a dose syringe may facilitate the flow of fluid. If this is not successful, approximately 1 l of warm water should be administered by gravity flow and the tube then should be lowered or aspirated using a dose syringe. The tube should be moved farther into the stomach and then out several inches and turned in an attempt to locate fluid within the stomach lumen. Gas escaping under pressure from the tube suggests that a significant quantity of ingesta or fluid is within the stomach, and attempts to decompress the stomach should continue.

If the horse is exhibiting severe pain or is fractious, slight sedation with xylazine will facilitate nasogastric tube passage and will cause lowering of the head, which decreases the chances of inhalation pneumonia if gastric reflux is profuse. The tube should be taped to the halter or sutured to the nostril if a large amount of fluid is obtained, and the horse will tolerate it. Administration of mineral oil or other substances following gastric reflux through the nasogastric tube is strongly contraindicated. Such substances will remain in the stomach and add

to distention, pain, and further predispose the stomach to rupture. Surgical intervention may be indicated if gastric dilatation cannot be relieved with a stomach tube but is rarely performed owing to the rapid systemic deterioration of the patient. Surgical approach to the evacuation of the equine stomach also poses significant technical problems.

Secondary gastric dilatation usually subsides when the intestinal obstruction or ileus is corrected. Ileus associated with peritonitis or intestinal surgery in the horse may last as long as 10 days. During this time, frequent decompression of the stomach is mandatory. If the horse will tolerate an indwelling nasogastric tube, this greatly facilitates management of such a patient. Usually horses with adynamic ileus require stomach decompression at two- to four-hour intervals. A slight increase in heart rate, evidence of abdominal pain, and ingesta at the external nares are indications for immediate stomach decompression. Other therapeutic measures for ileus include analgesics for intestinal pain (p. 221) and intravenous electrolyte supplementation as needed (p. 202). Intravenous nutritional support should be an adjunct to therapy, but it is extremely difficult if not impossible to meet the nutritional requirements of an adult horse by intravenous hyperalimentation (p. 111).

Secondary gastric dilatation due to intestinal obstruction is considered an indication for surgical exploration in the acute abdominal crisis patient. Gastric reflux in such cases must be regarded as only one sign of intestinal blockage, and findings from other diagnostic procedures (physical examination, rectal examination, and abdominocentesis) must be taken into consideration in making a decision as to the need for surgical intervention.

PROGNOSIS

Prognosis for primary gastric dilatation is dependent upon the severity and duration of the disease. Prognosis for secondary gastric dilatation due to ileus is fair to good and depends primarily on maintaining fluid and electrolyte balance as well as gastric decompression.

GASTRIC RUPTURE

A grave complication that is not uncommon in severe cases of gastric distention is rupture. Besides following gastric dilatation, gastric rupture can occur spontaneously. A study of horses with gastric rupture revealed that in 10 of 23 cases no predisposing cause was detected at necropsy. Rupture may occur secondary to a horse falling to the ground in severe abdominal pain or during attempts to vomit when the cardiac sphincter fails to relax. Sudden relief of pain in a horse that has exhibited severe colic and now exhibits an anxious facial expression and skeletal muscle fasciculations suggests that gastric rupture has occurred. The horse will also exhibit a profound tachycardia and evidence of severe hypovolemic shock with cyanotic mucous membranes and prolonged capillary refill time. Death rapidly follows. Antemortem diagnosis of gastric rupture can be aided by detection of gritty ingesta free in the abdominal cavity and on serosal linings of bowel felt during rectal palpation. Abdominocentesis in such cases usually yields abdominal fluid mixed with free ingesta. Ingesta obtained during abdominocentesis is not diagnostic for gastric rupture, as normal intestine can be punctured during the procedure. Accidental puncture of bowel during abdominocentesis is not uncommon and is usually harmless. At necropsy, an antemortem rupture of the stomach is characterized by diffuse peritonitis and hemorrhage. The antemortem rupture almost always occurs along the greater curvature, whereas postmortem ruptures occur anywhere, and hemorrhage and diffuse seeding of the abdominal cavity with ingesta is usually absent. Therapy for gastric rupture in the horse has been universally unsuccessful.

ULCERS

Gastric ulceration in horses is rarely reported but can result in serious clinical complications. Rooney[2] described eight cases of perforated gastric ulcers in foals. Two types of ulcers were observed, one involving the esophageal or nonglandular region of the stomach and the other involving only the pyloric region. Most ulcers that occur in the nonglandular region are located near the margo plicatus. Superficial ulcers and areas of irregular cornification of the esophageal portion, especially along the margo plicatus, are common incidental postmortem findings. *Gasterophilus intestinalis* larvae and foreign bodies have been incriminated as the cause of such ulcers. Stress has also been incriminated as the cause of ulceration that occurs in the pyloric region.

Phenylbutazone, a nonsteroidal anti-inflammatory agent widely used in horses, has also induced gastric ulceration in the horse. However, prolonged administration in performance horses for up to two years has been free of apparent adverse effects. Certain pony breeds (Shetlands and Welsh pony crosses) are particularly susceptible to toxic effects of phenylbutazone. Therapy for a period as short as five days at a dose above recommended levels has led to serious complications and even death. Phenylbutazone appears to affect the mucosal lining of

the gastrointestinal tract, which leads to a protein-losing gastroenteropathy. Interference with the mucosa progresses to ulceration. Other complications of phenylbutazone therapy include renal papillary necrosis, ulceration of oral mucosa, necrotizing phlebitis of the portal vein, and epistaxis. Clinical signs of toxicity include depression and anorexia. Total plasma protein levels are usually subnormal (less than 6.5 gm per dl). Other nonsteroidal anti-inflammatory agents (meclofenamic acid, naproxen, acetylsalicylic acid, and flunixin meglumine) may exert similar effects, although these drugs have not been evaluated to the same extent as phenylbutazone.

Prolonged antibiotic or steroid therapy has also been incriminated as a cause of gastric ulcers. Gastric ulcers in young foals have been associated with the occurrence of toxicoinfectious botulism (Shaker foal syndrome) (p. 367). Swerczek[3] proposed that mares on an excessively nutritious diet secrete increased corticosteroid in the milk when stressed. These steroids may be ulcerogenic or may predispose existing ulcers in the foal's stomach to overgrowth by *Clostridium botulinum* with liberation of the potent botulinum toxin.

CLINICAL SIGNS

Gastric ulceration results in one of three syndromes: (1) clinically silent or inapparent ulceration, (2) perforation of the gastric wall resulting in acute peritonitis, or (3) healing of the ulcer with scar tissue and secondary gastric stenosis.

As previously mentioned, superficial ulceration in the equine stomach especially in the nonglandular portion, is not an infrequent incidental finding at necropsy. Foals or adult horses with perforated ulcers commonly exhibit depression, profuse salivation, odontoprisis, abdominal pain, and regurgitation of ingesta at the external nares. Secondary reflux esophagitis can occur and result in dysphagia. Signs of endotoxemia and hypovolemic shock rapidly develop as the peritoneal cavity becomes contaminated with ingesta. Ulcers may heal with scar tissue and induce secondary gastric stenosis, which often involves the pylorus. A foal exhibiting mild to moderate abdominal pain, increased salivation, odontoprisis, and depression for longer than four to five days is more likely to have gastric (pyloric) stenosis than acute severe ulceration with perforation. The need for frequent decompression of the stomach via nasogastric tube is important in the diagnosis of gastric stenosis. Medical management of such cases also requires repeated decompression. Successful bypass surgery has been performed in foals with severe gastric ulceration prior to perforation and in foals with pyloric stenosis. Postoperative therapy with metoclopramide (10 mg intravenously four times a day), a derivative of procainamide, which stimulates gastric emptying in humans, has been beneficial in one foal that developed an atonic stomach following surgical intervention.

Medical management of gastric ulcers is supportive. Changing from a high grain diet to a total hay diet may be beneficial. Cimetidine, a histamine H_2 receptor antagonist that decreases gastric acid secretion, is used in treating peptic ulceration in humans and has been used in several foals with gastric ulceration. The dose used has been similar to that used in humans (800 to 1000 mg divided twice a day or three times a day). To date, too few foals have been treated to establish proper dosage and benefit in this species.

NEOPLASIA OF THE STOMACH

The most important neoplasm affecting the equine stomach is squamous cell carcinoma, which is described on page 259.

References

1. Drudge, J. H., Lyons, J. T., and Tolliver, S. C.: Parasite control in horses: A summary of contemporary drugs. Vet. Med. Small Anim. Clin., p. 1479, October, 1981.
2. Rooney, J. R.: Gastric ulceration in foals. Pathol. Vet., *1*:497, 1964.
3. Swerczek, T. W.: Experimentally induced toxicoinfectious botulism in horses and foals. Am. J. Vet. Res., *41*:348, 1980.
4. Tennant, B.: Intestinal obstruction in the horse: Some aspects of differential diagnosis in equine colic. Proc. 21st Annu. Meet. Am. Assoc. Eq. Pract., pp. 426–439, 1975.
5. Whitlock, R. H.: The stomach and forestomach. *In* Anderson, N. (ed.): Veterinary Gastroenterology, Part 1, Equine Stomach Diseases. Philadelphia, Lea & Febiger, 1980, pp. 392–395.

COLITIS-X

Catherine W. Kohn, COLUMBUS, OHIO

Colitis-X, a disease that occurs sporadically in horses, is a noncontagious, often fatal hemorrhagic enteritis that is usually most severe in the cecum and colon. The onset of clinical signs is typically sudden and associated with a history of stress (such as exhaustive exercise or respiratory disease) 10 days to three weeks prior to illness. After an initial short febrile interval, horses have normal or subnormal temperatures. Marked depression, tachycardia, hyperpnea, rapidly developing intense dehydration, hypotensive shock, neutropenia, and a degenerative left shift with or without explosive watery diarrhea and/or colic characterize the disease. Immediate supportive therapy is necessary, as many horses will die in 3 to 24 hours; a few may survive for 48 hours. Mortality in untreated horses is as high as 90 to 100 per cent.

As the name colitis-X implies, the cause of the disease is unknown. Indeed, hemorrhagic enteritis may represent a nonspecific response of the horse to several pathogenic stimuli. At least four possible pathogeneses have been suggested. Rooney et al.[8, 9] proposed that colitis-X is a manifestation of "*exhaustion shock*," total decompensation after prolonged exposure to stressful stimuli (chronic debilitating diseases, for example) that eventually overwhelm the horse's natural resistance. Although this theory correlates well with the history of stress in these cases, colitis-X often occurs in otherwise healthy, athletic horses, and the incidence of disease is not known to be higher in debilitated, low-resis-

tance horses. Experimental *endotoxic shock* in ponies mimics colitis-X. The role of endotoxin in naturally occurring disease is unknown; however, it is likely that gram-negative endotoxemia plays an adjuvant role. Experimental *anaphylaxis* in horses results in a disease that resembles colitis-X. The theory that exposure to an antigen to which the horse was previously sensitized may result in a systemic allergic reaction characterized by hemorrhagic colitis is attractive but unproven. *Enterotoxemia* caused by an intestinal pathogen, such as *Clostridium perfringens* type A, or enterotoxemic-like disease caused by Salmonella may be the most likely pathogenesis. Peracute salmonellosis is clinically indistinguishable from colitis-X; however, the diagnosis of salmonellosis must ultimately be based on recovery of the organism from stool or organ cultures. Most colitis-X cases do not yield positive Salmonella cultures either antemortem or postmortem.

Exhaustion shock, anaphylaxis, endotoxemia, and enterotoxemia are each characterized by a marked and acute decrease in effective circulating blood volume. This absolute decrease in blood volume evokes a sympathetic nervous system response resulting in venous and arteriolar vasoconstriction. Blood volume decrease and sympathetic vasoconstriction lead to a redistribution of blood flow with ischemia of splanchnic viscera. Bowel wall ischemia stimulates the local release of vasoactive substances, such as histamine, kinins, and prostaglandins, as well as adrenal secretion of catecholamines. These mediators

TABLE 1. SUBJECTIVE ASSESSMENT OF DEHYDRATION

	Body Wt (%)	Liter Deficit, 500 kg Horse	Clinical Signs
Mild dehydration	4	20	Decreased skin turgor
Moderate dehydration	6	30	Depressed, sunken eyes, ambulatory or in sternal recumbency
Severe dehydration	≥10	≥50	Subnormal temperature, moribund, lateral recumbency

cause increases in splanchnic capillary permeability, arteriolar dilatation, and venous constriction, and they inhibit the release of norepinephrine from sympathetic postganglionic nerves. Therefore, the pressure in arterioles is transmitted directly to capillary beds, and loss of plasma through capillary walls is extensive. Local tissue and systemic coagulation processes are activated. Sludging of blood flow in capillaries, formation of microthrombi, disseminated intravascular coagulopathy, irreversible shock, and death may rapidly follow.

Therapeutic efforts must initially be directed toward increasing the effective circulating blood volume and alleviating intestinal hypoxia before ischemic necrosis of the mucosa and walls of the cecum and colon is widespread. Since one cannot direct therapy toward a specific etiologic agent, the success of treatment depends on broad-based supportive care.

DIAGNOSIS

Diagnosis is based on typical clinical signs. Packed cell volume (PCV) may be as high as 80 per cent, with total protein (TP) elevations up to 8 to 10 mg per dl. Total white blood cell counts initially may be as low as 1500 cells per mm^3. Initial leukopenia may be followed by leukocytosis if the horse lives. Mild to moderate hyponatremia (120 to 135 mEq per l) and hypochloremia (80 to 90 mEq per l) are often present. Because metabolic acidosis may be severe (bicarbonate levels of 10 mEq per l), initial hyperkalemia may be present. However, potassium depletion occurs rapidly owing to absolute electrolyte loss in bowel contents, and hypokalemia (1.5 to 2.5 mEq per l) soon develops. Elevated BUN levels may reflect systemic dehydration or renal compromise resulting from decreased renal blood flow. Blood glucose levels three times normal may be present. Serum lactate levels may be elevated, reflecting increased anaerobic metabolism and tissue ischemia. Marked hypoalbuminemia (1.0 to 2.5 mg per dl) may rapidly develop because of intestinal albumin loss. Complications of colitis-X include laminitis, superinfections, and disseminated intravascular coagulopathy.

TREATMENT

DEHYDRATION

An estimate of fluid needs may be based on clinical signs (skin turgor, pulse rate and character, appearance of mucous membranes, and temperature of extremities) and on a subjective evaluation of the degree of dehydration (Table 1). Colitis-X may rapidly induce moderate to severe dehydration. A 500 kg horse with 8 per cent dehydration would require 40 l of fluid to replace existing deficits.

Fluids should be administered through two aseptic, nonreactive, indwelling venous catheters. When dehydration is intense and acute, rapid fluid administration is essential; a fluid pump* may be helpful initially. Twenty to 30 l of fluid can be administered without obvious complications in the first hour of therapy. If the horse urinates excessively during fluid infusion, the rate of administration should be decreased, as this indicates either overhydration or too rapid rehydration. Care must be taken when giving intravenous fluids to horses in lateral recumbency, as even when the extracellular fluid volume is significantly contracted, rapid intravenous fluid administration may induce pulmonary edema. Once the effective circulating blood volume has been augmented and the horse is over the hypotensive crisis, the rate of intravenous fluid administration may be decreased to 3 to 5 l. per hour or gravity flow. The rate of fluid administration should be adjusted to the patient's needs based on the response to therapy.

Assessment of response to fluid therapy is another means of estimating fluid losses and is essential for formulating the treatment regimen. When fluid loss is acute, approximately 90 per cent of body weight change in an anorectic horse is caused by fluid deficit. Therefore, if the horse can be weighed initially and periodically as therapy progresses, weight change serves as a guide to continuing fluid needs. For example, a horse with acute diarrhea is estimated to be 8 per cent dehydrated. If x equals the horse's normal body weight and the horse weighs

---

*Variable speed Masterflex pump, Cole Parmer Instrument Co., 7425 N. Oak Park Ave., Chicago, IL 60648

450 kg before fluid therapy, then the horse's predisease weight is determined as follows.

$$x = \frac{450}{(1 - 0.08)} = 490 \text{ kg}$$

After treating the horse with 40 l of intravenous fluid, the horse's measured weight is 475 kg. This means that the horse is still 15 kg under its normal weight. Therefore, the current estimated fluid deficit is 15 kg × .9 = 13.5 liters.

Unfortunately, a scale for horses may not always be at hand in the field situation. Serial estimations of PCV and TP represent a more practical means of monitoring the balance between response to fluid therapy and ongoing fluid loss. Table 2 indicates interpretations of relative changes in PCV and TP in horses undergoing fluid therapy. After heparinizing the intravenous catheter, a 10- to 15-minute equilibration period should precede collection of an anticoagulated venous blood sample for PCV and TP determinations.

After administration of the initial estimated fluid needs or when the horse responds clinically (decreasing pulse rate, improved pulse pressure, better capillary perfusion, more alert attitude), the infusion may be discontinued.

The intravenous fluid of choice for rapid administration is an isotonic balanced electrolyte solution that does not contain lactate or glucose. Glucose-containing solutions are inappropriate for two reasons: Hyperglycemia is present in the early stages of colitis-X, and rapid administration of solutions with glucose concentrations as low as 5 per cent results in osmotic diuresis. Tissue anoxia and increased anaerobic metabolism are accompanied by lactic acid production and may result in diminished metabolic conversion of lactate to bicarbonate.

ELECTROLYTE IMBALANCE

SODIUM AND CHLORIDE

Serum sodium (Na) and chloride (Cl) concentrations may be depressed. The existing sodium deficit may be calculated from the patient's measured Na level and the normal Na concentration.

Since Na is primarily an extracellular ion, its volume of distribution is the extracellular fluid (ECF), which is about 30 per cent of body weight in horses. Therefore, for a 500 kg horse with a Na concentration of 125 mEq per l:

$$500 \text{ kg} \times .3 = 150 \text{ l of ECF}$$

$$\underset{\text{Normal}}{140 \text{ mEq per l}} - \underset{\text{Patient}}{125 \text{ mEq per l}} = \underset{\text{sodium deficit}}{15 \text{ mEq per l}}$$

$$150 \times 15 \text{ mEq per l} = 2250 \text{ mEq total Na deficit}$$

To replace this horse's entire Na deficit with isotonic NaCl would require infusion of 15 to 16 l of fluid. When the initial volume deficit has been replaced with isotonic fluids, 2N Na solutions (approximately 300 mEq per l) may be infused to treat the remaining Na deficit. If the horse in the above example is given 10 l of isotonic saline (154 mEq per l Na) to replace the volume deficit, 1540 mEq of the Na deficit have been simultaneously replaced. The horse still needs 2250 − 1540 = 710 mEq Na. It can now be treated with an additional 5 to 6 l of isotonic saline or 2 to 3 l of 2N NaCl to completely replace the sodium losses. Hypertonic fluids are especially useful in horses in which volume overload may occur (concurrent renal or heart disease) and in horses with large salt deficits. The tonicity of the fluid should not exceed two times isotonic (2N).

A similar calculation may be made to determine

TABLE 2. INTERPRETATION OF RELATIVE CHANGES IN PACKED CELL VOLUME AND PLASMA PROTEIN IN PATIENTS UNDERGOING FLUID THERAPY

Plasma Protein	Packed Cell Volume	Possible Interpretations
Increasing	Increasing	Continuing dehydration occurring at a greater rate than fluid replacement
Unchanged	Unchanged	Rehydration keeping pace with fluid loss
Decreasing	Decreasing	Effective circulating blood volume is increasing; fluid therapy is effective
Decreasing*	Increasing	Continuing fluid loss with possible loss of capillary integrity and leaking of plasma protein out of the vascular space (e.g., pulmonary edema, shock, effusion)

*When plasma proteins are significantly decreased, colloid osmotic pressure in the blood decreases, and infused fluids will not remain in the vascular space. Under these conditions, the use of plasma colloid expanders such as dextrans, plasma, or whole blood should be considered.

(From Kohn, C. W.: Preparative management of the equine patient with an abdominal crisis. Vet. Clin. North Am. (Large Anim. Pract.), 1(2):301, 1979. With permission of the publisher.)

Cl deficit. The volume of distribution of Cl is the ECF.

POTASSIUM

In the initial hours of colitis-X, metabolic acidosis may be accompanied by hyperkalemia as K ions shift out of cells in exchange for hydrogen ions moving in. When acid-base status is corrected, K shifts back into cells, and if absolute K losses have been extensive (decreased total body K), hypokalemia may result. Thus, alkalinizing therapy must be accompanied by appropriate K replacement. Some horses have a low serum K in the face of metabolic acidosis; this indicates a significant total body K deficit, which must be treated with K replacement. Although the best ratio of K to bicarbonate (HCO_3) in replacement fluids for hyperkalemic acidotic horses is not known, K may be safely added at the rate of 10 mEq per l. K should not be given faster than 100 to 150 mEq per hour to adult horses.

When hypokalemia is present, the K deficit may be estimated by comparing the patient's measured serum K concentration to normal serum K levels. The total body K deficit is difficult to accurately estimate, since K is primarily an intracellular ion. Practical tests for evaluating intracellular K levels are not currently available. When the measured serum K level is low and metabolic alkalosis is not present, a conservative estimate of the K deficit can be made by empirically estimating the K volume of distribution at 40 per cent body weight. This percentage of body weight represents a volume of distribution larger than the ECF but smaller than the total body water, which clinically provides a "safe" estimate of K deficit.

Body wt in kg $\times$ .4 = volume of distribution of K

$$500 \text{ kg} \times .4 = 200 \text{ l}$$

$$3.5 \text{ mEq/l} - 2.5 \text{ mEq/l} = 1.0 \text{ mEq/l}$$
Normal   Patient   Deficit

$$200 \text{ l} \times 1.0 \text{ mEq per l} = 200 \text{ mEq total K deficit}$$

ACID-BASE IMBALANCE

Almost all horses with colitis-X have metabolic acidosis; however, it is difficult to predict the severity of bicarbonate loss without laboratory assessment of acid-base status. Whenever possible, acid-base status should be evaluated by using a blood gas machine or Harleco CO_2 analyzer.* When blood gas data are available, the actual HCO_3 deficit may be

*Harleco CO_2 Apparatus, American Scientific Products, Obetz, OH 43207

calculated. HCO_3, in one form or another, is present in all body water; therefore, its volume of distribution is 60 per cent of body weight. For a 500 kg horse with a measured HCO_3 of 14 mEq per l:

$$500 \text{ kg} \times .60 = 300 \text{ l } HCO_3 \text{ space}$$

$$24 \text{ mEq per l} - 14 \text{ mEq per l} = 10 \text{ mEq per l}$$
Normal   Patient   Deficit

$$300 \text{ l} \times 10 \text{ mEq per l} = 3000 \text{ mEq } HCO_3 \text{ deficit}$$

The *base excess* (a negative number in metabolic acidosis), calculated from the Sigaard-Anderson alignment nomogram or computed by a blood gas machine, may be used in a similar calculation. When the Harleco CO_2 determination is used, the difference between the patient's measured total CO_2 and normal total CO_2 is approximately equal to the base deficit in mEq per l.

A decrease in total CO_2 usually reflects a decrease in HCO_3. It should be noted that the total CO_2 value does not distinguish metabolic and respiratory components of acid-base imbalances, and this value must therefore be carefully interpreted in the context of a complete physical examination.

For horses with colitis-X, bicarbonate therapy should be initiated immediately. One half of the total calculated deficit should be replaced over a one-hour period; the example horse needs 1500 mEq HCO_3. Since 1 gm of $NaHCO_3$ contains 12 mEq, this horse requires 125 gm of $NaHCO_3$ immediately. The balance of HCO_3 needed should be given slowly (in 3 to 24 hours) with other fluids and considering the horse's response to therapy.

Concentrated solutions of bicarbonate may not be added to calcium- or lactate-containing fluids, as precipitates form. If the fluid is not clear, it should not be administered. It is important to remember that adding sodium bicarbonate to replacement fluids increases the tonicity of the fluids. The addition of 150 mEq of $NaHCO_3$ to 1 l. of isotonic fluid results in a solution that is 2N for Na. Administration of large volumes of such solutions may induce detrimental hypernatremia in patients that have relatively normal serum Na concentrations before fluid therapy. Also, isotonic solutions are preferred for rapid administration, and this must be taken into account when formulating fluids. For example, 150 mEq of $NaHCO_3$ added to distilled water forms an isotonic solution to which other electrolytes (K, Cl) may be added as needed.

If blood gas data are not available, 1.0 to 2.5 mEq per kg, or 50 to 100 gm of $NaHCO_3$ (600 to 1200 mEq) may be safely given empirically in compatible fluids. Decreasing respiratory rate and lessening signs of shock constitute a favorable response to therapy. If hyperventilation, rising pulse rate, and signs of shock appear again, another 50 gm of $NaHCO_3$ may be given. In colitis-X, continuing intestinal HCO_3 losses may be substantial, and almost constant infusions of dilute bicarbonate solutions may be required.

A number of balanced electrolyte solutions are commercially available. Liquid and powder sources of KCl and $NaHCO_3$ are also available as supplements for replacement fluids. The per liter cost of commercial intravenous fluids may be prohibitive for horses with diarrhea. Nonsterile "clean" fluid may be homemade from double distilled water and reagent-grade chemicals. Homemade fluids should be mixed in sterilized containers for administration, and every care should be taken to minimize contamination during formulation.

ORAL FLUIDS

Oral electrolyte solutions may be utilized as an adjunct to intensive intravenous therapy. Oral fluids should not have a tonicity exceeding 500 mOsm per l. Some useful commercially available oral electrolyte preparations developed for use in calves are listed in Table 3.

In colitis-X, the relatively normal small bowel should be capable of absorption of some water and electrolytes. Since K can be safely administered orally (up to 1000 mEq per dose), this route of therapy may be especially useful in horses with large K deficits.

The oral route is also particularly attractive for horses with large HCO_3 deficits. For example, up to 95 mEq of $NaHCO_3$ could be added to each liter of Electroplus B without making this solution excessively hypertonic. After oral bicarbonate therapy, alkalinization of the blood should occur when $NaHCO_3$ is neutralized by HCl in the stomach lumen. For each equivalent of hydrogen so consumed, it is postulated that one equivalent of HCO_3 is resorbed. Since the stomach should be relatively normal in colitis-X, correction of metabolic acidosis may be facilitated by oral therapy. Care must be taken to estimate the patient's total Na, K, and HCO_3 needs; administration of excessive Na, K, or HCO_3 *orally* may worsen signs of diarrhea, and when large overdoses occur, may induce salt poisoning and metabolic alkalosis.

Free choice oral electrolyte solutions should be available to horses with diarrhea. Voluntary intake aids the rehydrating process. A source of fresh water should also always be available.

COLLOID EXPANSION

When hypoalbuminemia is present, plasma colloid depletion may result in edema, which may worsen with fluid therapy. Plasma colloid expansion may be a necessary prerequisite for efficacious fluid therapy.

Low molecular weight dextran preparations transiently increase plasma volume. The high cost and risk of side reactions, as well as the transient nature of beneficial effects, combine to limit their clinical application.

Plasma from a healthy, Coggins test–negative, compatible donor is a more practical colloid expander. The approximate volume of plasma needed may

TABLE 3. ORAL ELECTROLYTE PREPARATIONS

Solute	Ion-Aid (Diamond) mM/l	Re-Sorb (Beecham) mM/l	Electroplus (Pittman Moore) mM/l A	B	C	Life Guard (Norden) mM/l
Glucose	135	129	60	0	60	168
Sodium	89	80	100	145	145	118
Glycine and imino amino acids	125	45	60	0	0	80
Other neutral amino acids	0	0	0	0	0	30
Bicarbonate	0	1.6 (as citrate)	40 (citrate)	55 (citrate)	0 (citrate)	80
Potassium	28	17	15	10	10	28
Osmolality	480	350	350	310	326	490

(Adapted from Lewis, L. D., and Phillips, R. W.: New information on fluid therapy for diarrheic calves. Norden News, 55(2):5, 1980.)

be estimated by comparing the patient's albumin level to the donor's albumin concentration:

$$3.0 \text{ mg per dl albumin} - 1.5 \text{ mg per dl albumin}$$
$$\text{Donor} \qquad\qquad \text{Patient}$$
$$= 1.5 \text{ mg per dl}$$
$$\text{Deficit}$$

Since plasma volume is 5 per cent body weight, a 500 kg horse has approximately 25 l of plasma. If each liter is 1.5 mg deficient in albumin, the total deficit is 37.5 mg of albumin. This means the horse requires 12.5 l of plasma containing 3.0 mg per dl of albumin to increase albumin to 3.0 mg per dl (assuming no further protein loss). It would be impossible to collect this much plasma from one donor. Several compatible donors may be used. In practice, even 4 to 6 l of plasma will benefit such a patient and may provide adequate support while intestinal protein loss is being controlled.

Possible side effects of plasma therapy include transfusion-like reactions, fever, sweating, muscle fasciculations, and laminitis. Plasma transfusions may be life-saving in some cases.

PHARMACOLOGIC SUPPORT OF THE FAILING CARDIOVASCULAR SYSTEM

Most horses with colitis-X become dehydrated so rapidly that emergency shock therapy is indicated. Large doses of corticosteroids, 2 to 5 mg per kg of aqueous dexamethasone,* or prednisolone acetate may be used. One quarter to one half of the dose of aqueous dexamethasone may be given intravenously. Corticosteroids have a protective effect in endotoxic shock, particularly when given early in the course of disease. At shock doses, corticosteroids may have a mild vasodilating effect. This emphasizes the need for concurrent effective fluid therapy.

Vasoactive drugs should be used with care, as blood pressure may be low. Alpha stimulants such as ephedrine sulfate should *not* be administered, as such drugs compound peripheral vasoconstriction and worsen already inadequate bowel capillary perfusion. The use of alpha blocking agents like phenothiazine tranquilizers seems theoretically justifiable; however, in practice, dose-dependent and therefore titratable hypotensive effects of these drugs worsen the problem of inadequate circulating blood volume by markedly expanding the capillary volume that must be perfused. Peripheral perfusion deficits are better corrected by volume expansion. Even when IV fluid administration is proceeding at a maximal safe rate, alpha blocking agents may cause

a hypotensive crisis. The same problem precludes the use of beta adrenergics like isoproterenol HCl,* which promote peripheral vasodilatation.

ANTIMICROBIAL THERAPY

As it is difficult or impossible to immediately exclude the possibility that colitis was caused by salmonellosis or intestinal clostridiosis, broad-spectrum antibiotic therapy is indicated. Further, decreasing replication of gram-negative bacteria in the bowel lumen should decrease endotoxin production. Death of gram-negative bacteria results in cell lysis and release of endotoxin; therefore, use of bacteriostatic agents is recommended. Chloramphenicol has a broad spectrum of action against anaerobic and aerobic bacteria, including most equine Salmonella isolates. To attain adequate blood levels, the drug should be given in the sodium succinate form† intramuscularly at a dose rate of 100 to 200 mg per kg in four doses. The extremely short half-life of chloramphenicol sodium succinate administered intravenously makes it almost impossible to maintain therapeutic blood levels of this preparation by the intravenous route in horses. This form of chloramphenicol is quite irritating in the muscle; however, the neutral form of the drug (chloramphenicol) achieves only very low blood levels after intramuscular administration. It should be noted that chloramphenicol sodium succinate is not approved for veterinary use in the United States. Both chloramphenicol‡ and chloramphenicol palmitate§ may be given orally at the same dose rate as above. The oral route is usually preferable when chloramphenicol is used.

Other choices for broad-spectrum antibiotic coverage are the combination of procaine penicillin G (10×10^6 IU per lb intramuscularly twice a day) and gentamicin‖ (1 mg per lb intramuscularly two or three times a day) or a sulfa-trimethoprim combination drug.** At present, sulfa-trimethoprim drugs are not approved for use in horses in the United States. A sulfamethoxazole-trimethoprim combination** has been used orally at the empirical dose rate of 10 ml per 100 lbs in some cases. The efficacy of this therapy cannot be determined at this time.

If the horse survives, antibiotic therapy should be

---

*Azium, Schering, Kenilworth, NJ

*Isuprel HCl, Breon Labs, New York, NY
†Chloromycetin sodium succinate, Parke Davis, Morris Plains, NJ
‡Chloramphenicol, Med-Tech, Inc., Elwood, KS
§Chloromycetin Palmitate, Parke Davis, Morris Plains, NJ
‖Gentocin, Schering, Kenilworth, NJ
**Bactrim, Roche Labs, Nutley, NJ

continued for three to five days after improvement occurs. As heavy antibiotic treatment may result in resistant enteric superinfections, the horse should be carefully monitored for development of secondary antibiotic-associated disease. Serial fecal cultures during antibiotic treatment help to identify resistant organisms.

ANTITOXIC THERAPY

The protective effects of large doses of adrenocorticosteroids have already been mentioned. Flunixin meglumine,* an antiprostaglandin, may help to control abnormal electrolyte secretion by diseased bowel. Electrolyte hypersecretion, while not documented in colitis-X, is seen with Na secretion in cholera in humans and chloride secretion in experimental salmonellosis. Abnormal secretion processes may be "turned on" by prostaglandin mediators. Banamine may be administered at a dose rate of 1.1 mg per kg intravenously.

The antipyretic effects of these drugs should be considered in evaluating the horse's overall response to therapy.

Bismuth subsalicylate† has antienterotoxic effects in toxigenic *E. coli* diarrhea in humans. This substance may be given by stomach tube at a dose of 2 to 4 quarts once or twice a day, as an empirical treatment. Alternatively, 2 to 4 quarts of Kaopectate‡ containing 2 to 4 ounces of activated charcoal may be given once or twice a day to horses with colitis-X. This preparation may help to absorb potential toxins in the bowel lumen.

CONTROL OF PAIN

Abdominal pain may be severe in some horses. Flunixin meglumine has potent visceral analgesic effects and may provide relief from pain for many horses. For horses that do not respond to flunixin meglumine, xylazine HCl§ is the drug of choice. In reasonable doses (0.4 to 0.6 mg per kg intravenously or 1.0 to 1.6 mg per kg intramuscularly), xylazine provides safe relief from abdominal pain. Single large doses may produce bradycardia and hypotension; however, in recommended doses, especially in conjunction with fluid therapy, decreases in peripheral blood pressure are not dangerous. The sedative effects of xylazine may be useful in controlling

horses that will not stand still for long-term intravenous fluid therapy. Narcotics are effective for visceral pain but less practical for routine use.

MODIFICATION OF MOTILITY

Diarrhea may be associated with normal, decreased, or increased bowel motility. Although parasympatholytic drugs (atropine) have often been used in attempts to slow intestinal ingesta transit and so improve diarrhea, such therapy usually fails in colitis-X. Static bowel acts as an unresisting conduit for liquid ingesta, and ingesta retention time may indeed be decreased after parasympatholytic therapy. The use of parasympatholytic drugs in the treatment of colitis-X is contraindicated.

MODIFICATION OF FECAL CONSISTENCY

Agents that promote forming of stools, such as Kaopectate, are usually ineffective in colitis-X. Kaopectate or mineral oil (2 to 4 quarts daily) may be given orally as intestinal soothants and protectants.

NUTRITIONAL SUPPORT

During the critical first 48 hours of treatment of a horse with colitis-X, little attention need be given to nutritional support of the patient. If the horse survives this crisis, then every attempt should be made to encourage some voluntary food intake (p. 112). Grass hay should be provided free choice. Most clinicians completely restrict concentrate intake, as highly fermentable substrates are thought to predispose horses to further enteritis and diarrhea. Since mucosal absorptive and digestive function in the cecum and colon will be limited or nonexistent, force feeding is not recommended in the first 10 days to 2 weeks of therapy.

As the horse begins to recover bowel function, appetite stimulants such as B vitamin injections* (10 to 20 ml subcutaneously or intramuscularly) or anabolic steroids† (.5 mg per kg intramuscularly, up to four doses one to two weeks apart) may help to promote increased voluntary intake. During the convalescent period, grass hay or grass, if available, should provide the bulk of the diet. Concentrates should not be introduced into the diet until recovery of digestive function is complete (three to six weeks).

*Banamine, Schering, Kenilworth, NJ
†Pepto-Bismol, Norwich-Eaton, Norwich, NY
‡Kaopectate, Upjohn Co., Kalamazoo, MI
§Rompun, Haver-Lockhart, Shawnee, KS

*Vitaplex, Vet-a-Mix, Shenandoah, IA
†Winstrol-V, Winthrop Labs., New York, NY

References

1. Anderson, N. V. (ed.): Veterinary Gastroenterology, Philadelphia, Lea and Febiger, 1980.
2. Burrows, G. E.: Equine Escherichia coli endotoxemia: Comparison of intravenous and intraperitoneal endotoxin administration. Am. J. Vet. Res., *40*:991, 1979.
3. Carlson, G. P.: Fluid therapy in horses with acute diarrhea. Symposium on Gastroenterology. Vet. Clin. North Am. (Large Anim. Pract.), *1*(2):313, 1979.
4. Ericsson, C. D., Evans, D. G., DuPont, H. L., Evans, D. J., Pickering, J. R., and Pickering, L. K.: Bismuth subsalicylate inhibits activity of crude toxin of *Escherichia coli* and *Vibrio Cholerae*. J. Infect. Dis., *136*:693, 1977.
5. Kohn, C. W.: Preparative management of the equine patient with an abdominal crisis. Vet. Clin. North Am. (Large Anim. Pract.), *1*(2):289, 1979.
6. McGavin, M. D., Gronwall, R. R., and Mia, A. S.: Patho-logic changes in experimental equine anaphylaxis. J. Am. Vet. Med. Assoc., *160*:1632, 1972.
7. Moore, J., Garner, H. E., Shapland, J. E., and Hatfield, D. G.: Lactic acidosis and arterial hypoxemia during sublethal endotoxemia in conscious ponies. Am. J. Vet. Res., *41*:1696, 1980.
8. Rooney, J. R., Bryans, J. T., Prickett, M. E., and Zent, W. W.: Exhaustion shock in the horse. Cornell Vet., *56*:220, 1966.
9. Rooney, J. R., Bryans, J. T., and Doll, E. R.: Colitis "X" of horses. J. Am. Vet. Med. Assoc., *142*:510, 1963.
10. Vaughan, J. T.: The acute colitis syndrome Colitis "X." Vet. Clin. North Am., *3*(2):301, 1973.
11. Whitlock, R.: Acute diarrheal disease in the horse. Proc. 21st Annu. Meet. Am. Assoc. Eq. Pract., December, 1975, pp. 390–401.
12. Wierup, M.: Equine intestinal clostridiosis. Acta Vet. Scand. (Suppl.), *62*:1, 1977.

ENTERIC SALMONELLOSIS

Bradford P. Smith, DAVIS, CALIFORNIA

Salmonella is the most commonly recognized agent that causes acute enteritis in the horse. Based on history and physical findings, it is usually impossible to determine whether Salmonella or another agent is responsible for severe diarrhea and subsequent circulatory derangements that occur in the horse. Thus, it is important that antemortem or postmortem cultures or both be performed in order to determine whether Salmonellae are present.

ETIOLOGY

The intestinal form of salmonellosis is one of four clinical forms of Salmonella infection in the horse. In addition to the toxic enteritis form of infection, horses infected with Salmonella may be (1) asymptomatic, with or without fecal shedding of the organism; (2) mildly ill with fever, anorexia, and depression; or (3) bacteremic, with generalized illness or localization of the infection into joints or certain organs. The reader is referred to the infectious diseases section for a more complete description of these forms of the diseases caused by Salmonella, since they may occur simultaneously or sequentially with the enteric form (p. 22).

More than 1800 serotypes of Salmonella exist, and while all are potential pathogens, relatively few serotypes are usually associated with severe diarrhea in the horse. These common serotypes include *Salmonella typhimurium*, *S. typhimurium* var. *copenhagen*, *S. enteriditis*, and *S. anatum*. In almost all reports, *S. typhimurium* (including var. *copen-*

hagen) is responsible for over 50 per cent of the cases and is associated with severe disease and a high mortality rate. Many other serotypes, including *S. heidelberg*, *S. newport*, and *S. infantis*, have also been associated with severe disease. Isolates from asymptomatic shedders appear to be composed in large part of serotypes such as *S. agona*, which are rarely associated with severe illness in the horse, but asymptomatic shedding of *S. anatum* and other relatively pathogenic serotypes is not uncommon. Fortunately, long-term asymptomatic shedding of *S. typhimurium* does not occur often, even in horses that have recovered from acute enteric salmonellosis.

Enteric salmonellosis is often preceded by a history of previous Salmonella infections on the premise or in a recently stressed horse. Stresses associated with salmonellosis include prolonged transport, fasting (either imposed or because of illness), worming, heavy parasite burden, and surgery, particularly abdominal surgery. A common factor, such as a change in the flora of the cecum and large colon, may allow Salmonellae to multiply and cause disease. When a diagnosis of salmonellosis has been made on a farm or in a clinic, isolation is important to prevent exposure of other animals.

CLINICAL SIGNS

Following infection, the organisms multiply in the bowel and penetrate the mucosa. The organism invades principally in the cecum and proximal large colon, but invasion may occur through any mucous membrane, including the conjunctiva and oropharynx. Following experimental oral exposure to *S. typhimurium*, clinical signs including fever and anorexia occur in 12 to 36 hours. At this point, a marked neutropenia usually occurs, resulting in a characteristically decreased total white blood cell count (<4000 per μl). Neutropenia is not specific for acute salmonellosis in the horse and may occur with a variety of other conditions, including acute toxic enteritis, which is not caused by Salmonella.

The pulse rate becomes progressively more rapid, and the pulse character becomes weaker as the disease progresses. The oral mucous membranes turn red, then a dark purple. Circulatory deterioration is also evidenced by poor capillary refill. At this time, the horse usually has projectile voluminous watery green to brown diarrhea. Both the frequency of defecation and the volume of fecal water are increased. The diarrhea has a fetid odor associated with mucosal necrosis in the cecum and large colon. Frank hemorrhage is rare. The character of the feces cannot be used to readily differentiate salmonellosis from other causes of acute toxic enteritis.

The initial hypovolemic shock is rapidly complicated by septic shock, which occurs when toxic material is absorbed from the gut lumen through the damaged mucosa of the cecum and colon. Salmonellae that have entered the body by invasion through the bowel wall also release endotoxins that contribute to the development of shock.

In any horse suffering from acute toxic enteritis, salmonellosis should remain on the list of differential diagnoses until culture results are available. Strict isolation procedures are indicated; it should also be kept in mind that *S. typhimurium* is the serotype most often responsible for enteric salmonellosis in humans. Horses experimentally infected with Salmonella that develop enteric disease excrete large numbers of Salmonellae in the feces, so that culture of the organism is relatively easily accomplished. Direct plating on an enteric agar such as brilliant green will give the most rapid results. Enrichment in selenite or tetrathionate broth is usually performed in addition to direct plating so that the presence of smaller numbers of Salmonellae in the feces may be detected. Enrichment techniques are usually required for the detection of asymptomatic shedders.

It appears that Salmonella is rarely the cause of chronic diarrhea (p. 216) unless it occurs as a sequel to an attack of acute Salmonella diarrhea. The findings of small numbers of Salmonella in the feces of a horse that does not have a history of a previous attack of acute diarrhea does not mean that the organism is the cause of the chronic diarrhea. On the contrary, a horse that is stressed by having chronic diarrhea may be infected secondarily with Salmonella because of the already altered bowel flora. Experimental oral exposure to small numbers of virulent Salmonella has not resulted in chronic diarrhea, even when the challenge organism can be readily recovered from fecal samples.

The postmortem changes observed in horses with enteric salmonellosis involve principally the cecum (typhlitis) and proximal portions of the large colon (colitis). The distal ileum may also be involved in severe cases. The serosal surfaces are usually a dark purple color, and some intramural edema may be obvious. The contents of the cecum and colon are watery and foul-smelling; often flecks of fibrin are floating in the diarrheic material. The mucosal surfaces are usually darkened and may be ulcerated or covered with fibrin.

TREATMENT

Treatment of enteric salmonellosis is aimed principally at replacing fluid and electrolyte losses and correcting acid-base abnormalities. This requires large volumes of sterile fluids prepared for intravenous administration and periodic monitoring of electrolyte (Na, K, Cl) and acid-base (pH, HCO_3) parameters.

The clinical assessment of the need for intravenous fluid replacement is based on skin elasticity, whether or not the eyes appear sunken, the character and rate of the pulse, the capillary refill time, mucous membrane color, and severity of the ongoing diarrhea. The packed cell volume (PCV) and total plasma proteins (measured on a refractometer) are also useful guides to determine the degree of dehydration. If the animal's normal weight is known, the percentage of dehydration can be determined most accurately. A useful, accurate, and inexpensive way to assess the total CO_2 (similar to HCO_3, and thus the metabolic acid-base component) is with the titration kit made by Harleco.*

In general, some degree of metabolic acidosis develops in horses with severe typhlitis and colitis, and bicarbonate therapy may be indicated once this has been determined. The reader should consult the section on fluid therapy (p. 311). Horses with Salmonella diarrhea are usually suffering from mixed water and electrolyte losses from both the extracellular and intracellular fluid compartments. Together with the lack of potassium intake due to anorexia, these losses can produce serious potassium deficits, and it may be beneficial to supply some potassium intravenously and the rest orally. Flow rates for intravenous fluids should be 3 to 5 liters per hour, although higher rates of flow may be indicated in

---

*Harleco CO_2 Apparatus, Gibbstown, NJ

TABLE 1. DOSAGES, INTERVALS, AND ROUTES FOR ANTIMICROBIALS USED IN THE TREATMENT OF SALMONELLOSIS

Drug	Dose (mg/kg)*	Interval	Route
Chloromycetin	25–50 mg/kg	Every 8 hours	IV, IM, or oral
Trimethoprim-sulfamethoxazole	4 mg/kg trimethoprim, 20 mg/kg sulfa	Every 12 hours	Oral, IV
Gentamicin	2–4 mg/kg	Every 8 hours	IM
Furazolidone†	4 mg/kg	Every 8 hours	Oral
Ampicillin	10–25 mg/kg	Every 8 hours	IV or IM

*Multiply this dose by the number of doses per day in order to determine the dose in mg/kg/day.

†Furazolidone administered orally will have an effect only on Salmonella within the gut, as it is poorly absorbed. Treatment with a parenterally administered systemic antimicrobial is therefore recommended in addition if furazolidone is used. Furazolidone is not recommended by this author.

patients with impending hypovolemic shock. Maximal flow rates for 5 per cent dextrose should be only 1 to 2 l. per hour, since higher flow rates exceed the rate of utilization and result in hyperglycemia and osmotic diuresis.

Oral intake can be voluntary or forced (by stomach tube). Loose KCl and NaCl can be offered, and many ill horses will voluntarily consume these salts. The drinking water can be spiked with KCl and the isotonic fluid offered to the horse. If the animal refuses to drink, isotonic fluids can be administered by stomach tube. Oral fluids are probably most beneficial during the recovery phase of illness when some net absorption is occurring in the cecum and colon.

In some horses, the administration of fluids, even by the intravenous route, does not appreciably alter the mucous membrane color, capillary refill, pulse rate, pulse character, or PCV, yet the horse may actually gain weight. It appears that these individuals are suffering from the effects of endotoxins (and perhaps other toxins absorbed from the gut) and that irreversible shock may have occurred. The therapy of endotoxic shock in the horse is currently based mainly on empirical observations of clinical cases and on information from other species. Fluid therapy is certainly the cornerstone of shock therapy, but drugs such as the adrenocorticosteroids also appear to be beneficial. Recommended doses of dexamethasone (or its equivalent) for the treatment of shock range from 0.2 mg per kg to 4.0 mg per kg. Plasma or plasma expanders such as dextran have been used and may be beneficial. Plasma is particularly indicated in horses in which the total plasma proteins decrease significantly, a relatively common finding in horses that have had severe diarrhea for several days. The major problems associated with plasma therapy are the time and expense incurred in collecting, preparing, and administering large volumes of plasma, but it is a relatively safe volume expander. Dextran* therapy must be undertaken

judiciously because of expense and the possibility of toxicity if an overdose is given or if it is used repeatedly. Probably no more than 8 gm per kg of a 6 per cent dextran (mol wt 40,000 to 70,000) solution should be given daily, and it should not be given for more than two or three days.

Although not all horses with enteric salmonellosis are bacteremic, most are susceptible because they are neutropenic and have a damaged mucosal barrier. Salmonellae produce disease by invasion through mucosal surfaces and by subsequently multiplying in the host tissues. The neutropenic horse with a damaged bowel is a high risk for the development of bacteremia. For these reasons, treatment with parenterally administered systemic antibiotics is indicated in an attempt to treat or prevent bacteremia. It does not appear that antimicrobial therapy significantly alters the course of the diarrhea once bowel damage has occurred. Excretion of Salmonella continues during and after treatment with either oral or parenteral antimicrobial drugs.

The choice of antimicrobial drug should be based on antimicrobial sensitivity of the isolate, achievable blood and tissue levels, route and interval required for proper dosage, untoward side effects, and cost (Table 1). Salmonellae frequently develop resistance to antimicrobial drugs by means of plasmids (or R factors), so that sensitivity testing is necessary in order to be sure that the drug being used in treatment is appropriate. Salmonella are usually sensitive to chloromycetin, trimethoprim-sulfa, gentamicin, and nitrofurazone. Pathogenic strains are often resistant to penicillin, streptomycin, sulfas, tetracyclines, neomycin, and many other commonly used antimicrobials. Unless previous isolates are available from the farm or until such time as isolates are tested and results reported back to the clinician, it is best to assume that this is the most likely pattern of resistance. It may be preferable to administer antimicrobials parenterally in order to be sure that adequate blood levels are achieved (especially when absorption is questionable owing to the damaged bowel) and to prevent undue resistance pressure on the enteric flora. There is one published

*Macrodex or Rheomacrodex, Pharmacia Labs., Piscataway, NJ 08854

report indicating that orally administered furazolidone* at a dose rate of 4 mg per kg three times a day was beneficial in a small number of foals that had been orally challenge-exposed with virulent *S. typhimurium*. The clinician should also be aware that the sensitivity patterns shown by Salmonella change frequently, and increased antimicrobial resistance should be expected when a particular drug is used on a premise repeatedly.

Intestinal adsorbants such as activated charcoal at a dose of 0.5 lb given twice a day can be given by stomach tube. These seem to be of some benefit, possibly by adsorbing endotoxins and other harmful material present within the gut lumen, thereby reducing the amounts available for absorption into the bloodstream. Kaopectate has been advocated as an intestinal protectant but has been of questionable benefit in treating salmonellosis.

Drugs that alleviate the cramping pain (associated with salmonellosis in humans) such as narcotic analgesics may be indicated. Prostaglandin synthetase inhibitors such as flunixin meglumine and other anti-endotoxin drugs have a theoretical place in the treatment of salmonellosis, but clinical experience has not demonstrated markedly beneficial effects following their use.

CONTROL

Control of the disease is based on minimizing exposure, reducing the incidence of concurrent diseases, and preventing stress. Salmonellosis occurs either sporadically in individually stressed horses or as an epidemic in a susceptible population such as a veterinary clinic or broodfarm with many foals. Overcrowding is to be avoided, and dispersing mares and foals to large sunny pastures is preferable to maintaining them in a barn where salmonellosis has recently occurred. Concurrent diseases such as rotavirus diarrhea may predispose foals to salmonellosis.

When a case of acute diarrhea does occur, the horse should be isolated, and all personnel should be required to wear boots and coveralls when entering the area. These should be removed when the area is left. Phenolic disinfectants are effective against salmonellae, which can persist in a cool, moist environment for months if a disinfectant is not applied (p. 24).

The value of vaccination for protection against enteric salmonellosis is unknown, but some authors report beneficial effects following the use of autogenous bacterins.

Supplemental Readings

1. Carlson, G. P.: Fluid therapy in horses with acute diarrhea. Symposium on Gastroenterology. Vet. Clin. North Am. (Large Anim. Pract.), *1*:313, 1979.
2. Morse, E. V., Duncan, M. A., Page, E. A., and Fessler, J. F.: Salmonellosis in equidae: A study of 23 cases. Cornell Vet., *66*:198, 1976.
3. Smith, B. P.: Salmonella infections in horses. Large Animal Supplement of the Compendium on Continuing Education, 3:S4, 1981.

*Furoxone, Norwich-Eaton, Norwich, NY

INTESTINAL CLOSTRIDIOSIS

Martin Wierup, UPPSALA, SWEDEN

Equine intestinal clostridiosis (EIC) was first described in the 1970s in Sweden and later in other countries, including the United States. The typical case is characterized by diarrhea and toxemia in stressed horses. An intestinal dysbacteriosis with abnormally high counts of *Clostridium perfringens* type A is pathognomonic for EIC. Strong evidence exists that EIC is an enterotoxemia caused by that microbe.

EPIDEMIOLOGY

The disease affects all ages but rarely occurs in horses less than one year of age. No sex or breed predisposition has been observed. Horses have often been subjected to stress, usually in the form of hard training but also in the form of infections, surgery, deworming, or recent antibiotic therapy. The disease is usually sporadic, but occasionally several cases may occur in one stable within a limited period of time. The prognosis is dependent on the degree of intoxication. In one study of 31 consecutive cases, 12 (39 per cent) died.

CLINICAL SIGNS

Typically the disease has a peracute onset, the most prominent signs being profound depression, diarrhea, and discolored mucous membranes. The diarrhea is often projectile, watery, dark-colored, and foul-smelling. Occasionally the first sign is depression followed by diarrhea a few hours later. Rarely diarrhea may not be present, but there may be colic. Conjunctival and scleral vessels may be congested as a result of the toxemia. Capillary refill is delayed accordingly. Severely affected horses stand or move only with great difficulty and usually lie down.

The heart rate varies with the severity of the illness. In severe cases, the heart rate is elevated to 75 to 140 beats per minute. Especially in severe cases, a decreased skin temperature indicates failing circulation (shock). The respiratory rate seems to be related to the severity of metabolic acidosis. The temperature may be normal but in most cases increases to 39 to 40° C. Dehydration is an important clinical feature. Laminitis may occur in prolonged cases. On rectal examination no abnormal observation is made apart from the watery rectal and intestinal contents.

The disease usually runs a rapid course. Occasionally death is apoplectic. Some horses have fallen dead during races. Among terminal cases, however, it is most common that the horse dies within 24 hrs after an acute onset with severe signs. Intensive therapy at an early stage of the disease may prolong the course. In milder cases, the course is often more prolonged. Horses surviving the disease appear to recover full health and racing capacity. Only in very few cases has recurrence been observed.

NECROPSY FINDINGS

Necropsy findings are characterized by widespread capillary damage with hyperemia, edema, and hemorrhages. The blood clots poorly. Acute inflammatory lesions are present in the intestinal tract. Acute hemorrhagic or necrotizing typhlitis and colitis of varying severity are consistent findings in subacute to chronic cases. The peracute cases may show only minor lesions. In the small colon and rectum, similar lesions are seen only in prolonged cases. In about two thirds of the patients, the small intestine is affected as well. Only in rare cases is the stomach the site of lesions. The intestinal contents of the cecum and large colon are watery, dark-colored, often mixed with blood, and usually foul-smelling.

Myocardial degeneration is occasionally observed histologically. The lungs consistently exhibit extensive hyperemia, edema, hemorrhage, and hyperinflation. Hemorrhage is also common in the adrenal glands, which may show necrosis. The liver is severely hyperemic in most cases and in horses with prolonged disease also has degenerative changes. The majority of the cases have hyperemic spleno-

megaly and congested intestinal lymph nodes. Bacteriologic examination of lymph nodes and organs reveals no specific aerobic or anaerobic organism.

CLINICAL PATHOLOGY

Increased serum levels of ornithine carbamyl transferase (up to 18.2 IU per l) and aspartate aminotransferase indicate liver damage. Liver injury and reduced liver function have also been verified by demonstration of extensive parenchymatous degeneration in liver biopsies and by increased retention of sulphobromophthalein. In the majority of the cases, there are high (up to 2004 IU per l) alkaline phosphatase levels, which mainly reflect lesions of the biliary tree. Elevated values of urea nitrogen can also be observed, most probably as a result of prerenal azotemia. Dehydration is indicated by elevated total protein values and by a rise in the hematocrit. Leukopenia (WBC down to 2.5×10^3) appears early, and leukocytosis occurs (WBC up to 25.9×10^3) later in the disease. ECG usually demonstrates abnormalities suggesting myocardial myopathy.

ETIOLOGY

Evidence clearly indicates that EIC is an enterotoxemia caused by *C. perfringens* type A. The disease is associated with an intestinal dysbacteriosis as shown by abnormally high counts of *C. perfringens*. Moreover, if the disease regresses, the *C. perfringens* counts decrease to normal levels. Numbers of *C. perfringens* in the feces are correlated with the severity of illness. In healthy horses in both Sweden and the United States, *C. perfringens* is not isolated or in rare cases is detected only in counts less than or equal to 10 colony-forming units (CFUs) per gm of feces.

The clinical and pathoanatomic findings resemble those characteristically seen during clostridial enterotoxemias in other animal species. Indeed, many of the prominent signs and the clinicopathologic changes can be construed as being indicative of physiologic disturbances or tissue damage caused specifically by toxins of *C. perfringens*. Immunologic investigations have revealed that EIC horses and those fed *C. perfringens* experimentally possess precipitating antibodies against an extracellular antigen elaborated by an equine isolate of *C. perfringens* type A. Although it has proved difficult to mimic enterotoxemias caused by *C. perfringens* under experimental conditions, horses given broth cultures of *C. perfringens* type A orally revealed signs similar to spontaneous cases of EIC, although usually less pronounced. It can be concluded that other predisposing factors must coincide with the rise in the *C. perfringens* counts in order to trigger the disease.

DIAGNOSIS

EIC should be suspected primarily in stressed horses developing acute signs of intoxication and diarrhea but also in cases of apoplectic deaths. However, for the confirmative diagnosis, clinical signs or pathologic changes must be found in connection with an abnormal rise in fecal or intestinal *C. perfringens* counts. The specimen, simply feces in a plastic bag, should be subjected to serial dilutions and *C. perfringens* identified primarily by Nagler reactions on egg yolk agar. Regularly, cultures should also be made for detection of Salmonella. Cultures should preferably be made within four hours of sampling, but within 24 hours is also acceptable when specimens are kept under cool conditions. *C. perfringens* counts greater than 10^2 CFUs per gm of feces in most types of horses can be judged as abnormal, but during the acute phase of EIC, the corresponding value usually is 10^4 to 10^5 CFUs. Bacteriologic examination thus is essential. If not performed, cases of EIC might be diagnosed as colitis-X, a term likely inclusive of various causes of acute colitis.

THERAPY

The primary treatment is directed at stopping the toxin production of *C. perfringens*. The basic therapy for this purpose is the immediate use of "sour milk." This milk product is derived from lactic acid–producing strains of Streptococcus and is available in every grocery store in Sweden.* A horse weighing 400 to 500 kg should be given 4 to 6 l by stomach tube. Treatment should be repeated at least once after six hours. Many cases of EIC are often dramatically improved within two hours. Though the clinical effect of sour milk is quite clear, its pharmacologic action is not fully understood. However, in vitro studies have demonstrated that sour milk has a strong antibacterial effect against *C. perfringens* but not against several other bacteria belonging to 12 genera, including Salmonella. As yet, research has not demonstrated a corresponding result for buttermilk or yogurt. It has also been reported that cases diagnosed as EIC have been successfully treated with *C. perfringens* types C and D antitoxin, 250 ml given intravenously diluted in 2 l of lactated Ringer's solution.

*Note: Sour milk is not generally available in the United States.

Treatment must also be directed to replacement of the loss of water and electrolytes and correction of the metabolic acidosis. This is done by intravenous infusions of lactated Ringer's and $NaHCO_3$ solutions (p. 203).

In severe cases, 40 to 60 l of fluid are needed. Conventional shock therapy with corticosteroids (1 to 4 mg per kg dexamethasone) may also be considered.

As no bacteremia occurs, any antibiotic used should be active in the intestine, but experience has shown antibiotics to be of little or no value. Neomycin and tetracycline must not be used because of the adverse effect on gut flora. If sour milk is not available or where such a therapy does not improve the condition, chloramphenicol may be used.

After recovery from severe EIC, a convalescence of at least one month is needed, and preferably no training should be started until an ECG examination has excluded myocardial lesions.

CONTROL

Clinical and experimental studies have clearly demonstrated that tetracycline therapy can result in an intestinal overgrowth of *C. perfringens* resulting in diarrhea and death, although a history of tetracycline therapy exists only for a minority of the spontaneous cases of EIC, and in the rest the underlying cause of the rise of the intestinal *C. perfringens* count is not known. Tetracycline should, therefore, be used with care, and long-term treatment with the drug should be avoided. It has been demonstrated experimentally that high doses of lysine and methionine can alter the intestinal flora of horses, as indicated by abnormally high, up to 10^5, *C. perfringens* CFUs per gm of feces. This observation should be kept in mind when these amino acids are included in feed additives given to intensively fed and trained racehorses.

References

1. Andersson, G., Ekman, L., Mansson, I., Persson, S., Rubarth, S., and Tufvesson, G.: Lethal complications following administration of oxytetracycline in the horse. Nord. Vet. Med., 23:9, 1971.
2. Anderson, N. V.: Veterinary gastroenterology. Philadelphia, Lea & Febiger, 1980.
3. Vaughan, J. T.: The acute colitis syndrome, colitis "X." Vet. Clin. North Am., 2:301, 1973.
4. Wierup, M.: Equine intestinal clostridiosis. An acute disease in horses associated with high intestinal counts of *Clostridium perfringens* type A. Acta Vet. Scand., Suppl. 62, AVSPAC, 62:1, 1977.
5. Wierup, M., and DiPietro, J. H.: Bacteriological examination of equine fecal flora as a diagnosis tool for equine intestinal clostridiosis. Am. J. Vet. Res., 42(12):2167, 1981.

FOAL HEAT DIARRHEA

Gary E. Rumbaugh, DAVIS, CALIFORNIA

Diarrhea is a frequently observed problem in foals and may or may not lead to serious consequences. Foals with diarrhea must be observed very carefully, as the condition may require prompt attention, depending upon its etiology. Resolution of any one case may occur with no treatment or only alterations in management or may proceed to an explosive septicemia terminating in death.

Foal heat diarrhea, or scours, is the most common diarrhea entity in the neonate. It often develops during the period when the mare's first postpartum estrus is expected, hence the name. The etiology is not well defined, and diarrhea has been observed in foals removed from their dams and raised in aseptic quarters during this time. Various contributing factors that have been suggested, although not definitively established, include (1) changes in milk composition during the heat period, (2) ingestion of genital discharges contaminating the mammary gland and teats, (3) ingestion of straw, hay, feces, grass, and other foreign matter, (4) overloading of the foal's digestive tract when the foal nurses after the mare returns from breeding, and (5) infestation with *Strongyloides westeri* acquired through intramammary transmission from the mare.

Johnston et al. reported no significant change in the pH, volume, lactose, protein, fat, ash, and estrogen content of mare's milk during the period when foal heat diarrhea occurs.[5]

In a large number of Thoroughbred, Standardbred, and Quarter horse mares and foals, there was no correlation between the onset of diarrhea in the foal and the onset of estrus in the mare. Additionally, orphaned foals and foals raised in aseptic isolation also appear to suffer from episodes of "foal heat" diarrhea. Extensive studies in Kentucky in 1973, while revealing that nearly all foals are infested with *Strongyloides westeri* parasites through intramammary transmission, showed the great majority of these infestations to be subclinical (p. 281). Diarrheas associated with Strongyloides infestations tend to occur somewhat later in life and to become chronic and difficult to treat.

The most plausible etiology seems to center on the suggestion that the ingestion of hay, straw, feces, grass, and other solid foreign matter and the associated gut flora changes that are occurring at this time of life are responsible for initiating diarrhea. Close observations of foals has revealed that the normal neonate is a very avid and experimental eater. By five to seven days of age, most foals are ingesting whatever solid matter is in their environment. Foals begin to eat hay by five to seven days of age and grain by 10 to 13 days. Apparently, all foals practice coprophagia to some extent beginning at three to six days of age. This activity, which appears to be a normal behavioral response, may introduce bacterial flora into the foal's gut and may supply certain vitamins that the foal is unable to synthesize.

THERAPY

Most instances of foal heat diarrhea are mild with a pasty yellow fecal discharge that may, on occasion, become watery enough to soil the tail and perineum. These foals remain bright and alert, nurse frequently, respond normally to their environment, and usually recover in two days to a week without treatment. A worried owner can be instructed to monitor the temperature daily and to keep the tail and perineum cleaned and covered with petrolatum to prevent hair loss. Routine use of antibacterial agents or drugs affecting gastrointestinal motility are not recommended for these foals. Any increase in body temperature and its persistence above 102° F, any signs of dehydration or depression, and anorexia manifested by a full udder on the mare should be subjected to more extensive diagnosis and therapeutic procedures.

The foal with a more profuse, watery diarrhea in association with some degree of anorexia represents a more serious clinical problem. These foals, like the newborn of other species, are in a precarious state of energy and water balance. The rapid development of dehydration and a weak, comatose state require rapid correction of developing deficits if recovery is to be effected. Not only are fluid losses higher than normal, but fluid replacement is well below normal. Signs of dehydration are obvious in foals when 10 to 15 per cent of their body weight in fluids is lost. Thus, a 50 kg foal may have a 5 l water deficit. This is most often accompanied by hypoglycemia, with blood glucose concentrations below 45 mg per dl. Conceding that accurate replacement of fluids should be integrated with laboratory determination of deficits, there are a few general observations that may be useful for immediate action (p. 311). Fluid loss from the lower gastrointestinal tract may result in significant losses of potassium and bicarbonate along with sodium. This results in hyponatremia and a metabolic acidosis and may or may not be accompanied by serum hyperkalemia.

Initial intravenous therapy can be initiated in the diarrheic foal with lactated Ringer's solution plus 5 per cent dextrose at a rate of 10 to 20 ml per kg until laboratory results are obtained. It has been our experience that many of the signs of dehydration and depression can be relieved by provision of an immediate energy source such as dextrose. Rapid and massive use of bicarbonate solutions is to be avoided at this stage because of its marked alkalinizing effects in an animal whose respiratory response may be reduced. It is well to remember that foals normally have a lower total protein concentration than older animals, and a laboratory value of 7 gm per dl may reflect dehydration when the normal value is 4.7 to 5 gm per dl. Once hydration is restored, whole plasma may be of benefit by providing trace minerals, essential fatty acids, and immunoglobulins. Administered intravenously, compatible plasma at a dosage of 20 ml per kg will also aid in raising total protein concentration and provide additional passive immunity to the foal.

A fecal culture should be done to rule out salmonellosis if diarrhea is profuse and especially if mucus or blood is present or if the temperature is elevated. Culture results may be of extreme importance in the management of this foal and other animals on the farm. If fever is present or salmonellosis is suspected, oral antibiotic therapy should be started with chloramphenicol or tribrissen.

The use of antidiarrheal drugs in these foals is a subject of considerable controversy, but morphine and loperamide may be of some value in slowing the passage of digesta through the tract, whereas atropine and the parasympatholytics are of little or no value and may even be contraindicated. The use of intestinal protectants such as kaolin-pectin, mineral oil, and milk of bismuth have not shown any efficacy in our practice and are not recommended in these foals, as most of them elevate water loss.

Once signs of recovery are seen, a change to oral administration of a mixed electrolyte and dextrose solution will most often meet the foal's needs (p. 204). At this point, withholding milk for 24 to 48 hours is often beneficial. This can be accomplished by muzzling the foal and milking out the mare. Because of reduced or absent intestinal lactase due to damaged mucosal cells, the digestion of the milk sugar, lactose, will be far below normal, resulting in indigestion and the addition of a fermentative, osmotic diarrhea on top of the mild diarrhea already present.

In summary, the condition known as "foal heat" diarrhea is most often a mild condition of loose feces that is generally best managed conservatively. If the diarrhea persists, and most particularly if it is accompanied by fever and depression, a more vigorous approach is indicated, as infectious etiologies may be involved.

References

1. Anderson, N. V. (ed.): Veterinary Gastroenterology. Philadelphia, Lea & Febiger, 1980.
2. Doll, E. R.: Diseases of Foals. Yearbook of Agriculture. U.S. Govt. Printing Office, Washington, DC, 1956.
3. Foal diarrhea seminar. Proc. 25th Annu. Meet. Am. Assoc. Eq. Pract., 1979, pp. 197–234.
4. Gideon, L.: Total nutritional support of the foal. Vet. Med. Sm. Anim. Clin., 72:1197, 1977.
5. Johnston, R. H., Kamstra L. D., and Kohler, P. H.: Mare's milk composition as related to "foal heat" scours. J. Anim. Sci., 31:549, 1970.
6. Udal, D. H.: The Practice of Veterinary Medicine, 4th ed. New York, Udall Pub. Co., 1943.

ANTERIOR ENTERITIS

Jill Johnson McClure, BATON ROUGE, LOUISIANA

The term anterior enteritis is used to describe an acute clinical syndrome characterized by abdominal pain, ileus, gastric distention, and toxic shock. The etiology is unknown, but Clostridium or other bacterial toxins are suspected to play a role in the disease pathogenesis.

The cardinal gross pathologic lesions associated with the clinical syndrome are multifocal areas of hemorrhage, congestion, and necrosis involving primarily the duodenum and proximal jejunum, but occasionally also involving the lower small intestine and colon. Thus, the terms hemorrhagic enteritis or duodenojejunitis may be more descriptive of the lesions. The condition has only been observed in adult horses. Whether any relationship between this condition and clostridum sp–induced hemorrhagic diarrhea in foals exists is presently undetermined.

HISTORY

Affected horses may initially show an acute onset of anorexia and depression but most often are discovered with abdominal pain. The condition is seldom violently painful. Grain engorgement has occasionally been associated with the onset of clinical signs.

CLINICAL FINDINGS

Ileus is a consistent physical finding. Gastric distention occurs secondary to the ileus and decreased absorption of fluids from the proximal small intestine, and characteristically affected animals reflux large volumes (gallons) of gastroenteric fluid following nasogastric intubation. The fluid is usually fetid, brownish-tinged, and occult blood–positive.

The horses generally present with signs of toxic shock. Pulse rates are elevated. Capillary refill time is prolonged. Mucous membranes are congested and injected. Dehydration estimated from loss of skin turgor usually ranges from 8 to 10 per cent. Body temperature is usually not elevated.

Rectal palpation findings are generally unremarkable. Small bowel distention is usually absent.

LABORATORY DATA

The packed cell volumes and total plasma protein values reflect severe dehydration and are often in excess of 55 per cent and 8.5 gm per dl, respectively. Consistent changes in the leukon have not been observed, and both leukopenia and leukocytosis with regenerative or degenerative left shifts have been observed. Blood glucose levels are often significantly elevated.

The majority of the cases present with a metabolic acidosis, which is somewhat remarkable considering the large volume of gastric reflux. Moderate hypochloremia is present in about 50 per cent of the cases. Serum potassium levels are generally within normal range, although total body potassium may be depleted in the presence of acidosis. Serum and peritoneal fluid amylase and lipase levels have been elevated in the few cases monitored and may indicate primary or secondary pancreatic involvement.

Abdominocentesis findings tend to be unremarkable unless mural necrosis has become advanced. This may be an important diagnostic feature in differentiating this syndrome from obstructive diseases of the small intestine such as strangulating obstructions. More dramatic peritoneal fluid changes might be expected in the same time frame if a strangulating lesion was present rather than the type of lesions associated with anterior enteritis.

THERAPY

Management of the syndrome is directed primarily at supportive therapy of the patient rather than at eliminating a specific etiologic agent.

One of the most important factors in the management of anterior enteritis is removal of the fluids that accumulate in the stomach. Either repeated or continuous nasogastric decompression is necessary to prevent rupture of the stomach or the affected small bowel. Suturing or taping a stomach tube in situ is advisable to prevent inadvertent displacement of the tube if the animal begins to struggle. Manipulation of the tube or siphoning may be necessary to initiate flow, but often large volumes of fluid are recovered once flow is initiated.

Administration of therapeutic agents via nasogastric tube is unrewarding, since normal intestinal flow is absent and most drugs are ultimately recovered in the reflux fluid.

Large-volume intravenous fluid therapy is needed to restore normal cardiovascular function. A balanced electrolyte solution such as lactated Ringer's solution is generally selected and supplemented with sodium bicarbonate as needed to combat the metabolic acidosis (p. 203).

Nonsteroidal anti-inflammatory/analgesic agents such as flunixin meglumine* (1.1 mg per kg, .5 mg per lb) are employed as needed to control pain, although continued decompression of the stomach often results in decreased visceral pain. These drugs may also be beneficial in reducing the inflammation of the affected bowel. Corticosteroids are generally reserved until an initial response to fluid therapy is evaluated and are not given if a favorable response is obtained.

Broad-spectrum antibiotics are administered.

Complications observed in recovered patients have included laminitis, pneumonia/pleuritis, hepatitis, and multifocal abscessation of peripheral lymph nodes. Thus, it is advisable to maintain the patient on soft footing, to monitor the feet carefully during therapy, and to place them in plaster casts if evidence of laminitis is detected (p. 104). Nasogastric decompression must be carefully performed to prevent contamination of the pharynx with foreign material and aspiration of materials into the lower respiratory tract. Antibiotic therapy is directed at preventing disseminated abscessation and hepatitis associated with septicemia.

Horses that recover generally do so within 48 hours. The mortality rate is approximately 50 per cent even with intensive therapy.

*Banamine, Schering Co., Kenilworth, NJ

CHRONIC DIARRHEA

A. M. *Merritt*, GAINESVILLE, FLORIDA

For the purposes of this discussion, chronic equine diarrhea is diarrhea that has continued unabated for at least one month. The classic case is characterized by soft ("cowflop") feces of about twice the normal volume and thin but not wasted body condition. Vital signs, demeanor, and appetite are normal. Such an animal may prefer to drink water laced with sodium and potassium chloride or may eat more salt than normal.

CLINICAL EVALUATION

PHYSICAL EXAMINATION

A thorough physical examination should be done on all horses with chronic diarrhea. No system should be overlooked, since occasionally a case has been associated, for instance, with an occult infection in something other than the gastrointestinal tract, such as sinusitis.

A rectal examination is absolutely essential. Pretreatment of the animal with 30 to 45 mg propantheline bromide* intravenously or 15 cc of lidocaine in 40 cc of water directly into the rectum may be necessary to promote rectal relaxation sufficient to perform a complete examination. A thorough rectal examination includes an attempt to palpate (1) any masses that might be within the gut lumen, wall, or mesentery, (2) the status of the lymph nodes and vessels within and around the cranial and caudal mesenteric root, and (3) the condition of the rectum itself. Any suggestion of a thickened rectal wall and friable rectal mucosa is an indication for proctoscopy and rectal biopsy. Shallow proctoscopy can be accomplished by the insertion of a vaginal pipe speculum into the rectum. Deep proctoscopy involves the manual instillation of a flexible fiberoptic instrument, although this may not be very useful unless the rectum is ballooned. Rectal biopsy is done by sampling a pinch of rectal mucosa with a uterine biopsy instrument.

ABDOMINOCENTESIS

Methods of abdominocentesis and interpretation of results of peritoneal fluid evaluation are described elsewhere (p. 227). Of particular interest in cases of chronic equine diarrhea are the number and type of white blood cells (WBC) and the total protein.

Most horses with chronic diarrhea studied by this author have had abdominal fluid with a normal WBC count (<5000 per mm^3); none have had a count greater than 15,000 per mm^3, and these higher counts, while primarily neutrophils, were not helpful in providing an etiologic diagnosis. However, this author has regarded a relative *eosinophil* count of greater than 2.5 per cent in the fluid to be very indicative of a high degree of strongyle larval migrans activity. An earlier observation that decreased peritoneal macrophage activity was a consistent component of the granulomatous enteritis syndrome needs further quantitative evaluation before it can be considered a real phenomenon.

DIRECT FECAL EXAMINATION

Protozoa. Some feces should be collected directly from the rectum and examined immediately for the presence of protozoa and WBC and for Gram staining characteristics. For protozoa, a drop of fecal liquor dispersed under a coverslip is used. Organisms are best seen under reduced condenser lighting. About 70 different species of ciliate protozoa live in the equine large intestine, and four or five of these (especially of the genuses *Blepharocorys* and *Cycloposthium*) are commonly found in small numbers in normal equine feces. In some cases of chronic diarrhea, ciliates of many species may abound, suggesting a washout phenomenon; in other cases, no protozoa of any kind may be found, indicating to this author a general reduction or absence of the ciliate population within the large intestines.

The small flagellate *Trichomonas equi* is also normally present, in small numbers to be sure, in large intestinal ingesta and feces. In a few cases of chronic diarrhea, the trichomonads may be found as the exclusive organism in the feces, sometimes in very large numbers. The finding of this organism prompted the etiologic diagnosis of "trichomonads-induced diarrhea" into which most, if not all, horses with chronic diarrhea used to be classed, whether the organism was present in the feces or not. The present, more tenable, impression is that excessive fecal trichomonads are indicative of a serious change in the intraluminal environment of the large bowel rather than being a cause of diarrhea. Whether this denotes a specific etiologic or pathophysiologic situation remains to be seen.

In summary, it is important to know the status of fecal protozoa in cases of chronic equine diarrhea, not because we can yet ascribe an etiologic diagnosis

---

*Pro-Banthine, Searle & Co., Chicago, IL

to a particular finding, but because what we find may be helpful in leading us to a therapeutic approach to the problem.

Leukocytes. Fecal leukocytes, if present, are quite easily demonstrated by mixing a drop of fecal liquor with a drop of new methylene blue, applying a coverslip, and examining the mixture microscopically under high dry objective. A second method involves drying a streak of liquid fecal material on a slide and staining the smear with "Diff-Quik."* Normally, no white blood cells should be found in the feces. Their presence, especially if they are neutrophils, is indicative of an active inflammation of the bowel (presumably within the colon of the horse). Classically, enteritis, a true inflammation of the bowel, is caused by an invasive bacterial agent such as Salmonella. The test for fecal leukocytes is generally more useful as a diagnostic tool in acute rather than chronic diarrheal disease but should always be done in evaluation of the latter, in spite of the fact that severe colitis is rarely found in association with chronic equine diarrhea.

Gram Stain. In general, gram-negative rods predominate in a Gram stain of feces from a horse with chronic diarrhea, but it is impossible to distinguish one genus of rod from another by this technique. A Gram stain should be done, however, to indicate if an abnormal preponderance of infrequently found organisms, such as Clostridium, is present, which can be significant.

ESSENTIAL CLINICAL LABORATORY PROCEDURES

Blood. Blood counts are infrequently contributory to making an etiologic diagnosis in chronic equine diarrhea. In a survey by this author of a substantial number of cases, 75 per cent had a total WBC count under 5000 per mm^3, whereas only 4 per cent had greater than 10,000. What may be more useful is the number of eosinophils present in the count, since an eosinophilia is indicative of parasitism, and this dictates a certain initial therapeutic approach.

Of particular interest in the blood chemistries are the serum protein values, including the electrophoretic pattern. Low serum albumin concentration without proteinuria is indicative of an excessive protein leak from plasma across the gut wall (a protein-losing enteropathy) or long-standing hepatocyte damage. A concurrent hyperglobulinemia, especially an increase in beta globulin concentration,

would be more indicative of chronic liver disease than protein-losing enteropathy, although this would have to be substantiated by more specific liver function studies. Alternatively, an increase in serum beta globulin concentration would also be consistent with a chronic strongyle larval migrans.

Serum electrolyte values are necessary, particularly in the initial evaluation of a case of chronic diarrhea, to decide whether forceful supportive fluid and electrolyte therapy is immediately indicated (p. 202). In most cases it is not. Serum electrolyte or enzyme values have not proved useful, however, in making a specific diagnosis.

Feces. Fecal culture is an essential component of the evaluation of a horse with chronic diarrhea. We are presently not exploiting this technique to its fullest potential to identify possible intestinal pathogens, purely out of ignorance, but it is important to know whether the patient is shedding Salmonella organisms.

In addition, fecal parasitology must also be done.

Finally, techniques such as measurement of fecal volatile fatty acids and in vitro fermentation procedures may be of use in classifying chronic diarrhea pathophysiologically but are not presently within the realm of routine laboratory procedures.

Absorption Studies. Adult horses with gastrointestinal disease confined to the small intestine may be unthrifty but are unlikely to have diarrhea. It seems that the large intestine must be damaged for diarrhea to be manifested. Strongyle larval migrans and granulomatous enteritis, which can cause chronic diarrhea, may also cause small intestinal mucosal disease that can be demonstrated by D-xylose malabsorption; thus, this test is useful in narrowing the differential diagnosis. The recommended diagnostic dose of D-xylose is 0.5 gm per kg body weight given by stomach tube as a 10 per cent solution. A heparinized blood sample is collected prior to xylose administration and every 30 minutes for at least two, preferably 3, hours postadministration. Normally the plasma xylose concentration peaks at 17 to 25 mg per dl between 60 and 90 minutes postdosing.

EXPLORATORY LAPAROTOMY

For the most complete clinical evaluation of a case of chronic diarrhea, especially where all other procedures already described yield no diagnostic information, an exploratory laparotomy, either in the standing or recumbent position, may be done. The abdomen and its contents can then be more thoroughly explored, followed by intestinal biopsy for histopathology and direct collection of large intestinal contents for microscopic examination.

---

*Harleco, Gibbstown, NJ

DIFFERENTIAL DIAGNOSIS AND TREATMENT

The most frustrating thing about working up a case of chronic equine diarrhea is that even after most or all of the procedures mentioned above have been done, the etiologic-pathophysiologic diagnosis is still often unknown. Of a large number of cases so examined by the author at the University of Pennsylvania between 1974 and 1978, 45 per cent fell into this undiagnosed or "open" category. That is, all they showed were some degree of weight loss and soft ("cowflop") to watery feces of two to three times the normal daily output. Patients having definitive findings of strongyle larval migrans (cranial mesenteric arteriopathy, histopathologic evidence of submucosal larvae via biopsy) comprised about 20 per cent, and those having indefinite findings of larval migrans (excess eosinophils in the peritoneal fluid, eosinophilia) made up about 15 per cent. Salmonella organisms were cultured from another 15 per cent, granulomatous enteritis was found in 3 per cent, and 2 per cent were associated with diseases of other organ systems.

"Open" Diagnosis

The "open" diagnosis cases show nothing of clinical significance except mild to moderate weight loss, persistent soft or watery feces of two to three times the normal daily output, increased water and salt consumption, and usually some change in the fecal protozoal numbers.

Therapeutically, 25 to 30 per cent of such cases will be resistant to anything that is tried. If ciliates or trichomonads are found swarming in a fecal specimen, the first order of therapy is iodochlorhydroxyquin (ICH)* at a dose of 10 gm (one bolus) per day. If there is no desirable response in two days, the ICH should be discontinued. If the feces begin to form up, the dose of 10 gm once a day should be continued for three to four more days and then slowly cut back until a minimal amount is needed to achieve the desired effect. This author feels that too much ICH will also cause diarrhea in some cases. After three to four weeks of therapy, the ICH may be discontinued to see if the effect is permanent. Some horses require it for the rest of their lives to maintain formed feces, which does not seem to be detrimental to the animal but is costly and annoying. When ICH is effective, it probably is not because of its apparent protozoacidal properties but because it somehow alters bacterial fermentative activity within the large intestine.

When no protozoa are found in the feces, transfaunation is recommended as the primary therapeutic approach. The time-honored way of accomplishing this was the fecal "cocktail," which is easy to prepare but quite weak in its concentration. A more potent but more difficult to obtain preparation is fresh colonic-cecal liquor from a horse with a normal gastrointestinal tract that is to be euthanatized. Five to six l of liquor are obtained by sieving colonic and cecal ingesta (pieces of large-diameter orthopedic stockinette tied off at one end with the open end draped over a bucket rim work very well) and transferring the liquor to the recipient by stomach tube as soon as possible. If the liquor is collected at a slaughterhouse or rendering plant, it should be kept warm and under a 2 to 3 cm layer of mineral oil while transporting it to the recipient. Animals that seem to respond best to this therapy are those whose feces were not too watery to begin with. Two or three treatments may be required to achieve the desired effect.

Oral drenching with cultured yogurt or buttermilk has had some testimonial success in certain cases of nonspecific chronic diarrhea in horses, and this approach deserves more study, especially with the use of some of the commercially available dried Lactobacillus preparations. The role of Lactobacillus in equine colonic function has not been investigated.

Large doses of oral mineral oil have been reported as successful in treating chronic diarrhea in horses. This therapy has not been successful in this author's hands, but this should not detract from its consideration if other forms of treatment are unsuccessful.

Unfortunately, too many horses in this "open" diagnostic category are unresponsive to any form of therapy that has a reasonable chance of effecting a cure. Opiates may firm up the feces while in use, but in contrast to ICH, their long-term application is not in the best interest of the patient. The atropine-like drugs fall into the same category. Antibiotic therapy cannot be applied with any good rationale without knowing more about its effects on colonic flora, and in this author's opinion, oral nonabsorbable antibiotics are absolutely contraindicated, since their chance of adversely disrupting colonic flora is much greater than is their chance of controlling or curing the disease. The advocacy of liters of horse serum given by stomach tube as an effective treatment of chronic diarrhea has not been substantiated by field experience.

Strongyle Larval Migrans

There is a clear impression from gut function studies and histopathology that certain horses react to migrating *Strongylus vulgaris* larvae in such a

*Reaform, Squibb, Princeton, NJ

way that results in severe diffuse gastrointestinal malfunction and chronic diarrhea. Certainly this group has to be small in relation to the total number of horses affected with larval migrans that do not have diarrhea, but it seemingly represents a considerable number of animals afflicted with the chronic diarrhea syndrome.

When there is clinical evidence of larval migrans, larvacidal therapy is recommended as the first step. Thiabendazole (TBZ) at 440 mg per kg (10 times the recommended vermifuge dose) given two days in succession, or fenbendazole at 60 mg per kg given once, have both been found to kill the early stages of migrating larvae. The avermectins, a new class of parasiticides, promise to have even greater larvacidal properties (p. 278). Of 14 animals with chronic diarrhea classified in the larval migrans group that were treated by this author with a "larvacidal" regimen of TBZ alone, seven responded satisfactorily; two others responded to follow-up ICH therapy, when before TBZ therapy they had not been responsive to ICH. If this therapeutic approach fails, those methods discussed under the "open diagnosis" category should be considered.

FECAL SALMONELLA SHEDDERS

In this author's experience, about 15 per cent of horses with chronic diarrhea shed Salmonella organisms in their feces. This shedding is continuous or intermittent and is unrelated to any changes in clinical signs or environment. In fact, most cases are clinically very similar to those classified in the "open" category. Some had a history of acute disease with fever and watery diarrhea signaling the onset of the chronic problem, but this was not a consistent feature. A few others were known to become more ill when exposed to a stressful situation or when given medications, such as oral antibiotics or iodochlorhydroxyquin.

Laboratory findings other than the presence of the Salmonellae in the feces were generally not remarkable. The question continually arises as to whether 10 to 15 per cent of any group of normal-appearing horses might be shedding Salmonellae in their feces, especially when they are under training conditions. Therefore, any consistent pathogenic relationship of the organism to the chronic diarrhea is presently unknown.

The diarrhea of animals in this category is difficult to control with any type of medication. Promoting hyperimmunization against the offending species of the organism has been unsuccessful. The fecal shedding may be stopped by appropriate antibiotic therapy (such as trimethoprim-sulfadiazine), but the diarrhea usually continues. Iodochlorhydroxyquin therapy has a very poor success rate, and there is

testimonial evidence that occasionally a horse will become more ill after receiving the ICH, which may suppress certain intestinal microflora that normally keep the Salmonellae in check.

Horses with chronic diarrhea that are shedding Salmonellae in their feces should be given a poor prognosis for recovery.

GRANULOMATOUS ENTERITIS (GE)

Most horses with granulomatous enteritis do not have diarrhea but have chronic weight loss, are hypoalbuminemic, and malabsorb D-xylose or D-glucose. "Granulomatous enteritis" is a broad term for a whole realm of protein-losing chronic enteropathies that can have some distinctive individual pathologic features along with granuloma formation. As time goes on, we may be able to distinguish specific etiologies for the distinctive pathologic manifestations. The disease basically appears to be an immunologic phenomenon, as it is in humans, the pathogenesis of which is poorly understood. In the horse it shows a preference for the small intestine, although those animals with diarrhea have had marked colonic lesions. Two cases studied by this author that were caused by avian tuberculosis also had diffuse rectal pathology that was demonstrated by rectal biopsy, although the rectum has been free of lesions in all but one case of GE of unknown etiology.

Two cases of GE under the care of the author and one case reported in the literature improved after long-term high-dose steroid administration. Prednisolone is recommended to reduce chances of causing laminitis, and it should be given at a dose of 400 to 500 mg per day parenterally rather than orally since these horses are malabsorbers. It should take three to four weeks before any strong evidence of benefit is seen, which commits the owner to considerable expense in the face of an extremely guarded prognosis. Antimetabolites and metronidazole, used in human medicine to treat Crohn's disease with varying success, have not been used in horses to treat granulomatous enteritis.

MISCELLANEOUS CAUSES

There are reported in the literature numerous other specific diseases, all of which are untreatable, in which chronic diarrhea has been one of the clinical signs in some but not all cases. These include an intestinal form of *Corynebacterium equi*, hepatic cirrhosis, lymphosarcoma, and malignant and benign gastric tumors (see article on gastrointestinal neoplasia, p. 259).

A final word on supportive therapy: for all horses

with chronic diarrhea, consider fluids (p. 202) and B vitamins. As indicated earlier, most horses with chronic diarrhea do not require intensive fluid therapy, although there is occasionally an animal that becomes so decompensated that intravenous therapy is required to get its system back on track. Free choice water with electrolytes mixed in is always indicated, however. Any of the commerical preparations that contain sodium, potassium chloride, and bicarbonate, mixed according to directions, will suffice (p. 204). Always provide a bucket of fresh water and a salt block as well.

Since needed B vitamins are manufactured by the equine colon, it is rational to include periodic (possibly weekly) B complex vitamin injections in the long-term supportive therapy for chronic diarrhea, which I think of as primarily a colonic disease. It should be stressed, however, that this recommendation is not supported to date by any experimental data.

Supplemental Readings

1. Argenzio, R. A.: Functions of the equine large intestine and their interrelationship in disease. Cornell Vet., 65:303, 1975.
2. Bach, L. G., and Ricketts, S. W.: Paracentesis as an aid to the diagnosis of abdominal disease in the horse. Eq. Vet. J., 6:116, 1974.
3. Bolton, J. R., Merritt, A. M., Cimprich, R. E., Ramberg, C. F., and Street, W.: Normal and abnormal xylose absorption in the horse. Cornell Vet., 66:183, 1976.
4. Damron, G. W.: Gastrointestinal trichomonads in horses: Occurrence and identification. Am J. Vet. Res., 37:25, 1976.
5. Manahan, F. F.: Diarrhea in horses with particular reference to a chronic diarrhea syndrome. Aust. Vet. J., 46:231, 1970.
6. Merritt, A. M.: Chronic equine diarrhea: Differential diagnosis and therapy . Proc. 21st Annu. Meet. Am. Assoc. Eq. Pract., pp. 401–404, 1975.
7. Merritt, A. M., Cimprich, R. E., and Beech, J.: Granulomatous enteritis in nine horses. J. Am. Vet. Med. Assoc., 169:603, 1976.
8. Merritt, A. M., and Smith, D. A.: Osmolarity and volatile fatty acid content of feces from horses with chronic diarrhea. Am. J. Vet. Res., 41:928, 1980.

MEDICAL MANAGEMENT OF COLIC

R. K. Shideler, FORT COLLINS, COLORADO
D. G. Bennett, FORT COLLINS, COLORADO

An intelligent approach to the medical management of colic requires an understanding of the causes and mechanisms of abdominal pain. Ultimately, the only painful stimulus to the gastrointestinal tract is an increase in intramural tension. This may be brought about by distention, which is associated with impactions, displacements, and excessive fermentation; or spasm, which is associated with irritation and ischemia. Vascular engorgement and inflammation reduce the pain threshold, so that an otherwise nonpainful increase in intramural tension may become painful. It is, therefore, essential in the treatment of colic to correct the cause of distention or spasm and, when necessary, to relieve associated pain until the correction has been accomplished. Drugs commonly used in colic therapy are listed in Table 1.

RELIEF OF PAIN

By far the most satisfactory method of pain relief is the correction of the cause of increased intramural tension. Frequently it is necessary to achieve temporary relief of pain chemotherapeutically, but the following points must be considered. Analgesics and tranquilizers may interfere with the assessment of the horse's condition and progress. Some analgesics depress the propulsive action of the intestine and increase sphincter tone and may predispose to further impaction or flatulence. Some tranquilizers cause vasodilatation, which may predispose to hypovolemic shock. Therefore, while recognizing that many horses in acute colic cannot be examined properly until some relief of pain has been accomplished, it is important to select drugs for control of pain that will accomplish the desired results without creating complications.

Once it has been determined that chemotherapeutic relief of pain is necessary or advisable, a choice of an agent must be made. The available groups of agents are the sedatives, the analgesics, the analgesic-sedatives, the antiprostaglandins, and the tranquilizers.

Chloral hydrate is an old standby and still an effective sedative for the horse. It is free from undesirable side effects in the cardiovascular and digestive systems. A 7 per cent solution given intravenously in a volume of 50 to 100 ml or to effect achieves standing sedation. The drug is extremely

TABLE 1. DRUGS AND MEDICATION USED IN THE MEDICAL MANAGEMENT OF COLIC

Trade Name	Generic Name	Manufacturer
Antiperistaltics		
Atropine	Atropine sulfate	Med-Tech, Inc.
Jenotone	Aminopropazine fumarate	Welcome Animal Health Products
Antiprostaglandins		
Banamine	Flunixin meglumine	Schering Corp.
Dipyrone (Novin)	Methampyrone	Haver-Lockhart
Butazolidin	Phenylbutazone	Welcome Animal Health Products
Intestinal Stimulants		
Stiglyn	Neostigmine methylsulfate	Pitman-Moore, Inc.
Panacol	d-pantothenyl alcohol	Western Serum Co.
Intestinal Lubricants		
Mineral oil		
Castor oil		
Cerusol-surfactant	Dioctyl sodium sulfosuccinate	Burns
Saline Cathartics		
Magnesium sulfate	Magnesium sulfate	
Sedatives and Tranquilizers		
Chloral hydrate		
Talwin	Pentazocine lactate	Winthrop Labs
Demerol	Meperidine	Wyeth Labs
Numorphan	Oxymorphone	Endo Labs
Rompun	Xylazine	Haver-Lockhart Labs
Promazine	Promazine hydrochloride	Ft. Dodge Labs
Acepromazine	Acepromazine maleate	Ayerst Labs
Antibiotics		
Neomycin sulfate		
Anthelmintics		
Omnizole	Thiabendazole	Merck & Co., Inc.

irritating if injected perivascularly. Given via nasogastric tube, chloral hydrate has a slower onset of action but may give more prolonged relief of pain. The usual oral dose is 50 to 60 gm.

The morphine derivatives are very effective analgesics for the colicky horse. They have no unfavorable cardiovascular side effects but may increase spastic contractions and decrease propulsive contractions of the intestine, which may not be desirable in some horses. Pentazocine (Talwin) is the mildest pain reliever in this group but has less of the undesirable effects on the intestinal tract. The usual dose is 0.4 mg per kg (0.2 mg per lb) body weight intravenously or intramuscularly. Meperidine (Demerol) and oxymorphone are controlled drugs requiring a narcotics license. They are very effective analgesics but occasionally produce undesirable excitement when given intravenously. The dosages are 4 mg per kg (2.0 mg per lb) for meperidine and .03 mg per kg (.015 mg per lb) for oxymorphone.

Xylazine (Rompun) is a very effective analgesic-sedative in the horse. When given intravenously, this drug produces its effect in approximately one minute, has no severe side effects on the cardiovascular or digestive system, and is very short-acting. The short action (15 to 30 minutes) is an advantage in most cases of colic, as it allows reevaluation of progress at more frequent intervals. This is especially important when vascular compromise and potential surgical intervention are anticipated. Failure of relief or extremely short relief of pain following the intravenous administration of xylazine is often an indication of a surgical colic. The dosage is 0.5 mg per kg body weight (0.25 mg per lb).

Tranquilizers are frequently used in the colicky horse. These drugs reduce anxiety but are not analgesics and, therefore, do not decrease pain. The phenothiazine tranquilizers have no undesirable effect on intestinal motility. However, as alpha blockers they cause peripheral vasodilation. This may, in the well-hydrated horse, increase perfusion of the intestine and visceral organs and may in fact help combat endotoxic shock and increase intestinal motility. However, if the horse is hypovolemic with indications of impending shock, the vasodilatation following administration of a phenothiazine tranquilizer is definitely contraindicated. The commonly used phenothiazine tranquilizers are promazine hydrochloride at 1.0 mg per kg (0.5 mg per lb) and acepromazine at .08 mg per kg (.04 mg per lb). These drugs, when given intravenously, are effective in 15 to 20 minutes and remain so for one to two hours.

The antiprostaglandins include aminopyrine (dipyrone), flunixin meglumine (Banamine), and phenylbutazone. These products have primarily an anti-inflammatory action. Dipyrone[2] is generally considered a mild pain reliever. In some controlled studies, it has had questionable effectiveness against visceral pain, although clinical impressions are that it is often valuable in mild pain. This drug may decrease nonpropulsive intestinal spasms but does not seem to decrease peristalsis, so side effects are minimal. Dipyrone may be given either intravenously or intramuscularly in dosages of 5 gm. Flunixin meglumine (Banamine) is reputed to have more effect on the gastrointestinal tract than the other antiprostaglandin drugs. It may be given intramuscularly or intravenously at the rate of 2 mg per kg (1 mg/lb) body weight. In our experience, this drug may be effective in 10 to 15 minutes and may provide relief of mild to moderate visceral pain for six to eight hours. Phenylbutazone is less effective in relieving pain from colic owing to its slower action. Peak effect may not be evident for two to three hours. This drug can be given only intravenously or orally. Perivascular injection results in a severe local reaction. Two gm per 450 kg is the recommended intravenous dose.

Different combinations of drugs for the relief of pain have been used to advantage. For example, a combination of acepromazine .04 mg per kg (.02 mg per lb) and pentazocine 0.3 mg per kg (0.15 mg per lb) has given both tranquilization and analgesia. Combining xylazine 0.5 mg per kg (0.25 mg per lb) and acepromazine .04 mg per kg (.02 mg per lb) has been shown to give relief for more than one hour. Acepromazine and chloral hydrate given intravenously provide prolonged relief in some cases. Xylazine 0.6 mg per kg (0.3 mg per lb) and flunixin meglumine 2 mg per kg (1 mg per lb) in combination have given prompt relief of pain with prolonged effect, especially in impaction colic. The drugs should not be mixed in the same syringe.

CORRECTION OF THE CAUSE OF DISTENTION OR SPASM

In correction of the cause of the increased intramural tension resulting in abdominal pain, it is first necessary to identify the cause as impaction, displacement, excessive fermentation, or spasm. A history of recent grain engorgement or dietary change

may be helpful. The duration, intensity, and persistence of pain along with the vital signs may be suggestive of the cause. Acutely developing, severe, unrelenting pain associated with increased heart rate and signs of impending shock suggests a displacement. However, excessive fermentation, especially gastric dilatation, may present a similar picture. Chronically developing, milder, intermittent pain suggests a large bowel impaction. Episodes of intense pain interspersed with periods of apparent normalcy suggest spasm as the cause. The patient's response to treatment and overall improvement are often rated on the abatement of pain. The inability to control pain is one of the most reliable criteria of the refractory intestinal obstruction that would indicate surgical intervention.

As a general rule, obstructions of the small intestine produce little abdominal distention, whereas obstructions in the large intestine produce great distention due to tympany in segments of the bowel.

Auscultation of the abdomen, rectal palpation, nasogastric tube passage, and abdominal paracentesis are important aids in determining the cause. Increased peristaltic sounds are more commonly associated with spasms and are less likely in displacements. Tinkling sounds associated with gas accumulation are more indicative of displacement or flatulence. The absence of sounds may be an initial response to pain and if continued, may point to a more serious condition. Rectal palpation may often confirm an impaction, displacement, or gastric dilatation. Reflux of an excess of gas or fluid from the nasogastric tube suggests gastric dilatation or high obstruction, such as volvulus of the small intestine. Changes in the peritoneal fluid may suggest arterial thromboembolism or venous occlusion, which is associated with displacement.

If a displacement is diagnosed, the only treatment is surgical intervention. The remainder of this discussion will deal with the treatment of nonsurgical colic.

IMPACTIONS

The primary goal in the treatment of impactions is to move the obstructing mass into a viscus with a larger lumen or out in the feces. Various substances are used to lubricate, moisten, or penetrate the impacting mass.

Mineral oil in a dose of 1/2 to 1 gal via stomach tube for a 450 kg horse has been a standard treatment. It is safer to give mineral oil by gravity rather than by stomach pump. In addition to lubricating masses and aiding the movement of ingesta, mineral oil has some protective action and may absorb some toxins. The use of mineral oil is seldom contraindicated in any colic. It is of no value in gastric dilatation or displacement but will cause little harm unless administered under pressure. Most surgeons do not feel that the presence of mineral oil in the intestinal tract interferes markedly should the horse become a surgical case. Reflux of mineral oil via nasogastric tube several hours after its administration is indicative of a high obstruction or ileus, and passage of oil in the feces generally indicates that there is no displacement, thus aiding in differential diagnosis. Patience and patient monitoring are essential requirements in treating large intestinal impactions, as several to many hours may be required to correct the problem.

Surface active agents such as dioctyl sodium sulfosuccinate (DSS) or dioctyl calcium sulfosuccinate (Surfak) act as stool softeners by lowering surface tension. This is thought to facilitate penetration of the fecal mass by water and fats. The dose is 8 oz of a 5 per cent solution in 1/2 gal water for a 450 kg horse. Surface active agents should not be mixed with mineral oil, as this may promote the absorption of oil emboli. To our knowledge, this has not been demonstrated in the horse but has been shown in humans.

Saline cathartics are soluble salts of poorly absorbed ions. Various proprietary preparations are combinations of several ions, but the total number rather than the variety of ions is what is important. Saline cathartics tend to hold water in the intestinal tract and may increase peristalsis. Their action is primarily in the small intestine. In horses that are in a preshock state, the action of surface active agents and saline cathartics in holding water in the lumen of the bowel may predispose to shock. Drastic purgatives are seldom used today and are contraindicated in horses with severe colic or signs of serious intestinal obstruction or both.

Warm water alone via stomach tube may help to soften an impaction and appears to encourage intestinal motility. In low impactions, such as those involving the transverse or small colon, warm saline enemas may be helpful. Saline solutions are preferred, as water enemas may cause edema of the intestinal wall.

After measures have been taken to soften an impaction, it may be desirable to stimulate peristalsis. However, intestinal stimulants are contraindicated in severe impactions and in displacements. Pain may be increased following the use of an intestinal stimulant.

Neostigmine combines with cholinesterase and exaggerates cholinergic stimuli. It will cause some cramping and is a potentially dangerous drug if there is a displacement. The action is dose-related, so repeated small doses may be used with some safety following lubrication of an impaction. The usual dose is 2 mg per 100 kg (1 mg per 100 lb); however, we have found 0.4 mg per 100 kg (0.2 mg per 100 lb) repeated at 30-minute intervals to be effective.

SPASM

Antiperistaltic drugs will decrease spasms to the intestine, but their use is quite limited and frequently contraindicated, as it is generally undesirable to decrease intestinal motility. Hypomotility always creates a potential for impaction or flatulent colic. Antiperistaltics that have been used are atropine and aminopropazine fumarate (Jenotone). Atropine is contraindicated in most cases. In addition to decreasing motility, it reduces secretions and definitely predisposes to impaction and flatulence. Jenotone, a smooth muscle relaxant, will decrease motility for several hours. Its usefulness is limited to unusual and specific instances.

In the great majority of spasmodic colic cases, it is best to relieve pain until the spasms pass without attempting to alter intestinal motility.

EXCESSIVE FERMENTATION

In the horse with severe flatulence and gas distention, it may be necessary to decompress the horse mechanically. This may be done via stomach tube if there is excessive gas buildup in the stomach, or it may be done by trocharization of the cecum or other distended bowel. Relieving gaseous distention reduces pain and decreases the potential for venous occlusion. It may be a life-saving procedure in severe distention (p. 237). Decompression via trocharization should be used only if the paralumbar fossae are obviously distended. It should be taken into consideration that the character of the abdominal fluid will be changed shortly after trocharization so that the value of abdominal paracentesis for diagnosis is decreased.

Antifermentatives are sometimes used in colicky horses. The goal is to reduce gas production, thus reducing distention, pain, and venous occlusion. These compounds break foam down into a single large bubble. In the ruminant, where eructation is possible, this may be of value; however, usefulness in the horse is questionable. Antibiotics are commonly used as antifermentatives with neomycin being the most popular. The mode of action is to eliminate or decrease the bacterial flora within the intestinal tract. Some clinicians question the use of antibiotics, as there is no way to control the numbers of bacteria eliminated for gas control or left viable for normal digestion.

In addition to their possible antifermentative action, there is evidence that the use of antibiotics may reduce the production of bacterial products (endotoxins) involved in the development of septic shock.

CHEMOTHERAPY OF VERMINOUS ARTERITIS

Most authorities agree that a very high percentage of colic is at least indirectly due to the effects of migrating larvae of *Strongylus vulgaris* in the mesenteric arteries. There has been intense interest in methods of killing these larvae or preventing the arterial reaction to them. Methods used to kill strongyle larvae are described on page 278.

EXERCISE

There is no evidence that walking a colicky horse increases intestinal motility or relieves pain. Walking the horse may occupy its attention and prevent injury and possibly displacement from rolling and thrashing. Contrary to a common lay conception, it is permissible to allow the horse to lie down. If the horse is more comfortable or at least not violent, recumbency and rest are advantageous. Exercise may predispose to shock in the hypovolemic animal.

Medical management of colic in the horse involves well over 90 per cent of all cases presented for treatment, with the remainder being surgical candidates. It becomes obvious, therefore, that a thorough clinical examination to determine the cause and location of abdominal pain is essential. Equally as important is the selection of medications that will act directly to alleviate the cause and relieve pain without untoward side effects. The methods and medications presented in this article do not include all drugs used now and in the past in the treatment of colic. It does, however, include those used with the greatest confidence and predictability by the authors and many other clinicians.

References

1. Anderson, N. V.: Veterinary Gastroenterology. Philadelphia, Lea & Febiger, 1980.
2. Drudge, J. H.: Clinical aspects of *Strongylus vulgaris* Infection in the Horse. Emphasis on diagnosis, chemotherapy and prophylaxis. Vet. Clin. North Am., Large Anim. Pract., 1:251, 1979.
3. Gray, G. W., and Yano, B. L.: A study of the actions of methampyrone and of a commercial intestinal extract on intestinal motility. Am. J. Vet. Res., 36:201, 1975.

SMALL BOWEL OBSTRUCTION

Eric P. Tulleners, KENNETT SQUARE, PENNSYLVANIA

Intestinal obstruction exists whenever the luminal contents of the gastrointestinal tract are prevented from passing distally.[2] Obstructions may result from mechanical occlusion (intraluminal, mural, or extraluminal lesions) or from adynamic ileus.

Simple obstruction is a compromise of the lumen of the bowel without compromise of its vascular supply. Fluids, electrolytes, and gases accumulate proximal to the obstruction, while distally the bowel is flaccid. Vascular compromise is limited to impairment of the intramural circulation caused by increased intraluminal pressure.[2] Sustained pressures, although seemingly small in magnitude, may produce changes in the bowel ranging from petechial hemorrhages to necrosis. Small bowel distention creates a vicious cycle of decreased intestinal absorption and increased secretion. Approximately half of the plasma volume may be sequestered in the lumen in 18 to 23 hours. As distention progresses, intestinal motility decreases progressively.

Strangulation obstruction results from a compromise of the vascular supply to the bowel with or without compromise of its lumen. Fluid and electrolyte losses still occur proximally; however, the cause of death revolves around pathologic changes in the closed loop itself. Intraluminal blood loss approaches 30 to 50 per cent of blood volume if one fifth to one third of the small intestine is strangulated. The gangrenous intestinal wall soon becomes permeable to bacteria and their byproducts, resulting in peritonitis, severe toxemia, and rapid death.

The incidence of mild abdominal pain (spasmodic, flatulent, or impactive colic) is unknown. Certainly it is high, and the vast majority of colic cases (85 to 90 per cent) respond to conservative medical therapy consisting of analgesics or cathartics or both. However, distention, alterations in motility, and pain may lead to more serious conditions. The animal's rolling may displace the bowel or initiate formation of a strangulating lesion such as volvulus, torsion, or intussusception. By virtue of its long mesentery and free-floating small intestine, the

TABLE 1. CLASSIFICATION AND EXAMPLES OF SMALL INTESTINAL OBSTRUCTIONS

I. Mechanical obstructions

Simple

A. Intraluminal
1. Ascarid impaction
2. Foreign bodies
3. Phytoliths
4. Polyps
B. Mural
1. Ileal hypertrophy
2. Hematomas, abscesses
3. Proximal duodenal strictures (foals)
C. Extraluminal
1. Congenital strictures
a. Atresias
b. Imperforations
c. Nonstrangulating mesodiverticular bands
d. Meckel's diverticulum
2. Acquired strictures
a. Inflammatory
—secondary to helminth larval migration
—peritonitis (usually bacterial)
b. Trauma
c. Neoplasia
3. Compression
a. Space-occupying tumors
b. Intra-abdominal abscesses
c. Displaced large bowel

Strangulating

A. Internal hernias
1. Mesentery of small intestine
2. Gastrosplenic mesentery
3. Epiploic foramen
4. Cecocolic mesentery
5. Mesentery of large colon
6. Broad ligament of uterus
7. Mesodiverticular bands
8. Meckel's diverticulum
9. Greater omentum
10. Nephrosplenic ligament
11. Diaphragmatic hernias
B. External hernias
1. Umbilical
2. Inguinal
C. Pedunculated lipomas
D. Intussusception
E. Volvulus
F. Inflammatory adhesions and fibrous bands
G. Arterial thrombosis

II. Paralytic ileus
A. Primary
B. Secondary
1. Surgery (esp. abdominal)
2. Peritonitis
3. Hypokalemia
4. After relief of a simple or strangulating obstruction

horse's bowel also has the ability to become obstructed (often with strangulation) in a wide variety of locations (Table 1).

Small intestinal impactions are rare and limited to ascarid impactions (p. 262) and phytoliths. The helminth *Strongylus vulgaris* infects virtually every horse, and anterior mesenteric arteritis resulting in arterial thrombosis is another cause of obstruction (p. 267).

CLINICAL EVALUATION

Potentially fatal small bowel obstructions are common enough to be included in the differential diagnosis of all cases of colic. Many owners are unwilling or unable to entertain the expense of surgery, but an accurate, *early* diagnosis is imperative if referral to a surgical facility is being contemplated. Cases that do not respond to initial medical therapy should be completely and critically reevaluated every three to four hours. A delay in surgical intervention of even 12 to 18 hours may be fatal in cases of strangulating obstructions.

DIAGNOSIS OF SMALL INTESTINAL OBSTRUCTION

Even in this era of the extensive use of sophisticated ancillary laboratory data, signalment, history, and physical examination remain the cornerstones of diagnosis.

SIGNALMENT

Breed differences in small bowel obstruction have not been observed. Sex-related incidence is confined to anatomic differences, namely, inguinal hernias in intact males and incarceration through tears in the broad ligament of the uterus in females. Population studies indicate that small intestinal obstructions occur equally in males, geldings, and females.

Age relationships are helpful but not conclusive. Epiploic foramen incarcerations are generally not observed before seven years of age. Pedunculated lipoma is a disease of older horses with a mean age of 15 years.[8] Rents in the gastrosplenic mesentery tend to occur in older horses. The majority of intussusceptions and ascarid impactions are seen in horses less than two years old. Atresias, meconium impactions (p. 260), and imperforations will become evident in the neonate, and duodenal strictures, although rare, are seen in suckling foals.

History

History includes the medical history and management practices. Management involves parasite control, nutrition, feeding practices, housing, use, and work schedule. Poor parasite control (including high stocking rates, poor sanitation, and infrequent or ineffective worming) can lead to ascarid impactions and infarctive diseases caused by *Strongylus vulgaris* at as early as four months of age. This problem appears to be particularly prevalent on large broodmare farms where numbers of mares and foals run together on contaminated pastures. Irregular feeding schedules, poor-quality feeds, and exhaustion from overuse or hard work have been incriminated in symptomatic colic. Well-managed farms where all these variables are controlled rarely have a problem with colic.

Prior medical history concerning illness (especially previous bouts of colic) or injuries may be important. For example, recurrent bouts of abdominal pain have been seen in horses with mesodiverticular bands, partial arterial thrombosis (p. 238), and inflammatory conditions producing fibrous bands, adhesions, and abdominal abscesses. Foaling mares may develop incarceration through holes in the broad ligament caused by the foal's foot during parturition. Stallions may develop inguinal hernias after breeding a mare. Several Standardbred colts have suffered from inguinal hernias following routine work or a race. Ascarid impactions in heavily infected foals have been seen following routine worming.

The immediate past history should include a discussion of the duration and intensity of pain, appetite, urination, defecation, and response to medication.

Pain resulting from spasmodic motility and distention, either proximal to a small bowel obstruction or in a closed loop, tends to be severe and unrelenting. Deterioration is rapid (6 to 12 hours). Many horses will become depressed and somnolent after several hours as vascular compromise becomes complete and the bowel suffers from ischemic necrosis. Intermittent (even for prolonged periods such as days) or mild and transient pain usually suggests a noninfarctive lesion and the possibility for medical therapy.

Horses with small bowel obstruction may exhibit a complete disregard for themselves and handlers. They attempt to relieve pain by throwing themselves on the ground, rolling violently, pawing incessantly, or assuming unnatural positions, such as dog sitting, lying on their backs, or leaning against solid structures. Rarely are mild signs observed, even in stoic individuals. It is often possible to correlate the severity of the lesion by how badly the horse has abused itself, as indicated by abrasions over bony prominences. Foals may be particularly difficult to deal with and may prefer to remain recumbent.

Water and feed intake usually falls to nearly zero. Some horses will "play" in the water bucket as an expression of pain. Many horses will posture to urinate and appear to strain, repeating this process over and over and yet will pass very little urine. As hypovolemia becomes more severe, the glomerular filtration rate decreases, and very little urine is produced. Defecation may occur but infrequently, and the volume of feces is decreased. Defecation may continue for 12 to 24 hours until the large colon empties or total ileus intercedes.

Commonly used analgesics may be ineffective or may only transiently control pain, especially in strangulating obstructions. Use of cathartics (such as mineral oil) may exacerbate the condition as the fluid pools in the stomach, increasing the distention and pain.

CLINICAL SIGNS

Temperature is usually normal to slightly elevated (<102.5° F) but may be subnormal in shock. An elevated temperature may warn of a bacterial peritonitis due to devitalized or ruptured bowel or an impending enteritis.

The pulse (rate and quality) reflects the cardiovascular status and amount of pain. A consistently elevated, weak pulse indicates hypovolemia and shock. Mucous membranes and capillary refill time (CRT) reflect the degree and quality of peripheral perfusion. A CRT of 1 to 2 seconds with pink, warm, moist mucous membranes is normal. Bright red mucous membranes with normal CRT is seen early in the vasodilatory stage of shock. Injected, muddy, dry mucous membranes with an elevated CRT reflect the vasoconstrictive phase of shock characterized by decreased peripheral perfusion and a toxemic state. Cool, blue, or ashen mucous membranes are seen terminally. A pale, washed-out color with an increased CRT may be seen in some strangulating lesions with extensive intraluminal loss of blood. The ocular sclera is injected. The extremities (ears and feet) become cool as conditions deteriorate. Respiration may be rapid and deep owing to metabolic acidosis.

TABLE 2. ANALYSIS OF EQUINE PERITONEAL FLUID (SUGGESTED GUIDELINES FOR ESTIMATING INFLAMMATORY RESPONSE IN THE PERITONEAL CAVITY)

Determination	Normal	Suspected Inflammation	Moderate Inflammation	Severe Inflammation
Total WBC	500–5000	5000–15,000	15,000–60,000	60,000 plus
Total protein (Gm/dl)	0.5–1.5	1.6–2.5	2.6–4.0	4.0
Color	Yellow	Yellow-red	Yellow-red	Yellow-red
Turbidity	Clear	Slightly cloudy	Cloudy	Cloudy

(From Nelson, A. W.: Analysis of equine peritoneal fluid. Vet. Clin. North Am., Large Anim. Pract., *1*(2):273, 1979.)

ABDOMINAL EVALUATION

Abdominal distention is not a feature of small bowel disease. Borborygmi are increased in spasmodic colic and in the early stages of small bowel obstruction, especially in foals. Hypomotility or total ileus generally indicates a more serious condition. As gas and fluid accumulate under tension, high-pitched tinkling sounds may be heard. External digital palpation of the abdomen is a useful technique only in young foals.

Nasogastric intubation will relieve fluid and gaseous distention. Generally, high obstructions (duodenum and proximal jejunum) produce large volumes of fluid reflux. Gastric pH is 4 to 5, while small intestinal reflux has a pH of 6 to 8. Bloody or malodorous brownish fluid may indicate a strangulating obstruction.

Rectal examination should be methodical and complete to avoid missing a life-threatening lesion. Straining may be at least partially overcome by sedation with xylazine (0.4 to 0.8 mg per kg intravenously), use of a twitch, having an assistant firmly pull the horse's tongue out, or by using lidocaine jelly on the obstetrical sleeve. In the normal horse, discrete loops of small bowel are not identifiable. In a high obstruction, distended loops will not be within reach. Lower, midjejunum to ileal obstructions result in distended loops of bowel. The small intestine is identified by its round, smooth exterior and 5 to 10 cm diameter, which is compressible to varying degrees depending on the amount of distention. A taut mesentery with even one loop of small intestine attached suggests an incarceration. Careful examination will often reveal a painful area where abnormalities can be identified. Bowel entering an inguinal ring can be palpated. Rarely can an exact diagnosis be made, but rectal findings will usually distinguish between a surgical and nonsurgical problem.

Abdominocentesis should be performed in nonresponsive cases, as abnormal peritoneal fluid appears within hours in strangulating lesions. A dependent site 5 to 10 cm to the right of midline may be preferable in order to avoid the spleen. An 18 gauge 1½ to 2 in needle using aseptic technique is usually effective. If multiple loops of tightly distended small intestine are palpated per rectum, it may be preferable to use a blunt metal teat cannula to prevent linear lacerations in a devitalized loop of intestine. Use of a twitch or xylazine or both is helpful in avoiding this problem. Accidental point penetration of bowel has not caused problems. The interpretation of abdominal fluid analysis is summarized in Table 2 and discussed in detail on page 233.

HEMATOLOGY

Serial monitoring of packed cell volume and total protein provide valuable information concerning the state of hydration and response to intravenous fluids. A total white blood cell count and differential are indicated if surgery is being considered (see relative contraindications to surgery).

Blood gases and electrolytes are used in nonresponsive or surgical cases in which it is important to identify and replace specific deficits, especially K^+, HCO_3^-, and Ca^{++}. In the absence of laboratory data, the following guidelines can be used.

A hypochloremic and hypokalemic metabolic alkalosis will result from a duodenal or proximal jejunal obstruction. Large amounts of fluid are lost into the bowel in lower bowel obstructions, but electrolytes are usually normal. If a serious disease proceeds without proper medication, a metabolic acidosis develops.

Fluid losses result in hemoconcentration, decreased glomerular filtration rate, and prerenal azotemia. Continued relative ischemia, potentiated by the use of halothane anesthesia and potentially nephrotoxic drugs such as aminoglycoside antibiotics and phenylbutazone warrant serial creatinine determinations in surgical cases.

THERAPY

An understanding of the pathophysiology of small intestinal obstructions allows for formulation of a rational therapeutic approach.[4]

Analgesics. Analgesics should be given to suppress pain. Ideally a diagnosis will have been reached prior to administering analgesics (as they alter vital parameters); however, this may not be possible in an animal suffering from extreme pain.

GROUP 1 (MILD TO MODERATE PAIN). In the majority of nonobstructed cases, dipyrone (50 per cent, 11 mg per kg, 5 mg per lb intravenously, and 11 mg per kg, 5 mg per lb intramuscularly)* appears clinically to be an effective spasmolytic. Nonsteroidal anti-inflammatory drugs such as phenylbutazone (4 to 9 mg per kg, 2 to 4 mg per lb intravenously)† or flunixin meglumine (1.1 mg per kg, 0.5 mg per lb intravenously)‡ are also effective in relieving mild to moderate visceral pain.

GROUP 2 (MODERATE TO SEVERE PAIN). As a general rule, if relief is not obtained in 30 to 60 min, then xylazine (0.5 to 1.0 mg per kg, 0.2 to 0.4 mg per lb intravenously or intramuscularly),§ pentazocine (0.4 mg per kg, 0.15 mg per lb intravenously)‖ or meperidine (1.1 mg per kg, 0.5 mg per lb intravenously with or without 1.1 mg per kg, 0.5 mg per lb intramuscularly)** are the next logical choices. Xylazine is the drug of choice in spite of its relatively short duration of action. It is usually extremely effective in providing sedation and may be repeated as needed (up to once an hour) to control intractable pain. Xylazine may also be given intramuscularly by clients. Xylazine may decrease an elevated heart rate back to the normal range, so caution must be exercised in evaluating clinical improvement.

GROUP 3 (SEVERE PAIN). Chloral hydrate (18 mg per kg, 8 mg per lb intravenously or to effect) may be used in severe, unrelenting pain to provide sufficient sedation and hypnosis to prevent the horse from self-mutilation and from injuring handlers. It is generally used as a last resort in intractable cases and must be given through a catheter or large-bore needle owing to the phlebitis produced by accidental perivascular injection.

If repeated doses of xylazine or other Group 2 drugs are required, then the animal should be carefully reevaluated for the possibility of an obstructing lesion. Continuous, severe pain is a warning that a life-threatening lesion exists.

Phenothiazine derivative tranquilizers (such as acepromazine) should *not* be given in an acute, undifferentiated abdominal crisis. They are potent peripheral vasodilators that will potentiate hypovolemic shock in an animal with a contracted extracellular volume.

---

*Novin, Haver-Lockhart, Shawnee, KS
†Butazolidin, Jensen Salsbery, Kansas City, MO
‡Banamine, Schering, Kenilworth, NJ
§Rompun, Haver-Lockhart, Shawnee, KS
‖ Talwin, Winthrop Labs, New York, NY
** Demerol, Winthrop Labs, New York, NY

Nasogastric Decompression. This procedure should be attempted in every case. Often fluid will reflux from the tube under pressure, indicating distention of the stomach. Unlike humans and most animals, certain anatomic features make it virtually impossible for the horse to regurgitate. Relieving gaseous and fluid distention will often make the horse more comfortable, improve vital parameters, and minimize the risk of a ruptured stomach. If fluid is not obtained, priming the tube with warm water followed by the application of vigorous suction from a large (16 oz) stainless steel dose syringe will create a siphon effect. This maneuver should be attempted several times before and after the tube is manipulated, as it often requires time and patience before fluid is retrieved. The tube may be left in place and taped to the halter. Continuous reflux of a volume of fluid, especially bloody or malodorous, signals intestinal obstruction. Failure to produce fluid does not rule out an obstructing lesion; if the pain continues, try again later. *No* oral medication of any kind should ever be given to a horse that is refluxing fluid, as this may exacerbate the condition and cause further deterioration.

Balanced Polyionic Solutions. Given intravenously, these solutions are effective in replacing fluids and electrolytes lost due to gastric reflux, sweating, urination, defecation, respiration, and cessation of oral intake of fluid during colic. Rapid extracellular volume expansion will combat dehydration, hemoconcentration, and hypovolemic shock and will improve tissue perfusion, venous return, cardiac output, and blood pressure. Normosol* or lactated Ringer's solution administered through a 14-gauge catheter secured to the neck with elastic tape may be given as rapidly as desired without deleterious effects. Volume adjustments are judged by clinical response, indicated by improving pulse, color, capillary refill time, PCV, total protein, skin turgor, and urine output. Slow intravenous administration of 50 gm (596 mEq per l) of sodium bicarbonate will buffer a mild acidemia. This amount of bicarbonate may be given empirically if blood gases are not available. If blood gases are available, replacement can be calculated in the following manner:

$$\text{bw (in kg)} \times 0.3 \times \text{base deficit} = \text{mEq NaHCO}_3$$

Equilibration in the extracellular fluid requires about 30 min. If measurements of serum electrolytes are available, specific deficiencies may be calculated in a similar fashion by taking into consideration the volume of distribution of each electrolyte (p. 202).

Gastrointestinal stimulants such as neostigmine or carbachol should not be used, as the intense con-

---

*Normosol, Abbott Labs, N. Chicago, IL

tractions of the intestine produced may cause additional pain or rupture in a distended, devitalized section of bowel. These drugs are of questionable efficacy even in cases of ileus.

Broad-Spectrum Antibiotics. These are indicated if an intestinal obstruction is suspected, especially if surgery is being considered. They must be effective against a wide range of gram-positive, gram-negative, and anaerobic organisms. Antibiotics will suppress bacterial growth, prolong the integrity of the bowel wall, and, therefore, delay the migration, absorption, and systemic manifestation of toxic factors.

Procaine penicillin G (22,000 units per kg, 10,000 units per lb intramuscularly twice a day), potassium or sodium penicillin (44,000 units per kg, 20,000 units per lb intravenously four times a day), or ampicillin (11 mg per kg, 5 mg per lb intramuscularly four times a day) and an aminoglycoside such as neomycin (5 mg per kg, 2.5 mg per lb intramuscularly three times a day),* kanamycin (5 mg per kg, 2.5 mg per lb intramuscularly three times a day),† or gentamicin (2.2 mg per kg, 1 mg per lb intramuscularly four times a day)‡ have been efficacious if begun prior to surgery and continued for five days. Chloramphenicol (10 to 25 mg per kg, 5 to 10 mg per lb intravenously four times a day)§ may also be effective. High levels of tetracycline, which have been incriminated in cases of enteritis due to alterations in gastrointestinal flora caused by enterohepatic excretion, should probably not be used.

Corticosteroids. These have been shown to have a beneficial effect in endotoxic shock and may be useful in cases in which a strangulating lesion is suspected. Doses are empirical; 1 gm of prednisolone sodium succinate intravenously‖ has been given with seemingly beneficial effects. Dexamethasone (100 mg intravenously) has also been used and repeated as conditions warranted.

SURGICAL TREATMENT

The decision to perform an exploratory celiotomy must be based on the composite clinical picture (Table 3). Careful consideration of signalment, history, physical findings, ancillary laboratory data, and response to medical therapy will lead to a rational decision. Mistakes are made when excessive weight is placed on one parameter (for example, the heart rate must be above 60?, 80?, 100?). The reverse,

however, is also true; sometimes the decision to perform surgery must be based solely on rectal findings, abdominocentesis, or a variety of other parameters. This is due to individual variations in expression of pain, response to medication, and other factors. The decision should not be delayed until the condition is hopeless.

Surgery should not be performed if severe peritonitis secondary to devitalized or ruptured bowel exists. Clinical warning signs include (1) somnolence, shaking, trembling, diffuse sweating, or suddenly becoming "quiet" after an extremely painful bout; (2) rigid, splinted abdomen; (3) reluctance to move or walk; (4) high fever and leukopenia—this may also warn of a nonsurgical lesion such as Salmonella enteritis; (5) ingesta and bacterial contamination on repeated abdominocentesis (beware of iatrogenic contamination); (6) grittiness, tears, or feces in the abdomen palpable on rectal examination.

Relative contraindications for surgery include (1) PCV of 60 to 65—extremely poor prognosis, 65 to 70, invariably fatal; (2) heart rate consistently greater than 100, usually accompanied by severely injected or cyanotic mucous membranes and a greatly elevated PCV and capillary refill time; (3) abdominocentesis—a white cell count of 80,000 to 100,000 may indicate peritonitis and not a surgical lesion; (4) rectal tears—unless a colostomy is indicated.

During transportation to a surgical facility, a stomach tube should be taped in place if reflux has occurred. The horse should be given ample room to lie down but should be given sufficient analgesics or sedatives to prevent rolling. Fluids may be continued and antibiotics begun.

Surgery should be performed under general (inhalation) anesthesia, utilizing positive pressure ventilation, in a clean room under conditions of asepsis. An adequate number of well-trained personnel (a minimum of two surgeons, one anesthetist, and two nurses) and adequate monitoring facilities (for blood gases, electrolytes, and routine hematology) are necessary for a successful effort. Aggressive, well-executed surgery is vitally important; however, many cases are saved or lost depending on the quality of postoperative care. Excellent descriptions of approaches, intraoperative technique, and postoperative care exist.[9]

PREVENTION

Prevention of small bowel obstruction is based on sound management. A parasite control program should be in effect on all farms (p. 276). Good-quality feed and hay should be fed at regular, nonvarying intervals. Fresh water and mineral supplements

---

*Biosol, Upjohn Co., Kalamazoo, MI
†Kantrim, Bristol Labs, Syracuse, NY
‡Gentocin, Schering, Kenilworth, NJ
§Chloromycetin, Parke Davis, Morris Plains, NJ
‖Solu-Delta-Cortef, Upjohn Co., Kalamazoo, MI

TABLE 3. THERAPEUTIC GUIDELINES FOR SMALL INTESTINAL OBSTRUCTIONS

Parameter	Indications for Surgery	Indications for Further Evaluation	Indications for Medical Management
Onset and course	Sudden with severe signs Rapid, abrupt deterioration in condition Refractory to treatment	Intermediate in onset and variable course—slow improvement, maybe chronic	Gradual onset with mild to moderate signs, but predictable, improving with time and therapy
Cardiovascular status Heart rate Pulse	Consistently elevated Weak, thready, not palpable	Cardiovascular status may be normal or only slightly abnormal early in the disease or after medication. Continue regular monitoring (at least every 2 hrs)	Normal to mildly elevated Strong, regular
Mucous membranes	Injected, cyanotic, red, or pale		Pink, pale pink, slightly injected or reddened
Capillary refill time	Usually elevated; may be normal in early vasodilatory stage of shock		Normal to slightly elevated
Extremities	Cold, poor skin turgor		Warm, normal turgor
Hematocrit	Usually elevated; may be radically elevated		Normal to mild elevation (splenic contraction)
Total protein	Usually elevated; may be normal or low in strangulating lesions due to protein sequestration		Normal to mild elevation
Nasogastric reflux	Positive; especially large volumes; bloody and foul-smelling; continuous small amounts of bloody fluid		Absent or very small
Pain	Severe or unrelenting; depression late in the disease	Low-grade, continued or intermittent pain	Relief provided by medication, improving with time
Intestinal motility	Hypomotile or ileus; abdominal distention (large colon)	Hypomotile or early hypermotility (spastic small bowel); not distended	Good or improving with time; not distended
Rectal signs	Palpable loops of small bowel or palpable lesion; scant feces	Suspect lesion; recheck later; get another opinion if possible	Feces in the rectum; no distention or palpable lesions
Abdominocentesis	Serosanguineous, increased volume, WBC, RBC, and protein	Normal early in disease process, recheck later or perform in a different site (regional disease)	Normal
Response to medication	Poor or continued deterioration; signs of shock worsening in spite of fluids, HCO_3^-, analgesics, and corticosteroids	Some relief but premonition of shock still exists or response transient (i.e., requires additional analgesics and intravenous fluids)	Improving with time

must be available. Avoid overuse, extreme stress, or exhaustion. Many types of strangulating lesions are simply chance occurrences and cannot be avoided.

References

1. Donawick, W. J.: Metabolic management of the horse with an acute abdominal crisis. J. South Afr. Vet. Assoc., 46(1):107, 1975.

2. Jones, R. S.: Intestinal obstruction. *In* Sabiston, D. C., Jr. (ed.): Textbook of Surgery, 10th ed. Philadelphia, W. B. Saunders Co., 1972, pp. 880–889.

3. Kohn, C.: Preparative management of the equine patient with an abdominal crisis. Vet Clin. North Am., Large Anim. Pract., 1(2):289, 1979.

4. Meagher, D.: Intestinal strangulations in the horse. Presented to the Second Annual Surgical Forum of the American College of Veterinary Surgeons, Chicago, IL, 1974.

5. Nelson, A. W.: Analysis of equine peritoneal fluid. Vet. Clin. North Am., Large Anim. Pract., *1*(2):267, 1979.
6. Smith, D.: Presurgical care of the equine colic patient. Cornell Vet., *68*(7):113, 1978.
7. Stashak, T.: Clinical evaluation of the equine colic patient. Vet Clin. North Am., Large Anim. Pract., *1*(2):275, 1979.
8. Tennant, B., Wheat, J. D., and Meagher, D. M.: Observations on the causes and incidence of acute intestinal obstruction in the horse. Proc. 18th Annu. Meet. Am. Assoc. Eq. Pract., pp. 251–257, 1972.
9. Vaughn, J. T.: Surgical management of abdominal crisis in the horse. J. Am. Vet. Med. Assoc., *161*:1199, 1972.

LARGE BOWEL OBSTRUCTION

James Orsini, KENNETT SQUARE, PENNSYLVANIA

Large bowel obstruction prevents transit of intestinal contents toward the rectum. A physical barrier obstructing the lumen of the bowel is classified as a mechanical obstruction. Physiologic abnormalities that impede normal transit, termed functional obstructions, are not commonly appreciated as a cause of intestinal obstruction. Mechanical obstructions are subclassified as either (1) simple mechanical obstruction, in which there is a single point of obstruction, or (2) closed loop obstruction, in which two points of obstruction are present so that a segment of bowel cannot be decompressed by either the normal aboral transit or by progressive dilation of intestine proximal to the obstructed segment.

ETIOLOGY

The causes of large bowel obstruction are given in Table 1. Congenital anomalies and meconium plugs (p. 260) are seen only in neonates, whereas neoplasms are seen most often in aged horses[5, 6] (p. 259). The other causes of obstruction occur in animals of all ages.

Causes of ileus are numerous, the most common being peritonitis and abdominal surgery. Hypokalemia, hypocalcemia, and vascular insufficiency also contribute to postoperative ileus.

PATHOPHYSIOLOGY

Storage and absorption of large volumes of fluid are the most important functions of the equine large bowel. The large intestine contains, on the average, 75 per cent of the total gastrointestinal water. Eight hours after feeding, the fluid content of the large bowel comprises one third of the animal's extracellular fluid. During a 24-hour period, the large bowel recovers a volume of water approximately equal to the total extracellular volume. Failure to recover this fluid volume leads to fatal hypovolemia and electrolyte and acid-base imbalances. The patho-

physiology of large bowel obstructions is greatly dependent on the cause of the obstruction. Impactions that may still allow passage of fluids distal to the site of obstruction result in a prolonged sequence of events that may last for several days. In contrast, complete obstruction of the bowel by herniation or volvulus produces peracute colic with rapid deterioration of the horse's condition.

Following obstruction, the bowel becomes progressively distended. Intraenteric pressure increases and causes a decreased flux of water and sodium from intestinal lumen to blood (insorption) and occasionally an increased flux from blood to lumen (exsorption). Increased intraluminal pressure also impairs venous drainage of the bowel, resulting in the edematous, boggy appearance of the tissues of the obstructed segment. A portion of this fluid

TABLE 1. ETIOLOGY OF LARGE BOWEL OBSTRUCTION

Congenital anomalies	Ileus (pseudo-obstruction)
Atresia of large or small colon	Flatulent
	Spastic (Ogilvie's syndrome)
Atresia ani	Meconium plug syndrome
Volvulus	Internal hernia
Large colon	Intussusception
Cecum	Cecocolic
Impaction/obstipation	Colonic
Cecum	Displacement
Pelvic flexure	Large colon (ascending colon)
Transverse colon	Cecum
Small colon	Organic causes
Vascular	Neoplasms
Thrombosis and embolic infarction of the mesenteric arteries	Adhesions
	Abscesses
	Fibrous bands
Intestinal concretions	Procidentia of the rectum (prolapse)
Enteroliths	Outflow obstruction
Phytotrichobezoars	Cecocolic valve
Trichobezoars	
Conglobates	
Foreign bodies	
Fibrous	
Sand	

exudes from the serosal surface of the large bowel into the peritoneal cavity. Fluid losses into the bowel lumen and parenchyma and into the peritoneal cavity can be extensive. In an acute large bowel obstruction, 36 per cent of the plasma volume may be lost intraluminally in four to six hours, and up to 50 per cent of the plasma volume may be lost after 18 to 24 hours. With prolonged large bowel obstruction, regurgitation may ensue, further contributing to fluid and electrolyte loss. The net effect of these losses is contraction of the extracellular fluid compartment. The resultant fall in plasma volume leads to hemoconcentration, decreased cardiac output, compensatory vasoconstriction, decreased central venous pressure, decreased glomerular filtration rate, prerenal azotemia, oliguria, tissue hypoxemia, and metabolic acidosis. The severity of the electrolyte and acid-base changes is directly related to the duration of the obstruction.

The distended bowel elevates the diaphragm, impairing portal circulation, central venous return, and respiratory function. This may contribute to the high incidence of pneumonitis, atelectasis, and respiratory failure observed in cases of prolonged bowel obstruction.

Bowel obstruction complicated by infarction usually results from a closed loop obstruction, which prevents decompression of the lumen retrograde; from a volvulus, which kinks the vascular supply; or from primary mesenteric arteritis. A simple obstruction, such as impaction, may on occasion result in volvulus of the edematous, heavy proximal bowel, converting it to a closed loop obstruction. In closed loop obstruction, there is leakage of bloody fluid from the bowel wall into the peritoneal cavity. This fluid is toxic owing to the presence of bacteria and bacterial endotoxins and exotoxins. The absorption of these substances and the resultant bacteremia lead to septic shock, characterized by hypotension, a decreased cardiac output, and metabolic acidosis.

The three most important factors that contribute to the death of patients with bowel strangulation are (1) fluid and electrolyte losses from bowel distention, (2) blood loss into the bowel lumen and peritoneal cavity, and (3) elaboration of toxic substances within the strangulated loop and their subsequent systemic absorption.

HISTORY

When examining a case of suspected bowel obstruction, the history should include the duration of the present illness, the number and frequency of recurrences, and the severity of signs. Impactions of the large bowel tend to be insidious in onset, as opposed to a volvulus, which is acute with constant pain. Environmental aspects of the history may reveal dietery, exercise, and stabling changes that could account for the presenting complaint. Congenital anomalies must be considered in a neonate.

CLINICAL SIGNS

The signs of large bowel obstruction depend on the nature of the obstruction and include abdominal pain, abnormal bowel sounds, constipation, obstipation (severe constipation) or diarrhea, and if the obstruction is of long duration, vomiting or regurgitation, weakness, dehydration, and occasionally dyspnea. Mechanical bowel obstruction characteristically elicits intermittent pain, which arises from a combination of stretching of smooth muscle in distended bowel segments and superimposed propulsive contractions. Constant, unrelenting pain is often associated with infarction. Necrotic segments of bowel should be suspected if fever and tachycardia accompany unrelenting pain. Paralytic ileus also produces constant pain, usually diffuse throughout the abdomen.

Constipation is evidenced by decreased fecal production and fecal balls that are coated with inspissated mucus, signifying delayed transport of the fecal material. A partial obstruction may result in small amounts of diarrhea because of passage of liquid stool past the obstruction. Complete obstruction of the bowel will result in obstipation.

Abdominal distention, which leads to domelike protrusion of the paralumbar fossae, is usually caused by gas accumulation and is a common sign of large bowel obstruction. The cecum is usually distended regardless of the level of the large bowel obstruction. Cecal distention is readily diagnosed by rectal examination and by the tintinnabulation heard during simultaneous auscultation and percussion in the right paralumbar fossa.

Rectal examination is an important part of the physical examination in cases of large bowel obstruction. One should note the character, appearance, and presence or absence of feces. An enlarged doughy cecum in the right caudal abdomen or a doughy pelvic flexure in the left caudal abdomen are indications of impaction. The taenia are important landmarks for identifying segments of bowel and should be examined for abnormal location or tenseness. In cases of volvulus-torsion, there is characteristically a large amount of gas distention proximal to strangulation. Evaluation of all pelvic and abdominal viscera is mandatory to rule out organic disease processes involving other organ systems that might mimic the signs of bowel obstruction.

Introduction of a nasogastric tube is essential to check for the development of gastric dilation. Unless the large bowel obstruction is of long duration, only small volumes of gas and fluid are obtained.

Trends in pain, temperature, pulse, respiratory rate, and color of the mucous membranes are important in differentiating an impaction that will respond to medical therapy from a condition such as volvulus-torsion that will require surgical intervention.

Impaction of the large bowel causes little abnormality of vital signs unless the impaction is prolonged. In contrast, volvulus or herniation of the bowel, which causes acute obstruction, results in unrelenting pain with tachycardia, tachypnea, fever, and brick red mucous membranes. As such cases deteriorate, the extremities become cold and the mucous membranes cyanotic.

LABORATORY EVALUATION

Laboratory evaluation should include a complete blood count, total plasma proteins, electrolytes, creatinine, blood urea nitrogen (BUN), acid-base status, and abdominal paracentesis.

Simple intestinal impaction leads to modest elevations of the number of circulating white blood cells. With strangulation obstruction, moderate rises in the white blood cell count occur with immature forms seen. Mesenteric infarction elevates the count further. These are only generalizations, however; a normal hemogram should not deter the clinician from making a diagnosis of strangulation obstruction if the history and other physical findings suggest it. A debilitated patient is less likely to respond to strangulation by increasing the number of circulating white blood cells. A low white blood cell count, with many immature forms (degenerative left shift), is common in overwhelming sepsis, such as in acute diffuse peritonitis.

Elevations in the packed cell volume and total plasma protein are indications of hemoconcentration and hypovolemia. A reduction in hematocrit may be caused by hemodilution due to splenic relaxation, intravenous fluid therapy, or the shifting of interstitial fluid into the intravascular space. A concurrent decrease in plasma proteins also indicates hemodilution or exudation of plasma intraluminally or intraperitoneally.

Hyponatremia, hypokalemia, and hypocalcemia occur in chronic obstruction. Creatinine and blood urea nitrogen are frequently elevated when hemoconcentration is present. This prerenal azotemia is a reliable indicator of reduction in glomerular filtration rate. The degree of elevation reflects the duration of decreased renal blood flow.

Metabolic acidosis occurs in cases of prolonged impaction or severe acute obstruction. Arterial blood samples should be obtained to accurately assess the metabolic and respiratory status prior to the institution of intensive fluid therapy. Arterial blood

samples are most easily obtained in the horse by puncture of the common carotid, dorsal metatarsal, or facial arteries. Adequate anticoagulation of samples can be easily achieved utilizing sodium heparin. Do not use more than 0.05 ml of sodium heparin for each milliliter of blood sample drawn. It is our practice to use only glass syringes for drawing blood gases. This eliminates absorption of oxygen by the plastic and allows detection of the ease with which the plunger goes back when the artery is entered. Air bubbles must be removed before the specimen is capped for transport to the laboratory.

ABDOMINOCENTESIS

Diagnostic paracentesis of the peritoneal cavity is a safe and invaluable technique for characterizing bowel obstruction. The nature of the fluid obtained often gives the earliest indication of the type of pathologic process that is occurring. Acute and chronic abdominal disease may be differentiated. Abdominocentesis is particularly useful in trajectory (direction and rate of change) evaluation.

Abdominocentesis is performed by use of a 2-in 18-gauge needle in the midline between the umbilicus and xyphoid cartilage. The area should be surgically prepared. Entrance into the peritoneal cavity is confirmed by movement of the hub of the needle with respiration. An alternate technique utilizes a teat cannula with local anesthesia to facilitate perforation of the skin with a scalpel. Normal peritoneal fluid is pale yellow and clear to slightly opalescent. Table 2 summarizes the normal composition of peritoneal fluid.

Fluid obtained by paracentesis may be normal in cases of impaction. In more acute cases of intestinal obstruction, the fluid may be pure blood, serosanguineous, purulent, or contaminated by ingesta. Blood that does not clot is indicative of intraperitoneal hemorrhage. Blood from inadvertent puncture of an abdominal blood vessel normally clots within a few minutes. Serosanguineous peritoneal fluid occurs in cases of strangulated hernia or infarction of bowel from a thromboembolic shower and is suggestive of a full-thickness bowel wall le-

TABLE 2. NORMAL PERITONEAL FLUID

Color	Clear pale yellow
WBC (per μl)	500–5000
WBC differential	Predominantly neutrophils and monocytes
Total protein (mg/dl)	0.5–1.5
Specific gravity	1.000–1.015
Cytology	Active phagocytosis; 50–60% of cells
Alkaline phosphatase (IU/l)	<20

sion. Purulent fluid with numerous polymorphs is indicative of inflammatory disease. Nonviscous, turbid fluid more often indicates a localized lesion, whereas viscous pus suggests generalized inflammation. A reddish-brown fluid that contains ingesta is obtained when the intestine is accidentally punctured or if rupture of an abdominal viscus has occurred. If a bowel lumen has been tapped, microscopic examination will reveal only intestinal bacteria and debris without polymorphs. No complications result from accidental entrance into the bowel lumen. There is no reason not to repeat the paracentesis with a fresh needle at a different site in the same quadrant.

Failure to obtain abdominal fluid has no significance. If laparotomy is indicated on clinical grounds, the fact that no fluid has been obtained from the peritoneal cavity must be completely disregarded. A normal paracentesis may justify continued conservative medical treatment until clinical and trajectory changes in the abdominal fluid warrant other more radical treatment.

RADIOGRAPHY

The roentgenographic examination of the abdomen may be extremely important in the diagnosis of intestinal obstruction in the neonate. Mechanical small bowel obstruction is characterized by air in the small intestine but not in the cecum or colon. Mechanical colonic obstruction is characterized by gas throughout the colon or a portion thereof with little gas in the small intestine. A barium enema is particularly useful in diagnosis of congenital atresias of the colon.

THERAPY

Management of large bowel obstruction requires removal of the obstruction and good supportive care consisting of relief of pain, nasogastric decompression, and fluid and electrolyte replacement[3] (p. 202). Surgical intervention may be essential.

RELIEF OF OBSTRUCTION

In cases of large bowel impaction, emollient laxatives, such as mineral oil, and surface-active agents, such as dioctyl sodium sulfosuccinate (DSS), promote defecation by softening the feces without either direct or reflex stimulation of peristalsis. Mineral oil, a liquid petrolatum, is absorbed to only a limited extent and softens the fecal contents by retarding reabsorption of water. Two to four liters are routinely administered orally to an adult horse.

Dioctyl sodium sulfosuccinate is an anionic deter-

gent agent, and its laxative effect is attributed to its surfactant properties, which facilitate penetration of the fecal mass by water. The recommended dose is 7.5 to 30 gm orally to an adult horse. Mixing DSS with mineral oil potentiates gut absorption of emulsified mineral oil and should be avoided.

Saline cathartics include a number of magnesium salts and various sulfates, phosphates, and tartrates. These salts are slowly and incompletely absorbed from the gastrointestinal tract and thus retain water in the intestinal lumen by osmosis. Peristalsis increases as a result of bowel distention. A dose of 0.5 to 1.0 gm per kg body weight is recommended. Enteritis and subsequent dehydration are seen when the use of these agents is prolonged or overzealous.

Anthraquinone cathartics are also known as the anthracene or emodin cathartics. The major constituents in this group are cascara sagrada and danthron. The cathartic effect is limited mainly to the large intestine. The precise mechanism by which peristalsis is increased is not known. It is believed to result from direct irritation of the bowel wall. Ten to 20 ml of a 20 per cent solution of cascara sagrada is administered subcutaneously to an adult horse. Fifteen to 30 ml of danthron orally is routinely employed. Response is expected within approximately 6 to 12 hours.

Bulk-forming laxatives include various natural and semisynthetic polysaccharides and cellulose derivatives. These dissolve or swell in the presence of water to form an emollient gel or viscous solution that retains water and maintains soft and hydrated feces. This bulk residue may stimulate peristalis reflexly. An initial dose of 0.25 to 0.5 kg of methylcellulose flakes in 8 to 10 l of warm water is given via a nasogastric tube. This is followed by half the original dose mixed with the feed. Bulk laxatives are used predominantly for the treatment of simple obstructions caused by impacted ingesta. Methylcellulose, in particular, is an effective laxative for the treatment of sand impactions, in which emollient, saline, and anthraquinone cathartics are ineffective.

Any drug that may interfere with normal bowel motility (such as atropine) should be avoided. Enemas may stimulate peristalsis, but the aggressive use of this mode of therapy is not warranted. Some clinicians favor the use of drugs that stimulate intestinal motility, such as carbachol (parasympathomimetic), neostigmine (cholinesterase inhibitor), and panthenol (smooth muscle stimulator). These medicaments must not be used indiscriminately; every effort should be made to uncover and correct the underlying etiology prior to their use.[3, 5]

ANALGESICS

Analgesics are useful in the treatment of the patient with obstruction. Efforts should be made to establish a working diagnosis prior to the administration of analgesics, which may otherwise confound the clinical picture.

Dipyrone is commonly used when signs of abdominal pain are first noted. It has analgesic, antispasmodic and antipyretic properties. A dose of 11 mg per kg intravenously and 11 mg per kg intramuscularly is routinely employed. Onset of action is approximately 10 minutes; the duration of action is about one hour.

Xylazine is consistently useful in the relief of visceral pain. The drug may be administered intravenously at 0.2 to 0.4 mg per kg or intramuscularly at 0.4 to 0.8 mg per kg. Duration of analgesia is variable but usually lasts from 30 to 60 minutes. Adverse effects include partial heart block, ileus, and hypotension. Repeated doses of xylazine are especially useful for sedation when transportation to a surgical facility is necessary.

Antiprostaglandin analgesic agents such as flunixin meglumine and phenylbutazone are additional drugs used for treatment of pain in colic cases. Flunixin meglumine (1.0 mg per kg intravenously or intramuscularly) is recommended for alleviation of visceral pain. Onset of action for the intravenous route is approximately 15 minutes and about two hours for intramuscular injection. Phenylbutazone is more useful in parietal pain. An intravenous dose of 2 to 4 mg per kg is initially used with prompt onset of action. Care must be taken to avoid extravasation, which results in severe tissue necrosis and inflammation.

Pentazocine, a narcotic partial agonist, is a synthetic analgesic that may provide more potent analgesia than non-narcotics. It causes minimal depression of gut motility and arterial blood pressure. Analgesic response in the equine patient is quite variable, and in some cases excitement may occur. An intravenous dose of 0.3 mg per kg is recommended with repetition of the same dose 5 to 15 minutes later intramuscularly.

Narcotic agonists meperidine hydrochloride, morphine sulfate, oxymorphone, and dolophine hydrochloride are used when the desired analgesic response is not attained with non-narcotic agents. Meperidine hydrochloride is recommended at a dose of 2.2 to 3.0 mg per kg intramuscularly; intravenous administration may cause CNS excitement. Doses of 0.5 to 1.0 mg per kg intravenously can be employed with great care. Morphine sulfate is given intramuscularly at 0.2 to 0.4 mg per kg, oxymorphone at 0.02 to 0.03 mg per kg intramuscularly, and dolophine hydrochloride at 0.1 to 0.2 mg per kg intramuscularly. Narcotics, especially meperidine and morphine, have the unwanted side effects of exacerbating bowel stasis, which must be weighed against their superior analgesic properties.

Narcotic antagonists will reverse the sedative and bowel stasis effects of narcotic analgesics. Levallorphan tartrate at the dose of 22 to 44 μg per kg and naloxone at 10 to 22 μg per kg are the two most commonly used.

Phenothiazine tranquilizers, such as acetylpromazine, are contraindicated because the alpha-adrenergic blocking activity can exacerbate shock.

FLUID AND ELECTROLYTE REPLACEMENT

Fluid and electrolyte replacement is a primary consideration in the management of large bowel obstruction. Monitoring of serum electrolytes (Na^+, K^+, Cl^-, HCO_3^-, Ca^{++}, and Mg^{++}), hematocrit, plasma proteins, central venous pressure, urinary volume and specific gravity, and the volume and composition of the fluid removed from the nasogastric tube are important in determining the volume and composition of fluids required and in determining the response to therapy.[1] Special emphasis should be given to obviating hypocalcemia and hypokalemia when obstruction or anorexia or both are prolonged.

Although metabolic alkalosis has been described, metabolic acidosis is the most common acid-base abnormality in large bowel obstruction. In obstruction of short duration, acid-base status may be normal. When blood gas analysis is not available, the empirical intravenous administration of 600 mEq (50 gm) sodium bicarbonate is suggested. This will not prove deleterious even in cases of metabolic alkalosis.

CORTICOSTEROIDS

Indiscriminate use of corticosteroids should be avoided. However, a single large dose or therapy for a few days may prove helpful in patients with septic and hypovolemic shock. Administration of glucocorticoids must be accompanied by intensive fluid, electrolyte, and acid-base therapy.

The two main groups of corticosteroids used are (1) those that have an appreciable sodium-retaining activity and (2) those that are practically devoid of this action. Hydrocortisone sodium succinate is an example of the first group. Intravenous administration in a drip at 1.0 to 4.0 mg per kg has an immediate onset but short-lived duration of action. Prednisolone sodium succinate is also routinely used at a dose of 0.25 to 1.0 mg per kg intravenously. The anti-inflammatory activity of prednisolone is at least four times that of hydrocortisone. Dexamethasone, a member of the second group, is administered together with prednisolone at the dose of 0.2 to 0.4 mg per kg intramuscularly for a more prolonged effect. Dexamethasone is contraindicated in cases with laminitis, in which instance prednisolone may be used.

ANTIMICROBIALS

Prophylactic antibiotics are not generally warranted in a patient with a simple obstruction that responds to medical therapy. In patients undergoing surgery with a risk of contamination, prophylactic institution of antibiotics should be considered. Unless earlier cultures and sensitivity dictate otherwise, personal preference and empiricism play a role in the choice of antibiotic(s).

SURGERY

Surgical intervention is warranted in cases of mechanical large bowel obstruction that do not respond to more conservative treatment or when there is evidence of devitalized bowel. The principal cause of high morbidity and mortality in closed loop obstruction is the transmural leakage and subsequent peritoneal absorption of toxic substances and bacteria. For this reason, surgery should be undertaken soon after recognition of this problem. Devitalized bowel should always be treated as a surgical emergency.

References

1. Donawick, W. J.: Metabolic management of the horse with acute abdominal crises. Arch. Am. Coll. Vet. Surg., 5(4):39, 1975.
2. Kohn, C. W.: Preparative management of the equine patient with an abdominal crisis. Vet. Clin. North Am., Large Anim Pract., 1(2):289, 1979.
3. Meagher, D. M.: Obstructive disease in the large intestine of the horse: Diagnosis and treatment. Proc. 18th Annu. Meet. Am. Assoc. Eq. Pract., pp. 269–380, 1972.
4. Nelson, A. W.: Analysis of equine peritoneal fluid. Vet. Clin. North Am., Large Anim. Pract., 1(2):267, 1979.
5. Robertson, J. T.: The digestive system. *In* Mansman, R. A., and McAllister, E. S. (eds.): Equine Medicine and Surgery, 3rd ed. Santa Barbara, CA, American Veterinary Pub. in press.
6. Tennant, B: Intestinal obstruction in the horse: Some aspects of differential diagnosis in equine colic. Proc. 21st Annu. Meet. Am Assoc. Eq. Pract., pp. 426–438, 1975.
7. Tennant, B., Wheat, J. D., and Meagher, D. M.: Observations on the causes and incidence of acute intestinal obstruction in the horse. Proc. 18th Annu. Meet. Am. Assoc. Eq. Pract., pp. 251–257, 1972.

FLATULENT COLIC

T. D. Byars, ATHENS, GEORGIA

Flatulent colic results from accumulation of excessive volumes of gases in the gastrointestinal tract. Synonymous terms include gastric tympany, wind colic, bloat, and tympanic colic. The overdistension of the viscera stimulates pain and pressure receptors, causing mild to severe signs of colic. The disease is usually due to increases in fermentation or ineffectual gastrointestinal motility or may be secondary to partial luminal obstruction.

Visceral distention inhibits vagal motility and propulsive intestinal activity while fermentation continues. Since the release of gases is normally dependent upon escape through the gastrointestinal tract, gas accumulates in the stomach, cecum, and large colon. Sources of the gases include aerophagia (wind cribbing) and the endogenous production of gases from the fermentation of feedstuffs. Accumulated gases are usually volatile fatty acids and other byproducts of fermentation. The accumulation of noxious gases is a reflection of a more severe change in fermentable substrate or the bacterial population.

FACTORS AFFECTING INCIDENCE

The signs of flatulent colic depend on the rate of gaseous accumulation and the portion of the gastrointestinal tract bearing the insult. Although gases may collect at normal flexures and stricture sites, gastric tympany is the most commonly encountered problem.

Causes of flatulent colic include (1) interruptions in gastrointestinal motility resulting from stress, excitement, pain, or parasympatholytic medication; (2) ileus secondary to uremia, liver disease, vascular compromise (thromboembolic colic), or surgical manipulation of the intestines; (3) late pregnancy; (4) impactions; (5) displacements; (6) constipation; or (7) space-occupying masses. Management-associated contributing factors include feeding highly fermentable substrate (grain overload), feeding when horses are exhausted or overheated, cold water engorgement, feeding grains before or after certain vermifuge medication (such as carbon disulfide), poor feed quality or texture, and feeding moldy hay or grains. Behavior-associated contributing factors include cribbing (aerophagia), inadequate mastication of feed, and rapid feed engorgement. Broad-spectrum antibiotics given orally may cause gas production by alteration of the normal bacterial population.

CLINICAL SIGNS

The clinical signs vary from merely being off feed to the acute distress that accompanies gastric distention. The temperature, pulse, and respiratory rate will usually be elevated in proportion to the severity of the clinical signs. The mucous membranes are pale. The respiratory pattern will shift to a more rapid and shallow effort as gases distend the viscera, occupy a greater percentage of the abdominal cavity, and place pressure against the diaphragm. Since the stomach is situated immediately adjacent to the diaphragm, this form of shallow respiration occurs more consistently with gastric tympany. With severe gastric dilation, retching and regurgitation of stomach contents can occur.

Rectal examination reveals gas-filled portions of the intestines. The fundic portion of the stomach can infrequently be felt as a large gas-filled structure in the cranial portion of the left upper quadrant; distended portions of the jejunum or ileum can be discerned as thin-walled loops without sacculations and taeniae; the distended cecum is fixed at the base and therefore can be located in the upper right caudal quadrant of the abdomen; the distended large colon can be felt to contain three antimesenteric bands except for the pelvic flexure, which lacks antimesenteric structures.

Auscultation of the abdomen is valuable in determining the presence or absence of intestinal sounds. Percussion aids in identifying the more precise region of gaseous accumulation.

Pain varies in intensity according to the rate and site of gas accumulation. Distention of the stomach results in severe signs of pain, and often the horse will be sweating, pawing, hyperactive, and resent nasogastric intubation. With distention of the cecum or large colon, the pain tends to be dull and intermittent.

The shape of the abdomen will change in response to the intra-abdominal distention. Cecal tympany often flattens and elevates the region of the right paralumbar fossa. Large colon tympany will usually result in bilateral abdominal distention.

THERAPY

The primary objective of treatment is relief of gaseous distention and prevention of further formation of gases. The effectiveness of treatment is directly related to the evacuation of the gases from the region of distention. Nasogastric intubation or trocarization of the cecum or large colon can provide immediate, although temporary, relief of clinical signs. Stomach tubing is always indicated as a diagnostic procedure in colic, and whenever gastric tympany is present, the elimination of gases through the tube is therapeutic.

Medical treatment should include supportive therapy to relieve pain and dehydration. Nonsteroidal anti-inflammatory drugs are used to decrease bowel inflammation and the incidence of laminitis. Parasympathomimetics should be used with caution, since asynchronous contracture of the viscera may increase the incidence of rupture (p. 223). Enemas can be used as an adjunct to rectal or small colon fecal evacuation.

Antifermentatives have long been accepted medications for flatulent colic; however, the efficacy of many of the conventional medicaments is questionable. Turcapsol is consided to be an irritant with only minimal value as an antifermentative. Mineral oil is often used to coat fermentable substrate and to lubricate the feed material within the gastrointestinal tract for easier passage. From one half to one gal of mineral oil should be given by stomach tube if gastric dilation is not present or after gastric distention has been relieved.

Cathartics are not directly indicated unless a need for intraluminal lubrication is suggested. Whenever cathartics are used, the horse should be in a hydrated state.

Trocarization of the cecum or large colon can be therapeutic and life-saving. The procedure can relieve distention prior to rupture, and deflation will often restore motility. Percussion is important for localization of the abdominal region in contact with the tympanic bowel. The cecum and right ventral colon can be percussed in the right paralumbar fossa and the left colon percussed in variable regions of contact with the left abdominal wall. The right side is more commonly used, although occasionally a patient will have to be bilaterally trocarized. The site of trocarization should be clipped, shaved, and surgically prepared. A local anesthetic is used to block the site, and a No. 15 scalpel blade is used to pierce the skin. A 14 cm trocar or 12 to 14 gauge biopsy needle is used to pierce the abdominal wall and to enter the abdominal cavity and proceed into the lumen of the bowel. A rush of gas from the needle will occur immediately, and the trocar should be left in place until gas is no longer free-flowing. From 10 to 20 cc of a broad-spectrum antibiotic is injected through the trocar as it is withdrawn as an aid to the prevention of local peritonitis. Systemic antibiotics may further suppress diffuse peritonitis or generalized infection.

PROGNOSIS

The prognosis for uncomplicated cases of flatulent colic is usually good. However, prolonged or recurrent cases may indicate a more serious underlying disorder affecting gastrointestinal motility or luminal patency. More intensive diagnostic tests and methods should be employed in cases of chronic colic.

The prognosis for horses developing local peritonitis after trocarization is good if early treatment has been performed. The sequelae of internal abscessation or adhesions can lead to chronic weight loss or recurrent colic. In cases in which the viscera rupture, the horse will usually succumb to diffuse peritonitis.

References

1. Argenzio, R. A.: Function of the equine large intestine and the interrelationship in disease. Cornell Vet., 65:3, 1975.
2. Coffman, J. R., and Garner, H. E.: Acute abdominal diseases of the horse. J. Am. Vet. Med. Assoc., *161*:1195, 1972.
3. Page, E. H., and Amstutz, H. E.: Gastrointestinal disorders. *In* Catcott, E. J., and Smithcors, J. S. (eds.): Equine Medicine and Surgery, 2nd ed. Wheaton, IL, American Veterinary Pub., 1972. pp. 258–260.
4. Tennant, B.: Intestinal obstruction in the horse. Proc. 21st Annu. Meet. Am. Assoc. Eq. Pract., pp. 426–438, 1975.

THROMBOEMBOLIC COLIC

Thomas J. Divers, ATHENS, GEORGIA
Nathaniel A. White, ATHENS, GEORGIA

ETIOLOGY

Thromboembolic colic (TE), nonstrangulating ischemia, or infarction results from the arterial lesions (verminous arteritis) produced by the migration of the fourth- and fifth-stage larvae of *Strongylus vulgaris*[5, 6] (p. 269). The number of migrating larvae, the horse's acquired resistance, and the extent of intimal damage determine the degree of thrombus formation.[6] The vascular insult results in hypoxia and ischemia with subsequent changes in intestinal motility and possibly devitalization of the intestinal wall. The production of ischemia is hypothesized to be either the result of thromboembolism with blockage of arterial branches or a low flow state produced by the major thrombus.

CLINICAL SIGNS

Thromboembolic colic is most common in yearlings and young adult horses (one to nine years), though it has occurred in foals less than two months of age[5, 16] and in aged horses. The disease is most prevalent in regions that favor the survival of *S. vulgaris* larvae.

The disease is most commonly identified by the recurrent episodes of abdominal pain. Recurrence is unpredictable and occurs days or weeks after a recent attack. Diarrhea and weight loss can be accompanying signs.

The location of the affected bowel and the degree of ischemia usually determine the clinical signs. Thromboembolism of the cecum and large colon most often results in moderate abdominal pain and a clinical course of up to seven days. Cecal or colonic tympany and abdominal distention may gradually develop from the thromboembolism, which then results in more severe, intractable abdominal pain. Horses with infarction may become less painful with time, only to develop severe depression that accompanies a developing peritonitis. Ischemic lesions of the small bowel can produce sudden small intestinal and gastric distention accompanied by severe pain and a rapidly deteriorating clinical course. Occasionally, horses with colic will have minimal intestinal distention but intense pain upon palpation of the mesenteric stalk and cranial mesenteric artery. Since the cecum and colon are the organs most commonly affected,[5] clinical signs are frequently suggestive of large bowel disease and may appear similar to large bowel impactions. There are no specific laboratory tests for the presence of thromboembolic colic; the diagnosis is based on the history, physical examination, and clinicopathologic findings. Rectal examination is helpful in determining other causes of large bowel disease such as displacement or intraluminal obstructions. Rectal examination of the cranial mesenteric artery is helpful in making the diagnosis only if pain is elicited on palpation of an enlarged artery. A tentative diagnosis of thromboembolic colic involving the small bowel is more difficult, as the condition resembles small intestinal obstruction (p. 224).

Physical examination and determination of packed cell volume and plasma protein often reveal hemoconcentration and dehydration, although plasma proteins may be lowered owing to fluid loss into the abdomen. This shifting of large amounts of protein into the abdomen warrants a poor prognosis. Inadequate tissue perfusion and endotoxemia lead to abundant anaerobic glycolysis, a metabolic lactic acidosis, and an increased anion gap.[11] Leukograms vary from stress leukograms to severe neutropenia with a left shift depending upon the amount of intestinal ischemia and resulting peritonitis. Plasma fibrinogen is often elevated above 600 mg per dl.

Peritoneal fluid evaluation (p. 233) is important in the diagnosis and management of thromboembolic colic. Elevation in peritoneal fluid protein is usually the first and most consistent abnormal laboratory finding. This is often followed by an increase in peritoneal white blood cells. With severe or prolonged ischemia or venous thrombosis, there may be diapedesis of red blood cells, producing a serosanguineous fluid. Bacteria will pass into the peritoneal cavity if intestinal infarction occurs. Alkaline phosphatase and lactic acid values may be elevated in the peritoneal fluid, but these findings do not separate thromboembolic colic from cases of strangulating intestinal ischemia.[12] Electrophoretograms of blood from horses with verminous arteritis frequently show an elevation in beta globulins and a decrease in albumin.[7] Fibrin degradation products and plasminogen values are not usually abnormal in horses with thromboembolism. Because of the long period of larval migration and the prepatent period of adults, fecal egg counts may not be indicative of parasite infection.

THERAPY

Surgical intervention in horses with thromboembolic colic has a mortality rate up to 90 per cent.[15] This can be attributed to the large portions of the colon or cecum that become involved, making resection impossible, a further decline in intestinal perfusion during anesthesia and the inability to accurately predict areas needing resection, resulting in a high incidence of reinfarction.

Medical therapy for suspected cases of thromboembolism results in a higher survival rate. The basis of therapy is the maintenance of normal cardiac output and tissue perfusion, prevention of further thrombus formation, and control of pain and peritonitis.[11] The maintenance of blood volume by administration of a pyrogen-free isotonic fluid is the single most important therapy. Fluids should be given intravenously in an amount and at a rate determined by degree of dehydration (percentage dehydration × body weight in kg = fluid deficit in liters) (p. 201), requirement for daily maintenance (15 to 25 ml per kg per day), capillary refill time, hematocrit, total proteins, and central venous pressure. In the absence of palpable small bowel distention or gastric reflux, water may be offered free choice. Sodium bicarbonate may be added to the intravenous fluids or ideally given as an isotonic solution. Sodium bicarbonate should be administered slowly as needed to maintain normal blood pH (p. 203). Acidotic horses will often have a dramatic improvement in cardiac function as blood pH returns to normal. Serum calcium and potassium should be evaluated in horses with intestinal disease, since absorption of these cations may be decreased and lack of food intake may produce an absolute daily loss. Hypokalemia and hypocalcemia diminish gastrointestinal peristalsis and may result in generalized body weakness. If serum potassium is low, 20 to 60 mEq of potassium chloride (KCl) may be added to each liter of intravenously administered fluids. Calcium chloride ($CaCl_2$, 0.5 to 1.0 mEq per kg) may be administered slowly intravenously if heart rate and rhythm are monitored carefully by auscultation or preferably with electrocardiography.

Antimicrobial therapy should be directed against gram-negative enteric organisms (including anaerobes) and Streptococcus sp. The administration of aqueous penicillin* (30,000 units per kg four times a day intravenously) or aqueous ampicillin† (11 mg per kg three times a day intravenously) in combination with an aminoglycoside such as kanamycin‡ (5 mg per kg three times a day intramuscularly), gentamicin§ (2 mg per kg three times a day intramuscularly) or neomycin‖ (10 mg per kg twice a day intravenously) is recommended. Aminoglycosides and penicillins should never be mixed in the same solution. Renal function (serum creatinine, urine specific gravity, and presence of granular urinary casts) should be evaluated before and during aminoglycoside therapy. The initiation and duration of antimicrobial therapy should be decided upon by the severity of peritonitis and the continued presence of gram-negative bacteria in the peritoneal fluid. Peritoneal lavage using 10 per cent prepodyne solution** in warm isotonic fluids may be used in severe cases of peritonitis to diminish bacteria and toxin buildup[16] within the peritoneal cavity.

*Pfizerpen, Pfizer Labs, New York, NY 10017
†Omnipen, Wyeth Labs, Inc., Philadelphia, PA 19101
‡Kantrim, Bristol Labs, Syracuse, NY 13201
§Gentocin, Schering Corp., Kenilworth, NJ 07033
‖Biosol, Upjohn Co., Kalamazoo, MI 49001
**Prepodyne Solution, West Chemical Products, Inc., New York, NY 11101

Analgesics are often necessary to alleviate the abdominal pain associated with thromboembolism. Xylazine hydrochloride* (0.4 to 0.8 mg per kg intravenously or 0.6 to 1.2 mg per kg intramuscularly) is reliable for the control of moderate pain when used in repeated small doses. Meperidine hydrochloride† (2.2 to 3.0 mg per kg intramuscularly) may be administered as an alternative, but repeated doses should be avoided. Cyclo-oxygenase inhibitors such as phenylbutazone and flunixin meglumine are useful analgesics and more importantly may depress further thrombosis in animals with vascular disease by inhibiting thromboxane production.[1] Flunixin meglumine‡ (1.1 mg per kg twice a day intravenously) is also known to reduce the clinical signs of endotoxemia in the horse when given prior to the endotoxin challenge.[10] When given prior to the endotoxin challenge, a single intravenous injection of dexamethasone§ (1.0 to 2.0 mg per kg intravenously) or methylprednisolone‖ (30 mg per kg intravenously) will stabilize lysosomal membranes and prevent endotoxin-induced mitochondrial dysfunction.[4] The administration of corticosteroids late in the clinical course of thromboembolic colic in horses will not produce the desired result.

Large bowel tympany should be relieved, since intestinal motility will not return as long as any portion of the gastrointestinal tract remains distended. Cecal tympany is best relieved by cecal trocarization using a 3½ to 6 in 14- to 16-gauge Vim-Silverman biopsy needle.** The trocarization site should be aseptically prepared at the most dorsal boundary of the cecum on the right side between the last rib and tuber coxae. The needle should be flushed with an antibiotic as it is withdrawn from the cecum to prevent leaving a trail of cecal contents in the peritoneum. Tympany of the large colon can be relieved by small dosages of neostigmine†† (0.004 to 0.008 mg per kg subcutaneously). Parasympathomimetic drugs can be used safely in treating large colon tympany, provided the tympany has resulted from a nonobstructive large bowel disease.

In the presence of small intestinal or gastric distention, gastric decompression should be attempted with a medium-size stomach tube. In the absence of gastric and small bowel distention, a mild laxative such as 5 per cent dioctyl sodium succinate‡‡ (4 to 6 oz per 450 kg once a day orally) will help avoid impaction formation. Mineral oil administered orally may help prevent endotoxin absorption in ischemic bowel. Neomycin (15 mg per kg once a day orally) can help reduce the enteric *Escherichia coli* population and experimentally has prolonged survival after colon infarction.[13] Anticoagulation therapy will not affect an existing thrombus but is utilized for the prevention of further fibrin deposition and thrombus formation. Minidose heparinization* (30 to 80 IU per kg twice a day subcutaneously) for prophylaxis of thrombosis is based upon its increased activity at the factor Xa level.[2] Bleeding complications due to heparin at this dosage are not reported.

Dextran 70† administered intravenously at a dosage of 5 to 15 ml per kg per day in a 6 per cent solution has been reported as being of benefit in treating thromboembolic colic in horses.[9] The dextrans are volume expanders and also have marked antithrombotic properties that result from decreased platelet adhesiveness and the coating of the vascular endothelium and red blood cells.[3] However, the expense of dextrans prevents their routine use.

Administration of chemotherapeutic agents effective against the migrating forms of *S. vulgaris* is recommended after intestinal function has returned to normal (p. 278). Thiabendazole‡ at the dose rate of 440 mg per kg administered orally on two successive days kills early fourth-stage larvae of *S. vulgaris*. Older larvae may not be killed by this dosage of thiabendazole. Repeated doses are believed to be advantageous because the action of benzimidazoles is effected through the energy utilizing mechanism of the parasite, which is a relatively slow process.[5] Albendazole§ administered at a dosage of 25 mg per kg three times daily for five days kills migrating larvae and resolves verminous thrombosis.[14] Although quite effective as an anthelmintic, Albendazole is known to have serious side effects at this dosage and is not yet approved for use in the horse. Fenbendazole‖ at 7.5 mg per kg daily for five days removed 80 per cent of migrating *S. vulgaris* larvae in one study, but others have questioned its efficacy.[5]

The most important consideration in TE colic is prevention. With proper parasite control programs (p. 276), this disease has been practically eradicated in certain parts of the country.

---

*Rompun, Haver-Lockhart, Shawnee, KS 66201
†Demerol, Winthrop Labs, New York, NY 10016
‡Banamine, Schering Corp., Kenilworth, NJ 07033
§Dexamethasone Injection, Pitman-Moore, Inc., Washington Crossing, NJ 08560
‖Solu-Medl, Upjohn Co., Kalamazoo, MI 49001
**Vim-Silverman, Physicians and Hospital Supply Co., Inc., Minneapolis, MN
††Stiglyn, Pitman-Moore, Inc., Washington Crossing, NJ 08560
‡‡Cerusol, Burns-Biotec, Oakland, CA 94621

References

1. Bell, T. G., Smith, W. L., Oxender, W. D., and Maciejko, J. J.: Biologic interaction of prostaglandins, thromboxane,

---

*Heparin, Elkins-Sinn, Inc., Cherry Hill, NJ 08034
†Dextran 70, Travenol, Deerfield, IL 60015
‡Omnizole, Merck Animal Health Division, Rahway, NJ 07065
§Albendazole, Smith Kline and French, Philadelphia, PA 19101
‖Panacur, American Hoechst Corp., Animal Health Division, Somerville, NJ 08876

and prostacyclin: Potential nonreproductive veterinary clinical application. J. Am. Vet. Med. Assoc., *176*:1195, 1980.

2. Byars, T., and Wilson, R.: Clinical pharmacology of heparin. J. Am. Vet. Med. Assoc., *178*:739, 1981.
3. Data, J., and Nies, A. C.: Dextran 40. Ann. Intern. Med., *81*:500, 1974.
4. DePalma, R. G., Glickman, M. H., Hartman, P., and Robinson, A. V.: Prevention of endotoxin induced changes in oxidative phosphorylation in hepatic mitochondria. Surgery, *82*:68, 1977.
5. Drudge, J. H.: Clinical aspects of *Strongylus vulgaris* infection in the horse. *In* Symposium on Gastroenterology, Vet. Clin. North Am., *1*(2):251, 1979.
6. Duncan, J. L.: Immunity to *Strongylus vulgaris* in the horse. Eq. Vet. J., *7*(4):192, 1975.
7. Duncan, J. L., and Dargie, J. D.: The pathogenesis and control of strongyle infection in the horse. J. S. Afr. Vet. Assoc., *46*:81, 1975.
8. Duncan, J., McBeath, D. G., and Preston, H. K.: Studies on the efficacy of fenbendazole used in a divided dosage regime against the strongyle infections in ponies. Eq. Vet. J., *12*:78, 1980.
9. Greatorex, J. C.: Diagnosis and treatment of "verminous aneurysm" formation in the horse. Vet. Rec., *101*:184, 1977.
10. Moore, J., Garner, H. E., Shapland, J. E., and Hatfield, D. G.: Prevention of endotoxin induced arterial hypoxia and lactic acidosis with flunixin meglumine in the conscious pony. Eq. Vet. J., *13*:95, 1981.
11. Moore, J. N., Traver, D. S., Garner, H. E., Coffman, J. R., Amend, J. R., and Tritschler, L. G.: A review of lactic acidosis with particular reference to the horse. J. Eq. Med. Surg., *1*:96, 1977.
12. Nelson, A. W.: Analysis of equine peritoneal fluid. *In* Symposium on Gastroenterology. Vet. Clin. North Am., *1*(2):267, 1979.
13. Nelson, A., Collier, J. R., and Griner, L. A.: Acute surgical colonic infarction in the horse. Am. J. Vet. Res., *29*(2):315, 1968.
14. Rendano, V., Georgi, J. R., White, K. K., Sack, W. O., King, J. M., and Bianchi, D. G.: Equine verminous arteritis. An arteriographic evaluation of the larvicidal activity of albendazole. Eq. Vet. J., *11*(4):223, 1979.
15. Valdez, H., Scrutchfield, W. L., and Taylor, T. S.: Peritoneal lavage in the horse. J. Am. Vet. Med. Assoc., *175*(4):388, 1979.
16. White, N. A.: Intestinal infarction associated with mesenteric vascular thrombotic disease in the horse. J. Am. Vet. Med. Assoc., *178*:259, 1981.
17. Wright, A. I.: Verminous arteritis as a cause of colic in the horse. Eq. Vet. J., *4*:169, 1972.

PERITONITIS

W. *Leon Scrutchfield,* COLLEGE STATION, TEXAS

Peritonitis in horses is associated with abdominal abscesses, verminous arteritis, uterine perforation at parturition, prolonged colon or cecal impaction, abdominal wall perforation, and rectal mucosal injury during palpation. Peritonitis may also develop following abdominal surgery and routine castration.

Since the peritoneum is capable of tremendous inflammatory reaction and absorption of toxic products, diffuse peritonitis affects all body systems. Local vasodilation and increased capillary permeability of the peritoneum result in effusion of fluid, electrolytes, and protein from the circulation into the peritoneal cavity. Additionally, absorption of toxins and bacteria from the peritoneal cavity may result in septicemia.

CLINICAL SIGNS

Clinical signs of peritonitis in the horse vary greatly, depending upon the etiology, severity, duration, and extent of the inflammatory process. The signs can vary from elevated rectal temperature (104 to 106° F), anorexia, reluctance to move, diarrhea, obvious signs of abdominal discomfort, and great depression to an animal that is "just not right" with slight elevation of rectal temperature, some decrease in appetite, and slight depression. Peritonitis

following abdominal surgery can be severe and life-threatening, and the animal may show minimal outward signs. Peritonitis should be suspected in an animal that is febrile, depressed, and anorexic following abdominal surgery, castration, or any traumatic perforation of the abdominal wall. To rule out the possibility of peritonitis, abdominocentesis should be included in the examination of any "poor-doing" horse and in any horse that is febrile for no apparent cause.

LABORATORY FINDINGS

The diagnosis of peritonitis must be made by examination of peritoneal fluid or exploratory laparotomy. The range of normal values for peritoneal fluid is presented in Table 1. Most horses with peritonitis have elevated peritoneal fluid white blood cell counts, particularly nucleated cells, elevated protein, and increased turbidity. The normal values of total protein vary from 0.1 up to 3.4 gm per dl; however, values above 2 gm per dl commonly suggest inflammation. Values above 3 gm per dl suggest sepsis. Cytologic examination will help differentiate peritonitis from verminous arteritis and neoplasia. Abnormal cells and an increase in mitotic figures may be seen with neoplasia. An increased number

TABLE 1. SUGGESTED NORMAL VALUES FOR PERITONEAL FLUID

	Mean (Bach and Rickets, 1974)	Range (Bach and Rickets, 1974)	Mean (McGrath, 1975)	Range (McGrath, 1975)
RBC (x/mm^3)			1.822	0.2 to 5.4
Nucleated cells/mm^3	3244	200 to 9000	2097	50 to 4600
Polymorphonuclear leukocytes (%)	59.5	36 to 78	90	80 to 98
Lymphocytes (%)	10.0	0 to 29	4.4	1 to 11
Mononuclear cells (%)	30.4	3 to 50	7.4	1 to 17
Eosinophils (%)	0.2	0 to 3	2.1	0 to 7
Protein (mg/dl)	1.1	0.1 to 3.4	1.05	0.1 to 2.5
Specific gravity	1.001	1.000 to 1.093	1.013	1.007 to 1.030
Color				Colorless, straw, or pale pink
Transparency				Clear or slightly turbid
Coagulation				Negative

of eosinophils may indicate the presence of Strongylus larva migrans. Rectal examination may be a further aid in differentiating these conditions.

It has been suggested that chronic bacterial peritonitis is frequently associated with peritoneal fluid total white cell counts of 20,000 per mm^3 to 60,000 per mm^3, but much higher counts may be present. Acute diffuse cases often have total white cell counts from 200,000 per mm^3 to 800,000 per mm^3 with a predominance of neutrophils. Toxic or degenerate cells are frequently present. Bacteria either free or ingested in leukocytes present in the peritoneal fluid are the best evidence of bacterial peritonitis. Failure to observe bacteria does not rule out a bacterial etiology.

There are reports that bacteria are seldom cultured from peritoneal fluid even when visible in Gram-stained smears. However, both aerobic and anaerobic cultures should be done on peritoneal fluid either with increased turbidity or from suspected peritonitis cases. Antimicrobial sensitivity testing should be done on all potential pathogens. Results of the sensitivity testing will be too late for the initial therapy, but when the results are available, they may indicate another more appropriate antimicrobial therapy than the one initially selected.

The results of the peritoneal fluid examination are evaluated in light of the history, clinical signs, physical examination findings, and other laboratory examinations, including hematology. For example, a white blood cell (WBC) count of 100,000 per mm^3 in peritoneal fluid three days after abdominal surgery may be due to inflammation and not infection. While this animal should be maintained on systemic antibiotics, more heroic measures such as peritoneal lavage are probably not indicated in this case. Clinical judgment is very important in the interpretation of peritoneal fluid examination results.

The hematologic findings in peritonitis vary considerably. The total WBC count may range from leukocytosis to leukopenia. Acute cases with sequestration of the white blood cells in the peritoneal cavity may have a peripheral leukopenia. A normal to elevated WBC count is usually accompanied by a relative and absolute neutrophilia. A left shift may be present and will probably be degenerative in horses with diffuse peritonitis. The plasma fibrinogen concentration is usually increased owing to the inflammatory response. A bone marrow depression anemia is often present in horses with chronic peritonitis.

Serum protein levels may be normal or elevated in chronic peritonitis but decreased in acute peritonitis with massive peritoneal effusions. Horses with chronic infectious peritonitis commonly have hyperproteinemia due to elevated gamma globulins in response to continual immunogenic stimulation.

TREATMENT

Treatment will not be successful unless the original insult causing the peritonitis is resolved. Treatment involves (1) measures to combat the systemic effects of the peritonitis that can lead to cardiovascular collapse and death, (2) systemic antimicrobial therapy, (3) peritoneal lavage if indicated, and (4) supportive care. Appropriate intravenous fluids should be given as needed. If acidosis develops, it should be corrected (p. 203). Attention must be given to serum potassium and protein levels, especially if peritoneal lavage is performed.

Systemic antibiotics should be administered. The antibiotic or antibiotic combination needs to be a broad-spectrum one because the etiology often involves multiple bacterial species (aerobic and anaerobic) and because antimicrobial therapy must be instituted before culture and sensitivity results are obtained. As aminoglycoside antibiotics are relatively ineffective against anaerobic bacteria, they should not be used by themselves. No single antibiotic or combination of antibiotics is clearly superior in the treatment of peritonitis in horses.

The combination of kanamycin sulfate* and penicillin provides a wide spectrum of activity. The recommended dose of kanamycin sulfate is 15 mg per kg per day divided into three 5 mg per kg injections.[4] Procaine penicillin G may be given at 20,000 to 100,000 units per kg every 12 hours. If more immediate effective blood levels of penicillin are desired, then potassium penicillin G may be given simultaneously intravenously; 10,000 to 50,000 units per kg is recommended.[4]

The use of chloramphenicol in horses is controversial because of the short serum half-life; however, it has been effective clinically in the treatment of peritonitis. Chloramphenicol has broad-spectrum activity, including obligate anaerobes. Chloramphenicol should be given orally at a dosage of 165 to 200 mg per kg divided into three or four doses per day.

The broad-spectrum activity of gentamicin sulfate† has made it highly regarded as a therapeutic agent, and it could be used to treat peritonitis at a daily dosage of 3 to 6 mg per kg intramuscularly divided into three doses.[4] However, aminoglycoside antibiotics are relatively ineffective against anaerobic bacteria; thus, gentamicin should not be used alone.

Other antibiotics and antimicrobial agents might be used to treat equine peritonitis. The antimicrobial treatment regimen should be based on the clinical signs, probable etiologic agent, economic aspects, and the results of sensitivity testing when available.

Nonsteroidal anti-inflammatory drugs such as phenylbutazone or flunixin meglumine‡ will relieve pain. This may enable the patient to move around more and may improve the appetite. Apparently these agents will not inhibit the movement of polymorphonuclear leukocytes into the abdominal cavity as will corticosteroids. Because of this inhibition of the movement of polymorphonuclear leukocytes and the adverse effects upon the immune system, corticosteroids should not be used in peritonitis cases unless given for shock.

PERITONEAL LAVAGE

If the peritonitis is life-threatening because of the rapid absorption of toxins, bacteria, and bacterial enzymes, then intermittent peritoneal lavage should be attempted. The decision to do peritoneal lavage will be based upon the patient's physical condition and laboratory results, especially the examination of peritoneal fluid. Clinical judgment must be used. Benefits of peritoneal lavage include the removal of toxins and bacterial enzymes, reduction in number of bacteria, and the removal of foreign material such as feces and gastrointestinal secretions.[7]

Several different types of catheters can be used for lavage in the horse. These include Foley catheters,* bubble tubing,† and even the cut-off end of a nasogastric tube, all of which must be sterilized before use. The ventral aspect of the abdomen is clipped, shaved, and scrubbed with povidone-iodine soap,‡ and then povidone-iodine solution§ is applied. The skin and rectus abdominis muscle are blocked with 2 to 3 ml of 2 percent lidocaine. An incision 1 cm long is made in the skin and extended deep enough to penetrate the external lamina of the rectus muscle. A curved intestinal forceps is pushed through the incision and peritoneum into the abdominal cavity. The forceps is pushed at an angle to the long axis of the body to reduce the potential of intestinal perforation. The forceps is withdrawn, and the tubing is placed between the jaws. The catheter is then carried into the abdominal cavity by the forceps through the previously made puncture, and the forceps is withdrawn. The catheter can be anchored in place with a tape butterfly sutured to the abdominal wall. A better method of securing the catheter involves continuous sutures placed around the catheter for a length of 4 to 5 cm. If a Foley catheter is used, a bulb can be inflated to retain the catheter.

The lavage fluid can be instilled into the abdomen by gravity flow or by using a hand pressure pump. Two gal of fluid at a time works well in the average-sized adult horse. The lavage fluid should be a balanced isotonic electrolyte solution such as Ringer's lactate to avoid electrolyte depletion and fluid shifts. The solution must be warmed to body temperature to help prevent discomfort. If the horse displays signs of discomfort, 100 to 200 mg of xylazine‖ given intravenously should alleviate the problem.

Povidone-iodine solution is a good antimicrobial agent to add to the lavage solution. The antibacterial spectrum of povidone-iodine far exceeds any currently available antibiotic. No peritoneal irritation or adhesion formation was evident following experimental intraperitoneal administration of povidone-iodine solution to rats or human patients. It was

*Kantrim, Bristol Laboratories, Syracuse, NY
†Gentocin, Schering Corp., Kenilworth, NJ
‡Banamine, Schering Corp., Kenilworth, NJ

*Foley Catheter, American Hospital Supply, Grand Prairie, TX
†Argyle Bubble Tubing, Sherwood Medical, St. Louis, MO
‡Betadine Scrub, Purdue Frederick Co., Norwalk, CT
§Betadine Solution, Purdue Frederick Co., Norwalk, CT
‖Rompun, Haver-Lockhart, Shawnee, KS

found that a maximal safe intraperitoneal dosage in rats is 2.5 ml per kg.[5] The author routinely adds 2 to 3 oz of povidone-iodine solution to each gallon of warmed, isotonic balanced electrolyte fluids. A 1000 lb horse is lavaged two to three times per day with 2 gal of fluids each time. This results in the patient's receiving a maximal amount of approximately 1 ml per kg per day of povidone-iodine solution. No adverse effects have been observed.

After the fluid is instilled into the abdominal cavity, the catheter is plugged and the horse is walked for a few minutes. Then the catheter is unplugged and the horse is walked again. A sterile absorbent bandage such as a government surplus abdominal field bandage is kept over the catheter between treatments.

If a specific antibiotic or combination of antibiotics is indicated by bacterial sensitivity testing, then they may be used in place of the povidone-iodine solution. There are reports of adverse effects from the intraperitoneal administration of different antibiotics. These include peritoneal irritation and adhesion formation from tetracycline, bacitracin, sulfonamides, erythromycin, oleandomycin, chloramphenicol, kanamycin, neomycin, and streptomycin. Intensified catabolic states with tetracyclines and allergic reactions due to penicillins have also been reported.

The addition of heparin to the lavaging solution may be beneficial. In experimentally induced peritonitis of both the dog and rat, heparin had a therapeutic effect by preventing the additional deposition of fibrin and rendering the bacteria more susceptible to cellular and noncellular clearing mechanisms.[3] In addition, heparin may decrease the plugging of the lavage catheter with fibrin. A dosage ranging from 10 to 20 units per kg body weight could be added to the lavaging solution. Larger doses might be more beneficial but would require monitoring the partial thromboplastin time.

The lavage catheter may become plugged with fibrin. The lavaging solution can usually be introduced but will not drain properly when the catheter is plugged. The plugged catheter should be removed and another catheter inserted if patency cannot be restored by flushing, suction, or other methods. The catheter is left in place and the lavaging continued until the peritoneal fluid appears normal. The catheter is then removed, and the patient is maintained on systemic antibiotics and appropriate supportive therapy.

If the laboratory and/or rectal examination indicates that verminous arteritis is present, then a larvicidal dose of anthelmintic should also be given (p. 278). There are several reports of concurrent peritonitis and verminous arteritis in horses. The migrating Strongyle larvae may play a role in inoculating the abdominal cavity with bacteria.

References

1. Bach, L. G., and Rickets, S. W.: Paracentesis as an aid to the diagnosis of abdominal disease in the horse. Eq. Vet. J., 6:116, 1974.
2. Coffman, J. R.: Clinical chemistry and pathophysiology of horses: Peritoneal fluid. Vet. Med. Sm. Anim. Clin., 75:1285, 1980.
3. Hau, T., and Simmons, R. L.: Heparin in the treatment of experimental peritonitis. Ann. Surg., 187:294, 1978.
4. Knight, H. D.: Antimicrobial agents used in the horse. Proc. 21st Annu. Meet. Am. Assoc. Eq. Pract., 131, 1975.
5. Lavigne, J. E., Brown, C. S., Machiedo, G. W., Blackwood, J. M., and Rush, B. F.: The treatment of experimental peritonitis with intraperitoneal Betadine solution. J. Surg. Res., 16:307, 1974.
6. McGrath, J. P.: Exfoliative cytology of equine peritoneal fluid. An adjunct to hematologic examination. Proc. First Internat. Sym. Eq. Hematol., Michigan State University, pp. 408–416, 1975.
7. Valdez, H., Scrutchfield, W. L., and Taylor, T. S.: Peritoneal lavage in the horse. J. Am. Vet. Med. Assoc., 175:388, 1979.

GRASS SICKNESS

John S. Gilmour, EDINBURGH, SCOTLAND

Grass sickness (grass disease) was first described as a clinical entity in horses following its appearance at a military training camp in Scotland in 1907. Since then it has been reported throughout the British Isles, much of northern Europe, and once in Australia.

CLINICAL SIGNS

The cause of the disease, which affects all species of Equidae and is usually fatal, is unknown. Therapeutic measures have been broadly symptomatic and largely unsuccessful. The severity of the disease ranges from acute to chronic. Acute cases usually die within 48 hours of being recognized and will have experienced an intractable stasis of the alimentary canal accompanied by depression, inability to swallow, patchy sweating, cutaneous fasciculation, and a markedly increased pulse rate. Episodes of colic are often surprisingly mild, though the stomach may be greatly distended by fluid, which in a large proportion of cases is regurgitated via the nasal passages. Further evidence of the stasis is found in the rectum, which may be empty save for sticky mucus and an occasional small hard fecal pellet, and in the large colon and cecum, where a mass of dehydrated digesta has accumulated, which provides a very striking necropsy finding. In cases of lesser clinical severity, the animal lives longer. The chronic case, however, rapidly loses body weight but retains some ability to eat and defecate. Occasionally cases of this type have been known to survive. Emaciation is the only consistent gross finding in chronic cases. Histologically, grass sickness is characterized by degenerative change affecting neurons of the peripheral autonomic ganglia and of specified nuclei in the central nervous system.[1, 5, 7]

TREATMENT

Records of successful therapy in grass sickness are few. The survival of some chronic cases appears attributable more to devoted nursing and the use of supportive therapy such as fluids and multivitamin injections than to a specific reversal of the disease process. A variety of treatments are recorded; a coaltar preparation and an infusion of the broom plant (*Cytisus scoparius*), potassium, and diluted formalin have been used to no good effect,[2] but recovery of a case of suspected grass sickness followed treatment with colloidal manganese.[3] The anticholinesterase

drug eserine and its synthetic analogue have been used (unpublished), as have other common purgatives, but none has appeared to relieve the gastrointestinal paralysis. The most successful treatment recorded involved the continuous withdrawal of stomach contents and the simultaneous intravenous administration of a large volume of saline.[8] This was applied to three cases, and although technically difficult, afforded spectacular relief. When, however, the complex procedures failed to operate, symptoms returned unabated and death resulted.

Many sources of toxins and types of infections have been investigated in an unsuccessful search for the cause of this disease. It is now known, however, that a circulating neurotoxic factor is present in acute cases of grass sickness,[4, 6] and this may be closely related to the etiology of the disease. Current research seeks to identify this factor, clarify its role, and trace its origin.

References

1. Barlow, R. M.: Neuropathological observations in grass sickness of horses. J. Comp. Pathol., 79:407, 1969.
2. Begg, G. W.: Grass disease in horses. Vet. Rec., 48:655, 1936.
3. Davidson, G. W. D.: Colloidal manganese in suspected grass disease. Vet. Rec., 25:699, 1932.
4. Gilmour, J. S.: Experimental reproduction of the lesions associated with grass sickness. Vet. Rec., 92:565, 1973.
5. Gilmour, J. S.: Observations on neuronal changes in grass sickness of horses. Res. Vet. Sci., 15:197, 1973.
6. Gilmour, J. S., and Mould, D. L.: Experimental studies of neurotoxic activity in blood fractions from acute cases of grass sickness. Res. Vet. Sci., 22:1, 1977.
7. Obel, A. L.: Studies on grass disease. The morphological picture with special reference to the vegetative nervous system. J. Comp. Pathol., 65:334, 1955.
8. Robertson, A., Burgess, J. W., Inglis, J. S. S., and Paver, H.: Observations on gastric decompression and intravenous saline administration in acute grass disease. Vet. Rec., 60:495, 1948.

MALABSORPTION SYNDROMES

Jonathan E. Palmer, KENNETT SQUARE, PENNSYLVANIA

Malabsorption, which may be a consequence of a number of diseases, is the failure of passage of products through the intestinal mucosa. It should be distinguished from maldigestion, which is the failure of intraluminal digestion of carbohydrates, proteins, or fats due to a defect in pancreatic exocrine function, bile acid content, or brush border enzymes. Since brush border digestion of disaccharides and peptides is intimately connected with

absorption of monosaccharides and amino acids, it is often difficult to distinguish the two syndromes. Pure maldigestion as a primary clinical syndrome has not been described in the horse.

PATHOGENESIS AND ETIOLOGY

Defects in the cellular phase or the delivery phase of absorption may result in malabsorption. The cellular defects need not be grossly evident. Metabolic abnormalities may result in a change in the structural polarity of the cell and a decrease in available energy for active transport and maintenance of the carrier proteins or brush border enzymes. Such changes have been postulated as the cause of malabsorption in Whipple's disease in humans, in which malabsorption occurs without histologic changes in the epithelium.[6]

Most malabsorption associated with cellular defects is associated with villus atrophy, which is the result of a decrease in epithelial cell production or an increase in cell loss. The decrease in cell numbers results in a decrease in absorptive ability and thus malabsorption. In humans, minimal villus atrophy represents a decrease in cell numbers of 25 per cent, whereas clubbing and fusing of villi and complete villus atrophy represent a decrease in cell numbers of 90 and 97 per cent, respectively.[6]

Malabsorption caused by defects in the delivery phase of absorption occurs when substances that are normally absorbed by epithelial cells are not delivered to the blood vessels or lymphatics. This is usually attributed to a diffusion block caused by the physical presence of inflammatory cells, tumor cells, or intracellular substances such as amyloid. It is difficult to find a pure delivery defect, since diseases associated with infiltration of the submucosa often also have villus atrophy, reflecting a concurrent epithelial cell defect. This occurs in granulomatous enteritis, in which the infiltration of inflammatory cells results in impaired diffusion and thus a delivery defect. However, it also causes an epithelial cell defect and villus atrophy, probably because of a change in the local metabolic environment.

Causes of the malabsorption syndrome in the horse have not been extensively studied. In other species, epithelial defects leading to malabsorption may be caused by viruses, local or generalized ischemia, protein malnutrition, and high doses of oral neomycin.[6] In the horse, it is likely that rotaviruses and other enteric viruses cause a transient malabsorption due to damage to epithelial cells. This is probably common and important in the pathogenesis of the resulting diarrhea but need not be treated, since it is a short-lived problem. *Strongylus vulgaris* may cause malabsorption because of local intestinal ischemia caused by the migration of larval stages. Protein malnutrition may also be an important cause of malabsorption in the horse. Since the clinical presentations of malnutrition and malabsorption are very similar, the role of secondary malabsorption in malnutrition may be overlooked. It is interesting to note that in humans, concurrent protein and carbohydrate malnutrition does not cause malabsorption, but protein malnutrition alone does.[9] Treatment of horses with diarrhea with high doses of oral neomycin is a common practice. This, in fact, may exacerbate the diarrhea by producing malabsorption through changes in the absorptive epithelial cells as well as by causing an imbalance in gastrointestinal tract flora.

The best documented cause of malabsorption in the horse is granulomatous enteritis.[11, 12] As noted earlier, this is an example of both an epithelial cell defect and a delivery block. The etiology of this disease is unknown, but it most closely resembles Crohn's disease in humans.[5] In the horse, a granulomatous reaction can result from infection by avian tuberculosis,[11] *Mycobacterium paratuberculosis*,[10] and intestinal histoplasmosis.[4]

Another documented cause of malabsorption in the horse is intestinal lymphosarcoma.[16] This disease is very similar to granulomatous enteritis in the horse, and the two may be confused without careful histologic examination. Intestinal amyloidosis is another possible cause of malabsorption; however, this is an exceedingly rare condition in the horse.

DIAGNOSIS

The diagnosis of malabsorption is usually made with the aid of monosaccharide (glucose and xylose) and fatty acid (tritiated oleic acid) absorption tests.[11–13] An etiologic diagnosis requires an intestinal mucosal biopsy. With the exception of a few cases that can be diagnosed with a rectal biopsy, major surgery is required to obtain the biopsy, but because of the poor nutritional state of the horse, wound healing is poor and dehiscence is often a problem. For these reasons, many cases of malabsorption are diagnosed solely with the aid of absorption tests.

Both glucose and xylose absorption tests are performed in a similar manner. The horse is fasted for 12 to 18 hours before and throughout the test period. Water is withheld for the first two hours of the test period. Half a gram of xylose per kg body weight as a 10 per cent aqueous solution or 1 gm of anhydrous glucose per kg body weight as a 20 per cent aqueous solution is given by stomach tube. Heparinized blood samples are taken for xylose determination, and potassium oxalate–sodium fluoride samples are taken for glucose determination. Samples taken before administration of the sugar and then every half hour for four hours are centrifuged, and the plasma is kept at $0°$ C until the determinations can be made. A maximum xylose blood level of 20.6 ± 4.8 mg per ml is expected at 60 minutes.[1] The zero time glucose level should be doubled by 120 minutes.[15] When graphing the results against time, a clear peak should be seen. The finding of a peak is as important as the absolute levels. The xylose and glucose absorption tests should not be run concurrently because of the competition between the two sugars for absorption.

Since carbohydrate absorption tests are often the only criteria for diagnosis of the malabsorption syndrome, their limitations should be noted. A common cause of a delayed peak in the absorption curve of both glucose and xylose absorption tests is a delayed gastric emptying resulting from hypertonicity of the glucose or xylose mixture, excitement, pain, or retained gastric contents. The stomach must be emptied of ingesta by fasting the horse in order to obtain an accurate test result. A 12-hour fast is often recommended. However, a longer fast is occasionally required to ensure a completely emptied stomach. The prolonged fast may cause problems for the glucose absorption test. A 0.5 gm per kg oral dose of glucose given after a 12-hour fast to a horse will result in 80 per cent absorption from the small intestine. However, after a 36-hour fast, only 40 to 50 per cent is absorbed.[2] Thus, prolonged fasting may give a false positive result with the glucose absorption test.

Other changes in gastrointestinal transit time that occur with changes in motility or partial obstruction may also cause a delayed peak in absorption. These delays are not usually confused with malabsorption unless the curve is not followed long enough to see the peak.

Several circumstances will cause a flat absorption curve to occur in a horse with normal absorptive capacity. A transient decrease in the intestinal blood flow may cause decreased absorption with normal mucosa. An equally confusing picture occurs when bacteria in the lumen of the small intestine metabolize the test sugar. This problem has been solved in human medicine by the recent introduction of the ^{14}C xylose absorption breath test. If there is a question of bacterial metabolism of xylose in a patient with a flat curve, the test is repeated using the radiolabeled sugar. If the bacteria are metabolizing the sugar, $^{14}CO_2$ is released early in the test and is found in the expired breath of the patient. Another problem with xylose is its tendency to rapidly equilibrate with many body fluids such as ascites. This lowers the blood level of xylose and gives a flat curve.[7] Similarly, since the glucose space and metabolism are controlled by the endocrine pancreas and the liver, an abnormality in glucose regulation may give an abnormal glucose absorption curve.

There are a few rare circumstances that cause a falsely high absorption curve. Fifty per cent of the absorbed xylose is secreted in the urine. Renal failure will cause an increase in blood xylose levels. About 13 per cent of the absorbed xylose is metabolized in the liver, and liver dysfunction can also raise blood xylose levels.[7]

Deciding whether to run a glucose or xylose absorption test is based on a number of factors. Glucose is a more readily available substrate for many practitioners, and the cost of the serum assay is low. However, the glucose absorption test is less specific than the xylose absorption test, since abnormalities of glucose regulation are also reflected in the test results. At least theoretically, the glucose absorption test is less sensitive than the xylose absorption test. Glucose is efficiently absorbed in the small intestine, and there is a large absorptive reserve capacity, even at high glucose levels. Thus, enough damage must be done to destroy this reserve before there is malabsorption of glucose. Xylose, on the other hand, is not effectively absorbed in the small intestine. Although it is actively absorbed using the same carrier as glucose, its affinity for the carrier is not great, and most of the xylose is absorbed passively. In humans, only 50 per cent of the 25 gm dose of xylose is absorbed.[6] It is also likely that the horse is not an efficient absorber of xylose, as reflected by the low blood levels found in normal horses given xylose.[13] Thus, it is likely that the absorptive mechanisms are saturated during the normal test and that there is no absorptive reserve. Therefore, a decrease in carbohydrate absorptive function of the intestine should be reflected in the xylose absorption test before the glucose absorption test.

THERAPY

All the information concerning the treatment of granulomatous enteritis in the horse is anecdotal, since no controlled treatment studies have been performed.

At this time, the most useful therapy seems to be anti-inflammatory agents, such as corticosteroids. Experience with a few cases suggests that the use of moderate doses of corticosteroids, such as 0.5 mg per kg of prednisolone twice daily, is indicated and may cause some regression of the lesion.[12] However, the response to therapy is inconsistent, and it often seems that by the time the horse begins to show clinical signs, it is beyond the time when treatment would be beneficial.

Another potentially useful drug that is best categorized as an anti-inflammatory agent is sulfasalazine (formally salicylazosulfapyridine).* The colonic bacteria split the azo bond in sulfasalazine, releasing 5-aminosalicylate and sulfapyridine. The mechanism of action is not thought to involve the antimicrobial activity of the drug, since sulfapyridine is rapidly

---

*Azulfidine, Pharmacia Laboratories, Piscataway, NJ 08854

absorbed after its release with no change in the gut flora. It is known that 5-aminosalicylic acid has antiprostaglandin activities, and this is thought to be its major beneficial action. Sulfasalazine at a dose of 15 mg per kg four times a day may have a beneficial effect in granulomatous enteritis in the horse.

Another approach to the treatment of granulomatous enteritis in the horse is the use of antimicrobial agents such as isoniazid (5 to 20 mg per kg per day). At least some cases have been associated with avian tuberculosis.[11] There is a possibility that the etiology may involve atypical mycobacteria that may be difficult to detect because of the presence of mycobacteriophages.[3] Although any horse shown to be infected by tuberculous organisms should be destroyed for public health reasons, the use of antituberculous agents such as isoniazid may have a place in treating granulomatous enteritis.

Specific therapy for other causes of malabsorption, with the exception of *Strongylus vulgaris*, which is covered elsewhere (p. 272), is not available. The use of DMSO for the treatment of renal amyloidosis has been reported, but its use in amyloidosis affecting the gastrointestinal tract has not.

SUPPORTIVE THERAPY

The general nutritional support of the horse with malabsorption is of prime importance. Although total parenteral hyperalimentation is the most rational approach, the cost (up to $500 per day in humans) and difficulty of maintaining intravenous catheters during long-term hypertonic fluid administration make this approach impractical. Malabsorption is nearly complete before clinical signs develop. However, there continues to be some absorption by the small intestine. Thus, ideally the horse should be fed small, frequent meals to take advantage of the limited remaining absorptive ability of the small intestine without overloading it. Unfortunately, most of the amino acids that are not absorbed in the small intestine will be lost to the horse. Even though the normal horse may be able to absorb a limited amount of amino acids from the large intestine,[8] it probably does not contribute significantly in these cases. On the other hand, since 25 to 30 per cent of the normal horse's energy requirements are met by volatile fatty acid production in the large intestine,[8] it is reasonable to assume that in malabsorption, some of the carbohydrates and fats that are not absorbed in the small intestine will be utilized for energy by the horse.

Nutritional therapy should be aimed at providing easily absorbed protein and carbohydrates, maintaining mineral balance, and supplementing with fat and water-soluble vitamins. The horse's diet should be supplemented with a high-quality, easily digested protein source. Milk protein is a high-quality source and is easily handled by the horse's small intestine; however, because horses over three years of age lack lactase,[16] whole milk should not be used. Easily absorbable carbohydrates may also be provided; however, glucose has no advantage over sucrose, since sucrose is more efficiently absorbed in the horse than glucose.[2, 16] Since Ca, Mg, Zn, Cu, and Fe are only absorbed in the small intestine of the horse[8] and since these minerals may be lost by binding to protein in a concurrent protein-losing enteropathy, their levels should be followed, and parenteral supplementation may be necessary. Although thiamine and B_{12} are absorbed in the large intestine of the horse to a certain extent,[8] large intestine absorption of vitamins should not be relied on. Fat-soluble vitamins may be retained in the intestinal lumen because of fat malabsorption. Thus, both water-soluble and fat-soluble vitamins should be supplemented parenterally.

References

1. Bolton, J. R., Merritt, A. M., Cimprich, R. E., Ramberg, C. F., and Street, W.: Normal and abnormal xylose absorption in the horse. Cornell Vet., 66:183, 1976.
2. Breukink, H. J.: Oral mono- and disaccharide tolerance tests in ponies. Am. J. Vet. Res., 35:1523, 1974.
3. Cimprich, R. E.: Equine granulomatous enteritis. Vet. Pathology 11:535, 1974.
4. Dade, A. W., Lickfeldt, W. E., and McAllister, H. A.: Granulomatous colitis in a horse with histoplasmosis. VM SAC, 68:279, 1973.
5. Donaldson, J. R., and Robert, M.: Crohn's disease of the small bowel. In Sleisenger, M. H., and Fordtran, J. S. (eds.): Gastrointestinal Disease. Philadelphia, W. B. Saunders Co., 1978, p. 1052.
6. Gray, G. M.: Maldigestion and malabsorption: Clinical manifestations and specific diagnosis. In Sleisenger, M. H., and Fordtran, J. S. (eds.): Gastrointestinal Disease. Philadelphia, W. B. Saunders Co., 1978, p. 272.
7. Hindmarsh, J. T.: Xylose absorption and its clinical significance. Clin. Biochem., 9:141, 1976.
8. Hintz, H. F., and Schryver, H. F.: Digestive physiology of the horse. J. Eq. Med. Surg., 2:147, 1978.
9. Jeffries, G. H., Weser, E., and Sleisenger, M. H.: Progress in gastroenterology: Malabsorption. Gastroenterology, 56:777, 1969.
10. Larsen, A. B., Moon, H. W., and Merkal, R. S.: Susceptibility of horses to *Mycobacterium paratuberculosis*. Am. J. Vet. Res., 33:2185, 1972.
11. Merritt, A. M., Cimprich, R. E., and Beech, J.: Granulomatous enteritis in nine horses. J. Am. Vet. Med. Assoc., 169:603, 1976.
12. Meuten, D. J., Butler, D. G., Thomson, G. W., and Lumsden, J. H.: Chronic enteritis associated with malabsorption and protein-losing enteropathy in the horse. J. Am. Vet. Med. Assoc., 172:326, 1978.
13. Roberts, M. C.: The D (+) xylose absorption test in the horse. Eq. Vet. J., 6:28, 1974.
14. Roberts, M. C.: Carbohydrate digestion and absorption studies in the horse. Res. Vet. Sci., 18:64, 1975.
15. Roberts, M. C., and Hill, F. W. G.: The oral glucose tolerance test in the horse. Eq. Vet. J., 5:171, 1973.
16. Roberts, M. C., and Pinsent, P. J. N.: Malabsorption in the horse associated with alimentary lymphosarcoma. Eq. Vet. J., 7:166, 1975.

ACUTE HEPATITIS

Bud C. Tennant, ITHACA, NEW YORK

Steve Dill, ITHACA, NEW YORK

CAUSES OF HEPATITIS

Acute hepatitis was recognized in large numbers of South African horses by Theiler following immunization against African horse sickness using simultaneous administration of live virus and immune serum of equine origin.[13] A disease similar to this was observed subsequently in the United States following immunization against western equine encephalomyelitis using live virus and equine antiserum simultaneously. Initially described as the "second disease" because hepatitis appeared in epidemics several weeks following initial outbreaks of encephalomyelitis, it was subsequently shown to occur almost exclusively in horses that had received equine serum.[4]

Since these original descriptions, epidemics of hepatitis have been recorded in horses following prophylactic administration of equine antiserum against equine encephalomyelitis virus, *Clostridium perfringens, C. botulinum, Streptococcus equi,* and the influenza virus.[12, 14] Sporadic cases also have been observed following the use of pregnant mare's serum and tetanus antitoxin,[3, 7] with a remarkably high frequency of hepatitis reported in southern California following tetanus antiserum administration.[8]

These observations taken collectively suggest that acute hepatitis in horses can result from an infection similar to that causing hepatitis associated with homologous serum administration or blood transfusion in humans. Large epidemics of acute hepatitis, however, have been reported in horses in which no association with equine serum administration could be made.

In a recent report of 40 cases of acute hepatitis, only six had histories of equine serum (tetanus antitoxin) administration prior to the onset of clinical signs. Two others developed hepatitis following contact with cases that had received injections of equine serum.[12]

Although most individual horses with acute hepatitis have no history of equine serum administration, this does not eliminate the possibility that many hepatitis cases are the result of a primary viral infection. If such an infection does exist, however, there must be modes of transmission in addition to serum injections. Our own experience and that reported by others during epidemics of postvaccinal hepatitis suggest that contact transmission can occur,[12, 14] but at this time, one can only speculate regarding the cause, incidence, or modes of transmission of suspected infectious hepatitis in horses.

It seems probable that dietary and other environmental toxins also play a role in the pathogenesis of acute equine hepatitis. Plants containing pyrrolizidine alkaloids typically produce a chronic liver disease that is characterized by megalocytosis, bile duct proliferation, and cirrhosis, differing significantly from the histopathology of acute hepatitis. Acute pyrrolizidine alkaloid poisoning has been reported in the horse,[6] however, and in the early stages, with massive hepatic necrosis, it would be impossible to distinguish with certainty the parenchymal damage induced by the pyrrolizidine alkaloids from other hepatotoxins or from the type of acute hepatitis that has been associated with serum administration.[7]

Several other hepatotoxins have been identified in the diet of horses. Alsike clover produces severe hepatic disease, although the clinical syndrome usually is chronic. Aflatoxin poisoning causes acute hepatic necrosis in horses similar to that observed in other species, and the toxin of *Penicillin rubrum* (rubratoxin), a frequent contaminant of corn, also causes acute hepatic necrosis in horses.[5, 12]

Outbreaks of acute hepatic disease in horses have been observed following application of waste oil to riding arenas for dust control and the poisonous principal identified as 2,3,7,8-tetrachlorodibenzodioxin (dioxin, TCDD).[1] These observations demonstrate that the improper disposal of toxic chemical waste must be kept in mind in the investigation of the cause of acute hepatitis. The possibility of two dietary or environmental toxins acting synergistically also must be considered.

A high seasonal frequency of acute hepatitis has been reported in the northeastern United States during the summer and fall.* Such a seasonal frequency was not, however, apparent in California.[12] Although the interpretation is not clear, these observations suggest that seasonal and associated environmental factors must also be considered in trying to identify the causes of acute equine hepatitis.[12]

CLINICAL SIGNS AND LABORATORY DIAGNOSIS

The presenting clinical signs of hepatic insufficiency in both acute and chronic forms of hepatic

---

*We are indebted to our colleague, Dr. John King, who first brought this to our attention.

249

disease may be similar.[2] The liver must lose more than half its functional reserve capacity before signs of failure become clinically apparent. Then, regardless of the cause and duration of the underlying hepatic disease, the onset of clinical signs may be abrupt with a fulminant clinical course. In acute hepatitis, this is the typical pattern. In cases of cirrhosis, there may be a variable pattern of malaise and weight loss for several weeks or months, then abrupt deterioration in the clinical course and development of signs of hepatic failure.[11]

When presented for examination, horses with acute hepatitis almost invariably are icteric, and signs of hepatic encephalopathy have been observed in more than 80 per cent of cases.[9, 11] Photodermatitis affecting unpigmented areas of skin, particularly the muzzle and extremities, and intravascular hemolysis[10] are seen less frequently. A combination of these clinical signs in association with elevations of serum bilirubin, aspartate aminotransferase (SGOT), gamma glutamyltransferase (γ-GT), sorbitol dehydrogenase (SDH), and alkaline phosphatase (AP) provide a basis for the presumptive diagnosis of acute hepatitis. Confirmation is usually based on percutaneous liver biopsy. These clinical, biochemical, and histologic data do not allow establishment of the actual cause of hepatitis. One must rely on historic or special chemical analyses for establishment of hepatotoxic causes. There are no specific tests at this time for suspected infectious viral agents, but because of rapid developments in human virus hepatitis research, we may anticipate advances in the equine field in the future.

TREATMENT

Treatment of patients with hepatic insufficiency is often difficult because of the degree of hepatic injury that has occurred before clinical signs are manifested. It is important to determine if the patient is affected with acute hepatitis or with chronic hepatic insufficiency because the prognosis associated with chronic hepatic insufficiency is so unfavorable that treatment may not be advisable.

Therapy of acute hepatitis is directed toward support of the patient for a sufficient period of time to allow spontaneous regeneration of hepatocytes. One of the most important considerations is the control of hepatic encephalopathy. Initial control of maniacal behavior in many cases can be provided by administration of the phenothiazine tranquilizers or xylazine, both of which may be required in reduced dosage because of hepatic insufficiency.

Measures directed toward decreasing blood ammonia levels also are indicated. Oral administration of a poorly absorbed antibiotic such as neomycin is recommended to decrease bacterial metabolism in the colon and the production of ammonia and other neurotoxic metabolites. The daily dose of neomycin is 40 to 60 gm per 400 kg horse divided in three to four doses. Cathartics such as dioctyl sodium sulfosuccinate or mineral oil also are indicated to reduce gastrointestinal stasis.

Providing the caloric needs of all anorectic patients is useful and is critical in those cases in which hepatic encephalopathy is associated with hypoglycemia.[11] Glucose can be given by nasogastric tube or by continuous intravenous drip as a 5 to 10 per cent solution. The resting (maintenance) energy requirement of a standard-sized horse is approximately 5 gm of dextrose per kg per 24 hours.

Photodermatitis in most cases is related to elevations in phylloerythrin, the porphyrin produced from dietary chlorophyll by the action of intestinal bacteria. Prevention of photodermatitis can be accomplished most readily by eliminating exposure to direct sunlight. Reduction in chlorophyll intake also may be beneficial.

Corticosteroid therapy has been suggested for treatment of certain types of hepatic failure.[11] In acute hepatitis in horses, there are no studies to demonstrate therapeutic efficacy, and we generally do not recommend steroid therapy. In horses receiving glucose therapy, supplementation with 100 to 200 mg per day of thiamine is indicated, and provision of other B complex vitamin supplementation also may be indicated.

In acute hepatitis cases in which central nervous system disturbances are either absent or minimal, response to supportive therapy is generally satisfactory, and recovery is usually complete. The mortality rate in horses with more fulminant signs of hepatic encephalopathy, however, exceeds 70 per cent in our experience, even with intensive care, and efforts should be directed toward prevention where possible. Care should be taken to prevent exposure to hepatotoxins, such as hepatotoxic plants or grains contaminated with mycotoxin-producing fungi. It is hoped that future research will provide the diagnostic procedures necessary for control and prevention of acute hepatitis of possible infectious etiology.

References

1. Carter, C. D., Kimbrough, R. D., Liddle, J. A., Cline, R. E., Zack, M. M., Jr., Barthel, W. F., Koehler, R.E., and Phillips, P. E.: Tetrachlorodibenzodioxin: An accidental poisoning episode in horse arenas. Science, *188*:738, 1975.
2. Fowler, M. E.: Clinical manifestations of primary hepatic insufficiency in the horse. J. Am. Vet. Med. Assoc., *147*:55, 1965.
3. Hjerpe, C. A.: Serum hepatitis in the horse. J. Am. Vet. Med. Assoc., *144*:734, 1964.
4. Marsh, H.: Losses of undetermined cause following an outbreak of equine encephalomyelitis. J. Am. Vet. Med. Assoc., *91*:88, 1937.
5. McGavin, M. D., and Knake, R.: Hepatic midzonal necrosis

in a pig fed aflatoxin and a horse fed moldy hay. Vet. Pathol., *14*:182, 1977.

6. McLintock, J., and Fell, B. F.: A case of acute ragwort poisoning in the horse. Vet. Rec., 65:319, 1953.

7. Robinson, M., Gopinath, C., and Hughes, D. L.: Histopathology of acute hepatitis in the horse J. Comp. Pathol., 85:111, 1975.

8. Rose, J. A., Immenschuh, R. D., and Rose, E. M.: Serum hepatitis in the horse. Proc. 20th Annu. Meet. Am. Assoc. Eq. Pract., 1974, p. 175.

9. Tennant, B., Baldwin, B. H., Silverman, S. L., and Makowski, C.: Clinical significance of hyperbilirubinemia in the horse. Proc. 1st Int. Symp. Eq. Hemat., May 1975, pp. 246–254.

10. Tennant, B., Evans, C. D., Kaneko, J. J., and Schalm, O. W.: Intravascular hemolysis associated with hepatic failure in the horse. Calif. Vet., 27:15, 1972.

11. Tennant, B., Evans, C. D., Schwartz, L. W., Gribble, D. H., and Kaneko, J. J.: Equine hepatic insufficiency. Vet. Clin. North Am., 3:279, 1973.

12. Tennant, B.: Acute hepatitis in horses: Problems of differentiating toxic and infectious causes in the adult. Proc. 24th Annu. Meet. Am. Assoc. Eq. Pract. 1978, p. 465.

13. Theiler, A.: Acute liver atrophy and parenchymatous hepatitis in horses. 5th and 6th Rep. Dir. Vet. Res., Dept. Agriculture, Union of South Africa, 1919, p. 15.

14. Thomsett, L. R.: Acute hepatic failure in the horse. Eq. Vet. J., 3:15, 1971.

CHRONIC LIVER DISEASE

Bradford P. Smith, DAVIS, CALIFORNIA

Chronic injury to the liver results in damage that may only become clinically evident when more than half of the functional capacity of the liver is destroyed. Once the reserve capacity of the liver is exceeded, clinical signs of hepatic failure may appear quite suddenly. Thus, clinical signs alone are insufficient to determine if the liver disease is acute or chronic.

CLINICAL SIGNS

The temperature, pulse, and respiratory rate of horses with chronic liver disease are usually normal, although in the terminal stages of failure, they may be elevated. Anorexia, variable depression, and some change in personality or behavior of the horse is often noted by the owner. Such personality aberrations include poor feed discrimination, excessive yawning, and general lethargy, which may progress to full-blown hepatoencephalopathy. Icterus is variable and may be absent in some horses with chronic liver disease.

Weight loss is usually present but may be noted simply as unthriftiness rather than emaciation. Photosensitization develops in nonpigmented areas that are exposed to sunlight in about 25 per cent of horses. In contrast to other species, edema and ascites rarely occur in horses with chronic liver disease. Defective blood clotting, manifested by hemorrhages on mucous membranes, bleeding, or hematoma formation at venipuncture sites, is seen only occasionally. The unthriftiness and other clinical signs noted in horses with chronic hepatic disease are related to loss of important liver functions. These include synthesis of albumin and some nonessential amino acids, gluconeogenesis, storage of lipid-soluble vitamins, and the metabolism and excretion of potentially toxic substances.

The clinical signs related to partial loss of these functions are rather nonspecific, and laboratory tests are often required to determine the presence of chronic liver disease. Once liver failure has occurred, it may be helpful to distinguish acute failure from chronic failure, since animals with chronic failure carry a very poor prognosis and are almost invariably dead within six months regardless of therapy. Although difficult to treat, acute liver failure carries a better prognosis, and if one is able to provide supportive therapy, regeneration may occur following acute failure.

CAUSES

The most common cause of chronic liver disease in many areas of the world is pyrrolizidine alkaloid toxicity. Plants containing pyrrolizidine alkaloids include *Amsinckia intermedia*, a number of Senecio species, several Crotolaria species, *Heliotropium europaeum*, and *Eschium lycopsis*. Most are unpalatable when green and are avoided in pastures if other feed is available. Problems arise mainly when hay, cubes, pellets, or grains are contaminated and the animal is unable to selectively avoid ingestion of these plants. In California, *Senecio vulgaris* is a common contaminant of first cutting alfalfa hay, while *Amsinckia intermedia* is most often found in grass hays such as oat hay cut in spring. Hay may be examined for evidence that it contains these weeds, or in the case of cubes or pellets, it may be necessary to submit samples for chemical analysis for pyrrolizidine alkaloids. Ingestion of large amounts of heavily contaminated hay may result in clinical signs within weeks. More commonly, low-level exposure occurs, often with a period of months before clinical signs of chronic liver disease become apparent. Clinical signs may appear long after all contaminated feed has been consumed, as the effects appear to continue once fibrosis begins.

The classical histologic features of chronic liver disease due to pyrrolizidine alkaloid toxicity are fibrosis, megalocytosis, and bile duct proliferation. A liver biopsy is the best means by which to confirm a diagnosis of pyrrolizidine toxicity.

LABORATORY TESTS

Laboratory tests can be divided into two major categories: (1) liver-derived serum enzymes, which provide an index of continuing liver damage; and (2) liver function tests. The concentration of liver-derived serum enzymes provides an indication of active liver damage but not necessarily of liver failure. Enzyme elevations may also occur secondary to other disease conditions such as severe anemia, anoxia, acute toxic enteritis, and with other severe systemic diseases. Liver-specific enzymes in the horse include sorbitol dehydrogenase (SDH) and ornithine carbamyl transferase (OCT). Nonspecific enzymes include lactic dehydrogenase (LDH) and aspartate amino transferase (AST), which was formerly called glutamic oxalacetic transaminase (GOT). Alkaline phosphatase (AP), although nonspecific, is particularly elevated in horses with chronic liver diseases involving the bile ducts (chronic biliary cirrhosis). Gamma-glutamyl transpeptidase (GGT) is liver-specific and very useful in the diagnosis of chronic liver disease. In many cases, the most active phase of hepatic destruction has passed before the problem is brought to veterinary attention, so that normal serum enzymes may be found in some horses with severe chronic liver disease, although GGT and AP often remain elevated.

Serum bilirubin is almost always markedly elevated in acute liver disease but commonly is only slightly elevated in chronic liver disease. Blood urea nitrogen (BUN) below 9 mg per dl is a fairly consistent feature of horses with severe chronic liver disease as well as horses with acute or chronic liver failure. Bilirubinuria is also seen in most horses with liver disease and imparts a green-brown color to the urine.

The sulfobromophthalein (BSP) clearance half-time provides an extremely useful assessment of hepatic function in the horse. The normal clearance ($T\frac{1}{2}$) is less than 3.7 min and when greater than 5 min indicates significant hepatic dysfunction. The test is useful if the total serum bilirubin is below 6 mg per dl, since above that level the half-time is invariably increased owing to competition of the dye with bilirubin for conjugation.

Once the clinician has determined that the clinical signs are due to liver disease, a liver biopsy can be an extremely useful diagnostic procedure to aid in determining the type of liver disease. It is safe, quick, easy, and provides otherwise unobtainable information. If the horse has evidence of a coagulopathy, a prothrombin time should be done prior to the biopsy. On rare occasions, the horse may exsanguinate following biopsy if a bleeding problem exists. In horses presented with liver failure, histopathologic examination allows the clinician to determine whether the disease is acute or chronic and whether massive supportive therapy is justified.

The prognosis for horses with chronic liver disease is generally unfavorable. It is grave if evidence of hepatoencephalopathy, intravascular hemolysis, or fever exists. Even when these grave signs have not yet appeared, supportive treatment of chronic liver disease is likely to be of only temporary benefit.

TREATMENT

Therapy for horses with chronic liver disease with failure is similar to that employed in horses suffering from acute liver disease (p. 249):

Horses should be housed out of direct sunlight.

A continuous intravenous infusion of 5 per cent dextrose at a rate of 1 l per hr will usually maintain blood glucose levels at 100 to 160 mg per dl. This amount of glucose will not supply the animal's total caloric requirements but helps to meet immediate glucose needs. A maintenance solution such as half-strength Ringer's lactate with 2.5 per cent dextrose may be used if intravenous therapy continues for more than two or three days.

A diet relatively low in protein but highly digestible is preferred to minimize the production of ammonia and other potentially neurotoxic substances by the intestinal microflora. A grass hay and grain (high-carbohydrate) may be the best diet. A nonabsorbable antimicrobial drug such as neomycin (10 gm two times a day) given orally should also help to minimize production of these products by decreasing the colonic microbial population. Protracted use of oral antimicrobial drugs may lead to changes in enteric microflora and the development of diseases such as salmonellosis. Oral antimicrobials should therefore be used cautiously in horses with severe liver disease.

Mild laxatives such as mineral oil may be helpful in keeping the feces soft. Horses with chronic liver disease often have small, hard fecal balls.

Corticosteroids are beneficial in horses with

chronic active hepatitis because of their anti-inflammatory effect. They do not appear to be beneficial in noninflammatory liver conditions such as chronic end-stage liver disease, nor are they useful for maintaining blood glucose levels, since the liver must be functional for corticosteroids to exert their gluconeogenic effect.

If the horse is not eating or drinking, stomach tubing with glucose and electrolyte solutions is indicated. Additional calories may also be supplied by other liquid dietary supplements in this way.

Dietary supplementation with branched-chain amino acids (leucine, isoleucine, and valine) may be beneficial. At present, the cost of these purified supplements is high. Sorghum grains (such as milo) have a relatively high content of branched-chain amino acids and may thus be useful supplements in horses with liver disease.

In addition to the forms of therapy discussed here, it is obvious that all horses should be prevented from ingesting more contaminated feed.

Contaminated feed may be economically difficult to dispose of. Since sheep appear to be relatively resistant to the toxic effects of pyrrolizidine alkaloids, the feed could be mixed with uncontaminated hay and fed to sheep. Cattle, especially young growing calves, are susceptible to the alkaloid.

Supplemental Readings

1. Carlson, G. P.: Liver disease in the horse. *In* Mansmann, R. A., and McAllister, E. S. (eds.): Equine Medicine and Surgery, 3rd ed. Santa Barbara, CA, American Veterinary Pub., Inc., in press, 1982.
2. Cornelius, C. E., and Wheat, J. D.: Bromosulfophthalein clearance in the horse: A quantitative liver function test. Am. J. Vet. Res., 18:369, 1957.
3. Gulick, B. A., et al.: Use of plasma amino acid patterns in liver disease of the horse. Calif. Vet., 33:21, 1979.
4. Qualls, C. W., and Segall, H. J.: Rapid isolation and identification of pyrrolizidine alkaloids (*Senecio vulgaris*) by use of high performance liquid chromatography. J. Chromatogr., 150:202, 1978.

CHRONIC PANCREATITIS

Debra Deem Morris, KENNETT SQUARE, PENNSYLVANIA

Chronic pancreatitis is rarely recognized clinically in the horse but is not an infrequent necropsy finding.[5] Chronic interstitial pancreatitis is the form usually seen and may arise by spread of an inflammatory process that begins in the ducts. The causes are nonspecific, and the microbes present are the normal inhabitants of the gastrointestinal tract. Since the biliary and pancreatic ducts enter the duodenum via a common papilla, cholangitis and mild hepatitis frequently coexist with pancreatitis. Pancreatitis that begins in the interstitial tissue is common in horses as a result of verminous migration. The larvae of *Strongylus equinus* pass part of their developmental cycle in and about the pancreas, and the larvae of *S. vulgaris* and *S. edentatus* sometimes reach the pancreas by aberrant migration.

Chronic pancreatitis is usually subclinical in horses and is only recognized when there has been sufficient disease to result in fibrotic replacement of the islets of Langerhans and subsequent hypoinsulinism (diabetes mellitus) (p. 169).

Signs referable to exocrine pancreatic insufficiency, notably steatorrhea and voluminous stool, do not occur in horses with chronic pancreatitis even though necropsy may reveal an absence of acinar tissue. Lack of steatorrhea is partially due to the fact that the equine diet contains very little fat, but there is evidence that pancreatic enzymes, amylase, lipase, trypsin, and the peptidases, are not essential for digestion in the horse. Microbial fermentation of substrate undigested in the small intestine takes place in the cecum and large colon, resulting in the production of volatile fatty acids that are absorbed and metabolized for energy.

Pancreatic secretion of the horse possesses certain unusual features that further support the concept that it is not highly important in digestion. The resting secretion is profuse and continuous but can be increased to even higher rates by nervous and hormonal stimuli. The content and output of digestive enzymes in the juice is extremely small.[1] Stimulation of the vagus nerves increases the amylase concentration to only 2 to 4 U per ml compared with 50 to 80 U per ml in the pig and dog.[2]

Another unique feature of equine pancreatic juice is that the bicarbonate concentration is low and does not exceed that of chloride at any rate of secretion. The content of sodium and potassium resembles that of plasma, but in contrast to cats, dogs, humans, and pigs, chloride, rather than bicarbonate, is the predominant inorganic anion.[2,4] This distinctive quality of equine pancreatic juice suggests that its most important function may be the provision of a medium for anionic exchange in the terminal ileum. It has been established in a number of species that bicarbonate is secreted into the terminal ileum and colon, probably in exchange for chloride.[3] It would be advantageous if this capacity were well developed in the horse, so an abundant supply of bicarbonate would be available to buffer the products of fermentation in the large intestine. The effect of pancreatic insufficiency on microbial fermentation in the equine large intestine has not been studied.

References

1. Alexander, F., and Hickson, J. C. D.: The salivary and pancreatic secretions of the horse. *In* Phillipson, A. T. (ed.): Physiology of Digestion and Metabolism in the Ruminant. Newcastle-on-Tyne, England, O'Riel Press Ltd., 1970, pp. 375–389.
2. Hickson, J. C. D.: The secretion of pancreatic juice in response to stimulation of the vagus nerves in the pig. J. Physiol., *206*:275, 1970.
3. Hubel, K. A.: Effect of luminal chloride concentration on bicarbonate secretion in rat ileum. Am. J. Physiol., *217*:40, 1969.
4. Janowitz, H. D.: Pancreatic secretion of fluid and electrolytes. *In* Handbook of Physiology, Vol 6., Sec. II. Washington, DC, The American Physiological Society, 1967, p. 925.
5. Jubb, K. V. F., and Kennedy, P. C.: Pathology of Domestic Animals, Vol. 2. New York, Academic Press, 1970, pp. 263–276.

RECTAL PROLAPSE

John A. Stick, EAST LANSING, MICHIGAN

DIAGNOSIS

Although there is normally some prolapse of mucous membrane through the powerful cone-shaped sphincter muscles at defecation, rectal prolapse does not occur with the same frequency in the horse as it does in pigs and cattle. Rectal prolapse usually occurs in young animals and can be classified by the severity of evagination and anatomic structures involved as (1) mucosal prolapse, (2) complete mural prolapse of the rectum, or (3) complete prolapse of the rectum and small colon. In all cases, the exposed mucosa of prolapsed structures may be edematous, congested, and even necrotic. Mucosal prolapse appears as a doughnut shape at the anus, while a complete mural prolapse involving the ampulla recti is more spherical and larger. Prolapse of the rectum and small colon appears as a large sausage-shaped structure and should be differentiated by palpation from colonic intussusception. A prolapse involving the rectum is continuous with the mucocutaneous junction of the anus, while an intussusception has a palpable circumferential trench of variable depth inside the rectum.

PATHOPHYSIOLOGY

Rectal prolapse may be the result of any prolonged tenesmus. Predisposing factors may include loss of anal sphincter tone or laxity of the submucosal connective tissue attachments or suspensory ligament of the rectum. Labor, foaling accidents, or any condition that results in proctitis, such as bot larvae infection of the rectal mucosa, diarrhea, constipation, or false copulation, can all produce tenesmus, which leads to prolapse of the rectum.

MEDICAL MANAGEMENT

Conservative therapy of rectal prolapse is possible only if the evagination can be reduced. Irreducible rectal prolapse of several days duration or colonic intussusception usually requires surgical intervention. Medical therapy should be aimed at removal of the source of intrapelvic pressure or pelvic irritation and early reduction of the prolapse. This can be accomplished by topical anesthesia of rectal mucosa and/or perirectal structures using epidural anesthesia, depressing sensibilities with frequent use of sedatives, maintaining the animal in a standing position, and providing supportive local therapy to the prolapsed tissues.

Local anesthesia of the rectal mucosa can be achieved by topical application of an ointment four or five times a day. Preparations with water-insoluble bases*† may provide a greater duration of anesthetic action than water-soluble creams and will have the added benefit of delaying dehydration of exposed tissues. In the event that an anesthetic ointment is not available, topical application of a 2 per cent lidocaine solution may be used to give short-term relief of straining. Should the animal continue

---

*Nupercainal anesthetic ointment, CIBA Pharmaceutical Co., Div. CIBA-GEIGY Corp., Summit, NJ 07901

†Surfacaine Ointment 1 per cent, Eli Lilly and Co., Indianapolis, IN 46225

to strain after topical anesthetics have been applied in and around the prolapse, an epidural anesthetic should be given. The epidural space is entered between the first and second coccygeal vertebrae with a 5 to 7 cm 19-gauge needle inserted at a 60° angle from the horizontal plane. Eight to 10 ml of local anesthetic* injected into the epidural space is sufficient to produce anesthesia of the perineum for 1½ to 2 hours. Difficulties encountered with repeated use of epidural injections include failure to obtain adequate analgesia and rear limb paralysis, so this technique should be reserved for the initial examination and treatment period.

Sedation of the animal can be used as a method of chemical restraint to permit handling and treatment of the prolapse or as an added method of reducing the frequency and violence of tenesmus. A phenothiazine tranquilizer† is the drug of choice because it will provide greater duration of action and safety for the operator than will xylazine.‡

Injury to the prolapse can occur as the animal lies down and rises. Therefore, the animal should be maintained in a standing position through the use of short cross-ties. This will also reduce the increased abdominal pressure that occurs in a recumbent animal.

Topical medical therapy of prolapsed tissues may be the most important factor in permitting early reduction of the prolapse. Exposed tissues should be cleansed with mild soap and water and thoroughly rinsed to remove any residual soap. The rectal mucosa should be kept moist through the application of antimicrobial dressings such as nitrofurazone,§ tolnaftate,‖ or silver sulfadiazine** cream four to five times a day. Petroleum jelly or mineral oil may be used to serve the same purpose but will not aid in reducing local bacterial populations. Edema can be reduced by applying hot compresses to the rectal mucosa using bath towels. This should be continued for 20 minutes three to four times a day followed by application of the wound dressings. In cases in which severe edema has caused the prolapse to approach the size of a volleyball, several parallel longitudinal incisions 3 cm apart can be made through the mucosa on the ventral surface of the prolapse. This decreases the tension on the mucous membrane, relieves venous congestion, permitting some edema to resolve through the normal hemolymphatic system, and allows drainage of some edema fluid through the incisions.

After several treatments, the prolapse usually can be reduced by gentle manipulation. A pursestring suture in the anus may be used to maintain the prolapsed tissues in the normal position. Most of the remaining edema is usually resolved within 24 hours, and the suture should be removed. This procedure is less successful in the horse than in other animals because the consistency of equine feces makes defecation through the pursestring suture difficult, often leading to impaction of the rectum. To avoid this problem, the consistency of feces should be altered to a more moist form by the feeding of a pelleted mash or green grass prior to placement of the suture. Some horses tend to strain against the anal irritation of the suture, and a more successful approach is to replace the prolapse four to five times a day at the completion of each treatment period. This can be continued until necrotic mucosa sloughs and edema resolves, permitting the prolapse to stay reduced. Mucosal prolapses and some complete mural prolapses benefit from four to five days of medical therapy, circumventing the necessity for surgery.

SURGICAL MANAGEMENT

Uncontrolled straining, extensive tissue necrosis, and failure to maintain reduction of the prolapse after conservative therapy are indications for surgery. Mucosal prolapses with persistent polypoid masses of edematous or devitalized mucosa can be removed by submucosal resection. Complete mural prolapses can be treated by submucosal resection, but extensive prolapses, especially where tearing of mesocolon and mesorectum with associated disruption of blood supply have occurred, should be resected. Amputation of the rectum can be performed by two methods: (1) staged resection and suture in which one quadrant of the rectum is divided and sutured before dividing the next quadrant, or (2) transfixation to a prolapse ring or tube. After surgery, fecal consistency should be kept soft to prevent further straining during the healing period.

*Lidocaine hydrochloride injection 2 per cent, Vedco, Inc., Omaha, NB 68127

†Acepromazine maleate, Fort Dodge Laboratories, Inc., Fort Dodge, IA 50501

‡Rompun, Haver-Lockhart, Bayvet Division, Cutter Laboratories, Inc., Shawnee, KS 66201

§Furacin Dressing, Norden Laboratories, Inc., Lincoln, NB 68501

‖Tinavet Cream 1 per cent. Schering Corp., Kenilworth, NJ 07033

**Silvadene Cream, Marion Laboratories, Inc., Kansas City, MO 64137

Supplemental Readings

1. Johnson, H. W.: Submucosal resection: Surgical correction of prolapse of the rectum. J. Am. Vet. Med. Assoc., *102*:113, 1943.
2. Levine, S. B.: Surgical treatment of recurrent rectal prolapse in a horse. J. Eq. Med. Surg., 2:248, 1978.
3. Turner, T. A., and Fessler, J. F.: Rectal prolapse in the horse. J. Am. Vet. Med. Assoc., *177*:1028, 1980.
4. Walker, D. F., and Vaughn, J. T.: Bovine and Equine Urogenital Surgery. Philadelphia, Lea and Febiger, 1980, pp. 222–224.

RECTAL TEARS

Dean W. Richardson, KENNETT SQUARE, PENNSYLVANIA

Although most equine practitioners are aware of the inherent dangers of rectal palpation, rectal tears result in over 13 per cent of the malpractice suits involving the veterinarian in equine practice. Tears can be rapidly fatal, and immediate recognition and treatment are required for successful management.

The majority of rectal tears are iatrogenic as a sequela to rectal palpation and can be produced by even the most careful and experienced examiner. Other causes include penile penetration of the rectum during breeding, enemas, forceps extraction of meconium, sadism, and dystocia. Arabian horses may be predisposed to tears by their size and temperament. A disproportionate number of tears occur in male horses during rectal palpation because males are unaccustomed to the procedure that is usually used to palpate structures deep within the abdomen.

CLINICAL SIGNS

Immediate recognition of a rectal tear is important. A sanguineous tinge to the lubricant and rectal mucus usually indicates mucosal irritation. When blood or clots are on the withdrawn arm, a rectal tear should be first on the list of differential diagnoses. Prior to removing the arm, the examiner is often unaware that a tear has occurred, although a sudden release in tension of the rectum may be noted. Because tears can occur undetected at the time of palpation, a tear should be suspected in any horse showing signs of abdominal pain or shock within a few hours following a rectal examination.

THERAPY

Peristalsis should immediately be halted to prevent contamination of the peritoneum or pelvic cavity by rectal contents. An epidural anesthetic should be given to relax the anal sphincter and distal rectum. Intravenous xylazine* (0.1 to 0.2 mg per kg) will induce a transient relaxation of the large bowel as well as sedation that will facilitate further examination. A parasympatholytic drug such as propantheline bromide† (0.014 mg per kg) or atropine‡

---

*Rompun, Haver-Lockhart, Shawnee, KS 66201

†Probanthine for injection, Searle & Co., Chicago, IL 60680 (Note: this drug is very difficult to obtain; when needed, an oral preparation [15 mg tablets, Lannett Co., Philadelphia, PA 19136] can be dissolved in sterile water and centrifuged and the supernatant administered intravenously.)

‡Atofate (15 mg per ml), W. A. Butler Co., Columbus, OH 43228

(0.1 mg per kg) should be given intravenously. In most horses, the former drug relaxes the rectal wall within three minutes of administration. It is also useful in preventing rectal tears in horses that are difficult to examine. The drug's action is relatively short-lived, however, and treatment with a longer-acting drug such as atropine may be indicated if definitive therapy cannot be carried out at once.

After peristalsis has been slowed and an epidural anesthetic administered, a tube speculum can be inserted into the relaxed rectum to allow safe visual identification of the lesion. The mucosal folds make visualization difficult, however, and a heavily lubricated bare hand is probably more sensitive in delineating the location and severity of the tear. Since tears are classified by their depth, it is important to determine the extent of the tear through the bowel wall as accurately as possible.[2] Grade 1 tears cause a mucosal or submucosal defect only; Grade 2 tears extend into the muscularis; Grade 3 tears traverse all layers except serosa; and Grade 4 tears perforate all layers of the bowel. Grade 2 tears are rarely recognized, and their clinical significance is minimal. Grade 3 and 4 tears may extend into the suspending dorsal mesentery, which initially limits the extent of peritoneal contamination. Most tears occur in the dorsal third of the bowel; this may be due to an inherent weakness in that area or to the constriction of the rectum over the knuckles of the pronated hand.

After the tear has been assessed, the owner should be immediately informed of the problem and the prognosis given according to the severity of the tear. Immediate, vigorous treatment not only is an important part of the therapy but also improves the defense of a malpractice suit.

GRADE 1 TEARS

Grade 1 tears that are close to the anus can be sutured directly with the use of a Caslick's speculum and long-handled instruments. A headlamp* is invaluable in this surgery. A simple continuous pattern of heavy (No. 1) chromic gut is recommended.

If a Grade 1 tear is not readily accessible to surgical repair, medical management is usually successful. Overly vigorous attempts at repair may only enlarge the lesion. The horse should be started immediately on broad-spectrum antibiotics and a laxative diet such as green grass and bran mashes. Broad-spectrum antibiotics are essential to therapy of rectal lacerations of any type, since the colonic

---

*Headlight #49003, Welch Allyn, Skaneateles Falls, NY 13153

flora includes a variety of pathogenic facultative and anaerobic bacteria. Chloramphenicol* (30 mg per kg orally four times a day) or a combination of procaine penicillin G (5000 IU per kg intramuscularly twice a day) and gentamicin† (0.5 mg per kg intramuscularly four times a day) are generally effective. If it can be administered, potassium or sodium penicillin (5000 IU per kg) intravenously four to six times daily is more effective than procaine penicillin. It is important to note that aminoglycosides alone are generally ineffective against anaerobes. Mineral oil (3 to 4 l per 450 kg), dioctylsodium sulfosuccinate‡ (5 mg per kg), or magnesium sulfate (150 to 300 gm per 450 kg) and water (12 to 15 l) via stomach tube should be given to keep the feces as loose as possible in order to prevent distention of the injured rectum.

The area should not be palpated except with extreme care for the next four to six weeks. The horse should be monitored closely for several days for signs of fever, abdominal pain, and dyschezia. Serial peritoneal fluid analyses are useful in assessing progression of the lesion. Grade 1 tears of the rectum must be managed carefully in all cases because of the possibility of their further development into full-thickness lesions.

GRADE 3 AND 4 TEARS

Rectal lacerations extending beyond the muscularis are surgical emergencies, and horses should be referred to a clinic with the capacity to perform a laparotomy under general anesthesia. Tetanus prophylaxis, antibiotics, and parasympatholytics must be administered prior to shipment. Fecal balls in the area of the tear should be removed as gently as possible and the area lightly packed with antiseptic-soaked cotton.

SURGICAL CORRECTION

Suture of an intraperitoneal tear is most easily accomplished by a prepubic laparotomy with the horse in dorsal recumbency and its hind quarters elevated. The incision can be either midline or paramedian ipsilateral to the tear. A tube speculum in the rectum can facilitate intra-abdominal exposure and suturing of the tear.[1] In young or thin horses, the rectum can be prolapsed through the anus with intra-abdominal assistance so the lesion can be sutured directly. The use of nonabsorbable suture material is generally recommended in the colon.

COLOSTOMY

Rectal tears are often too friable and edematous to hold sutures well, and repeated attempts to place sutures may be harmful. For this reason, a diverting colostomy is indicated in many third- and fourth-degree tears.[1-6] Two major techniques are the end-on colostomy and the loop colostomy. The former technique (Fig. 1) involves transection of the small colon proximal to the tear, the distal segment being oversewn and carefully lavaged with an antiseptic solution. The proximal bowel is brought through the skin of the lower left flank at approximately the level of the stifle and sutured in place to allow complete diversion of fecal contents. The bowel should be sutured with interrupted sutures to each layer of the body wall to prevent herniation. Minimal body wall tissue should be removed in order to avoid subsequent peristomal herniation. Correct placement of the stoma to allow adequate emptying without herniation is important. The major disadvantage of the end-on technique is that reanastomosis is difficult because the distal segment undergoes atrophy.

A loop colostomy (Fig. 2) can be performed more rapidly, allows adequate fecal diversion when properly constructed, and also facilitates colostomy closure. Management of the stoma includes daily flushing of the functional and nonfunctional limbs and protection of the skin from scalding.

The severe peritonitis that follows Grade 3 or Grade 4 rectal tears may be life-threatening, despite successful closure of the tear and/or creation of a colostomy. Bacterial contamination also can lead to dehiscence of a sutured laceration or a colostomy. Peritoneal lavage is useful in the management of these cases. Lavage with large volumes (20 to 30 l) of a balanced electrolyte solution* containing antibiotics reduces the number of bacteria and amounts of toxins and adjuvant substances in the peritoneal cavity and presents high levels of antibiotics to the site of infection. Lavage in the horse is performed by infusing fluid through 14-gauge intravenous catheters† placed in both paralumbar fossae. Fluid is retrieved through one or two ventrally placed large-bore Foley catheters.‡ These drains are easily placed at the time of abdominal surgery or can be inserted in the standing horse using a blunt-ended instrument and local anesthesia. The ventral drains should be intermittently occluded and the horse walked to distribute the lavaging fluid. Heparin (50 units per kg) may be added to the lavage fluid to help prevent the formation of intra-abdominal ab-

*Anacetin, Bioceutic Labs, St Joseph, MO 64502

†Gentocin, Schering Corp., Kenilworth, NJ 07033

‡Aerosol OT 75 per cent; Fisher Scientific Co., Pittsburgh, PA 15219 (Note: This is a much more concentrated solution than other available products.)

*Normosol R, pH 7.4, Abbot Laboratories, North Chicago, IL 60064

†Abbocath-T 14 G × 5½″, Abbot Laboratories, North Chicago, IL 60064

‡Bardex 26F 75 cc balloon, C. R. Bard, Inc., Murray Hill, NJ 07974

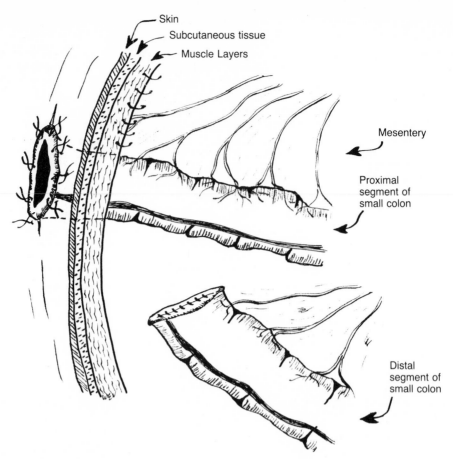

Figure 1. An end-on colostomy allows complete diversion of fecal material but is time-consuming to construct.

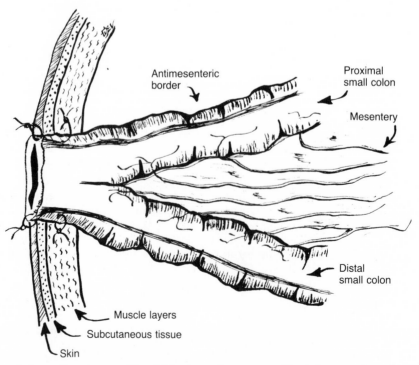

Figure 2. A loop colostomy allows lavage of the distal colon and rectum, resulting in less atrophy and easier reanastomosis.

scesses and adhesions. Serum electrolytes should be monitored carefully to avoid any disturbances caused by the dialyzing effect of lavage. Intravenous fluids must be administered for the correction of any abnormalities.

Retroperitoneal injuries of the rectum often lead to perirectal abscesses. Dyschezia is often the first sign, although abscesses near the peritoneal reflection may rupture into the abdomen and present with a peracute fulminant peritonitis. Dorsally positioned abscesses can often be drained into the rectum and ventral abscesses into the vagina. Extensive perirectal abscesses are best treated by external drainage where possible and repeated packing with iodine-soaked gauze.

The grave consequences associated with rectal tears demand that great care be taken during rectal palpation. Adequate physical and chemical restraint, proper facilities, copious lubrication with a gel lubricant, and, above all, a yielding hand are essential in preventing rectal tears.

References

1. Arnold, J. S., and Meagher, D. M.: Management of rectal tears. J. Eq. Med. Surg., 2:64, 1978.
2. Arnold, J. S., Meagher, D. M., and Lohse, C. L.: Rectal tears in the horse. J. Eq. Med. Surg., 2:55, 1978.
3. Azzie, M. A. J.: Temporary colostomy and the management of rectal tears in the horse. J. S. Afr. Vet. Assoc., 46:121, 1975.
4. Herthel, D. J.: Colostomy in the mare. Proc. 20th Annu. Meet. Am. Assoc. Eq. Pract., 1974, pp. 187–191.
5. Speirs, V. C., Christie, B. A., and vanVeenendaal, J. C.: The management of rectal tears in horses. Aust. Vet. J., 56:313, 1980.
6. Stashak, T. S., and Knight, A. P.: Temporary diverting colostomy for the management of small colon tears in the horse: A case report. J. Eq. Med. Surg., 2:196, 1978.
7. Stauffer, V. D.: Equine rectal tears: A malpractice problem. J. Am. Vet. Med. Assoc., 178:798, 1981.

GASTROINTESTINAL NEOPLASIA

A. M. Merritt, GAINESVILLE, FLORIDA

There are only two gastrointestinal neoplasms of the horse that are worthy of note: gastric squamous cell carcinoma and intestinal lymphosarcoma. The outstanding clinical sign of both for which the veterinarian is usually called is progressive weight loss. Both are seen almost exclusively in horses over six years old, and both are incurable.

SQUAMOUS CELL CARCINOMA

The squamous cell carcinoma is much more common than the intestinal lymphosarcoma, and while it is seen worldwide, there is some impression of increased incidence in certain regions. As well as losing weight, horses with gastric squamous cell carcinoma tend to become anorectic, depressed, and quite anemic as the disease progresses. Hyperpnea has been noted in a few cases and ptyalism in one. Rectal examination is generally, although not always, very helpful; irregular, odd-sized masses may be palpated around the cranial mesenteric root or within the mesentery itself. Rectal palpation of a very large smooth mass deep in the anterior lower left abdomen (that is, the enlarged stomach) should, along with the signs described above, make the diagnosis of gastric carcinoma highly likely. A more definitive diagnosis may be obtained by cytology of gastric lavage or peritoneal fluid, although problems can arise is accomplishing both of these procedures.

With gastric lavage, it may be impossible to get a tube into the stomach because of the tumor, and thus any washing fluid obtained may not be representative. With paracentesis abdominis, the tumor may not be sufficiently metastatic to be exfoliative, or it may be so metastatic that it lies along the ventral abdominal wall and makes intraperitoneal needle penetration impossible. Finally, exploratory laparotomy may be done; a standing left flank approach is appropriate, through which the stomach and mesenteric lymph nodes can be directly palpated and metastatic nodules can be appreciated and biopsied.

INTESTINAL LYMPHOSARCOMA

Intestinal lymphosarcoma seems to demonstrate itself clinically primarily through its malabsorptive effects in the small intestine—namely, progressive weight loss in spite of an extremely good or voracious appetite. As the horse's condition becomes terminal, its appetite decreases, and it develops a lethargic attitude. Short of laparotomy and biopsy, intestinal lymphosarcoma may be difficult to differentiate clinically from granulomatous enteritis (see article on chronic diarrhea); both cause mesenteric lymphadenopathy, anemia, and sugar malabsorption. In both, chronic diarrhea is a variable sign, most likely dependent upon the degree of colonic pathology. Some published reports would suggest that hypoalbuminemia is a consistent finding in intestinal lymphosarcoma, as it is in granulomatous enteritis, but the unpublished experience of some clinicians would not support this. The small intestinal histopathology of some cases of granulomatous enteritis can very closely resemble lymphosarcoma, and this whole issue needs further clarification by future careful case studies.

Certain non-neoplastic tumors of the equine gastrointestinal tract have the potential to present clinically like lymphosarcoma or granulomatous enteritis. For instance, MacKay et al.[1] have described a case of exuberant granulation of the squamous portion of the gastric mucosa that entirely filled the stomach, causing persistent weight loss, a palpable intra-abdominal mass, hypoalbuminemia, and xylose malabsorption. Intra-abdominal abscesses must also be considered in the differential diagnosis of such cases, although recurrent fever spikes, persis-

tent neutrophilia, hyperglobulinemia, and hyperfibrinogenemia would be more consistent with abscessation than neoplasia.

Supplemental Readings

1. MacKay, R. J., Iverson, W. O., and Merritt, A. M.: Exuberant granulation tissue in the stomach of a horse. Eq. Vet. J., *13*:119, 1981.
2. Meagher, D. M., Wheat, J. D., Tennant B., and Osburn, B. I.: Squamous cell carcinoma of the equine stomach. J. Am. Vet. Med. Assoc., *164*:81, 1974.
3. Neufeld, J. L.: Lymphosarcoma in the horse: A review. Can. Vet. J., *14*:129, 1973.
4. Roberts, M. C., and Pinsent, P. J. N.: Malabsorption in the horse associated with alimentary lymphosarcoma. Eq. Vet. J., 7:166, 1975.
5. Titus, R. S., Leipold, H. W., and Anderson, N. V.: Gastric carcinoma in a mare. J. Am. Vet. Med. Assoc., *161*:270, 1972.
6. Wiseman, A., Petrie, L., and Murray, M.: Diarrhea in the horse as a result of alimentary lymphosarcoma. Vet. Rec., 95:454, 1974.

RETAINED MECONIUM

Roy V. Bergman, COCHRANVILLE, PENNSYLVANIA

The failure of a newborn foal to pass meconium, the first gastrointestinal excretion, is a common disorder seen in equine practice. The severity of the condition varies greatly from a simple accumulation in the rectum immediately following birth to a more complex disorder of foals several days of age that includes impaction of the small colon.

Aristotle was the first to use the word meconium to describe the fetal feces. He suggested that this substance maintained the fetus in a sleeping state in the mother's womb and, therefore, used the Greek word meconium-arion, meaning "from poppy" or "like opium," to describe it.[1]

Meconium consists of gastrointestinal and glandular secretions, digested amniotic fluid, and cellular debris. Swallowing and peristaltic movements propel the meconium through the bowel and subsequently store it in the colon and rectum. The accumulating material in the fetal intestine changes in character as water is absorbed from the greenish, viscous liquid of the small intestine to the firm, dry fecal balls found in the small colon.

Normal foals pass meconium shortly after birth. In a survey of healthy newborn pony foals, initial passage of feces occurred within one hour of birth.[3] Normally, all the meconium is passed within the first few hours of life, and during the next three days, the excrement gradually assumes the characteristics of normal foal feces.

INCIDENCE

Approximately 1.5 per cent of all foals born experience meconium retention that is serious enough to require veterinary assistance.[3] Many mild cases probably resolve without treatment and are unreported.

The condition is commonly thought to occur more frequently in male foals, presumably related to their smaller pelvic canal diameters. Mares that carry their foals longer than term or are stall-fed during pregnancy produce foals that have a higher incidence of the disorder. In addition, the problem seems to be recognized more frequently during the colder months and occurs in certain years more than others. Some farms tend to experience the disorder with higher frequency than others, suggesting that management factors may be involved in the etiology.

CLINICAL SIGNS

The clinical signs of mild discomfort related to meconium retention may first be recognized shortly after birth as straining and lifting or "flagging" of the tail. They reflect a rectum full of firm, dry feces and result from the foal's efforts to evacuate them. Usually the foal achieves this without assistance, though occasionally an enema is required.

Of greater concern is the situation seen 12 to 48 hours after birth in which the foal exhibits more severe signs of colic such as pollakiuria, squatting, looking around at its flanks, turning its head back when recumbent, getting up and then lying down, and lying in dorsal recumbency with a foreleg extended over the head. Some foals may refuse to suck, although anorexia is not a constant feature.

Such nonspecific signs of abdominal distress result in this instance from intestinal obstruction produced by the simple accumulation of firm, dry meconium. The pain is caused by gas and/or fluid distention of the bowel proximal to the obstruction. Animals exhibiting these signs require vigorous treatment to relieve the situation.

ETIOLOGY AND PATHOGENESIS

The cause of the disorder is unknown, although theories abound. Some observers have tried to implicate deficiencies of maternal nutrition, especially Vitamin A, during the last third of pregnancy.[3] As of this writing, no definitive answer is available.

In human babies, a similar syndrome occurs, sometimes in normal babies but more often associated with cystic fibrosis. In the former group, the pathogenesis is unknown, but in the latter there is found to be depletion or absence of pancreatic enzymes that limit normal digestive activities in the intestine. Also, the intestine has been shown to have an increased secretory activity of mucoproteins, which causes the meconium to attain a viscid mucilagenous state. The meconium clings to the intestinal wall, and peristaltic movements are partially or totally unable to move it.[4] Whether any of these factors plays a role in the condition in the horse has not been investigated.

DIFFERENTIAL DIAGNOSIS

The diagnosis is usually based upon the history and clinical findings. Digital palpation may or may not reveal the presence of firm fecal balls in the rectum, thereby helping to differentiate this disorder from other causes of abdominal distress.

The condition most commonly confused with meconium retention is rupture of the urinary bladder. Abdominal paracentesis is usually sufficient to differentiate a ruptured bladder, as the fluid obtained has the characteristic ammoniacal odor when heated. Additional evidence can be obtained by passing a urethral catheter into the bladder and infusing a sterile dilute solution of methylene blue in saline. A second abdominocentesis performed 30 to 60 minutes later will yield a dye-stained fluid. In addition, simultaneous serum and peritoneal fluid creatinine levels should reveal a higher peritoneal fluid level when compared to serum, thus confirming the diagnosis. In cases of meconium retention, the characteristics of the peritoneal fluid are within normal limits.

The list of differential diagnoses must also include atresia coli, which may be distinguished by the absence of rectal fecal staining, and a variety of internal bowel derangements, including torsions, volvuli, intussusceptions, and internal hernias involving the mesentery and diaphragm. These conditions are usually unresponsive to treatment and result in progressive deterioration with the expected accompanying clinical signs.

THERAPY

The initial goals of therapy are to provide analgesia, thus protecting the foal from self-inflicted injury, and to relieve the obstruction. Dipyrone (44 mg per kg, 20 mg per lb intravenously or intramuscularly)* has long been the analgesic drug of choice because it is effective, safe, and inexpensive. Furthermore, it produces a minimal degree of central nervous system depression. Flunixin meglumine† (2.2 mg per kg, 1 mg per lb intravenously) is as effective as dipyrone and has the added advantage of acting slightly faster and for a longer period of time. As a general rule, if more potent analgesics are required to provide relief, the diagnosis and treatment regimen should be reevaluated.

After providing analgesia, relief of the impaction may be obtained by administration of a warm soapy water enema by gravity flow through a well-lubricated soft flexible rubber tube. This type of enema is much more effective than the commercially available phosphate enemas, which do little more than facilitate evacuation from the rectum. Mineral oil or glycerine may be added to the 1 to 1½ quarts of soapy water and seem to assist passage of especially hard or large fecal balls. This writer has not found the addition of dioctyl sodium succinate (DSS) to improve the effectiveness of the enema. It is extremely irritating to rectal mucosa and is not recommended. The length of the enema tube that can be safely introduced into the rectum varies with the skill of the operator. The tube may be inserted as far as 12 to 18 inches if it passes very easily.

Enemas may have to be repeated either immediately or after several hours of rest before complete relief is achieved. Local applications of an antibiotic-corticosteroid cream inside the rectum will prevent it from becoming excessively edematous during these procedures.

Pediatricians have had very good results using an

---

*Dipyrone, Med-Tech, Inc., Elwood, KS 66024
†Banamine, Schering Corp., Kenilworth, NJ 07033

enema of meglumine diatrizoate (Gastrografin) diluted with an equal amount of saline. This material is a radiopaque liquid used in contrast radiography of the bowel that stimulates accumulation of fluid within the lumen of the gut. In humans, a single Gastrografin enema is usually effective. However, its strong hygroscopic effect necessitates monitoring of electrolyte and fluid balance. The procedure warrants consideration for use in foals, as the time, effort, and trauma saved in minimizing the number of enemas would more than cover the increased cost of the drug.

If all of the firm fecal matter cannot be removed by the enemas, oral laxatives or lubricants should be administered via stomach tube to provide additional assistance in relieving the obstruction. Many agents have been used alone and in combination with good results. One very effective combination is 4 oz milk of magnesia, 8 oz mineral oil, and 2 oz castor oil. The castor oil is particularly helpful because it stimulates small intestinal peristalsis and is much safer and less traumatic to the foal than parasympathomimetic drugs.

Clients may be advised to administer 2 to 4 oz of milk of magnesia orally in combination with a mild systemic analgesic to a foal that they suspect has a meconium retention while awaiting the arrival of the veterinarian. The response time to subsequent therapy is often reduced, and even if the client's diagnosis is incorrect, this therapy is extremely safe.

Once proper symptomatic treatment has been instituted, supportive therapy such as fluid replacement, nutritional supplements, or antibiotics may be indicated in isolated cases but are usually unnecessary. Close monitoring of affected animals is essential, and enemas or analgesics may have to be repeated. Clinical signs can persist for as long as a day or two, but if the diagnosis is correct, patience and gentle treatment will be rewarded. Client education with regard to these aspects is important.

In an extremely stubborn case, surgical intervention may be required. The technique is described in standard surgical texts, and the prognosis is favorable.

PREVENTION

Prevention of meconium impaction is based on early ingestion of colostrum to stimulate elimination and the administration of a soapy water enema to the newborn shortly after birth. The enema may be given by either the veterinarian or the foaling person, depending on the skill and reliability of the latter. It is prudent to wait until the foal is standing steadily on its feet before attempting to administer the enema, rather than to try treating the foal struggling to rise. Also, it permits the foal to establish a bond with its mother without the interference of additional external stress. However, occasionally even those foals that have had early colostrum and a properly administered enema may still develop meconium impaction.

References

1. Antonowicz, I., and Shwachman, H.: Meconium in health and in disease. Adv. Pediatr., 26:275, 1979.
2. McGee, W. R.: Care of newborn foals. Lectures of the Stud Managers Course, Lexington, KY, 1970.
3. Rossdale, P. D., and Ricketts, S. W.: The Practice of Equine Stud Medicine. London, Bailliere Tindall, 1974.
4. Vaughan, V. C., McKay, R. J., and Behrman, R. E. (eds.): Nelson Textbook of Pediatrics, 11th ed. Philadelphia, W. B. Saunders Co., 1979.

ASCARIASIS

J. H. Drudge, LEXINGTON, KENTUCKY

E. T. Lyons, LEXINGTON, KENTUCKY

OCCURRENCE

Infections of *Parascaris equorum* occur mainly in suckling and weanling foals. Yearlings are infected to a lesser extent, and thereafter, incidence decreases to a point, generally validating the hypothesis that ascarid infection does not occur in mature horses. *P. equorum* infection is worldwide in distribution and is usually present wherever horses and other Equidae are raised.

Once contaminated with ascarid eggs, premises remain contaminated for a prolonged period, providing the source of infection in successive crops of foals. Ascarid eggs are very resistant to adverse environmental factors. Longevity of the eggs is a matter of years, and it has been contended that a patent infection of the horse has to occur only once every few years to perpetuate this parasite. The transmission potential of *P. equorum* is enhanced by the persistence of the infective eggs in the environment. Also, this may explain the unexpected appearance of *P. equorum* in a crop of foals in situations in which horses have been absent for prolonged periods.

DEVELOPMENT

Foals acquire infections of *P. equorum* through the ingestion of infective eggs in contaminated food and water. The most common source of infective eggs is the paddock or pasture on which the foal and dam are placed within a few days after birth of the foal. Usually ascarid eggs have been deposited on the paddock and pasture by the previous crops of foals. Once voided in the feces, ascarid eggs require about two weeks to develop to the infective stage, after which they may remain viable for very long periods of time. Under negligent hygienic and management conditions, the infection may occur in stables or sheds in which contaminated bedding has been allowed to accumulate.

In the infection process, ingestion of embryonated eggs by the foal is followed by hatching and penetration of larvae into the gut wall in the small intestine. Larvae migrate by the portal circulation to reach the liver in two days and then proceed onward to the lungs during the 7- to 14-day period after ingestion.[3, 14] During the 15- to 23-day postinfection interval, a rapid course of events ensues. Larvae invade the alveoli of the lungs, which is followed by their ascent of the bronchial tree to the pharynx and descent via the esophagus to return to the lumen of the gastrointestinal tract. Larvae tend to accumulate in the proximal portion of the small intestine, where growth and development proceed to sexual maturity in 10 to 12 weeks after the ingestion of infected eggs.[1, 2, 14]

Development of *P. equorum* infection under natural conditions does not proceed in the orderly fashion just described for experimental infections. Natural exposure of foals is on a continuous, daily basis as opposed to one or a limited number of doses given experimentally; thus, a variety of stages and sizes of *P. equorum* may be present concurrently in a foal. In the small intestine, forms ranging in length from less than 10 mm to 25 cm may be encountered. Maximal size and total number present appear to be interrelated. Ascarids tend to be larger when fewer specimens are present and vice versa. Sexual maturity has been observed by the authors for male and female *P. equorum* 10 cm and 15 cm and longer, respectively. Female ascarids are prolific egg producers, and daily output of 100,000 per female has been estimated.

Ascarid infection in foals tends to be labile. Spontaneous discharge in the feces is a normal feature of this infection. Either mature or immature forms may be voided. Mature ascarids can be readily recognized by their large size. Immature ascarids may be confused with female pinworms, which are also discharged spontaneously. Mature female pinworms have a long, tapering, sharp-pointed tail that contrasts with the more uniform body diameter and blunt-ended tail of immature ascarids. An infection may be entirely expelled within a short span of time, or only one worm may occasionally be passed. Factors associated with the expulsions are not well understood. Dietary factors and immune mechanisms are doubtlessly involved in the apparent spontaneous elimination, and the authors have observed that a febrile condition in a foal is quite efficacious for the removal of *P. equorum*.

PATHOGENESIS

Migration of the larvae of *P. equorum* through the lungs has been credited by many observers as a common cause of coughs in foals. Coughs from other causes frequently afflict foals; hence, the role of ascarid larvae has not been clearly established. Recent observations on experimental infections indicate that infective doses with large numbers of ascarid eggs results in severe lung damage manifested by coughing and nasal discharge during the two- to three-week postinfection interval.[4, 22] Experimental infections with small numbers of larvae were not associated with these pulmonary signs.[14] Thus, under natural conditions, ingestion of infective eggs is variable and accounts for the apparent discrepancies in the evaluation of the clinical significance of the pneumonic phase of the infection.[10, 20]

Interrelationships between migrating ascarid larvae and infective agents do not appear to have clinical significance in foals[18] similar to that recognized in swine for simultaneous infections with enzootic pneumonia and *Ascaris suum*.[24]

The primary danger of ascarid infection is rupture of the small intestine, which results in a fatal peritonitis. Rupture appears to be a result of the balling-up tendency of the ascarids, which stimulates a strong peristaltic wave of the intestine, causing a tear along the mesenteric attachment. Ruptures are not necessarily related to the numbers of ascarids present, except that more than a few worms are required and large numbers are more hazardous. These fatal ascarid infections are usually seen in the fall and early winter in late suckling or weanling foals in which the ascarid worm burdens have accumulated. Other manifestations of abnormal peristalsis triggered by ascarids include telescoping and twists in the small intestine.

Unthriftiness is commonly associated with ascarid infection. Retarded growth and disproportionate distention of the abdomen result in the classical term "pot-belly." These effects can be experimentally induced in foals by either small or large doses of infective ascarid larvae.[2, 22]

DIAGNOSIS

Flotation examination of feces and the demonstration under the microscope of ascarid eggs indicates the presence of mature ascarids in the intestinal tract. Typical eggs of *P. equorum* are round with a thick shell that is colored a medium dark brown. Some ascarid eggs are devoid of the roughened brown outer layer of the shell and appear as smooth hyaline-like, thick-walled eggs. In comparison with eggs of other equine parasites, those of *P. equorum* are quite dense and do not rise as readily in the flotation medium. Hence, in quantitative techniques, ascarid egg counts (EPG) are less reliable than stronglye EPGs as an index of the number of worms harbored. Presence of ascarid eggs in a flotation examination justifies treatment. In exceptional cases, ascarids may be present in a foal in which the EPG is negative, and conversely, a positive EPG may be associated with a failure to detect passage of worms in feces following treatment or during postmortem examination.

Ascarid eggs do not appear in feces until foals are about three months of age because of the 10-week period required for intrinsic development. Older sucklings and weanlings are the age groups in which ascarid infection has the highest incidence. Frequency of patent infections decreases in yearlings and two-year-olds, and thereafter only rarely are ascarids encountered in a mare or other mature horse.

Clinically, foals exhibiting an unthrifty physical condition, including poor weight gain and the characteristic pot-bellied, roughened hair coat appearance, may be presumed to be harboring an ascarid infection. A fecal examination will assist in verifying this. Also, the spontaneous discharge of ascarids will be observed from time to time in the feces of such poorly performing foals as well as others. Usually only a part of the ascarid infection is eliminated; hence, it is safe to presume that additional ascarids are in these foals.

TREATMENT

A number of compounds are quite efficacious for the removal of *P. equorum*. Ascarid removal activity may be only one of several factors involved in the selection of a compound for use at a given time in a given situation.

PIPERAZINES

Anthelmintic action of piperazines in the horse was explored in the early 1950s.[6, 19, 21] The spectrum of action included *P. equorum,* and piperazines were quickly recognized as the drug of choice for removing 100 per cent of *P. equorum* from the intestinal tract. Chemically, piperazine is a base, and a variety of acid radicals such as chloride, adipate, phosphate, sulfate, and citrate or carbon disulfide are combined to yield a variety of salts and formulations. Activity of the acid salt formulations is based on the piperazine base content, which varies widely among the salts as well as the products formulated and has caused some confusion as to the proper dosage to use. The standard dose for the piperazines is 88 mg base per kg body weight, which is equivalent to 40 mg per lb. Usually the piperazine concentration in a formulation is expressed in terms of the piperazine base, which facilitates the computations. There is some evidence[7, 13] that some piperazine products are efficacious for ascarids at lower dose rates. Picadex or piperazine–carbon disulfide complex* is quite active at 44 mg piperazine base per kg, and the piperazine and thiabendazole mixture† delivers piperazine base at 55 mg per kg. In these two instances, the carbon disulfide and thiabendazole components, respectively, are independently active to some degree on *P. equorum* and, thus, contribute to the total action achieved by these two products.

Mixtures of piperazine with phenothiazine (PPZ-PTZ) also provide effective removal of *P. equorum.* These preparations‡§ or ad hoc mixtures are designed for primary action against strongyles and usually deliver full therapeutic doses of piperazine. Thus, whenever the PPZ-PTZ mixtures are administered, ascarids are effectively removed.

Spectrum of action of piperazine base includes the pinworm (*Oxyuris equi*) and small strongyles, including those populations or strains that are resistant to phenothiazine and the benzimidazoles. Large strongyles are not effectively removed by piperazine, and *Strongyloides westeri* is completely refractory to piperazine.

Piperazine administration is generally free of untoward side effects. Sixfold increases in the dose rate of piperazine base resulted in toxicosis.[11, 17] Clinically, piperazine toxicosis, manifested primarily by a typical neurologic syndrome,[17] is a rare event and is associated with accidental overdosing or occurs in an animal with impaired kidney function that inhibits the excretion of piperazine. Prolonged handling of piperazine by veterinarians or their aides is apt

---

*Parvex, UpJohn Co., Kalamazoo, MI 49001
†Equizole A, Merck and Co., Rahway, NJ 07065
‡Dyrex T. F., Ft. Dodge Labs, Ft. Dodge, IA 50501
§Parvex Plus, Upjohn Co., Kalamazoo, MI 49001

to result in an acquired sensitivity manifested by a severe urticaria. This type of sensitivity to piperazine has not been observed in the horse, even those that have received repeated doses of piperazine over a span of years.

Methods of administering piperazine are limited by the large volume. Thus, stomach tube administration is the method of choice. Paste formulations are cumbersome, and feed administration is not reliable. Drenching may be satisfactory in the young suckling in which the total dose volume is small.

BENZIMIDAZOLES

Antiascarid activity varies widely in this group of compounds. Mebendazole*, cambendazole†, and oxibendazole‡ are consistently quite efficacious for *P. equorum* at the regular therapeutic dose levels of 8.8 mg per kg, 20 mg per kg, and 10 mg per kg, respectively. Fenbendazole§ requires a doubling of the regular 5 mg per kg dose rate to 10 mg per kg for effective removal of ascarids. Likewise, thiabendazole‖ is labeled at the double rate of 88 mg per kg, especially for ascarids, but even this level does not achieve consistently effective removal of *P. equorum*. Oxfendazole** required 10 mg per kg for efficacious ascarid activity, even though effective strongyle action was manifested at much lower levels.[15]

Benzimidazoles also vary in activity against *Strongyloides westeri*, which may be an important consideration in treating foals likely to be infected simultaneously with ascarids. Thiabendazole at 44 mg per kg, cambendazole at 20 mg per kg, and oxibendazole at 10 mg per kg are quite effective for enteric strongyloides. In contrast, mebendazole, fenbendazole, and oxfendazole are generally ineffective or of limited activity against *S. westeri* at the regular therapeutic dose levels of 8.8 mg per kg, 10 mg per kg, and 10 mg per kg, respectively, that would be given to foals for ascarids.

Antistrongyle activity is overall the most important segment of the spectrum of action of benzimidazoles. However, in foals, only small strongyles are present in the intestinal tract and are effectively removed when any of the benzimidazoles are used unless resistant strains or populations are present (p. 274).[12]

Benzimidazoles lend themselves to the various types of formulation and methods of administration. Traditionally, the stomach tube has been the

method of choice for foals because of the assurance that the prescribed dose is in fact delivered. Recent development of paste formulations ensures easy, accurate dosage. Drench administration of the suspension formulations of fenbendazole and oxibendazole by dose syringe is also quite feasible because the administration of only 5 ml per 45.45 kg (100 lb), respectively, results in a small total dose volume.

PHENYLGUANIDINES

Febantel* is the only representative of this group. It is very effective against *P. equorum* at the lowest dose rate (6 mg per kg) of any compound except the recently developed avermectins.[16] Febantel is not very active against *S. westeri* at 6 mg per kg, and twofold to fourfold increases in the dose rate are only partially effective. Febantel parallels the benzimidazoles in its antistrongyle activity; it exhibits quite efficacious removal of both large and small strongyles, but benzimidazole-resistant strains of the latter are usually also refractory to febantel. The toxicosis potential of febantel is low, and the paste formulation was favored in the development, so treatment of foals as well as all age groups is easily accomplished.

TETRAHYDROPYRIMIDINES

Pyrantel pamoate†‡ is the only salt or analogue in this group marketed in the United States. Pyrantel has a high order of activity against *P. equorum* at 6.6 mg of base per kg body weight. It is ineffective against strongyloides. Strongyle action is generally characterized as good, and a very important aspect is the effectiveness of pyrantel against the populations of small strongyles that are resistant to benzimidazoles and febantel. Pyrantel pamoate has a relatively wide margin of safety. The suspension formulation is administered at 6 ml per 45.45 kg, so dosing of foals can be accomplished by stomach tube, drenching, or top dressing on grain. A paste formulation has been in use for several years in other countries.

ORGANIC PHOSPHATES

This group is represented by two ascarid-active compounds: trichlorfon§‖ and dichlorvos.** Primary

*Telmin, Pitman-Moore, Washington Crossing, NJ 08560
†Camvet, Merck and Co., Rahway, NJ 07065
‡Anthelcide EQ, Norden Labs, Lincoln, NB 68521
§Panacur, American Hoechst, Somerville, NJ 08876
‖Equizole, Merck and Co., Rahway, NJ 07065
**Benzelmin, Diamond Labs, Des Moines, IA 50303

*Rintal, Haver-Lockhart, Shawnee, KS 66201
†Strongid T, Pfizer, New York, NY 10017
‡Imathal, Beecham, Bristol, TN 37620
§Dyrex, Ft. Dodge Labs, Ft. Dodge, IA 50501
‖Combot, Haver-Lockhart, Shawnee, KS 66201
**Equigel, Shell/Squibb, Princeton, NJ 08540

use of the organic phosphates has been for bot removal, but the action spectrum also includes *P. equorum*. Early formulations of trichlorfon were powders before the liquid was developed. Both were most effectively administered to foals by stomach tube at the dose rate of 35 to 40 mg per kg. Initially, dichlorvos was developed as a resin pellet formulation given at about 35 mg per kg in the feed, which was not satisfactory for foals. More recently, gel formulations of both compounds have been developed, and effective dose levels for ascarids are 35 mg per kg for trichlorfon and 20 mg per kg for dichlorvos. Neither compound has shown activity against *S. westeri*. Likewise, the gel formulations are not active on strongyles, so the question of activity against benzimidazole-resistant small strongyles is moot. However, it should be noted that the pellet formulation of dichlorvos is effective in removing the resistant strongyles. The margin of safety for organic phosphates is generally characterized as low, but they can be used in foals with no cause for alarm, provided the dosage and other label instructions are followed.

CONTROL

Control of *P. equorum* has the objective of achieving and maintaining a low level of infection in the foals on the farm. This intermediate, subclinical point in the control scale is a feasible objective rather than the total eradication of the infection. Suppression of the level of infection requires a sustained schedule of periodic treatments with ascarid-active compounds. Treatment of foals once or twice a year may reduce infections temporarily in the animals, but such a practice is generally inadequate to reduce the infection level for most nursery situations involving an appreciable number of foals. Furthermore, such a practice may indeed endanger the lives of the foals if the infections of *P. equorum* are allowed to build up in the foals (during the suckling period) and if treatment is not administered until late in the suckling period or delayed until after weaning. The killing of large numbers of ascarids by the anthelmintic may produce a large mass of deteriorating worms with the hazard of a blockage of the intestinal tract or a toxemia from the absorption of substances from the disintegrating parasites.

Successful control of *P. equorum* requires periodic treatment of foals throughout the suckling and weaning periods and the repetition of the schedule of treatments on each successive crop of foals from year to year. Design of the treatment schedule[8, 9, 23] is based on the inherent enzootic nature of ascarid infection. The first treatment is administered when the foals average about eight weeks of age. This aborts the initially acquired infections before the worms become sexually mature. Thereafter, repeating treatments at eight-week intervals prevents subsequent infections from maturing. Regular removal of the ascarids before maturation prevents further contamination of paddocks and pastures with eggs and gradually reduces the exposure of foals to infection. This schedule of treatments is continued until the foals become yearlings, when emphasis is shifted to the control of strongyles. Most of the antistrongyle compounds are also active against ascarids (see Strongylosis, p. 267); thus, the continuation of the schedule of treatments for strongyles also serves to remove the ascarid infections that occur with decreasing frequency in adolescent and mature horses.

Treatment schedules may vary from the foregoing. Some equine practitioners advocate treatment of sucklings more frequently than the eight-week interval, such as six- or four-week intervals. This practice appears to be a holdover from the carbon disulfide era. Carbon disulfide is only partially effective for removal of ascarids from sucklings,[7] whereas its efficacy is usually complete in weanlings and older animals. This foal age–related activity differential does not obtain for piperazines and the more recently introduced compounds, so ascarid removal is not a basis for the four- to six-week treatment schedules. At the outset of the institution of a control program in a heavily contaminated situation, treatments at intervals less than eight weeks perhaps can be justified.

There is no evidence of resistance of *P. equorum* to anthelmintics. Piperazines have been used for over 25 years with no loss of effectiveness. Carbon disulfide was used for a much longer period, but its lower order of activity was not attributed to drug resistance. Experience with benzimidazoles and other modern compounds is relatively less, but resistance of ascarids has not become apparent.

References

1. Bello, T. R., Amborski, G., Torbert, B. J., and Greer, G. J.: Anthelmintic efficacy of cambendazole against gastrointestinal parasites of the horse. Am. J. Vet. Res., 34:771, 1973.
2. Clayton, H. M., and Duncan, J. L.: Experimental *Parascaris equorum* infection of foals. Res. Vet. Sci., 23:109, 1977.
3. Clayton, H. M., and Duncan, J. L.: The migration and development of *Parascaris equorum* in the horse. Int. J. Parasitol., 9:285, 1979.
4. Clayton, H. M., and Duncan, J. L.: The development of immunity to *Parascaris equorum* infection in the foal. Res. Vet. Sci., 26:383, 1979.
5. Clayton, H. M., Duncan, J. L., and Dargie, J. D.: Pathophysiological changes associated with *Parascaris equorum* infection in the foal. Eq. Vet. J., 12:23, 1980.
6. Downing, W., Kingsbury, P. A., and Sloan, J. E. N.: Critical tests with piperazine adipate in horses. Vet. Rec., 67:641, 1955.
7. Drudge, J. H., Leland, S. E., Jr., Wyant, Z. N., Elam, G. W., and Hutzler, L. B.: Field studies comparing pipera-

zine–carbon disulfide complex with carbon disulfide for parasite control in the horse. Am. J. Vet. Res., *21*:397, 1960.

8. Drudge, J. H., Leland, S. E., Jr., Wyant, Z. N., and Hutzler, L. B.: Field studies with piperazine–carbon disulfide complex against parasites of the horse. J. Am. Vet. Med. Assoc., *131*:231, 1957.
9. Drudge, J. H., and Lyons, E. T.: Control of internal parasites of the horse. J. Am. Vet. Med. Assoc., *148*:378, 1966.
10. Drudge, J. H., and Lyons, E. T.: Pathology of infections with internal parasites in horses. The Blue Book, 27:267, 1977.
11. Drudge, J. H., Lyons, E. T., and Swerczek, T. W.: Critical tests and safety studies on a levamisole-piperazine mixture as an anthelmintic in the horse. Am. J. Vet. Res., *35*:67, 1974.
12. Drudge, J. H., Lyons, E. T., and Tolliver, S. C.: Benzimidazole resistance of equine strongyles—critical tests of six compounds against population B. Am. J. Vet. Res., *40*:590, 1979.
13. Drudge, J. H., Lyons, E. T., Wyant, Z. N., and Elam, G.: Anthelmintic activity of low doses of piperazine in horses. J. Am. Vet. Med. Assoc., *140*:678, 1962.
14. Lyons, E. T., Drudge, J. H., and Tolliver, S. C.: Studies on the development and chemotherapy of larvae of *Parascaris equorum* (Nematoda Ascaridoidea) in experimentally and naturally infected foals. J. Parasitol., *62*:453, 1976.
15. Lyons, E. T., Drudge, J. H., and Tolliver, S. C.: Critical tests of oxfendazole against internal parasites of horses. Am. J. Vet. Res., 38:2049, 1977.
16. Lyons, E. T., Drudge, J. H., and Tolliver, S. C.: Antiparasitic activity of ivermectin in critical tests in equids. Am. J. Vet. Res., *41*:2069, 1980.
17. McNeil, P. H., and Smyth, G. B.: Piperazine toxicity in horses. J. Eq. Med. Surg., 2:321, 1978.
18. Nicholls, J. M., Clayton, H. M., Pirie, H. M., and Duncan, J. L.: A pathological study of the lungs of foals infected experimentally with *Parascaris equorum*. J. Comp. Pathol., 88:261, 1978.
19. Poynter, D.: Piperazine adipate as an equine anthelmintic. Vet. Rec., 67:159, 1955.
20. Russell, A. F.: The development of helminthiasis in Thoroughbred foals. J. Comp. Pathol., 58:107, 1948.
21. Sloan, J. E. N., Kingsbury, P. A., and Jolly, D. W.: Preliminary trials with piperazine adipate as a veterinary anthelmintic. J. Pharmacol., 6:718, 1954.
22. Srihakim, S., and Swerczek, T. W.: Pathologic changes and pathogenesis of *Parascaris equorum* infection in parasite-free pony foals. Am. J. Vet. Res., 39:1155, 1978.
23. Todd, A. C., and Doherty, L. P.: Treatment of ascariasis in horses in central Kentucky. J. Am. Vet. Med. Assoc., *119*:363, 1951.
24. Underdahl, N. R., and Kelley, G. W.: The enhancement of virus pneumonia of pigs by the migration of *Ascaris suum* larvae. J. Am. Vet. Med. Assoc., *130*:173, 1957.

STRONGYLOSIS

J. H. Drudge, LEXINGTON, KENTUCKY
E. T. Lyons, LEXINGTON, KENTUCKY

OCCURRENCE

Strongyle infection is a common cause of illness and impaired performance of horses of all ages throughout the world.

The term *strongyle* refers to a large group of rather closely related roundworm or nematode parasites.[27] They occur in the sexually mature stage within the large intestine of the horse. Herein, they are arbitrarily divided into two subgroups: large strongyles and small strongyles.

The large strongyle group is composed of only three species of general importance; however, large strongyles are much more important than the small strongyles because of their greater pathogenic potential. *Strongylus vulgaris* is the causative agent of "verminous aneurysms" involving the large arteries supplying blood to the major portion of the digestive tract. *S. vulgaris* is not only the most harmful of all of the strongyles but also the most damaging of any of the internal parasites of the horse. *S. vulgaris* occurs very commonly and is worldwide in distribution. The second large strongyle, *Strongylus edentatus*, is also common but less pathogenic. The third species, *Strongylus equinus*, is more sporadic in occurrence than *S. vulgaris* and *S. edentatus*, and its pathogenicity is intermediate between *S. vulgaris* and *S. edentatus*.

Small strongyle morphology is rather heterogeneous, and this arbitrary grouping of about 35 species is based more upon common biologic characteristics than on taxonomic considerations. Small strongyles are the most common of the parasites of horses, and infections of large numbers (greater than 10^5) in the aggregate of the species represented are not unusual in a single animal. Within the group, some species characteristically occur in relatively large numbers (greater than 10^4), whereas other species are represented by relatively few (less than 10^2) specimens. Even though infections of small strongyles may be large in number, the harmful effects of the small strongyles as a group are generally less than those caused by the large strongyles.

DEVELOPMENT

Factors affecting the transmission of strongyle infections have been recently reviewed[2, 7, 32-34] and can be categorized into three broad areas: (1) source of the infections; (2) environmental factors, especially the climatic conditions; and (3) receptive state of exposed animals.

Life cycles of both large and small strongyles are "direct," no intermediate host or vector being required for transmission. Although the spread is direct, a lag period is required for extrinsic development.

Foals are born free of infections of both large and small strongyles. Sexually mature strongyles inhabiting the large intestine of Equidae that are several months of age and older provide the residual sources of the infections because the female worms lay eggs that are eliminated into the environment in the feces. These eggs are not immediately infective but must develop on the pastures or paddocks. Time requirements vary for the development of strongyle eggs to the infective larval stage, but under favorable temperature and moisture conditions, about one week is required. Infective larvae are free-living and are quite actively motile on the herbage. They are enclosed in the thin skin or sheath that affords protection against unfavorable climatic and environmental conditions. Thus, in temperate regions, infective larvae may survive over the winter, and those developing during the grazing season may remain viable for several months. Infective larvae do not feed, so their life span is limited by the amount of food stored in their intestinal cells. Although larval viability may be prolonged, newly developed larvae are quite vigorous and, thus, are relatively more infective than older larvae that have depleted their stored energy. Larvae are quite active, and their random though limited migrations on herbage place them in a position to be ingested as the foal or horse grazes. The bulk of the transmission probably occurs within a matter of a few weeks after the eggs contaminate the pastures. In temperate regions, this is reflected in seasonal variation in transmission, wherein the infection potential is greater during the warm months than during the cold months of the year. Under tropical or subtropical conditions, the transmission may not show these seasonal changes. With either geographic situation, the highly susceptible foals tend to be introduced in springtime when the hazard of infection is great.

Daily egg production of female large strongyles is on the order of 5000; whereas that of female small strongyles is much less, ranging from less than 100 for the small species to several hundred for the larger species. These rather modest figures assume added impact when the aggregate total daily output is projected. A mare with an "average" infection, producing 1000 eggs per gm in a daily total of 15 kg of feces, contaminates the pasture with 15 million eggs per day. Further compounding this by the number of horses grazing the pasture demonstrates the necessity of an effective control program to suppress pasture infestation.

Strongyles infect horses of all ages and, for all practical purposes, a horse is never entirely free of infection under natural conditions. Exposure to infection starts during the first few days of life of the foal or when it is first placed on an infected paddock or pasture. Both large and small strongyle larvae are in the exposure mix, but specific biologic features result in different time period requirements for maturation to the adult worm stage in the host. Developmental periods for large strongyles are lengthy: six months for *S. vulgaris*, nine months for *S. equinus*, and 11 months for *S. edentatus*. Prepatent periods for the small strongyles range from 5 to 10 weeks. In terms of epizootiology, these data indicate that foals two to three months of age contaminate the environment with eggs of small strongyles. In contrast, dissemination of large strongyle infections requires foals ranging in age from six to eight months for *S. vulgaris* and adolescents of 12 months or more for *S. edentatus*.

Strongyle and other worm parasite infections are inherently different from infectious diseases of viral or bacterial origin. In general, infectious diseases are spread by contact, and only one exposure is needed. Viral and bacterial agents multiply rapidly within the infected animal, fulminating to a climax wherein the animal either succumbs or the defense mechanisms overcome the invaders by achieving an immune or refractory state. Strongyle infection can only be disseminated after a lag period for development of extrinsic stages. Strongyles do not multiply in the body; only one worm can develop for each infective larva ingested, so infections develop slowly unless exceptionally large numbers of infective larvae are ingested within a short period of time. Exposure to infection or reinfection is on a continual daily basis, and the animals achieve only a relative state of immunity or refractivity to strongyle infections.

PATHOGENESIS

Migrations of the strongyle larvae begin soon after infective larvae are ingested and account for the most serious of the pathogenic effects of strongyle infections. Large strongyle larvae travel extensively in parenteral tissues for extended periods of time and cause serious, often fatal, consequences. In comparison, migrations of small strongyle larvae are limited to the walls of the alimentary tract; so the adverse effects are less.

STRONGYLUS VULGARIS

S. *vulgaris* is the most harmful of the large strongyles and is especially dangerous because of the predilection of S. *vulgaris* larvae to enter and migrate inside the arteries supplying blood to the digestive organs. These migrations induce a prompt and severe reaction manifested by thrombosis and embolism, especially in susceptible foals. The extent and type of the resultant arterial occlusions depends on the number and concentration of the migrating larvae in the vessel(s), the size of the vessel(s), the immune state of the animal, and other unknown factors. The reactive process reduces the blood flow to the organ normally supplied by the affected vessel(s). Complete blockage of the vessel(s) frequently occurs and results in death or gangrene of the tissue(s). Principally affected organs are the posterior portion of the small intestine, the cecum, and the ventral colon. Lesions and dysfunction also occur in the liver and kidneys and other organs.

Small numbers of S. *vulgaris* larvae can be lethal. Experimentally, larval doses between 800 and 8000 caused the death of greater than 90 per cent of foals within three weeks after administration.[13, 19–21] Other characteristics of the acute clinical syndrome induced by S. *vulgaris* infection include (1) fevers of 40.0 to 41.1° C, (2) loss of appetite, (3) rapid loss of 20 per cent of body weight, (4) mental depression and lethargy, and (5) colic and other abdominal distress. Concurrent changes in blood components include (1) moderate normocytic anemia, (2) neutrophilic leukocytosis, (3) increased total serum protein values, and (4) marked changes in serum protein profiles.

During the rapid sequence of the foregoing clinical events, the migrating larvae proceed rapidly (2.5 cm per day) upstream in the iliac, medial cecal, lateral cecal, and ventral colic branches of the mesenteric artery. They reach their apparent destination for further development, the cranial mesenteric artery, in about two weeks and are only 1 to 2 mm long.

Under natural conditions, repeated ingestion of small numbers of infective larvae is typical. Multiple doses of larvae produce the same types of injury to the arteries and tissues and are manifested by many of the same clinical signs but to a lesser degree. There is a slower tempo to the course of events, and the death rate is of a reduced order when ingestion of larvae is spread over a period of time simulating the natural condition.

Migration of S. *vulgaris* larvae is not necessarily restricted to the cranial mesenteric artery. Wanderings of smaller numbers may be found in the aorta and the coeliac, hepatic, splenic, iliac, renal, and coronary arteries. Their ramifications are clearly demarcated by the threadlike tortuous tracks on the arterial intima.

Aneurysms of the cranial mesenteric artery are the primary pathologic process associated with S. *vulgaris* infection. The larvae stimulate a reactive thrombosis made up of fibrin deposits, infiltrations of inflammatory cells, and accumulations of necrotic debris. Larvae tend to accumulate and may remain in the aneurysm for maturation to the adult (fifth) stage, which occurs three to four months after infection. Developing larvae and the agamous adult worms are embedded in the thrombotic accumulations that vary in size from small clusters to large accumulations that measure 10 to 20 cm or more in diameter. There is an accompanying expansion in the diameter of the cranial mesenteric artery that is the basis for the term *aneurysm*. By strict definition, this is a misnomer because the arterial wall does not become thinner. Instead, the wall actually thickens and becomes tougher because of fibrosis. Rupture of these verminous aneurysms and a consequent fatal hemorrhage is a rare event, but embolism is an ever-present danger because the thrombotic processes tend to be vegetative.

After about five months, the larvae of S. *vulgaris* return to the intestine for further development. Characteristic nodules are found on the mucosa of the cecum and ventral colon. They are small cysts that usually contain agamous S. *vulgaris*.

Adult, sexually mature S. *vulgaris* are attached principally to the mucosa or lining of the cecum and to the ventral colon to a lesser extent. The bulbous-type mouth provides a sucker for holding on, and the teeth at the base of the mouth capsule scarify the mucosa, and together these make up the blood-sucking mechanism of the worms. Some hemorrhage also occurs when the worms detach and reattach themselves from time to time. This loss of blood joins with a depressive effect of the migrating larvae of S. *vulgaris* on the erythrocytes and the blood-letting activity of other strongyles to produce anemia.

Immunity of varying degrees is acquired to infection with S. *vulgaris*. Experimental infections, mainly in pony foals, induced an acquired immunity.[1, 16, 21, 35, 39] The present investigators[13] have reported that multiple doses of small numbers of larvae (250 larvae twice a week for 16 weeks) were devoid of a protective reaction and proved to be fatal; however, an unpublished repeat of this experiment resulted in an immune response, and the foal did not succumb.

Natural infections result in a relative degree of

resistance in most horses. The acute *S. vulgaris* syndrome occurs under natural conditions only in young animals, mainly suckling and weanling foals, whereas the mares or other mature horses grazing the same pasture concurrently remain tolerant of a proportionate level of exposure to infection. This naturally acquired immunity is not absolute or permanent. Thus, the various developmental stages of *S. vulgaris* and/or the adverse effects are seen in horses of all ages. Surveys of the prevalence of *S. vulgaris* in horses of all ages indicate an infection rate of 70 to 100 per cent for mature worms in the digestive tract[34] and a similar high incidence of verminous aneurysms. Persistence of the infection in horses of all ages results in adverse clinical signs, especially recurrent colic. Thus, a long-term control program is necessary not only to protect the foals from the hazard of an acute infection but also to reduce the incidence of colic in the older horses.

STRONGYLUS EDENTATUS

Prevalence and geographic distribution of *S. edentatus* are similar to *S. vulgaris*, but the migrating pathway taken by larvae is distinctly different. The pathogenic potential of *S. edentatus* is less even though the parenteral migrations are extensive and prolonged.[31, 47] Infective larvae of *S. edentatus* penetrate the intestinal mucosa, principally the cecum, soon after ingestion and travel via the cecal veins and the portal circulation to invade the liver in two days. Experimental infections of 3000 to 75,000 larvae result in acute or subacute illness and death within two weeks to two months. The liver is swollen and discolored with a bluish-red cast. Contrasting with this color are the stark white larvae under the capsule of the liver. Several weeks after infection, subcapsular hemorrhages and tortuous track-like swellings, demarcating the meanderings of the larvae, give the liver surface an uneven appearance. Peritonitis is also present, and serosanguineous fluid accumulates in the peritoneal cavity. Serosal surfaces of abdominal organs, particularly the cecum, ventral colon, and omentum, are inflamed and roughened with diffuse fibrin deposits. Adhesions between these organs and the abdominal wall may occur. Perivascular thickening, especially around the cecal veins, suggests that this is the primary route of the early larval migrations.

Survival of the acute effects results in the onset of chronic inflammatory changes. The liver becomes fibrotic, especially at the borders, with a characteristic waxy texture or appearance. Calcium deposits develop on the serosal surfaces of the cecum and ventral colon, in the omentum, and in the tissues around and in the walls of the cecal and portal veins.

Clinical signs of *S. edentatus* infection include an undulating low-grade fever, depression, intermittent inappetence, colic, constipation, and diarrhea. Blood changes consist of moderate anemia and leukocytosis with an eosinophilia that may increase to 20 to 30 per cent and persist for a prolonged period of time. The total serum protein may increase to twice the normal level, and the relative decrease in the albumin component is more than counterbalanced by marked increases in the alpha and beta globulins. Subcutaneous edema in the brisket and ventral abdomen may result from depletion of serum albumin. These clinical manifestations correspond with many of those described for *S. vulgaris*, but the dynamics of their development are slower.

Chronic infections are continued by further migrations of *S. edentatus* larvae. They are deflected under the liver capsule and proceed dorsad to the hepatic ligaments, followed by invasion of the subperitoneal tissues in the flanks. These retroperitoneal lesions are characteristically blood-tinged and edematous and usually contain agamous adult *S. edentatus*. The next lesion of the migratory pathway is a submucosal cyst, mainly in the ventral colon and cecum, that is diffusely edematous, blood-tinged, and also inhabited by agamous adult worms. Erupting from these lesions, the worms develop to sexual maturity to complete their development 11 months after infection.

Natural infections generally are not recognized by a unique clinical manifestation. The chronic type of liver lesions were not recognized by our diagnostic personnel before the experimentally infected animals were examined at necropsy.

STRONGYLUS EQUINUS

Geographic distribution of *S. equinus* is also worldwide, but it is not a prevalent infection like *S. vulgaris* and *S. edentatus*. Thus, the pathogenic potential of *S. equinus* under natural conditions is low.

Experimental infections with 4000 larvae of *S. equinus* resulted in severe illness and a high mortality rate.[46] Thus, in terms of numbers of infective larvae, pathogenicity of *S. equinus* is closer to *S. vulgaris* than *S. edentatus*. Ingested larvae penetrate the mucosa of the cecum and ventral colon and encyst in the submucosa. Emerging from these small hemorrhagic nodules after 10 to 11 days, they break out into the peritoneal cavity and penetrate into the liver. Migration in the liver for six to seven weeks results in necrosis and hepatitis. Larvae return to the peritoneal cavity and invade the pancreas about two months after infection. Development to agamous adults requires four to five months. They return to the intestinal lumen, mainly the cecum, where they attach as blood-sucking mature worms about nine months after infection.

Clinical signs during the migrating phase of *S. equinus* infection include fever, colic, inappetence, depression, and rapid deterioration of body condition. Detection of prepatent *S. equinus* infection as a specific disease entity is not possible at the present time.

SMALL STRONGYLES

Small strongyles are probably the most common parasitic infection of horses of all ages. Even though large numbers may be present, the deleterious effects in the aggregate are less than the harm from large strongyles because larval migrations are limited to the mucosa and submucosa of the cecum and large colon. Many larvae encyst superficially in the cecal and colonic mucosa and do not provoke a tissue reaction; others penetrate deeper and stimulate nodule formations of various sizes. Rupture of these nodules by escaping larvae causes small ulcerations in the mucosa. One species causes characteristic large, craterlike ulcers in the dorsal colon. Large numbers of encysted larvae may accumulate and impair the normal digestive function of the mucosa of the large intestine. Severe diarrhea has been associated with these infections. Changes in serum proteins similar to those described for *S. vulgaris* and *S. edentatus* have been found in experimental infection of mixed species of small strongyles.[39] Larvae may remain encysted for prolonged periods of time; their encystment and maturation is inhibited by influences emanating from adult worms already present in the lumen and from other sources. Thus, completion of development may require a longer period of time than the 5 to 10 weeks observed in experimental infections.

The bulk of the mature small strongyles inhabit the interface between the mucosa and the mass of the ingesta. Only a few species are attached to the mucosa and ingest blood.

DIAGNOSIS

Several methods may be used to determine the presence of mature strongyle infections and to ascertain their clinical significance during the prepatent period.

FECAL EXAMINATIONS

Mature strongyle infections can be verified by using levitation methods to separate eggs for microscopic examination. Qualitative flotation examina-tion is the easiest to perform, but the information provided is limited, and interpretations should be made with caution. Quantitative methods to determine eggs per gram (EPG) of feces are more difficult to complete, but the value of the data derived usually justifies the effort. Egg counts at periodic intervals indicate the general level of strongyle infections in the animals on a farm, thereby indicating the effectiveness of a control program. Completion of a count at the time of treatment with an anthelmintic and again 7 to 14 days after treatment will monitor the effectiveness of the drug administered. This may detect the presence of drug-resistant strongyles. Strongyle EPGs have a limited value, because both large and small strongyles produce thin-walled, hookworm-type eggs that cannot be differentiated by microscopic examination. Feces can be cultured to derive the third-stage infective larvae, which can be differentiated by microscopic examination. Larvae of *S. vulgaris*, *S. edentatus*, and *S. equinus* have distinctive morphologic features and can be differentiated from larvae of small strongyles. Specialized techniques and personnel are required for the culture examinations, so they are not routinely done except in research laboratories.

For practical purposes, EPG examinations to verify the presence of strongyle eggs can be regarded as presumptive evidence of the presence of large strongyles because they occur very commonly along with small strongyles. Several qualifications of interpretation of EPG data by the clinician should be kept in mind. EPG examinations do not reflect the presence of immature large strongyles during the long prepatent period. Thus, only animals 6 to 11 months of age and older may show evidence of infection with the mature stages of one or more of the three species of large strongyles. In yearlings and older animals, large strongyle eggs ordinarily constitute less than 10 per cent of the strongyle EPG. This ratio may not always be constant, particularly after treatment, depending on the spectrum of activity achieved. Thus, a drug such as piperazine that is relatively more effective in removing small strongyles than large strongyles will result in low posttreatment EPGs, but the residual eggs are predominantly large strongyle eggs, which have a dangerous potential. In contrast, benzimidazole-resistant small strongyles may cause a high post-treatment EPG composed only of eggs of small strongyles. This situation probably has less clinical impact than the low count cited for postpiperazine treatment. Aside from the exceptional situations, experience indicates that average strongyle EPGs on the order of 100 or less are associated with subclinical infections and indicate that the antistrongyle measures applied are providing effective control.

The number of animals from which fecal samples

are collected for EPG examinations may vary depending on the situation and the judgment of the attending veterinarian. In cases where only a few (five or less) horses are involved, it is probably advisable to collect samples from each one. When larger groups (10 or more) are involved, it is not necessary to sample all of the animals. As a general rule, one can obtain a reliable readout on the effectiveness of a treatment by taking samples from a minimum of five animals or about 10 per cent of the animals in an age group treated with the same preparation.

It is important when sampling a portion of a total group of animals that the same animals are sampled both before and after treatment. Also, in sampling, one should be mindful of other factors, such as a broodmare band that is stabled and/or pastured in two or more barns and weanlings or yearlings in which the fillies are separated from the colts. These and similar situations dictate the advisability of taking samples representative of each barn, pasture, sex, or other factor subgroup.

HISTORY AND CLINICAL SIGNS

Definitive diagnosis of acute syndromes that accompany migrations of large strongyles is difficult and must be based on the clinical situation. A history of no strongyle control program coupled with detection of high egg counts in a given group of horses provides a likely setting. Because foals are the most susceptible, the acute syndromes usually occur in sucklings and weanlings. Favorable conditions for buildup of pasture contamination with infective larvae occur in the summer and fall in temperate regions, and these are the seasons when acute syndromes are most apt to be observed.

Clinical signs are also substantial criteria for diagnosis. The acute syndrome attributed to *S. vulgaris* is characterized by high fever, inappetence, depression, and moderate leukocytosis with a shift to the left. These are also signs of some bacterial infections. Intermittent diarrhea and constipation have been attributed to larval migrations of large strongyles, and colic is probably the most common clinical manifestation of strongyle infections, particularly *S. vulgaris*. In fact, the incidence of colic in a group of horses is a good index of the effectiveness of the strongyle control program.

BLOOD STUDIES

Blood studies are helpful in establishing a causal relationship between migrating larvae and the clinical signs. A moderate normocytic anemia is present, and moderate leukocytosis is also typical. Besides the neutrophilia in acute *S. vulgaris* infections,

eosinophilia is generally indicative of parasitism. Circulating eosinophils increase considerably in subacute and chronic types of prepatent strongyle infections. An increase in total serum protein and a decrease in the albumin:globulin ratio due to a relative decrease in albumin and increases in alpha and beta globulins are also indicative of both large and small strongyle infections.

THERAPY

A large number of compounds or products that are quite effective for the removal of both large and small strongyles are currently available. Selection and use are dependent upon a number of factors that should be taken into account by the clinician. The compounds will be discussed more or less in the order of the chronologic development rather than on a relative efficacy basis, because it is impossible for all practical purposes to compile an order of choice strictly on removal activity.[2, 6, 11, 23, 32, 40, 43]

PHENOTHIAZINE

Phenothiazine (PTZ) ushered in the modern era of anthelmintics, beginning in 1940.[24] PTZ was the first compound of demonstrated effectiveness against strongyles, and thus, PTZ was the drug of choice for strongyle therapy for nearly 20 years. The horse is relatively more susceptible to the toxic effects of PTZ than other species; early experience with dose levels comparable to those used in sheep (550 mg per kg) were accompanied by toxic reactions, principally a hemolytic anemia and the sequelae of icterus or hematuria. Much lower dose rates retained effectiveness against strongyles and were much less toxic, so the therapeutic dose rate of 55 mg per kg became established. This required 2 oz (60 ml) for a mature (454 kg) horse of the standard suspension of PTZ formulated to contain 12.5 gm per 30 ml.

The therapeutic dose of PTZ is relatively more effective for removal of small strongyles (85 to 95 per cent) than the large strongyles, *S. vulgaris* (50 to 75 per cent) and *S. edentatus* (20 to 40 per cent). Recognition of the problem of drug resistance of strongyles to PTZ coupled with the advent of more efficacious compounds has led to the marked decline in the use of therapeutic doses of PTZ either alone or in mixtures.

Present-day use is largely limited to mixtures of PTZ with piperazine (PPZ) in such products as Parvex Plus,* Dyrex T. F.,† or in preparations made

---

*Parvex Plus, Upjohn Co., Kalamazoo, MI 49001
†Dyrex T. F., Ft. Dodge Labs, Ft. Dodge, IA 50501

up by the clinician. These mixtures were developed to deliver a reduced level of PTZ, averaging about one half the therapeutic dose rate of PTZ or 27.5 mg per kg. The advantages offered by these PTZ-PPZ mixtures include (1) enhancement of the removal activity against both large and small strongyles, (2) mitigation of the problem of PTZ resistance, and (3) reduction of the toxicosis hazard of PTZ.

The low-level system of medication was also developed for PTZ.[5] The regimen consists of feeding 2.0 gm PTZ as a top dressing on the daily grain ration during the first 21 days of each month on a year-round basis in mares and other adolescent and mature horses. A lower level of 1.0 gm is fed to suckling and weanling foals. This method of administering PTZ is much more efficacious than therapeutic doses, providing a level of control approaching 100 per cent for both large and small strongyles. The use life of this system was short, extending from mid-1940 to mid-1950 and fell into disfavor for ill-defined reasons. It was purported to induce a hypothyroidism, thereby impairing the performance of racing animals, and the feeding of a noxious substance on a daily basis was deemed to be more detrimental than a therapeutic dose of the same substance administered periodically. Later, the drug resistance problem of strongyles to PTZ was recognized,[14, 36] and this is a valid basis seriously limiting the use of low-level PTZ.

PIPERAZINES

Piperazines are already established as one of the most valuable of the anthelmintics developed for use in the horse. Antistrongyle activity of PPZ at the dose rate of 88 mg base per kg (4 gm base per 45.45 kg) is inadequate for effective strongyle control. It is relatively more effective for removal of small strongyles (90 to 100 per cent) than the large strongyles, S. vulgaris (40 to 60 per cent) and S. edentatus (0 to 100 per cent) and therefore gives good reductions in post-treatment EPGs, but these are misleading. Various salts derived from PPZ base and common acid radicals (adipate, hydrochloride, citrate, phosphate, and sulfate) or carbon disulfide are available as powder or solution formulations under a variety of trade names. Effectiveness of anthelmintic action of the various piperazines is related to the base content, which varies with the salt as well as the particular formulation, so the label is very important in determining that the desired dosage of 88 mg base per kg is being administered. Stomach tube dosing is generally the most satisfactory for PPZ, because the relatively large total dose volume and the unpalatable nature of PPZ salts make dosing by feed and water unsuccessful. The toxic hazard of PPZ is relatively low for all ages of horses. Recent

evidence indicates that the margin of safety is lower than previously thought, and doses exceeding three times the therapeutic rate of 88 mg per kg should not be administered.

Two factors prompted the development and usage of mixtures of PPZ with PTZ. First, such mixtures[14, 36] result in a synergistic action on the large strongyles, increasing the average removal of S. vulgaris to 90 to 100 per cent and S. edentatus to 40 to 60 per cent. Dose rates of such mixtures* and ad hoc preparations by clinicians retained the level of PPZ at 88 mg base per kg but reduced the PTZ level by 50 per cent to 27.5 mg per kg. The PPZ-CS_2 (picadex) mixture with PTZ† is an important exception to other PPZ-PTZ mixtures in the enhancement of S. edentatus removal to 70 to 90 per cent in addition to the bot removal derived from the carbon disulfide component.[14]

Simultaneously, it was also discovered that the problem of strongyle resistance to PTZ was effectively overcome by the PPZ component mixtures with PTZ.[14, 36] Resistance of the strongyles to these mixtures does not appear to be a likely event because in a long-term clinical trial, picadex-PTZ has maintained effective strongyle control for 18 years and the PPZ-PTZ-trichlorfon mixture for 14 years.[12]

Mixing of PPZ with thiabendazole‡ was begun to overcome the shortcoming of thiabendazole (TBZ) for removal of *Parascaris equorum*, but this mixture is also efficacious for removal of benzimidazole-resistant small strongyles. Dosages of this mixture deliver TBZ at the regular therapeutic rate of 44 mg per kg (2 gm per 45.45 kg) and PPZ at the intermediate rate of 55 mg base per kg (2.5 gm base per 45.45 kg). This mixture has also been observed to retain effective strongyle control for a long period of time—13 years in one clinical trial.[12]

Current strongyle control programs utilize PTZ-PPZ and PPZ-TBZ mixtures as very important components. Toxicosis incidents appear to be minimal. Occasionally a horse that has an idiosyncrasy to PTZ will react even to the reduced level of PTZ in the mixture, and treatment of such horses with PPZ-PTZ should be avoided. Treatment with a PPZ-TBZ mixture is generally devoid of toxic reactions except when the chemotherapy of migrating stages of S. vulgaris is attempted and the mixture is used as the source of TBZ. This chemotherapy requires a dose of TBZ 10 times the normal strength, or 440 mg per kg on two successive days. This delivers PPZ base in excess of 500 mg per kg or six times the dose rate of PPZ base that was noted previously, and a piperazine toxicosis is apt to be produced; thus, *the PPZ-TBZ mixture should not be used for the chemotherapy of acute* S. vulgaris *syndrome.*

*Dyrex T. F., Fort Dodge Labs, Fort Dodge, IA 50501
†Parvex Plus, Upjohn Co., Kalamazoo, MI 49001
‡Equizole-A, Merck and Co., Rahway, NJ 07065

BENZIMIDAZOLES

Thiabendazole (TBZ) was the first (1961) of the benzimidazoles. A decade later, a burst of development resulted in a number of products currently available, including mebendazole (MBZ)* cambendazole (CBZ)† fenbendazole (FBZ)‡ oxfendazole (OFZ)§, and oxibendazole (OBZ)‖, a very recent introduction.

Broad-spectrum anthelmintic activity, low order of toxicity, relatively low dose rate requirements, amenability to diverse formulations, and methods of dosing are the primary features presented by the benzimidazoles. Benzimidazoles as a class are highly effective (90 to 100 per cent) against all three species of large strongyles.[2] Mature small strongyles in the intestinal lumen are quite efficaciously removed (98 to 100 per cent), and the immature small strongyles (fourth-stage larvae) in the lumen are removed to a lesser degree. Parenteral migrating stages of large strongyles and small strongyle larvae embedded or encysted in the wall of the intestine are not affected by the regular therapeutic dose rates of the benzimidazoles. Higher dose levels and repeated administration regimens of benzimidazoles are active against these immature forms of strongyles, and this aspect will be discussed later (see Chemotherapy of Migrating Larvae).

Therapeutic dose levels of the various benzimidazoles are itemized in Table 1. In the evolution of this class of compounds, there has been an increase in activity and reciprocal trend in dose level. Ninety per cent reduction now occurs with 5 mg per kg of FBZ compared with 44 mg per kg of TBZ. This differential could be extended to 98 per cent by comparing the efficaciousness of OFZ at 1.1 mg per kg against both large and small strongyles[28] rather than the 10 mg per kg dosage in Table 1, which is prescribed to achieve effective removal of *P. equorum* rather than the strongyles.

Benzimidazoles are generally regarded as unusually safe products to use in the horse, and there is a wide margin of safety ranging from 10 times to 100 times (Table 1) when administered alone. Widespread clinical use of the benzimidazoles has been generally accompanied by a lack of untoward side effects. Attempts to produce toxicosis have been limited in several instances by the failure to administer sufficient quantities of the drugs to the horse rather than the induction of toxicosis; hence, a specific acute benzimidazole toxicosis syndrome has not been reported in the horse.[43]

Mixtures of or simultaneous administration of benzimidazoles with other compounds such as piperazine,* trichlorfon,† dichlorvos,‡ and carbon disulfide are generally compatible, and specific contraindications are not known when therapeutic dosages are given. However, toxicosis potentials are modified markedly (Table 1) because of the limitations of the alternate component rather than the benzimidazole component or a specific untoward result of a combination effect. Special care should be exercised so that recommended dosages of organic phosphates, especially trichlorfon with less than a twofold margin of safety, are used for the adjunctive purpose of bot removal, or that the mixture of PPZ with TBZ *is not used* as the source of TBZ for the chemotherapy of acute *S. vulgaris* syndrome at the tenfold dose rate of 440 mg per kg on two successive days.

Some concern for the teratogenic potential has attended the usage of benzimidazoles in domestic animals. Deformed lambs were associated with treatment with parbendazole (PBZ)§ for parasite control in ewes in South Africa.[4] PBZ was the second of the benzimidazoles, so this event occurred early in the course of development of those compounds. Development of PBZ for use in horses[29] and other domestic animals was discontinued, and special attention to this detrimental aspect of usage was focused on subsequent anthelmintics.

In rats, teratogenic effects are produced by CBZ, MBZ, OFZ, ABZ, and PBZ but not by TBZ, OBZ, or FBZ.[2, 4, 43] During the research and development of the newer benzimidazoles, the possibility of adverse effects on breeding stock has been investigated, and at the present time, only CBZ has a label restriction that cautions against administration of CBZ to mares during the first trimester of pregnancy. The widespread and prolonged clinical use of benzimidazoles for parasite control in the horse has not been associated with harmful effects on reproduction.

Relatively low dose requirements and the chemical nature of benzimidazoles permit a variety of formulations of proprietary products, including powders, pellets, suspensions, and pastes. Thus, various methods of administration may be used except the parenteral route, which is not viewed as especially advantageous for administration of routine dosages of anthelmintics in blooded horses. Efficacy is the same regardless of the dosing method used, provided that the prescribed dosage is administered. Development of the paste formulations is deemed to be one of the most important advances made in parasite control because treatment can be accom-

*Telmin, Pitman-Moore, Washington Crossing, NJ 08560
†Camvet, Merck and Co., Rahway NJ 07065
‡Panacur, American Hoechst, Somerville, NJ 08876
§Benzelmin, Diamond Labs, Des Moines, IA 50317
‖Anthelcide-EQ, Norden Labs, Lincoln, NB 68501

*Equizole B, Merck and Co., Rahway, NJ 07065
†Telmin Plus, Pitaman-Moore, Washington Crossing, NJ 08560
‡Equigel, Squibb, Princeton, NJ 08540
§PBZ, SmithKline Corp., Philadelphia, PA 19101

TABLE 1. COMPARISON OF THERAPEUTIC DOSES OF BENZIMIDAZOLES

Compound	Proprietary Product	Therapeutic Dose Levels (mg/kg)	Safety Margin	Remarks
Thiabendazole	Equizole	44	25×	Generally free of side effects;
	Equizole A	44 + 55 PPZ*	5× PPZ*	PPZ toxicosis at >250 mg/kg;
	Equizole B	44 + 40 TCF†	1× TCF†	Organophosphate toxicosis at 80 mg/kg
Cambendazole	Camvet	20	30×	Do not use in 1st trimester of pregnancy
Oxfendazole	Benzelmin	10	10×	Generally free of side effects
Oxibendazole	Anthelcide-EQ	10	60×	Generally free of side effects
Mebendazole	Telmin	8.8	40×	Generally free of side effects;
	Telmin B	8.8 + 40 TCF	1× TCF	Organophosphate toxicosis at 80 mg/kg
Fenbendazole	Panacur	5	100×	Generally free of side effects

*Piperazine
†Trichlorfon

plished with minimal restraint of the horse and effort by the administrator.

Small strongyle populations may be resistant to benzimidazoles, but the three species of large strongyles are not.[15] Of more than 30 species in the small strongyle group, only five species exhibit the resistance, and the other species are susceptible. Resistance of strongyles to thiabendazole was first documented in 1965.[8, 25] As the newer benzimidazoles became available, TBZ-resistant populations were also resistant to the new products, which gave rise to the present axiom that resistance to one benzimidazole is tantamount to resistance to the other benzimidazoles, with one exception—oxibendazole (OBZ). The exception of OBZ is not understood, but it may be a transient phase in the selection process interrelated with differences in the mechanisms of action involved. Resistant populations of small strongyles are very common in central Kentucky horses and are now present on nearly every farm. Feedback indicates that the benzimidazole resistance problem is widespread in the United States and other countries. Clinically, use of a benzimidazole should be monitored for effectiveness. Failure of treatment to result in marked reductions in post-treatment strongyle egg counts is suggestive that drug-resistant parasites are present.

ORGANOPHOSPHATES

Organophosphates are represented by two compounds, trichlorfon and dichlorvos, which are active against strongyles.

TRICHLORFON

Trichlorfon is used primarily for bot control (p. 285), but the bolus formulation* was developed for effective removal of strongyles in addition to bots, ascarids, and pinworms.[45] This was achieved by (1) treating at the dose level of 80 mg per kg, or two times the regular therapeutic rate of 40 mg per kg for trichlorfon, which is not active on strongyles, and (2) sufficient compression of the bolus to permit slow disintegration during passage through the digestive tract, which delivers concentrations of trichlorfon in the cecum and colon sufficient to affect the strongyles. Activity is acceptable against both large strongyles, *S. vulgaris* (85 to 100 per cent) and *S. edentatus* (35 to 45 per cent), and small strongyles (85 to 95 per cent). Administration of these boluses results infrequently in a choke from lodging of the bolus in the esophagus and occasionally in organophosphate toxicosis, manifested primarily by diarrhea. Hence, this product is not widely used.

DICHLORVOS

Dichlorvos in the resin pellet formulation,* is efficacious for strongyles. Dosing at the rate of 35 mg per kg removes *S. vulgaris* (95 to 100 per cent), *S. equinus* (95 to 100 per cent), *S. edentatus* (70 to 80 per cent), and small strongyles (85 to 95 per cent). The formulation was designed for administration by mixing in the daily grain ration. Consumption of medicated grain is quite unpredictable among horses, and this variable factor in successful administration has limited the use of this product. This is unfortunate because it has a broad spectrum of activity in the horse and it is effective against strongyles that are resistant to PTZ, benzimidazoles, and febantel. Special inducements for consumption indicated on the label should be followed, and each animal should be checked to be certain that the pellets in the medicated grain are in fact eaten along with the grain. Many horses can selectively con-

---

*Dyrex Cap-Tabs, Ft. Dodge Labs, Ft. Dodge, IA 50501

*Equigard, Squibb, Princeton, NJ 08540

sume the grain and leave the dichlorvos pellets in the feed box.

Pelleted dichlorvos is generally safe to use in horses of all ages; however, the label indicates that it should not be administered to foals under six months of age. This is in deference to a lack of data in suckling and young weanling foals because of the consumption factor rather than evidence of a selective toxicosis for foals, which is implied by the exclusion on the label.

FEBANTEL

Febantel (Rintal)* is classified as a phenylguanidine and is quite efficacious for strongyles, ascarids, and pinworms in the horse. At the dose level of 6 mg per kg, febantel removes 98 to 100 per cent of *S. vulgaris, S. edentatus, S. equinus,* and small strongyles. Paste and suspension formulations permit intraoral, drench, stomach tube, or top-dress feed types of administration. The margin of safety is about 40 times, and it can be administered to horses of all ages and types. Febantel and trichlorfon are compatible and can be administered together.

Benzimidazole-resistant strongyles are also resistant to febantel. The cross-over of benzimidazole resistance to febantel[12] is explained by the latter's being an "open ring benzimidazole" that becomes closed in the body to function as a benzimidazole for its anthelmintic action.

PYRANTEL

Pyrantel is a tetrahydropyrimidine that is active against strongyles, ascarids, and pinworms in the horse. The pamoate salt of pyrantel†‡ is available in the United States as a suspension for stomach tube, drench, or top-dress feed types of administration. A paste formulation has been in use for several years in other countries. At the dose rate of 6.6 mg base per kg of body weight, strongyle removal rates are 95 to 100 per cent for *S. vulgaris,* 65 to 75 per cent for *S. edentatus,* 100 per cent for *S. equinus,* and 90 to 100 per cent for small strongyles. There is a wide margin of safety (20 times). Pyrantel pamoate can be used in horses of all ages, including stallions and pregnant mares. Strongyles that are resistant to PTZ, benzimidazoles, or febantel are fully responsive to the action of pyrantel.

AVERMECTINS

Avermectins are a new class of compounds that are chemically complex fermentation products derived from *Streptomyces avermitilis.* Their broad spectrum of action includes arthropods as well as nematodes. In the horse, preliminary reports[26, 30] indicate that relatively low dose rates (0.2 mg per kg) are quite efficacious for strongyles as well as other internal parasites. Limited data indicate that avermectins* are effective against benzimidazole-resistant strongyles. Avermectins are effective by either enteral or parenteral routes of administration, but further experience is necessary to determine the feasibility of the methods of administration.

CONTROL

Strongyle control is the number one priority in the overall parasite control program for a horse farm operation. The measure of success of controlling strongyles, especially the large strongyle, *S. vulgaris,* is the state of health reflected in the enhanced growth of the foals and the low order of adverse effects on horses of all ages. Strongyles in particular, but with other internal parasites contributing, pose the most common and important everyday threat to the health and well-being of horses. Control should be a cooperative venture among the equine practitioner, the owner, and the farm manager. The veterinarian should participate in the development of a program of control suitable for the individual farm situation, and in most operations, the practitioner's professional services are indispensable to the application of the program.

Effective control is achieved by continuous efforts applied over a prolonged period of time. The task is a year-round and year-to-year undertaking because the parasites are inherently insidious and tenacious. Management and sanitation practices that reduce contamination of the pastures and paddocks with strongyle eggs and larvae are valuable adjuncts to specific drug treatments and should be applied to the maximal degree feasible in keeping with other factors.

Contemporary control of strongyles relies heavily on the proper application of anthelmintics.[2, 6, 9, 11, 23, 32, 34, 40] There is no means of biological control, and no vaccine or method of immunization has been developed. With the current availablity of the foregoing array of compounds or mixtures, the means

*Rintal, Haver-Lockhart, Shawnee, KS 66201
†Strongid-T, Pfizer, New York, NY 10017
‡Imathal, Beecham, Bristol, TN 37620

*Equalan, Merck & Co., Rahway, NJ 07065

to achieve effective control of these important parasites is at hand.

A control program should emphasize preventing or minimizing the infections through long-term sustained efforts because the large strongyles especially produce their primary damage by the migrations of the immature stages. Furthermore, the migrating stages are in the tissues outside the gut lumen and are not affected by the anthelmintics as they are routinely used to remove the stages from the digestive tract. However, removal of the gut lumen stages relieves the horse of the damage, such as blood-sucking, being inflicted by these forms. More important from the control standpoint is the interruption or breaking of the life cycle of the parasites that is effected by the removal of the worms from the gut lumen. This stops or reduces the contamination of the environment with eggs and larvae, thereby stopping or limiting the spread of the infections, which indirectly protects the same or associated horses or foals from infection or reinfection. One or two treatments a year, although beneficial to the treated animals, do not provide much impact on the transmission potential of the parasite populations and cannot be expected to achieve effective strongyle control on most farms, especially nursery operations.

GENERAL FEATURES OF CONTROL PROGRAMS

Several universally applicable measures should be practiced to render success from a program employing antiparasitic drugs. These follow.

1. All horses on the farm should be included in the program. Little is accomplished if some horses, such as barren mares or ponies, are not treated and are allowed to contaminate pastures, paddocks, and other areas grazed by horses to which control measures are applied.

2. Transient or boarded horses and any newly added animal should be quarantined or isolated and dewormed before being turned out with resident horses. Much effort can be wasted in a few days by introducing an untreated animal onto a farm where regular treatments are given.

3. Foals are protected against infection, particularly from strongyles, by regular treatment of the mares. Treatment of the foal itself has no bearing on the acquisition and damage caused by large strongyles.

4. Laboratory examination of fecal samples should be made periodically to maintain surveillance of the effectivenesses of the drugs being used and on the program's application. Drug efficacy can be determined by comparing an examination one to two weeks after treatment with the worm egg count

on the day of treatment. The pretreatment count is also usually the best index of the effectiveness of the overall program. An effective drug is expected to reduce strongyle egg counts to very low levels (0 to 20 per gm of feces, EPG) that are maintained through five weeks post-treatment.

5. No single drug or mixture should be used exclusively for strongyle control. This has been advocated for a number of years now in the belief that it would obviate or delay the selection or development of drug-resistant strains or populations of parasites. However, recent deliberations,[37] based mostly on drug-resistant populations of nematodes in sheep, recommend the repeated use of the same compound for each generation of parasites and changing compounds between generations. Whether this practice would apply to strongyles of horses, where generations are not as well demarcated, remains to be determined. Regular alternation of anthelmintics also compensates for activity differences, and this practice is deemed to render beneficial complementary effects.

6. Feed administration is effective only if the medicated feed is consumed by the horse. The advent of several of the newer anthelmintics permits this method of dosing because the compounds are inherently less disagreeable, and relatively small amounts compose the total dose. However, the farm manager or veterinarian should check to be certain that the medicated grain is actually consumed, and grooms should not be relied upon unless they are absolutely trustworthy.

7. Labels should be read and completely understood before an anthelmintic is administered. All dosage recommendations and special preparatory procedures should be followed. Abide by any precautions or contraindications indicated on the label. In the event that there are discrepancies between the label and the dosages given in this discussion, those on the label should be followed. This will compensate for possible future changes and other unforeseen eventualities.

CONTROL SYSTEMS

Two basic systems or programs of drug administration are used for controlling strongyles. They are (1) the "low-level" system, in which small daily doses are given on a continuing basis; and (2) single dose programs, in which single therapeutic doses are given at periodic intervals.

Low-Level System. The low-level regimen has been used only to a limited extent and on a practical basis; only phenothiazine has been applied in this manner[5, 44] (p. 273).

Periodic Therapeutic Dose System. This system is currently used extensively, and the effectiveness is related to (1) the efficacy of the drug against the parasites and (2) the spacing of treatments at appropriate intervals. Both of these serve to keep the number of parasites in the intestinal lumen at minimal levels.

The most important criterion for selecting an antistrongyle compound is its effectiveness against the large strongyles, *S. vulgaris* and *S. edentatus*. Overall, experiences indicate that *S. equinus* responds similarly to *S. vulgaris*. Efficacy of various compounds was described before.

The interval between treatments is extremely important and is related more to the biology of the parasites and dynamics of the infections than to the effectiveness of the drugs. Even with the most efficacious compounds, the marked reductions in fecal egg counts following treatment, which characteristically persist for four to five weeks, are followed by small increases at six weeks and greater increases at eight weeks. Thus, treatments at intervals of six to eight weeks are required for effective control. In the central Kentucky region, six treatments per year are sufficient to minimize the adverse effects of strongylid infections. This is especially significant because of the many intensive nursery operations where highly susceptible foals are present and must be protected. In general, this treatment schedule would be appropriate in comparable operations under similar conditions in other areas. With greater concentrations of animals or in locations favoring higher levels of parasitism, more frequent treatment may be needed, perhaps at six-week or even four-week intervals. Conversely, fewer treatments than six per year may suffice where only a few horses or no foals are involved and where conditions are unfavorable for development and transmission of parasites.

METHOD OF ADMINISTRATION

For a number of years, the physical nature of the available compounds, large volume of therapeutic doses, or the unpalatable nature of the chemicals made it necessary to administer anthelmintics to the horse via stomach tube. This ensured the administration of the desired dosage. In the evolution of new products, more active agents requiring lower dosage levels and greater palatability have been developed, so that such products as CBZ, dichlorvos, febantel, FBZ, MBZ, OBZ, pyrantel, and TBZ may be given on the feed. Most recently, paste types of formulations for oral administration have been developed, and these can be handily administered with no loss of expected activity. Currently, several compounds are available as pastes, including TBZ, MBZ, CBZ, OBZ and febantel, so it is unfortunate

that benzimidazole resistance is exhibited against all of these compounds except OBZ. With the recent advent of the avermectins, the parenteral route of administration has been revived. Levamisole showed some promise in this regard but was found wanting in activity, and it was prone to induce a local tissue reaction. Further clinical experience will determine whether parenteral administration of avermectins is feasible for routine use in parasite control in the horse.

DRUG RESISTANCE

This phenomenon was discussed earlier. The constant threat of the appearance of resistant forms makes surveillance of any drug imperative. The value of the benzimidazoles in an overall parasite control program should not be entirely discredited by the resistance of the small strongyles. Indeed, if a judicious selection is made in their use, a significant contribution to parasite control can still be gained. Benzimidazoles as a group are highly effective against the large strongyles (*S. vulgaris* and *S. edentatus*), the most harmful of all the internal parasites and, thus, the primary targets of control. Certain parasites are efficiently removed only by certain benzimidazoles, for example, *Strongyloides westeri* infection of foals by TBZ, OBZ, and CBZ. As a group, the benzimidazoles are quite safe to use, and thus, untoward effects on the horse are not apt to occur. Effective antiparasitic activity at low dose rates adds up to small total dose volumes that are pliable to a variety of treatment formulations and methods of administration.

CHEMOTHERAPY OF MIGRATING LARVAE

The quest for a chemotherapeutic agent effective against the parenteral migrating forms has been motivated by a desire to kill all of the parasites in the body at one treatment, thereby achieving an improved measure of control. Success in this search was first met with *S. vulgaris* through the use of high doses of TBZ in experimental infections in foals raised helminth-free.[8] In the model system used, a lethal dose of larvae was administered, and after symptoms of the acute *S. vulgaris* syndrome developed, the curative value of the drug was tested. Because of the rapid course of events in the disease, the drug had to be administered during the first two weeks after infection, usually between days 7 and 14.

Radical and clinical cures are the two types of responses described for chemotherapeutic agents effective against *S. vulgaris* larvae in the early stages.[8] A radical cure is defined as a response in which the clinical signs are abated and a marked killing action on the larvae is effected. A clinical cure represents only a remission of the signs without any appreciable lethal effect on the larvae.

In the early tests, only TBZ produced a radical cure.[10] The optimal treatment regimen of TBZ was two doses, each at the rate of 440 mg per kg (10 times the dewormer rate) administered orally on two successive days for an aggregate total dose of 880 mg per kg. Other treatment regimens, including a single dose of TBZ at 880 mg per kg and two doses at 220 mg per kg on successive days, resulted in clinical cures but not radical cures. Neither type of cure was achieved by either a single dose of thiabendazole at 440 mg per kg or two doses at 110 mg per kg on successive days. Other compounds, including diethylcarbamazine, parbendazole, pyrantel, and ±-tetramisole, produced positive clinical responses, but radical cures were not accomplished by any or these compounds at any dose used. Treatments generally included repeated administration of each compound at higher than usual therapeutic (anthelmintic) dose rates. In recent tests, radical cures of early (seven- to nine-day-old) fourth-stage larvae of S. vulgaris were elicited by multiple daily doses of fenbendazole (3 × 50 mg per kg) and by single doses of nitramisole at 8 mg per kg or ivermectin at 0.1, 0.3, and 0.8 mg per kg.[41] Against 28-day-old larvae, albendazole (ABZ)* in multiple doses of 25 mg per kg three times a day for five days[38] or 50 mg per kg twice a day for three days (unpublished data) effects a radical cure. Ivermectin in a single dose at 0.2 mg per kg also was efficacious against eight-week-old larvae of S. vulgaris in experimental infections.[42] These findings indicate the development of compounds and treatment regimens that produce radical cures with relatively low dosages.

Successful chemotherapy with high doses of TBZ in clinical cases of chronic S. vulgaris infection accompanied by colic has been reported.[3] Personal communication with other equine practitioners indicates that no benefit was derived from this treatment regimen in horses with recurrent colic; however, this variation is predictable from the experimental evidence. If colic is secondary to a thromboembolic arteritis in which appreciable numbers of young migrating larvae are the cause, a clinical response would be expected. However, cases of colic arising from arteritis from older larvae, embolisms, or adhesions would not be responsive to the chemotherapeutic effect of high doses of TBZ. A recent report indicated that a single dose of FBZ at a rate of 30 to 60 mg per kg reduced the numbers of intra-arterial fourth-stage larvae of various ages in naturally infected ponies by 76 and 83 per cent, respectively.[17] Such favorable results (unpublished) were not seen in our controlled tests of FBZ using a single dose of 60 mg per kg or two daily doses of 50 mg per kg in yearling horses naturally infected with late fourth- and fifth-stage S. vulgaris. A similar lack of effect on natural infections was also recorded for ABZ following two daily doses at 50 mg per kg.

The rationale for the use of repeated high doses of benzimidazoles as the regimen of chemotherapy for migrating S. vulgaris larvae is the difficulty with which requisite concentrations of drug come into contact with the parasites that are protected by embedment in varying amounts of thrombotic deposits. Also, the fifth-stage forms are usually encased in the retained sheath of the fourth-stage larvae. Repeated doses are also deemed to be advantageous because the action of benzimidazoles is effected through the energy utilization mechanisms of the parasites, which is a relatively slow killing process. This is reflected in the recent report that FBZ at 7.5 mg per kg daily for five days was quite efficacious for migrating S. vulgaris in aneurysms, retroperitoneal S. edentatus, and small strongyles encysted in the intestinal mucosa.[18] Activity of ivermectin against natural infections remains to be evaluated; however, its potential appears quite formidable.

These favorable developments in the chemotherapy of migrating strongyle larvae indicate the feasibility of achieving radical cures of strongyle infections and forecast probable changes in control concepts and practices.

References

1. Amborski, G. F., Bello T. R., and Torbert, B. J.: Host response to experimentally induced infections of *Strongylus vulgaris* in parasite-free and naturally infected ponies. Am. J. Vet. Res., 35:1181, 1974.
2. Arundel, J. H.: Parasitic diseases of the horse. Vet. Rev. No. 18, 83 pp., University of Sydney, The Post-Graduate Foundation in Veterinary Science, Sydney, NSW, Australia, 1978.
3. Coffman, J. R., and Carlson, K. L.: Verminous arteritis in horses. J. Am. Vet. Med. Assoc., 158:1358, 1971.
4. Delatour, P., Lorgue, G., and Courtot, D.: Teratogenicity of benzimidazole anthelmintics. World Vet. Congr., Thessaloniki Summaries, 1:107, 1975.
5. Dimock, W. W.: The two gram daily dose of phenothiazine for strongylosis of the horse. Vet. Med., 44:99, 1949.
6. Drudge, J. H.: Metazoal diseases, endo-parasitisms. *In* Catcott, E. J., and Smithcors, J. F. (eds.) Equine Medicine and Surgery, 2nd ed., Chap. 5. Wheaton, IL, American Veterinary Pub., 1972, pp. 157–179.
7. Drudge, J. H.: Clinical aspects of *Strongylus vulgaris* infection in the horse: Emphasis on diagnosis, chemotherapy, and prophylaxis. Vet. Clin. North Am. (Large Anim. Pract.), 1(2):251, 1979.
8. Drudge, J. H., and Lyons, E. T.: Newer developments in

---

*Valbazen, SmithKline Corp., Philadelphia, PA 19101

helminth control and *Strongylus vulgaris* research. Proc. 11th Annu. Meet. Am. Assoc. Eq. Pract., 1965, pp. 381–389.

9. Drudge, J. H., and Lyons, E. T.: Control of internal parasites of the horse. J. Am. Vet. Med. Assoc., *148*:378, 1966.

10. Drudge, J. H., and Lyons, E. T.: The chemotherapy of migrating strongyle larvae. *In* Bryans, J. T., and Gerber, M. (eds.): Equine Infectious Diseases (Proceedings of the Second International Conference on Equine Infectious Diseases, Paris, 1969). Basel, Switzerland, S. Karger, 1970, 2:310–322 (Discussion 323–325).

11. Drudge, J. H., and Lyons, E. T.: Control of equine parasites. Lectures, Stud Manager's Course, Lexington, KY, 1976, pp. 139–148.

12. Drudge, J. H., and Lyons, E. T.: Drug resistance in parasites. The Blood-Horse, *104*:1178, 1980.

13. Drudge, J. H., Lyons, E. T., and Szanto, J.: Pathogenesis of migrating stages of helminths, with special reference to *Strongylus vulgaris. In* Soulsby, E. J. L. (ed.): Biology of Parasites: Emphasis on Veterinary Parasites. New York, Academic Press, 1966, pp. 199–214.

14. Drudge, J. H., Lyons, E. T., and Szanto, J.: Critical tests of piperazine–carbon disulfide complex and phenothiazine mixtures against internal parasites of the horse. Am. J. Vet. Res., *30*:947, 1969.

15. Drudge, J. H., Lyons, E. T., and Tolliver, S. C.: Benzimidazole resistance of equine strongyles — critical tests of six compounds against population B. Am. J. Vet. Res., *40*:590, 1979.

16. Duncan, J. L.: Immunity to *Strongylus vulgaris* in the horse. Equine Vet. J., 7:192, 1975.

17. Duncan, J. L., McBeath, D. G., Best, J. M., and Preston, N. K.: The efficacy of fenbendazole in the control of immature strongyle infections in ponies. Equine Vet J., 9:146, 1977.

18. Duncan, J. L., McBeath, D. G., and Preston, N. K.: Studies on the efficacy of fenbendazole used in a divided dosage regime against strongyle infections in ponies. Equine Vet. J., *12*:78, 1980.

19. Duncan, J. L., and Pirie, H. M.: The life cycle of *Strongylus vulgaris* in the horse. Res. Vet. Sci., *13*:374, 1972.

20. Enigk, K.: Zur Entwicklung von *Strongylus vulgaris* (Nematodes) im Wirtstier. Z. Tropenmed. Parasit., 2:287, 1950. (English version in Cornell Vet., *63*:223, 1973.)

21. Enigk, K.: Weitere Untersuchungen zur Biologie von *Strongylus vulgaris* (Nematodes) im Wirtstier. Z. Tropenmed. Parasitol., 2:523, 1951. (English version in Cornell Vet., *63*:247, 1973.)

22. Enigk, K.: The development of the three species of *Strongylus* of the horse during the prepatent period. *In* Bryans, J. T., and Gerber, H. (eds.): Equine Infectious Diseases (Proceedings of the Second International Conference on Equine Infectious Diseases, Paris, 1969). Basel, Switzerland, S. Karger, 2:259–268 (Discussion 323–325), 1970.

23. Gibson, T. E.: Veterinary anthelmintic medication. Technical Communication No. 33, 3rd ed. Commonwealth Institute of Helminthology, Farnham Royal, UK, Commonwealth Agricultural Bureaux, 1975, p. 348.

24. Haberman, R. T., Harwood, P. D., and Hunt, W. H.: Critical tests with phenothiazine as an anthelmintic in horses. North Am. Vet., *22*:85, 1941.

25. Kelly, J. D., and Hall, C. A.: Resistance of animal helminths to anthelmintics. *In* Advances in Pharmacology and Chemotherapy, s3616:89, New York, Academic Press, 1979.

26. Klei, T. R., and Torbert, B. J.: Efficacy of ivermectin (22, 23-dihydroavermectin B₁) against gastrointestinal parasites in ponies. Am. J. Vet. Res., *41*:1747, 1980.

27. Lichtenfels, J. R.: Helminths of domestic equids. Illustrated keys to genera and species with emphasis on North American forms. Proc. Helm. Soc. Wash., *42* (special issue), 92 pp., 1975.

28. Lyons, E. T., Drudge, J. H., and Tolliver, S. C.: Critical tests of oxfendazole against internal parasites of horses. Am. J. Vet. Res., *38*:2049, 1977.

29. Lyons, E. T., Drudge, J. H., and Tolliver, S. C.: Antiparasitic activity of parbendazole in critical tests in horses. Am. J. Vet. Res., *41*:(1):123, 1980.

30. Lyons, E. T., Drudge, J. H., and Tolliver, S. C.: Antiparasitic activity of ivermectin in critical tests in equids. Am. J. Vet. Res., *41(12)*:2069, 1980.

31. McCraw, B. M., and Slocombe, J. O. D.: Early development of and pathology associated with *Strongylus edentatus*. Can. J. Comp. Med., *38*:124, 1974.

32. McCraw, B. M., and Slocombe, J. O. D.: *Strongylus vulgaris* in the horse. A review, Can. Vet. J., *17*:150, 1976.

33. Ogbourne, C. P.: Pathogenesis of Cyathostome infections of the horse. A review. Misc. Pub. No. 5, Commonwealth Institute of Helminthology, Farnham Royal, Bucks, England, 25 pp., 1977.

34. Ogbourne, C. P., and Duncan, J. L.: *Strongylus vulgaris* in the horse: Its biology and veterinary importance. Misc. Pub. No. 4, Commonwealth Institute of Helminthology, Farnham Royal, Bucks, England, 40 pp., 1977.

35. Patton, S., and Drudge, J. H.: Clinical response of pony foals experimentally infected with *Strongylus vulgaris*. Am. J. Vet. Res., *38*:2059, 1977.

36. Poynter, D., and Hughes, D. L.: Phenothiazine and piperazine—an efficient anthelmintic for horses. Vet. Rec., 70:1183, 1958.

37. Prichard, R. K., Hall, C. A., Kelly, J. D., Martin, I. C. A., and Donald, A. D.: The problem of anthelmintic resistance in nematodes. Aust. Vet. J., *56*:239, 1980.

38. Rendano, V. T., Georgi, J. R., White, K. K., Sack, W. O., King, J. M., Bionchi, D. G., and Theodorides, V. J.: Equine verminous arteritis. An arteriographic evaluation of the larvicidal activity of albendazole. Equine Vet. J., *11*:223, 1979.

39. Round, M. C.: The development of strongyles in horses and associated serum protein changes. *In* Bryans, J. T., and Gerber, M. (eds.): Equine Infectious Diseases. (Proceedings of the Second International Conference on Equine Infectious Diseases, Paris, 1969). Basel, Switzerland, S. Karger, 2:290–303 (Discussion 323–325), 1970.

40. Scott, P.: A review of some modern equine anthelmintics. N. Z. Vet. J., *25*:373, 1977.

41. Slocombe, J. O. D., and McCraw, B. M.: Evaluation of pyrantel pamoate, nitramisole and avermectin B₁ against migrating *Strongylus vulgaris* larvae. Can. J. Comp. Med., *44*:93, 1980.

42. Slocombe, J. O. D., McCraw, B. M., Pennock, P. W., and Llewellyn, H. R.: Anthelmintic treatment of migrating stages of *Strongylus vulgaris*. Proc. 26th Annu. Meet. Am. Assoc. Eq. Pract., 1980, pp. 37–44.

43. Theodorides, V.: Antiparasitic drugs. *In* Georgi, J. R. (ed.): Parasitology for Veterinarians, Chap. 20. Philadelphia, W. B. Saunders Co., 1980, pp. 397–448.

44. Todd, A. C.: Control of strongyle parasites in horses. Kentucky Agricultural Experimental Station Bulletin 582, 22 pp., 1952.

45. Trace, J. C., Hepperle, W. H., Eppley, R. J., Sender, L., and Edds, G. T.: New broad spectrum anthelmintic for horses. Vet. Med., 57:144, 1962.

46. Wetzel, R.: Zur Entwicklung des grossen Palisadenwurmes (*Strongylus equinus*). im Pferd. Arch. Wiss. Prakt. Tierheilk, 76:81 1940.

47. Wetzel, R.: Die Entwicklungsdauer (Prapatenzperiode) von *Strongylus edentatus*. im Pferde. Dtsch. Tierarztl. Wsch., 59:129, 1952.

STRONGYLOIDOSIS

J. H. Drudge, LEXINGTON, KENTUCKY

E. T. Lyons, LEXINGTON, KENTUCKY

OCCURRENCE

The intestinal threadworm *Strongyloides westeri* is a very common parasite of young foals throughout the world. Stronglyloides is the first of the worm infestations to mature in foals. Eggs of *S. westeri* commonly appear in feces of sucklings during the second week after birth. Intestinal infections are self-limiting, and egg-bearing forms tend to disappear after a few months, so patent infections characteristically decrease by the time foals are six months old, and a low incidence is typical for older weanlings and yearlings. Feces of mature horses are devoid of Strongyloides eggs.

DEVELOPMENT

Source of *S. westeri* infection in foals during the early postpartum period remained an enigma until infective larvae were discovered in the milk of the mare.[6, 8, 11] Presence of infective larvae in milk four days postpartum and persistence in the milk of some mares for 47 days[9] provide the source of infection for very young foals when environmental conditions are unfavorable for extrinsic development of the fragile infective larvae. They also account for the perennial appearance of *S. westeri* infection when each crop of foals typically undergoes a self-cure before weaning and the mares do not have patent enteric infections. Infective larvae do develop from the eggs shed by infected foals when environmental conditions are favorable. These larvae invade by skin penetration or by ingestion, but the epizootiologic role played by these extrinsically derived larvae has not been elucidated. They probably enhance the enteric infections in the foals and are the source of the tissue-dwelling forms that eventually appear in the milk. Factors that mobilize the larvae in the mammary tissues for discharge in the milk have not been determined.

PATHOGENESIS

Diarrhea is the most common clinical manifestation of strongyloides infection in foals.[6, 12, 13] However, evidence of the causal relationship is equivocal. Infection, development, and maturation of *S. westeri* occur at the same time that foals are afflicted by the nine-day scours syndrome. Therapy with anthelmintics such as thiabendazole or cambendazole may appear to be curative, but 9-day scours tends to be self-limiting if untreated. The syndrome is associated with the foaling heat period in the mare, which implies a causal relationship with lactogenic factors. However, the scouring may occur in orphaned foals, and inhibition of the foaling heat period by hormone therapy of the mare does not obviate the diarrhea syndrome in the foal.[4] Heavy enteric infections of *S. westeri* as indicated by high fecal egg counts may not be associated with diarrhea, while in contrast, a low egg count may be determined in the presence of severe scouring.

Experimental infections of worm-free foals with large numbers of larvae (4.5 to 13.0 million) produced severe diarrhea, pyrexia, and death in foals.[9] Infections with lesser numbers of larvae have not been associated consistently with diarrhea.[7, 9]

DIAGNOSIS

Presence of intestinal infections of *S. westeri* can be determined by demonstration of the typical eggs in the feces. Microscopic examination at 100× magnification of salt, sugar, or other flotation preparations reveals the thin-walled eggs, each containing a larva that may be weakly motile. The shape of *S. westeri* eggs tends to be more round than that of strongyloides of other animals. Only freshly voided feces should be used because (1) eggs of *S. westeri* hatch within a few hours, releasing the first-stage larvae, which are quite fragile and do not float readily; and (2) strongyle eggs also undergo development to vermiform stages within a matter of hours after passage and may be misdiagnosed as strongyloides by the inexperienced observer. The latter may be the derivation of reports of strongyloides infection in adolescent and mature horses.

Suckling foals (two to four weeks of age) are commonly infected with *S. westeri* and are voiding embryonated eggs in their feces. These young foals may also consume fresh feces from their dams, which results in the passage of strongyle eggs through the digestive tract of the foal and their appearance in the feces of the foal. Older foals (two to three months of age) commonly have maturing infections of small strongyles, and thus, both types of eggs may be present in their feces concurrently.

Detection of *S. westeri* larvae in milk or tissues is not a feasible procedure for clinicians or clinical pathology laboratories. Recovery of larvae from milk or tissue samples is best accomplished by sedimentation in Baermann funnels, which requires specialized personnel. Ordinarily, the tissue-dwelling larvae are not found in necropsy examinations unless a specific search is made.

Clinically, strongyloides infection should be considered as the possible etiologic agent in all episodes of diarrhea in foals. Differentiation from scouring due to bacterial, viral, nutritional, and idiopathic causes may be difficult. Typically, feces associated with the nine-day scouring syndrome are green. Strongyloides-induced diarrhea is not characterized by the fetid odor associated with bacterial types such as Salmonella, and febrile reactions usually do not appear as with bacterial and viral diseases. Demonstration of eggs of *S. westeri* in feces may be helpful in the diagnosis; however, the likelihood of concurrent nonparasitic infections and strongyloides infection should not be overlooked. Many clinicians routinely administer the anthelmintic thiabendazole early in the course of events, and a prompt remission of the diarrhea is presumptive evidence of the involvement of *S. westeri* in the episode.

TREATMENT

Thiabendazole*†‡ has been the mainstay for treatment of foals for the intestinal stage of *S. westeri* infection. Both controlled tests on experimental infections in worm-free foals (author's unpublished data) and clinical trials on naturally infected foals[5] demonstrated the efficacy of a single dose of thiabendazole at the rate of 44 mg per kg against *S. westeri* in the small intestine. More recently, cambendazole§ has been introduced, and it also is quite efficacious[1, 2] for *S. westeri* infection at the rate of 20 mg per kg as a single dose. These products are available in a variety of formulations, including powder, suspension, and paste, that provide for administration to foals by stomach tube, drench, or oral deposition, depending on the preference of the clinician. Equal therapeutic activity is derived from the various types of dosing, provided the administration is successful. Toxicosis of these products is of a low order, and the regular therapeutic dose rates can be administered safely to sucklings of all ages.

Other products possessing significant activity against *S. westeri* include fenbendazole*[3, 14] and oxibendazole.†[3] However, fenbendazole requires a dose of 50 mg per kg or 10 times the therapeutic dose for strongyles. Oxibendazole is effective for *S. westeri* at the regular therapeutic dose rate of 10 mg per kg,† but the clinical experience is limited.

CONTROL

Treatment schedules for thiabendazole and cambendazole for control of strongyloides infection in foals vary. The usual practice in central Kentucky entails periodic treatments of suckling foals with a thiabendazole piperazine mixture‡ or cambendazole,§ primarily for ascarid control (see Ascariasis, p. 262), which provides simultaneous removal of strongyloides from the small intestine. The first treatment is given when foals are about eight weeks old and is repeated at eight-week intervals. Episodes of diarrhea caused by strongyloides in very young foals are treated on an individual case basis. Some clinicians advise treatment of seven-day-old foals routinely with a therapeutic dose of thiabendazole as a prophylactic measure against diarrhea. The merit of this practice is empirical. Justification for treatment of two-week-old foals has a basis in being timed with the maturation of the first *S. westeri* infections. Repeating treatments at two-week intervals during the next six weeks would coincide with the maturation of subsequent infections of *S. westeri*. Application of such a rigorous schedule of treatment with these benzimidazoles may be called for in situations in which strongyloides pose an unusually serious problem.

Chemotherapy of the tissue-dwelling stages of *S. westeri* or effecting a radical cure is a theoretical goal for equine parasitologists in the quest for improved control of strongyloides.[10] Daily administration of cambendazole at 10 or 20 mg per kg to the mare during the early postpartum period delayed maturation of *S. westeri* in the nursing foal during the medication period. The paste formulation of cambendazole at 30 mg per kg daily was the most consistently effective regimen. Lower daily dose rates of the paste, given intraorally or as a pelleted formulation on the feed, were not consistently effective in all mares. Suspension of treatment resulted in the appearance of strongyloides eggs in the feces of foals after the usual time for prepatent development, which indicated that the tissue stages in the mares were not killed. In this model system,

*Equizole, Merck & Co., Rahway, NJ 07065
†Equizole A, Merck & Co., Rahway, NJ 07065
‡Omnizole, Merck & Co., Rahway, NJ 07065
§Camvet, Merck & Co., Rahway, NJ 07065

*Panacur, American Hoechst, Somerville, NJ 08876
†Anthelcide-EQ, Norden Labs, Lincoln, NB 68501
‡Equizole A, Merck & Co., Rahway, NJ 07065
§Camvet, Merck and Co., Rahway, NJ 07065

thiabendazole paste* at 44 mg per kg or 88 mg per kg was not active. Unpublished data from similar trials with paste formulations of oxibendazole and mebendazole† indicate that oxibendazole at 10 mg per kg is not effective, whereas mebendazole at three, four, and eight times the basic dose rate of 8.8 mg per kg exhibited activity. Treatment with the paste formulations of these two compounds induced diarrhea in the mares, so their potentials have not been fully explored.

References

1. Bello, T. R., Amborski, G. F., Torbert, B. J., and Greer, G. J.: Anthelmintic efficacy of cambendazole against gastrointestinal parasites of the horse. Am J. Vet. Res., *34*:771, 1973.
2. Drudge, J. H., Lyons, E. T., and Tolliver, S. C.: Critical tests of suspension, paste, and pellet formulations of cambendazole in the horse. Am. J. Vet. Res., *36*:435, 1975.
3. Drudge, J. H., Lyons, E. T., Tolliver, S. C., and Kubis, J. E.: Critical tests and clinical trials on oxibendazole in horses with special reference to removal of *Parascaris equorum.* Am. J. Vet. Res., *40*:758, 1979.
4. Drudge, J. H., Lyons, E. T., Tolliver, S. C., and Kubis,
5. J. E.: Clinical trials with fenbendazole and oxibendazole for *Strongyloides westeri* infection in foals. Am. J. Vet. Res., *42*:526, 1981.
5. Drudge, J. H., Szanto, J., and Wyant, Z. N.: Studies on the anthelmintic thiabendazole in the horse. II. Field studies. Seminar on parasitic diseases with special reference to thiabendazole. Proc. Pan-Am. Congr. Vet. Med. Zootech, *4*:81, 1962.
6. Enigk, K., Dey-Hazra, A., and Batke, J.: Zur klinischen Bedeutung und Behandlung des galaktogen erworbenen Strongyloides-Befalls der Fohlen. D. T. W., *81*:605, 1974.
7. Greer, G. J., Bello, T. R., and Amborski, G. F.: Experimental infection of *Strongyloides westeri* in parasite-free ponies. J. Parasitol., *60*:466, 1974.
8. Lyons, E. T., Drudge, J. H., and Tolliver, S. C.: Parasites from mare's milk. The Bloodhorse, 95:2270, 1969.
9. Lyons, E. T., Drudge, J. H., and Tolliver, S. C.: On the life cycle of *Strongyloides westeri* in the equine. J. Parasitol., *59*:780, 1973.
10. Lyons, E. T., Drudge, J. H., and Tolliver, S. C.: Observations on development of *Strongyloides westeri* in foals nursing dams treated with cambendazole or thiabendazole. Am. J. Vet. Res., *38*:889, 1977.
11. Mirck, M. H.: *Strongyloides westeri* Ihle, 1917 (Nematoda: Strongyloididae). I. Parasitologische Aspecten van de Naturrlijke Infectie. Tijdschr, Diergeneesk, *102*:1039, 1977.
12. Poynter, D.: Some observations on the nematode parasites of horses. Proc. 2nd Internatl. Conf. Equine Infect. Dis., 1969–1970, pp. 269–289.
13. Russell, A. F.: The development of helminthiasis in Thoroughbred foals. J. Comp. Pathol., *58*:107, 1948.
14. Tiefenbach, B.: Panacur—weltweite klinische Prufung eines neuen Breitband-Anthelminthikums. Die Blauen Hefte, *55*:204, 1976.

*Omnizole, Merck and Co., Rahway, NJ 07065
†Telmin S.F., Pitman-Moore, Inc., Washington Crossing, NJ 08560

BOTS

J. H. Drudge, LEXINGTON, KENTUCKY
E. T. Lyons, LEXINGTON, KENTUCKY

OCCURRENCE

Virtually every horse is infected with bots. It is unusual to perform a necropsy on a horse or foal at any time of the year and find the stomach free of bots.[8, 9, 13] Four species of bots are included in the check list[2] of parasites of horses in the United States and Canada. Two of these species, *Gasterophilus intestinalis* and *Gasterophilus nasalis*, are prevalent throughout this country as well as other parts of the world.[1] The third species, *Gasterophilus hemorrhoidalis*, is also recorded on a worldwide basis, but its occurrence was quite rare (in 2 of 629 horses) in a recent survey.[9] Distribution of this species was previously recorded[17] as somewhat restricted to the North Central states, and these were not included in the latest survey.[9] The fourth species, *Gasterophilus inermis,* has not been found recently.

DEVELOPMENT

Bots are insects and undergo four stages—egg, larva, pupa, and adult—in the cycle of development. The adults are honeybee-like in general appearance, and the female flies deposit eggs on the hairs of the horse. Female *G. intestinalis* prefers to put the eggs on the hairs of the forelimbs but also uses hairs on the neck, chest, flanks, and the mane. In contrast, *G. nasalis* females limit the deposit of eggs to hairs under the jaws or in the throat region, hence, the common name of "throat bot" for this species.

In temperate zones, the season of botfly activity and egg deposition is prolonged, extending from late spring until late fall. The transmission season of *G. intestinalis* is further extended for several weeks into early winter by the persistence of viable larvae in egg cases on the animal's hair.[8, 14] Development of the egg into a first-stage larva requires about one week. Embryonated eggs of *G. intestinalis* do not hatch spontaneously but must be stimulated by the warmth, moisture, and action of the horse's lips. In contrast, the eggs of *G. nasalis* hatch after one week of development when they contain infective first-stage larvae, and these larvae crawl to the lips. In either case, the first-stage larvae invade the oral tissues, and after three weeks of growth and development, they emerge and pass to the stomach as second-stage larvae. Further growth and development to third-stage larvae take place in the stomach within three to four weeks. Third-stage larvae remain as such in the stomach for variable periods up to 10 months before they detach and pass in the feces. It is not known whether this prolonged time spent as third-stage larvae is necessary for maturation.

Typical clusters are formed by second- and third-stage larvae, with *G. intestinalis* preferring the white-lined area of the stomach and *G. nasalis* the duodenum just beyond the pylorus. In temperate zones, bot larvae spend the winter in the stomach of the horse. There is only one generation per year. Departure of third-stage larvae is spontaneous, and the requisite factors triggering their release are not known. Discharge is not en masse as formerly thought but is spread out over a prolonged period of time, starting in the spring and extending into the summer, providing an additional mechanism for perpetuation of the species.

Pupae develop from the larvae discharged in the feces. Pupation takes place in the soil and requires three to four weeks or longer, depending on the temperature. Adult flies emerge from the pupae, and females soon start the egg laying process. Egg production varies from 150 to 750 per female.[17]

PATHOGENESIS

Egg laying activities of the female flies are annoying to horses. Reactions include head tossing, running, and congregation to gain protection from the flies.

First- and second-instar larvae of *G. intestinalis* and *G. nasalis* produce periodontal ulcerations mainly involving the upper molars and to a lesser extent the lower molars.[16] Poor growth and unthriftiness have been ascribed to these mouth lesions.[3, 9]

In the stomach, bots produce deep pits at the points of attachment, and occasionally these perforate the wall and result in fatal peritonitis. Stomach rupture has also been attributed to heavy bot infections. Other adverse effects, such as digestive disturbances, colic, and obstructions, have been ascribed to bot infections, but these signs are more

obscure and have not been produced experimentally.

DIAGNOSIS

Definite diagnosis of bot infection cannot be made by fecal flotation unless a bot larva happens to be found in the sample. The presence of eggs on the animal's hair is usually sufficient evidence to indicate internal infections. Otherwise, the prevalence of bots is such that infection can be presumed in most horses, particularly during the fall, winter, and spring seasons in temperate zones.

TREATMENT

Development of compounds efficacious for the removal of bots has not kept pace with that of drugs for the other internal parasites of the horse; however, several products are currently available.

Carbon Disulfide

Carbon disulfide was the traditional drug for bot removal over the span of years between World War I[10] and the early 1960s. During the first part of this period, carbon disulfide was formulated in gelatin capsules for administration by balling gun, but in more recent years, the liquid form administered by stomach tube became the exclusive method of treatment. A dose rate of 2.4 ml per 45 kg or the total dose of 24 ml (6 drams) is the standard dose for the 454 kg horse. For larger mares, a total dose of 30 ml (1 oz) is commonly used. A pretreatment fast of 18 hours was a part of the treatment ritual with carbon disulfide, but this was reduced to withholding the grain ration on the morning of treatment. This mollified the digestive disturbances that commonly followed treatment of fasted horses without reducing the efficacy against bots.[15] Activity of carbon disulfide is limited to the second and third instars in the stomach, and removal expectancy is 90 to 100 per cent. Ascarids are also effectively removed by carbon disulfide, but other internal parasites are not affected. Usage of carbon disulfide has been phased out, but it is still used by some clinicians to treat mares. It can be administered at the same time as other anthelmintics that lack bot activity. Specific contraindications are not known for combination treatment with products tested thus far. It is customary in the tubing process to administer the carbon disulfide after the anthelmintic preparation has been introduced, and water is used to flush the tube to complete the operation.

PICADEX

Picadex* was the first of the broad-spectrum antiparasitic agents because the carbon disulfide component provided bot removal to add to the anthelmintic activity of the piperazine. Later, strongyle activity was enhanced by the addition of phenothiazine (PTZ) to the piperazine–carbon disulfide complex,† and its use has largely replaced the straight picadex.[6] With either product, bot activity is dependent upon the release of carbon disulfide in the stomach, which is facilitated by a low pH. Bot removal by picadex is unpredictable owing to the variation in the acidity of the stomach among horses; so the bot activity is enhanced and stabilized at 75 to 85 per cent on the average by the administration of 600 ml of 0.5 per cent hydrochloric acid along with picadex. After several years, dosage of the picadex-PTZ suspension was reduced by 33 per cent from 1.5 oz, or 45 ml per 45 kg, to 1.0 oz, or 30 ml per 45 kg, which lowered bot removal expectancy to 70 to 80 per cent on the average.

TRICHLORFON

Trichlorfon was the first of the organophosphates developed for the horse. It is the most commonly used compound for bot control. At the dose rate of 35 to 40 mg per kg, trichlorfon is quite efficacious (90 to 100 per cent) for the removal of both species of bots from the stomach as well as the first and second instars in the mouth.

A variety of proprietary products are currently available and provide for a selection of methods of administration.[7] A liquid formulation‡ is given by stomach tube alone or along with other anthelmintics. Trichlorfon is generally compatible with the benzimidazoles, pyrantel, and febantel (see Strongylosis, p. 275). A gel formulation‡ is administered intraorally, and a bolus form§ is given by balling gun. A mixture of trichlorfon with PPZ and PTZ‖ is administered by stomach tube. Mixtures of trichlorfon with benzimidazoles include thiabendazole** and mebendazole††, which are preferably given by stomach tube, although feed administration is possible.

Trichlorfon has a narrow margin of safety, about 2 times. Therapeutic doses of 35 to 40 mg per kg

---

*Parvex, Upjohn Co., Kalamazoo, MI 49001
†Parvex Plus, Upjohn Co., Kalamazoo, MI 49001
‡Combot, Haver-Lockhart, Shawnee, KS 66201
§Dyrex Cap-Tabs, Ft. Dodge Labs, Ft. Dodge, IA 50501
‖Dyrex, T. F., Ft. Dodge Labs, Ft. Dodge, IA 50501
**Equizole B, Merck & Co., Rahway, NJ 07065
‡‡Telmin Plus, Pitman-Moore, Washington Crossing, NJ 08560

---

may induce transient loosening of feces because of the increased peristalsis of the gastrointestinal tract resulting from the pharmacologic blocking action on cholinesterase. Increasing the dose rate to 60 to 80 mg per kg enhances the severity of the reaction to a profuse, watery diarrhea. Atropine is antidotal. In spite of this toxicosis potential, trichlorfon has been in clinical use on a widespread basis for a prolonged period of time, and the untoward side effects have been incidental for the most part. Recently, administration of trichlorfon after a portion of the grain ration is consumed has been advocated to increase the tolerance of the drug without reducing therapeutic activity.

DICHLORVOS

Dichlorvos (DDVP) is also an organophosphate that is efficacious for the removal of bots. The resin pellet formulation* was developed as a broad-spectrum agent in the horse that inherently was limited to administration in the grain ration.[4] At the dose rate of 35 mg per kg, removal of bots averages only slightly less (80 to 100 per cent) than trichlorfon, but the delayed release provides efficacious removal of large and small strongyles as well as ascarids and pinworms. Mouth-dwelling stages of bots are also removed by these formulations.

Palatability of the pelleted formulation of DDVP is the primary limitation for the usage of this product. Consumption of medicated grain is unpredictable, so special attention should be directed to ensure that the dosage is, in fact, consumed. Label instructions restricting water consumption for a period of time before and after consumption are very important because the presence of water in the stomach interferes with the bot removal action. Untoward side effects are unusual because it is difficult to have a horse consume a sufficient quantity of the pellets to be harmful. The delayed release of the dichlorvos from the pellets and the rapid metabolism of DDVP in the body are further safeguards against toxicosis.

The gel formulation of DDVP† provides for the quick release of the dichlorvos, which restricts the spectrum of action to exclude strongyles.[5] Bot removal is quite effective (90 to 100 per cent), including the first and second instars in the mouth as well as the second and third instars of both *G. intestinalis* and *G. nasalis* from the stomach. Bot removal is achieved by the gel at the dose rate of 10 mg per kg, whereas a higher rate (20 mg per kg) is required for ascarid and pinworm removal. The gel formula-

---

*Equigard, Squibb, Princeton, NJ 08540
†Equigel, Squibb, Princeton, NJ 08540

tion of DDVP is generally free of toxicosis, and it can be given at the same time that other anthelmintics are administered.

AVERMECTINS

Avermectins are a new class of compounds in the horse. Preliminary reports[11, 12] indicate that relatively low dose rates (0.2 mg per kg) are quite efficacious for bots in the stomach as well as other internal parasites. Effects on the stages of bots in the mouth have not been determined. Avermectins are effective by either enteric or parenteral routes of administration, but further experience is necessary to determine the feasibility of the methods of administration.

CONTROL

Specific grooming measures can be helpful in reducing the intake of larvae of the common bot *G. intestinalis*. These procedures include clipping or plucking the hairs containing the attached egg cases or sponging the forelimbs and other body areas where the eggs are located with warm water. The former procedure removes the egg cases as well as the developing larvae so that newly deposited eggs are readily evident. In contrast, sponging causes artificial hatching to release the larvae, which are wiped off, but the egg cases are left and cannot be readily differentiated from newly laid eggs. Repeating these procedures at weekly intervals or more frequently will minimize infections of *G. intestinalis*. The throat bot, *G. nasalis*, does not lend itself to these grooming procedures. The eggs are deposited on the short hairs under the jaws and are not readily seen like those of the common bot on the longer hairs. Furthermore, hatching of *G. nasalis* cannot be induced by warm water rinses.

Treatment to remove the bots supplements or supplants the foregoing grooming procedures. It has been traditional practice to treat horses in the late fall or early winter to remove the bots. Timing this treatment about a month after the first heavy frost, which stops fly activity, provides for removal when the accumulation of bots in the stomach is maximal. This waiting period is important when carbon disulfide or picadex are used because they are not active on the bot larvae in the mouth. However, the organophosphates, trichlorfon or dichlorvos, obviate this delay because they are efficacious against the larvae in the mouth as well as those in the stomach. Coordinating this organophosphate treatment with a grooming procedure to eliminate the viable eggs of *G. intestinalis* will enhance the control because this residual source of larvae is eliminated. The or-

ganophosphates tend to effect a radical cure because of the removal of all bot larvae in the body, thereby presenting an advantage over carbon disulfide or picadex, whether used for the yearly treatment or more frequently during the year for broad-spectrum parasite control.

References

1. Arundel, J. H.: Parasitic diseases of the horse. Vet. Rev., No. 18, The University of Sydney, The Post-Graduate Foundation in Veterinary Science, Sydney, 83 pp., 1978.
2. Becklund, W. W.: Revised check list of internal and external parasites of domestic animals in the United States and possessions and in Canada. Am. J. Vet. Res., 25:1380, 1964.
3. Bello, T. R., and Seger, C. L.: Antiparasitic efficacy of dichlorvos paste formulation against first-instar *Gasterophilus intestinalis* in the tongues of Shetland pony foals. Am. J. Vet. Res., 33:39, 1972.
4. Drudge, J. H., and Lyons, E. T.: Critical tests of a resin-pellet formulation of dichlorvos against internal parasites of the horse. Am. J. Vet. Res., 33:1365, 1972.
5. Drudge, J. H., Lyons, E. T., and Swerczek, T. W.: Activity of gel and paste formulations of dichlorvos against first instars of *Gasterophilus spp.* Am. J. Vet. Res., 33:2191, 1972.
6. Drudge, J. H., Lyons, E. T., and Szanto, J.: Critical tests of piperazine–carbon disulfide complex and phenothiazine mixtures against internal parasites of the horse. Am. J. Vet. Res., 30:947, 1969.
7. Drudge, J. H., Lyons, E. T., and Tolliver, S. C.: Critical and controlled tests of the antiparasitic activity of liquid and paste formulations of trichlorfon in the horse. VM SAC, 70:975, 1975.
8. Drudge, J. H., Lyons, E. T., Tolliver, S. C., and Wyant, Z. N.: Occurrence of second and third instars of *Gasterophilus intestinalis* and *Gasterophilus nasalis* in stomachs of horses in Kentucky. Am. J. Vet. Res., 36:1585, 1975.
9. Haas, D. K.: Equine parasitism. VM SAC, 74:980, 1979.
10. Hall, M. C., Smead, M. J., and Wolf, C. E.: Studies on anthelmintics. II. The anthelmintic and insecticidal value of carbon disulfide against gastrointestinal parasites of the horse. J. Am. Vet. Med. Assoc., 55:543, 1919.
11. Klei, T. R., and Torbert, B. J.: Efficacy of ivermectin (22, 23-dihydroavermectin B₁) against gastrointestinal parasites in ponies. Am. J. Vet. Res., 41:1747, 1980.
12. Lyons, E. T., Drudge, J. H., and Tolliver, S. C.: Antiparasitic activity of ivermectin in critical tests in equids. Am. J. Vet. Res. 41:2069, 1980.
13. Schooley, M. A., Marsland, W. P., and Fogg, T. J.: Monthly distribution of *Gasterophilus* species in horses in the United States—implications on treatment schedules. VM SAC, 66:592, 1971.
14. Sukhapesna, V., Knapp, F. W., Lyons, E. T., and Drudge, J. H.: Effect of temperature on embryonic development and egg hatchability of the horse bot, *Gasterophilus intestinalis* (Diptera: Gasterophiladae). J. Med. Entomol., 12:391, 1975.
15. Todd, A. C., and Brown, R. G., Jr.: Critical tests with toluene for ascarids and bots in horses. Am. J. Vet. Res., 13:198, 1952.
16. Tolliver, S. C., Lyons, E. T., and Drudge, J. H.: Observations on the specific location of *Gasterophilus spp* larvae in the mouth of the horse. J. Parasitol., 60:891, 1974.
17. Wells, R. W., and Knipling, E. F.: A report of some recent studies on species of *Gasterophilus* occurring in horses in the United States. Iowa State Coll. J. Sci., 12:181, 1938.

CESTODE INFECTION

J. H. Drudge, LEXINGTON, KENTUCKY

E. T. Lyons, LEXINGTON, KENTUCKY

OCCURRENCE

Three species of tapeworms occur in the digestive tract of horses in North America[3] and in other parts of the world.[1] Of these three species, *Anoplocephala perfoliata* and *Anoplocephala magna* are more common than *Paranoplocephala mamillana*. *A. perfoliata* locates in the cecum with the tendency to form clusters at the ileocecal valve area, whereas *A. magna* and *P. mamillana* prefer the distal and proximal portions of the small intestine, respectively. *A. perfoliata* occurs more commonly than *A. magna*. Occurrence of these two species tends to be cyclic; *A. magna* appears every few years, and *A. perfoliata* is seen more consistently from year to year. There is a tendency, however, for the incidence of *A. perfoliata* to peak every few years with recessive periods in between.

Tapeworms occur in horses of all ages, but yearlings and two-year-old horses are more commonly infected. Data on the prevalence of tapeworms in North America are sparse. A recent survey of necropsy data[2] derived from eight states in the United States indicated average infection rates of 18 and 26 per cent for foals and horses, respectively. Similarly, fecal examinations for tapeworm eggs revealed 13.6 per cent samples positive for *A. perfoliata* in Ontario.[5]

DEVELOPMENT

The life cycle of these tapeworms involves an intermediate host, orbatid mites, which exist as free-living forms on pastures. The prevalence of tapeworm infections in horses is related to the geographic distribution of the mites. Development of cysticercoids in the mites requires two to four months after the eggs voided in the feces of the horse are ingested by the mites. Horses become infected while grazing by eating the cysticercoid-infested mites. Development of the tapeworms to maturity in the horse requires two to four months.

PATHOGENESIS

Clustering of *A. perfoliata* at the ileocecal orifice results in severe ulcerations of the mucosa. A few of these tapeworms may be present without causing definite clinical signs, but heavier infections are accompanied by digestive disturbances and unthriftiness. Perforation of the cecum has been attributed to *A. perfoliata;* granulomatous tissue builds up, which along with the mass of tapeworms, may occlude the opening.

Catarrhal inflammation of the small intestine has been attributed to small numbers of *A. magna*, while greater numbers may result in a hemorrhagic inflammation.

DIAGNOSIS

Definitive diagnosis of tapeworm infection can be made by finding the typical angular-shaped eggs in a fecal flotation sample. In light infections, the discharge of proglottids is sporadic. Hence, a single examination may fail to disclose an infection, so examinations should be made on several samples.

Discharge of gravid proglottids may be observed. However, they are usually voided singly and resemble a grain of rice in appearance, so a close inspection of the feces is necessary.

TREATMENT AND CONTROL

Anthelmintic treatment of light infections is not a routine practice in many areas. This is due at least in part to the little research aimed at developing taeniacidal agents for the horse. As a consequence, there is no specifically labeled product for removing equine tapeworms in the United States.

Niclosamide* at the dose rate of 100 mg per kg has been advocated as efficacious and safe to use. More recently, pyrantel pamoate at twice the usual therapeutic rate or 13.2 mg base per kg was quite effective (98 per cent) for *A. perfoliata*.[5]

Neither of these compounds is labeled for treatment of horses for tapeworms; however, pyrantel†‡ is labeled for strongyles, ascarids, and pinworms, so the use of pyrantel pamoate at 6.6 mg base per kg for the control of these nematodes also removes some of the tapeworms.[4]

---

*Yomesan, Haver-Lockhart, Shawnee, KS 66201
†Strongid-T, Pfizer, New York, NY 10017
‡Imathal, Beecham Labs, Bristol, TN 37620

References

1. Arundel, J. H.: Parasitic diseases of the horse. Vet. Rev., No. 18, The University of Sydney, The Post-Graduate Foundation in Veterinary Science, Sydney, 83 pp., 1978.
2. Haas, D. K.: Equine parasitism. VM SAC, 74:980, 1979.
3. Lichtenfels, J. R.: Helminths of domestic equids. Proc. Helm. Soc. Wash., 42:1, 1975 (special issue).
4. Lyons, E. T., Drudge, J. H., and Tolliver, S. C.: Critical tests of three salts of pyrantel against internal parasites of the horse. Am. J. Vet. Res., 35:1515, 1974.
5. Slocombe, J. O. D.: Prevalence and treatment of tapeworms in horses. Can. Vet. J., 20:136, 1979.

OXYURIS INFECTION

J. H. Drudge, LEXINGTON, KENTUCKY

E. T. Lyons, LEXINGTON, KENTUCKY

OCCURRENCE

Oxyuris equi is a common parasite of horses throughout the world.[1] Adult pinworms are commonly found in weanling foals and adolescent horses but are relatively rare in mature horses. However, seemingly heavy infections of immature or larval oxyurids, numbering in excess of 10^4, can occur in horses of all ages.[4]

Oxyuriasis is more of a problem in stabled horses because the eggs tend to accumulate on feeders and waterers by the tail-rubbing inclinations of infected animals, which enhances the chances of completing the life cycle. Pasturing tends to reduce the infections because depositories of the eggs are widespread and they are quite susceptible to drying.

DEVELOPMENT

Adult pinworms live in the posterior portion of the gastrointestinal tract, i.e., the dorsal and small colons. Gravid females migrate to the rectum and anus. Because they are quite fragile, they rupture easily, and their eggs and other contents are deposited on the host's perineum. Some adult worms are voided intact in the feces.

Pinworm eggs are sticky, and they adhere to stable walls and fixtures, fences, bedding, and other objects in the horse's environment. Their development is rapid, requiring only three to five days to contain infective larvae. The infective eggs in contaminated bedding, water, or on walls and fences are then ingested. The larvae develop in the colon to the fourth stage in 3 to 10 days without invading the mucosa. The adult stage is reached in about 50 days, but the worms do not reach sexual maturity until five months following infection.[3]

PATHOGENESIS

The principal effect of pinworm infection is anal irritation caused by the deposits of ruptured females. The pruritus may be intense, causing the horse to rub its rear quarters on any available object. This results in loss of hair from the tail, giving it the characteristic "rat-tailed" appearance. Otherwise, oxyuris infection does not cause any specific clinical signs.

Heavy burdens of the larval oxyurids may cause erosions of the mucosa of the large colon because of the feeding habits of the larvae.[3, 5] However, this irritation of the colon may not be noticed clinically or by gross inspection at necropsy because surprisingly large numbers of fourth-stage larvae are found in horses that do not exhibit these untoward effects.

DIAGNOSIS

Oxyurid eggs are not ordinarily seen in routine fecal flotations, even in animals known to be infected. Use of transparent tape to collect eggs in the perineal region helps to detect their presence. The female worms are passed spontaneously and are frequently seen in fresh feces. Their gray-white color and sharp-pointed tails are distinguishing features. Tail rubbing and loss of hair from the tail provide presumptive evidence of pinworm infection.

TREATMENT AND CONTROL

Pinworms do not ordinarily require specific anthelmintic treatment because nearly all of the compounds that are efficacious for strongyles and ascarids are also active against pinworms[1, 2] (see

Strongylosis, p. 267, and Ascariasis, p. 262). A number of compounds are effective at the same dose rates against *O. equi,* including the various piperazine salts, all of the benzimidazoles, the organophosphates, pyrantel, febantel, and the avermectins.

The primary use of these drugs in strongyle or ascarid control programs automatically provides the supplementary benefit of efficacious control of pinworms.

References

1. Arundel, J. H.: Parasitic diseases of the horse. Vet. Rev., No. 18, The University of Sydney, The Post-Graduate Foundation in Veterinary Science, Sydney, 83 pp., 1978.
2. Drudge, J. H., and Lyons, E. T.: Control of equine parasites. Lecture, The Stud Manager's Course, Lexington, KY, 1976, pp. 139–148.
3. Enigk, K.: Zur Biologie und Bekampfung von *Oxyuris equi.* Z. Tropenmed. Parasitol., *1:*259, 1949.
4. Haas, D. K.: Equine parasitism. VM SAC, 74:980, 1979.
5. Lichtenfels, J. R.: Helminths of domestic equids. Proc. Helm. Soc. Wash., *42:*1, 1975 (special issue).

Section 6

DISEASES OF THE HEMATOPOIETIC AND LYMPHATIC SYSTEMS

Edited by Gary P. Carlson

EVALUATION OF THE HEMATOPOIETIC SYSTEM 293

BLOOD LOSS ANEMIA 297

HEMOLYTIC ANEMIA 299

ANEMIA AS A RESULT OF INSUFFICIENT ERYTHROPOIESIS 303

LYMPHOPROLIFERATIVE AND MYELOPROLIFERATIVE DISEASES 305

HEMOSTASIS 306

DISSEMINATED INTRAVASCULAR COAGULATION 309

FLUID THERAPY 311

MEDICAL MANAGEMENT OF THE EXHAUSTED HORSE 318

IMMUNOLOGIC DISEASES 321

BLOOD TRANSFUSION 325

EVALUATION OF THE HEMATOPOIETIC SYSTEM

Joseph G. Zinkl, DAVIS, CALIFORNIA

Gary P. Carlson, DAVIS, CALIFORNIA

The hematopoietic system consists of the circulating blood cells, precursors in the bone marrow and lymphatic tissue, and the plasma constituents such as protein and fibrinogen. The hematopoietic system may be affected by diseases directly involving its components, or it can manifest responses to diseases and conditions of other organ systems. Evaluation of the hematopoietic system begins with the performance of a complete blood count (CBC). For proper utilization of results for diagnostic, prognostic, and therapeutic purposes, it is important to understand normal values and the factors that may affect them.

NORMAL VALUES

Hematologic parameters vary according to age, sex, breed, and conditioning of the animal. Geographic location may cause some variation in data. Animals at high elevations usually have a higher red blood cell (RBC) count, hemoglobin (Hb) concentration, and packed cell volume (PCV). It is unfortunate that data matched for all possible sources of variation are not always available. Some of the variables are known, however, and these should be kept in mind when evaluation of the hematopoietic system is undertaken.

Hematologically, horses are divided into two broad categories, "hot-blooded" and "cold-blooded." The term "hot-blooded" generally refers to light breeds, while "cold-blooded" refers to draft types of horses and pony breeds. Hematologic values for adult light breed horses are given in Table 1. The most significant differences between these values and those of heavy breed animals (Table 2) are the lower erythrocyte parameters (PCV, Hb, RBC count). Heavy breed animals also have slightly lower leukocyte counts (Table 2). Differential leukocyte counts do not differ enough between these groups to cause a problem in interpretation. Significant hematologic variations occur in the postnatal period. Packed cell volume, Hb, and RBC count are high at birth but fall rapidly during the first two weeks of life (Table 3). Thereafter they begin to slowly increase toward adult values. Young horses have a low mean corpuscular volume (MCV). The erythrocytes are particularly small in one- to three-month-old foals. This occurs in all horses and should not be regarded as a sign of iron deficiency.

Most young animals have low plasma protein concentrations because they have low levels of immunoglobulins. Very low plasma proteins in the newborn foal suggest a failure of transfer of colostral antibody. Estimation or quantification of serum immunoglobulin levels is indicated. The serum of newborn foals is often dark yellow, and the icteric index is elevated in these foals, probably because of incomplete development of the bilirubin metabolism mechanisms. The icteric index drops rapidly to adult values within a few days after birth.

Leukocyte parameters are also influenced by age (Table 4). Total leukocyte count is slightly elevated in young horses. Leukocyte counts continue to rise in growing foals and reach their highest values at about 18 months. This increase is primarily due to an increasing lymphocyte count. Other leukocyte numbers in foals are not markedly different from those in adults. A left shift of slightly greater magnitude than that of adult horses may be found in the

TABLE 1. NORMAL HEMATOLOGIC VALUES FOR ADULT, LIGHT BREED HORSES

	Range	Mean
Erythrocytes ($\times 10^6/\mu$l)	6.8–12.9	9.0
Hemoglobin (gm/dl)	11.0–19.0	14.4
Hematocrit (%)	32.0–53.0	41.0
Mean corpuscular volume (MCV) (fl)	37.0–58.5	45.5
Mean corpuscular hemoglobin concentration (MCHC) (mg/dl)	31.0–38.6	35.2
Mean corpuscular hemoglobin (MCH) (pg)	12.3–19.7	15.9
Plasma protein (gm/dl)	5.8–8.7	6.9
Plasma fibrinogen (mg/dl)	100–400	—
Platelets ($\times 10^3/\mu$l)	100–350	—
Icteric index (units)	7.5–20	—
Leukocytes (/μl)	5400–14,300	9050

	%		Absolute Numbers (/μl)	
	Range	Mean	Range	Mean
Neutrophils				
Band	0.0–8.0	0.5	0–100	20
Mature	22.0–72.0	52.5	2260–8580	4745
Lymphocytes	17.0–68.0	38.5	1500–7700	3500
Monocytes	0.0–14.0	4.5	0–1000	400
Eosinophils	0.0–10.0	3.5	0–1000	300
Basophils	0.0–4.0	0.5	0–290	50

(Data from Schalm, O. W., Jain, N. C., and Carroll, E. J.: Veterinary Hematology, 3rd ed. Philadelphia, Lea and Febiger, 1975.)

TABLE 2. DIFFERENCE BETWEEN LIGHT AND HEAVY BREEDS IN HEMATOLOGIC VALUES

	Light Breeds		Heavy Breeds	
	Range	*Mean*	*Range*	*Mean*
RBC ($\times 10^6/\mu l$)	6.8–12.9	9.0	5.5–9.5	7.5
Hb (gm/dl)	11.0–19.0	14.4	8.0–14.0	11.5
PCV (%)	32.0–53.0	41.0	24.0–44.0	35.0
WBC (/μl)	5400–14,300	9050	6000–12,000	8500

(Data from Schalm, O. W., Jain, N. C., and Carroll, E. J.: Veterinary Hematology, 3rd ed. Philadelphia, Lea and Febiger, 1975.)

first two weeks of life. The aged horse appears to have a lower lymphocyte count than young adult horses.

The major effect of stress or corticosteroid administration in horses is to increase mature neutrophils in the blood, presumably by mobilization of the storage pool of mature neutrophils from the bone marrow into the circulation. Leukocyte counts may increase to 20,000 per μl or slightly higher for 12 to

24 hours following the initial dose of a potent glucocorticoid such as dexamethasone. Long-term steroid therapy with less active preparations such as prednisolone has few effects on the total or differential leukocyte count.

Hematologic parameters are influenced by excitement to a greater degree in horses than in any other domestic animal because of the large splenic reserve of cells. Strenuous exercise also produces similar changes. The greatest change is in the PCV, Hb, and RBC counts, which increase markedly. There is also a modest increase in WBC count due to increase in lymphocytes as well as neutrophils. Conditioning and type of training also influence erythrocyte parameters. Thoroughbreds in race training usually have PCV, Hb, and RBC counts at the upper range of normal, while Standardbreds in training maintain marginally lower erythrocyte parameters. A large erythrocyte mass is believed to facilitate the transfer of oxygen during vigorous exercise, which may minimize the anaerobic conditions that occur when racing at maximal effort over relatively short distances. In contrast, horses trained for endurance events usually have relatively low erythrocyte pa-

TABLE 3. ERYTHROCYTE PARAMETERS, ICTERIC INDEX, PLASMA PROTEINS, AND FIBRINOGEN IN YOUNG HORSES

Age	RBC ($\times 10^6/\mu l$)	Hb (gm/dl)	PCV (%)	MCV (fl)	Icteric Index (units)	Plasma Protein (gm/dl)	Fibrinogen (mg/dl)
1 day	10.5 ± 1.4	14.2 ± 1.3	41.7 ± 3.6	40.1 ± 3.8	40 ± 30	6.2 ± 0.9	260 ± 60
2–7 days	9.5 ± 0.8	12.7 ± 0.9	37.1 ± 2.8	39.2 ± 2.8	29 ± 21	6.4 ± 0.5	330 ± 130
8–14 days	9.0 ± 0.8	11.8 ± 1.2	34.9 ± 3.7	39.1 ± 2.2	19 ± 6	6.1 ± 0.6	300 ± 50
21–30 days	11.2 ± 1.3	13.1 ± 1.1	37.8 ± 3.3	34.0 ± 2.4	12 ± 6	6.2 ± 0.4	400 ± 50
1–3 months	11.9 ± 1.3	13.4 ± 1.6	38.3 ± 4.1	32.4 ± 1.9	15 ± 5	6.4 ± 0.4	460 ± 70
8–18 months	8.6 ± 0.6	11.8 ± 1.6	34.5 ± 3.8	40.1 ± 2.9	—	7.3 ± 0.9	280 ± 40

(Data from Schalm, O. W., Jain, N. C., and Carroll, E. J.: Veterinary Hematology, 3rd ed. Philadelphia, Lea and Febiger, 1975.)

TABLE 4. TOTAL LEUKOCYTE, NEUTROPHIL, AND LYMPHOCYTE COUNT IN YOUNG HORSES

		Neutrophils				Lymphocytes	
		Band		*Mature*			
Age	Total WBC (/μl)	%	*Number (/μl)*	%	*Number (/μl)*	%	*Number (/μl)*
1 day	9602 ± 3372	7.5 ± 1.8	138 ± 198	69.8 ± 10.7	6824 ± 2757	25.1 ± 10.3	2192 ± 891
2–7 days	9300 ± 2346	0.3 ± 0.4	29 ± 37	68.2 ± 9.4	6448 ± 2128	27.0 ± 9.8	2420 ± 739
8–14 days	9483 ± 2196	0.5 ± 1.1	48 ± 125	66.2 ± 9.0	6338 ± 1849	28.5 ± 9.4	2653 ± 933
21–30 days	9688 ± 1940	0.2 ± 0.3	19 ± 33	56.8 ± 7.4	5501 ± 1346	39.6 ± 6.5	3823 ± 863
1–3 months	10893 ± 2977	0.1 ± 0.3	10 ± 28	46.9 ± 12.1	5315 ± 2437	48.5 ± 11.5	5086 ± 1419
8–18 months	10812 ± 1874	0.1 ± 0.2	16 ± 28	43.8 ± 7.0	4658 ± 745	47.9 ± 6.0	5210 ± 1250
2 years	9678 ± 1883	0.4 ± 1.1	39 ± 81	50.1 ± 10.1	4805 ± 1196	41.4 ± 10.5	4059 ± 1456

(Data from Schalm, O. W., Jain, N. C., and Carroll, E. J.: Veterinary Hematology, 3rd ed. Philadelphia, Lea and Febiger, 1975.)

rameters. This effect is believed to be a response to long-term aerobic exercise and may be related to an expanded plasma volume. Total oxygen-carrying capacity is probably not significantly different from that of pleasure horses. The expanded plasma volume may represent an adaptive mechanism to dehydration, which frequently occurs from sweating during these rides. Endurance horses are rarely exercised at levels likely to result in anaerobic metabolism.

HEMATOLOGIC RESPONSE TO DISEASE

ANEMIA

Anemia is defined as a decrease in the oxygen-carrying capacity of the blood below accepted normal values. Clinical signs of anemia are largely referable to a deficit in this vital erythrocyte function and the physiologic responses to this deficit. These signs include exercise intolerance, elevated heart and respiratory rates, pale mucous membranes, low-grade systolic murmurs, lassitude, and depression. Exercise intolerance is an early presenting sign in performance horses. In quiet sedentary horses, anemia may be more advanced before a problem is recognized and veterinary assistance is sought. Clinical signs become progressively more obvious as the PCV decreases, and a PCV of 10 per cent or below should be considered a critical anemia. Additional clinical signs that may provide an indication of the type of anemia are icterus and rarely hemoglobinuria associated with hemolytic disorders and petechial or ecchymotic hemorrhages and melena seen with certain bleeding disorders. Before any therapeutic intervention, efforts should be made to classify the anemia as to type and if possible to determine the cause. Additionally, the severity of the anemia and indications of progression or response are critically important. The administration of iron-containing hematinics is of little benefit in a hemolytic anemia or anemia secondary to chronic disease. Blood transfusions may be life-saving after acute blood loss and impending hypovolemic shock but may be of limited lasting value in mild depression anemia. Clinical recognition of anemia and the initial confirmation by low erythrocyte parameters may not always provide sufficient information to make intelligent therapeutic decisions. The primary objectives of hematologic evaluation are (1) confirmation of the presence of anemia and its severity, (2) determination of whether an effective erythropoietic response is being mounted, and (3) determination of the type and, when possible, the cause of the anemia.

There are three basic types of anemia. These are blood loss anemia, increased erythrocyte destruction, or hemolytic anemia, and decreased erythrocyte production, or depression anemia. Using sound clinical judgment and hematologic tools available to most practicing veterinarians, it is possible to differentiate these types of anemia and at times to determine the cause.

In the light breeds of horses, anemia is considered to be present when the PCV is below 30 per cent, the hemoglobin concentration below 10 gm per dl, and the erythrocyte count less than 6.5×10^6 per μl. For the cold-blooded or heavy breeds, values 25 per cent lower than these would be indicative of anemia (for example, hemoglobin less than 7.5 gm per dl). Except for massive acute blood loss where hypovolemia may produce irreversible shock prior to the full hematologic manifestations of anemia, a PCV between 20 and 30 per cent should be considered a moderate anemia. At this stage, serial hemograms are indicated to determine if the anemia is progressive.

Blood loss or hemolytic anemia normally produces an active proliferative response in the bone marrow. Anemia due to these causes is thus referred to as responsive anemia. In all species except the horse, this erythropoietic response is manifested by the appearance of significant numbers of young large erythrocytes in the peripheral blood. However, polychromasia, hypochromasia (decreased mean corpuscular hemoglobin concentration—MCHC), macrocytosis (increased MCV), reticulocytosis, and nucleated erythrocytes are rarely seen in horses responding to even severe anemias. Bone marrow evaluation provides the most reliable index of response to anemia. An active proliferative response is indicated by increased numbers of polychromatic erythrocytes and reticulocyte percentage (i.e., 5 per cent or greater). With an active erythropoietic response, the myeloid to erythroid (M:E) ratio is generally less than 1 and frequently less than 0.5. With marrow depression anemia, there is generally an inadequate erythropoietic response for the degree of anemia.

Blood loss anemias are responsive anemias, often associated with hypoproteinemia, and frequently there is clinical evidence or a history of blood loss. Hemolytic anemias are also responsive anemias, frequently but not invariably associated with clinical icterus. It is possible to establish an etiologic diagnosis of some hemolytic anemias on the basis of morphologic characteristics or special hematologic procedures. Depression anemias are nonresponsive anemias, frequently are mild and slowly progressive, and are often secondary to some systemic disease process. Therapeutic approaches for each type of anemia will be discussed in the following articles in this section.

INFECTIOUS OR INFLAMMATORY DISEASE

The hematologic responses to infectious or inflammatory diseases serve as both diagnostic and prognostic indicators and aid in the evaluation of the response to therapy. The normal range of variation and the influences of age, excitement, and stress have been discussed. More detailed explanations of these factors and the alteration in leukocyte kinetics in response to disease have been published elsewhere.[1, 5]

Most infectious or inflammatory diseases cause an increase in the leukocyte count (leukocytosis) and plasma fibrinogen concentration. When the demand for neutrophils exceeds the marrow's capacity to supply cells from its reserve of mature cells, there is a release of immature cells into the circulation. The appearance of these young or immature cells (band neutrophils, some metamyelocytes, and rarely myelocytes) in the blood is termed a left shift. A left shift is commonly seen in the initial or active response phase to an infection. If the leukocyte count remains elevated and the mature neutrophils exceed the total immature neutrophils, the response is termed a regenerative left shift. This indicates a marked and active response to the infection and depending upon the nature of the primary medical problem, is a reasonably good prognostic indicator. A degenerative left shift applies to the situation in which there are more immature neutrophils than mature neutrophils in the peripheral blood. This occurs when the demand for neutrophils exceeds the ability of the marrow to produce them. At these times, some of the neutrophils may manifest toxic morphologic changes as described in Table 5. A "toxic degenerative left shift" is an unfavorable prognostic indicator and may be seen with acute toxic enteritis, salmonellosis, acute peritonitis or pleuritis, and septicemia. Prompt, vigorous therapy with appropriate antibiotics or other forms of therapy may be indicated.

Chronic infections and inflammatory or granulomatous processes such as foreign body reactions following penetrating wounds, internal abscesses, or pleuritis are characterized by a persistent but at times modest neutrophilia with little left shift. Monocytosis may be noted at this time. The plasma fibrinogen concentration is often markedly elevated and may be greater than 1000 mg per dl in some cases. As these chronic inflammatory processes invoke an immune response, there may be a marked increase in serum immunoglobulins over a period of weeks or months. The total serum protein concentration may increase to 9 to 12 gm per dl with virtually all of the increase due to increases in the globulin fraction. At times the site of the chronic inflammatory lesion is clinically obvious. With some frequency, however, these horses present with

TABLE 5. CHARACTERISTICS OF TOXIC NEUTROPHILS

Characteristic	Morphology and Cause
Basophilia	Persistence of the bluish cytoplasm usually found in immature neutrophilic cells such as metamyelocytes and myelocytes
Toxic granulation	Primary granules retain some of their ability to stain azurophilic or reddish in mature cells. Blue-black granules may also occur.
Foamy or vacuolated cytoplasm	Toxic products cause lysosomal release and development of vacuoles.
Döhle bodies	Small (up to 1 μm) areas of basophilia representing aggregates of endoplasmic reticulum
Giant neutrophils, bands, and metamyelocytes	Very large cells, perhaps polyploidal, that may represent skipped cell division

chronic weight loss, intermittent low-grade fever, and little else. The hematologic picture just described should alert the clinician that a serious medical problem is present, and a vigorous diagnostic effort is indicated to determine the nature and location of the lesion.

The hematologic response can be a helpful guide to the effectiveness of therapy for infectious or inflammatory diseases. The drainage of an abscess or the institution of appropriate antibiotic therapy for bacterial infections is often associated with a prompt and progressive return toward normal for the total and differential leukocyte counts and the fibrinogen concentration. These hematologic changes, when associated with clinical evidence of recovery, are indications for continuation of the present course of treatment until the problem is resolved. In certain toxemic or septic conditions, the hematologic findings provide evidence as to whether host defenses appear adequate or are about to be overwhelmed. These findings should always be considered in relation to other clinical findings but can be helpful for evaluation of the response to supportive therapy and in providing a prognosis.

BONE MARROW BIOPSY

Collection of bone marrow for the assessment of response to anemia is a relatively simple procedure that can be done in field situations. Aspiration sites include the ribs, the iliac crest, and the sternum. The site is shaved and surgically prepared, and a small amount of local anesthetic is infused under the skin and down to the periosteum overlying the bone. Using aseptic techniques, a small skin incision is made, and the bone marrow needle,* consisting of a stylet and tight-fitting cannula, is introduced. These needles are 16 to 18 gauge and should be between 1½ and 3 inches in length. The marrow cavity is penetrated by drilling the needle into the bone using pressure and rotation. Examination of the beveled edge of the stylet for the presence of blood-tinged marrow at intervals will ensure proper placement. Aspiration of marrow with a 20 ml syringe may require some pressure to initiate flow, but great care should be taken to avoid excessive blood contamination. Aspiration should be terminated once 0.5 to 1 ml of marrow has been obtained. This small marrow sample is quickly transferred to a 2 ml EDTA tube. To avoid shrinkage of the cells, it is advisable to remove some EDTA from these evacuated tubes prior to the transfer. When the tube is rotated, small spicules of bone and fat globules in this bloodlike material may be visible and indicate marrow. Either the sample or smears made from the sample are submitted for staining and cytologic evaluation. The normal M:E ratio in the horse varies from 0.5:1 to 1.5:1. An active marrow response is indicated when the M:E ratio is 0.5:1 or less and when the marrow reticulocyte percentage is greater than 5 per cent.

*Wasterman-Jensen Biopsy Needle, Becton-Dickinson, Rutherford, NJ

References

1. Archer, R. K., and Jeffcott, L. B.: Comparative Clinical Hematology. London, Blackwell Scientific Pub., 1977.
2. Osbaldiston, G. W., Coffman, J. R., and Kruckenberg, S. M.: Biochemical differentiation of equine anemias. J. Am. Vet. Med. Assoc., 157:322, 1970.
3. Rumbaugh, G. E., Ardas, A. A., Ginno, D., and Tromershausen-Smith, A.: Identification and treatment of colostrum-deficient foals. J. Am. Vet. Med. Assoc., 174:273, 1979.
4. Schalm, O. W.: Bone marrow erythroid cytology in anemias of the horse. First International Symposium on Equine Hematology, Michigan State University, 1975, p. 17.
5. Schalm, O. W., and Carlson, G. P.: Diseases of the blood and blood forming organs. In Mansmann, R., and McAllister, S. (eds.): Equine Medicine and Surgery. Santa Barbara, American Veterinary Pub., 1982, in press.
6. Schalm, O. W., Jain, N. C., and Carroll, E. J.: Veterinary Hematology, 3rd ed. Philadelphia, Lea and Febiger, 1975.

BLOOD LOSS ANEMIA

Gary P. Carlson, DAVIS, CALIFORNIA
Joseph G. Zinkl, DAVIS, CALIFORNIA

Major blood loss is often obvious, as with wire cuts, lacerations, or surgical complications. However, bleeding may be less obvious with internal bleeding into body cavities, the gastrointestinal tract, or from muscle masses following trauma. Both internal and external parasitism may lead to blood loss, but clinically significant anemia is generally not seen unless there is massive infestation by blood-sucking parasites. Post-race pulmonary hemorrhage seen in performance horses is generally not severe enough to produce anemia. Vascular disorders, platelet abnormalities, or coagulopathies may result in petechiation or ecchymosis and in some cases frank bleeding and are discussed in a subsequent section.

For clinical therapeutic reasons, it is convenient to consider three blood loss situations: acute massive hemorrhage of less than one day's duration, acute blood loss that may occur over several days to a week, and chronic blood loss that may occur over several weeks or months.

HEMORRHAGE

The blood volume of horses ranges from 6 to 10 per cent of body weight. An average blood volume of 8 per cent in a 1000 lb (454 kg) horse would be just over 36 l. Rapid loss of 25 to 30 per cent of the blood volume (9 to 11 l) can generally be tolerated, although syncope may be seen in some instances. Acute losses of substantially larger volumes of blood are likely to produce hypovolemic shock, which may become irreversible if not promptly treated. Acute massive blood loss thus represents an emergency situation.

Blood loss results in decreases of all components of the blood (plasma, erythrocytes, and leukocytes). During the initial posthemorrhage period (i.e., up to four to six hours), there may be little hematologic evidence of anemia. However, clinical signs of hypovolemia develop rapidly. These signs include elevated heart and respiratory rates, weak thready pulse, poor jugular distensibility, and blanched pale mucous membranes. In time, various homeostatic responses will result in increased plasma volume in order to partially restore effective circulating blood volume. This response may take 12 to 24 hours. Until this time, the packed cell volume (PCV), erythrocyte count, and hemoglobin concentration will not accurately reflect the degree of blood loss or anemia. With acute and massive blood loss, therapeutic decisions must largely be based on evidence of hemorrhage and clinical signs of hypovolemia.

THERAPY

Whenever possible, the initial therapeutic step should be to stop or decrease the rate of blood loss. This may be done in some circumstances by pressure bandages, intermittent tourniquets, or ligation. Phenothiazine derivative tranquilizers or other peripheral vasodilator compounds should be avoided, as they may aggravate the hypotensive state and lead to collapse. Horses with signs of impending hypovolemic shock require rapid restoration of effective circulating blood volume. Fresh whole blood is the obvious therapeutic choice in this situation. However, the availability of suitably typed blood donors, collection apparatus, and assistance often precludes blood transfusion (see Blood Transfusion, p. 325). Another approach in an emergency situation is the rapid administration of saline or one of the sodium-containing polyionic replacement fluids (lactated Ringer's solution, Hartman's solution, or Normosol). These fluids will transiently expand the plasma volume and thus the effective circulating blood volume. With either blood transfusions or sodium-containing fluids, the volume administered should vary in relation to the volume and rate of blood loss and whether the blood loss has been stopped or is continuing. Thus, blood or fluids are given to effect. The volume of blood required may vary from 6 to 10 l or more. Sodium-containing fluids should be administered in volumes between two and three times greater since only a third of the administered fluid will be retained within the plasma volume. The remainder of such fluids is distributed to the rest of the extracellular fluid volume.

ACUTE BLOOD LOSS

The hematologic manifestations of acute blood loss after the first 24 hours are anemia (decreased PCV, erythrocyte count, and hemoglobin concentration) and decreased plasma protein concentration. Evidence of erythropoietic response in the peripheral blood is rarely evident in horses. The therapeutic approach should be directed at halting additional blood loss or removing the offending cause. As an example, with warfarin poisoning, removal from access to the poison, provision of Vitamin K_1, and perhaps a fresh plasma or whole blood transfusion may correct the coagulopathy and stop the blood loss. If this is accomplished, the normal bone marrow should begin the process of replacing the erythrocyte deficit by its proliferative response in four to seven days. The provision of iron-containing hematinics, preferably as oral preparations, is extremely helpful in this regenerative process.

Sequential measurements of PCV or, preferably, a complete blood count (CBC) will allow determination of whether the blood loss has been controlled or the anemia is progressive. Abdominal paracentesis, rectal palpation, and examination of the feces for occult blood provide useful information when there has been internal blood loss, as with postparturient mares with ruptured uterine arteries or iatrogenic puncture of the spleen during abdominocentesis. Alteration in the hemostatic mechanism, vascular integrity, platelets, and coagulation factors may result in internal as well as external hemorrhage and should be considered as a causative or contributing factor.

Although the clinician should be concerned when the PCV decreases to 20 per cent or perhaps as low as 15 per cent, there is often no immediate need for transfusion. Careful and close hematologic monitoring is indicated. Transfusion is considered when the PCV reaches 10 per cent or below. However, the rate at which the anemia appears to be progressing and the clinical status of the horse are more important determining factors than some fixed value for PCV when transfusion is being considered. Undue excitement should be avoided in horses with critical anemia, and the benefits of diagnostic or therapeutic procedures must be weighed against potential risks.

CHRONIC BLOOD LOSS

Chronic blood loss can exist as a slow, insidious process, and anemia may be well advanced before a problem is recognized. This type of blood loss is often associated with erosive lesions in the bowel. With continual blood loss, there is a gradual depletion of the body's iron reserves. When sufficient iron depletion has occurred, the blood loss anemia is complicated by iron-deficient erythropoiesis. Iron deficiency is not a common problem in horses, and evaluation of this problem is reasonably straightforward. The classically described hematologic features of iron deficiency (hypochromic, microcytic anemia) represent severe depletion and are not common in the horse. Determination of serum iron and iron-binding capacity can be performed by most commercial laboratories. Serum iron normally ranges from 70 to 140 μg per dl, and the total iron-binding capacity ranges from 240 to 400 μg per dl. Iron deficiency may be reflected by a decrease in serum iron concentration and an increase in total iron-binding capacity. An earlier and perhaps more reliable indication of iron depletion can be obtained by subjective evaluation of marrow iron using the Prussian blue stain.

THERAPY

The treatment of iron deficiency secondary to chronic blood loss is the provision of supplemental iron. A wide variety of iron-containing hematinics are available for oral administration. If iron is to be given parenterally, iron cacodylate should be employed. Iron dextran preparations used for the treatment of anemia in baby pigs should not be injected into horses, as there is a significant risk of adverse, even fatal, reactions. Aside from the treatment of chronic blood loss, efforts should be made to determine the primary cause. Treatment of anemia may be unrewarding if the primary process is neoplasia or another progressive disease with an unfavorable prognosis.

References

1. Carlson, G. P.: Evaluation of responsive anemias in horses. First International Symposium on Equine Hematology, Michigan State University, 1975, p. 327.
2. Dixon, J. B., and Archer, R. K.: Interpretation of equine anaemias. Vet. Ann., *15*:185, 1975.
3. Lumsden, J. H., Valli, V. E., McSherry, B. T., et al.: The kinetics of hematopoiesis in the light horse. II. The hematological response to hemorrhagic anemia. Can. J. Comp. Med., 39:324, 1975.

HEMOLYTIC ANEMIA

Gary P. Carlson, DAVIS, CALIFORNIA
Joseph A. Zinkl, DAVIS, CALIFORNIA

Hemolytic anemia is generally the result of an increased rate of erythrocyte destruction and thus a shortened red cell life span. In some instances, intravascular hemolysis may occur, resulting in hemoglobinemia and hemoglobinuria. In addition to clinical signs of anemia, icterus is a frequent but not invariable feature of hemolytic anemia. Clinical icterus is due to an increase in the prehepatic, unconjugated, or indirect-reacting bilirubin resulting from accelerated erythrocyte destruction. Although all visible mucous membranes reflect icterus, the sclera tends to provide the most reliable clinical guide. The degree of clinical icterus accompanying hemolytic anemia depends upon the rate of erythrocyte destruction and the liver's ability to take up, conjugate, and excrete bilirubin. Liver disease and other systemic diseases resulting in anorexia also produce icterus in the horse. Clinicopathologic evaluation is generally necessary to clearly differentiate hemolytic anemia from other causes of icterus (p. 16).

Hemolytic anemias are characterized as responsive anemias in other species, since there is usually an active proliferative response by the erythroid marrow. In the horse, hematologic evidence of this response is usually lacking. The erythrocyte indices (mean corpuscular volume [MCV], mean corpuscular hemoglobin [MCH], and mean corpuscular hemoglobin concentration [MCHC]) generally remain normal, and reticulocytes and nucleated erythrocytes are rarely seen in peripheral blood smears. Bone marrow evaluation can be most helpful in assessing the response to hemolytic anemias. In icteric horses, the plasma is dark yellow and there is an increase in the icterus index. Plasma protein concentration is variable but generally remains within the normal limits, and serum haptoglobin concentration decreases. With hemolytic anemia, red cells are not lost from the body, and most of the components of these destroyed erythrocytes are salvaged by the reticuloendothelial system. Body iron stores generally remain normal, and there is little response to iron-containing hematinics.

A number of specific disease entities may produce a clinically significant hemolytic anemia. These include infectious causes such as equine infectious anemia, equine piroplasmosis, and equine ehrlichiosis, toxic or metabolic causes due to exposure to oxidizing agents such as phenothiazine, wild onions, red maple leaves, and liver failure, and immune-mediated hemolytic anemias such as neonatal isoerythrolysis and autoimmune hemolytic anemia. More detailed accounts of these diseases are presented elsewhere, and this discussion will be confined to the salient diagnostic and therapeutic features of these causes of hemolytic anemia.

EQUINE INFECTIOUS ANEMIA

Equine infectious anemia (EIA) (p. 7) is a complex, immunologically mediated viral disease. The anemia is, in part, due to immunologic damage to erythrocyte membranes. EIA may manifest itself in acute, subacute, chronic intermittent, or inapparent forms. The hematologic features seem to depend upon the form of the disease. The anemia is largely due to IgG, IgM, or complement binding to the erythrocyte membranes and subsequent removal from the circulation. Heinz bodies have been reported during hemolytic episodes. In addition to hemolytic anemia, the bone marrow response may be ineffective. During the active febrile stages of the disease, there is usually a marked increase in the rate of erythrocyte destruction. The features at this time include anemia, increased icteric index, thrombocytopenia, and leukopenia, primarily due to a low neutrophil count. Autoagglutination of erythrocytes may be noted. During remission, between active episodes of the disease or during the chronic inapparent form, few hematologic abnormalities except borderline anemia may be found. The Coggins agar gel immunodiffusion (AGID) test for the presence of antiviral serum immunoglobulins is the most useful and specific diagnostic procedure. Few false positive reactions occur; false negative reactions may be found early in acute fulminating forms. Foals of AGID-positive mares may give positive tests during the first four to six months of life because of passive transfer of antibody in colostrum. AGID-positive horses represent a hazard to horses in close association with them. State and federal regulations place some restrictions on the shipment of AGID-positive horses of which owners and veterinarians must be aware. There is at present no effective treatment for EIA. However, some therapeutic regimens may exacerbate the disease. Immunosuppressive therapy such as with corticosteroids has been associated with activation of the disease. Mechanical transmission by needles, syringes, and surgical equipment from carrier to normal horses can occur, and normal precautions should be taken. The isolation of AGID-positive horses from normal horses is an effective method for prevention of spread of the disease, since no biologic vectors or nonequine reservoirs have been detected. Biting insects are the principal means of natural transmission.

EQUINE PIROPLASMOSIS

A tick-borne protozoal disease of horses caused by *Babesia caballi* or *Babesia equi* has been reported from Florida and many tropical areas of the world where there are suitable tick vectors. Clinical signs of varying severity include fever, depression, weakness, icterus, petechial hemorrhages, edema, and transient hemoglobinuria (with *B. equi* infections). Clinical signs are more severe in horses first exposed as adults, and a persistent carrier state confers resistance to clinical babesiosis. Hematologic features during the acute phase include anemia, thrombocytopenia, leukopenia, and intracellular organisms within erythrocytes. *B. caballi* presents as paired pyriform bodies in 3 to 7 per cent of the erythrocytes, whereas *B. equi* is smaller and appears as groups of four inclusions in the form of a Maltese cross in 60 to 85 per cent of the erythrocytes. The number of parasitized red cells depends upon the stage of the disease and is demonstrated on blood films stained with Giemsa or fluorescent antibody. A variety of serologic tests have been employed for the identificaiton of carrier horses. Treatment consists of isolation, tick control, and chemotherapy. Amicarbalide diisethionate (8 mg per kg intramuscularly) and imidocarb dihydrochloride (2 mg per kg intramuscularly or intravenously) as a single dose are reported to alleviate symptoms and reduce parasitemia when given early in the clinical course. Chemosterilization for the elimination of *B. caballi* in carrier horses is possible where elimination of the disease is desired.

EQUINE EHRLICHIOSIS

Ehrlichiosis (p. 13) is an infectious noncontagious disease of horses caused by a rickettsia-like agent. The disease at present has a limited geographic distribution in the foothill areas of California and is believed to be transmitted by ticks. The disease is characterized by an acute onset of high fever, severe depression, and developing icterus. Edema of the distal extremities and petechial and ecchymotic hemorrhages may be seen. Hematologic features in acute infecitons include leukopenia, thrombocytopenia, mild to moderate anemia, and the presence of cytoplasmic inclusion bodies or morulae in the neutrophils and eosinophils. Preparation of buffy coat smears provides an opportunity to examine a large number of polymorphonuclear cells and enhances the prospect for positive diagnosis. Although most horses recover spontaneously in 7 to 10 days, daily intravenous administration of tetracycline administered at a rate of 5 mg per kg alleviates clinical signs and hastens this process. Although horses are extremely ill in the acute phases of this disease, response to therapy is generally prompt and complete.

HEINZ BODY ANEMIA

Ingestion or administration of certain oxidizing agents such as wild onions, phenothiazine as vermifuge, or phenothiazine-impregnated salt blocks may result in an acute and severe hemolytic anemia. These agents result in oxidation of hemoglobin and the formation of intracorpuscular globin aggregates. These structures are seen on routinely stained blood smears as small round refractile inclusions projecting from or breaking away from the surface of the erythrocytes. These structures are most easily detected with the new methylene blue stain with which they stain blue. As these damaged erythrocytes are removed from the circulation, an acute and severe anemia may develop with hemoglobinuria in some cases. The development of Heinz bodies in response to phenothiazine is thought to be dose-dependent, but some horses may be particularly susceptible, since they develop Heinz bodies when given the recommended dose of 20 to 30 gm per 450 kg body weight. Renal disease may increase susceptibility, and debilitated horses or horses receiving inadequate diets appear to be more sensitive. Treatment is largely supportive and includes blood transfusion if the anemia is severe. Fluids should be administered to ensure an adequate urine flow, since impaired renal function secondary to hemoglobin nephrosis is an unfavorable complication.

Recently, a seasonally occurring acute and severe hemolytic anemia with methemoglobinemia and Heinz body formation has been associated with ingestion of red maple leaves. Although the poisonous principle has not been identified, it appears to develop in the summer and early fall. In most instances, toxicity occurred when trees or tree limbs blew down in storms or were cut down and horses were allowed to browse the withered leaves. Affected horses have an acute onset of depression, hemoglobinuria, marked icterus, and often progressive anemia. At times the visible mucous membranes and blood samples have a brown color due to methemoglobinemia. During the hemolytic episode, some horses may be febrile. Treatment at this time is largely supportive, including transfusions, but the fatality rate may be high in horses with severe anemia. An important consideration is the removal of the offending cause before multiple cases occur.

IMMUNE-MEDIATED HEMOLYTIC ANEMIA

Hemolytic anemias mediated by immunologic abnormalities include autoimmune hemolytic anemia (AIHA) and neonatal isoerythrolysis (NI). Destruction of transfused erythroctyes also occurs by way of immune mechanisms when incompatible transfusions are given. AIHA occurs when an individual forms antibodies directed at its own erythrocytes. This may occur because the erythrocyte surface is altered and the animal forms antibodies to what are recognized as foreign proteins. Alternatively, an ab-

normal clone of cells may arise that produces antibodies directed toward normal (erythrocyte) self protein. The immunoglobulins may be either IgG or IgM. The former are also called "warm reacting" antibodies, whereas the latter are called "cold reacting." Complement may also sensitize erythrocytes during the disease. Diagnosis of AIHA is dependent upon detecting antibodies directed toward antibodies on the erythrocytes, or in serum. Classically, the Coombs' antiglobulin tests, direct and indirect, are used to detect these antibodies. Although Coombs' reagents have been developed for use in horses, none are currently available commercially.

Lacking specific diagnostic means of detecting immunoglobulins directed toward erythrocytes, diagnosis of AIHA in the horse is presumptive and largely based upon hematologic findings. AIHA should be considered in horses with a responsive hemolytic anemia and autoagglutination and erythrophagocytosis. Spherocytosis may be seen, although this abnormality is difficult to recognize because the erythrocytes of the horse are small and normally lack a clear area of central pallor.

AIHA may be seen as a secondary process in association with neoplasia, bacterial infections, purpural reactions, drug reactions, and as a primary idiopathic process. A major mechanism for the anemia in EIA is immune-mediated erythrocyte destruction, and during acute phases such horses will be Coombs positive. EIA should be ruled out by a negative Coggins test prior to the institution of therapy in horses with suspected AIHA. Although documented data are sparse, the anemia of some horses with AIHA will respond to corticosteroids. These anemias may be more correctly called steroid-responsive anemias until it is possible to accurately document the causal factors. Dexamethasone, 20 to 40 mg per day for several days with decreasing dosage in response to therapy, has worked well in such cases. Treatment and resolution of the primary disease process are essential in the case of secondary AIHA.

NEONATAL ISOERYTHROLYSIS

Neonatal isoerythrolysis (NI) is an immune-mediated hemolytic condition of newborn foals that develops owing to blood group incompatibilities between the foal and its dam. Since prior sensitization of the mare to red cell antigens must occur, the condition develops most frequently in foals born to multiparous dams. The risk is particularly high if previous foals of the mare have developed this disorder. While a number of blood group incompatibilities between dam and foal can occur, the Aa and Qa systems are most frequently implicated when serious hemolytic problems develop. When Aa- or

Qa-negative mares that have been previously sensitized to these erythrocyte antigens are carrying Aa- or Qa-positive foals, the potential for NI is established. This sensitization may occur through transplacental exposure to erythrocyte antigens during previous pregnancies, through unmatched blood transfusions, and possibly as the result of exposure to equine tissue culture vaccines. Antibodies directed against the foal's erythrocytes tend to accumulate during the last month of pregnancy and are passively transferred to the foal with ingested colostrum. Blood group incompatibilities may occur without clinical consequence if the mare does not become sensitized or if the antibodies formed are nonhemolytic or present in low concentrations in the colostrum. Although agglutinating and hemolytic antibodies may be produced, the hemolytic antibodies are of primary clinical concern.

Clinical signs in the foal vary depending upon the nature and concentration of the isohemolytic antibody and the amount of colostrum and antibody ingested and absorbed. Foals may die acutely in 24 hours or less with severe depression, anemia, and hemoglobinuria. More commonly, foals are born normally, nurse well, and develop clinical signs 24 to 48 hours or more later. In these foals, hemoglobinuria may be transient, but marked clinical icterus and progressive anemia and depression are characteristic features. Death is related to the degree of anemia and associated complications. Some foals recover without treatment, and mild cases may be unrecognized.

While clinical signs of anemia, hemoglobinuria, and icterus are important diagnostic features, hematologic evaluation provides a quantitative guide to the degree of anemia, the rate of progression, and thus, the need for replacement or exchange transfusion. Newborn foals normally have a PCV of 40 per cent and an erythroctye count of 10.5×10^6 per μl. Anemia should be considered when the PCV is less than 30 and the erythrocyte count less than 6.5×10^6 per μl. Agglutination or hemolysis of erythrocytes may be evident in blood collection vials or on blood smears. The icteric index is generally 100 or greater, and total serum bilirubin may be markedly elevated to 20 to 30 mg per dl. In some cases, there will be a marked elevation in the direct-reacting bilirubin as well as the anticipated elevation in indirect-reacting bilirubin. The urine is often dark and may be positive for hemoglobin and bilirubin. Transfusion should be considered in severely depressed foals in which the PCV drops below 15 per cent or the erythrocyte count falls below 3×10^6 per μl. The need for transfusion depends on the foal's clinical status as well as the apparent rate of decline in the erythrocyte parameters.

Treatment of severely affected foals is generally performed in one of two ways. When there is a pro-

gressively developing anemia and persistence of circulating maternal antibody in the foal's blood, the most effective treatment is the transfusion of washed erythrocytes from the mare. Since the mare's plasma contains isoantibodies, whole blood from the mare cannot be used. The plasma must be removed after centrifugation of acid citrate dextrose (ACD) anticoagulated blood and the erythrocytes washed several times with sterile saline. The administration of 1 to 2 l of washed erythrocytes from the mare may be life-saving in foals with critical anemia. The objective is the maintenance of red cell volume until erythrocyte production by the foal's marrow can replace the deficit.

The other means of treatment employed in seriously affected foals is an exchange transfusion with a compatible blood donor. Finding compatible blood donors may be difficult if the level of circulating isohemolytic antibodies in the foal's serum is high. A total of 3 to 4 l of sterile, warm anticoagulated blood is administered slowly (1 to 2 l per hour) by intravenous catheter while a similar amount of blood is simultaneously withdrawn from the opposite jugular vein. This procedure can be particularly helpful in foals with life-threatening anemia and marked bilirubinuria. If a randomly selected donor is used and the level of circulating isohemolytic antibodies is high, most of the transfused erythrocytes may be destroyed.

Supportive care for the foal should include warm, dry housing, and undue exercise and excitement should be avoided. Severely affected foals that are not nursing may benefit from intravenous maintenance fluids that contain dextrose. This provides energy and water to ensure adequate urine flow. After the first 24 to 48 hours, there is no benefit in withholding the mare's milk. The immunoglobulin concentration in the milk decreases fairly rapidly, and the intestinal absorption of immunoglobulin by the foal is essentially negligible by this time.

Treatment of NI can be unrewarding in severe cases, and when possible, prevention is more beneficial than treatment. A variety of preventive steps can be taken. Sire selection based on blood type could be employed in mares with previous NI foals or mares with Aa- and Qa-negative blood types. However, for many breeds, 80 to 96 per cent of the horses will be positive for either or both of these blood types, and sire selection would be extremely limited. Alternatively, all mares on a brood farm could be blood typed. This involves submission of a 10 ml ACD blood sample and 10 ml of clotted blood for serum to a typing laboratory.* Mares positive for both Aa and Qa blood are unlikely to ever

---

*Serology Laboratory, School of Veterinary Medicine, University of California, Davis, CA 95616

develop a problem. The serum of Aa- and Qa-negative mares should be checked against the erythrocytes of the stallion or a panel of control horses for the detection of alloantibodies several weeks prior to parturition. It has been suggested that an agglutinin or hemolysin titer of 1:32 or greater at this time is indicative of significant risk. Alternatively, the serum or colostrum of this mare could be cross-matched with washed presuckle erythrocytes from the foal. This test generally evaluates the agglutination reaction and may be an unreliable indicator, since the hemolytic component is of greater significance. If blood typing or cross-matching indicates significant risk, the colostrum can be withheld. To accomplish this, the foaling must be attended and the foal promptly muzzled. It is essential that the foal receive passively transferred protective antibodies normally found in colostrum. Foals should be given 500 to 1000 ml of colostrum or as much as is available from another mare. Colostrum can be collected from mares that have lost foals at birth and stored frozen for long periods of time. The colostrum can be evaluated for the presence of isohemolytic antibody by sending a sample to the Serology Laboratory at the University of California at Davis or by cross-matching with the foal's erythrocytes. If suitable colostrum is unavailable, the foal should receive 1 to 2 l of plasma from a selected donor (but not the mare). Plasma can be collected from donor horses found to be free of antierythrocyte antibodies and stored frozen. Sterile pyrogen-free plastic containers with transfer packs* are very convenient but expensive. Centrifugation of large volumes of blood requires special equipment. A reasonable separation of plasma and erythrocytes can be obtained by allowing the blood to settle for one to two hours.

The prognosis for foals that develop NI must be guarded. Prompt and vigorous therapy must be instituted early with close monitoring of progress to achieve a favorable outcome.

References

1. Becht, J. L., and Page, E. H.: Neonatal isoerythrolysis in the foal: An evaluation of predictive and diagnostic field tests. Proc. 25th Annu. Meet. Am. Assoc. Eq. Pract., 1979, pp. 247–259.
2. Collins, J. D.: Autoimmune haemolytic anemia in the horse. Proceedings of the First International Symposium on Equine Hematology, Michigan State University, 1975, p. 342.
3. Issel, C. J., and Coggins, L.: Equine infectious anemia: Current knowledge. J. Am. Vet. Med. Assoc., 194:727, 1979.
4. Lumsden, J. H., Valli, V. E., McSherry, B. J., Robinson, G. A., and Claxton, M. J.: The kinetics of hematopoiesis in the light horse. III. The hematological response to hemolytic anemia. Can. J. Comp. Med., 39:332, 1975.
5. Tennant, B., Dill, S. G., Glickman, L. T., Mirra, E. J., King, J. M., Polok, D. M., Smith, M. C., and Kradel, D. C.: Acute hemolytic anemia, methemoglobinemia, and Heinz body formation associated with ingestion of red maple leaves by horses. J. Am. Vet. Med. Assoc., 179:143, 1981.

*Fenwal Laboratories, Division of Travenol Laboratories, Inc., Deerfield, IL 60015

ANEMIA AS A RESULT OF INSUFFICIENT ERYTHROPOIESIS

Bernard F. Feldman, DAVIS, CALIFORNIA

Anemia as a result of insufficiency in the production of red cells, so-called depression or nonresponsive anemia, is the most common type of anemia encountered in equine practice. These anemias are confusing diagnostically and are often refractory to therapy. Included in this group are anemias resulting from iron deficiency, chronic or inflammatory disease, renal disease, bone marrow intrinsic disorders, tumor invasion of the bone marrow, and dyserythropoiesis.

Anemia as a result of insufficiency of red cell production is usually more modest and less rapidly progressive than anemia resulting from blood loss or hemolysis (p. 297, 299). In horses, erythropoiesis is completed in the bone marrow even under conditions of severe blood loss or hemolytic anemia. Therefore, it is difficult to ascertain from erythrocyte morphology in the stained blood film and the erythrocyte values in the hemogram whether or not there is a response to existing anemia through intensification of erythropoiesis. Though anisocytosis may be present, red cells are normochromic, and mean corpuscular volume increases only slightly. Nucleated red cell precursors rarely appear in circulating blood. Reticulocyte counts made on aspirated bone marrow provide the most reliable index of erythrocyte response in the horse.

Insufficient red cell production is characterized by bone marrow reticulocyte counts of less than 5 per cent and bone marrow myeloid:erythroid ratios of more than 0.75. A consistent and productive approach to these types of anemia includes a hemogram, bone marrow aspirate (for cell morphology, myeloid:erythroid ratios, and reticulocyte counts), serum iron, and total iron-binding capacity (TIBC, transferrin). These data, in concert with a good history and physical examination, provide the clinician with the tools to differentiate anemias of various causes.

IRON DEFICIENCY ANEMIA

Iron deficiency anemia, though infrequent in the horse, may be seen in association with chronic blood loss. Chronic blood loss is seen primarily with gastrointestinal diseases, including parasitism, ulcerative neoplasia, and coagulation disorders. As anemia develops, increasing fatigue, exercise intolerance, and tachycardia develop. Occasionally horses with iron deficiency may develop depraved appetite (pica). The anemia is initially normocytic and normochromic. Only rarely are microcytic hypochromic cells, the hallmark of moderate or severe iron depletion, seen in the horse. A modest thrombocytosis is often noted. The distinguishing laboratory features are low serum iron and increased total iron-binding capacity (TIBC). Bone marrow iron stores as measured with the Prussian blue stain are depleted. Therapy should be directed at the primary problem. A variety of iron-containing hematinics are commercially available. Iron cacodylate is the only safe parenteral preparation available for use in the horse.

ANEMIA OF INFLAMMATORY DISEASE

Anemia of inflammatory disease (AID, anemia of chronic disease) is associated with long-standing inflammatory, infectious, or malignant disease. This form of anemia is modest and may be so innocuous as to be clinically unrecognizable. AID mimics iron deficiency anemia in that it may be normocytic and normochromic initially and then, with extreme chronicity, microcytic and hypochromic. Serum iron is decreased, but in contrast to iron deficiency anemia, TIBC is normal to decreased. Prussian blue stain of bone marrow aspirates reveals adequate iron stores in reticuloendothelial cells but little or no iron in developing red cell precursors. Injections of iron and other hematinics are valueless in AID because the inflammatory process, through a complex series of biochemical interactions, sequesters iron in the reticuloendothelial system. Therapy directed at the underlying primary disorder must be undertaken to resolve this form of anemia.

APLASTIC PANCYTOPENIA

Intrinsic marrow disease, or aplastic pancytopenia, is a condition in which the bone marrow contains diminished numbers of hematopoietic precursors and therefore cannot produce adequate numbers of circulating erythrocytes, granulocytes, and platelets. This illness is frequently called aplastic anemia in spite of the fact that the most important clinical manifestations are not caused by the deficiency of erythrocytes but are the result of granulocytopenia and thrombocytopenia. Aplastic pancytopenia is an acquired disorder. The syndrome is most frequently caused by a toxic insult to the bone marrow. There is no age predilection for this form of the disease, which is frequently fatal. The importance of a careful history to determine a possible etiology cannot be overemphasized. It is important for the veterinary clinician to determine whether the patient has been exposed to a myelotoxin. Successful reversal of a marrow aplasia is dependent upon elimination of the offending agent. Aplastic pancytopenia may result from organic solvents, trichloroethylene-extracted soybean oil meal, heavy metals, diuretics, insecticides, and ionizing radiation. Recent reports have suggested that toxic marrow suppression occurs in horses from phenylbutazone administration. Adverse reactions to phenylbutazone are associated with a high dose rate. There may be an individual or breed susceptibility to phenylbutazone. Bone marrow aspirate and core biopsies are most helpful in diagnosing intrinsic marrow disease. Aplastic pancytopenia has been treated with corticosteroids and splenectomy, but there is no proof of the effectiveness of either of these modalities. Androgens have been tested, but reports of clinical studies have yielded conflicting results as to their benefits. Corticosteroids should be used with caution, as they may compromise neutrophil function in a patient already granulocytopenic and susceptible to infection.

MYELOPHTHISIS

The marrow microenvironment provides a unique site for the proliferation of normal hematopoietic cells. Metastasizing cancer cells may also localize and proliferate in the marrow. The proliferation of abnormal cells occurs at the expense of normal hematopoiesis and may result in anemia, leukopenia, and thrombocytopenia. This form of marrow invasion is termed myelophthisis and is confirmed by bone marrow aspiration or biopsy. Lymphoma and rarely myeloproliferative diseases have been reported to invade equine bone marrow.

DYSERYTHROPOIETIC ANEMIA

Dyserythropoietic anemia refers to abnormal erythroid maturation in the marrow. This may be characterized by multiple nuclei, nuclear fragmentation, and megaloblastic nuclear morphology. There is no evidence that vitamin B_{12} deficiency occurs in the horse, but folic acid deficiency has been associated with lowered racing performance and mild anemia. Folic acid deficiency is difficult to ascertain owing to testing inadequacies. Horses inadvertently fed low-folate diets had macrocytic anemia after several months. These horses responded well to parenteral but not oral folate therapy.

Supplemental Readings

1. Archer, R. K., and Jeffcott, L. B.: Comparative Clinical Haematology. London, Blackwell Scientific Pub., 1977, p. 165.
2. Dunovant, M. L., and Murray, E. S.: Clinical evidence of phenylbutazone-induced hypoplastic anemia. First International Symposium on Equine Hematology, Michigan State University, 1975, p. 383.
3. Rumbaugh, G. E., Smith, B. P., and Carlson, G. P.: Internal abdominal abscesses in the horse: A study of 25 cases. J. Am. Vet. Med. Assoc., 172:304, 1978.
4. Smith, B. P.: Pleuritis and pleural effusion in the horse: A study of 37 cases. J. Am. Vet. Med. Assoc., 170:208, 1977.
5. Williams, D. L., Lynch, R. E., and Cartwright, G. E.: Drug-induced aplastic anemia. Semin. Hematol., 10:195, 1973.

LYMPHOPROLIFERATIVE AND MYELOPROLIFERATIVE DISEASES

Joseph G. Zinkl, DAVIS, CALIFORNIA

The tumors of the hematopoietic system of the horse include malignant lymphoma, plasma cell myeloma, and myelocytic or myelomonocytic leukemia. Of these neoplastic diseases, malignant lymphoma is the most common. However, hematopoietic neoplasia in horses is relatively rare compared with the occurrence in dogs, cats, and cattle.

Malignant lymphoma may involve the lymph nodes, the skin, or the body cavities. There is no sex predilection for malignant lymphoma in horses. The disease appears to be more common in older horses, although it has been seen in immature and young adult horses as well. The clinical signs of the disease are related to the location of the neoplastic lesions and their effect on body organs or lymphatic drainage. Malignant lymphoma develops insidiously in most cases, leading to progressive weight loss and the gradual appearance of other signs. Malignant lymphoma should be suspected when nonpainful cutaneous masses or lymphadenopathy is detected, even though only a single node may be involved. Lymphadenopathy of internal nodes may alter organ function or may produce edema and ascites. Ventral edema is a common sign. Fluid effusions in the pleural cavity may be massive and may cause dyspnea. Repeated episodes of choke may indicate that the mediastinum near the thoracic inlet is involved. Subcutaneous tumor masses, which at times may be numerous and rapidly enlarging, may also remain unchanged for years.

Diagnosis is made through cytologic examination of tumor masses or effusions and only rarely the peripheral blood. Lymph nodes and body cavity fluids contain large numbers of immature lymphoid cells. These cells are large and pleomorphic, varying in size and shape. The nucleus is usually large and irregular and may contain a large nucleolus. Mitotic figures may be present. Bone marrow may occasionally be massively involved to such an extent that the production of leukocytes, erythrocytes, and platelets is compromised.

Although rapid progress is being made in the treatment of lymphoid neoplasia in humans and small animals, there have been few attempts at therapy in horses. The cost of anticancer drugs and the relative rarity of the disease have precluded such treatment. Transient regression of subcutaneous masses may occur in response to potent glucocorticoids. Although no dosage regimen has been established, dexamethasone given at 20 to 40 mg once a day followed by a decreasing dose rate has been of temporary benefit. The prognosis of malignant lymphoma should be based upon the signs and the organs involved. For example, horses with subcutaneous involvement may live for years with the disease, whereas horses with a generalized disease or leukemia are unlikely to survive long.

Another lymphoproliferative disease of horses that is rarely seen is plasma cell myeloma, or multiple myeloma. This disease occurs when a clone of plasma cells becomes neoplastic. In reported cases, the bones and the lymph nodes were commonly invaded by neoplastic plasma cells. Lameness and weakness due to lytic bone lesions occurred. Anemia due to myelophthisis was present. Although lymph nodes were not usually enlarged, most of the cells within them were neoplastic plasma cells. Diagnosis of the condition was made by finding a high concentration of a monoclonal protein on electrophoresis. Treatment of the condition has not been attempted, and the prognosis should be regarded as grave.

Even more rarely, a myeloproliferative condition resembling myelocytic or myelomonocytic leukemia occurs in horses. Horses may manifest anemia and thrombocytopenia. Leukocytosis is accompanied by immature, bizarre myeloid or monocytoid cells. Hemorrhage after minor trauma or foaling was the immediate cause of death in these horses and was believed to be related to the thrombocytopenia. In one horse, many tissues, including lymph nodes, spleen, liver, bone marrow, and adrenal glands, were infiltrated by the neoplastic cells. Treatment was not attempted in any of these horses except in a pregnant mare, which was supported with transfusions until she foaled.[1]

References

1. Brumbaugh, G. W., Stitzel, K. A., Zinkl, J. G., and Feldman, B. F.: Myelomonocytic myeloproliferative disease in a horse. J. Am. Vet. Med. Assoc., *180*:313, 1982.
2. Miller, J. M.: Animal model: Lymphosarcoma in cattle, sheep, horses, and pigs (malignant lymphoma, leukosis, leukemia). Am. J. Pathol., *75*:417, 1974.
3. Neufeld, J. L.: Lymphosarcoma in the horse: A review. Can. Vet. J., *14*:129, 1973.
4. Schalm, O. W., and Carlson, G. P.: Diseases of the blood and blood forming organs. *In* Mansmann, R., and McAllister, S. (eds.): Equine Medicine and Surgery. Santa Barbara, American Veterinary Pub., Inc., 1982, in press.

HEMOSTASIS

Bernard F. Feldman, DAVIS, CALIFORNIA

The function of the normal hemostatic mechanism is to prevent blood loss from intact vessels and to stop excessive bleeding from severed vessels. The mechanism by which blood is prevented from being shed from intact vessels is uncertain, but the structural integrity of the vessels and the presence of normal platelets are necessary for this function. Arrest of bleeding following trauma is controlled by three interrelated factors. These factors are the reaction of blood vessels to injury, the formation of the platelet plug at the site of injury, and the coagulation of blood. Hence, coagulopathies in the horse may be caused by vascular disorders, thrombocytopenia, platelet function defects, coagulation defects, or excessive fibrinolysis.

There are some common manifestations of bleeding seen in clinical equine practice. Petechiae represent blood that has extravasated from intact blood vessels and are seen in patients with vascular disorders, thrombocytopenia, and platelet function defects. When petechiae become confluent they are known as purpura. They are larger and are caused by the same abnormalities that produce petechiae. An ecchymosis or bruise is a large area of extravasated blood that may occur in patients that have vascular or platelet disorders. A hematoma is a large bruise that has infiltrated subcutaneous tissue or muscle. Hematomas and hemarthrosis (hemorrhage into a joint) are seen in patients with trauma or severe coagulation defects such as hemophilia. These signs, as well as hematuria, may be seen in association with hemophilia, anticoagulant therapy, or drugs that interfere with platelet or coagulation function.

The approach to a patient with a suspected diagnosis of generalized bleeding includes obtaining an accurate history, careful physical examination, and selection of appropriate screening tests of hemostasis. Answers to the following four questions should be sought. (1) Does the patient have a generalized hemostatic defect? (2) Is it inherited or acquired? (3) Is it likely that it is due to a vascular or platelet abnormality, a coagulation abnormality, or a combined problem? (4) What is the precise nature and extent of the abnormality? The answers to the first three questions can often be obtained by careful evaluation of the patient's bleeding manifestations, whereas the answer to the fourth question can only be evaluated by performing tests of hemostasis.

Generalized defects are usually recognized by bleeding from multiple sites or by spontaneous bleeding in the form of petechiae, hematomas, or joint bleeding. Patients with inherited disorders usually have difficulties as young animals, though some patients with mild hemostatic defects may not be recognized until adulthood. Whether the bleeding problem is caused by a vascular, platelet, or coagulation abnormality may often be predicted by the type of bleeding manifestation discussed before. Petechial and ecchymotic hemorrhages are generally seen with vascular or platelet defects, whereas bleeding into joints, body cavities, or orifices may be seen with coagulopathies.

SCREENING TESTS FOR VASCULAR OR PLATELET DISORDERS

Screening tests for vascular or platelet disorders include the bleeding time, platelet count, and clot retraction. The bleeding time is an unsophisticated test in which a standardized cut is made and blotted with filter paper at 30-second intervals. The time to clot is the bleeding time. Platelet numbers may be estimated by examining a blood film or may be enumerated by actual count. The ability of a whole blood sample to clot and retract from the sides of a test tube is a measure of platelet numbers and platelet function. Clot retraction in the horse is slower than in other domestic species.

SCREENING TESTS FOR COAGULATION DISORDERS

Screening tests for coagulation disorders include the activated clotting time (ACT), the partial thromboplastin time (PTT), the prothrombin time (PT), and the thrombin time (TT). The ACT tests the intrinsic and common pathways (Fig. 1) for a clotting

factor deficiency. It is not a very sensitive measure of coagulation defects. Abnormal prolongations in ACT indicate a severe factor or platelet deficiency. The PTT tests the same pathways as the ACT but is more sensitive to modest factor deficiencies and is not affected by thrombocytopenia. The PT tests the integrity of the extrinsic and common pathways and has a sensitivity range similar to the PTT. The TT tests for fibrinogen quantitatively and qualitatively. It is possible to have a normal fibrinogen (Factor I) quantity but a prolonged TT if the fibrinogen is functionally compromised. Laboratory findings are depicted in Table 1.

PURPURA HEMORRHAGICA

Bleeding disorders may be manifested when vessels have been structurally altered by disease processes. Most often, vascular disorders are mediated by inflammatory or immune processes affecting the vessel wall. Bleeding is usually not severe, is mainly into the skin, and occurs immediately after trauma. Purpura hemorrhagica is a condition seen in mature horses that occurs most frequently as a sequela to respiratory infections two to three weeks previously. Purpura in the horse is almost always due to immune or inflammatory vasculitis and is not associated with thrombocytopenia. Several investigators believe that purpura should be classified as a thrombotic disorder with hemorrhage secondary to necrotizing vasculitis. In addition to immune vasculitis, vascular inflammatory disorders may be initiated by bacterial, fungal, or viral pathogens or drugs. Treat-

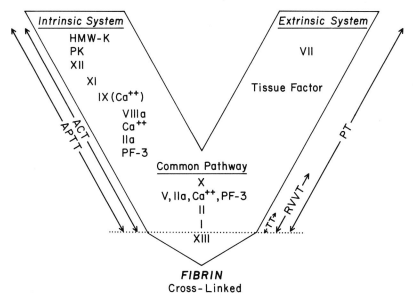

Figure 1. Coagulation cascade and coagulation screening tests. HWM-K, high molecular weight kininogen; PK, plasma prekallikrein; PF-3, platelet factor 3; Ca^{++}, calcium; ACT, activated coagulation time; APTT, activated partial thromboplastin time; PT, prothrombin time; RVVT, Russell's viper venom time; TT, thrombin time. (From Feldman, B. F.: Coagulopathies in small animals. *J. Am. Vet. Med. Assoc.*, 179(6):559, 1981.)

TABLE 1. EQUINE HEMOSTASIS—SCREENING TESTS AND THERAPY

Disorder	PT	PTT	TT	BT	ACT	Fibrino-gen	FDPs	Platelets	Therapy
*Thrombocytopenia	N	N	N	N ↑	N ↑	N	N	↓	Platelet-rich plasma, steroids
†Vascular disease	N	N	N	N ↑	N	N ↑	N	N	Steroids, diuretics
Warfarin toxicosis	↑	↑	N	N	↑	N ↑	N	N ↓	Vitamin K$_1$
Hemophilia A or B	N	↑	N	N	↑	N	N	N	Transfusion (fresh plasma)
Disseminated intravascular coagulation	↓N↑	↓N↑	↑	N ↑	N ↑	↓	↑	↓	Volume expansion; fluids; subcutaneous heparin; heparin incubated with whole blood
Thrombosis	↓N	N ↓	N ↓	N	N ↓	N ↓	N ↑	N ↓	
‡Normal Values	9.7–11.7 sec	28–44 sec	13–16 sec	<5 min	<2 min	100–400 mg/dl	<10 μg/ml	100,000–400,000/μl	

PT = one-stage prothrombin time; PTT = partial thromboplastin time; TT = thrombin clotting time;
BT = bleeding time; FDPs = fibrin degradation products; ACT = activated coagulation time; N = normal; ↑ = prolonged or increased; ↓ = decreased
*Bone marrow aspirate, PF-3 and Coombs' antiglobulin test recommended
†Lesional biopsy recommended to confirm diagnosis
‡Veterinary Medical Teaching Hospital, School of Veterinary Medicine, University of California, Davis, CA 95616

ment consists of systemic antibiotics when bacterial infections are involved. Penicillin is the drug of choice for streptococcal infection and should be given at a rate of 20,000 units per kg twice a day. Steroids are recommended in relatively high doses initially (i.e., 20 to 50 mg dexamethasone) with gradual decrease as there is response. Diuretics such as furosemide are helpful in the initial stages when there is substantial edema. Diuretics should not be used for more than the first few days. Supportive care and bandaging of draining lesions on the legs may be necessary in some cases. The prognosis should be guarded until response to therapy is noted. It may be necessary to continue steroid therapy for several weeks.

ACQUIRED COAGULATION DISORDERS (WARFARIN TOXICITY)

Acquired coagulation disorders may be associated with vitamin K deficiency, liver disease, or disseminated intravascular coagulation. Warfarin is a rodenticide that is antagonistic to vitamin K but has been recommended as a therapeutic agent in navicular disease. Moldy sweet clover poisoning, which results in vitamin K deficiency, is seen mostly in cattle, although the condition has been recorded in horses. Vitamin K is essential to the production of functional Factors II, VII, IX, and X. Deficiencies in these factors prolong the ACT, PT, and PTT. The hemogram may reveal a marked anemia and hypoproteinemia. Early signs may include epistaxis, hematoma formation, and rectal bleeding. Severe bleeding into the gastrointestinal tract, body cavi-

ties, and between large muscle masses may occur. Since the half-lives of the vitamin K–dependent factors are quite short (VII, less than 6 hours; IX, less than 14 hours; X, less than 16 hours; and II, less than 41 hours), therapy must be aggressive and continuous. Fresh plasma or whole blood transfusion, which supplies clotting factors in addition to volume and cellular replacement, may be life-saving in acute cases. Vitamin K$_1$ at a twice daily dosage of 75 mg subcutaneously is suggested. Intravenous vitamin K$_1$ has no therapeutic advantage. An initial dose of 0.3 to 0.5 mg per kg has been suggested. Adverse reactions, some of which may be severe or fatal, may occur when using this route of administration. Evidence of remission is based on clinical signs and the return of the PT and PTT to normal. Vitamin K$_3$ is not recommended in warfarin poisoning.

The anticoagulant response to warfarin varies widely from horse to horse and during the course of the therapy. Intercurrent hepatic disorders or infectious diseases and the concurrent use of a multitude of drugs may influence the coumarin activity. Drugs that may enhance warfarin toxicity include phenylbutazone, salicylates, penicillin, streptomycin, heparin, phenothiazine, ACTH, and corticosteroids. These anti-inflammatory drugs and antibiotics displace warfarin from plasma albumin.

Liver disease, as manifested by elevation of direct-acting bilirubin, hepatic enzymes, and an increased Bromsulphalein half-life, may result in bleeding manifestations, since all factors, with the exception of Factor III (tissue thromboplastin), Factor IV (calcium), and Factor VIII (antihemophilic factor), are produced in the liver. All factors have short half-lives, with fibrinogen having the longest (96 hours).

HEMOPHILIA

Hemophilia can be manifested by post-traumatic bleeding that can continue for days. Classical hemophilia (hemophilia A) is a deficiency in Factor VIII and has a prolonged PTT but a normal PT and TT. This deficiency has been reported in Thoroughbreds and Standardbreds. The author is also aware of a case of hemophilia A in a quarter horse. Factor IX deficiency (hemophilia B) has not been reported in horses. Multiple clotting defects (VII, IX, and XI) have been reported in an Arabian colt. Hemophilia is seen only in young males with the clinical presentation of a bleeding tendency, especially into joints. Most foals die or are killed before six months of age. Treatment with fresh plasma to replace Factor VIII or IX or correction of a prolonged PTT by plasma containing one of these factors is both diagnostic and therapeutic. There is no long-term therapy for these disorders, and the prognosis is highly unfavorable. Genetic counseling is advisable, since the mare remains a carrier and has the potential to pass this trait to her female offspring.

Supplemental Readings

1. Dodds, W. J., and White, J. G.: Coagulation and platelet function. 1st International Symposium on Equine Hematology, Michigan State University, 1975, p. 197.
2. Franco, D. A.: Thrombocytopenia and its relationship to sporadic idiopathic epistaxis in Thoroughbreds. VM SAC, *64*:1071, 1969.
3. Hinton, M., Jones, D. R., and Lewis, I. M.: A clotting defect in an Arab foal. Eq. Vet. J., 9:1, 1977.
4. Scott, E. A., Sandler, G. A., Byars, T. D.: Warfarin: Effects on anticoagulant, hematologic and blood enzyme values in normal ponies. Am. J. Vet. Res., *40*:172, 1979.
5. Smith, M. S.: Diagnosis and control of idiopathic thrombocytopenia in a horse. J. Eq. Med. Surg. 2:257, 1978.

DISSEMINATED INTRAVASCULAR COAGULATION

T. D. Byars, ATHENS, GEORGIA

Disseminated intravascular coagulation (DIC), although well recognized in some species, is poorly documented in the horse. The horse possesses an inhibited coagulation mechanism that rarely completes the processes of clotting and clot dissolution rapidly enough to allow for an accurate laboratory diagnosis. Horses appear to be particularly prone to low-grade forms of the syndrome commonly associated with ischemic and thrombotic disorders. The occurrence of DIC has been described in conjunction with colic and laminitis.[1-3, 5-7] Its existence is also clinically suspected but seldom documented in shock, septicemia, endotoxemia, renal failure, liver disease, and postoperative hemorrhage.

PATHOPHYSIOLOGY

Disseminated intravascular coagulation refers to an exaggeration of the clotting system with the subsequent consumption of the clotting proteins (factors) and platelets. Activation occurs in response to an increase in a systemic procoagulant substance(s), and a hypercoagulable state precedes the blood clotting. Intravascular coagulation results in fibrin deposition in the general microcirculation, including that of many of the vital organs. Microthrombi decrease perfusion, and vascular ischemia initiates the enzymatic degradation (secondary fibrinolysis) of fibrinogen and fibrin. Fibrinogen and fibrin degradation products (FDPs) are breakdown products of clot dissolution, which when they enter the systemic circulation, act as potent anticoagulants to prevent ongoing fibrin formation. DIC is therefore a consumptive coagulopathy that may present clinically as a thrombotic crisis or a hemorrhagic diathesis. The syndrome may occur in a generalized, local, acute, or chronic (low-grade) form.

PREDISPOSING CAUSES

DIC is always a disorder secondary to an underlying primary disease. It can be associated with any generalized or local disorders that result in an insult to the blood components or vasculature (Table 1). Since DIC may present in variable forms, the clinical and laboratory findings may not determine which primary entity results in certain forms of the syndrome.

CLINICAL PRESENTATION

The presentation of profound hemorrhage with DIC is rare in the horse. The clinician should at-

TABLE 1. CONDITIONS THAT MAY CAUSE DISSEMINATED INTRAVASCULAR COAGULATION

Abdominal crisis	Postoperative hemorrhage
Adrenal crisis	(e.g., castration)
Endotoxemia	Respiratory hemorrhage
Exhaustion syndrome	Respiratory distress (hypoxia)
Hemolytic crisis	Renal disease
Laminitis	Septicemia
Liver disease	Shock
Obstetrical complications,	Transfusions
including abortion and	Trauma
retained placenta	Vasculitis

tempt to make a clinical diagnosis on the basis of subtle lesions of thrombosis and hemorrhage in conjunction with a suitable predisposing cause. Petechiation and ecchymosis are most frequently found on the mucous membranes, nictitating membranes, sclera, and inner pinna. Epistaxis is a rare and unexpected finding. Hematoma formation after venipuncture occasionally occurs, but more often, rapid thrombosis of either veins or arteries follows a perforating procedure. Spontaneous thrombosis is often associated with a severe primary systemic disease. DIC should be suspected in cases of advanced disease whenever the sequelae indicate that microvascular thrombosis is responsible for the deterioration of vital organ function. Laminitis, colic, and dysfunction of the adrenals, kidneys, liver, and reticuloendothelial system can be considered as clinical sequelae to DIC as well as predisposing causes.

DIAGNOSIS

The confirmation of a clinical diagnosis must be made in the laboratory or at necropsy. In order for a precise diagnosis to be made, at least three of the laboratory tests should be abnormal in a hemostatic profile (Table 2). Since changes in coagulation are subtle in the horse, DIC is seldom diagnosed.

Tests of clotting function are frequently within normal limits even in the face of a consumptive coagulopathy owing to the hypercoagulable status of the patient. The activated coagulation time (ACT) test

TABLE 2. RECOMMENDED HEMOSTATIC PROFILE*

Prothrombin time (PT)	Thrombin time (TT)
Partial thromboplastin time	Platelet count
(PTT)	Fibrinogen concentration
Activated coagulation time	Fibrinogen/fibrin degradation
(ACT)	products (FDPs)

*A control sample must be analyzed with tests of clotting time. Normal values will vary and must be established for each laboratory.

will allow for an initial assessment of clotting function under field conditions and serves as an indicator for further testing.[3, 8] Although the ACT may be within normal limits, clot formation with DIC is sluggish, and clots are poorly formed and often show evidence of clot lysis within the tube.

Platelet counts are usually lowered in acute DIC. An absolute platelet count is recommended, although a scan for adequate platelets under a high-powered field usually correlates well with the actual number of platelets. Horses with a thrombocyte count of less than 20,000 per mm^3 are clinically prone to spontaneous hemorrhage.

Although decreases of fibrinogen concentration might be anticipated, hypofibrinogenemia is not common in horses with DIC. In chronic cases, the fibrinogen content may be elevated owing to overcompensation or the erroneous measurement of substances other than fibrinogen, which may interfere with conventional fibrinogen estimation.

Fibrin degradation products (FDPs) are best detected and quantified using a commercially available standard kit.* Fibrin degradation products are rapidly cleared by an intact reticuloendothelial system and may not be present in detectable quantities in the systemic circulation of low-grade cases of DIC. False positives can be encountered in normal horses. If FDPs are elevated above the control, the amount of elevation should be considered irrelevant, since their presence ensures that fibrinolysis as a component of DIC has occurred. In order to separate the FDPs generated from fibrinogen (primary fibrinogenolysis) from those of fibrin, the protamine sulfate test can be used to detect the soluble monomers of fibrinogen degradation. Other laboratory tests that offer future diagnostic potential include the euglobulin lysis time test, plasminogen/plasmin quantification, and circulating antithrombin III levels.

At postmortem examination, DIC can be suspected whenever diffuse thrombosis and hemorrhage are both evident. Histologic confirmation is difficult, since fibrinolysis continues in the postmortem state.

THERAPY

The treatment of DIC involves three basic courses of therapy: (1) treatment of the primary disorder, (2) treatment of DIC, and (3) treatment of sequelae.

Treatment of the primary disorder responsible for the initiation of DIC is essential. An accurate diagnosis of the inciting cause and evaluation of the se-

---

*Thrombo-Wellcotest, Burroughs-Wellcome Co., Research Triangle Park, NC 27709

verity of the DIC should influence the clinician's decision on treatment. For example, if sepsis due to bacterial infection were to cause DIC, treatment with the appropriate antibiotic and supportive care may be all that are required to control the syndrome.

The direct treatment of DIC is aimed at the inactivation of the procoagulant activity. This can be accomplished by volume expansion to prevent hemoconcentration in the microvasculature, drugs to stabilize the endothelial lining to decrease contact activation and production of inflammatory procoagulants, and anticoagulants to inhibit the consumptive process.

Volume dilution is achieved by appropriate balanced fluid therapy to restore cardiovascular integrity and acid-base homeostasis. Restoration of fluid volume will increase perfusion of the microvasculature and will decrease capillary sludging. Drugs that stabilize the endothelium and increase capillary perfusion act as adjuncts to fluid therapy. The nonsteroidal anti-inflammatory agents (such as phenylbutazone and flunixin meglumine*) are useful in these regards, and they have the added benefit of inhibition of platelet function. Steroids, although potent anti-inflammatory compounds, should be avoided, as they can exacerbate DIC by reducing the procoagulant clearance activity of the reticuloendothelial system.

Use of systemic anticoagulants in a potential bleeding disorder is a paradoxical treatment that is utilized to inhibit the consumptive process. Heparin is the most commonly used anticoagulant. In therapeutic doses, it offers varying degrees of success. Since antithrombin III is required for heparin to function as an anticoagulant, failure of heparin can occur in cases of DIC due to decreased levels of antithrombin III. If heparin therapy is employed, 80 to 100 IU per kg intravenously is recommended every 4 to 8 hours, or it can be added to fluids as a continuous drip. The low-grade form of DIC is

*Banamine, Schering Corp., Kenilworth, NJ 07033

treated with 25 to 40 IU per kg subcutaneously two or three times daily. Other anticoagulants have not been investigated sufficiently to recommend their use in place of heparin.

Blood transfusions and/or plasma and platelet concentrates are considered controversial without prior heparinization. Transfusions may provide additional substrate for ongoing DIC and may be contraindicated. Since massive hemorrhage due to DIC is rare to nonexistent in the horse, transfusions are not warranted unless fulminant blood loss has occurred (for example, postsurgical hemorrhage).

The treatment of sequelae will vary according to the organ involvement. Liver and kidney function should be assessed whenever DIC has been suspected.

References

1. Coffman, J. R.: Acute abdominal disease of the horse. J. Am. Vet. Med. Assoc., *161*(11):1197, 1972.
2. Garner, H. E.: Pathophysiology of equine laminitis. Proc. 21st Annu. Meet. Am. Assoc. Eq. Pract., 1975, p. 386.
3. Gentry, P. A., Woodbury, F. R., and Black, W. D.: Comparative study of blood coagulation tests in the horse and pony. Am. J. Vet. Res., 39(2):333, 1978.
4. Hood, D. M.: Current concepts of the physiopathology of laminitis. Proc. 25th Annu. Meet. Am. Assoc. Eq. Pract., 1979, pp. 13–20.
5. Hood, D. M., Gremmel, S. M., Amoss, M. S., et al.: Equine laminitis. III. Coagulation dysfunction in the development of acute disease, J. Equine Med. Surg. 3:355, 1979.
6. Kociba, G. J., and Mansmann, R. A.: Acquired hemostatic defects in horses. Proc. First International Symposium on Equine Hematology, Michigan State University, 1975, pp. 554–559.
7. McClure, J. R., McClure, J. J., and Usenik, E. A.: Disseminated intravascular coagulation in ponies with surgically induced strangulation obstruction of the small intestine. Vet. Surg., 8(3):78, 1979.
8. Rawlings, C. A., Byars, T. D., and Van Noy, M. K.: Activated coagulation test in normal and heparinized ponies and horses, Am. J. Vet. Res., 36:711, 1975.
9. Schalm, O. W., Jain, N. C., and Carroll, E. J.: Blood coagulation and fibrinolysis. *In* Schalm, O. W., Jain, N. C., and Carroll, E. J. (eds.): Veterinary Hematology, 3rd ed. Philadelphia, Lea and Febiger, 1975, pp. 295–300.

FLUID THERAPY

Gary P. Carlson, DAVIS, CALIFORNIA

Fluid therapy is an important and often critical component of medical management of horses with serious systemic disorders. The evaluation of dehydration in the horse and the development of rational therapeutic plans have been the subjects of a number of reviews. Emphasis in recent years has

been placed on evaluation of the individual patient and formulation of flexible plans to meet variable and changing needs of the patient.

Response to fluid therapy will primarily depend upon (1) the accumulated net fluid and electrolyte deficits, (2) the physiologic responses to these defi-

TABLE 1. COMPOSITION OF INTRAVENOUS FLUIDS

	Na (mEq/l)	K (mEq/l)	Ca (mEq/l)	Mg (mEq/l)	Cl (mEq/l)	Bicarbonate Precursor (mEq/l)	Calories (Kcal/l)
Polyionic replacement solution							
Lactated Ringer's	130	4	3		109	28 (Lactate)	9
Polysal*	140	10	5	3	103	55 (Acetate)	18
Isolyte E†	140	10	5	3	103	47 (Acetate)	18
Multisol-R‡	140	5		3	98	50 (Acetate, gluconate)	18
Normosol-R‡	140	5		3	98	50 (Acetate, gluconate)	18
Dilusol-R§	140	5		3	98	50 (Acetate, gluconate)	18
Physiologic saline	154				154		0
Five per cent dextrose							170
Five per cent bicarbonate	600					600	0

*Cutter Laboratories, Berkeley, CA
†McGraw Laboratories, Santa Ana, CA
‡Abbott Laboratories, North Chicago, IL
§Diamond Laboratories, Modesto, CA

cits, (3) the composition of the administered fluid, and (4) the rate and route of fluid administration. The objective of fluid therapy is the restoration or partial restoration of homeostasis so that resolution of the primary disease process can occur with a minimum of systemic organ damage or dysfunction.

Since this book is concerned with therapy, it may be advisable at the outset to discuss some of the common therapeutic fluids and to consider their physiologic effects. The chemical composition of a number of commonly available intravenous fluids is presented in Table 1. With few exceptions, these fluids are isotonic with the body fluids. Although the characteristics of each fluid or group of fluids will be discussed individually, fluids are often used in combination, and the physiologic effects of these combinations depend upon the total solute content as well as the volume administered. Oral intake, either voluntary or administered, must also be considered, as this is a major but often overlooked component in the restoration and maintenance of fluid balance.

POLYIONIC REPLACEMENT FLUIDS

The most widely recommended and commonly used fluids are the polyionic or balanced replacement fluids. The composition of these fluids is similar to that of the extracellular fluid (ECF). They differ from one another principally in the amount and composition of the available bicarbonate precursor. When administered intravenously, these fluids are largely confined to the ECF volume owing to their electrolyte composition. The initial response is transient expansion of the plasma volume and, thus, the effective circulating blood volume. These fluids are, thus, particularly useful when there is loss or compartmentalization of sodium-containing fluids (diarrhea, excessive sweating, or obstructive bowel disease) and signs of developing hypovolemia. Fluids of this composition distribute to all components of the ECF volume. Response to these fluids is one of volume expansion and is manifested by decreases in packed cell volume (PCV) and total plasma protein (TPP) concentration. These fluids normally have minimal direct effects on electrolyte concentration or acid-base status. Improved tissue perfusion may ameliorate a pre-existing metabolic acidosis.

0.9 PER CENT SALINE

Although sometimes referred to as physiologic saline, this fluid is simply isotonic and is not exactly similar to the body fluids. Saline contains an excess of chloride relative to sodium when compared to the concentrations present in the ECF. This fluid contains no bicarbonate precursors and is the fluid of choice for treatment of horses with hypochloremic metabolic alkalosis. The physiologic response to this isotonic sodium-containing fluid is very similar to that of the polyionic fluids, i.e., expansion of plasma and ECF volume reflected in decreases in PCV or TPP concentrations. A transient hyperchloremia and mild dilutional acidosis may also occur.

FIVE PER CENT SODIUM BICARBONATE

Hypertonic solutions of sodium bicarbonate should be reserved for the treatment of serious metabolic acidosis. When this acid-base disturbance occurs, it is usually secondary to hypovolemia and inadequate tissue perfusion. Severe metabolic acidosis is *not* an invariable finding in horses with diarrhea, obstructive bowel disease, or exertional myopathies.

The presence or probable presence of metabolic acidosis should be established prior to the administration of any substantial amounts (i.e., over 2 l) of 5 per cent sodium bicarbonate. Each liter of 5 per cent sodium bicarbonate contains nearly 600 mEq of sodium as well as bicarbonate. This sodium input must be considered when formulating fluid plans for horses with combined electrolyte and acid-base alterations. Aside from increasing bicarbonate concentration and blood pH, this hypertonic sodium-containing solution causes a transient expansion of plasma and ECF volume. This response is similar to that with other sodium-containing fluids. Volume expansion is manifested by transient but significant decreases in PCV and TPP concentration. If hypertonic bicarbonate solutions are administered to horses with a normal acid-base balance or horses with significant chloride and potassium deficits, a persistent metabolic alkalosis may result. Adverse effects on the physiologically important cations potassium, calcium, and magnesium as well as respiratory depression may be noted.

FIVE PER CENT DEXTROSE

Dextrose as a 5 per cent solution is an approximately isotonic but electrolyte-free fluid that supplies 50 gm of dextrose per liter. Dextrose solutions provide free water and energy. Approximately 4 kcal of energy are produced by the oxidative metabolism of each gram of dextrose. Dextrose-containing fluids are particularly indicated in those horses that develop dehydration and relative water deficit due to an inability to eat or drink. These energy-containing fluids could be effectively employed in horses with serious systemic diseases and associated anorexia. This is particularly true of neonatal foals that have limited energy reserves. Despite the hyperglycemia seen in certain types of shock, the glucose utilization rate is actually increased so that maintenance of glucose concentration by parenteral administration in addition to volume replacement has beneficial effects. Dextrose provides readily metabolizable energy required by the brain, erythrocytes, and other tissues and tends to have a protein-sparing effect. Although it would be difficult to supply all of a horse's energy needs with 5 per cent dextrose,

administration at a rate as low a 1 l per hour would provide 4.8 Mcal per day. This is approximately equal to the estimated irreversible glucose utilization rate and approximately one third of the basal metabolic energy expenditure for a 1000 lb horse. If dextrose-containing fluids are administered at a rate sufficient to produce hyperglycemia (i.e., greater than 100 gm dextrose per hour), the clinicopathologic effects would be decreased plasma sodium concentration, normal to increased osmolality, and minimal effect on PCV or TPP concentration. Once the glucose is metabolized, the remaining free water will distribute proportionally between the intracellular and extracellular fluid volumes.

EVALUATION OF DEFICIT

Recommendations for fluid therapy in horses have largely been based on data generated in other species. The most frequently used approaches are standardized treatment regimens designed to correct anticipated alterations or deficits. As an example, massive volumes of polyionic fluids and sodium bicarbonate have been recommended for routine treatment of horses with acute diarrhea, colic, or exertional myopathies. Indeed, hypovolemic shock and an accompanying metabolic acidosis are likely to occur in the later, terminal stages of these disease processes. This approach focuses on those horses with the most severe alterations and least favorable prognosis. It may be more appropriate to consider the larger group of horses with milder, developing alterations that are apt to be responsive to appropriate fluid therapy. Even more importantly, the anticipated deficits for most forms of dehydration of horses are not accurately known. Net fluid and electrolyte deficits occur as a result of alteration of both intake and output by all routes. Accumulated fluid and electrolyte deficits, thus, vary from case to case depending upon these factors and the staging or time course of the disease process.

A more flexible approach is based on evaluation of the individual patient to meet its specific and often changing needs. This may not be as difficult or impractical as it may seem. A wide variety of clinical and clinicopathologic data are available to assist in this evaluation and are listed in Table 2. In

TABLE 2. CLINICOPATHOLOGIC FEATURES OF DEHYDRATED HORSES

	Body Wt (kg)	PCV (%)	TPP (gm/dl)	Na (mEq/l)	K (mEq/l)	Cl (mEq/l)	Blood pH	HCO₃ (mEq/l)	Pco₂ (mm Hg)	BB (mEq/l)
Normal	450	40	7.0	138	4.0	100	7.40	24	40	+2
Horse A	425	55	9.5	120	2.5	94	7.20	14	39	−10
Horse B	400	46	7.9	147	3.5	105	7.38	21	38	0
Horse C	440	60	9.0	138	3.8	102	7.30	20	42	−6

some cases, however, the clinician must reach a decision alone in a cold and dark stall aided only by a flashlight. Fortunately, most clinical situations lie somewhere between the most and the least ideal. While appreciating that some of the diagnostic information to be discussed may be unavailable in certain instances, it is important that the clinician effectively utilizes all available information. The critical element is not the number of laboratory samples analyzed but is the exercise of clinical judgment correlating the history, clinical signs, and any available additional information.

FLUID AND ELECTROLYTE BALANCE

A useful place to start the evaluation of fluid balance is a consideration of the input and output. Homeostasis is associated with a balance between these factors that may vary widely. Alterations occur when intake is inadequate to balance normal to increased output. Input and output may vary substantially in response to various physiologic or pathologic processes. Simple anorexia, a sign that accompanies many systemic diseases, normally results in a marked diminution in fecal and to a lesser extent urinary water output and, thus, decreased voluntary water consumption. Water consumption is ordinarily adjusted to meet output and may vary from less than 5 l per day with food restriction to more than 100 l per day, depending on losses. Body size, quantity and composition of feed, environmental temperature, exercise, and lactation all have an impact on water intake. In most clinical situations, fecal losses are the largest single component of water output. Fecal water losses may vary from complete absence with anorexia to over 100 l per day with chronic diarrhea. Urinary losses may vary from approximately 2 l per day with anorexia to over 45 l in horses with Cushing's syndrome. Insensible water loss may decrease from 8.5 l to 1 to 3 l per day in certain circumstances. Normally sweat losses are negligible but may reach 10 to 15 l per hour with protracted exercise in hot climates.

Strict sodium economy is observed in normal resting horses on sodium-deficient all-roughage diets. Free choice salt or salt supplementation of 25 to 75 gm per day is recommended. Horses on all-roughage diets have an enormous potassium intake (2000 to more than 5000 mEq per day). Potassium is largely absorbed in the small intestine and colon, and excesses are eliminated by renal excretion. This high dietary potassium intake is the principal reason that potassium depletion is generally unrecognized in horses recovering from dehydration that begin eating normally, However, substantial potassium deficits may develop in horses with anorexia owing to continued renal excretion. Inappropriate fluid therapy may also contribute to increased potassium losses and unrecognized potassium depletion in some circumstances. These great variations in input and output make accurate prediction of anticipated deficits extremely difficult in most clinical circumstances. Fortunately, accumulated fluid and electrolyte deficits have predictable clinical and clinicopathologic manifestations.

CLINICAL EVALUATION

Although not always available or completely reliable, an accurate history can be an invaluable diagnostic aid. The duration and severity of the primary problem responsible for dehydration should be noted and, when possible, resolved. Appetite and water consumption during this period are exceedingly important. Horses that continue to eat normally and have access to water and salt are not likely to develop severe imbalances requiring parenteral therapy. If input is adjusted to meet output, fluid balance will be maintained even in the face of excessive losses. Inability to eat or drink in the face of increased losses may lead to the development of serious dehydration.

When sodium depletion is associated with dehydration, profound and rapidly developing physiologic effects may be observed. The sodium content is the principal determinant of ECF volume. Sodium deficits result in decreases in ECF volume, which are always reflected by decreased plasma volume. Clinical signs of sodium depletion are, thus, those of developing hypovolemia. Sodium depletion is not normally produced by dietary restriction but most often occurs when there has been an excessive loss of sodium-containing fluids. Acute diarrhea, massive sweat losses, or excessive use of diuretics produce similar effects that are related to sodium depletion. Obstructive bowel disease or acute peritonitis may produce similar effects by a compartmentalization of sodium-containing fluids. The common clinical signs associated with sodium depletion are elevated heart rate, decreased pulse pressure, decreased jugular distensibility, increased capillary refill time, and decreased urine output. Edema is the clinical indicator of sodium excess.

Clinical signs of dehydration include altered skin turgor, dry mucous membranes, drawn-up abdomen, and sunken eyes. It is generally said that these signs are first recognizable with fluid deficits of 4 to 5 per cent of body weight and become progressively more severe with fluid deficits of 10 per cent of body weight or more. While this clinical assessment is important and most experienced clinicians are comfortable using it, there is little accurate documentation of this relationship. Measured change in body weight provides a much more accurate estimate of net change in fluid balance during dehydration and in response to therapy. It should be noted that it is possible to have dehydration with or without sodium depletion and vice versa.

CLINICOPATHOLOGIC EVALUATION

Clinical and laboratory data, when used appropriately, provide a quantitative as well as qualitative guide for the assessment of fluid and electrolyte imbalances and response to therapy. Each of the diagnostic procedures will be discussed in relationship to specific deficits.

Body Weight. In acute situations, 90 per cent or more of weight change is related to change in fluid balance. The total body water (TBW) of a 450 kg horse is approximately 300 l. A weight loss of 50 kg represents a fluid loss of 45 l, leaving a postdehydration TBW of 255 l, a 15 per cent reduction in body water. There is a relationship between electrolyte losses and the compartmental distribution of the fluid loss. If large amounts of sodium are lost as with acute diarrhea, the extracellular fluid volume will bear most of the decrease. With food and water deprivation and developing potassium depletion, most of the fluid deficit will be from the intracellular compartment.

Sodium Concentration. Plasma sodium concentration does not always provide a reliable guide to sodium depletion or excess. The serum sodium concentration reflects the relationship between the exchangeable sodium content of the ECF, the exchangeable potassium content of the ICF, and the TBW:

$$\text{Serum Na} \simeq \frac{\text{Exchangeable Na} + \text{Exchangeable K}}{\text{TBW}}$$

Hypernatremia (Na greater than 146 mEq per l) indicates a decrease in body water in relation to the exchangeable cations sodium and potassium (i.e., a relative water deficit). This is an indication for volume replacement using electrolyte-free fluids. Hyponatremia (Na less than 132 mEq per l) occurs when the combined loss of both sodium and potassium exceeds water loss (i.e., a relative water excess). This most commonly occurs when there has been both fluid and electrolyte loss as with diarrhea followed by partial to complete replacement of the water deficit by water consumption. The therapeutic implications of hyponatremia are that all fluids administered can be electrolyte-containing. The persistence of hyponatremia in some horses given volumes of sodium-containing fluids underscores the importance of replacement of the coexisting potassium deficit. If the combined losses of sodium and potassium relative to water are 140 to 150 mEq per l, there will be little change in sodium concen-

tration. Thus, the combined loss of sodium and potassium of 6300 mEq in our horse with a 45 l fluid deficit may have profound physiologic effects, but the plasma sodium concentration is likely to remain unchanged. Sodium concentration is a guide to relative water balance and when used as such is an exceedingly useful therapeutic indicator.

Packed Cell Volume and Total Plasma Protein Concentration. The availability of the microhematocrit and refractometer have made determination of PCV and TPP concentration the two most commonly employed laboratory tests for evaluation of dehydration. Although it is widely believed that increases in PCV and TPP concentration reflect the degree of dehydration (i.e., water loss), available experimental data have not supported this conclusion (Table 3). Changes in PCV and TPP concentration are much more closely correlated to changes in sodium balance than water balance. Sodium deficits cause decreases in ECF volume, which are always reflected by changes in plasma volume. The reverse is not always true. To use PCV and TPP concentration as indexes of change in plasma volume, initial volumes must be known, and blood or protein loss must be minimal. In dehydrated horses, increases in PCV and TPP concentration indicate sodium depletion. The percentage increase provides a crude quantitative index of the deficit and is a useful indicator of the adequacy of volume replacement with sodium-containing fluids. The foregoing discussion applies indirectly to third space problems associated with obstructive bowel disease. In some of these instances, marked decreases in plasma volume may occur with resultant increases in PCV and TPP concentration, while the ECF volume may remain un-

TABLE 3. PERCENTAGE CHANGE IN PACKED CELL VOLUME (PCV) AND PROTEIN CONCENTRATION AS INDICES OF CHANGE IN BODY WEIGHT AND SODIUM BALANCE

	Body Weight % Δ	Sodium Balance	PCV % Δ	TPP % Δ
Carlson,[2] saline infusion	+3.7%	+3000	−13%	−16%
Carlson,[2] water ingestion (following 72 Hr NPO)*	+7.4%	0	+5%	+1%
Tasker,[4, 5] NPO 7 days	−9.5%	−746	−3%	+13%
Carlson,[2] NPO 72 hours	−10.7%	−1800	+14%	+14%
Carlson,[2] Lasix infusion	−8.1%	−2400	+25%	+28%
Tasker,[4, 5] diarrhea 7 days	−9.4%	−4445	+34%	+40%

*NPO indicates non per os, i.e., complete food and water deprivation.

changed or actually increased. This is due to a redistribution of sodium-containing fluid from the rest of the ECF into the gastrointestinal tract.

Potassium Concentration. Potassium is the principal intracellular cation, and plasma potassium concentrations may not always accurately reflect net potassium balance. As an illustration, horses held without food and water developed a measured potassium deficit of nearly 4500 mEq. The serum potassium of these horses decreased from 4.3 to 3.5 mEq per l. Horses with induced diarrhea had a decrease in serum potassium from 4.3 to 2.1 mEq per l with a net potassium deficit of approximately 2000 mEq.[4, 5] These seemingly contradictory findings can be resolved in part by a consideration of potassium content as related to potassium capacity. With appropriate consideration for acid-base effects, alterations in serum or plasma potassium concentration reflect intracellular potassium content as related to intracellular capacity or volume. Hyperkalemia (potassium greater than 5.5 mEq per l) is not a common finding in dehydrated horses and when present is often associated with impaired renal function. Hypokalemia (potassium less than 3.0 mEq per l) is much more common and may produce adverse physiologic effects. Fluids administered to hypokalemic horses should contain potassium, but unless exceedingly careful monitoring is employed, the potassium concentration of these fluids should not be higher than 15 to 20 mEq per l. This is particularly true when large volumes of such fluids are administered rapidly. It is difficult to replace significant potassium deficits (i.e., 2000 to 5000 mEq) via the intravenous route. Fortunately, even large potassium deficits are rapidly replaced when horses begin to eat substantial amounts of hay or other potassium-rich forage. Potassium depletion is thus principally a problem of horses with anorexia.

Acid-Base Balance. Acid-base alterations are frequently but not invariably associated with fluid and electrolyte alterations in the horse. Primary respiratory problems of acidosis or alkalosis are reflected by alterations in P_{CO_2}. Severe pneumonia, obstructive lung disease, and general anesthesia may induce respiratory acidosis. Chronic hypercarbia may initiate a metabolic response with increases in bicarbonate, which dampen the effect of the increased CO_2 concentration on blood pH. Arterial blood gas evaluation is preferred in horses with respiratory problems, since the P_{O_2} and P_{CO_2} are of primary importance. Venous blood samples are easier to obtain than arterial samples and are reliable indicators of acid-base status of horses in most other disease states.

Metabolic acid-base alterations are of more common occurrence in the horse and are reflected by changes in bicarbonate concentration. Hypochloremic metabolic alkalosis occurs with some frequency in horses and may be associated with protracted exercise in hot environments, the initial stages of bowel obstruction, and iatrogenically following inappropriate bicarbonate administration. Blood pH, bicarbonate, and buffer base (BB) will be elevated. There is often a compensating increase in P_{CO_2}. Therapy for hypochloremic metabolic alkalosis is aimed at replacement of the chloride and potassium deficits with sodium or preferably potassium chloride salts.

Metabolic acidosis is the anticipated response in many serious systemic disorders, including acute diarrhea, obstructive bowel disease, exertional myopathies, and chronic renal failure. This acid-base alteration is not an invariable feature of these diseases, and blood gas evaluation should always precede bicarbonate administration. Metabolic acidosis is characterized by decreased blood pH, bicarbonate, and buffer base. Respiratory compensation may be noted with a decrease in P_{CO_2}. Estimates of bicarbonate requirements necessary to restore pH to normal levels can be calculated using the base deficit:

$$HCO_3^- \text{ (mEq/l)} = 0.4 \text{ body wt (kg)} \times \text{base deficit}$$

A 450 kg horse with a base deficit of 10 mEq per l would require approximately 1800 mEq of bicarbonate. This could be supplied in 3 l of 5 per cent $NaHCO_3$, which provides approximately 600 mEq of bicarbonate per l. It should be noted that 5 per cent $NaHCO_3$ is hypertonic and also supplies sodium at a concentration of 600 mEq per l.

Reliable acid-base data can be obtained from sealed heparinized blood samples for two to four hours after collection if stored in ice. When full laboratory facilities are not available, the simple Harleco procedure for total CO_2 estimation provides a good index of metabolic acid-base alterations. Approximately 95 per cent of the total CO_2 content is bicarbonate, which will be decreased in metabolic acidosis and increased in metabolic alkalosis. This procedure is an extremely valuable index of acid-base balance for after-hours clinical evaluation.

Renal Function. It is advisable to evaluate renal function in horses that require massive fluid therapy. Prerenal elevations of blood urea nitrogen (BUN) and creatinine are frequently noted with serious dehydration. These elevations are generally modest and decline as normal urine flow is established. When there are marked elevations in these parameters or a failure to decrease in response to therapy, or if there are abnormal findings in the urinalysis, close monitoring and control of fluid therapy are warranted.

Dehydration is generally associated with decreased urine production and increased urine specific gravity. Restoration of urine flow and decreasing urine specific gravity are good indexes of volume replacement in response to therapy. Urine electrolyte excretion is dependent upon a variety of factors, among which dietary intake is extremely important. Low urine sodium or chloride concentration may simply reflect renal conservation on salt-deficient diets. Low urine sodium and chloride concentrations may be seen in sodium depletion but are not always reliable indexes of ECF volume depletion. Low urine chloride may actually be noted when the extracellular fluid volume is expanding, as in heart failure, since sodium accumulation is generally the result of increased renal sodium retention. The greatest value of urine sodium and chloride concentration is the exclusion of extracellular fluid volume depletion as a primary problem. With a few uncommon exceptions, in horses with normal renal function, the finding of substantial urine sodium and chloride concentrations (i.e., 50 mEq per l or more) essentially excludes depletion of these ions as a primary problem. As an example, urine sodium and chloride concentration is high in horses held without food and water when the primary problem is a water deficit. In Tasker's study,[4, 5] there was nearly a hundredfold increase in urine sodium concentration in horses held without food or water for seven days. In our own studies, urine sodium and chloride concentration were generally greater than 90 mEq per l, with dehydration up to 10 per cent of body weight following food and water deprivation. Saline infusion in these horses resulted in nearly quantitative renal excretion of all the sodium and chloride infused at urine concentrations exceeding 200 mEq per l. Clearly, saline is not the fluid of choice for a primary water deficit, and urine sodium and chloride concentrations could have been used to predict this response.

FORMULATION OF PLANS FOR FLUID THERAPY

The initiation of fluid therapy as early as possible, prior to the development of massive deficits, enhances the probability of a favorable response. While this is not always possible, it may be unwise to make rapid and complete correction of all estimated deficits when large losses have occurred. A reasonable approach is to formulate a plan for fluid therapy designed to replace a portion of the estimated deficits in a specific period of time. The more critical the patient's condition, the shorter this time period should be. The patient should be monitored at frequent intervals, the response to therapy evaluated, and the plan adjusted as indicated.

The intravenous route of fluid administration should be employed in horses with serious dehydration, signs of hypovolemia, or diseases that may impair alimentary absorption (such as acute toxic

enteritis or obstructive bowel disease). The oral route should be used whenever it is felt that there will be adequate absorption. Isotonic or hypotonic solutions should be used in volumes no larger than 5 to 10 l given every 30 minutes to one hour. Voluntary water consumption should be monitored if at all possible, and this fluid should be counted as intake. In certain selected cases in which it may not be possible to use other routes of fluid administration, rehydration enemas may be beneficial. Unless the horse has a fever or diarrhea or the environmental temperature is high, maintenance water requirements for horses are probably 10 to 15 l per day.

The evaluation plans for fluid therapy of the three horses listed in Table 2 illustrate the approach taken. In each instance, a combination of clinical and clinicopathologic data is considered. The normal values listed should be taken as the predehydration data for these three horses.

Horse A was presented with acute diarrhea of two days' duration. Fecal losses had been massive, and although the horse was eating little, large volumes of water had been consumed. The horse was depressed and had an increased capillary refill time, increased pulse rate, decreased pulse pressure and jugular distensibility, and slight to moderate dehydration. The changes in body weight and sodium concentration indicate that the net fluid deficit is between 20 and 25 l, but there is a relative water excess. History of diarrhea, the signs of hypovolemia, and marked increase in PCV and protein concentrations indicate substantial sodium depletion. Additionally, there is a significant metabolic acidosis. The plan for fluid therapy during the initial eight-hour period was 22 l of balanced polyionic replacement fluid intravenously with an initial flow rate of 5 to 10 l per hour. Additionally, the horse received 3 l of 5 per cent sodium bicarbonate. These fluids provide nearly 4800 mEq of sodium in 25 l. Although the potassium concentration of these fluids could be fortified up to 15 to 20 mEq per l, the total amount of potassium administered would be less than 500 mEq, while probably the potassium deficit may exceed 3000 mEq. The potassium deficit will not be fully replaced until the horse begins to eat. Should the horse remain anorectic, oral supplementation with potassium chloride 40 gm three times a day should be considered. At the end of the initial treatment period, the horse should be reevaluated, and the plan for the next period should be based on the response to therapy. Renal function should be evaluated, as this horse may have a prerenal azotemia.

Horse B has been unable to eat or drink for a least three days. The horse was depressed and moderately dehydrated, and the abdomen was drawn. The change in body weight indicates a fluid deficit of 45 to 50 l, and the increased serum sodium concentration indicates that most of the fluid loss was as water (relative water deficit). Water depletion appears to be the major problem, and the modest increases in PCV and protein concentration suggest minimal sodium depletion. It is probable that urine sodium and chloride concentrations would be high. Administration of balanced polyionic replacement fluid to this horse would be inappropriate. Simple provision of drinking water in graded amounts may be the treatment of choice. If this is not possible and there are no other contraindications, water may be given by stomach tube in amounts of 5 to 10 l every two to three hours. Electrolyte supplementation of this water should be in small amounts. Commercially available packets of electrolytes and glucose* are most convenient and should be diluted to provide sodium at a concentration of 20 to 40 mEq per l. It may be advisable to add supplemental potassium to this mixture. If the horse must be treated parenterally, the fluid of choice may be potassium-fortified 5 per cent dextrose or one of the commercially available dextrose-containing polyionic maintenance solutions. Obviously the major therapeutic effort should be directed at resolution of the process responsible for the inability to eat or drink.

Horse C was presented with colic of 12 to 24 hours' duration. Pulse and respiratory rates were elevated, capillary refill time was increased, and pulse pressure and jugular distensibility were diminished. The horse was in moderate pain, and the abdomen was distended. The clinical signs and elevated PCV and plasma protein suggest developing hypovolemia. This is probably the result of a com-

partmentalization of fluid within the intestinal tract. The abdominal distention and minimal change in body weight support this view. Therapy in this horse is aimed at a physiologic effect, restoration of effective circulating blood volume, rather than replacement of specific deficits. Polyionic sodium-containing fluids should be administered initially at a fairly rapid rate—10 l per hour or more with close monitoring of the response to therapy. Volume replacement will probably correct the mild metabolic acidosis, but administration of sodium bicarbonate should be considered if the base deficit increases. Restoration of hydration and fluid volume is particularly helpful in the treatment of impaction colic. While sodium-containing fluids result in transient expansion of plasma volume, in time these fluids will distribute to all of the ECF, including the intestinal tract. Unless the process responsible for the third space problem is resolved, some of the administered fluid will also enter this space. With rapid progression and severe changes noted in this horse, surgical intervention may be necessary.

References

1. Carlson, G. P.: Fluid therapy in horses with acute diarrhea. Vet. Clin. North Am., *1*:313, 1979.
2. Carlson, G. P.: Unpublished data, Equine Disease Research Laboratory, University of California, Davis, CA.
3. Rose, R. J.: A physiologic approach to fluid and electrolyte therapy in the horse. Eq. Vet. J., *13*:7, 1981.
4. Tasker, J. B.: Fluid and electrolyte studies in the horse. IV. The effects of fasting and thirsting. Cornell Vet., *57*:658, 1967.
5. Tasker, J. B.: Fluid and electrolyte studies in the horse. V. The effects of diarrhea. Cornell Vet., *57*:668, 1967.
6. Waterman, A.: A review of the diagnosis and treatment of fluid and electrolyte disorders in the horse. Eq. Vet. J., 9:43, 1977.

*Eltrad 4000, Haver-Lockhart, Shawnee, KS 66201

MEDICAL MANAGEMENT OF THE EXHAUSTED HORSE

Gary P. Carlson, DAVIS, CALIFORNIA

The role of the veterinarian during endurance rides is the preservation of the health and well-being of these remarkable equine athletes. This consists of three major phases: (1) prevention of medical problems, (2) early recognition of potential problems, and (3) prompt and vigorous therapy when problems develop.

PREVENTION

Adequate training and sound experienced horsemanship are essential for the prevention of serious medical problems. Training schedules vary considerably but generally range from 100 to 200 miles per week. Successful competitors begin such training three to four months before the endurance season. This long period of training is necessary to condition the cardiovascular and musculoskeletal systems, in which a variety of adaptive responses are invoked. The extended training and conditioning period also provides a noncompetitive period in which the horseman develops an understanding of what his horse can and cannot do. Experienced horsemen who know their mounts are often able to recognize impending problems and by providing extra rest, altering the pace, or getting off the horse and walking, prevent such problems. On rugged uphill climbs, many riders will tail their horses up the slope. In hot weather most riders carry plastic containers or sponges and cool their horses down whenever water is available.

Feeding regimens vary considerably, but most endurance horses are fed a larger proportion of hay in relation to grain than most performance horses. A number of outstanding performers are fed high-quality alfalfa hay and no grain at all. Supplemental salt should always be available, and many riders provide salt supplementation during the rides. The horse should be allowed a drink at every opportunity, and the course of the ride should be arranged so as to provide frequent drinking places. Although some excitable and competitive horses will refuse to drink on the shorter rides of 50 miles or less, they should be encouraged and trained to do so. At rest stops, the horses should be provided with shade, fresh water, and feed. This is usually handled by the "pit crew" who travel ahead, make appropriate arrangements, and look after the horse and rider when they arrive. This is exceedingly important, since the rider is often more fatigued than the horse.

On particularly hot days, ride officials should warn competitors of potential heat-related problems. At times, the number of veterinary checkpoints are increased, or the time that horses must remain at those checkpoints is extended to slow the pace of the ride. There should be an adequate number of veterinarians on the ride to ensure close and careful examination of every horse before, during, and after the ride. In addition, a separate treatment crew should be available for horses requiring treatment. Radio communications, which are usually provided by local radio clubs, allow for close control of ride progress and the provision of prompt veterinary service where needed. A suitable trailer should be available for the transport of any ill or injured horses to an area where appropriate treatment can be administered.

RECOGNITION OF EXHAUSTION

The clinical signs of exhaustion are presented in Table 1. There are variations and gradations of severity of signs in individual horses. Aside from those horses that are forced to stop on the trail, most problems are recognized at the veterinary checkpoints or at the mandatory rest stops. All competing horses will have elevated rectal temperatures, pulse, and respiratory rates and variable dehydration on arrival at rest stops and checkpoints. The most reliable quantitative guide to impending exhaustion is the rate of recovery of normal pulse and respiratory rates. At the mandatory rest stops, the 30-minute

TABLE 1. CLINICAL SIGNS OF EXHAUSTION

Depression	Poor jugular distensibility
Elevated rectal temperature	Increased capillary refill time
Persistently elevated pulse and respiratory rates	Decreased pulse pressure
Dehydration	Intestinal atony
Anorexia	Dilated anus
Lack of thirst	Spasmodic colic
Ineffective sweating response	Muscle cramps, spasms
	Synchronous diaphragmatic flutter

postarrival pulse and respiratory rates must return to acceptable levels, usually 60 to 70 per minute and 40 per minute, respectively. At the veterinary checkpoints, which have shorter mandatory rest periods of 10 to 15 minutes, slightly higher values may be used. No horse should be allowed to proceed until pulse and respiratory rates have recovered sufficiently. Riders are informed of specific criteria to be used on the individual ride, and many riders will monitor the pulse and respiratory rates to pace their ride and to avoid problems at the veterinary inspection. Unless these horses are showing other signs of the exhaustive disease syndrome, most will respond to cooling, rest, feed, and water. They should, however, be closely watched until recovery is complete.

Recognition of the severely exhausted horse presents few diagnostic problems. These horses are usually severely depressed with little interest in food or water despite obvious dehydration. Most of these horses will continue to sweat, although at apparently reduced rates. Pulse and respiratory rates generally remain elevated despite the period of rest. Pulse pressure and jugular distensibility are usually decreased, and cardiac irregularities may be noted. Some horses will maintain a respiratory rate in excess of the heart rate. This so-called inversion is more common in warm, humid climates than in arid climates and is usually transient. Except for those horses that develop spasmodic colic, there is usually a marked diminution or absence of intestinal sounds and a lack of anal tone. These horses require prompt and vigorous therapy with careful monitoring to ensure that they respond. Some horses will also develop synchronous diaphragmatic flutter. This contraction of the diaphragm is recognized as a tic or spasm in the muscles of the flank that is synchronous with the heartbeat. It may occur on either the right or left side and in some instances is bilateral. The condition often develops during the rest period, and although not serious by itself, it generally indicates derangement of acid-base and electrolyte balances and is grounds for elimination from competition. This condition in endurance horses is generally self-limiting and responds promptly to therapy.

Horses manifesting depression and persistently elevated pulse and respiratory rates as their only problems may respond to rest, cooling, access to salt, and clean feed and water. A return of appetite and water consumption is a good indication of recovery. Horses should be closely watched, and if there is no improvement in 30 minutes, they should receive oral and/or intravenous fluids.

Rectal temperatures normally begin to return to normal 15 to 30 minutes after exercise. Horses with markedly elevated rectal temperatures (i.e., in excess of 105° F) or with persistently elevated rectal temperatures should be cooled with a spray of cold water in an area with free air movement. This is usually effective, and most horses will respond. Cold water enemas may be beneficial in severe cases of hyperthermia. Rapid cooling of horses with marked hyperthermia and signs of altered CNS function is essential. Antipyretics such as phenylbutazone or dipyrone may be of some benefit.

THERAPY

INTRAVENOUS FLUIDS

Horses with signs of severe exhaustion require prompt and vigorous fluid therapy. The aim of fluid therapy is the restoration of the volume deficit, correction of electrolyte deficits, and the provision of readily metabolizable energy as glucose. Since the principal problems in these horses are dehydration and sodium depletion, rapid restoration of the plasma and extracellular fluid (ECF) volume with sodium-containing replacement fluids is essential. Polyionic replacement solutions such as Ringer's solution would be an excellent fluid choice. Saline, although not a physiologically balanced solution, contains sodium and chloride in proportions that are appropriate to the likely deficits. Potassium should be added to these solutions to provide at least 10 mEq per l. Energy as glucose can be supplied as 5 per cent dextrose and may be extremely beneficial in horses with marked hypoglycemia. The suggested flow rate for 5 per cent dextrose is 2 l per hour. Horses with synchronous diaphragmatic flutter almost invariably have intestinal atony. These horses generally respond promptly to calcium solutions given intravenously. A 20 per cent solution of calcium borogluconate can be administered to effect with careful monitoring of the heart. Many veterinarians prefer to use one of the milk fever preparations that contain magnesium and glucose in addition to calcium. Intravenous administration of calcium solutions should be at a relatively slow rate to effect and should be discontinued if cardiac irregularities develop.

ORAL FLUIDS

Intravenous fluids can be supplemented or, in some cases, supplanted by fluids administered by a stomach tube. Fluids administered by this route appear to be well tolerated and fairly rapidly absorbed. This route of fluid administration offers the advantages of speed and convenience but probably should not be used in horses that are recumbent or manifesting signs of colic. Volumes administered at any one time should range from 5 to 10 l and may be repeated every 30 minutes to an hour as required. Fluid administration by this route should be discontinued if there is evidence of gastric reflux or abdominal discomfort. Either water alone or electrolyte-supplemented water may be administered. The addition of 40 gm of sodium chloride and 30 gm of potassium chloride to 10 l of water will provide 680 mEq of sodium, 400 mEq of potassium, and 1080 mEq of chloride with an approximate concentration of 68, 40, and 108 mEq per l, respectively. Hypertonic saline solutions should not be administered to these horses, since the osmotic gradient created may draw water into the bowel from an already compromised extracellular fluid volume.

RATE OF FLUID ADMINISTRATION

The volume, rate, and route of fluid administration should vary with the severity of the presenting problems. Since under field conditions, absolute losses are unknown, quantitative estimates provide a guide to the fluid and electrolyte requirements. Volume requirements may range from 20 to 40 l or more. In severely affected horses, sodium-containing fluids should be administered intravenously at a rate of 5 to 10 l per hour. In some instances, it may be necessary to catheterize both jugular veins or to use a pressure bulb to achieve flow rates required. Fifteen l of Ringer's solution or 13 l of saline will provide approximately 2000 mEq of sodium. Severely dehydrated horses with probable sodium deficits in excess of 4000 mEq may require twice this amount or more. The therapeutic emphasis in these horses is on the replacement of plasma and ECF volume with sodium-containing fluids. Responses to therapy include improvement in capillary refill time, pulse pressure, and jugular distensibility. The packed cell volume (PVC) and total plasma protein (TPP) concentrations will decline toward normal values in response to this form of therapy, but sodium concentration is usually unaltered. There may be a marked improvement in attitude and appetite. Establishment of normal urine flow is also a good indicator of the adequacy of volume replacement.

It will be noted that while all intravenous fluids should contain potassium, there is little prospect of replacing deficits of 1500 to 3000 mEq with intravenous fluids containing 10 mEq per l. Deficits of this magnitude may produce physiologic effects, especially if hypokalemia is pronounced, but are generally not so serious as the sodium depletion. Once the horse begins to eat substantial quantities of hay, the potassium deficit is readily replaced from this potassium-rich source.

The principal objective of fluid therapy in these horses is the partial restoration of homeostasis so that the horse recovers sufficiently to replenish its accumulated deficits by voluntary consumption. The provision of 50 to 100 gm of glucose as 5 per cent dextrose per hour will not provide for all the body's energy needs. It will, however, elevate blood glucose to normal levels or above and will provide the brain and other glucose-dependent organs with essential energy substrates at a critical time when body reserves may be depleted.

There appears to be little ground for the administration of sodium bicarbonate to horses with the exhaustive disease syndrome. Most of these horses have a normal acid-base balance or a mild metabolic alkalosis. Additionally, horses with chloride depletion and hypochloremia are more sensitive to bicarbonate administration, and a profound and persistent metabolic alkalosis may be created with adverse effects on ionized calcium and magnesium concentration as well as potassium. Contrary to popular belief and practice, we have not found metabolic acidosis to be a consistent feature with exertional rhabdomyolysis in horses. In fact, many of these horses have a mild metabolic alkalosis. Use of diuretics such as furosemide to promote urine flow is also unwise until fluid deficits have been replaced. Phenothiazine derivative tranquilizers have been recommended for the treatment of exertional rhab-domyolysis for their peripheral vasodilatory effects. The use of such hypotensive drugs in dehydrated horses manifesting signs of hypovolemia is definitely contraindicated. Some horses manifesting signs of muscle cramps or spasms do not appear to have major muscle destruction. The muscle cramps in these horses may be related to the fluid and electrolyte alterations, and many of these horses respond to walking. Horses with severe muscle damage and myoglobinuria are reluctant to move and should remain where they are. If dehydrated, these horses should receive fluids, and treatment generally includes vitamin E and selenium, B vitamins, and in some instances, corticosteroids or phenylbutazone (p. 101). Response to therapy is variable.

References

1. Carlson, G. P., Ocen, P. O., and Harrold, D.: Clinicopathologic alterations in normal and exhausted endurance horses. Theriogenology, 6:93, 1976.
2. Carlson, G. P.: Physiologic responses to endurance exercise. Proc. 25th Annu. Conv. Am. Assoc. Eq. Pract., 1979, p. 459.
3. Fowler, M. E.: Veterinary problems during endurance trail rides. Proc. 25th Annu. Conv. Am. Assoc. Eq. Pract., 1979, p. 469.
4. Hinton, M. H.: The biochemical and clinical aspects of exhaustion in the horse. Vet. Ann. 18:169, 1978.
5. Rose, R. J., Ilkiw, J. E., and Martin, I. C. A.: Blood-gas, acid-base and haematological values in horses during an endurance ride. Eq. Vet. J., 11:56, 1979.
6. Rose, R. J.: A physiological approach to fluid and electrolyte therapy in the horse. Eq. Vet. J., 13:7, 1981.

IMMUNOLOGIC DISEASES

Gary E. Rumbaugh, DAVIS, CALIFORNIA

Alex A. Ardans, DAVIS, CALIFORNIA

The domestic horse is immunocompetent at birth and is capable of reacting in several ways to exposure to foreign protein. These immune reactions may be responsible for resistance to infection, recovery from infection, or the imposition of immune-mediated disorders having an adverse affect on the animal.

ONTOGENY

It is now generally accepted that these immune reactions are mediated by at least two major classes of lymphocytes that are derived from a common stem cell precursor that arises in the yolk sac during fetal development. Postnatally, the bone marrow is the major source of lymphocyte precursor cells.

Developing lymphoid precursor cells may follow one of two maturational pathways. Those cells destined to become T lymphocytes migrate to the thymus as early as 11 to 12 weeks of gestation, where mitotic division and maturation occur. The equine thymus consists of left and right lobes and lies along the trachea. They then migrate to peripheral lymphoid tissues of the body, arriving as early as 13 weeks of gestation. T lymphocytes comprise the majority of lymphocytes in peripheral blood and play three major roles in immune responses: (1) they interact with B lymphocytes in the production of specific antibody, in which case they are referred to as helper T cells; (2) they may suppress immune responses and, in those cases, are classified as suppressor T lymphocytes; (3) finally, these lymphocytes are responsible for cell-mediated immunity, which is important in host defense against neoplastic cells, fungi, protozoa, intracellular bacteria, and some viral infections. Responsive T cells have been detected in the equine thymus at 80 days and the peripheral blood at 120 days of gestation.

B lymphocytes derived from similar lymphoid stem cells may require a similar intervening maturational phase. In birds, the bursa of Fabricius provides the maturational environment for B lymphocytes, but the mammalian counterpart of this tissue has never been conclusively identified. B lymphocytes express significant amounts of immunoglobulin (Ig) on their surfaces and can synthesize and secrete IgM, IgA, or IgG. On appropriate stimulation, B cells differentiate to plasma cells, which have a short life span and a remarkable capacity to synthesize and secrete immunoglobulin. Specific antibodies secreted by these cells play an important role in host defense against extracellular bacteria and some viral infections. Immunoglobulins have been detected in equine fetuses prior to 200 days of age.

Neutrophils and macrophages are significantly involved in host defense through the phagocytosis and enzymatic digestion of microorganisms. This process involves the ingestion of the agent, the joining of the phagosome with cytoplasmic lysosomal granules, and the release of degradative enzymes into the phagosome.

Under normal conditions, the interaction of antigen with immunologically specific and functionally mature lymphocytes results in an immune response. In brief, antigen interaction with T lymphocytes produces lymphokines, which may (1) augment or suppress the activity of T and B lymphocytes, (2) chemotactically attract lymphocytes, monocytes, or granulocytes, (3) inhibit the migration of leukocytes, and (4) cause cytolysis of cells bearing new surface antigens. Upon interaction with specific antigen, B lymphocytes secrete antibodies, which may directly neutralize some microbial agents, or more typically, antibody and components of the complement system interact to neutralize or lyse microbial agents. In addition, the interaction of antigen, antibody, and complement can augment the phagocytosis of infectious agents by neutrophils.

Occasionally this reaction becomes detrimental to the host through overproduction of antibody, antigen-antibody complex deposition in tissues rather than destruction, or the interaction and destruction of the body's own tissues instead of the microbial agent. These are often referred to as immune-mediated diseases, pemphigus vulgaris and purpura hemorrhagica (p. 307) being two of the more common examples.

EVALUATING THE EQUINE IMMUNE SYSTEM

When continuing and persistent clinical signs, unusual infecting agents, and conditions not responsive to appropriate therapy suggest a defect in the animal's defenses, a search for the immune system involved is initiated. The diagnosis of immune disorders in the horse is based on clinical and laboratory measurement of the components of the immune system.

COMPLETE BLOOD COUNT

Routine performance of CBCs in all cases of neonatal infections or persistent problems in older animals will often detect cases that should be more closely evaluated. An animal with unexplained marked and persistent lymphopenia should be evaluated for the possibility of an immunodeficiency syndrome.

B CELL FUNCTION

Serum Electrophoresis. As a tool for diagnosis of immunologic disorders, serum electrophoresis has very limited use, namely the detection of monoclonal or polyclonal gammopathies. Immunoglobulin deficiencies are not readily recognized unless they are absolute, because of the relatively wide range of values for gamma globulins in the horse and because IgM and IgA are found in the region in which other serum globulins would conceal their presence or absence.

Single Radial Immunodiffusion (SRID). While requiring the use of specialized equipment and trained personnel, SRID has the advantage of sensitivity and of being quantitative. The most common use of this procedure is in the quantification of immunoglobulins and complement components in the serum or secretion of affected animals. It serves as the most reliable method to detect an immunoglobulin (humoral) immunodeficiency disease. Because elevations in IgG, IgM, and IgA are seen in a myriad of infectious and noninfectious diseases, a definitive diagnosis based solely on SRID can be made only for absolute immunoglobulin deficiencies.

Simple Evaluation of Immunoglobulin Content. The use of the zinc sulfate turbidity test as an assessment of immunoglobulin content is discussed in the following section on passive transfer of immunoglobulins in the foal.

SPECIAL PROCEDURES

Immunofluorescence. This technique is a histochemical or cytochemical procedure most often used to locate or identify antigens in tissue (direct technique) or detect specific antibody in serum or other secretions (indirect technique). While this procedure has proved valuable in our laboratory in the diagnosis of certain dermatologic and renal conditions, it is a highly sophisticated technique and is only performed upon request by specialized laboratories.

Lymph Node Biopsy. The lymph nodes are placed on lymphatic channels in such a way that they can trap antigen being carried from the periphery of the body to the bloodstream. The interior of the lymph node is divided into a peripheral cortex containing predominantly B lymphocytes arranged in nodules. The next layer is the paracortical zone, consisting mainly of T lymphocytes. In athymic animals, this area is devoid of cells and can be considered a thymic-dependent area. The cells of the medulla include B lymphocytes, macrophages, reticular cells, and plasma cells arranged in cellular cords between the lymphatic sinuses.

T CELL FUNCTION

T Lymphocyte Evaluation. The majority of tests of equine T cell function require expensive, specialized equipment not readily available to clinicians. As mentioned later, the absence of T cells in a lymph node biopsy in the paracortical areas suggests a T cell deficiency.

Rejection of allogenic skin grafts is a well-recognized test of T cell response. Normal rejection time ranges from 11 to 14 days for the first graft. Retention beyond this time represents defective T cells.

Lymphocytes isolated from peripheral blood or from lymph nodes can be cultured. The ability of these cells to undergo DNA synthesis when stimulated with phytohemagglutinin (PHA) or concanavalin A (Con A) is a reflection of T lymphocyte function.

The absence of cells in the cortex indicates a deficiency in the B cell population, while decreased numbers or the absence of cells in the paracortical area points to a T cell deficiency. In the CID syndrome, there is almost a complete lack of cells in the peripheral lymph nodes.

IMMUNOLOGIC DISORDERS

IMMUNE DEFICIENCIES

In recent years, several immunologic disorders of foals have been described. While these are often exciting to diagnose and treat, one must be cautious in ensuring that ill foals are appropriately examined and treated adequately for the more common foalhood infectious problems before looking for the unusual problems.

PASSIVE IMMUNE TRANSFER

It has been said that the greatest single factor contributing to the maintenance of the newborn foal's health is the assurance that the foal gets an adequate quantity of colostrum.

The mare has a diffuse epitheliochorial type of placenta that does not allow transplacental passage of immune proteins during gestation; however, the dam gives the foal, through colostrum, temporary passive protection against a range of common microorganisms with which she has previously been challenged.

Absorption of these colostral immunoglobulins occurs via the epithelial cells of the foal's small intestine by an active process called "pinocytosis," or cell drinking. These cells have a rapid turnover rate and are replaced by more mature cells within 24 to 36 hours of life, ending absorption. No appreciable difference in the termination of this absorption has been observed in foals not fed colostrum, although the effects of complete starvation have not been investigated.

Peak values of passively acquired immunoglobulins are attained by approximately 18 hours of life and are usually equal to or slightly below that of the dam's serum. These passive antibody molecules gradually decline until they are completely absent by about five months of age.

Many reasons have been postulated for failure of this passive transfer mechanism, but premature onset of lactation in the mare is the most common. Its exact cause is obscure but is presumably associated with hormonal changes in association with placentitis, placental separation, or twinning. Since colostrum is secreted by the mammary gland only once during gestation, a steady drip from the udder over a few days can materially reduce the amount of immunoglobulin available to the foal. Failure to produce useful colostrum has been said to occur in some mares, but only one reference to this condition has been found in the literature. Other factors may involve malabsorption in the neonatal small intestine and undue stress of parturition. Prematurity does not appear to impair the ability of the neonatal intestine to absorb the large molecules, but mares foaling before approximately 320 days' gestation may not have had sufficient time or hormonal stimulus for colostrum production to take place.

Since the amount of immunoglobulin required for protection against infectious organisms depends on several factors, including environmental and management conditions, invading organisms, and effective titers of antibodies absorbed, it is difficult to define the level of protection needed by the young foal. The estimation of serum immunoglobulin concentrations in early life is, therefore, of clinical importance if failures of transfer or insufficient colostral immunoglobulins are to be identified in time to preclude neonatal disease through the use of immunoglubulin supplementation.

The zinc sulfate turbidity test is a rapid, acceptable method for determining failure of transfer of colostral immunoglobulins. The results from zinc sulfate turbidity examinations can be utilized in two ways. When time and equipment permit, the results can be correlated with a curve prepared from serum of known IgG concentrations. If a spectrophotometer is not available when the neonatal foal serum is examined, as may be the case in many field situations, the detection of cloudiness or opacity in the test tube is sufficient indication that the foal has suckled and absorbed colostral IgG. In practical field situations, we have often made use of the zinc sulfate turbidity test by comparing samples from the foal and the mare, since, according to previous reports, the newborn foal 18 to 24 hours of age should have circulating passively acquired immunoglobulin levels equal to or slightly lower than that of the adult (800 mg per dl IgG), making the dam an excellent reference point for visual assessment of the zinc sulfate turbidity test.

This test has limitations in that it is primarily qualitative, results vary with extremes of temperature, and the solution decays over time. New solutions should be made periodically and stored in a closed bottle.

Early recognition of failure of colostral immunoglobulin transfer is essential so that protection by supplementation of immunoglobulin can be timely. In the foal of less than 18 to 24 hours of age, oral colostral supplementation is preferable. Giving by bottle or nasogastric intubation 200 to 250 ml of frozen colostrum screened for anti–red blood cell (RBC) activity has produced satisfactory levels of serum immunoglobulin and should not overdistend the foal's stomach. Intravenous administration of anti-RBC alloantibody-free plasma from a locally selected equine donor is the recommended therapy for the older foal. A dosage rate of 20 ml per kg body weight, freshly thawed and warmed equine plasma has proved adequate in our practice. At this dosage, the average neonate receives approximately one liter.

If the precaution of serologic screening has not been taken, pooled plasma from three to four locally available geldings that have never received a blood transfusion is an acceptable alternative source of immunoglobulins.

COMBINED IMMUNODEFICIENCY

The combined (B and T lymphocyte) immunodeficiency (CID) syndrome has been recognized and partially characterized in foals of Arabian or part Arabian ancestry as a genetic defect transmitted as an autosomal recessive trait. Affected foals are markedly lymphopenic (less than 1000 per μl), possess only a rudimentary hypoplastic thymus, and the lymph nodes are devoid of lymphocytes. Such foals are incapable of responding to immunization and produce no immunoglobulin on their own. Presuckle serum samples lack IgM, and this is an important diagnostic feature of this disorder. CID foals

will absorb colostral immunoglobulin from the mare, and the quality and quantity of colostral immunoglobulins determine to a large extent the life expectancy of these foals. CID foals develop clinical infections from 2 to 65 days of age, and all identified CID foals to date have died by five months of age, regardless of antimicrobial therapy or thymic or lymphoid tissue transplants.

The emergence of several immunodeficiency disorders in foals emphasizes the need for differential diagnostic criteria so that a prognosis can be given and appropriate therapy can be instituted if indicated. Furthermore, as a diagnosis of immunodeficiency implicates both the dam and the sire as carriers of a possible genetic trait, accuracy of diagnosis is important. The minimal information required for a diagnosis of combined immunodeficiency is the age of the foal, a total lymphocyte count that is repeatable and stays below 600 cells per μl, a negative serum IgM presuckling value, and the status of cell-mediated immunity as measured by in vitro tests.

AGAMMAGLOBULINEMIA

Agammaglobulinemia has been identified in only two horses that had a complete absence of functional B lymphocytes but demonstrated normal T lymphocytes and cell-mediated immunity. Both horses were male, and both were over 15 months of age. Recurring bacterial infections that failed to respond or responded incompletely to standard therapy were seen in both cases. The mechanism whereby B cells were preferentially not produced in these animals remains to be elucidated, but their surviving longer than CID foals attests to the importance of T lymphocytes.

IgM DEFICIENCY

Several foals of Arabian and quarter horse breeding have been detected with low or absent IgM levels. This has been the only apparent immunologic deficit, as lymphocyte counts, immunoglobulins other than IgM, B and T cell numbers, and lymphocyte responses to in vitro stimulation have all been within normal limits. These animals have all presented with persistent respiratory infections that eventually resulted in their death over a period of four months to two years.

TRANSIENT HYPOGAMMAGLOBULINEMIA

Hypogammaglobulinemia as a result of delayed production of gamma globulins in a foal has been reported. This one foal did not reach normal levels of antibody until about four months of age. The foal had developed systemic infections resulting in abscesses.

References

1. MacKenzie, C. D.: Histological development of the thymic and intestinal lymphoid tissue of the horse. J. S. Afr. Vet. Assoc., *46*:47, 1975.
2. Perryman, L. E.: Primary and secondary immune deficiencies of domestic animals. Adv. Vet. Sci. Comp. Med., *33*:22, 1979.
3. Perryman, L. E., McGuire, T. C., Poppie, M. J., et al.: Pri-
mary immunodeficiency disorders in foals. Pathogenesis and differential diagnosis. Proceedings of the Fourth International Conference on Equine Infectious Diseases, Lyon, France. J. Equine Med. Surg., Suppl. 1, Princeton, NJ, Vet. Pub., Inc., 1978.
4. Rumbaugh, G. E., Ardans, A. A., Ginno, D., and Trommershausen-Smith, A.: Identification and treatment of colostrum-deficient foals. J. Am. Vet. Med. Assoc., *174*:273, 1979.

BLOOD TRANSFUSION

Paul G. Morris, MANHATTAN, KANSAS

INDICATIONS

Blood transfusions may be required when significant loss of whole blood, red blood cells, plasma, or platelets occurs. Clinically, the use of whole blood may be indicated in severe lacerations and certain surgical operations when both erythrocyte and volume losses occur. Red blood cells alone are needed in some cases of hemolytic anemia. Plasma can be beneficial in hypogammaglobulinemia caused by a failure of passive transfer, in hypoproteinemia as from severe diarrhea, or in warfarin poisoning where vitamin K–dependent clotting factors (II, VII, IX, and X) are low.[8] Platelets may be indicated in certain clinical conditions in which there are quantitative or qualitative platelet defects. Usually, though, most thrombocytopenias are successfully managed by administering steroids, and thrombopathias by removing the cause, such as phenylbutazone, aspirin, anti-inflammatory drugs, antihistamines, local anesthetics, promazine tranquilizers, phenothiazines, nitrofurans, sulfonamides, penicillins, estrogens, plasma expanders, and live virus vaccines.[5]

LABORATORY TESTS

Diagnostic laboratory tests that can aid in establishing the degree of blood or blood component loss have been discussed in previous sections (p. 293). A packed cell volume (PCV) declining to values of 15 per cent or less and hemoglobin values of less than 5 gm per 100 ml are indicative of deficient oxygen-carrying capacity for which transfusion should be considered. When whole blood loss occurs, the actual need for red blood cells and plasma may not be truly apparent until 12 to 24 hours posthemorrhage owing to the release of erythrocytes by splenic contraction, but a history of massive blood loss and clinical signs of hypovolemia are indications for transfusion. Serum protein concentrations of less than 3.0 gm per 100 ml or albumin values less than 1.5 gm per 100 ml are indications for plasma transfusion, particularly if edema is present.

Plasma transfusion should be considered in foals one day old or older in which a failure of passive transfer is suspected. The zinc sulfate turbidity test provides a simple estimate of globulin content, while more accurate estimates of immunoglobulin concentration can be made using commercial immunodiffusion kits. Plasma transfusion is definitely indicated if globulin concentration is less than 200 mg per dl and should strongly be considered in foals with concentrations between 200 and 400 mg per dl, depending upon clinical signs and management conditions.[3]

In cases of suspected or observed bleeding disorders, a coagulation profile should be requested. Prolonged clotting times or platelet counts less than 20,000 per μl support the need for plasma or platelet-rich plasma, respectively.

Whenever possible, compatibility testing should be done prior to transfusion. Preselection of suitable donors on a large brood farm or in the practice locale is possible using blood typing procedures.* The preferred donor is one whose blood is negative for A, C, and Q red blood cell antigens and contains no common antierythrocyte antibodies. Major and minor agglutination and lysis cross-matching tests can be performed before transfusion to further ensure compatibility. Lysis tests are performed by adding rabbit absorbed serum† to the donor-recipient mix-

---

*Serology Laboratory, University of California, Davis, CA 95616
†Pel Freez Biologicals, Inc., P.O. Box 68, Rogers AR 72756

tures, providing the complement necessary to activate lytic antibodies.[1, 11] These tests should reduce the likelihood of any immediate systemic reactions or later complications such as hemoglobinuric nephrosis.

In situations in which tests cannot be performed, a healthy male that has never had a transfusion is the most suitable donor. Multiparous mares should be avoided as donors, since previous sensitization to red blood cell antigens may have occurred.[11]

DOSAGE

The total dose of whole blood, red blood cells, or plasma required can only be estimated. When gamma globulin or coagulation factors are deficient, dosage formulas are more applicable. The blood volume of a 500 kg horse should be approximately 8 per cent of the body weight, or 40 l. The plasma volume is approximately 5 per cent or 25 l, and the red cell mass approximately 16 l. With massive acute blood loss, signs of hypovolemia may be evident before there are full hematologic manifestations of the extent of the anemia. The development of these signs depends upon the rate of blood loss as well as the volume lost. Volume deficits in a 500 kg horse with moderate signs of hypovolemia may exceed 8 l. The body's initial response to blood loss or hemolytic anemia is an expansion of plasma volume in an effort to restore blood volume. This contributes to the decline in measured PCV, red blood cell count, and hemoglobin concentration. Using the 500 kg horse as an example, a decrease in PCV from 40 per cent to 10 per cent implies a loss of 12 l of erythrocytes or more. If the entire deficit were to be replaced, it would require 30 l of blood with a PCV of 40 per cent. Such an approach would be impractical as well as inappropriate, leading to volume overload. The objective of blood transfusion is the preservation of blood volume and the oxygen-carrying capacity of the blood until the marrow's regenerative response can repair the deficits. In most cases, replacement of 20 to 40 per cent of the deficit, in the previous example 6 to 12 l, appears adequate. Since there are potential problems with unmatched transfusions, particularly in fillies and mares with breeding potential, blood transfusions should be reserved for those situations in which they are essential. The survival of transfused red cells in horses is only four to six days when compatibility tests are utilized.[7] Longer survival of transfused cells may be possible if donors are selected by more careful blood typing procedures. In spite of the short red cell life, whole blood or red blood cell transfusions are clinically effective, even life-saving in certain cases, and should be administered when indicated.

Protein deficits can be estimated based upon the plasma volume rather than the blood volume. If the normal plasma protein value is approximately 7 gm per 100 ml and the recipient's plasma protein concentration has decreased to 3 gm per 100 ml, a protein deficit of 4 gm per 100 ml, or 40 gm per l, exists. In a 500 kg horse with a plasma volume of 25 l and a plasma protein deficit of 40 gm per l, the total protein deficit is at least 1000 gm. Replacement of 100 per cent of this deficit would require 14.3 l of plasma; 50 per cent replacement would be 7.2 l. These calculations provide only a crude estimate, since the volume distribution of plasma proteins is nearly twice the plasma volume.

Gamma globulin requirements can generally be met by providing 20 ml per kg of donor plasma or 1 to 2 l of plasma to the foal. Replacement of coagulation factors may require 3 to 5 l per 500 kg, although dosage should be adjusted depending upon clinical and clinicopathologic responses.

COLLECTION

Anticoagulants. Anticoagulants that can be employed if blood is to be used immediately include sodium citrate, which acts by chelating calcium or heparin, which interferes with the action of thrombin and certain other activated coagulation factors. Sodium citrate solutions* in concentrations of 2.5 to 4 per cent are added as one part to nine parts of blood. Heparin† is an effective anticoagulant when used at 4.5 to 5 units per ml of blood. If heparinized blood is not used immediately, it should be stored at 1 to 6°C and used within 48 hours. When transfusion volumes of greater than 10 to 20 ml per kg are anticipated, heparin should be avoided, since bleeding problems could be associated with heparinizing dosages of 50 to 100 units per kg. Consequently, heparin should be utilized only when small volumes are needed and when sodium citrate is not available.

Although most equine blood for transfusion is used immediately, blood can be stored, but an anticoagulant storage medium is required. In human blood centers, CPDA-1 (citrate-phosphate-dextrose adenine) is preferred, since greater than 70 per cent of the red blood cells are viable at the end of five weeks. Other anticoagulant storage media, such as CPD (citrate-phosphate-dextrose) and ACD (acid-citrate-dextrose), provide only a three-week life span. A laboratory prepared storage medium for

---

*Sodium citrate solution, 2.5 per cent, Veterinary Laboratories, Inc., Lenexa, KS 66215

†Heparin sodium injection, 1000 units per ml, Elkins-Sinn, Inc., 2 Easterbrook Lane, Cherry Hill, NJ 08034

blood containing CPD with trisodium ascorbate-2 phosphate allows a six-week life span for dog blood[10] but is not commercially available. The best medium for horse blood has not been established, but based upon the preceding information, CPDA-1 may be the one of choice.

Containers. Plastic containers are preferred over glass for blood collection. These containers do not activate platelets or Factor XII and do not cause red cell injury associated with nonsiliconized glass containers.[5] In addition, they are unbreakable. Plastic collection bags offer distinct advantages of convenience, requiring little storage space and coming in prepared sterile packages. Plastic carboys* (polypropylene) in 4 or 8 l sizes can be reused and sterilized. This may be an advantage in practices where large blood volumes are collected more frequently.

Plastic bags† come either in blood pack units with CPDA-1 medium‡ or transfer pack units to which an anticoagulant, generally sodium citrate or ACD, can be added. In most cases, utilization of 1 or 2 l transfer packs§ is the most economical. If the blood pack units are used, integral donor tubing is attached to the bag, avoiding the need for an additional collection set. If the transfer pack units are used, it becomes necessary to utilize a transfer set, since the integral tubing has a coupler end rather than a needle adapter end. A transfer set‖ having a needle adapter end is connected to a 9- to 12-gauge needle that has been passed into the animal's jugular vein. At the opposite end, a coupler is inserted into one of the ports in the transfer pack. If a plastic carboy is utilized, the coupler end can be placed inside a tubulation port, or the two can be connected with tubing. After collection, the port opening can be closed with a sampling site coupler** or by clamping the tubing.

SEPARATION

Unless whole blood is required, erythrocytes and plasma may be separated by centrifuging or sedimentation. Large container centrifuges are available for this purpose and may be found in large clinical laboratories or human blood banks. These facilities should be utilized if they are nearby and cooperative arrangements can be made. Otherwise, sedimentation is the method used. Equine red blood cells usually settle within two hours. If only red blood cells are needed, they can be given intravenously to the animal as they drain from the bottom of the container. Plasma can be obtained by draining the red cells off the bottom or removing the plasma from the top either by squeezing the plastic bag, aspiration, or siphoning. Squeezing the plastic bag generally results in a more sterile transfer. A commercial plasma extractor,* which has a back and a spring-loaded plate, can be used to put pressure on the plastic bag, forcing plasma out of the top tubing into a connected transfer pack. The flow is stopped by clamping metal clips† over the tubing. This method is fast and maintains sterility.

STORAGE

Whole blood or packed red blood cells, if not used immediately, should be refrigerated (4°C) and used as soon as possible. Since the need for blood transfusion is limited in most practices, there is little need for blood banking or prolonged storage. Fresh plasma is generally preferred for the correction of coagulation factor deficits.

Plasma can be frozen. At household freezer temperatures (-15 to $-20°C$), it should not be kept for more than two to four months; at $-40°C$ or colder it can be kept up to one year. These restrictions apply to plasma for preserving coagulation factors.[5] Whether this applies to plasma used for replacing protein or immunoglobulin deficits is not known, but plasma stored up to one year at $-20°C$ has been used successfully for these purposes.[3]

ADMINISTRATION

Before administering blood or any of its components, the fluid should be warmed to near body temperature. When giving whole blood, red blood cells, or plasma, an administration set with an inline filter should always be used to prevent the infusion of clots. When platelet-rich plasma is administered, it is best not to use a filter; otherwise, platelets will aggregate on the filter and will not be delivered to the patient.

Before administering any significant quantity of whole blood, red blood cells, or plasma, it is good practice to give a small test dose over a period of five minutes to check for an early reaction. Ideally, prednisolone sodium succinate as well as an antihistamine should be available for such emergencies.

The rate of administration will vary with the clinical problem. In acute, severe blood loss, flow rates

---

*Nalge Co., Division of Sybron Corp., Rochester, NY

†Fenwal System, catalog #4R4414, Division of Travenol Laboratories, Inc., Deerfield, IL 60015

‡Fenwal catalog #4R6102

§Fenwal catalog #4R2031 and 4R2041

‖Fenwal catalog #4R2240

**Fenwal catalog #4R2406

---

*Fenwal catalog #4R4414

†Fenwal catalog #4R4418

can be up to 20 ml per kg per hr in an adult 450 kg horse or up to 40 ml per kg per hr in a young foal. Similar rates are often used in administering a liter of plasma to foals that have failure of passive transfer, although preferably and particularly if a second liter is given, the flow rate should be reduced to 20 ml per kg per hr. When plasma is administered for treating hypoproteinemia, flow rates of 5 ml per kg per hr are less likely to cause problems of volume overload.

When replacing red blood cells, the option exists to use either whole blood or packed red blood cells. If whole blood is utilized, the risk of volume overload may be avoided by performing an exchange transfusion. The procedure is accomplished easily by putting a catheter in each jugular vein, one for giving and the other for removing blood. Instead, if one can wait a few hours after collecting blood, sufficient time will have transpired to allow the red cells to settle in the container. Subsequently, the red blood cells can be administered from the bottom of the container. The advantages of the exchange transfusion are that there is no time delay and the possible problem of volume overload with whole blood is avoided. The advantage of the latter method is that the patient receives just the red blood cells, which is the only blood component needed.

In some situations in which a compatible donor is not available, it may be possible to collect the patient's own blood in advance of surgery. Autologous red blood cells remain viable much longer than homologous blood cells. For elective operations in which excessive bleeding can be expected as in a nasal septum resection, collection of the animal's blood two to three weeks before surgery for administration during surgery is quite feasible. The retrieval and readministration of the patient's own lost blood is not feasible and has limited application in the horse.[2, 4]

References

1. Becht, J. L., and Page, E. H.: Neonatal isoerythrolysis in the foal: An evaluation of predictive and diagnostic field tests. Proc. 25th Annu. Conv. Am. Assoc. Eq. Pract., 25:247, 1979.
2. Brzica, S. M., Pineda, A. A., and Taswell, H. F.: Autologous blood transfusion. Mayo Clin. Proc., 51:723, 1976.
3. Crawford, T. B., and Perryman, L. E.: Diagnosis and treatment of failure of passive transfer in the foal. Equine Pract., 2:17, 1980.
4. Crowe, D. T.: Autotransfusion in the trauma patient. Vet. Clin. North Am. (Small Anim. Pract.), 10:581, 1980.
5. Dodds, W. J.: Bleeding disorders. In Ettinger, S. J., (ed.): Veterinary Internal Medicine: Diseases of the Dog and Cat, Vol. 2. Philadelphia, W. B. Saunders Co., 1975, pp 1679–1698.
6. Gimlette, T. M. D.: Transfusion of autologous and allogeneic chromium-51 labelled red cells in ponies. J. R. Soc. Med., 71:576, 1978.
7. Kallfelz, F. A., Whitlock, R. H., and Schultz, R. D.: Survival of ^{59}Fe-labeled erythrocytes in cross-transfused equine blood. Am. J. Vet. Res., 39:617, 1978.
8. Scott, E. A., Byars, T. D., and Lamar, A. M.: Warfarin anticoagulation in the horse. J. Am. Vet. Med. Assoc., 177:1146, 1980.
9. Smith, J. E., and Agar, N. S.: Studies on erythrocyte metabolism following acute blood loss in the horse. Equine Vet. J., 8:1, 1976.
10. Smith, J. E., Mahaffey, E, and Board, P.: A new storage medium for canine blood. J. Am. Vet. Med. Assoc., 172:701, 1978.
11. Stormont, C.: Positive horse identification. Part 2. Blood typing. Equine Pract., 1:48, 1979.

Section 7

NEUROLOGIC DISEASES

Edited by I. G. Mayhew

CEREBROSPINAL FLUID COLLECTION AND ANALYSIS 331

BEHAVIORAL ABNORMALITIES 335

HEAD TRAUMA 339

SEIZURE DISORDERS 344

EASTERN EQUINE ENCEPHALOMYELITIS 350

WESTERN EQUINE ENCEPHALOMYELITIS 352

SPINAL CORD TRAUMA 355

CERVICAL VERTEBRAL MALFORMATION 359

EQUINE HERPESVIRUS-1 MYELOENCEPHALITIS 362

EQUINE PROTOZOAL MYELOENCEPHALITIS 365

BOTULISM SYNDROMES: SHAKER FOALS AND FORAGE POISONING 367

POSTANESTHESIA MYOPATHY-NEUROPATHY 370

CEREBROSPINAL FLUID COLLECTION AND ANALYSIS

Carolyn R. Beal, GAINESVILLE, FLORIDA
Ian G. Mayhew, GAINESVILLE, FLORIDA

Cerebrospinal fluid (CSF) analysis can be an important diagnostic tool in the evaluation of diseases of the central nervous system. Although not diagnostic in itself, when used in conjunction with the physical and neurologic examinations and other diagnostic tests, CSF analysis may be the key to solving a difficult diagnosis. Several disorders of the central nervous system produce alterations in the cerebrospinal fluid that can be detected by a few simple analytical procedures that may be performed in any practice laboratory.

COLLECTION TECHNIQUES

Cerebrospinal fluid can be collected from the atlanto-occipital (AO) and lumbosacral (LS) sites. Collection from the LS site is usually the method of choice in the ambulatory adult horse because general anesthesia is unnecessary. However, if an intracranial or cranial cervical lesion is suspected, an AO tap may be indicated.

ATLANTO-OCCIPITAL SITE

With the adult horse under general anesthesia or the foal under physical and/or chemical restraint and in lateral recumbency, the neck is flexed so that the median axis of the head and the cervical vertebrae are at right angles to each other. The nose is elevated to maintain the head in a horizontal plane. A styletted 18- or 20-gauge, 9 cm spinal needle* is used in adult horses. For foals, a 4 cm, 19- or 20-gauge disposable needle with a plastic hub or a 6 cm, 23-gauge styletted spinal needle can be used. The advantage of the disposable needle is that CSF appears in the hub immediately when the subarachnoid space is penetrated, but obviously there is more risk of removing CNS tissue if such an unstyletted needle penetrates the medulla. The needle is inserted through the skin of the aseptically prepared site into the subarachnoid space at the intersection of imaginary lines drawn between the cranial borders of the wings of the atlas and along the dorsal midline, aiming toward the lower jaw (Fig. 1–1).

The depth of the subarachnoid space is between 5 and 8 cm in adult horses and 2 to 4 cm in foals. Upon entry, a popping sensation may be felt as the atlanto-occipital membrane and cervical dura mater are penetrated, usually simultaneously. The stylet can then be removed, and success is indicated by the presence of CSF at the needle hub. Cerebrospinal fluid pressure may be measured with a sterile manometer* when the dura is first penetrated (opening pressure) and after withdrawal of a 2 to 5 ml CSF sample (closing pressure). Penetration of the medulla during an AO CSF tap is a risk. Also, if there is increased CSF pressure, relieving this pressure by removing fluid from this site should be done with extreme care because herniation of the cerebrum and cerebellum caudally under the bony ridges of the calvarium is a possibility. This can cause damage to the brain stem, even to the extent of respiratory arrest.

LUMBOSACRAL SITE

In the standing horse, the spinal needle is inserted, after local analgesia and appropriate restraint, into the aseptically prepared site through a small stab incision made with a sterile surgical blade. The site is depicted and landmarks are explained in Figure 2. In animals standing up to 12 hands (120 cm) high, a 9 cm 18- or 20-gauge spinal needle can be used. In horses from 12 to 17 hands (175 cm) tall, a 15 cm 18-gauge spinal needle is used. A special 20 or 23 cm needle with a stylet may be needed in horses over 17 hands. The average depth of the subarachnoid space at this site in a 450 kg horse is approximately 13 cm, and the lumbosacral space diameter is approximately 1 cm. Penetration through the LS interarcuate ligament, dura mater, and arachnoid membrane often gives a characteristic sensation of change in resistance. Tail movement and some slight response by the patient usually accompanies this penetration. CSF can even be obtained from the ventral subarachnoid space by advancing the needle to the vertebral canal floor and withdrawing slightly without overt clinical problems.

*Becton, Dickinson and Co., Rutherford, NJ

*Manometer Tray, Pharmaseal Laboratories, Glendale, CA 91201

331

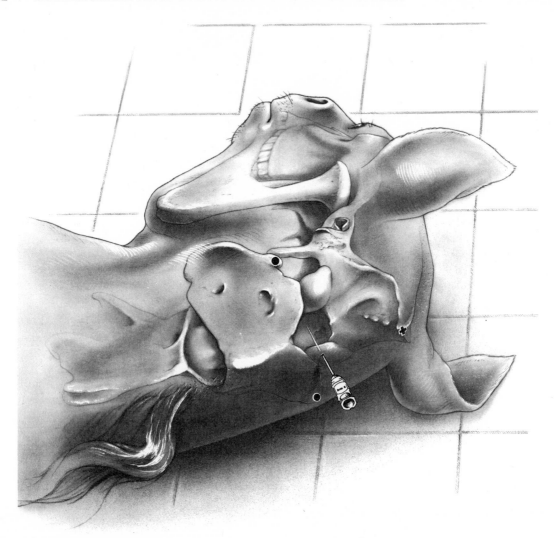

Figure 1. Atlanto-occipital cerebrospinal fluid collection from the recumbent horse. Spinal needle in position with stilette removed. Palpable landmarks are the cranial borders of the atlas (●——●) and the external occipital protuberance (+) on the dorsal midline. (From deLahunta, A.: Veterinary Neuroanatomy and Clinical Neurology. Philadelphia, W. B. Saunders Co., 1977, p. 44.)

ANALYSIS TECHNIQUES

Cells in CSF degenerate rapidly, presumably because of the minimal amount of protein present for support. Without fixation, cells may become morphologically undifferentiable within less than one hour. Thus, for optimal results, the cytologic analysis needs to be completed within 30 minutes of collection. The total cell count should be performed first and the 25-minute sedimentation started immediately if leukocytic pleocytosis is evinced to ensure the least amount of degeneration of the cells.

Increased numbers of white cells signifies an inflammatory reaction. An extremely turbid sample indicates very high amounts of protein and/or cells. Either of these indications suggests the advisability of saving some of the sterile sample for culture. Normal horse CSF has a cellular population of less than 8 mononuclear leukocytes per μl, usually with a higher percentage of lymphocytes than monocytes. When a mononuclear pleocytosis occurs, a viral cause may be suspected. An important exception to this rule is noticed in acute alphaviral encephalitides, especially eastern equine encephalomyelitis (EEE). These diseases typically produce a profound neutrophilic response in the first few days, which later becomes the expected mononuclear leukocytosis. Virus isolation attempts from CSF may be helpful if EEE is one of the differential diagnoses. In acute, subacute, or chronic stages of diseases such as western equine encephalomyelitis (WEE) and equine herpesvirus-1 (EHV-1) myeloencephalitis, CSF viral antibody titer determinations may be valuable.

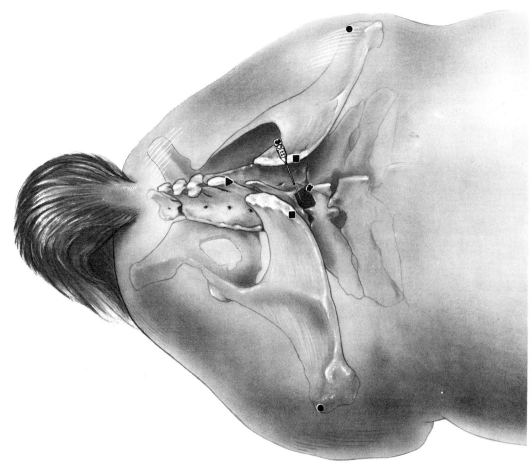

Figure 2. Lumbosacral cerebrospinal fluid collection from the standing horse. Spinal needle in position with stilette removed. Palpable landmarks are the caudal borders of each tuber coxae (●——●), the caudal edge of the spine of L6 (✛), the cranial edge of the second sacral spine (▲), and the cranial edge of each tuber sacrale (■——■). (From deLahunta, A.: Veterinary Neuroanatomy and Clinical Neurology. Philadelphia, W. B. Saunders Co., 1977, p. 45.)

CYTOLOGY

TOTAL CELL COUNT

Evenly distribute the cells in undiluted CSF by gentle inversion and apply to one side of a dual improved Neubauer hemocytometer chamber.* Counting all cells in five of the nine 1 sq mm areas and multiplying by 2 equals the total number of cells per μl: ten 1 sq mm areas contain 1 μl of fluid.

Sometimes differentiating between red blood cells (RBCs) and white blood cells (WBCs) can be difficult, so the other side of the counting chamber is filled with CSF that has been mixed in a 1:10 WBC dilution pipet with one part in 10 of diluting fluid (0.2 gm crystal or methyl violet dissolved in 10 cc of glacial acetic acid to yield 100 ml with distilled water). This dilution fluid lyses RBCs and stains

WBC nuclei in approximately two minutes. Once again, five of the 1 sq mm areas are counted, and the result is multiplied by 2.2 (derived by multiplying 2 × the dilution factor 10:9). This product equals the number of WBC per μl. In formula form, this is represented as

$$WBC/\mu l = \text{leukocytes counted} \times \text{dilution}$$
$$\times \frac{10}{\#1 \text{ mm}^2 \text{ areas counted}}$$

Total cells per μl minus WBC per μl equals RBC per μl. Normal CSF contains no RBC, so any present are due to either recent hemorrhage or contamination of the sample with peripheral blood. The number of WBCs in the CSF due to peripheral blood contamination can be estimated by using the approximate ratio of 1 WBC per 500 RBC in peripheral blood and subtracting this value from the CSF WBCs. Caution should be utilized in interpreting results procured using this estimation tech-

---

*Fisher Scientific Co., Fairlawn, NJ

nique because it has been shown to be unreliable. Another tap may be performed in 24 hours, but interpretation of subtle abnormalities in such a sample is difficult. To assist in distinguishing between iatrogenic blood contamination and previous hemorrhage, the remaining CSF can be centrifuged after the cytologic examination has been performed. If the supernatant becomes clear, this indicates a bloody tap, while if xanthochromia persists and the patient is not icteric, this is more consistent with injury or vascular leakage. With preexisting subarachnoid hemorrhage, red cells will usually be crenated or lysed, depending on the amount of time that has passed, because of the rapid degeneration of cells in CSF. Hemorrhage 48 hours prior to CSF collection results in a xanthochromia due to RBC breakdown products, which may take three to four weeks to disappear in the absence of further hemorrhage.

DIFFERENTIAL CELL COUNT

A differential count should be made whenever the WBC count is elevated. Up to 1 ml of freshly collected CSF is placed in a sedimentation chamber (Fig. 3). After 25 minutes, in which time the cells settle, the supernatant is aspirated (and saved for protein estimation), and the glass cylinder is removed by breaking the paraffin seal. Any excess CSF is removed by touching the center with absorbent paper. The slide is now lightly sprayed with fixative* or air dried and fixed in methanol for two minutes, allowed to dry, and then stained with any commercial WBC stain. A coverslip can be applied with mounting medium.†

PHYSICAL APPEARANCE

COLOR

Normal CSF from adult horses is transparent and grossly identical to distilled water when compared against a white background. Pink to red to brown coloration represents either iatrogenic blood contamination or recent hemorrhage. Xanthochromia (yellow coloration) usually represents older hemorrhage or leakage of blood pigments. A subtle pale yellow color with normal clarity may be acceptable in an icteric horse or a young foal.

CLARITY

Normal CSF is clear, as can be indicated by reading black print through the sample. If the CSF is

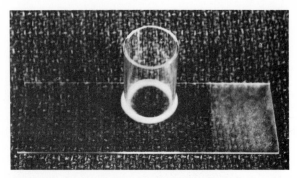

Figure 3. Sedimentation chambers are prepared by cutting the top inch off of a plain Vacutainer tube and sealing the smooth edge of this to a slide with paraffin.

opaque, the turbidity can be caused by large increases in the number of cells and/or in protein content. Color and clarity can be graded on a scale from +1 to +4 according to the intensity of the change noted.

PRELIMINARY SCREENING PROCEDURES

These methods are rapid but not necessarily accurate. They are useful as a quick indication of results to come and for accuracy comparisons.

REFRACTIVE INDEX

Refraction can be read on a refractometer,* which measures the deviation of light when it passes obliquely between media of different densities. Normal refraction values are from 17 to 20 (equivalent to refractive index values of 1.3347 to 1.3350). Elevated values represent increases in the quantity of total solids in the form of cells, protein, or other particles.

URINARY REAGENT STRIPS

Any of the available rapid test urinary reagent strips† may be useful in grossly quantifying blood pigment, protein and glucose contents, and the pH value. Normal values in the horse are blood, negative; glucose, trace to positive; pH, 8 ± 1. A protein value of 100 on the reagent strip is usually found in normal horse CSF, but this could also represent an elevated value. Values above this are to be considered elevated.

PANDY TEST

In this rapid test for protein, to 1 ml of Pandy reagent (10 mg carbolic acid crystals, to yield 100

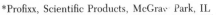

*Profixx, Scientific Products, McGraw Park, IL
†Permount, Fisher Scientific Co., Fairlawn, NJ

*Goldberg Refractometer, American Optical, Buffalo, NY
†Hemocombistix, Ames Co., Elkhart, IN

ml with distilled water) in a test tube, a few drops of CSF are added and shaken thoroughly. Normal CSF develops a faint turbidity, whereas pathologic CSF may develop a white turbidity. This turbidity can be graded +1 to +4 and is proportional to the globulin content. Normal CSF protein is composed almost entirely of albumin, which is normally capable of passing across the blood-CSF barrier in very small amounts. Globulins (which are larger molecules) can pass through in many pathologic conditions.

QUANTITATIVE PROTEIN CONTENT

To 1 ml or less (adjusted to 1 ml with distilled water) of fresh or frozen CSF, 3 ml normal saline and 1 ml 12.5 per cent trichloroacetic acid (TCA) are added and mixed. If less than 1 ml is used, this must be compensated for later in the calculations. This is left to stand for 5 to 10 minutes, and then the percentage transmittance is read from a standard laboratory spectrophotometer* set at a wave length of 420 nm. A distilled water blank is used. The mg per dl concentration of total protein can be determined from a previously prepared human protein standard curve. A protein standard close to the value determined on the urinary reagent strip should be run with every protein determination. If this standard is within ±5 per cent of the curve, the determination can be considered valid.

Values between 20 and 80 mg protein per dl

---

*Bausch and Lomb Spectronic 70, Fisher Scientific Co., Fairlawn, NJ

(mean ± 2 standard deviations) are regarded as normal. However, horses with no detectable CNS lesions and normal neurologic examinations have been found to have up to 120 mg per dl protein in their CSF on multiple occasions. Also, foals less than one week of age have been reported[6] to have CSF protein contents ranging from 90 to 250 mg per dl, but these authors suggested that these levels dropped toward normal adult levels within two weeks of birth. In light of this, it has been found useful to draw CSF simultaneously from the AO and LS sites and to compare the protein contents. A difference of more than 25 mg per dl between these indicates an elevated protein content, with the higher value probably being in the sample taken closest to the lesion.

Normal values for protein content should be determined for each laboratory.

References

1. de Lahunta, A.: Veterinary Neuroanatomy and Clinical Neurology. Philadelphia, W. B. Saunders Co., 1977, Ch. 3.
2. Hoerlein, B. F.: Canine Neurology: Diagnosis and Treatment, 3rd ed. Philadelphia, W. B. Saunders Co., 1978, pp. 138–148.
3. Kaneko, J. J., and Cornelius, C. E.: Clinical Biochemistry of Domestic Animals, 2nd ed. New York, Academic Press, 1971, Ch. 6.
4. Mayhew, I. G.: Collection of cerebrospinal fluid from the horse. Cornell Vet., 65:500, 1975.
5. Mayhew, I. G., and Beal, C. R.: Techniques of analysis of cerebrospinal fluid. Vet. Clin. North Am. (Small Anim. Pract.), 10(1):155, 1980.
6. Rossdale, P. D., Falk, M., Jeffcott, L. B., Palmer, A. C., and Ricketts, S. W.: A preliminary investigation of cerebrospinal fluid in the newborn foal as an aid to the study of cerebral damage. J. Reprod. Fertil., Suppl. 27:593, 1979.

BEHAVIORAL ABNORMALITIES

T. D. Byars, ATHENS, GEORGIA

Domestication of the horse has allowed selective breeding to increase the athletic potential of the species and training methods to overcome the unpredictable flight response described by horse owners and handlers as "spooking" or "shying." Breeds of horses have been developed that have differing degrees of athletic ability as well as differences in their normal psyche. The Thoroughbred is noted for its speed and "flighty" mentality, whereas draft breeds have been successfully bred for strength and a docile disposition at the expense of speed. Training capitalizes upon a particular breed's physical qualities while reinforcing predictable behavior.

NORMAL VARIATIONS IN BEHAVIOR

Normal behavior is influenced by the breed, age, sex, sexual and social status, environment, diet, management, and previous experiences.[4, 5, 7, 8] Shying, striking, kicking, and bucking are normal defensive responses. Veterinarians must give ample consideration to normal and abnormal horse behavior, since the administration of painful procedures is often essential to diagnosis and therapy. Restraint is vital to the safety of the practitioner, client, and horse and requires a reasonable degree of caution in order to avoid any excessive defensive behavior by the patient. Removing escape pathways and applying excessive restraint to normal horses can result in sulking. A sulking horse presents with a sleepy-eyed appearance as if unresponsive to external stimuli. Since sulking horses may suddenly react violently, the veterinarian may resort to chemical restraint, minimal physical restraint, or returning to the horse at a later time. Chronic sulking in horses should be considered either as a problem of disposition or as a response to improper training.

The social status or "peck-order" identifies either a dominant or submissive personality within a group. In crowded conditions, the submissive horse is often a poor doer owing to an unwillingness to compete for food. Recurring evidence of kick and bite wounds from the other horses suggests a submissive horse that should be segregated from the group. Snapping of the teeth and jaws in foals and yearlings is normal submissive behavior.[4] Orphan foals have the reputation of being submissive to other horses and obnoxious toward people. These problems are usually overcome when the orphan foal is introduced into a population of its peers at the appropriate time.[11]

STALLIONS

Stallions are particularly subject to variations in normal behavior due to excessive confinement, isolation, and inappropriate discipline or handling. Changes in sexual behavior include excessive aggression, loss of libido, and the inability to copulate.[8] Excessive aggression is influenced by the level of testosterone and sexual anxiety, especially in young stallions. In the United States, castration is the usual treatment for horses exhibiting this behavior.

MARES

Mares often exhibit changes in behavior during their estrous cycle, which can affect their success in racing, work, or show competition. Occasionally, veterinarians will be requested to control the estrous cycle by the use of progesterone injections (p. 405) to keep the mare out of heat. Some ill-tempered mares may require ovariectomy. Aggressive masculine behavior sometimes seen in mares may be due to androgen-secreting ovarian tumors. Surgical removal is required to correct the condition. Early postparturient mares are aggressive in order to protect the foal.[5]

REJECTION OF THE FOAL

Rejection of a foal by its dam is relatively rare but most commonly occurs with nervous maiden mares,

especially those that foal at pasture in the presence of older barren mares. An abundance of strangers or visitors at the time of or immediately following foaling can result in foal rejection.[5] In all such cases, the mare should be tranquilized in a quiet environment and encouraged to accept the foal. Failure to allow the foal to suckle may be due to a painful or engorged udder and, more rarely, mastitis. Proper treatment for these mares consists of tranquilization and the use of anti-inflammatory drugs such as the nonsteroidal analgesics.*† Physical restraint with a twitch may also be needed. Mastitic milk should be cultured and the mare treated with the appropriate antimicrobial agent. Agalactic mares frequently demonstrate a lack of maternal behavior.

VICES

Vices are objectionable to owners and handlers. The horse's social or physical environment is probably responsible for the majority of bad habits (Table 1). Crowding or intensive housing of animals that have been bred for locomotion is an invitation to abnormal mental and physical habits. Vices occurring in stalls include weaving, stall kicking, bucking, digging, nipping, savaging, masturbating, and cribbing. Vices occurring outdoors include fence pacing (rutters), masturbating, cribbing, dirt eating, and coprophagy. Fecal consumption in adolescent and mature horses is usually considered a vice, although improper feed texture, trace nutrient deficiencies, and hunger are often considered to be responsible. Coprophagy is normal in foals during the second to fifth weeks of life. Dirt eating is more commonly observed in foals than adults and is thought to be due to mineral, especially salt, deficiencies. Pica refers to a depraved appetite and is usually due to dietary deficiencies or metabolic disorders.

Cribbing is a vice in which bored horses of any age engage in intermittent aerophagia. They seldom start as wood chewers. The use of pelleted feeds is associated with cribbing and increases the incidence of wood chewing.[10] Treatment includes a change in environment, cribbing collars, hay fed free choice, increased pasture time, electrified fencing, and surgical intervention (p. 181). The most recent surgical procedure, the accessory neurectomy, even when combined with a myotomy is only partially successful.

Tail wringing is a vice of unknown etiology observed primarily in young show fillies. Because prolonged estrus has been suggested as a cause, pro-

---

*Sterile Phenylbutazone Injection, Med-Tech, Inc., Elwood, NJ 66024
†Banamine, Schering Corp., Kenilworth, NJ 07033

TABLE 1. CLINICAL BEHAVIOR AND TREATMENT OF COMMON VICES IN THE HORSE

Vice	Clinical Behavior	Treatment
Cribbing	Wood chewing.	Treat wood with repellents, remove pelleted diet, provide free choice hay or pasture, remove wood.
Cribbing (windsucking)	Grasps inanimate objects such as fences with the incisor teeth and sucks or gulps air (aerophagia). A grunting sound is heard.	Provide devices for mental diversion; cribbing collars, accessory neurectomy, sternocephalicus myotomy; electrify fences.
Coprophagy	Manure eating in horses from 6 months and older.	Adjust diet, increase pasture grazing.
Dirt eating	Eating dirt or sand; colic, obstipation, chronic diarrhea.	Adjust diet, provide salt, place feed up off the ground; routine catharsis.
Masturbation	Forcing the erect penis against the ventral abdomen until ejaculation occurs.	Stallion rings, abdominal wire brush harness.
Savaging	Violent or aggressive behavior toward humans or other horses usually exhibited by vicious biting, striking, and pawing.	Retraining, decrease isolation and confinement; muzzling, sedation, euthanasia for unresponsive cases.
Stall digging, bucking, weaving	Fractious stall behavior; sidesteps continually in the stall doorway.	Decrease confinement, provide companionship or devices such as a tire or hanging plastic jug for mental distraction.
Tail wringing	Tail held high over the back and then waved in windmill fashion when working.	Progesterone injections, epidural anesthesia, coccygeal myotomy.
Tongue sucking	Tongue is held outside the commissure of the mouth.	Change bits or tie the tongue in a normal position with gauze.
Head shaking or throwing	The horse throws its head upward toward the rider.	Check the ears for mites, inflammation, or neoplasia; check the teeth, change bridles, use of "tie-down on the tongue."

gesterone* and megestrol acetate† can be tried for prevention of estrus (p. 405). Trainers may request alcohol epidurals for long-term desensitization of the tail. Complications such as tail sloughing outweigh the benefits of this procedure.

Other less well-defined vices of performance horses include chronic sulking, tongue sucking, and head shaking. A thorough physical examination for evidence of a painful condition and for defective vision should be performed on sulking horses. A complete otoscopic examination should be performed on head shakers to rule out the presence of ticks or mites.[1] The teeth should also be examined to determine if there is a painful site associated with bridling (p. 186). The actual cause of head shaking will usually be elusive even after a thorough diagnostic work-up.

*Progesterone, Philadelphia Labs, Inc., Philadelphia, PA
†Ovaban, Schering Corp., Kenilworth, NJ 07033

PROBLEM BEHAVIOR

Self-mutilation, such as the aggressive gnawing of a limb or the abdomen, is fortunately a rare syndrome in horses. Violent biting or chewing of the skin occurs in stallions. The cause is unknown. The use of a companion animal or a change in housing and management practices is worth trying therapeutically, although a muzzle or neck cradle may eventually be required. Vicious behavior, such as chronic savaging and aggression, is relatively rare and is associated with isolation and excessive confinement, abuse, androgenic stimulation, and sexual anxieties. An extremely vicious horse is referred to as a rogue and is to be considered a dangerous animal. In Europe, the surgical procedure of leukotomy or frontal lobotomy has been used on rogue horses. The operation has not been proven consistently acceptable, since the centers of the brain responsible for aggression have not been defined.

A "dark-hole" syndrome, or fear of excessive confinement, occurs in horses and may be analogous to claustrophobia in humans. The problem most frequently occurs in horses being stalled or transported. The result of confinement during transport is a bout of frantic escape behavior known as "van fits." Treatment consists of stopping the vehicle, changing the horse to another box or stall, tranquilization, or a combination of these.

DISEASE ENTITIES AFFECTING THE BEHAVIOR OF HORSES

Many medical conditions alter the behavior of horses. Behavioral changes characteristically accompany diseases of the forebrain, such as viral and bacterial inflammation, CNS hemorrhage, encephalopathies, toxicity, space-occupying masses, aberrant parasite migration, vascular lesions, hematoma formation, and plant- and mycotic-induced leukoencephalomalacia. These diffuse or local diseases create variable changes in behavior depending upon the site of CNS involvement.

Some horse owners believe that chronic pruritus is a psychological problem, but a complete medical work-up will usually determine an etiology. Horses that suffer from any form of chronic pruritus should be examined thoroughly to rule out itching secondary to contact dermatitis, mycosis, allergic hypersensitivity to insect or parasite infestation, liver disease, or viral encephalitides. Pruritus is initiated by noxious stimuli and is perceived by the somesthetic cortex via the spinothalamic tract and ventral lateral nucleus of the thalamus. Lesions of the neurons in these central nervous system (CNS) pathways may be responsible for pruritus of an inapparent or insidious origin.

Toxic diseases such as endotoxemia and renal or liver failure cause profound depression and lethargy. Liver disease caused by plant toxicosis, infectious hepatosis, serum sickness, and idiopathic fibrosis is frequently encountered in equine practice. Behavioral changes seen include depression, lethargy, violent behavior, belligerence, somnolence, yawning, aimless walking, head pressing, and seizures. The prognosis is generally poor in advanced cases even with intensive supportive therapy.

Many chemical toxins are either stimulants or depressants. The stimulants that cause behavioral changes such as anxiety, hyperexcitability, belligerence, and "mindless" behavior include chlorinated hydrocarbons, lead poisoning, tremorgenic fungal toxins, and plant alkaloids. Depressants include opiates, bromide intoxication, strychnine-like plant alkaloids, and plants such as bracken fern (Pteridium sp) and horsetails (Equisetum sp), which contain thiaminase.

Vestibular disease may present with profound behavioral changes. A horse that is recumbent due to acute vestibular disease will often make frantic and sometimes futile attempts to regain a normal posture; this behavior may be confused with a convulsive syndrome.

Convulsive syndromes in foals may result from perinatal anoxia or vascular accidents as well as being an important clinical occurrence with severe neonatal isoerythrolysis. Therapy for these disorders requires intensive nursing and supportive care. The neonatal maladjustment syndrome, which often includes convulsions, occurs in foals from a few hours to days after birth. Recumbency, failure to suckle, wandering, and lack of mare recognition are other common clinical features of this neonatal syndrome.[9]

A partial or complete loss of vision can affect behavior by causing a transient reluctance to work or an increase in the frequency of shying, stumbling, and falling. A reluctance to move is often misinterpreted as belligerence. Abnormal head postures occur to allow for visual accommodation. A head tilt may be observed in horses with unilateral blindness, although in time most horses will adjust to this disability. There is a visual disturbance termed night blindness in Appaloosa horses in which vision is impaired in the twilight hours.

Clients regard excessive stall wetting as a vice but should be aware that brood mares with suckling foals and some stallions urinate excessively. These cases should be differentiated from true cases of polydipsia or polyuria caused by renal disease, Cushing's syndrome (p. 164), adrenal gland dysfunction, diabetes mellitus (p. 169), or diabetes insipidus. Horses with Cushing's syndrome may exhibit changes in behavior as the hypothalamus is impinged upon by a pituitary adenoma. Psychogenic diabetes insipidus may occur in horses owing to excessive water consumption secondary to boredom. An idiopathic increase in salt consumption may result in excessive diuresis.

Acute or chronic pain can significantly alter the behavior of horses. Pain can cause inappetence, weight loss, increased recumbency, alterations in recumbent posture (such as shifting sternal or lateral or dog-sitting), and sudden changes in the social hierarchy of horses.[3] Reluctance to perform can be a reflection of a painful stimulus. In cases of breeding stallions, a painful experience can result in psychological impotence, and the stallion may require retraining.[8] Mares suffering similar experiences may become nervous or timid in the breeding shed and will usually require tranquilization or breeding by artificial insemination. Acute pain, as seen with abdominal disease, can result in immediate changes in behavior such as an intractable response to restraint or violent rolling and kicking. The veterinarian's objective is to determine the site or cause of the pain and prescribe the proper course of therapy.

Certain lamenesses are often thought by owners to be learned or psychological in origin. Owners often request advice on therapy or accept the condition as a ploy by the animal and continue to use the horse. Veterinarians should inform their clients that a psychological lameness is probably non-existent, and a diagnostic evaluation will usually reveal a painful or functional cause of the lameness.

MEDICATION-INDUCED CHANGES IN BEHAVIOR

Medications are frequently used in horses to alter their attitude, disposition, and performance. Changing the attitude and disposition aids the owner or trainer in controlling the particularly fractious and hyperactive horse or in altering the aggressiveness of the competitive horse. The drugs used for these purposes fall into two general categories: stimulants and depressants. The use of these drugs is prohibited in racing and in show events and is restricted to training. However, the indiscriminate use of controlled substances should never become part of any routine training program. Sedation is commonly employed for problem horses during training and allows these animals to be schooled properly or to become more suitable for work or pleasure use. Occasionally, sedation is utilized to help move a horse into a different level of competition. The drugs most commonly employed are chloral hydrate, promazine hydrochloride, acetylepromazine, reserpine, various barbiturates, and morphine derivatives.

The use of placebos in horses that have been preconditioned to drugs during training may have an effect. For example, a hyperactive horse used to tranquilization may respond to a saline injection on the day of competition as if it was a tranquilizer.

Horses that perform below expectations are sometimes treated with behavior-altering drugs that supposedly enable them to outperform other horses. The use of these drugs is questionable on legal and ethical grounds. Drugs used for this purpose include morphine, meperidine hydrochloride, cocaine, caffeine, pemoline, methadone, propoxyphene, fentanyl, antihistamines, apomorphine, and amphetamines. After such treatment, these horses eat more frequently and exhibit increased motor activity. Androgenic steroids are used nonspecifically to boost the lazy horse both physically and mentally; however, the success of such medication for these purposes has not been adequately studied.

References

1. Cook, W. R.: Head shaking in horses. Equine Pract., *1*(5):9, *1*(6):36, *2*(1):31, *2*(2):7, 1979–1980.
2. Francis-Smith, K., and Wood-Gush, D. G. M.: Coprophagia as seen in Thoroughbred foals. Equine Vet. J., *9*(2):155, 1977.
3. Fraser, J. A.: Some observations on the behavior of the horse in pain. Br. Vet. J., *125*:150, 1969.
4. Houpt, K. A.: Horse behavior: Its relevancy to the equine practitioner. J. Equine Med. Surg., *1*:87, 1977.
5. Houpt, K. A., and Wolski, T. R.: Equine maternal behavior and its aberrations. Equine Pract., *1*(1):7, 1979.
6. Kiley, M.: A review of the advantages and disadvantages of castrating farm livestock with particular reference to behavioral effects. Br. Vet. J., *132*(3):323, 1976.
7. Obeig, F. O., and Francis-Smith, K.: A study on eliminative and grazing behavior: The use of the field by captive horses. Equine Vet. J., *8*(4):147, 1976.
8. Pickett, B. W., Voss, J. L., and Squires, E. L.: Impotence and abnormal sexual behavior in the stallion. Theriogenology, *8*(6):329, 1977.
9. Rossdale, P. D.: Modern concepts of neonatal disease in foals. Equine Vet. J., *4*:117, 1974.
10. Willard, J. G., Willard, J. C., Wolfram, S. A., and Baker, J. P.: Effect of diet on cecal pH and feeding behavior of horses. J. Anim. Sci., *45*(1):87, 1977.
11. Williams, M.: The effect of artificial rearing on the social behavior of foals. Equine Vet. J., *6*(1):17, 1974.

HEAD TRAUMA

Stephen M. Reed, PULLMAN, WASHINGTON

Head trauma with or without skull fractures is not uncommon in horses. Commonly recognized injuries include fractures of the mandible, maxilla, and incisive bone, although fractures of the basisphenoid and basioccipital bones have also been reported.[10, 14] The latter fractures are associated with a high morbidity and mortality and often result from the horse falling over backwards, striking the poll.

Fractures of the skull often heal by means of dense connective tissue and are functionally stable and satisfactory even without osseous union.[12] Rarely are the fracture fragments themselves life-threatening, although the associated neurologic problems may be fatal. It is essential, therefore, that a rapid diagnosis be made and damage to the central nervous system be accurately assessed in order to initiate early medical or surgical therapy.

PATHOPHYSIOLOGY OF CRANIAL TRAUMA

The types of cranial trauma progressing from least to most severe include concussion, contusion, laceration, and hemorrhage. Concussion is usually associated with a short loss of consciousness but without brain damage and has a favorable prognosis. A contusion of the brain indicates both vascular and nervous tissue damage without a major disruption of architecture. Contusions may be either on the same side or on the side away from the site of the injury and result from sudden acceleration or deceleration injuries or severe blows to the head. These injuries may result in intraparenchymal hemorrhage and subsequent cavitation injury within the brain.[13] Cerebral concussion or contusion may be seen without the presence of skull fractures. The prognosis for cerebral contusions must be guarded and primarily is dependent upon the lesion's location. Cerebral lacerations and hemorrhages may also result from acceleration or deceleration injuries but may be produced by penetrating wounds, such as gunshots or skull fractures. The prognosis with these injuries is governed by the same general rules as for concussions and contusions and is significantly worse only when the lesions are large and situated in the brain stem. Intracranial hemorrhages may occur in epidural, subdural, intracerebral, and subarachnoid sites.[3, 9] However, subdural hematomas (i.e., between the dural and arachnoid membranes), as occur in humans, are uncommon in the horse. The more common hemorrhage in the horse appears to be subarachnoid, which reportedly results in aseptic meningitis rather than compression of brain tissues and intracerebral bleeding.[3]

Intracerebral hematoma formation with loss of brain parenchyma may result in focal neurologic signs although these may be difficult to identify because of signs of diffuse brain disease caused by the commonly associated cerebral edema. The greatest concern with intracranial hematomas is their potential for expansion within the intact skull. With such expansion, as with cerebral edema, the resulting brain swelling causes a redistribution of brain tissue within the calvarium. Herniation of brain tissues can thus occur through natural foramina. Thus, one cerebral hemisphere may bulge to the opposite side, both hemispheres may move caudally under the tentorium between the cerebrum and cerebellum, or the cerebellum may herniate caudally into the foramen magnum (cerebellar coning). Such herniations result in additional compression of parts of the brain stem because of the presence of a rigid calvarium.

Signs of midbrain damage or compression include profound depression or coma, asymmetric pupils, and delayed pupillary light reflexes.

Strabismus, along with other vestibular signs, may accompany brain herniation and may indicate involvement of the medulla oblongata. The cause of death in patients with severe cranial injury includes cardiac and respiratory arrest, which result from brain stem involvement. Medical complications, including septic and aseptic meningitis, may be seen and should be considered when evaluating therapy.

A general scheme of events following traumatic head injury is membrane disruption, cellular swelling (especially glial cells), tissue hypoxia, cerebral edema, and, finally, increased intracranial pressure.[6] After membrane disruption and loss of selective permeability, there is an increase in extracellular potassium, a change in bicarbonate levels due to ischemia, and an accumulation of sodium (Na^+), chloride (Cl^-), and water into the cells with resultant swelling.[2, 6] Glial swelling further results in tissue hypoxia because of increased distance for the diffusion of oxygen (O_2) and carbon dioxide (CO_2), as well as mechanical obstruction of small vessels. As the tissues become more hypoxic, further membrane disruption and cellular swelling occur, establishing a vicious cycle. Barbiturates, glucocorticoids, dimethyl sulfoxide, and loop diuretics may have a protective effect against cell membrane disruption.[5, 6, 11]

As the brain tissue swells in response to trauma, a concomitant increase in intracranial pressure occurs. Recent experimental evidence suggests that the use of diuretics, which decrease extracellular water, and barbiturates, which produce vasoconstriction, may reduce intracranial pressure, blocking this vicious cycle.[6]

INITIAL EVALUATION AND TREATMENT

Management of a cranial trauma patient is dependent upon the degree of disability. This must be evaluated rapidly to begin with, then by a complete neurologic examination. Immediate attention must be given to establishing and maintaining a patent airway, control of blood loss, and management of shock. The latter does not appear to be a frequent component of uncomplicated traumatic head injuries.

PHYSICAL EXAMINATION

A history that includes an accurate account of the accident may be helpful in establishing the type of injury and locating a depressed skull fracture. A physical examination should be performed to identify injuries such as fractures of the axial or appendicular skeleton, as well as trauma to the abdomen or thorax. The identification of blood from the mouth, nose, ears, or other body orifices may direct therapy to areas in need of immediate attention. Respiratory rate, heart rate, and an estimate of blood pressure (i.e., pulse strength and capillary perfusion) must be monitored in order that cardiovascular collapse and inadequate ventilation may be detected and rapidly corrected.

NEUROLOGIC EXAMINATION

Following stabilization of the patient and completion of a physical examination, attention is directed toward the neurologic status. A complete neurologic examination is important; techniques for this are described elsewhere.[1] A record of the findings from neurologic examinations is important, since serial changes in neurologic status help to predict a prognosis and to modify therapy. Performance of the neurologic examination may be limited by the patient's condition, resulting in omission of some parts. It is optimal to perform this examination without the influence of sedative drugs, although for protection of one's self and the client, as well as the patient, it may be necessary to use analgesics or sedatives, such as xylazine. One reason to avoid use of xylazine is the initial hypertension caused by the drug. This hypertension may accentuate intracranial hemorrhage. However, the author uses this drug at a dose of 0.1 to 0.15 mg per kg intravenously and 0.2 to 0.5 mg per kg intramuscularly to achieve a calming effect.

General guidelines for localizing the lesion are given in Table 1. The important features of the neurologic examination in cranial injury are level of consciousness, cranial nerve examination (especially pupil size, symmetry, and response), posture and motor function, and respiratory patterns. The patient's level of consciousness is dependent upon the extent of damage to the cerebrum and the ascending reticular activating system in the brain stem. Further definition of the site of a focal brain stem lesion is possible, and an outline of the clinical findings helpful to achieve this is given in Table 2.

The presence of voluntary movements of the limbs in a recumbent patient should be evaluated along with spinal reflexes. The loss of a reflex may indicate concurrent spinal cord or peripheral nerve damage (p. 355). If the patient has rigid extension of all four limbs with opisthotonos, one should suspect a severe brain stem or cerebellar lesion. Damage in the region of the pons and medulla oblongata may result in a head tilt or abnormal torsion of the neck and body and nystagmus if the vestibular apparatus is damaged. In patients that are ambulatory,

TABLE 1. GENERAL SYNDROMES RESULTING FROM TRAUMA TO THE VARIOUS SITES IN THE BRAIN

Sites of Injury	Major Signs
Cerebrum	Behavioral changes Blindness Circling Depression/coma
Midbrain	Anisocoria Depression/coma Gait abnormalities/tetraplegia
Pons, medulla oblongata, inner ear	Abnormal nystagmus Abnormal respiratory patterns Head tilt Gait abnormalities/tetraplegia
Cerebellum	Intention tremor Menace response deficit without blindness Ataxia and hypermetria

it is often very difficult to separate paresis and ataxia resulting from caudal brain stem injury from a cervical spinal cord injury, unless depression or dysphagia is apparent, in which case the lesion is in the brain.

Severe brain stem injuries may also result in abnormal respiratory patterns. The development of apneustic or ataxic breathing indicates a poor prognosis.

Brain stem injury can result in bilateral miotic, bilateral mydriatic, or asymmetric pupils (Table 2). The finding of bilaterally dilated pupils that do not respond to light is associated with a grave prognosis, since this usually indicates a nonreversible midbrain lesion. A change in pupil size from bilateral constriction to bilateral dilation with no pupillary light reflexes is an indication that prompt medical or surgical treatment is necessary to combat a progressive midbrain lesion. The finding of asymmetric or bilaterally miotic pupils in a horse sustaining cranial injury is not uncommon, and such a patient should be observed closely for change in pupil size and responsiveness of pupils to light. The return of normal pupillary size and response is a good indication of a favorable trend.

Cranial nerve examination can be particularly helpful in localizing a lesion (Table 2). If the function of a cranial nerve is determined to be deficient, this may indicate that the nerve has been severed from its brain stem attachment, somewhere along its peripheral course, or that damage to the cranial nerve nucleus in the brain stem has occurred. If cranial nerve function is intact at the initial examination but lost on subsequent examinations, it indicates a progressive lesion and a less favorable prognosis.

TABLE 2. SIGNS CHARACTERISTIC OF FOCAL BRAIN STEM INJURY AT VARIOUS LEVELS

Levels	Consciousness	Motor Function	Pupils	Other Cranial Nerve Signs
Diencephalon (thalamus)	Depression to stupor	Normal to mild tetraparesis, "adversive syndrome"*	Bilateral, nonreactive pupils with visual deficit	None
Midbrain	Stupor to coma	Hemiparesis, tetraparesis, or tetraplegia	Nonreactive pupils, mydriasis	Ventrolateral strabismus
Pons	Depression	Ataxia and tetraparesis or tetraplegia	Normal	Head tilt, abnormal nystagmus, facial paralysis, medial strabismus
Rostral medulla oblongata (including inner ear)	Depression	Ataxia or hemiparesis to tetraplegia	Normal	Same
Caudal medulla oblongata	Depression	Ataxia, hemiparesis to tetraparesis, abnormal respiratory patterns	Normal	Dysphagia, flaccid tongue

*Deviation of the head and eyes with circling all toward the side of a unilateral lesion.[1]

MEDICAL THERAPY

Initial therapy must be prompt, followed by careful monitoring of clinical signs to evaluate progress and thus the effectiveness of therapy. Table 3 is a guide to therapy based on changes in clinical signs of the patient. Serial neurologic examination is an essential tool in decision-making. Tracheal intubation may be the most important initial consideration and has been shown to reduce mortality in humans and dogs.[5] Its use in the horse needs further investigation. One important group of therapeutic agents is the glucocorticoids. They are helpful in combating shock, as well as for reduction of cerebral edema associated with trauma. The author recommends using dexamethasone at a dose of 0.1 to 0.2 mg per kg body weight intravenously repeated every six to eight hours for the first 24 hours. A favorable response should be seen within the first 8 to 12 hours.

The use of osmotic diuretics, such as mannitol, is advocated to reduce cerebral edema. One of the major benefits of such compounds is the rapidity of onset of action, which experimentally has been shown to begin approximately 30 minutes following administration.[3] The dosage of 2 gm per kg of a 20 per cent solution of mannitol intravenously was formerly recommended; however, more recent work has indicated that a dose of 0.25 gm per kg may be adequate.[7] Caution must be used when administering hypertonic fluids, especially if one is uncertain about the presence of intracranial hemorrhage, since a decrease in brain edema allows additional space for further hemorrhage, and leakage of mannitol into an area will draw body fluids with it. The use of mannitol should be repeated no more than three times to avoid complications associated with hypertonic fluids, such as systemic hypotension and dehydration. These complications are monitored by evaluating skin elasticity, packed cell volume, plasma total solids, urine output, and central venous pressure. Overhydration can result in increased intracranial pressure following the administration of hypertonic solutions.

A more controversial agent for management of cranial and spinal cord trauma is dimethyl sulfoxide.*,[8],[11] Its use has been questioned because of the lack of adequate controlled experimentation. Notwithstanding, the author has found this agent to be helpful at a dosage of 0.9 to 1.0 gm per kg given intravenously as a 30 to 40 per cent solution in saline, once a day for three days, followed by once every other day for three further treatments. Other clinicians recommend its use at a dose of 1.0 gm per kg as a 10 per cent solution in 5 per cent dextrose in water. The theory of action of dimethyl sulfoxide is that it reduces the production of arachidonic acid and its conversion to prostaglandins, thus resulting in stabilization of membrane phospholipids.[11] In addition, dimethyl sulfoxide may act as a scavenger of toxic byproducts generated during cranial trauma. Further investigation is necessary to explain the effects of this drug. Therefore, its use on patients suffering from cranial trauma should be considered experimental at this time.

Additional therapeutic agents that may have ben-

*Domoso, Diamond Labs, Des Moines, IA 50303

TABLE 3. FLOW CHART FOR MANAGEMENT OF CRANIAL TRAUMA

LEVEL OF CONSCIOUSNESS	Alert ⟷	Lethargic Depressed ⟷	Stupor ⟷ Coma
PUPILS	Normal	Small, reactive or unilaterally dilated	Bilateral nonresponsive, miotic — Bilateral nonresponsive, mydriatic
MOTOR FUNCTION	Normal	Hemiparetic or tetraparetic	Hemiparetic or tetraparetic — Decerebrate rigidity / Flaccid paralysis
TIME COURSE (HOURS TO DAYS)	Static	Static / Progressive	Static / Progressive — Static (from time of accident) / Progressive
PROGNOSIS	Good	Guarded / Guarded	Poor — Grave
SPECIFIC MANAGEMENT	Observe	Corticosteroids / Corticosteroids, mannitol, dimethyl sulfoxide	Corticosteroids, mannitol, dimethyl sulfoxide — Corticosteroids, dimethyl sulfoxide, mannitol, assisted ventilation
SURGERY	Not indicated	Not indicated / Progressive → Exploratory craniotomy	Progressive → Exploratory craniotomy — Progressive → Craniotomy

(Modified with permission from Oliver, J. E.: Intracranial injury. *In* Kirk, R. W. (ed.): Current Veterinary Therapy VII: Small Animal Practice. Philadelphia, W. B. Saunders Co., 1980, p. 819.)

eficial effects in cranial trauma patients include barbiturates and loop diuretics, such as furosemide.[6] Until further studies have proved the efficacy of these compounds, their use must be questioned.

The use of antimicrobial therapy and tetanus prophylaxis is also an important consideration when treating head injury patients. Antimicrobial agents are especially important in conditions such as basilar skull fractures, in which blood and blood-tinged cerebrospinal fluid may be observed in the nasal passages or ear canals. Chloramphenicol at a dose of 25 to 50 mg per kg orally four times a day may be used, although with disruption of the blood-brain barrier, most antimicrobial agents should achieve therapeutic levels at the site of injury. Also, agents administered by parenteral routes may be safer because there is less danger of further trauma caused by manipulation of the head.

Some animals that have experienced head trauma may convulse or be violent. Attempts to control these actions with diazepam* should be made. The dose for foals is 25 mg, and for adult horses 100 mg, intravenously, repeated as necessary.

SURGICAL MANAGEMENT

Deterioration of neurologic signs in the face of medical therapy indicates progressive cerebral edema or hemorrhage, and an exploratory craniotomy should be considered. Craniotomies have been performed at large institutions on horses suffering from brain trauma; however, it is the opinion of this author that a veterinarian desiring to perform this procedure would benefit from seeking the advice of a practitioner of human neurosurgery and must have access to a high-quality, well-equipped equine surgical suite. Surgical intervention must be undertaken with caution but may provide hemostasis and relief of intracranial hypertension and may allow elevation of depressed bony fragments, evacuation of hematomas, and débridement of contaminated tissue. The evacuation of intracranial hematomas may be accomplished through trephines or

*Valium, Roche Labs, Nutley, NJ 07110

twist drill openings, although clotted blood may be difficult to remove through a very small opening and may necessitate larger incisions.

The use of general anesthesia for craniotomy is essential, since complete immobility is necessary. Inhalation anesthetics such as halothane* may cause vasodilation and may increase intracranial expansion; however, they are the compounds of choice, since assisted ventilation is often necessary. If these agents are not available, then glyceryl guaiacolate or chloral hydrate may be satisfactory. During surgical exploration, complete surgical débridement is important. This may be assisted by use of normal saline as a flushing agent. Possible complications include the formation of brain abscesses or development of meningitis.

References

1. deLahunta, A.: Veterinary Neuroanatomy and Clinical Neurology. Philadelphia, W. B. Saunders Co., 1977, p. 344.
2. Fishman, R. A.: Brain edema. N. Engl. J. Med., 293:706, 1975.
3. Holliday, T. A.: Trauma to the central nervous system. *In* Catcott, E. J., and Smithcors, J. F. (eds.): Equine Medicine and Surgery, 2nd ed. Wheaton, IL, American Veterinary Pub., pp. 466–470, 1972.
4. Mayhew, I. G., and Ingram, J. T.: Neurological examination of the horse. Proc. 24th Annu. Conv. Am. Assoc. Eq. Pract., 1978, pp. 525–541.
5. McQueen, J. D.: Treatment of craniocerebral injuries. *In* Zuidema, G. P., Rutherford, R. B., and Bollinger, W. F. (eds.): The Management of Trauma, 3rd ed. Philadelphia, W. B. Saunders Co., 1979, pp. 218–226.
6. Miller, S. M., Cothell, J. E., and Turndorf, H.: Cerebral protection by barbiturates and loop diuretics in head trauma: Possible modes of action. Bull. NY Acad. Med., 56:306, 1980.
7. Oliver, J. E.: Intracranial injury. *In* Kirk, R. W. (ed.): Current Veterinary Therapy VII: Small Animal Practice. Philadelphia, W. B. Saunders Co., 1979, p. 819.
8. Parker, A. J., and Smith, C. W.: Lack of functional recovery from spinal cord trauma following dimethyl sulfoxide and epsilon amino caproic acid therapy in dogs. Res. Vet. Sci., 27:253, 1979.
9. Selcer, R. R.: Trauma to the central nervous system. Vet. Clin. North Am. (Small Anim. Pract.), 10(3):619, 1980.
10. Stick, J. A., Wilson, J. and Kunze, D.: Basilar skull fractures in three horses. J. Am. Vet. Med. Assoc., 176:228, 1980.
11. Torre, J. C. de la, Kawanga, H. M., Rowed, D. W., Johnson, C. M., Goode, D. T., Kajinhara, K., and Mullan, S.: Dimethyl sulfoxide in central nervous system trauma. Ann. NY Acad. Sci., 243:362, 1975.
12. Turner, A. S.: Surgical management of depression fractures of the equine skull. Vet. Surg., 8:29, 1979.
13. Walker, A. E., and Youmans, J. R.: Mechanism of cerebral trauma and the impairment of consciousness. *In* Youmans, J. R. (ed): Neurological Surgery. Philadelphia, W. B. Saunders Co., 1973, Ch. 43, pp. 936–949.
14. Wheat, J. D.: Fractures of the head and mandible of the horse. Proc. 21st Annu. Conv. Am. Assoc. Eq. Pract., 1975, pp. 223–228.

*Fluothane, Ayerst Labs, New York, NY 10017

SEIZURE DISORDERS

Ian G. Mayhew, GAINESVILLE, FLORIDA

This chapter considers all types of seizure disorders. Seizures are regarded as intracranial paroxysmal disturbances. These episodes begin and end abruptly, are associated with characteristic alterations in brainwaves on an electroencephalogram (EEG), and are usually accompanied by clinical signs. Various terms are used to describe one of these events, including *fit*, *attack*, *stroke*, and *ictus* as well as *seizure*. Obvious from this list is the aura of hobgoblin connotations that surrounds these disorders.

For this discussion, *convulsion* refers to any seizure accompanied by tonic and clonic muscular activity with some loss of consciousness, while *epilepsy* refers to recurrent seizures or, most frequently, convulsions that result from the presence of nonprogressive intracranial alterations of either an acquired or inherited nature. For the most part, a horse showing isolated or repetitive convulsions occurring as a result of a disease process that requires some specific therapy, in addition to anticonvulsive therapy, should not be regarded as having epilepsy. Thus, the large majority of horses with recurrent seizures resulting from space-occupying cerebral lesions, encephalitis, meningitis, and metabolic and toxic conditions do not have epilepsy. Neurologic examination of most of these patients between seizures (i.e., in the interictal period) will reveal some abnormality. Epilepsy may be inherited or acquired; however, true inherited epilepsy has not been reported in horses.

Seizures occur much less frequently in horses than in other species such as dogs and humans. Adult horses are less likely to exhibit seizures than foals for the same "level" of seizure stimulus; adult horses are thus said to possess a *high seizure threshold*.

DESCRIPTION OF SEIZURES

Seizures are conveniently divided into those that are generalized and those that are partial. In horses, *generalized seizures* are more common than partial seizures. A generalized seizure involves the whole cerebral cortex and the whole body musculature. There is a period of unconsciousness that is followed by symmetric clonic contractions of body parts, then a period of symmetric, generalized tonic muscular spasm. The horse usually falls to the ground if standing and may show deviations and abnormal movements of the eyeballs, dilated pupils, excessive salivation, trismus or jaw clamping, opisthotonus, lordosis or kyphosis, violent paddling movements of the limbs, uncontrolled urination and defecation, and excessive sweating. Most generalized seizures in the horse last from 5 to 60 seconds, with the animal regaining its feet in several minutes. A preictal aura consisting of subtle changes in behavior is not usually demonstrated by horses, although postictal depression and blindness may be seen for variable periods of time.

Partial seizures occur when one part of the cerebrum is affected, the signs depending on the part affected. Types of partial seizures that have been seen in horses include contralateral (to the lesion) twitching of the limbs and particularly the face, compulsive running in a circle, and possibly self-mutilation (asymmetric). Most often there is secondary generalization of such a partial seizure with signs as described before; these are known as *partial seizures with secondary generalization.* All forms of partial seizures should be regarded as originating from focal lesions that are therefore probably acquired either in utero or postnatally.

Status epilepticus is the term reserved for repeated generalized seizures occurring one after the other. This phenomenon is not common in horses.

CAUSES OF SEIZURES

A list of diseases that have been associated with or suspected as being associated with isolated or repeated seizures in horses is given in Table 1. It is convenient to divide these processes into extracranial and intracranial categories. As a general rule, the extracranial causes are more amenable to therapy.

APPROACH TO THE PATIENT WITH A SEIZURE DISORDER

A single seizure observed in a foal may be the signal of a recurrent seizure disorder, though in almost all cases it is not. An isolated seizure in a healthy foal, unaccompanied by concurrent illness that requires specific therapy, does not require an expensive laboratory investigation and treatment. On the other hand, when faced with a horse in status epilepticus, the veterinarian should ensure a patent airway, supply oxygen if needed, and sedate the animal immediately with intravenous diazepam* at 0.1 to 0.4 mg per kg or pentobarbital,† phenobarbital,‡ chloral hydrate–MgSO₄§ or even guaifenesin‖ given to effect. Also, xylazine** at 0.5 to 1 mg per kg intravenously may be tried.

Major aims of the initial approach to the patient should be to determine whether or not there is a treatable extracranial or intracranial disease process that is causing the seizure and to determine whether the seizures have been increasing, stabilizing, or decreasing in duration, severity, or frequency. The latter information is vitally important in determining a prognosis for the seizure disorder. For example, if a horse begins having idiopathic seizures and their frequency is decreasing over a period of weeks, it is likely that this frequency will continue to decrease, that any causative process is not progressing, and that the horse probably does not require chronic anticonvulsant therapy. On the other hand, a case involving an aged horse with a history of many seizures occurring at an increasing frequency over a few weeks probably warrants a poor to bad prognosis. This would be particularly so if some localizing neurologic deficit was detected and if the seizures were partial, and then became partial with secondary generalization. Even if anticonvulsant therapy were successful in such a case, ultimately the frequency of seizures would probably increase unless something could be done about the irritating, probably space-occupying, intracranial lesion.

HISTORY

At this stage, a thorough review of the history is in order. On most occasions, the veterinarian will not witness a seizure and must rely on the owner's description. Consequently, this is possibly the most important part of evaluation of the patient. An important aspect of the history is the number, duration, and frequency of the seizures. If they are clearly increasing in duration and/or frequency, the prognosis is less favorable than the converse. Historic evidence of localizing signs should be sought. These indicate partial seizures as described earlier and, consequently, an acquired disorder. Indications of trauma or access to toxins and clinical evi-

---

*Valium, Roche Labs, Division of Hoffmann-La Roche, Inc., Nutley, NJ 07110

†Pentobarbital, 65 mg per ml, W. A. Butler Co., Columbus, OH 43228

‡Phenobarbital, 120 mg IV ampules, Eli Lilly and Co., Indianapolis, IN 46206

§Chloral-Thesia, Med-Tech, Inc., Elwood, KS 66024

‖Guaifenesin, Burns-Biotec Lab, Division of Chromalloy Pharmaceutical, Inc., Omaha, NB 68103

**Rompun, Haver-Lockhart, Inc., Shawnee, KS 66201

TABLE 1. KNOWN AND SUSPECTED CAUSES OF SEIZURES

Mechanism	Extracranial	Intracranial
Injury	—	BRAIN TRAUMA
Infections	Septicemia, endotoxemia, febrile seizures Tetanus Botulism	BACTERIAL MENINGITIS ARBOVIRAL (TOGAVIRAL) ENCEPHALITIDES Cerebral abscess Rabies Mycotic encephalitis Verminous encephalitis (larva migrans) (?)Equine protozoal myeloencephalitis
Malformation	—	(?)Hydrocephalus
Toxicity	Acute organophosphate (?)Strychnine (?)Metaldehyde (snail bait) Miscellaneous*	Moldy corn (Fusarium sp) Locoweeds (Oxytropus sp, Astragalus sp) Bracken fern (?)Lead, arsenic, mercury (?)Ryegrass, Phararis, Paspalum Miscellaneous*
Metabolic	HEPATOENCEPHALOPATHY Hypomagnesemia Hypocalcemia Hyperkalemia Hypoxia (?)Hypoglycemia (?)Uremic encephalopathy (?)Gastrointestinal disease (?)Hyperlipidemia	—
Vascular	—	NEONATAL MALADJUSTMENT SYNDROME—VASCULAR ACCIDENTS STRONGYLUS VULGARIS CEREBRAL THROMBOEMBOLISM INTRACAROTID INJECTION
Tumor	—	Neoplasm Hamartoma (?)Cholesterol granuloma
Idiopathic	—	(?)Epilepsy

Tabulated according to causative mechanisms and the principal location or target inside or outside the cranium. Diseases that more frequently result in seizures are indicated in capital letters.

*See Blood, D. C., Henderson, J. A., and Radostits, O. M.: Veterinary Medicine, 5th ed. Philadelphia, Lea and Febiger, 1979, for additional organic and inorganic intoxications resulting in seizures in horses.

dence of recent or concurrent illness are of significance.

PHYSICAL AND NEUROLOGIC EXAMINATIONS

The physical and neurologic examinations that follow history-taking assist in detecting extracranial reasons for seizures. These examinations also should identify any permanent neurologic signs that may assist in localizing an intracranial lesion. The presence of postictal depression and blindness, which may be regarded as temporary neuronal exhaustion, can be confusing at this stage.

If there are clues of an intracranial disease process from the neurologic examination, then further work-up as outlined later may be modified. For example, additional signs of depression, aimless wandering, head pressing, and blindness indicate a diffuse cerebral lesion, and the further work-up should be aimed at differentiating such diseases as the viral encephalitides, hepatoencephalopathy, bacterial meningitis, and the neonatal maladjustment syndrome. Alternatively, circling in one direction, asymmetric blindness, asymmetric pupils, and unilateral facial hypalgesia in addition to seizures are indicative of diseases such as cerebral abscess, cerebral hematoma, intracarotid injection reaction, *Strongylus vulgaris* cerebral thromboembolism, and cerebral tumors. Further evaluation should be directed at determining which of these diseases is present.

Appropriate therapy for any associated intracranial or extracranial cause for seizures can be instituted at this stage.

TABLE 2. ANTICONVULSANT DRUGS USED TO TREAT SEIZURE DISORDERS

Stage of Treatment	Drug	50 kg Foal	450 kg Horse
Initial therapy (including status epilepticus)	Diazepam*	5–20 mg IV per dose	25–50 mg IV per dose
	Phenobarbital† or pentobarbital‡	150–1000 mg IV to effect	—
	Phenytoin††	200–500 mg IV per dose	?
	Primidone‡‡	1–2 gm orally per dose	—
	Chloral hydrate–MgSO₄§ (± barbiturate)	3–10 gm chloral hydrate IV to effect	15–60 gm IV to effect
	Xylazine**	25–50 mg IV or IM per dose	300–500 mg IV or IM per dose
	Guaifenesin‖ (± barbiturate)	—	40–60 gm IV to effect
Maintenance therapy	Phenobarbital†	25–50 mg orally twice a day or to effect	250–1000 mg orally twice a day or to effect
	Phenytoin††	50–250 mg IV or orally every 2 to 4 hours Reduce to 50–250 mg orally every 12 hours	(?)500–1000 mg orally 3 times a day
	Primidone‡‡	1 gm orally once or twice a day	—

Included are suggested dose ranges for both initial therapy of acute convulsions (including status epilepticus) and maintenance therapy in an average-sized foal (50 kg) and an adult horse (450 kg). The drugs are listed in suggested order of preference. Although all these drugs have been used with success, several are not licensed for use in the horse. These doses should be regarded as guidelines only; lower doses may be equally effective.

*Diazepam, Valium, 5 mg per ml, 10 ml multidose vial. Roche Laboratories, Division of Hoffmann-La Roche, Inc., Nutley, NJ 07110. Note: Diazepam is denatured by contact with plastic for more than a few minutes.

†Phenobarbital, 120 mg IV ampules, Eli Lilly and Co., Indianapolis, IN 46206. 100 mg tablets, Purepac Pharmaceutical Co., Division of Kalipharma, Inc., Elizabeth, NJ 07207

‡Pentobarbital, sodium pentobarbital injection, 65 mg per ml, 100 ml vial. W. A. Butler Co., Columbus, OH 43228

§Chloral hydrate–MgSO₄, Chloral-Thesia, 30 and 25 per cent (respectively), 250 ml vials. Med-Tech, Inc., Elwood, KS 66024

‖Guaifenesin, Glycodex, 5 per cent solution, 1000 ml. Burns-Biotec Laboratories, Division of Chromalloy Pharmaceutical, Inc., Omaha, NB 68103

**Xylazine, Rompun, 100 mg per ml multidose vial. Haver-Lockhart, Bayvet, Division of Cutter Laboratories, Inc., Shawnee, KS 66201

††Phenytoin, Dilantin, 100 mg Kapseals and 250 mg injection vials. Parke-Davis and Co., Detroit, MI 48232

‡‡Primidone, 250 mg tablets. Ayerst Laboratories, Inc., New York, NY 10017

INITIAL ANCILLARY AIDS

The first ancillary aids that should be employed in further evaluating the patient should include a complete hemogram and blood chemistry analyses, including liver function tests, renal function tests, and glucose, calcium, magnesium, potassium, sodium, and chloride concentrations, blood gas determinations, and blood lead level. Also, storage of frozen serum for later serologic determinations is a sensible step to take at this stage. A cerebrospinal fluid (CSF) sample may be analyzed at this stage, particularly if evidence of an intracranial process is found.

INITIAL THERAPY

By this stage of evaluating the patient, it should be clear if there is a treatable extracranial disease process occurring. If economically practical, such diseases should be treated appropriately.

Under these circumstances, convulsions may not require specific therapy if they are of short duration, only occur up to a few times a day, and the patient can be prevented from sustaining injury while convulsing. If convulsions persist, then anticonvulsants may be required (Table 2).

It is almost always unwise to attempt to physically restrain an adult horse that is convulsing. However, foals can be restrained successfully from injuring themselves during convulsions while medication is being administered and the anticonvulsive effects are being awaited. This is achieved best by having the handler sit with the foal on the lap and holding the head extended by cradling it with one arm while restraining the upper hind limb with the other hand.

If a seizure is occurring or has just occurred, the author usually uses diazepam* at 0.05 to 0.4 mg per kg intravenously, repeated in 30 minutes if necessary, after ensuring adequate ventilation and oxy-

*Valium, Roche Labs, Division of Hoffmann-La Roche, Inc., Nutley, NJ 07110

genation (p. 475). Rossdale[6] recommends phenytoin (Dilantin, diphenylhydantoin)* for convulsing foals at an initial dose of 5 to 10 mg per kg intravenously or orally, reducing to 1 to 5 mg per kg every two to four hours. May and Greenwood[4] report that primidone† at 2 gm orally successfully stops seizures in foals within 20 minutes. They follow this with 1 gm doses orally twice a day. Several authors[1, 4] have used acetylpromazine in foals, but this drug and the related phenothiazine tranquilizers are not recommended, as they lower the seizure threshold. For foals that show continuing convulsions, the author will usually follow one or two initial doses of diazepam with phenobarbital‡ (approximately 1 to 10 mg per kg) or pentobarbital§ (approximately 3 to 15 mg per kg intravenously) given to effect. In adult horses, chloral hydrate–MgSO₄ mixture‖ or guaifenesin** all given to effect, also have been used. In all cases the minimum quantity of drug to control seizure activity is best. A guide to anticonvulsant drug therapy is outlined in Table 2. Hypoglycemia seems to cause depression rather than seizures in horses; however, intravenous glucose should be given if prolonged seizures have occurred.

Further Evaluation and Treatment

If the diagnosis is made or if seizures have ceased, then further ancillary investigations need not be pursued. If, however, an aggressive approach to confirmation of the diagnosis is required or if the diagnosis is still nebulous, some or all of the following procedures may be undertaken.

Cerebrospinal Fluid Collection. CSF samples, preferably taken from the cisterna magna or from both cisterna magna and lumbosacral collection sites, are analyzed (p. 331). In this way, evidence of a viral, bacterial, or parasitic encephalitis may be obtained, and cultural, serologic, and therapeutic procedures can be initiated. Brain trauma and vascular diseases can result in xanthochromic CSF with an elevated protein content. Sometimes red blood cells, neutrophils, and particularly mononuclear cells showing erythrophagocytosis may be present. Space-occupying masses of all types may result in elevated CSF pressure (greater than 450 mm of H₂O in lateral recumbency) and can result in leakage of blood pigments and protein into the CSF.

Radiography. Radiographs of the head and neck

---

*Dilantin, Parke-Davis and Co., Detroit, MI 48232
†Primidone, Ayerst Labs, Inc., New York, NY 10017
‡Phenobarbital, Eli Lilly and Co., Indianapolis, IN 46206
§Pentobarbital, W. A. Butler Co., Columbus, OH 43228
‖Chloral-Thesia, Med-Tech, Inc., Elwood, KS 66024
**Guaifenesin, Burns-Biotec Labs, Division of Chromalloy Pharmaceutical, Inc., Omaha, NB 68103

may be of value in patients suspected of having sustained head injury. Air ventriculography may be used to confirm the presence of hydrocephalus. However, in the horse this malformation is most frequently secondary to some other disease process destroying cerebral tissue (such as hydrocephalus ex vacuo), and horses with only hydrocephalus are not usually presented because of a seizure disorder. Cerebral angiography, radioisotope scans, and computerized axial tomography still must be regarded as too invasive, too expensive, or too impractical to be recommended for use in evaluating horses with seizure disorders, except for academic interest.

Electroencephalography. EEG in the horse is in its infancy as a diagnostic tool. Paroxysmal dysrhythmias, often occurring as spike and wave complexes on the EEG tracing, almost certainly occur in equine seizure disorders, as they do in other species.[3] Ideally an EEG performed on a patient with a seizure disorder may reveal evidence of any focal lesion indicating an acquired disease. Also, a marked asymmetry in the EEG tracing may help localize a lesion. It is suggested that if an EEG is performed, one or more control recordings should be taken from normal horses of similar age and under the same conditions.

Prolonged Treatment. Extended treatment of seizures is rarely indicated in the horse. In the majority of cases, the patient will succumb to the inciting disease, or seizure activity will desist with resolution of the process, making continued treatment unnecessary. Initially, while medicating a horse for a seizure disorder, it is necessary to slowly decrease the dosage of anticonvulsant drugs to determine whether continuous therapy is necessary. The stage at which this is attempted can be partly governed by the severity of the seizure disorder and the disappearance of signs of any associated disease in response to specific therapy.

For continuous anticonvulsant therapy, the following suggestions are offered (Table 2). If intravenous pentobarbital* or phenobarbital† has successfully reduced seizure activity, then oral phenobarbital should be tried because this is the cheapest and possibly the safest anticonvulsant drug. The dose can be extrapolated from the effective intravenous dose, and may be 0.5 to 2.0 mg per kg orally twice a day. Phenytoin‡ at 1 to 5 mg per kg orally twice a day has been used successfully in foals,[6] as has primidone§ at 0.75 to 1.0 gm orally twice a day.[4] Both these latter drugs are considerably more expensive than phenobarbital, and as a cautionary note, these drugs have not been licensed for use in horses. Doses of up to 2500 mg per day orally of

---

*Pentobarbital, W. A. Butler Co., Columbus, OH 43228
†Phenobarbital, Eli Lilly and Co., Indianapolis, IN 46206
‡Dilantin, Parke-Davis and Co., Detroit, MI 48232
§Primidone, Ayerst Laboratories, Inc., New York, NY 10017

phenytoin* have been used by the author in yearling horses with no noticeable side effects.

As with most neurologic diseases in the horse, the prognosis accompanying seizure disorders must be tempered by consideration of the future use of the animal and the potential risks to those associated with the animal.

NOTES ON SOME SPECIFIC SEIZURE DISORDERS IN THE HORSE

NEONATAL FOALS

Convulsions occur quite frequently in foals affected with the neonatal maladjustment syndrome (NMS).[1, 4, 6, 7] This syndrome is probably caused by various combinations of subarachnoid, parenchymal, and intraventricular hemorrhages and edema and necrosis of brain tissue. Collectively, these changes can be regarded as resulting from vascular or anoxic accidents occurring in the perinatal period. Anticonvulsant drug therapy as outlined earlier, along with physical restraint of these foals during convulsions and intensive nursing care, results in at least a 50 per cent survival rate with no detectable long-term problems.[5]

Acute head injury and infections (Table 1) possibly account for most of the other convulsions seen in neonatal foals.

ADOLESCENT FOALS

The whole spectrum of diseases producing seizures listed in Table 1, except tumors, may be encountered in adolescent foals.

There does appear to be a syndrome of idiopathic convulsions in foals from several weeks to several months of age. This syndrome may be more common in weanling foals of the Arabian breed. It is characterized by a sudden onset of recurrent seizures that may increase in frequency over a period of days to weeks so that the foal is convulsing many times per day. The seizures are generalized but may not proceed to generalized tonic muscular spasm, leaving the foal standing with the head and neck extended in a semiconscious state and showing various other signs of a generalized seizure, as described earlier.

These seizures respond well to anticonvulsant drugs. Notwithstanding, chronic therapy should not be undertaken unless several attempts at reducing the drug doses have been made because this syndrome appears to be self-limiting, with the foals "growing out" of the disorder. The etiology is not known, but metabolic and toxic causes along with febrile seizures should be considered.

ADULT HORSES

All causes of seizures outlined in Table 1, including tumorous growths, can occur in adult horses.

The general work-up of an adult horse with a seizure disorder is as described earlier, with the primary aims of defining any associated diseases and determining whether or not the disorder is progressing or regressing. In cases in which the frequency of seizures is increasing, the prognosis is guarded to poor, and evidence of an interictal neurologic deficit should be searched for to confirm a morbid disease process.

In mares that are cycling, there is very often an increase in the frequency or severity of seizures at the time of estrus. A hormonal association with seizure threshold has been documented in humans.[2] This fact should be kept in mind when treating a mare with a seizure disorder, and progesterone injections may be tried to reduce the frequency of seizures, or the dosage of anticonvulsant drug may be increased prior to estrus. If such treatments were successful, ovariectomy could be considered if the inciting disease appeared to be progressive. It should be remembered that such an approach would have no effect on the inciting cause.

Occasionally other stimuli, such as noise, lights, or sexual activity, have been observed to trigger a convulsion in an adult horse known to have a seizure disorder.

References

1. Baird, J. D.: Neonatal maladjustment syndrome in a thoroughbred foal. Aust. Vet. J., 49:530, 1973.
2. Bäckström, T.: Epileptic seizures in women related to plasma estrogen and progesterone during the menstrual cycle. Acta Neurol. Scand., 54:321, 1976.
3. Holliday, T. A.: Seizure disorders. Vet. Clin. North Am. (Small Anim. Pract.), 10(1):3, 1980.
4. May, C. J., and Greenwood, R. E. S.: Recurrent convulsions in a thoroughbred foal: Management and treatment. Vet. Rec., 101:76, 1977.
5. Palmer, A. C., and Rossdale, P. D.: Neuropathological changes associated with the neonatal maladjustment syndrome in the thoroughbred foal. Res. Vet. Sci., 20:267, 1976.
6. Rossdale, P. D.: Differential diagnosis and treatment of equine neonatal disease. Vet. Rec., 91:581, 1972.
7. Rossdale, P. D., and Leadon, D.: Equine neonatal disease: A review. J. Reprod. Fert. Suppl., 23:685, 1975.

Supplemental Readings

1. Blood, D. C., Henderson, J. A., and Radostits, O. M.: Veterinary Medicine, 5th ed. Philadelphia, Lea and Febiger, 1979.
2. deLahunta, A.: Veterinary Neuroanatomy and Clinical Neurology. Philadelphia, W. B. Saunders Co., 1977.

---

*Dilantin, Parke-Davis and Co., Detroit, MI 48232

EASTERN EQUINE ENCEPHALOMYELITIS

Julia H. Wilson, GAINESVILLE, FLORIDA

Eastern equine encephalomyelitis (EEE) is an acute, often fatal disease of horses and humans. The causative agent is an RNA virus classified as alphavirus within the Togaviridae family. The disease's incidence is sporadic and seasonal. Its life cycle is sylvatic, involving bird and rodent reservoirs and insect vectors. Transmission to horses is by mosquitoes, primarily *Aedes sollicitans* and *Aedes vexans*. The horse is considered a "dead-end" host owing to the low level of viremia in the disease. Epizootics of EEE have been reported in the United States, primarily along the Eastern seaboard, Gulf coast, and around the Great Lakes, and also in Alberta, the Caribbean, and Central and South America.[2]

PATHOGENESIS AND CLINICAL SIGNS

After an infective mosquito bites a susceptible horse, proliferation of the virus in regional lymph nodes is followed by viremia. This may result in one of the following syndromes: (1) mild fever, lymphopenia, and neutropenia, which often are subclinical; (2) a generalized febrile illness with signs of anorexia, depression, tachycardia, and high fever (up to 41°C) with severe lymphopenia and neutropenia; or (3) encephalomyelitis. The clinical signs of the classic encephalitic form typically begin as changes in behavior with loss of appetite and fever, progressing in 12 to 24 hours to dementia with head pressing, circling, and often blindness. Intense pruritus has also been reported. Cranial nerve dysfunctions may produce signs such as nystagmus, facial paralysis, and dysphagia. Progressive ataxia and weakness from brain stem and spinal cord involvement result in an inability to stand. Seizures may occur and progress in severity. Respiratory arrest two to three days after the onset of clinical signs is the usual terminal event. Mortality varies from 75 to 90 per cent, so a guarded prognosis must be given. Surviving cases may be left with residual central nervous system (CNS) damage such as visual deficits and behavioral and learning disabilities and frequently are referred to as "dummies."[3]

Peripheral blood analysis frequently reveals lymphopenia and neutropenia. Cerebrospinal fluid (CSF) may have increased protein content and white cell counts. Neutrophils are often found in CSF in the acute disease; mononuclear cells predominate in later stages. At necropsy the gross lesions may mimic those of brain trauma, with patchy discoloration of the brain and spinal cord, edema, and hemorrhage. A diffuse meningoencephalomyelitis is seen histologically, affecting primarily gray matter, with neuronal degeneration, gliosis, and perivascular infiltrates. These perivascular cuffs consist of neutrophils in the acute stage, later consisting of neutrophils and large and small mononuclear cells.

DIAGNOSIS

Clinical diagnosis of EEE is based on the season, locale, clinical signs and their progression, and ancillary aids. Clinical differentiation from western equine encephalomyelitis (WEE) or Venezuelan equine encephalomyelitis (VEE) is very difficult and usually is based on the outcome of the case. Confirmation by serologic testing, utilizing either hemagglutination inhibition (HI) or complement fixation (CF) titers, requires demonstration of at least a fourfold rise in antibody titer in samples taken 7 to 10 days apart or a very high single titer in an unvaccinated animal. (Definition of a single high titer is controversial. Titers of greater than or equal to 1:160 for EEE and greater than or equal to 1:40 for WEE and VEE are considered diagnostic in Florida.) At postmortem examination, virus isolation from preferably fresh, refrigerated, or deep frozen portions of the brain should be attempted if facilities are available, and routine histologic examination will define the presence or absence of meningoencephalomyelitis. Other conditions causing diffuse or multifocal neurologic deficits that should be considered in the differential diagnosis include WEE, VEE, head trauma, hepatoencephalopathy, rabies, leukoencephalomalacia, bacterial meningoencephalitis, protozoal myeloencephalitis, and verminous encephalitis.

TREATMENT

If EEE is strongly suspected and the horse is recumbent, then any attempts at therapy should be tempered by the bad prognosis for survival and the great risk of residual signs. In early or mild cases, the mode of therapy is identical to that for WEE, for which there is a better prognosis (p. 352).

No specific antiviral agents are available currently; hence, supportive measures and symptomatic therapy are the primary modes of therapy. To minimize the complications of recumbency and self-induced trauma, a very well bedded area should be provided, and the horse should be kept as clean and dry as possible. The recumbent horse should be rolled several times a day and maintained in a sternal position if possible to minimize pulmonary congestion and prolonged weight-bearing on skin surfaces over bony prominences. Slinging should be attempted if feasible to decrease muscle damage, increase limb use and circulation, and decrease the likelihood of the development of decubital ulcers. Any skin sores or abrasions should be treated meticulously with antiseptic or antibiotic ointments to avoid secondary infections. If spontaneous urination is not observed, the bladder should be manually expressed per rectum or catheterized aseptically. An indwelling urinary catheter may be advisable if prolonged recumbency is anticipated, at which time prophylactic antimicrobial agents should be considered because of the high risk of ascending infection. Urine scald should be prevented by application of petrolatum or other water-repellent ointments to areas likely to become wet with urine. Manual evacuation of feces several times a day may also be necessary.

Adequate food and water intake should be ensured. Nasogastric tube feeding can be employed to maintain hydration and provide energy if the horse cannot eat or drink. If nasogastric intubation is used for more than a few days, rhinitis and pharyngitis may develop, in which case an esophagostomy can be employed. Intravenous fluids, though more costly, can also be used. Hydration and electrolyte levels should be monitored if inanition lasts for more than a few days.

Signs of progressing depression, and particularly dilated pupils that become unresponsive to light, suggest potentially fatal cerebral edema. Intravenous mannitol* (20 per cent) may be given by slow intravenous infusion at 0.25 to 0.5 gm per kg. Furosemide† at 0.5 to 1.0 mg per kg intravenously alternatively could be used, although this is perhaps less effective for such purposes than mannitol. Mannitol is usually not repeated unless following an initial clinical response there is a relapse in 6 to 24 hours. Furosemide can be repeated at six- to eight-hour intervals with close monitoring of hydration and serum potassium levels.

Anti-inflammatory drugs such as dexamethasone‡ at levels of 0.1 to 0.25 mg per kg may be indicated to reduce the inflammatory component of the CNS tissue damage. Their use is controversial but is accepted as current practice. If elected, this therapy should be continued at tapering dosages for several

days, initially on a twice a day schedule and then once a day.

High fevers can be treated with antipyretics such as dipyrone* (10 to 20 ml intravenously) and phenylbutazone† (4 to 8 mg per kg intravenously), though these sometimes are ineffective. Alcohol baths usually will markedly reduce fevers and can be repeated as necessary.

Seizures should be controlled with barbiturates (pentobarbital or phenobarbital), diazepam, chloral hydrate, or guaifenesin to prevent self-trauma and myositis (p. 347). Head padding with foam helmets is advisable to minimize risks of corneal abrasions and skull fractures.

The duration of immunity following natural infection is unknown; therefore, recovered animals should be vaccinated in a routine manner.

PREVENTION

In the face of an EEE outbreak, vaccination may be beneficial, as protective levels of antibody have been demonstrated as soon as three days postvaccination in VEE studies. Strict mosquito control measures should be instituted. Current recommendations for routine EEE vaccinations are two injections three to four weeks apart with inactivated EEE-WEE (with or without VEE) vaccine one month prior to the mosquito season followed by yearly revaccinations. Clinical experience in areas with long mosquito seasons strongly suggests that semiannual revaccination is necessary. Both intradermal and intramuscular vaccines are available, some in combination with tetanus toxoid and influenza. The inactivated vaccines are safe for use in pregnant mares. Serum antibody levels in foals that have received colostrum are similar to those of the dams, and the half-life of maternally derived antibodies in the foal is 20 days.[1] The presence of such maternal antibodies blocks active immunization in foals; consequently, foals of mares vaccinated against EEE should be given a series of two to three monthly vaccinations beginning at two to four months of age. Colostrum-deprived foals should be vaccinated earlier.

PUBLIC HEALTH SIGNIFICANCE

Equine cases of EEE do not pose a threat to humans, as circulating virus levels are not high enough to transmit the disease via mosquitoes. Notwithstanding, sufficient viral titers may be present in

---

*Manni-ject, 20 per cent solution, Hart-Delta, Inc., Baton Rouge, LA 70805

†Lasix, 5 per cent solution, National Labs, Somerville, NJ 08876

‡Azium, 2 mg per ml, Schering Corp., Kenilworth, NJ 07033

*Dipyrone (methampyron), 500 mg per ml, Med-Tech, Inc., Elwood, KS 66024

†Phenylbutazone, 200 mg per ml, Haver-Lockhart Labs, Shawnee, KS 66201

infected tissues, especially CNS; therefore, appropriate precautions should be undertaken at the time of necropsy examination of EEE cases. In humans, the EEE virus causes an acute encephalitis with a mortality rate of approximately 50 per cent. Outbreaks of human cases often coincide with or are preceded by equine epizootics; hence, strict mosquito control in affected areas is necessary to prevent both human and equine cases, and all equine cases should be reported to state health officials.

References

1. Ferguson, J. A., Reeves, W. C., and Hardy, J. L.: Studies on immunity to alphaviruses in foals. Am. J. Vet. Res., 40:5, 1979.
2. Gibbs, E. P. J.: Equine viral encephalitis. Equine Vet. J., 8(2):66, 1976.
3. Walton, T. E.: Eastern, western, and Venezuelan equine encephalomyelitis. *In* Gibbs, E. P. J. (ed.): Virus Diseases of Food Animals—A World Geography, Vol. 2. New York, Academic Press, 1981, Chap. 24.

WESTERN EQUINE ENCEPHALOMYELITIS

Dean E. Goeldner, VAN NUYS, CALIFORNIA

Western equine encephalomyelitis (WEE or "sleeping sickness") is the mildest and most common of the three equine arboviral encephalitides (eastern, western, and Venezuelan) encountered in North America. Like the others, it is characterized clinically by varying degrees of altered consciousness, ataxia, and paralysis. Because the disease also affects humans, it has public health significance.

ETIOLOGY

The causative agent is the WEE virus, an arthropod-borne virus, or arbovirus. It is a small, enveloped RNA virus and is morphologically similar to but antigenically distinct from the EEE and VEE viruses.[4] All three are now classified as alphaviruses of the togavirus family (formerly group A arboviruses). Several strains of the WEE virus are known to exist, and their antigenicity and virulence vary geographically.

EPIZOOTIOLOGY

WEE occurs in the United States from the Mississippi River Valley westward and in western Canada.[8] Occasional outbreaks occur in the eastern part of North America. Mexico and Central and South America also experience the disease.

In nature, WEE is primarily an infection of wild birds that is transmitted by the mosquito vector *Culex tarsalis*.[4] The birds act as reservoirs for the virus and usually do not exhibit clinical signs. The mosquito becomes infected by taking a blood meal from a viremic avian host. If the virus is able to penetrate the "gut barriers" of the mosquito, it passes through the hemolymph to the salivary glands, where it multiplies. In 4 to 10 days, virus is being shed in the saliva. The mosquito remains infected for life, and its longevity does not appear to be affected by the presence of the virus.[5]

Toward the end of the vector season, *Culex tarsalis* becomes more opportunistic and begins to feed on other hosts, including horses and humans. It is in this incidental way that these species become infected. This pattern also accounts for the distinct seasonality of WEE, which occurs in most temperate climates between June and November, peaking in late summer and early autumn when the mosquito populations are highest. In warmer regions where the vector season is longer, the disease problem may be more continuous. The horse is considered a "dead-end" host, as the viremic stage is not of sufficient magnitude to allow for further transmission.

The incidence of WEE in horses is generally sporadic, although epizootics do occur periodically. The morbidity is highly variable, depending on the climatic conditions and the prevalence of the vectors. All ages are susceptible, but the young are affected more often and more severely. Mortality of 10 to 30 per cent is common but may run as high as 50 per cent.

The reduced incidence of WEE in horses in the eastern United States, despite the presence of the virus in reservoir avian hosts, is interesting. Geographic variation in the virulence of the virus may be a factor; however, the vector in this region is a different mosquito, *Culiseta melanura*. Unlike its western counterpart, this vector feeds exclusively on passerine birds and tends to live and breed deep in wooded, fresh-water swamps. Thus, the opportunity for a second, mosquito vector to transmit the disease to horses or humans is more remote.[6]

How the virus is able to survive the winter or nonvector season is uncertain. Increasing evidence, however, points to its persistence within the avian population.

PATHOGENESIS AND PATHOLOGY

After inoculation of the virus by the vector into the equine host, there is local multiplication in the muscle, subcutaneous tissues, and regional lymph nodes. The virus then spreads via the bloodstream to vascular endothelial cells and highly vascular organs such as the liver and spleen. This is the period of extraneural amplification and is characterized by viremia and fever. At this point, the reticuloendothelial system begins to rapidly clear the virus from the body.[7] If completely successful, no further clinical signs will be manifested, although neutralizing antibodies will develop.

In spite of immunologic efficiency, several mechanisms, such as erythrocyte adsorption, transportation in leukocytes, or rapid multiplication in vascular tissues, may allow the virus to persist. In these cases, the central nervous system comes under attack either by penetration of the cerebral capillaries (crossing the "blood-brain barrier") or via the choroid plexus into the cerebrospinal fluid.[7] The gray matter of the cerebral cortex, thalamus, and hypothalamus are most often affected, with occasional involvement of the medulla and spinal cord. Cortical lesions usually account for the pronounced clinical signs. Invaded cells are usually destroyed, and sufficient irreversible brain damage can lead to death. The WEE virus is rather fragile and disappears from infected tissues within a few hours after death.

There are no gross lesions and no inclusion bodies histologically. Tissue sections reveal degenerating neurons and perivascular cuffing with some leukocytic infiltration and hemorrhage. These lesions tend to be milder than those of the other alphavirus encephalitides.

CLINICAL SIGNS

After receiving an infective dose of the WEE virus, there is a one- to three-week incubation period. The first manifestation of the disease is a fever, which may reach 105° F (41° C), and an accompanying viremia. This stage is transient (24 to 48 hours) and often goes undetected, as there are few obvious clinical signs. Some cases do not progress beyond this point and would rarely be seen by a clinician.[2]

As the fever wanes (or in some cases as a second episode of fever ensues), characteristic CNS signs may become apparent. The hallmark here is altered consciousness. In the early stages, the animal often seems restless and excitable. There may be periods of compulsive walking and circling, with the horse sometimes crashing blindly into walls and objects. This is followed by extreme mental depression. There is reluctance to move, and standing postures may be abnormal. The head hangs low, the lips droop, the eyes close, and there may be tremors of the face and shoulders. In severe cases, the legs buckle, and younger animals may actually sink to the ground. More commonly, however, this loss of balance is sufficient stimulus for the animal to catch itself before falling. Indeed, the affected horse can usually be aroused, and temporary periods of more normal consciousness may cause the condition to appear episodic in nature. However, if left unstimulated, the animal will relapse into somnolence. If forced to walk, the gait at this time is quite ataxic, particularly in the rear legs and especially when circling. There is generally a concomitant dysphagia. During stuporous periods, the animal shows no interest in food or water.

The most severe signs generally last only a few days, but the entire course of the disease may be two weeks or more. If the horse remains standing and the clinical course is not prolonged or complicated, complete recovery is often possible. For animals that progress to paralysis and recumbency, the prognosis is grave. Some victims that survive will sustain permanent cerebral damage that renders them unable to respond to normal stimuli and, therefore, unusable.

LABORATORY FINDINGS

There are no specific hematologic or biochemical changes associated with WEE. Alterations that do occur may relate to secondary problems such as anorexia, dehydration, or respiratory infection. The changes in the cerebrospinal fluid are not entirely diagnostic. There is a modest pleocytosis (40 to 200 cells per mm^3) of small mononuclear cells with a protein content generally in excess of 100 mg per dl. Slight xanthochromia may also be present.

DIAGNOSIS

A presumptive diagnosis of WEE can be made on the basis of clinical signs and compatible conditions (seasonality, prevalence of vectors, poor vaccination history, and other confirmed cases in the area). Definitive diagnosis requires confirmation. In acute, fatal cases, the virus must be isolated from affected brain tissue. Samples from the cerebral cortex, diencephalon, and midbrain should be quickly harvested, cooled, and submitted, as the virus disappears rapidly after death. Sections should also be preserved and examined histologically. In prolonged or convalescent cases, serologic studies are necessary to establish the diagnosis. Paired serum samples should be collected in the early acute phase and 10 to 14 days later. A rising complement fixation or hemagglutination titer, especially fourfold or greater, is considered diagnostic.

Because many conditions of the central nervous system have a similar clinical appearance, the differential diagnosis can be frustrating. The other arbovirus encephalitides may be identical clinically, but geographic distribution, severity, CSF changes, serology, and cultures will help to distinguish among them. Early cases of dumb rabies are similar in many respects, including CSF findings. These animals, however, progress rapidly to recumbency in two to four days and die in one week or less. In botulism, peripheral paralysis occurs with no alteration in mental status, and the CSF is also unaffected. In hepatoencephalopathy, the primary disease is in the liver. There is generally no fever and no alteration of the CSF. Routine evaluation of liver enzymes is often diagnostic. Trauma, neoplasia (including cholesterol granulomas), and brain abscesses should also be considered. The clinical course, presence or absence of fever, and CBC and CSF analysis should be of help in differentiating these problems.

TREATMENT

As no specific antiviral drugs are available, treatment for WEE is primarily supportive. The effort is worthwhile, however, as many affected horses recover. From the beginning, protective leg wraps should be used to prevent injury. Antipyretics such as phenylbutazone (4 to 6 mg per kg intravenously) may be helpful in reducing the initial fever.

The diet should be nutritious and somewhat laxative in nature to minimize the chance of impaction. If anorexia persists for more than 48 hours, feeding by stomach tube should be implemented. A convenient regimen for short-term maintence utilizes 1½ pounds of alfalfa pellets per 100 pounds of body weight per day, divided into four or more feedings. The pellets for each feeding should be soaked in water to form a thick slurry, the volume of which should not exceed 2 gal for a mature horse. This mixture can be pumped through a large nasogastric tube with a marine bilge pump. If the tube is to be left in place between feedings, it should be sutured to the false nostril and flushed with water after each administration. Hydration should also be monitored

and dehydration treated orally or intravenously as needed with balanced fluid solutions.

If the horse is unable to stand, attempts should be made to support it with a sling. If this apparatus is not tolerated or if it is impossible to implement, the recumbent animal should be bedded heavily and rolled frequently.

Secondary bacterial infections may occur, and each should be evaluated and treated with appropriate antibiotics. For example, streptococcal respiratory infection is an occasional sequela in younger animals, and in such cases intramuscular procaine penicillin G (20,000 units per kg twice daily) is recommended.

The use of corticosteroids in viral infections is controversial. While providing beneficial short-term effects, they probably do not alter mortality and may contribute to the development of secondary bacterial disease. Nevertheless, in cases of coma due to severe encephalitis, intravenous dexamethasone (0.1 to 0.2 mg per kg four to six times daily) may be indicated to help relieve the associated edema.

PREVENTION AND CONTROL

The vaccines currently marketed against WEE are very effective. Most are killed (formalin-inactivated) virus of chick tissue culture origin. All are at least bivalent (WEE and EEE), and some are trivalent[1] (WEE, EEE, and VEE). Dosage and administration schedules vary by manufacturer. If VEE vaccine is to be given, it is recommended that all three be administered simultaneously, as the response to VEE vaccination alone is poorer in horses previously vaccinated against WEE and EEE.[9] Annual vaccination should be completed in late spring or several months prior to the beginning of the encephalitis season.[2] In areas where the mosquito problem is prolonged or continuous, biannual vaccination is suggested. Vaccination of susceptible horses in the face of an outbreak is also recommended.

The optimal time to begin vaccinating foals for WEE remains unclear. Passive immunity to WEE is obtained via the colostrum, and this protection will interfere with the foal's ability to mount an antibody response to routine vaccination.[3] The amount and duration of the passive immunity can vary considerably. Thus, vaccination may begin at six to eight weeks of age, but boosters should be given at six months and one year to ensure adequate protection. Vaccinating mares one month prior to foaling will enhance the colostral antibody levels.

Environmental management practices that eliminate standing water where mosquitoes breed are also important. In endemic areas or outbreak situations, further mosquito control measures can be extremely beneficial. Wide-scale spraying, screened stalls, and topical treatment for individual animals should all prove helpful if indicated. Because of the reservoir population of wild birds, it is unlikely that WEE will ever be completely eradicated.

PUBLIC HEALTH SIGNIFICANCE

Human cases of WEE occur every year, and a small percentage are fatal. Clinical signs include fever, headache, confusion, and stupor. Both humans and horses are incidental "dead-end" hosts for WEE. The horse serves as a sentinel for humans in that equine cases in a given area generally precede human cases by two to five weeks. Therefore, it is important that suspected equine cases be verified and, if positive, reported to state officials. Contact between humans and infected horses does not pose a transmission problem, but personnel involved in removing the brain from a horse that has died of WEE should take precautions to avoid inoculations or punctures with infected tissue.

References

1. Barber, T. L., Walton, T. E., and Lewis, K. J.: Efficacy of trivalent inactivated encephalomyelitis virus vaccine in horses. Am. J. Vet. Res., 39:621, 1978.
2. Byrne, R. J.: The control of eastern and western arboviral encephalomyelitis of horses. Proceedings of the Third International Conference on Equine Infectious Diseases. Paris, 1972–1973, pp. 115–123.
3. Ferguson, J. A., Reeves, W. C., and Hardy, J. L.: Studies on immunity to alphaviruses in foals. Am. J. Vet. Res., 40:5, 1979.
4. Gibbs, E. P. J.: Equine viral encephalitis. Eq. Vet. J., 8:66, 1976.
5. Hanson, R. P.: Virology and epidemiology of eastern and western arboviral encephalomyelitis of horses. Proceedings of the 3rd International Conference on Equine Infectious Diseases. Paris, 1972–1973, pp. 100–114.
6. Hayes, C. G., and Wallis, R. C.: Ecology of western equine encephalomyelitis in the eastern United States. Adv. Virus Res., 21:37, 1977.
7. Johnson, R. T.: Pathophysiology and epidemiology of acute viral infections of the nervous system. Adv. Neurol., 6:27, 1974.
8. Sekla, L. H. (ed.): Western encephalomyelitis. Can. J. Pub. Health, 67, Suppl. 1, 1976.
9. Vanderwagen, L. C., Pearson, J. L., Franti, C. E., Tamm, E. L., Reimann, H. P., and Behymer, D. E.: A field study of persistence of antibodies in California horses vaccinated against western, eastern and Venezuelan equine encephalomyelitis. Am. J. Vet. Res., 36:1567, 1975.

SPINAL CORD TRAUMA

Stephen M. Reed, PULLMAN, WASHINGTON

One of the most incapacitating nonfatal injuries of the horse is spinal cord trauma. Such trauma may or may not be accompanied by fractures of the vertebral column and lesions of the ligaments. The indications for surgical exploration of traumatic spinal injuries are controversial,[1, 10] but prevention of further damage to neural tissue is the major aim of both medical and surgical management. In addition to prevention of further neural damage, one must be aware of life-threatening injuries to the head, thorax, or abdomen, which often occur concurrently. Early rehabilitation with a more favorable prognosis for the horse is dependent upon correct management at the time of injury and during preparation and shipment to the veterinary hospital for further diagnostic evaluation and on prevention of complications. This chapter will be concerned with types of vertebral trauma, the pathophysiology of spinal cord trauma, performance and interpretation of the neurologic examination, and current medical and surgical management of spinal cord trauma.

TYPES OF VERTEBRAL TRAUMA

Vertebral trauma most commonly occurs as a result of a horse falling or colliding with a relatively immovable object, considerable force being necessary for vertebral displacement. The age of the animal may contribute to the location of spinal cord trauma, foals appearing to be more susceptible to vertebral trauma than adults and frequently suffering fractures of the cranial cervical (C), and caudal thoracic (T) regions. Adult horses are susceptible to injury of the middle (fifth [C5] through seventh [C7]) cervical vertebrae, as well as the caudal thoracic region.[4] The higher incidence of luxations, subluxations, and epiphyseal separations in young animals may be because closure of the cervical vertebral (C2-C6) epiphyseal growth plates occurs at four to five years of age.

A summary of the common types of vertebral injuries, their locations, and the resulting clinical syndromes is given in Table 1. The types of injuries

TABLE 1. COMMON TYPES OF VERTEBRAL TRAUMA

Level of Injury	Age	Type of Vertebral Trauma	Common Traumatic Incident	Syndrome
Cervical	Foal to yearling	Fracture of dens, luxation C1-C2	Hyperflexion (e.g., somersault)	Tetraparesis, respiratory depression, death
Cervical	Young adult	Epiphyseal fracture	Hyperextension	Tetraparesis to tetraplegia
Cervical	Adult	Compression fracture	Head-on collision	Tetraparesis to tetraplegia
Cranial thoracic	Usually young	Fracture of dorsal spinous process	Flipping over backwards	Often none
T2-S1	Any	Transverse fracture of vertebral arch, with dislocation	Somersaulting or falls	Paraparesis
Sacroiliac subluxation	Adult	Subluxation	Falls or slipping on ice	None
Sacral fracture	Any	Compression	Fall over backwards or dog-sitting when backed	Urinary and fecal incontinence with or without posterior paresis; paralysis of the tail and anus

include hyperextension, hyperflexion, dislocation, and compression and result in syndromes varying from tetraplegia to no neurologic deficit. Hyperextension injuries often affect the cervical vertebrae and may result from a failure to negotiate a jump with the horse landing on the chest and ventrum of the neck. Hyperflexion injuries of the neck may result from a horse stumbling and falling in a somersault fashion. These injuries often result in vertebral fractures with impact to the spinal cord by dislocated osseous fragments. With very severe injury, soft tissue structures supporting the vertebral column may be disrupted, resulting in dislocation of the cervical vertebrae. When dislocations occur, the spinal cord may be seriously damaged. Notwithstanding this, one should remember that the vertebral canal is of larger diameter than the spinal cord itself, which undoubtedly accounts for sparing of the spinal cord with some severe vertebral injuries. Both luxations and subluxations have been reported in horses.[4] Luxations of the vertebra frequently occur between the atlas and axis and atlas and occiput as well as in the thoracolumbar region. Subluxations have been recognized as a part of the cervical vertebral malformation syndrome (p. 359) and may result in signs of paresis, ataxia, and spasticity. Compression injuries are associated with a shortening of the vertebral body and usually result from a head-on collision with an immovable object or another horse.

PATHOPHYSIOLOGY OF SPINAL CORD TRAUMA

The pathophysiologic response of the spinal cord to injury is the subject of much debate and study.

Discussion has centered around types of injury, the acuteness of the injury, whether the vasculature is affected more than the nervous tissue, and finally the importance of inflammatory mediators such as biogenic amines and prostaglandins in the production of hemorrhagic necrosis following the initial insult.[7]

Impact injuries appear to be most damaging to the gray and central white matter, affecting the neuropile more than the microvasculature, although with severe impact injuries damage occurs to both nervous and vascular tissues. The release of biogenic amines may result in vasospasm and hypoxia, subsequently leading to tissue necrosis.[2, 5] In addition, prostaglandins I_2 and F_2 appear to play a role in the propagation of spinal cord trauma. The effect appears to be related to the development of ischemia, which further complicates the structural and functional alterations. The rate of development of compression appears to be important, and from a clinical point of view, the more rapidly progressive the compression, the more rapidly one needs to decompress the spinal cord.[10]

NEUROLOGIC EXAMINATION

Initial evaluation of any patient suspected of receiving spinal cord injury must be directed toward the most life-threatening factors, including obstruction of the airway, cardiovascular collapse, potentially fatal hemorrhage, and concurrent head injuries. Following stabilization of these problems, the veterinarian should seek an accurate account of the injury, as this can help localize the injured site.

A systematic evaluation should proceed from the head to the tail, and a technique for this has been described.[6] The examination for head trauma is described elsewhere (p. 341). Attention is now directed at evaluation of the gait and posture, neck and forelimbs, trunk and hindlimbs, and tail and anus. A recumbent patient should be observed for its ability to rise. If only the head can be raised, there is probably a cranial cervical lesion (C1-C3). If the horse is able to raise the head and neck off the ground but is unable to use the thoracic limbs well, it is likely the lesion is more caudal, such as C4-T2. Animals so affected may be able to maintain sternal recumbency but are unable to effectively use forelegs when attempting to rise. A horse that can achieve a dog-sitting posture and use the thoracic limbs fairly well probably has a lesion caudal to T2.

Flaccid paralysis is characteristic of a lower motor neuron lesion. Evaluation of these lesions may be assisted by reflex testing. Signs resulting from an upper motor neuron lesion in the cervical region include loss of voluntary motor function, while muscle tone may be increased and spinal reflexes may be normal to hyperactive. Spinal reflexes of the thoracic limbs may be evaluated by pinching the distal extremity and observing for flexion of the joints of the forelimb. This tests the integrity of the peripheral sensory nerve, spinal cord segments C6-T2, and the motor fibers of the peripheral nerves. If the patient also demonstrates a cerebral response, one can assume that the sensory pathways to the forebrain are intact. A lesion cranial to C6 may result in a loss of the upper motor neuron influences, and the patient should show a hyperactive reflex.

Localization of a lesion caudal to T2 may be aided by identification of a loss of sensation over the truck or hindlimbs at the level of the lesion. In addition, diffuse sweating may be seen as a result of a lesion in the descending sympathetic tracts of the spinal cord, while patchy sweating may be seen with damage to specific preganglionic or postganglionic sympathetic nerve fibers. Decreased panniculus response suggests a lesion in the region of C8-T1 or damage to the lateral thoracic spinal nerve. The use of spinal reflex testing of the hindlimbs in recumbent animals is limited to the patellar and flexor reflexes. These reflexes test the femoral nerve and spinal cord segments L4-L5 and the sciatic nerve and cord segments L5-S5, respectively. A release of these reflexes from upper motor neuron modulation results in hyperactive reflexes and suggests a lesion cranial to L4.

The final regions to be examined are the tail and anus. The tone of the tail, as well as the perineal reflex, should be examined. The nerves responsible are the pudendal nerve, caudal rectal nerve, and the sacrococcygeal spinal cord segments. Abnormalities resulting from lesions in the region of L4 through the caudal sacral segments include ataxia and paresis to paralysis of the hindlimbs, poor tail and pelvic limb tone, hypalgesia to analgesia of the affected area, urinary incontinence, and obstipation.

Ancillary diagnostic aids in evaluation of spinal cord trauma should include radiography and sometimes myelography. Some benefit may be derived from cerebrospinal fluid (CSF) analysis (p. 331) and electromyography, if available. On CSF analysis, the most common findings associated with spinal cord trauma are xanthochromia (yellow color) and slight to moderate elevation in protein content. If the injury is severe enough, a bloody sample may be obtained. In some instances with a severe fracture-dislocation, collection of CSF from the lumbosacral space may not be possible because of complete obstruction to flow of CSF (i.e., spinal block).

MEDICAL THERAPY

The management of vertebral injuries in the horse is dependent upon the amount of vertebral displacement and in particular the attending neural damage. Vertebral displacement may be obvious if there is a significant malformation of the neck or back. In cases of damage to the cervical region, radiographs may be helpful to determine if a fracture is present as well as to show the amount of vertebral displacement. Therapy should be governed by the patient's response as determined by serial neurologic examinations. Some horses with few or no neurologic abnormalities may require only stall rest and observation.

The author's drug of choice for immediate management of acute spinal cord trauma is dexamethasone* at a dosage of 0.1 to 0.2 mg per kg body weight intravenously, although some controversy exists over its beneficial effects.[9] The dosage may be repeated every six to eight hours with a favorable response expected within four to eight hours. Following initial improvement, the patient may be placed on oral prednisolone at a dose of 0.2 mg per kg once a day for three to five days followed by gradual reduction in dosage. In steroid-treated horses, caution must be used to prevent infection if open wounds are present.

Failure to achieve a favorable response within four hours or deterioration of signs indicates the need for more aggressive treatment. Osmotic diuretic agents, such as mannitol,† at a dose of 3 gm per kg as a 20 per cent solution may be helpful. In fact, these agents may have beneficial therapeutic effects at dosages as low as 0.25 gm per kg. A favorable response to mannitol treatment is expected within 30 to 60 minutes. Intravenous mannitol may be repeated at least two times, although continued use of hypertonic solutions intravenously may be complicated by severe dehydration.

---

*Azium, Schering Corp., Kenilworth, NJ 07033
†Osmitrol, Travenol Labs, Deerfield, IL 60015

A less conventional and somewhat controversial therapy is dimethyl sulfoxide.* The intravenous dosage is 1 gm per kg body weight diluted in saline at concentrations of 10 to 45 per cent; all of these concentrations have an osmolality greater than plasma. This drug has been reported to decrease edema, prevent platelet aggregation, maintain spinal cord vascular integrity, and increase the availability of oxygen to tissues.[12, 13] Some authors have failed to identify a beneficial effect of the drug either alone or in combination with other drugs in treatment of spinal cord trauma in dogs.[8]

SURGICAL INTERVENTION

The decision for surgical intervention is made when there is a lack of response to medical treatment or when radiographs indicate the need for decompression or stabilization. In many instances, the use of medical treatment is necessary to stabilize the patient prior to performing surgery. The technique for decompression of compressive lesions has been described in the dog.[3] The same procedures may be utilized in the horse when a lesion is demonstrated radiographically, when there is failure to respond to medical management, or when there is progression of signs such as a change in the location of a sensory deficit along the axial skeleton or a further loss of motor function.

At the time of decompression, it may be prudent to avoid surgical incision of the dura because of its close adherence to the spinal cord. The use of normothermic saline for irrigation and flushing appears to be a beneficial adjunct to decompression.[11] If the trauma has resulted in loss of stability between vertebrae, the technique of ventral fusion of the vertebrae (p. 361) may be useful, especially for treatment of cervical vertebral injuries.[14]

Paraplegic and tetraplegic patients that have lost all response to deep pain caudal to the spinal cord lesion have a functional or anatomic spinal cord transection and are candidates for euthanasia unless response to medical or surgical therapy is noted in 24 hours or less.

NURSING MANAGEMENT

The management of horses that are recumbent is fraught with complications such as the development of pressure sores over the elbow, tuber coxae, and other bony prominences, as well as urinary bladder atony and obstipation. Daily catheterization of the

bladder with aseptic technique appears more beneficial in the author's hands than application of an indwelling catheter. The use of an indwelling urinary catheter often leads to ascending infection and cystitis. Caution must be used when evacuation of the rectum is performed to avoid applying too much pressure to a distended bladder.

The use of antimicrobial therapy is important because recumbent patients frequently develop pneumonia, cystitis, and occasionally meningitis. The author uses chloramphenicol at a dose of 25 to 50 mg per kg orally four times a day or other antimicrobial agents based on culture and sensitivity testing of material from the infected region.

A final consideration in nursing care for recumbent horses is the use of a sling. It is important to have a sling with both a breast and butt strap in order to maintain the horse in position. Proper positioning of the recumbent patient in the sling is difficult and must be done carefully. A commercially available sling* is the most satisfactory one this author has used.

References

1. Black, P.: Injuries of the spine and spinal cord: Management in the acute phase. In Zuidema, G. D., Rutherford, R. B., and Ballinger, W. F. (eds.): Management of Trauma, 3rd ed. Philadelphia, W. B. Saunders Co., 1979, pp. 226–252.
2. Griffiths, I. R., McCulloch, M., and Crawford, R. A.: Ultrastructural appearance of the spinal microvasculature between 12 hours and 5 days after impact injury. Acta Neuropathol., 43:205, 1978.
3. Hoerlein, B. F.: Spinal fractures, luxations, and fusions. In Hoerlein, B. F. (ed.): Canine Neurology: Diagnosis and Treatment, 3rd ed. Philadelphia, W. B. Saunders Co., 1978, pp. 561–590.
4. Jeffcott, L. B.: Disorders of the thoracolumbar spine of the horse—a survey of 443 cases. Vet. J., 12:197, 1980.
5. Kobrine, A. I., Evans, D. E., and Rizzoli, H. V.: The effects of ischemia on long tract neural conduction of the spinal cord. J. Neurosurg., 50:639, 1974.
6. Mayhew, I. G., and Ingram, J. T.: Neurologic evaluation of the horse. Proc. 24th Annu. Conv. Am. Assoc. Eq. Pract., 1978, pp. 525–541.
7. Osterholm, J. L.: The pathophysiological response to spinal cord injury. J. Neurosurg., 40:5, 1974.
8. Parker, A. J., and Smith, C. W.: Lack of functional recovery from spinal cord trauma following dimethyl sulfoxide and epsilon amino caproic acid therapy in dogs. Res. Vet. Sci., 27:253, 1979.
9. Rucker, N. C., Lumb, W. V., and Scott, R. J.: Combined pharmacologic and surgical treatments for acute spinal cord trauma. Am. J. Vet. Res., 42:7, 1981.
10. Selcer, R. R.: Trauma of the central nervous system. Vet. Clin. North Am. (Small Anim. Pract.), 10(3):619, 1980.
11. Swain, S. F., Vandevelde, M., Sammons, W. C., Baine, L.,

*Domoso, Diamond Labs, Des Moines, IA 50303

*Liftex Sling, Inc., 204 Railroad Dr., North Hampton Industrial Park, Ivyland, PA 18974

and McGuire, J. A.: Comparison of hypothermic and normothermic spinal cord perfusion in the dog. Vet. Surg., 8:119, 1979.

12. Torre, J. C. de la, Johnson, C. M., Goode, D. J., and Mullan, S.: Pharmacologic treatment and evaluation or permanent experimental spinal cord trauma. Neurology, 25:508, 1975.

13. Torre, J. C. de la, Kawanga, K. M., Rowed, D. W., Johnson, C. M., Goode, D. J., Kajihara, K., and Mullan, S.: Dimethyl sulfoxide in central nervous system trauma. Ann. NY Acad. Sci., 243:362, 1975.

14. Wagner, P. C., Grant, B. D., and Bagby, G.: Evaluation of cervical spine fusion as a treatment in the equine wobbler syndrome. Vet. Surg., 8:84, 1979.

CERVICAL VERTEBRAL MALFORMATION

Pamela Carroll Wagner, CORVALLIS, OREGON

Cervical vertebral malformation (CVM) refers to abnormalities in the vertebral bodies, articular processes, and vertebral foramina that ultimately result in functional or anatomic stenosis of the vertebral canal. Such abnormalities are not uncommon, and one study estimated the incidence to be 10 per cent in the Thoroughbred population.[5] The condition often goes unrecognized unless impingement of the vertebrae on the spinal cord causes focal compression and neurologic signs. Focal spinal cord compression results in gait abnormalities that have been described as part of the wobbler syndrome.[3] The condition has also been referred to as equine sensory ataxia and equine incoordination.

Several types of osseous malformations may be responsible for stenosis of the vertebral canal and pressure-induced lesions of the spinal cord.[9] For the purpose of a therapeutic approach, they may be loosely grouped as follows.

Functional Stenosis. When the neck is flexed or hyperextended, the vertebrae move in such a manner as to cause compression of the spinal cord. This has been referred to as spondylolisthesis. Seen most frequently in weanlings and yearlings, the abnormal angulation is often accompanied by articular process changes as well as remodeling of the caudal vertebral epiphyses. With the neck in a neutral position, compression of the spinal cord is reduced; however, the vertebral canal may still be narrowed owing to the remodeling changes.

Absolute Stenosis. Osseous changes in the vertebrae that cause spinal cord compression not altered by neck positioning have been described.[3, 9] These include stenosis of the cranial vertebral foramina, medial ingrowth of the cranial articular processes, and arthropathy of the cranial and caudal articular processes.

CLINICAL SIGNS

Most horses are affected in the first two years of life, usually as weanlings or yearlings. Onset of signs may be sudden and related to a traumatic incident or insidious with slowly progressive and debilitating incoordination. Several authors have noted a sexual predisposition, with colts being affected more often than fillies. Most affected horses are in good flesh and have been on an excellent plane of nutrition.[3]

The presenting clinical signs are those of a focal pressure-induced lesion of the cervical spinal cord.[3] Damage to the ascending spinal cord tracts results in proprioceptive deficits of all four limbs that manifest clinically as ataxia and occasionally hypermetria. Damage to the descending spinal cord tracts is evidenced by tetraparesis and degrees of stiffness or hypometria.

If the malformation exerts pressure on the cranial cervical spinal cord, the proprioceptive deficits will be more severe in the pelvic limbs than the thoracic limbs. The ataxia is most noticeable at a walk or when the horse is turned in small circles. If the animal is able to gallop, it does so with a characteristic "bunny hop." The rear legs will circumduct, and the toes may drag. The hocks have little flexion, and the stride appears to be prolonged. In general, the rear quarters of the horse seem stiff and unbalanced. If the horse is turned sharply, it may pivot on the inside leg, while a normal horse steps around briskly. While the pelvic limbs appear most involved, subtle signs of foreleg involvement may be noted on close examination. The front legs may be more obviously affected if the vertebral malformation occurs at C5-C7. The horse may step abnormally wide and cross its forelegs while moving. If the legs are placed in abnormal postures, the horse may not correct its stance.

These signs can be exaggerated by leading the horse downhill or with the head elevated. In general, focal cervical spinal cord compression will result in a horse that has more pronounced signs of ataxia in the pelvic limbs than in the thoracic limbs. Backing the horse may elicit signs of ataxia; however, this is variable. When led over obstacles, the horse may drag its feet and stumble. Usually the proprioceptive signs are bilateral and symmetrical; however, one pelvic limb may appear more affected than the other.

Signs of paresis are elicited by pressure over the withers and loins and by sway tests. If pressure is exerted over the withers or loins, the horse may move downward and may fall if paresis is severe. The sway test should be performed while the horse is moving. The handler pulls the tail firmly to one side as the horse is being walked away. A weak horse will be readily pulled to the side, and the severely affected horse may stumble and fall down. Paresis reflects damage to the descending tracts of the upper motor neuron pathways.

Some horses show rapid onset of signs with stabilization at variable levels of disability. Signs in some horses never stabilize and slowly get progressively worse, while in others signs may be present for some time and then may appear to improve. Reports of spontaneous full recoveries of confirmed cases of CVM are uncommon.

DIAGNOSIS

Other causes of ataxia such as vertebral trauma, equine degenerative myelopathy, equine protozoal myeloencephalitis, and equine herpesvirus 1 infection must be ruled out. Definitive diagnosis is accomplished by obtaining radiographs and myelograms of the cervical vertebrae to demonstrate focal spinal cord compression. Radiographs should be made with the horse under general anesthesia in lateral recumbency. The cervical spine should be visualized from the base of the skull to the intervertebral space of C7-T1. After radiographs are made of the neck in the neutral position, the neck should be flexed by gently pulling the horse's muzzle toward the carpus and securing it in this position. This provides adequate flexion of all articulations of the cervical vertebral column. Care should be taken not to overflex the neck, as further damage to the cord may occur if there is a severe subluxation. Areas of apparent stenosis may be confirmed with myelography. The use of metrizamide* as a myelographic agent has made the procedure safe and accurate.[3]

Dynamic cord compression occurs when there is an abnormal relationship of one vertebra to another, which has been referred to as a subluxation, functional stenosis, or spondylolisthesis. Radiographically, the vertebral canal narrows significantly when the neck is flexed. A myelogram is essential to confirm functional stenosis. In these cases, the myelographic dye columns are visible both dorsally and

*Accurate Chemical Co., Hicksville, NY 11801

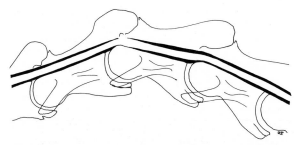

Figure 1. Diagram of a cervical myelographic study of a horse with CVM and functional stenosis. There is dramatic attenuation of the ventral dye column and obliteration of the dorsal dye column at the level of the C3 and C4 vertebral articulation when the neck is in a flexed position.

ventrally when the neck is extended, but both columns narrow or disappear with flexion (Fig. 1).

Many cases of functional stenosis resulting in spinal cord compression also have some degree of absolute stenosis. However, this stenosis does not, in itself, result in spinal cord compression. Dorsal protrusion of the caudal vertebral epiphyses as well as remodeling of the articular processes is often seen in horses with functional stenosis.

Absolute stenosis causes a static compression of the spinal cord that can be noted on the myelogram when the cervical vertebrae are in extended, neutral, and flexed positions. Compression is due to bony changes of the vertebrae that include absolute stenosis of the cranial or the caudal orifice of the vertebral foramina, remodeling of the articular processes, and exostoses and degeneration of the articular surfaces indicative of degenerative joint disease. An example is shown in the diagram of a myelogram in Figure 2. While the compression may be exaggerated by flexion or hyperextension, it is present at all times.

Cerebrospinal fluid (CSF) analysis has been useful in ruling out other causes of ataxia and paresis. Cerebrospinal fluid from the horse with CVM is usually normal.

Electromyography (EMG) has been employed to differentiate lower motor neuron (LMN) disease from upper motor neuron (UMN) disease. Most ste-

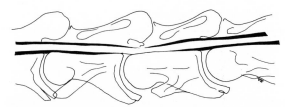

Figure 2. Absolute stenosis of the vertebral canal at the caudal orifice of C5 and the cranial orifice of C6 is evident in this line drawing of a myelogram of a horse with CVM. Many horses with functional stenosis, as depicted in Figure 1, have some degree of absolute vertebral canal stenosis at the site of spinal cord compression.

notic cervical vertebral lesions result in compression of myelinated fibers, including those in the descending tracts, i.e., UMN damage. The EMG in upper motor neuron disease is essentially normal, and thus an EMG of the cervical muscles of horses with stenotic lesions is usually within normal limits. In some cases of absolute stenosis with static cord compression at C5-C7, some EMG changes have been noted. This has been attributed to pressure on the ventral roots as they leave the vertebral canal.

PATHOGENESIS OF BONY LESIONS

The cause of cervical vertebral malformation is unknown but is probably a result of a combination of factors. An early study reported the condition to be hereditary,[1] but more recent work disputes that theory.[2] In most cases, the articular processes and vertebral foramina are malformed, causing cord compression directly or allowing malarticulation that causes compression of the cord during movement that some authorities have interpreted as evidence of instability.

Osteochondrosis-like lesions have been seen in the articular surfaces as well as in the vertebral body growth plates in some horses affected with CVM. It has been reported that the primary etiologic factors causing osteochondrosis are a genetic predisposition for rapid growth combined with a large intake of high-energy food.[6] The effect of hormonal factors has not been analyzed; however, a reported sex predilection indicates such studies may be helpful.

In all probability, many factors are involved. A horse selected for rapid growth being fed on a high plane of nutrition is certainly the most likely candidate for this syndrome.

TREATMENT

Cervical spinal cord compression carries a guarded prognosis. Because the course of the clinical syndrome is variable, some treatments may appear to be successful for a period of time and then fail.

MEDICAL MANAGEMENT

Medical treatment is aimed at reducing inflammation at the site of compression. Dexamethasone* at a dosage of 0.1 mg per kg has been used, and some improvement of clinical signs has been noted for the duration of the therapy. Phenylbutazone† at a dosage of 8 to 10 mg per kg has also been used. Some veterinarians have obtained good results using 1 cc per kg of 50 per cent dimethylsulfoxide* in 1 liter of saline intravenously every other day until improvement is noted. With all of these medical treatments, stall rest and feeding and watering the horse from an elevated position to discourage extensive neck movement is recommended. The severely affected horse will be prone to lacerations of the bulbs of the heels of the forelimbs due to overreaching as well as cuts of the head and body due to hitting objects and falling. Good nursing care is imperative; however, the outcome is usually not rewarding. Some horses will stabilize enough to be used as breeding animals, but many improved horses will worsen when medical therapy is discontinued.

SURGICAL MANAGEMENT

Arthrodesis of the Cervical Spine. The surgical approach to relieve cord compression depends on the nature of the lesion. *Functional stenosis* that results in maximal cord compression during flexion may be treated by fusion of the affected vertebrae to prevent movement at that site.[7] The Cloward technique of anterior cervical fusion as used in humans has been modified for horses to achieve osseous bridging between two vertebrae, maintaining the vertebrae in the extended position.[7, 8] This technique entails drilling out the intervertebral space and using a bone dowel to stabilize and fuse the vertebrae in extension.

In the experience of the author, the majority of improvement is seen in the first year postoperatively. In most of the cases, clinical improvement is seen; however, the degree of improvement is dependent upon several factors: (1) The duration of time the horse has shown signs prior to surgery. Most surgical cases are not identified and scheduled for surgery less than one month following the onset of signs, and in many the time elapsed is much greater. In general, the horses that are operated upon early after the onset of signs do improve to a greater extent than those that show signs for months prior to surgery. (2) The severity of signs prior to surgery. While hores with very severe signs will respond to surgery, the residual level of ataxia still remaining may be greater than that present in the horse with milder signs presurgically. (3) The age of the horse. In general, younger horses appear to improve the most. This may, in fact, reflect the duration of time that signs have existed. Ataxia may be overlooked until the horse is required to work.

Complications of this surgical procedure include

---

*Dexasone, Med-Tech, Inc., Elwood, KS 66024
†Westazon, Western Medical Supply, Inc., Arcadia, CA 91006

*Domoso, Diamond Labs, Des Moines, IA 50304

spinal cord trauma, hemorrhage, and damage to the recurrent laryngeal nerve, all of which may be avoided by careful surgical technique. Postsurgical complications include trauma during recovery as well as failure of the dowel after implantation.

Subtotal Dorsal Decompressive Laminectomy. *Absolute stenosis* causing a static compression of the spinal cord in both the extended and flexed positions is best treated by a subtotal dorsal decompressive laminectomy. The surgery requires proper equipment for positioning and operation.[10] The procedure is fraught with complications related to the surgical approach and the postanesthetic recovery and should not be undertaken without considerable preparation and practice.

The prognosis for return to usefulness of horses with CVM is guarded. Most surgically treated horses with functional stenoses are able to be used for breeding animals, and some can be used in hard work such as racing, show, and pleasure. Those horses with anatomic stenoses requiring subtotal dorsal decompressions have a much more guarded prognosis. Much of the return to function depends on the degree of spinal cord damage, and the extent of improvement cannot be evaluated realistically for many months after surgery.

References

1. Dimock, W.: "Wobbles"—an hereditary disease in horses. J. Hered., *41*:319, 1950.
2. Falco, M. J., Whitewell, K., and Palmer, A. C.: An investigation into the genetics of "wobbler disease" in thoroughbred horses in Britain. Equine Vet. J., 8:165, 1976.
3. Mayhew, I. G., deLahunta, A., Whitlock, R. H., Krook, L., and Tasker, J. B.: Spinal cord diseases in the horse. Cornell Vet., *68*, Suppl. 6:1, 1978.
4. Nyland, T. G., Blythe, L. L., Pool, R. R., Helphrey, M. G., and O'Brien, T. R.: Metrizamide myelography in the horse: Clinical radiographic and pathologic changes. Am. J. Vet. Res., *41*:204, 1980.
5. Rooney, J. R.: Biomechanics of Lameness in Horses. Baltimore, Williams and Wilkins, 1969, p. 222.
6. Stromberg, B.: A review of the salient features of osteochondrosis in the horse. Equine Vet. J., *11*:211, 1979.
7. Wagner, P. C., Bagby, G. W., Grant, B. D., Gallina, A., Ratzlaff, M., and Sande, R.: Surgical stabilization of the equine cervical spine. Vet. Surg., 8:7, 1979.
8. Wagner, P. C., Grant, B. D., Bagby, G. W., Gallina, A., Sande, R., and Ratzlaff, M.: Evaluation of cervical spinal fusion as a treatment in the equine "wobbler" syndrome. Vet. Surg., 8:84, 1979.
9. Whitwell, K. E.: Causes of ataxia in horses. In Practice, *2*(4):17, 1980.
10. Wagner, P. C., Grant, B. D., Gallina, A., and Bagby, G. W.: Ataxia and paresis in horses. Part III. Surgical treatment of cervical spinal cord compression. Compendium of Continuing Education for the Practicing Veterinarian, 3(5):S192, 1981.

EQUINE HERPESVIRUS-1 MYELOENCEPHALITIS

Robert J. MacKay, GAINESVILLE, FLORIDA

Neurologic disease (myeloencephalitis) in horses due to infection with equine herpesvirus-1 (EHV-1) has been recognized with increasing frequency in recent years. The disease occurs sporadically, but morbidity may be quite high, approaching 100 per cent in certain groups of horses. There does not appear to be any breed or sex predisposition to EHV-1 myeloencephalitis, although mares in early to midgestation may be more susceptible. Horses more than a year old are usually affected, although a recent report described neurologic signs in a group of young foals infected with EHV-1.[2]

Myeloencephalitis, like other EHV-1 associated diseases (rhinopneumonitis, abortions, and perinatal infections), occurs most commonly where there are aggregations of horses as in racing, breeding, or boarding stables.

Virus and host factors that determine why neurologic disease develops in some horses or groups of horses and not others have not been defined clearly. There is as yet no evidence for a distinct neurotropic strain of EHV-1.

CLINICAL FINDINGS

Experimentally, neurologic disease may be seen about 7 days after infection by either nasal or subcutaneous routes.[3] Clinical observations suggest a similar incubation period in naturally occurring cases. Fever (39 to 40°C) develops three to four days after infection, followed by signs of neurologic disease two to three days later. Horses may also show signs of upper respiratory disease such as cough and nasal discharge. Horses in contact with other affected horses may be infected and febrile without developing central nervous system (CNS) disease.[4]

Signs of myeloencephalitis develop acutely. There is weakness and ataxia in one to all of the limbs, but typically the pelvic limbs are most severely affected. The deficits may be worse on one side than on the other and can vary in severity from slight pelvic limb incoordination (swaying of the hips and circumduction) to peracute tetraplegia. Characteristically, there is urinary incontinence and bladder distention at the onset, accompanied sometimes by penile or vulvar flaccidity. Reduced tail tone and perineal hypalgesia are inconsistent findings. Neurologic deficits may become worse during the first 48 hours, although many mildly affected horses begin to improve within hours of the onset of signs. If recumbency occurs, it is usually within the first 24 hours, and paralysis may become so complete that the horse is unable to raise its head from the ground.

Surprisingly, despite the name, clinical signs of encephalitis are seldom seen. Depression, when it occurs, is more likely due to complications of fever and secondary infection than to primary brain disease.

Most horses with EHV-l myeloencephalitis that remain standing recover completely within one to three weeks, although more protracted recoveries (up to several months) may occur. In general, the time to recovery depends on the initial severity of signs. There are reports of horses regaining their feet after several weeks of recumbency, although most horses that become tetraplegic do not recover. Many of these deaths are due to complications of paralysis and recumbency such as respiratory, urinary tract, or decubital infections and starvation or dehydration.

LABORATORY FINDINGS

Blood samples taken during the initial febrile period may show mild leukopenia with moderate lymphopenia (less than 1000 lymphocytes per mm³).

Samples of cerebrospinal fluid (CSF) from either cisternal or lumbosacral sites are markedly xanthochromic (yellow). Protein levels are elevated to 100 to 500 mg per dl (normal range is 30 to 80 mg/per dl), although cell numbers are usually normal (less than 5 cells per mm³). In an exceptional series of cases recently reported, cell counts were elevated (up to 400 cells per mm³) in postmortem CSF samples of six of eight horses with EHV-l myeloencephalitis.[5] The possible effects of postmortem changes on these cell counts are unknown. The typical CSF abnormalities reflect the diffuse vascular inflammation and leakage characteristic of the disease.

Attempts at viral isolation from nasopharyngeal swabs or buffy coat cultures are only successful if performed early in the disease or during the prodromal febrile period.

A fourfold rise in serum neutralizing (SN) or complement fixing (CF) antibody titers can be demonstrated between acute and convalescent sera. Horses in contact with other affected horses not showing neurologic signs may also have a significant rise in antibody titer.

PATHOLOGIC FINDINGS

The characteristic lesion throughout the spinal cord and brain is vasculitis, especially involving arterioles. Changes due to vasculitis may be evident grossly as brownish patchy discolorations on the cut surface of spinal cord sections. These discolored areas represent the hemorrhagic and ischemic infarction of gray and particularly white matter of the spinal cord that results from the vesicular lesion. Similar histologic lesions are usually evident in the brain, and a trigeminal (gasserian) ganglioneuritis is rather consistent.

Virus is seldom isolated from the CNS of horses with histologic findings typical of EHV-1 myeloencephalitis. This may be a consequence of the high SN titer usually present at the time of death.

DIAGNOSIS

EHV-1 myeloencephalitis must be distinguished from other diseases that may cause similar signs such as the arboviral encephalitides, equine protozoal myeloencephalitis, verminous myelitis, vertebral malformations, and rabies.

A suitable diagnostic plan for suspected cases of EHV-1 myeloencephalitis in a racing or breeding stable is as follows:

1. Submit sera from affected horses to a diagnostic laboratory at the onset of the disease and two to three weeks later for SN or CF titers.

2. Also submit paired sera from a sample of contact horses and any mares that have aborted during the previous month.

3. The brains (and spinal cords if possible) of horses submitted for necropsy should be fixed in formalin for histologic examination.

4. Tissues from any aborted foals and tracheal and lung tissue from horses dying following respiratory signs should be examined histologically and submitted for viral isolation.

TREATMENT

Slightly affected horses that remain standing usually recover uneventfully if confined in a stall and rested for two to four weeks. Those horses with pronounced ataxia and weakness that have difficulty standing may need careful nursing care to recover. The aim of this supportive therapy is to prevent the complications of prolonged recumbency and bladder atony such as external trauma, pressure sores, and secondary bacterial infections. Deep bedding must be kept under the horse and must be cleaned and changed frequently. Clean straw is preferred, but wood shavings or shredded paper may be adequate. If possible, horses should be assisted to stand every four to six hours to improve skin circulation and encourage urination and defecation. Those horses with a placid nature and reasonable strength may be able to stand and rest in a sling. Sling support may be used intermittently to assist standing or continuously until the horse is ambulatory. It is imperative that the animal not hang in the sling, or severe respiratory embarrassment and even death may result.

Recumbent horses should be assisted to the sternal position if possible. Those animals unable to maintain sternal recumbency should be rolled every two hours during the day and at least twice during the night. Pressure sores will inevitably develop over bony prominences and may need to be soaked frequently and protected with additional cotton padding taped or sutured to the skin. A towel or other soft padding should be placed under the downside eye to prevent corneal abrasion and ulceration. Necrotic pressure-induced cystitis develops quickly, and atonic bladder distention must be relieved twice daily by careful, clean urethral catheterization. Broad-spectrum antibiotics, such as ampicillin trihydrate,* 10 mg per kg every 8 to 12 hours, should be used prophylactically during periods of urinary bladder catheterization. Bacterial bronchopneumonia may develop as a complication of EHV-1 rhinopneumonitis due to hypostatic lung congestion, poor chest movements, and aspiration of foreign materials. Such respiratory infections must be treated vigorously with appropriate antimicrobials. Water and nutrients (such as alfalfa meal gruel) must be provided via nasogastric tube if voluntary intake is inadequate owing to weakness or secondary complications.

There is a tendency to recommend euthanasia for humane reasons in horses severely paralyzed with EHV-1 myeloencephalitis. It is worth emphasizing, however, that an intensive supportive effort as outlined before may be rewarding even in these horses.

Considerable controversy exists regarding the use of corticosteroids in horses with EHV-1 myeloencephalitis. Many clinicians feel that rates of survival and recovery are improved by early treatment with a high dose (or doses) of corticosteroids. There is some evidence that lesions of EHV-1 myeloencephalitis are immune mediated and therefore potentially steroid-responsive. However, it is important to remember that immunosuppression may cause

exacerbation of any viral disease and may increase the severity of secondary infections. The author's recommendation is to give a single dose of 0.1 to 0.2 mg per kg dexamethasone* (or its equivalent) intramuscularly or intravenously at the onset of the disease and to consider repeating the dose the following day.

CONTROL

EHV-1 infection spreads very rapidly among horses in close contact. In some cases, more than 50 per cent of a group of horses have developed neurologic disease within three weeks. All horses within the immediate vicinity of an affected horse are assumed to be infected with EHV-1 until proved otherwise. All movement or contact between this group of horses and other horses should be stopped. Breeding operations may have to be suspended.

The virus is spread between horses by aerosol. This spread is favored by close contact between horses and poor ventilation. The most effective method of preventing spread of infection, therefore, is to separate all horses or groups of horses. Stabled horses should be turned out over as large an area as possible even if this disrupts the farm routine. The virus is not persistent in the environment, but stable personnel should dip or clean all potential fomites (such as boots, clothes, and grooming instruments) in a virucidal disinfectant such as Nolvasan.† Any aborted fetuses must be quickly removed and the area thoroughly disinfected and rested.

Both modified live and killed vaccines against EHV-1 are commercially available in the United States. The efficacy of these vaccines in preventing myeloencephalitis has not been critically evaluated. The use of such vaccines in the face of an outbreak of myeloencephalitis associated with EHV-1 infection cannot be recommended at this stage.

References

1. Dinter, Z., and Klingeborn, B.: Serological study of an outbreak of paresis due to equine herpesvirus 1 (EHV-1). Vet. Rec., 99(1):10, 1976.
2. Greenwood, R. E. S., and Simson, A. K. B.: Clinical report of a paralytic syndrome affecting stallions, mares and foals on a Thoroughbred stud farm. Equine Vet. J., 12:113, 1980.
3. Jackson, T. A., Osburn, B. I., Cordy, D. R., and Kendrick, J. W.: Equine herpesvirus 1 infection of horses. Studies on the experimentally induced neurologic disease. Am. J. Vet. Res., 38:709, 1977.
4. Pursell, A. R., Sangster, L. T., Byars, T. D., Divers, T. J., and Cole, J. R.: Neurologic disease induced by equine herpesvirus 1. J. Am. Vet. Med. Assoc., 175:473, 1979.
5. Platt, H., Singh, and Whitwell, K. E.: Pathological observations on an outbreak of paralysis in broodmares. Equine Vet. J., 12:118, 1980.

*Polyflex, Bristol Laboratories, Syracuse, NY 13201

*Azium, Schering Corp., Kenilworth, NJ 07033
†Nolvasan, Fort Dodge Labs, Fort Dodge, IA

EQUINE PROTOZOAL MYELOENCEPHALITIS

W. Kent Scarratt, GAINESVILLE, FLORIDA

Equine protozoal myeloencephalitis (EPM) is an inflammatory disease of the brain and particularly the spinal cord of horses that has been recently associated with a coccidian parasite.[9] EPM is also known as focal myelitis-encephalitis,[8] equine toxoplasmosis, and toxoplasma-like encephalomyelitis. This disease has been reported in Ohio, Illinois, Florida,[9] New York,[6, 7] and Pennsylvania,[1] but histopathologic evidence from many other states, especially in the eastern, southern, and midwestern regions, suggests widespread occurrence in the continental United States. EPM is usually sporadic, but several horses from one location may be affected over a period of several years.

CLINICAL FINDINGS

This disorder commonly affects young to adult horses (two to seven years old), especially of Standardbred or Thoroughbred breeding.[1, 2, 6–8] EPM is frequently noted in racing and breeding animals, often during warmer months of the year. Males and females are affected equally.

The most common first signs are ataxia, stumbling or falling, lameness, weakness, disorientation, and muscle wasting.[1, 6, 7] These signs have a gradual or sudden onset, but the course is usually progressive with horses often being unable to rise after a few weeks to months. Closer inspection often reveals an asymmetric gait abnormality consisting of ataxia, spasticity, and weakness in one or more limbs. Lameness may be intermittent, progressive, nonresponsive to therapy, difficult to localize, and suspected to arise from the proximal (upper) part of the limb. Weakness is seen as limb dragging, difficulty in rising, and decreased resistance to wither or loin pressure and lateral tail pull. Signs of gray matter disease are common and include loss of cranial and spinal nerve reflexes, muscle atrophy, and sensory deficits. Other signs of brain lesions include dullness, blindness, ear, eyelid, or lip droop, head tilt, circling, and dysphagia. Muscle atrophy is most commonly noted in the gluteal, suprascapular, and masseter areas. In some cases, the progression of signs may be arrested, but affected animals rarely recover fully.

LABORATORY FINDINGS

As there is no unequivocal antemortem test to diagnose EPM, a definitive diagnosis is obtained by microscopic examination of the central nervous system (CNS). Of the ancillary aids, cerebrospinal fluid (CSF) evaluation contributes most to a clinical diagnosis of EPM.[6] CSF may (in up to half of the cases) have mild xanthochromia, a slight increase in protein (80 to 100 mg per dl), and moderate pleocytosis (10 to 100 leukocytes per μl) consisting primarily of mononuclear cells, with neutrophils and eosinophils in the minority.[1, 6, 7] A complete blood count (CBC) often reveals a stress hemogram. An electromyogram (EMG) should help to distinguish disuse muscle atrophy from neurogenic atrophy. Indirect hemagglutinating (IHA) serum antibodies to *Toxoplasma gondii* are low (less than 1:64), and titers to Sarcocystis sp. are inconclusive.

DIFFERENTIAL DIAGNOSIS

A number of syndromes have been noted with EPM. Though a few horses may develop peracute tetraplegia, the majority of horses have a progressive, asymmetric gait abnormality of one or more limbs that must be distinguished from other neurologic diseases. These include cervical vertebral malformation (CVM), equine degenerative myeloencephalopathy (EDM), equine herpesvirus-1 myeloencephalitis (EHV-1), trauma, and cerebrospinal nematodiasis.[6, 7] Horses with CVM are commonly young (six months to three years old) male Thoroughbreds that are large for their age and breed.[2, 7] Their abnormal gait consists of ataxia, weakness, and spasticity, is slightly worse in the rear limbs than in the forelimbs, and is usually symmetrical. In horses with EPM, the gait abnormality is usually asymmetric and may be restricted to the rear limbs. In cases of CVM, lateral cervical radiographs may reveal vertebral abnormalities with a narrowed vertebral canal. In horses with CVM, CSF may have slight xanthochromia, mild elevations in protein, and a subtle increase in mononuclear cells. EDM is a disease of young horses (mean age at onset is five months) that has a gradual onset and progression of neurologic signs.[2, 7] The gait is symmetrically abnormal, and signs of gray matter disease are absent. CSF examination is unremarkable. Horses with EHV-1 myeloencephalitis usually have an acute onset of fever, bladder paralysis, and essentially symmetric gait abnormalities that fail to progress significantly after a few days.[2, 6, 7] Several animals may be affected, often after exposure to horses with respiratory disease or abortions. CSF examination usually reveals moderate xanthochromia and protein elevation without pleocytosis. Paired serum samples showing a rise in EHV-1 serum neutralization (SN) titers contribute to a diagnosis. Horses with spinal cord trauma usually have an acute onset of neurologic signs, often referable to a focal lesion, which rarely progress after the first day and tend to remain stable or improve.[2, 6, 7] If a fracture has occurred, a line of hypalgesia or analgesia may be present, and radiographs may be diagnostic. CSF may be xanthochromic and may have a slight increase in leukocytes. Parasite migrations through the brain or spinal cord often produce an acute onset of asymmetric signs that have a variable course[2] and often are referable to a focal lesion. CSF examination may reveal moderate pleocytosis consisting primarily of eosinophils.

As EPM can produce profound disease of the spinal cord gray matter, severe atrophy of the gluteal muscles may result, which could resemble hip trauma. When EPM affects the brain stem, vestibular signs and dysphagia often occur. Signs of unilateral vestibular disease include ataxia, circling, head tilt, and nystagmus.[2] Central vestibular disease, seen with EPM, will result in dullness, weakness, and the previously stated signs. Horses with otitis media and otitis interna have vestibular signs and abnormal otoscopic or radiographic findings in the middle ear. Rabid horses often have a rapid progression of symmetrical signs and become dysphagic and recumbent.[2]

TREATMENT

Specific therapy for horses suspected of having EPM is unavailable. The use of folic acid antagonists in EPM has been extrapolated from their efficacy against Toxoplasma sp. in humans and experimental animals.[1, 6] Oral pyrimethamine* (1 mg per kg as a loading dose followed by 0.05 mg per kg twice a day) and trimethoprim-sulfadiazine† (15 mg per kg twice a day) have arrested the progression of signs in some cases of EPM.[6] Depending on the severity and progression of signs, horses may receive these medications for a few weeks to a few months. In human toxoplasmosis, the dose of pyrimethamine may be halved after three to four weeks and continued for an additional four to five weeks. As horses on prolonged therapy potentially may develop folic acid deficiency, hemograms should be evaluated periodically. If hematopoiesis is reduced, the dose of folic acid antagonists should be reduced and folic acid supplementation* begun. Although pyrimethamine and trimethoprim-sulfadiazine are not licensed for horses, many horses have received these compounds for several weeks with no ill effects or alterations in hemograms. However, one horse developed profound leukopenia after receiving 1 mg per kg of pyrimethamine daily for six weeks. The cost of medication is variable but will approximate $7.00 per day for a 450 kg horse.

As large doses of pyrimethamine may produce teratogenic effects in laboratory animals, folic acid supplementation is recommended when pyrimethamine is used to treat toxoplasmosis in pregnant women. No adverse fetal effects have been detected when pregnant mares with EPM have received folic acid antagonists without folic acid supplementation.

Levamisole† (2.5 mg per kg per day) given for three days every two weeks for two months to human toxoplasmosis patients increased T lymphocyte numbers and markedly improved the patients' clinical status.[5] The efficacy of levamisole in cases of EPM has not been reported.

Horses with peracute EPM may benefit from osmotic diuretics such as mannitol‡ (0.25 to 2.0 gm per kg, 20 per cent solution intravenously). Dimethyl sulfoxide (DMSO)§ (1 to 2 gm per kg, 45 per cent solution) given intravenously to experimental animals subjected to CNS trauma markedly improved motor recovery and survivability.[3] As DMSO has been used to reduce intracranial pressure in horses with cranial trauma, it may be helpful in the treatment of peracute EPM. Intravenous sulfonamides‖ (50 mg per kg twice a day) may also be effective in these instances.

It is difficult to assess the efficacy of various medications used to treat horses suspected of having EPM, as the definitive diagnosis is made only postmortem.

Human toxoplasmosis is commonly associated with immunosuppression, and corticosteroids reactivate toxoplasmosis in humans and animals.[1, 5, 6] Corticosteroids failed to improve the course of EPM, and in some cases, appeared to exacerbate the clinical signs.[7] Hence, the use of corticosteroids should be avoided in horses with neurologic signs suggestive of EPM. The author recommends that folic acid antagonists be given during stressful events such as transportation and parturition to horses surviving an episode of suspected EPM to minimize exacerbation of signs.

---

*Daraprim, Burroughs Wellcome Co., Research Triangle Park, NC 42615
†Tribrissen, Burroughs Wellcome Co., Research Triangle Park, NC 42615

*Folvite, Lederle Laboratories, Division of American Cyanamid Co., Wayne, NJ 07470
†Levasole, Pitman-Moore, Inc., Washington Crossing, NJ 08650
‡Mannitol, Med-Tech, Inc., Elwood, KS 66024
§Domoso, Diamond Laboratories, Des Moines, IA 50304
‖Triplesulfa Injectable, Med-Tech, Inc., Elwood, KS 66024

In addition to chemotherapy, recommendations for uncoordinated horses include stall confinement and protective helmets and leg wraps to reduce self-trauma. Dysphagic horses should receive an alfalfa slurry fed free choice or given by stomach tube. Recumbent animals should be slung or rolled frequently and bedded deeply. Nursing care should prevent or treat decubital sores, constipation, and overdistention of the bladder.

PATHOLOGIC FINDINGS

Gross necropsy findings are restricted to the CNS. On cut section, focal areas of hemorrhage, discoloration, or softening may be seen in the white and gray matter of the spinal cord and brain.[1, 7-9] Histologic examination of lesions reveals a multifocal, necrotizing, nonsuppurative myeloencephalitis associated with protozoal organisms, which are seen in half the cases. These coccidian parasites are similar to *Toxoplasma gondii* but lack specific staining properties. Electron microscopic studies have shown that asexual reproduction of the organism in the horse CNS has many of the characteristics of the genus Sarcocystis.[9] In acute sarcocystosis of cattle, sheep, and swine, protozoal organisms are detected in peripheral blood smears and in endothelial cells of extraintestinal veins and capillaries. In EPM, protozoal organisms are noted most frequently in capillary pericytes and within circulating neutrophils within CNS capillaries. This suggests that the putative Sarcocystis organism of EPM may have a hematogenous phase of infection.[9] Hence, a thorough postmortem examination of all tissues should be performed in cases of EPM.

References

1. Beech, J.: Equine protozoan encephalomyelitis. Vet. Med. Small Anim. Clin., *69*:1562, 1974.
2. deLahunta, A.: Veterinary Neuroanatomy and Clinical Neurology. Philadelphia, W. B. Saunders Co., 1977.
3. de La Torre, J. C., Kawanaga, H. M., Rowed, D. W., Johnson, C. M., Goode, D. J., Kajihara, K., and Mullan, S.: Dimethylsulfoxide in central nervous system trauma. Ann. NY Acad. Sci., *243*:362, 1975.
4. Dubey, J. P.: A review of Sarcocystis of domestic animals and of other coccidia of cats and dogs. J. Am. Vet. Med. Assoc., *169*:1061, 1976.
5. Fegies, M., and Guerrero, J.: Treatment of toxoplasmosis with levamisole. Trans. R. Soc. Trop. Med. Hyg., *71*:178, 1977.
6. Mayhew, I. G., deLahunta, A., Whitlock, R. H., and Pollock, R. V. H.: Equine protozoal myeloencephalitis. Proc. 22nd Annu. Conv. Am. Assoc. Equine Pract., 1976, pp. 107-114.
7. Mayhew, I. G., deLahunta, A., Whitlock, R. H., Krook, L., and Tasker, J. B.: Spinal cord disease in the horse. Cornell Vet., 68, Suppl. 6:1, 1978.
8. Rooney, J. R., Prickett, M. E., Delaney, E. M., and Crowe, M. W.: Focal myelitis-encephalitis in horses. Cornell Vet., *60*:494, 1970.
9. Simpson, C. F., and Mayhew, I. G.: Evidence for *Sarcocystis* as the etiologic agent of equine protozoal myeloencephalitis. J. Protozool., *27*:288, 1980.

BOTULISM SYNDROMES: SHAKER FOALS AND FORAGE POISONING

James P. Klyza, PARIS, KENTUCKY

SHAKER FOALS

The shaker foal syndrome was first reported in the literature in 1967.[8] However, the disease has been observed for years in central Kentucky. It occurs sporadically on numerous farms in the area.

ETIOLOGY

Conjecture as to the etiology has varied from metabolic aberrations to an enterotoxemia. Recent work by the author and others[1, 2, 9] appears to show that the etiology of the disease is the colonization of the young foal's intestinal tract with *Clostridium botulinum* type B, with subsequent in vivo toxin production similar to that shown in infant botulism. Thus, the disease may be regarded as toxicoinfectious botulism.

The high incidence of the disease in central Kentucky may be due to the large population of susceptible foals each spring, along with a heavy concentration of *Cl. botulinum* type B found in the soil of the area.[9]

The age at which the foal is exposed to the organism appears critical. Most cases involve young foals around three weeks of age. Recent work in gnotobiotic mice has shown that their gastrointestinal tract will become colonized by the organism only when they are between 10 and 13 days old.[5] Another study has shown that in mice, removal of the cecum prevented development of the disease.[4]

Botulinum toxin has an affinity for the neuromuscular junction, where it alters the release and/or binding of acetylcholine. This results in neuromuscular blockade and diffuse muscle weakness.

CLINICAL SYNDROME

The typical patient is a foal of about three weeks of age.[9] On rare occasions, however, older foals and even adults may be affected. Until the onset of clinical signs, the foal usually has been a vigorous, rapidly growing animal. The owner's chief complaint is often that the foal has been found lying down or that it walks with a stilted gait. When forced to rise, it can stand for only a few minutes before generalized muscle trembling begins and it drops to the ground, often rolling into lateral recumbency. Often the foal has not been taking all of the dam's milk and shows evidence of dysphagia, with milk running from its mouth or nostrils.

Physical examination usually reveals a well-nourished foal that is bright and alert with normal vital signs. The pupils are often dilated and respond sluggishly to light. The foal can stand when assisted but usually remains standing for only three to five minutes before it begins to shake and eventually collapses. Mildly affected foals may be able to stand for 30 or more minutes. As the disease progresses, the length of time that foals can stand decreases.

Constipation and ileus are consistent findings. The respiratory rate increases, with the thorax taking on a slab-sided appearance owing to paralysis of the intercostal muscles. The heart rate escalates as death becomes imminent. Inhalation pneumonia often ensues in the terminal stages of the disease.

PROGNOSIS

In the majority of cases, death occurs within 24 to 72 hours of the onset of signs. Mild cases do occur, and in those situations the foal recovers over a period of three or more weeks. There have been no sequelae in foals that recover. Even with conscientious therapy and nursing care, however, the mortality rate for the disease is about 90 per cent.

DIAGNOSIS

In practice, clinical diagnosis is based on both the age of the foal (two to four weeks, with the majority of cases occurring at approximately 22 days) and the typical clinical presentation outlined earlier. To date, laboratory tests have not been beneficial in confirming this diagnosis, as serum samples have not shown evidence of toxin. Hemograms and blood chemistries are invariably normal.

In a recent study by the author, *Cl. botulinum* type B was isolated from antemortem fecal specimens of shaker foals but was not found in any of the specimens taken from healthy foals. Because of the time and specialized technique required to culture the organism, however, the results of these cultures would normally not be available until after the foal had succumbed. Thus, its major use would be as postmortem confirmation of the clinical diagnosis.

Autopsy findings include a contracted dorsal and ventral colon that contains a small amount of dry, hard ingesta. Mucosal hyperemia and hemorrhage are also reported. In the descending colon, the ingesta is similar but is also coated with thick, tenacious mucus. There is usually an excess of pericardial fluid and diffuse petechiation of the epicardium.[8]

Gastric ulcers are reported as a postmortem finding in shaker foals, and it is hypothesized that *Cl. botulinum* colonizes the ulcers, which serve as the portal of entry for the toxin.[10] The presence and significance of the gastric ulcers in the pathogenesis of the shaker foal syndrome need to be clarified for the following reasons: (1) Gastric ulcers are often found in foals that have been sick and have succumbed to any of a variety of illnesses and are not pathognomonic in the shaker foal syndrome; (2) if the ulcers do serve as a portal for the *Cl. botulinum* organism and toxin, then the shaker foal syndrome is an example of wound botulism and would not be comparable to the infant botulism syndrome, in which the organism colonizes the infant's gastrointestinal tract and produces toxin without the presence of ulcers.[1]

TREATMENT

Treatment of an affected foal depends primarily upon supportive care. The following principles should be addressed: elimination of toxin, destruction of the organism, alimentation, nursing care, promotion of muscle function, and respiratory support.

Elimination of Toxin. Mineral oil (12 oz) or milk of magnesia (2 oz in enough water to make 1 l) is administered via stomach tube. This serves to empty the gastrointestinal tract. Activated charcoal* (4 to 8 oz) can be administered in a slurry via stomach tube to adsorb toxin in the gastrointestinal tract. A warm water enema can also be given as an aid in

---

*Activated charcoal, Humco Laboratory, W. A. Butler Co. Columbus, OH

obtaining a fecal specimen for culture and to further stimulate evacuation of the colon and rectum.

In theory, botulinum antitoxin might be of benefit, since type B toxin takes a period of time to become irreversibly bound to the neuromuscular junction. The antitoxin, however, is difficult to obtain, the proper dosage is as yet undetermined, and untoward reactions may occur with its use.

Destruction of the Organism. Use of antibiotics in botulism remains controversial.[1] It is best to avoid aminoglycosides because they may act synergistically with botulinum toxin at the neuromuscular junction and cause a worsening of the clinical signs. Parenteral potassium or sodium penicillin (40,000 units per kg intravenously twice a day) is the most commonly used antibiotic in these foals. Oral penicillin therapy has the concomitant danger that it may result in the rapid release of a large amount of toxin into the intestinal tract, as botulinum toxin is released when death of the vegetative cells occurs. Indiscriminate use of oral antibiotics may further alter the intestinal flora and permit overgrowth of *Cl. botulinum.*

Alimentation. A Harris flush tube* may be passed into the stomach and sutured to the nares, and the foal may be fed with a milk replacer, the mare's milk, or an oral electrolyte preparation. Balanced electrolyte solutions and glucose can also be administered as supportive therapy, especially in those cases that are protracted and in which gut motility is slow to return to normal.

Nursing Care. Catheterization of the bladder will relieve distention. As with any patient that is recumbent, the animal should be turned from side to side frequently to prevent decubital sores and hypostatic congestion of the lungs.

Promotion of Muscle Function. Neostigmine† administered at a dose of 2 mg intramuscularly every two hours has been used to stimulate gut motility and to increase the length of time that the foal can stand. It is not given initially in mild shakers because improvement is transient, and the condition becomes refractory to the drug.

Guanidine hydrochloride‡ has been used in cases of food-borne botulism in humans with some response, but this experimental drug has not been of any benefit at the human dosage of 35 mg per kg per day in the few foals on which it has been tried.

Other experimental drugs used in the treatment of the disease include 4-aminopyridine and 3,4-diaminopyridine. 4-Aminopyridine,§ when adminis-

tered at a dose of 0.75 to 1.00 mg per kg, produces a mild but transient response. There is an observable though undramatic reversal of clinical signs, and effectiveness of the treatment appears to diminish with subsequent doses. This drug is extremely toxic; 2 to 3 mg per kg have been reported as a lethal dose in the horse.[7]

3,4-Diaminopyridine* is three to four times less toxic than 4-aminopyridine. In laboratory animals, the drug has been successful in treating experimentally induced botulism and has reversed clinical signs for periods of two to three hours (George Lewis, personal communication, 1980). The drug has been tried at a dose of 1 mg per kg on a foal that was severely affected by the syndrome. After treatment the foal was able to urinate independently, its pupils contracted readily in response to light, the depth of respiration increased, and peristalsis increased. The length of time the foal was able to stand was not increased, however. Mild signs of toxicity, including teeth grinding and head shaking, were also noted. It appears, therefore, that a decreased dose of perhaps 0.75 mg per kg would be more efficacious. As with 4-aminopyridine, the effect of the treatment was transient, lasting only two to three hours. The degree of response decreased with subsequent doses, and the foal eventually succumbed. These drugs are not approved for use in horses in the United States.

Respiratory Support. Death in infants hospitalized with infant botulism is rare because of the ability to maintain the infant on a respirator.[1] We have tried this approach on one foal, but the logistics and expense of intensive care in the horse are such that this was not a practical solution.

PREVENTION

A successful vaccination program against *Cl. botulinum* type B should be the most efficacious way to control this disease. A pilot study is under way to vaccinate pregnant mares with type B toxoid and subsequently to protect their foals through passive transfer of antibodies to *Cl. botulinum* type B through the colostrum.[4] If this proves effective, then control of the disease in problem areas should be possible.

FORAGE POISONING

Classically, the term "forage poisoning" has been used to refer to botulism in adult horses. This is an infrequent disease. It has been associated with the feeding of silage to horses, and recent work has

---

*Harris flush tube, Size 24 French, Bard Hospital Division, C. R. Bard, Inc., Murray Hill, NJ 07074

†Neostigmine-Stiglin, Pitman-Moore, Washington Crossing, NJ 08560

‡Guanidine hydrochloride, Key Pharmaceuticals, Miami, FL

§4-Aminopyridine, Sigma Chemical Co., St. Louis, MO

---

*3,4-Diaminopyridine, Sigma Chemical Co., St. Louis, MO

shown that wilted grass silage serves as a medium for the growth of the organism.[3, 6, 9]

CLINICAL SYNDROME

The disease may affect one horse or a group of horses, with common signs being dysphagia, weakness of gait, and eventual recumbency and respiratory arrest.

PATHOPHYSIOLOGY

The disease is thought to be due to the ingestion of preformed *Cl. botulinum* toxin from contaminated feedstuff. Toxin is absorbed through the gastrointestinal tract and then is bound to the neuromuscular junctions, resulting in irreversible neuromuscular blockade. *Cl. botulinum* type C is most commonly responsible for forage poisoning.[9, 10]

DIAGNOSIS

Diagnosis should be based on a history of feeding silage to the horse or on finding toxin in the feedstuff, fecal samples, or serum samples. When confronted with a botulism-like syndrome in a group of horses, it is often best to contact your state veterinarian or the National Centers for Disease Control (CDC) in Atlanta, Georgia, for advice on proper sample selection and shipment for the isolation of the suspected *Cl. botulinum* toxin.

DIFFERENTIAL DIAGNOSIS

Differential diagnoses should include organophosphate toxicity, hypocalcemia or hypomagnesemia, and rabies.

THERAPY

As with the shaker foal, therapy is primarily supportive. The difference is in management, focusing upon the fact that forage poisoning is often seen as a herd outbreak. In this case, the source of the toxin is exogenous rather than in vivo production. This necessitates finding the source of the toxin. Since this source is usually the feedstuff, removal from the pasture involved and changing the source of concentrate and hay being fed until culture and toxin studies can be performed are indicated.

References

1. Arnon, S. S.: Infant botulism. Ann. Rev. Med., *31*:541, 1980.
2. Klyza, J. P.: Shaker foals. *In* Mansman, R., and McAllister, E. S. (eds.): Equine Medicine and Surgery, 3rd ed. Santa Barbara, CA, American Veterinary Pub., 1983.
3. Knight, H. D.: Other bacterial infections. *In* Catcott, E. J., and Smithcors, J. F. (eds.): Equine Medicine and Surgery, 2nd ed. Wheaton, IL, American Veterinary Publ., 1972, pp. 98–99.
4. Lewis, G.: Prevention of shaker foal syndrome through brood mare immunization. 27th Annu. Conv. Am. Assoc. Eq. Pract., 1981, in press.
5. Moberg, L. J., and Sugiyama, H.: Microbial ecological basis of infant botulism as studied with germ free mice. Infect. Immun., 25(2):653, 1979.
6. Notermans, S., Kozaki, S., Dufrenne, J., and Van Schothorst, M.: Toxin production by *Clostridium botulinum* in grass. Appl. Environ. Microbiol., 38(5):767, 1979.
7. Ray, A. C., Dwyer, J. N., Fambro, G. W., and Reagor, J. C.: Clinical signs and chemical confirmation of 4-aminopyridine poisoning in horses. Am. J. Vet. Res., 39(2):329, 1978.
8. Rooney, J. R.: Shaker foal syndrome. Mod. Vet. Pract., 48:44, 1967.
9. Smith, L. D. S.: Botulism, the Organism, Its Toxins, the Disease. Springfield, IL, Charles C Thomas, 1977, pp. 92, 201–203.
10. Swerczek, T.: Toxicoinfectious botulism in foals and adult horses. J. Am. Vet. Med. Assoc., *176*:217, 1980.

POSTANESTHESIA MYOPATHY-NEUROPATHY

N. A. White, ATHENS, GEORGIA

CLINICAL SIGNS

Radial nerve paralysis in the horse is associated with long periods of recumbency. In early reports, the disease was thought to be a myopathic paralysis of the triceps due to compression of the muscle, which interfered with circulation.[2] With the advent of equine anesthesia, this disease has been termed postanesthesia forelimb lameness,[15] radial paralysis,[1] and postoperative myopathy.[6] The disease is reported to primarily affect the triceps muscle group, although the quadriceps, other hindlimb extensor muscles, the longissimus muscles, lumborum muscles, masseter muscle, and gluteal muscles can be affected.

The postanesthesia syndrome can be identified clinically in two forms. The first is local myopathy or nerve paralysis, seen more often when the horse is on a hard surface without padding or is recumbent for more than two hours under general anesthesia.[6, 15] The muscles involved are the triceps muscles or the extensors of the hindlimb, which are ventral during lateral recumbency, or the gluteal muscles, which are ventral during dorsal recumbency. The muscles may be flaccid or hard, severely swollen, and hot. The horse is weak or unable to support weight on the affected limbs. Triceps paralysis causes a dropped elbow with normal forelimb extensor function. Paralysis of extensors of the rear digit produces knuckling of the hind fetlock with inability to extend the digit. Quadriceps weakness or paralysis causes a loss of weight support at the stifle and results in an inability to stand. After lateral recumbency, the muscles of the upper limb may also be affected with varying degrees of weakness.[6] Signs may appear immediately on recovery or 30 to 60 minutes after standing.

The horse with single muscle group myopathy usually recovers within 24 hours. Many horses improve greatly two to three hours after standing. The act of standing can be difficult for the horse with limb dysfunction, and, therefore, recovery from anesthesia can be violent and may result in additional injury.[1]

The second clinical syndrome is the generalized myopathy or "myositis." Increased incidence of a generalized myopathy has been reported when unexpected arousal, movement, or severe cardiovascular depression has occurred during anesthesia.[6, 14] This disease can affect both pectoral and pelvic girdle muscles. The affected horse can rarely rise upon recovery from anesthesia owing to severe weakness of the hindlimbs. Muscles over the hindquarters and along the back can become rigid or remain flaccid. The horse appears anxious, sweats, and has colic. Horses attempt to rise and roll or throw themselves from sternal recumbency to lateral recumbency, traumatizing themselves repeatedly. Horses that do rise tend to stumble, show generalized weakness or paraparesis, and are prone to fall when attempting to walk. A horse having extensive muscle necrosis will have myoglobinuria. Struggling to get to a standing position appears to worsen the disease, producing muscle rigidity and an increased effort to remain standing.

Clinicopathologic changes include elevations in serum creatine phosphokinase (CPK) and serum aspartic amino transferases (SGOT).[6] Serum CPK levels of up to 300 IU can be detected in horses unaffected after recumbency and anesthesia and may be as high as 2000 IU after violent recovery. Horses with localized myopathy will have CPK levels greater than 300 IU. Generalized myopathic horses will have levels greater than 1000 IU, and levels have exceeded 30,000 IU. Lactic acidosis is not present unless another problem is present.[4, 15]

PATHOPHYSIOLOGY

Limb dysfunction after anesthesia appears clinically as nerve and/or muscle damage. The localized postanesthesia myopathy includes muscle degeneration. Muscle lesions seen using transmission electron microscopy include swollen mitochondria with loss of matrix and a reduction in numbers of cristae.[16] These lesions are similar to lesions from long-term pneumatic tourniquet application,[12] and experimental muscle ischemia.[5] Similar lesions have been reported in muscles from horses with acute rhabdomyolysis.[7] Histochemical examination of triceps muscle from limbs with postanesthesia dysfunction shows initial degeneration and necrosis of type II muscle cells and is similar to the lesions and sequence of early type II cell degeneration reported in both experimental ischemic myopathy[8] and in muscle from horses with acute exertional rhabdomyolysis.[7]

One form of the disease has also been described as a compartmental syndrome,[8] which is defined as an increase in pressure in osteofascial compartments.[13] Muscle pressure has been measured by wick catheter, direct needle measurement, or catheter placement in muscle.[8, 9, 17] Reduced blood flow was detected after muscle pressure exceeded 50 mm Hg and was reduced to 5 per cent of normal with a pressure of 80 mm Hg.[3] Muscular damage resulting from the pressure-induced ischemia produced muscle dysfunction and induced fibrous replacement and permanent contracture. The same pressure that produced a reduction in blood flow produced a nerve block. Decreased action potential progressed to a complete nerve block within two hours at muscle compartment pressures of 80 to 120 mm Hg in dogs.[3] Complete block was also obtained at pressures of 50 mm Hg,[13] but at pressures of 20 mm Hg for eight hours, conduction remained normal.[13] Triceps muscle pressures greater than 80 mm Hg have been recorded in large muscular horses placed on a flat, unpadded surface.[8, 16] Nerve conduction blockade in the horse may be an important part of limb dysfunction after anesthesia. Whether osteofascial compartments have an increased pressure after recovery has yet to be determined.

The local ischemic myopathy-neuropathy can be explained by increases in intracompartmental pressure with subsequent ischemia. The generalized form of the myopathy, appearing as an episode of postanesthesia "tying up," cannot be explained by pressure alone. In a generalized myopathy, the same biochemical changes may occur but may be generalized owing to stress, lowered blood pressure during anesthesia, excessive use of muscle relaxants, or muscle sensitivity to anesthetics. Hypothetically, if ATP is depleted by uncoupling of oxidative phosphorylation or blockade of glycolysis, the normal retention of calcium at the sarcoplasmic reticulum fails, and calcium can overload mitochondria and myofibrils.[18] The resultant calcium release and lack of energy production may produce segmental hypercontraction of individual muscle fibers. If enough fibers are affected, muscle dysfunction occurs. If combined with nerve block, the affected muscle group may be paralyzed, producing muscle flaccidity.

The degeneration of muscle can continue if damage is sufficient to produce an inflammatory response with edema and cellular infiltrates. Muscles become swollen, hot, and painful to touch, simulating the compartmental syndrome observed in humans.[11] In humans, the increased pressure reduces perfusion needed by the muscle.[11] Dysfunction then becomes prolonged, and increased compartmental pressure with subsequent damage can continue even after recovery from anesthesia.[17]

THERAPY

Therapy for postanesthesia myopathy-neuropathy is symptomatic. Very mild cases of triceps or hindlimb extensor paralysis can be treated successfully by administration of a nonsteroidal anti-inflammatory agent such as flunixin meglumine* (1 mg per kg once a day intravenously or intramuscularly) or phenylbutazone† (4.0 mg per kg twice a day intravenously) to reduce pain and prevent excessive inflammation. Massage and external heat supplied by hot towels may help effect more normal limb function. The opposite limb should have a support wrap placed at the fetlock. Such horses can usually support weight on the affected leg within 24 hours, and there appears to be no permanent muscle damage (Trim, C. R.: personal communication).

Severe muscle group myopathy or a generalized acute rhabdomyolysis requires both local therapy and systemic support. A recumbent horse that is unable to rise should not be urged to move. A horse remaining recumbent for more than three hours should be provided with food and water and should be assisted to sternal recumbency hourly to allow muscle movement. The horse should be kept calm and tranquilized if necessary and provided relief from pain. Acetylpromazine* (0.04 to 0.07 mg per kg as required intravenously) is a satisfactory tranquilizer that may also allow muscle vasodilation by alpha-adenergic blockade. Combinations of narcotic agents such as meperidine† (1.0 to 2.0 mg per kg as required intramuscularly) or morphine (0.5 to 1.0 mg per kg intramuscularly) with low dosage of acetylpromazine or chloral hydrate (7.0 mg per kg as required intravenously) provide excellent pain relief. Xylazine‡ can be used as an analgesic, but the muscle relaxation produced may result in considerable instability in the horse that has limb dysfunction. Nonsteroidal anti-inflammatory agents such as phenylbutazone (4.0 mg per kg twice a day intravenously or orally) or flunixin meglumine (1.0 mg per kg once a day intravenously or intramuscularly) are helpful in reducing the inflammation that can occur as a result of muscle necrosis. If pain is not reduced using this therapy, an increased dosage is not indicated.

Methocarbamol§ (10 to 20 mg per kg four times a day or as required intravenously) is a central-acting muscle relaxant that helps reduce pain by relieving muscle spasm. Following administration, the horse may become ataxic and depressed. The dosage can be reduced to control spasm and avoid the weakness or ataxia that can accompany higher dosages. Guaifenesin,‖ another central-acting muscle relaxant, can be used, but careful administration is essential. There is a slim margin between the dose needed to relieve muscle spasm and the dose that will induce muscle weakness. Guaifenesin is short-acting, which makes its use as a muscle relaxant difficult to control. Dantrolene** (1.0 to 2.0 mg per kg orally as a preventive dose) is a muscle relaxant that acts on the muscle cell by slowing the release of calcium from the sarcoplasmic reticulum. This reduction of calcium release even during the period of muscle stimulation weakens the contraction and helps to prevent spasm. The drug is most effective as preventive therapy and may be indicated for the horse at risk (Klein, L., personal communication) or under stress.[14] Pretreatment of all horses prior to anesthesia is not indicated unless there is a history of exertional myopathy, suspected risk, or if a halothane or caffeine muscle sensitivity test predicts a generalized muscle problem.

Glucocorticosteroids can reduce inflammation and muscle damage by stabilizing lysosomal mem-

---

*Banamine, Schering Corp., Kenilworth, NJ 07033
†Sterile phenylbutazone 20 per cent, Med-Tech, Elwood, KS 66024

---

*Acepromazine, Ayerst Labs, Inc., New York, NY 10017
†Demerol, Winthrop Labs, New York, NY 10016
‡Rompun, Bayvet Division, Cutter Laboratories, Shawnee, KS 66201
§Robaxin, A. H. Robins Co., Richmond, VA 23220
‖Guaifenesin NF XIV, Ames Chemical Co., Pennsville, NJ 08020
**Dantrium, Norwich-Eaton, Norwich, NY 13815

branes. In mild cases, nonsteroidal anti-inflammatory agents are sufficient. In cases of massive muscle damage, glucocorticosteroids are *probably* indicated using anti-inflammatory doses of dexamethasone (0.02 to 0.05 mg per kg twice a day intravenously or intramuscularly). Such treatment is controversial, since corticosteroid use is thought to predispose to exertional rhabdomyolysis,[9] and dramatic improvements are not seen when corticosteroids are used. Higher doses may be indicated to prevent edema of muscle or nerves.

When swelling from edema is present, furosemide* can help reduce the edema. Little clinical improvement is produced in severe cases of muscle damage, and long-term use of furosemide is not recommended.

Sodium bicarbonate (NaHCO$_3$) has been recommended to treat postanesthesia myopathy and acute rhabdomyolysis theoretically owing to production of lactic acid during muscle spasm and ischemia. Acidemia is not reported in clinical cases or in cases of experimentally produced postanesthesia myopathy; thus, physiologic fluid administration may not be needed in mild cases of myopathy. However, since myoglobin can pass in the urine at levels that injure the proximal tubules, even without being seen as a brown discoloration, prophylactic fluid administration is indicated any time myoglobinuria is detected or suspected. Bladder catheterization may be helpful in the recumbent horse to monitor urine output and to detect changes in urine color. A balanced electrolyte solution such as Ringer's solution or a lactated Ringer's solution (20 to 25 ml per kg intravenously) is satisfactory. Monitoring blood urea nitrogen and serum creatinine levels will help determine the presence of kidney damage and whether continued fluid therapy is necessary. Furosemide is of benefit to promote diuresis if spontaneous diuresis does not occur following fluid administration.

Other therapeutic agents that have been used include dimethylsulfoxide (DMSO)† and Vitamin E and selenium. DMSO has been used topically with massage without dramatic results reported. Vitamin E and selenium have been given at the time of myopathy but are of little benefit in the acute crisis. In cases of animals living in areas where feedstuffs are grown in selenium-deficient soils, the blood selenium or glutathione levels[10] may indicate a mild degree of white muscle disease. This disease could present as a generalized weakness and could have signs similar to generalized postanesthesia myopathy. In these cases, vitamin E and selenium therapy is indicated.

PREVENTION

The prevention of postanesthesia muscle disease is just as important as treatment. If the anesthetic protocol includes tranquilization with acetylpromazine, induction of anesthesia with an ultrashort-acting barbiturate combined with guaifenesin and maintenance with halothane,* triceps dysfunction or hindlimb extensor dysfunction can easily result. Muscle pressures are usually in excess of 40 mm Hg in the triceps muscle on a flat, unpadded surface. When the muscle pressure is greater than the capillary perfusion pressure (25 to 30 mm Hg), perfusion of the muscle ceases and ischemia occurs.[3, 9]

Positioning and padding are critical in reducing dependent muscle pressure. Appropriate positioning and padding can reduce muscle pressure in the triceps group by 50 per cent. Foam mattresses,† air mattresses,‡ and water mattresses have been used successfully to reduce the incidence of postanesthesia limb dysfunction. If air mattresses or water mattresses are used, inflation should be adequate to lift the patient off the hard surface, but mattresses must not be overinflated at the risk of producing another "hard" surface. If a foam mattress is used, it should be at least 4 in thick and able to support the entire body. Inner tubes can be used for the triceps area, but they leave the chest and hindlimb unsupported and susceptible to pressure ischemia.

Raising the upper limbs is also helpful during positioning in lateral recumbency. The lower limb muscle pressure can be reduced from 5 to 10 mm Hg by simply maintaining the upper limb level with the body. This reduces lower limb dysfunction and also improves upper limb function. Blood flow to the lower limb is greater than that to the upper limb when the upper limb is left unsupported. If the upper limb is supported level with the body, the blood flow becomes at least equal to that of the lower limb, indicating the importance of level positioning. Limb elevation should be practiced on both front and rear limbs. Pulling the lower limb forward to an advanced position can also markedly lower pressure in the dependent triceps muscle and should be practiced whenever possible. Cycling inflation in air mattresses has also been used to produce a change in local pressures and may be effective. Care must be taken to have enough buoyant padding during all phases of the cycles, or the result may be simple displacement of pressure within the muscle.

Dorsal recumbency requires exact positioning. Patients must be balanced on the dorsal midline

---

*Lasix, National Lab Corp., Somerville, NJ 08876
†Domoso, Diamond Labs, Des Moines, IA 50304

*Fluothane, Ayerst Laboratories, New York, NY 10017
†Neurogard Poly, Columbia Mattress Co., Chicago, IL 60623
‡Goodyear Dunnage Bay, Goodyear Aerospace Corp., Rockmart, GA 30153

and, as with lateral positioning, should be lifted just off the table or floor surface with mattresses. Front limbs can be extended but should not be abducted or adducted excessively. The hindlimbs must not be moved in a cranial or caudal direction. A "frog-sitting" position with no restraint or a vertical extension of the limbs is preferred. Padding under the shoulders or hips to support the animal's position must be used carefully to prevent leaning on padding and increased pressure development at one site.

Repositioning the horse after initiation of halothane and 100 per cent oxygen appears to reduce the incidence of a localized myopathy. Horses that are never moved after the initial induction may have a rapid onset of hypoxia owing to the combination of immediate rise in muscle pressure and lack of perfusion due to the lowered blood pressure common with barbiturate induction.

The mixture of thiamylal sodium and guaifenesin for induction of anesthesia may predispose to a generalized myopathy and should be avoided in the horse considered a high risk, (Heath, B.: Personal communication). With deepening of anesthesia, blood pressure falls, decreasing the difference between muscle compartment pressure and diastolic pressure. Hypotension from generalized cardiovascular depression or associated with ventilatory inadequacy is associated with stress-related myopathy.[4] Anesthesia protocols should include methods to maintain adequate systemic blood pressure and cardiac output.

Diet control should also be considered prior to anesthesia. The generalized form of postanesthesia myopathy appears to occur more often in the horse fed grain up to the time of anesthesia compared to the horse whose grain has been withheld for at least 24 hours. Owing to the association of acute rhabdomyolysis with continued energy intake and lack of exercise, especially in fit horses, patients about to have elective anesthesia should be withdrawn from all grain for 24 to 72 hours prior to surgery.

In conclusion, prevention of generalized postanesthesia myopathy is difficult. Methods of identifying the horse that may be predisposed to myopathy need to be developed. Muscle sampling prior to surgery to identify horses with halothane muscle sensitivity may also become a means of identifying horses that are particularly susceptible to the generalized postanesthesia myopathy. Dantrolene needs to be evaluated as a preventive agent. The use of muscle pressure catheters during recumbency may prove valuable to indicate positioning

that offers the least tissue pressure, as well as identifying high-risk horses in which tissue pressure is high owing to weight and conformation.

References

1. Adams, O. R.: Lameness in Horses, 3rd ed. Philadelphia, Lea and Febiger, 1974, p. 165.
2. Dollar, J. A.: Regional Veterinary Surgery and Operative Technique. Chicago, American Veterinary Pub. Co., 1920, pp. 775–776.
3. Hargens, A. R., Romine, J. S., Sipe, J. C., et al.: Peripheral nerve-conduction block by high muscle-compartment pressure. J Bone and Joint Surg., 61A:192, 1979.
4. Johnson, B. D., Heath, R. B., Bowman, B., Phillips, R. W., Rich L. D., and Voss, J. L.: Serum chemistry changes in horses during anesthesia: A pilot study investigating the possible causes of postanesthetic myositis in horses. J. Equine Med. Surg., 2:109, 1978.
5. Karpati, G., Carpenter, S., Melmed, C., and Eisen, A. A.: Experimental ischemic myopathy. J. Neurol. Sci., 23:129, 1974.
6. Klein, L.: A review of 50 cases of postoperative myopathy in the horse—intrinsic and management factors affecting risk. Proc. 23rd Annu. Meet. Am. Assoc. Eq. Pract., 1978, p. 89.
7. Lindholm, A., Johansson, H. E., and Kjaersgard, P.: Acute rhabdomyolysis ("tying up") in Standardbred horses. Acta Vet. Scand., 15:325, 1974.
8. Lindsay, W., McDonnell, W., and Bignell, W.: Equine postanesthetic forelimb lameness: Intra-compartmental muscle pressure changes and biochemical patterns. Am. J. Vet. Res., 41:1919, 1980.
9. Matsen, F. A., Mayo, K. A., Sheridan, G. W., and Krugmire, R. B.: Monitoring of intramuscular pressure. Surgery, 79:702, 1976.
10. Maylin, G. A., Rubin, D. S., and Lein, D. H.: Selenium and vitamin E in horses. Cornell Vet., 70:272, 1980.
11. Owen, C. A., Mubarak, S. J., Hargens, A. R., Rutherford, L., Garelto, L. P., and Akeson, W. H.: Intramuscular pressures with limb compression: Clarifications of the pathogenesis of the drug-induced muscle-compartment syndrome. N. Engl. J. Med., 300:1169, 1979.
12. Patterson, S., and Klenerman, L.: The effect of pneumatic tourniquets on the ultrastructure of skeletal muscle. J. Bone Joint Surg., 61B:178, 1979.
13. Sheridan, G. W., and Matsen, F. A.: An animal model of the compartmental syndrome. Clin. Orthop., 113:36, 1957.
14. Short, C. E., and White, K. K.: Anesthetic/surgical stress induced myopathy (myositis). Part I. Clinical occurences. Proc. 23rd Annu. Meet. Am. Assoc. Eq. Pract., 1978, p. 101.
15. Trim, C. M., and Mason, J.: Postanesthetic forelimb lameness in horses. Equine Vet. J., 5:71, 1973.
16. White, N. A.: Postanesthetic recumbency myopathy in horses. Compend. of Contin. Ed., 4(2):844, 1982.
17. Whitesides, T. E., Haney, T. C., Morimoto, K., and Harada, H.: Tissue pressure measurement as a determinant for the need of fasciotomy. Clin. Orthop., 113:43, 1975.
18. Wrogemann, K., and Pena, S. D. J.: Mitochondrial calcium overload: A general mechanism for cell-necrosis in muscle diseases. Lancet, 1:672, 1976.

Section 8

OCULAR DISEASES

Edited by Gretchen M. Schmidt

APPROACH TO OPHTHALMIC PROBLEMS 377

ADMINISTRATION OF OCULAR THERAPY 378

RED, PAINFUL EYES (UVEITIS) 382

OCULAR DISCHARGE IN YOUNG HORSES 385

CORNEAL OPACITIES 388

CATARACTS 390

OCULAR FUNDUS AND CENTRAL NERVOUS SYSTEM CAUSES OF BLINDNESS 393

APPROACH TO OPHTHALMIC PROBLEMS

Gretchen M. Schmidt, BERWYN, ILLINOIS

The following chapters describe methods of diagnosing and treating common ocular problems in the horse. The authors do not attempt to include every diagnostic possibility but have limited their discussions to the most common problems encountered. Table 1 defines common physical findings in equine ophthalmic disease and is intended to provide easy reference for diagnostic considerations. The veterinarian should then consult the appropriate article for the discussion of the ocular abnormality in question. Additional references are listed in each chapter, and should the veterinarian still have questions, he or she is encouraged to seek the advice of specialists.

Once the diagnosis is made, administration of medication to the eye is often the greatest challenge in the case. For this reason, an entire chapter is devoted to this topic.

TABLE 1. DIAGNOSIS OF OPHTHALMIC PROBLEMS

Client Observation	Basic Problem	Initial Approach	Differential Diagnosis	Page
Swollen eyelids Eye closed Ocular discharge	Painful, inflamed eye	A complete ocular exam is often impossible because of eyelid swelling and blepharospasm. Sedation and/or lid blocks are necessary to assess the problem. Nonsteroidal anti-inflammatory drugs are useful in reducing periocular swelling so that a later exam can be more complete. Key observations would be (1) integrity of cornea, (2) pupil size and response to light, and (3) presence of foreign bodies.	Uveitis Conjunctivitis Ulcerative keratitis	382 385 389
Film over eye Cloudy eye	Corneal opacity	Determine location of cloudiness: cornea or lens. Corneal opacity will obscure portions of the iris, while cataracts will be obscured by the iris. Corneal opacities are most commonly corneal edema (a diffuse, bluish haze) that will vary in transparency.	Cornea: Ulcerative keratitis Uveitis Congenital opacities Lens: Chronic uveitis	389 382 391 382
	Cataract	Cataracts may be focal or generalized opacities of the lens.	Congenital cataracts	391
Blindness Abnormal behavior	Loss of vision in a quiet eye: Light not reaching retina Retinal dysfunction Optic nerve dysfunction Central nervous system dysfunction	Determine if light is able to reach retina by looking for fundic (tapetal) reflection with penlight in darkened area. Also check pupillary responses to bright light, both direct and consensual responses. Perform funduscopic examination and observe retinal and optic disc anatomy. Observe horse's neurologic responses to environment and simple visual stimuli.	Quiet eye: Opaque cornea Mature cataract Retinal atrophy Retinal detachment Optic nerve hypoplasia Optic nerve atrophy Optic nerve ischemia Encephalitis Encephalopathy	388 390 394 394 395 394 395 395 395
	Loss of vision in a red eye: Light not reaching retina Retinal dysfunction		Red eye: Uveitis Retinal detachment	382 394

ADMINISTRATION OF OCULAR THERAPY

Joyce M. Murphy, ANCHORAGE, ALASKA

Ocular therapy can be administered by topical, subconjunctival, subpalpebral, retrobulbar, intraocular, and systemic routes. The most common methods of treatment are topical and subconjunctival. A combination of administration routes is often necessary to maintain constant and effective levels of many drugs in the eye. This usually involves topical, subconjunctival, and systemic methods.

TOPICAL ADMINISTRATION OF DRUGS

Topical administration of drugs includes application of solutions or ointments around the eyelids and into the conjunctival cul-de-sac. Topical therapy is most effective for simple blepharitis, conjunctivitis, and keratitis; however, this method requires an animal that can be handled several times a day and that is not fractions when touched around the head. It also requires an owner who has the time and ability to treat the horse several times daily.

Ointments are in an oily or petrolatum base and therefore provide longer contact time, resulting in fewer treatments. Ointments are sometimes more difficult to administer than solutions, especially to a nervous animal. Ointments can be used for blepharitis and conjunctivitis. They can be rubbed around the lids with a cotton swab or a clean finger. Ointments can be administered to the upper or lower conjunctival cul-de-sac by everting the upper or lower lid and placing a ⅛ to ¼ in ribbon of ointment across the conjunctival surface. If the animal is nervous and will not allow eversion of the lids, then ointment can be placed on a clean finger and spread across the upper eyelid margin around the base of the eyelashes. The ointment then will warm with body temperature, dissolve, and flow into the palpebral aperture. Satisfactory amounts of the drugs can thus reach the conjunctival and corneal surfaces.

Solutions may be used for conjunctivitis and keratitis; however, because of their liquid vehicle, the contact time is decreased and more frequent applications are necessary. Solutions usually come in plastic dropper bottles and may be used directly from these, or they may be used with an eye dropper. Both of these methods require the horse to allow the veterinarian or owner to manipulate the eyelids for proper placement of the drops into the lower conjunctival cul-de-sac. A tuberculin syringe is helpful on nervous animals. The syringe can be filled with the medication, which can be squirted into the upper or lower conjunctival cul-de-sac or directly at the cornea when the eyelids are open.

Ocular inserts are a new drug delivery system that give slow release of medication by sustained-release devices. The most promising system for use in animals is the Ocusert.* Ocular inserts are effective in the horse for antifungal therapy. They are placed in the lower conjunctival cul-de-sac between the lower lid and the anterior surface of the nictitans. If the insert tends to be displaced from the fornix by the movement of the nictitans, it can be sutured to the loose palpebral conjunctiva with fine gut suture.

Topical administration of drugs can cause corneal damage in the fractious animal, and other routes may have to be chosen.

SUBCONJUNCTIVAL INJECTIONS

Subconjunctival injections are indicated (1) when intraocular penetration is desirable, (2) when long-term effects are needed, (3) when the owner cannot give frequent treatments, or (4) when the animal will not allow daily topical treatment. Subconjunctival injections can usually be administered with topical anesthetic and with the aid of a nose twitch. The injection is best made in the dorsal bulbar conjunctiva with a 26- or 28-gauge needle. It is not necessary to inject under Tenon's capsule, but the injection should be placed in the loose bulbar conjunctiva about 3 to 4 mm from the limbus. The injection bleb will slowly release the medication into the tear film, and this will be absorbed through the ocular tissues. Part of the injected material is also absorbed directly into the intraocular structures by scleral diffusion. Subconjunctival injections can be repeated frequently, but certain drugs can cause scleral plaquing and necrosis.

EYELID BLOCKS

In order to properly examine the ocular structure or to medicate the eye, it may be necessary to anesthetize or block the lids. This results in hypokinesia of the palpebral musculature and facilitates observation of the ocular structures. The frontal, lacrimal, zygomatic, and infratrochlear nerves supply sensation to the eyelids (Fig. 1). The nerves can be blocked by injecting local anesthetic at specific sites for each nerve.

---

*Alza Pharmaceuticals, Palo Alto, CA.

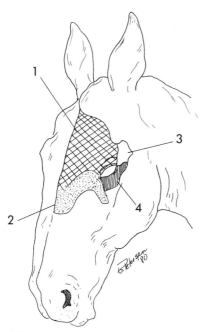

Figure 1. Diagram depicting the sensory innervation of the upper and lower eyelids. 1; area supplied by frontal nerve; 2, area supplied by infratrochlear nerve; 3; area supplied by lacrimal nerve; and 4, area supplied by zygomatic nerve. Modified from Manning, J. P., and St. Clair, L. E.: Palpebral, frontal and zygomatic nerve blocks for examination of the equine eye, VM SAC, 71:187, 1976.

To anesthetize the frontal nerve and the medial portion of the palpebral branch of the auriculopalpebral nerve, the supraorbital foramen is identified by grasping the supraorbital process between the middle finger and thumb. As the finger and thumb are moved medially, the space between them begins to widen. At that point, the index finger is pushed against the skin, and the supraorbital foramen can be felt. A 1-in 22-gauge needle is inserted into the foramen to a depth of ¾ in. A syringe containing 5 ml of lidocaine hydrochloride is attached to the needle, and 2 ml are injected. As the needle is slowly withdrawn, another 1 ml is injected. The last 2 ml are injected subcutaneously over the foramen.

The zygomatic nerve is anesthetized by placing the index finger on the ventral rim of the orbit against the supraorbital portion of the zygomatic arch. The needle is placed medial to the finger, directed medially along the rim of the orbit, and 2 ml of anesthetic solution are injected.

The lacrimal nerve is anesthetized by directing the needle medially along the dorsal rim of the orbit just medial to the lateral canthus. Two to 3 ml of anesthetic are injected just under the rim of the orbit.

The infratrochlear nerve is identified by finding the notch of the upper rim of the orbit near the medial canthus. This can be felt by firm pressure

with a finger. Two to 3 ml of anesthetic agent are given by deep injection slightly rostral to the notch.

Adequate immobilization of the lids is usually attained by injecting the supraorbital foramen and the zygomatic sites. The eyelids can then be manipulated for examination or medication of the eye. These blocks may be repeated at frequent intervals without untoward side effects.

SUBPALPEBRAL AND NASOLACRIMAL RETENTION CATHETERS

Application of topical medications to the eye of a fractious horse is difficult and dangerous even if the animal is adequately restrained. The cornea may be damaged by dropper bottle or tube tip, and the medication itself may become contaminated. The subpalpebral medication retention tube has been shown to be a very effective method for daily treatment of nervous animals and those animals with temporary tarsorrhaphies needing daily medication for the eye. The subpalpebral methods ensure delivery of the medication directly to the conjunctival and corneal surfaces. Several subpalpebral systems have been described. The following is a description of several systems that have proved to be very safe and effective in the horse. These systems can usually be placed in the horse using local lid blocks, topical anesthetic, and tranquilization or after blepharoplastic procedures before the horse awakens from general anesthesia. The subpalpebral systems will not produce ocular damage when properly positioned in the conjunctival fornix and can be used for long periods of time. These systems permit continuous delivery of medications to the corneal and conjunctival surfaces without hazard to the horse, client, or veterinarian.

A simple technique is to insert a 12-gauge needle without its hub into the lid at the dorsomedial aspect and penetrate into the conjunctival fornix. Polyethylene tubing (PE 160 or 200) is then inserted through the needle lumen and pulled out through the lid. This positions the tubing nasally. The needle is then placed through the lid of the dorsolateral area. The tubing is then passed through the needle, and the needle is removed. A knot is tied in the end of the tubing at the nasal side, and two or three holes are cut in the tubing so that when the tubing is pulled tight the knot is secure against the skin and the holes in the tubing are underneath the lid in the upper fornix. The tubing is sutured to the skin, and the long end of the tubing is then secured to the neck or withers with adhesive tape. Medicated solutions can be administered manually intermittently or continuously by a pump (Fig. 2B). After flushing the catheter with the medication, air is pushed through the catheter with the syringe in or-

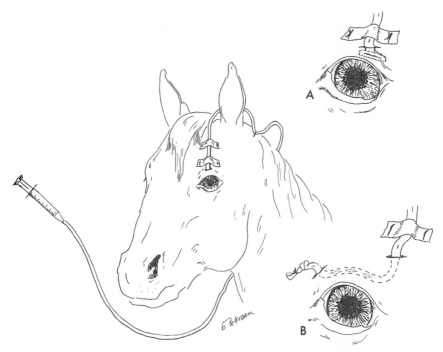

Figure 2. Subpalpebral catheter placed in the upper conjunctival fornix. *A*, Use of a footplate; *B*, Use of a retention catheter.

der to flush all medication through the tubing. An 18-gauge needle may be left in the distal end of the tubing to facilitate easier flushing of the tubing. In order to keep this needle clean, it can be placed inside a syringe casing and taped to the side of the neck.

Another modified subpalpebral technique uses silicon tubing and a 4 to 6 mm diameter footplate made from a piece of 2 mm silicon sheeting.* The tubing is made 30 cm long, and the hole in the sheet for the footplate is punched with a 22-gauge needle. The footplate is attached to the tubing with special glue.† Maintain the needle through the footplate and into the tubing until the glue dries. Another piece of silicon sheeting is fashioned into a disc with a 10 mm diameter. The center of this disc should have a hole the size of the tubing. The disc or stabilizer is glued to the tubing after the system is positioned in the conjunctival fornix. The tubing is positioned in the dorsolateral conjunctival fornix by inserting a 12- to 14-gauge needle through an anesthetized eyelid from the fornix. The tubing is placed into the needle, and the needle is withdrawn. The footplate is positioned in the fornix, and the stabilizer is glued to the tubing external to the eyelid. The stabilizer and footplate prevent movement and migration of the subpalpebral system within the eyelid. The tubing may be sutured to the skin and secured around the neck with adhesive

tape. Additional tubing may be added to the subpalpebral unit to administer medication at a distance from the eye. Flushing and maintaining the catheter is as previously described.

A nasolacrimal retention catheter is another method of administering medication to the eye and nasolacrimal system. Polyethylene tubing (PE 90 or 160) is passed retrograde through the nasal puncta well up into the nasolacrimal duct but not passing through the lower palpebral punctum. A 12-gauge needle is then inserted through the lateral fold of the nasal meatus above the nasal punctum. The distal end of the tubing is then drawn through the needle, and the needle is pulled out of the nasal meatus. A piece of tape is placed around the tubing at the nasal punctum and is sutured to the nasal mucosa. The tubing is also secured with tape and sutured at the lateral nasal meatus. The tubing is then drawn up along a head halter and secured with tape. Additional tubing may be added and secured at the neck for more distance from the eye. Medication may then be flushed retrograde through the nasolacrimal system onto the cornea.

The major complication with the subpalpebral medication method has been ulcerative keratitis due to migration of the tubing within the conjunctival fornix onto the cornea. The modified subpalpebral method prevents this problem. The nasolacrimal retention tubing also does not cause corneal damage, and it allows for medication to be administered to the nasolacrimal system when there is a need to treat chronic dacryocystitis.

Catheters are also useful in flushing the nasolac-

---

*Silastic Sheeting, Dow Corning, Midland, MI
†Medical Adhesive, Dow Corning, Midland, MI

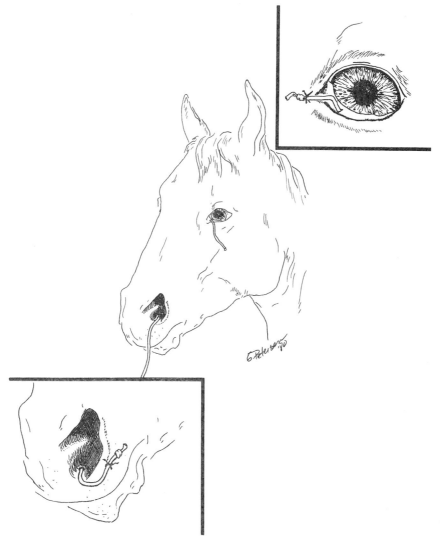

Figure 3. Nasolacrimal retention catheter in position and sutured at the medial canthus and lateral area of the nasal meatus.

rimal system in the horse. Polyethylene tubing (PE 90 or 160) is prepared with a point by putting tension on the length of tubing as it is held over a match or flame. The tubing starts to melt and is stretched to a point. The point is then smoothed with scissors. This facilitates passage and reduces damage to the duct. This tubing then can be passed through the lower palpebral punctum, which is the largest and easiest to penetrate. The catheter is attached to a syringe containing the irrigating solution. This procedure can be easily accomplished with topical anesthetic and a nose twitch. Nervous animals may be given tranquilizers or sedatives such as xylazine.* This type of catheter may be easily passed retrograde from the nasal punctum, and retrograde flushing of the nasolacrimal system is accomplished. Na-

sal stomach feeding tubing (size 8 French)* is also satisfactory as a catheter for flushing the lacrimal system and has the advantage of already being prepared for use.

In cases of chronic dacryocystitis with complete obstruction, the PE tubing can be passed from the lacrimal punctum or retrograde from the nasal punctum. Most obstructions in the horse occur near the nasal punctum, and the terminal nasolacrimal duct may be completely scarred so that tubing cannot be forced through the scarred punctum. Usually the tubing can be palpated beneath the nasal skin near the punctum. Using local anesthesia, a Bard-Parker blade is used to dissect the scar tissue down to the tubing. The tubing is then sutured at the medial canthus and at the ventrolateral nasal meatus (Fig. 3).

*Rompun, Haver-Lockhart Laboratories, Shawnee, KS 66201

*Pharmaseal, Inc., Toa Alta, Puerto Rico

RETROBULBAR INJECTIONS

Retrobulbar injections into the postorbital fat or into the postorbital socket have few indications for use in ocular therapy of the horse. The primary indication is for infiltration anesthesia. An 18-gauge 4½-in needle is used to inject the retrobulbar area. The needle is inserted at the level of the supraorbital foramen immediately caudal to the zygomatic process of the frontal bone. The needle is inclined 40° from the vertical and is advanced medioventrally and caudal to the orbital foramen. Retrobulbar injections can be dangerous. Possible complications are penetration of the globe, damage to the optic nerve, and retrobulbar hemorrhage. Horses lack scleral rigidity, and retrobulbar injection may predispose to loss of vitreous humor during intraocular surgery.

INTRAOCULAR INJECTIONS

Intraocular injection cannot be recommended unless there is immediate danger of losing an eye or if all other methods of therapy have proved ineffectual. Intraocular injections are uncommon in veterinary medicine, but drugs may be injected into the anterior chamber or the vitreous body or both. Intraocular injections give high drug concentrations, but the eye only tolerates small volumes.

For intracameral injections, the globe is immobilized with fixation forceps. A 25- or 26-gauge needle is inserted through the bulbar conjunctiva 3 to 4 mm from the limbus, and the needle is directed subconjunctivally to the limbus. The needle is inserted through the limbus into the anterior chamber at the angle between clear cornea and iris. The needle pathway through the limbus is angled so that the punctured area will be self-sealing. The volume of drug placed in the anterior chamber should equal the amount of aqueous removed. Care must be taken to avoid damaging corneal endothelial cells, iris, and lens. For intravitreal injection, a 25- or 26-gauge needle is inserted 5 to 6 mm from the limbus through the sclera and lateral pars plana of the ciliary body. This will minimize intraocular hemorrhage and retinal damage.

SYSTEMIC ADMINISTRATION

Systemic drugs may penetrate certain regions of the blood-aqueous barrier in a normal eye. The ciliary body processes are probably most permeable to medications by active transport or simple diffusion. Diseases of the eyelids, orbit, and anterior and posterior segment are effectively treated with systemic drugs. Other routes of administration are often combined with the systemic route.

References

1. Gelatt, K. N.: The eye. *In* Catcott, E. J., and Smithcors, J. F. (eds.): Equine Medicine and Surgery, 2nd ed. Wheaton, IL, American Veterinary Pub., 1972, pp. 399–432.
2. Gelatt, K. N.: Veterinary Ophthalmic Pharmacology and Therapeutics, 2nd ed. Bonner Springs, KS, Veterinary Medical Pub., 1979.
3. Gelatt, K. N.: A modified subpalpebral system for the horse. J. Equine Med. Surg., 3:141, 1979.
4. Manning, J. P., and St. Clair, L. E.: Palpebral, frontal and zygomatic nerve blocks for examination of the equine eye. VM SAC, 71:141, 1976.
5. Severin, G. A.: Veterinary Ophthalmology Notes, 2nd ed. Ft. Collins, CO, Colorado State University Press, 1978.

RED, PAINFUL EYES (UVEITIS)

Mary B. Glaze, BATON ROUGE, LOUISIANA

The uveal tract is composed of three intraocular structures—the iris, ciliary body, and choroid. Uveitis is defined as an inflammatory process involving one or, more commonly, a combination of these components. Although the primary structures involved in most instances of equine uveitis are the iris and ciliary body, secondary effects on the cornea, lens, vitreous, choroid, and retina are commonly seen, both acutely and as chronic sequelae.

Unfortunately, such an inflammatory disease is seldom as simple to treat successfully as it is to define.

What obstacles are encountered in the therapy of equine uveitis? Probably of most significance is the inability to recognize the signs of either acute or chronic intraocular inflammation. Obviously without the correct diagnosis, a rational therapeutic plan cannot be formulated or executed. Secondly, the initiating cause of uveal inflammation is often difficult if not impossible to identify; the stimulus may then persist despite symptomatic therapy, ultimately resulting in chronic disease and blindness. Even when the correct diagnosis is made and the cause is known, therapy may not be sufficiently aggressive initially or may be terminated prematurely so that optimal control of the uveitis is never achieved.

CLINICAL SIGNS

The chief complaint of owners in cases of equine uveitis is that of a "red," "cloudy," "half-closed," "painful" eye or that of a "blind" animal. A thorough ophthalmic examination should be performed in the assessment of these blind red eyes, both to ascertain the degree of ocular involvement and if possible to detect the initiating cause. Because of pain, lid blocks (p. 378) may be necessary to thoroughly evaluate the ocular structures. Corneal ulcers and lacerations should be ruled out, since these too produce red, painful eyes. History of prior ocular disease is an important consideration and may support clinical evidence of recurrent uveitis. These findings will subsequently dictate the therapy as well as the prognosis.

The lesions observed in equine uveitis vary, based on the severity and duration of the disease. Active uveitis is often heralded by severe blepharospasm, epiphora, and photophobia, though these signs may be negligible in chronic inflammatory disease. Conjunctivitis is usually observed, as is ciliary vessel injection circumcorneally and deep to the conjunctival tissue.

Corneal edema is a frequent finding in uveitis; cellular precipitates on the inner corneal surface result in altered endothelial function, fluid imbibition by the corneal stroma, and a characteristic cloudy, blue appearance. Vascularization of the cornea proceeds from the limbus circumferentially and is either superficially located, characterized by tree-like branching, or more deeply situated, appearing in a straight "paintbrush" pattern.

Alterations in the anterior chamber are due to aqueous flare (increased protein), hypopyon (accumulations of inflammatory cells), and hyphema (blood), all arising from altered vascular permeability in the course of the inflammatory disease. The anterior chamber may appear shallow because of iris swelling.

Edema contributes to the iris' lackluster appearance, as will adherent inflammatory debris on the iris surface. Chronic or recurrent disease results in iris depigmentation and atrophy of the corpora nigra.

Iridal spasm produces miosis, an important diagnostic observation in uveitis and one of therapeutic

concern. Characteristically, the inflamed iris responds poorly to mydriatics. The close contact of the miotic iris with the lens favors the formation of posterior synechiae; cataracts may form at these adhesions, or iris bombé and secondary glaucoma may result if the synechiae occur circumferentially.

Digital palpation of the affected eye reveals decreased intraocular pressure stemming from diminished aqueous production by the inflamed ciliary body. Severe chronic uveitis results in permanent hypotony and phthisis bulbi, a shrunken, enophthalmic globe with concomitant nictitans prolapse and a notched appearance of the upper lid owing to loss of its support by the eye.

Altered lens metabolism associated with posterior synechiae or accumulations of inflammatory debris on the anterior capsule may result in cataract formation. Pigment flecks may remain on the lens capsule following either spontaneous or therapeutic resolution of the synechiae. Effects on the ciliary processes and zonules predispose the lens to subluxation or luxation as well.

Vitreal involvement is characterized by debris ("floaters") and linear traction bands extending toward the retina. Liquefaction of the normally gel-like vitreal substance also occurs.

Active chorioretinitis with exudation or edema causes dullness and loss of detail in these tissues when observed ophthalmoscopically. Lesions are commonly reported adjacent to the optic disc, both nasally and temporally. Inactive lesions of chorioretinitis appear as peripapillary depigmented foci, commonly referred to as "butterfly" lesions. Retinal detachment can occur in chronic uveitis owing to loss of support by the liquefied vitreous or as a result of anterior traction by fibrous vitreal bands.

ETIOLOGY

Identification of etiologic factors in equine uveitis is often a difficult task. A list of differentials to be considered is found in Table 1.

TABLE 1. ETIOLOGIC FACTORS IN EQUINE UVEITIS

Exogenous Factors	Endogenous Factors
Corneal ulceration	Infectious agents
Infectious agent	Leptospirosis
Trauma	Onchocerciasis
Concussive blow	Strangles
Foreign body	Viral arteritis
Postsurgical response	Immune-mediated disease
	Autoimmune phenomena
	Hypersensitivity reactions
	Idiopathic disease

THERAPY

The therapeutic goal in acute uveitis is to maintain visual function by reducing intraocular inflammation and preventing irreversible sequelae. In many instances, this is accomplished through symptomatic therapy alone, utilizing anti-inflammatory agents and mydriatics, though specific therapy may be instituted against etiologic factors such as fungi and bacteria. Table 2 presents a therapeutic approach to uveitis.

Steroids. Steroidal anti-inflammatory agents may be administered via several routes; severe uveitis requires a combination of these. An acetate-derivative steroid, such as prednisolone acetate,* designed for ophthalmic administration and chosen for its corneal penetrability, should be applied topically at one- to four-hour intervals, dictated by the severity of the disease. The potent anti-inflammatory action of dexamethasone† preparations makes these useful agents for topical administration as well. Consideration should be given to the use of a subpalpebral or nasolacrimal lavage apparatus, since frequent and prolonged therapy usually meets with resistance by the patient (p. 380).

Ophthalmic solutions and ointments are both acceptable formulations, the latter requiring direct application to the eye but at less frequent intervals. If both are used, the solution should be applied first. Ointments should not be used if perforation of the globe has occurred, since the oil base will cause inflammation upon entering the eye. In general, therapy should be continued at least two weeks beyond resolution of clinical signs. If corneal ulcers occur in conjunction with uveitis, topical steroids should be used only with extreme caution and careful monitoring of the eye (p. 389).

An alternative to frequent topical administration of steroids is the subconjunctival injection of methylprednisolone acetate.‡ Twenty to 40 mg in a volume of 0.5 to 1.0 ml injected beneath the bulbar conjunctiva may be therapeutically effective for up to 10 days. Clinical judgment will indicate whether a second injection is necessary before that time.

Systemic corticosteroid administration is warranted in addition to topical therapy in extreme or resistant inflammation. Intramuscular injection of 20 mg dexamethasone§ twice daily is recommended for up to five days but should not be used for long-term maintenance.

Antiprostaglandins. Nonsteroidal anti-inflammatory agents with antiprostaglandin activity may be substituted for systemic steroids because prostaglandins

---

*Pred-Forte, Allergan Pharmaceuticals, Irvine, CA 92713
†Maxitrol, Maxidex, Alcon Labs, Fort Worth, TX 76134
‡Depo-Medrol, Upjohn Co., Kalamazoo, MI 49001
§Azium, Schering Corp., Kenilworth, NJ 07033

TABLE 2. THERAPEUTIC PLAN FOR ACUTE UVEITIS OF UNKNOWN ETIOLOGY

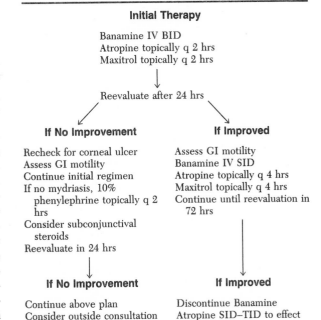

Initial Therapy

Banamine IV BID
Atropine topically q 2 hrs
Maxitrol topically q 2 hrs

↓

Reevaluate after 24 hrs

If No Improvement

Recheck for corneal ulcer
Assess GI motility
Continue initial regimen
If no mydriasis, 10% phenylephrine topically q 2 hrs
Consider subconjunctival steroids
Reevaluate in 24 hrs

If Improved

Assess GI motility
Banamine IV SID
Atropine topically q 4 hrs
Maxitrol topically q 4 hrs
Continue until reevaluation in 72 hrs

If No Improvement

Continue above plan
Consider outside consultation

If Improved

Discontinue Banamine
Atropine SID–TID to effect
Maxitrol q 4–6 hrs

---

are an important mediator of intraocular inflammation.

Phenylbutazone* intravenously or orally at a dosage of 3 to 5 mg per kg twice a day has analgesic and anti-inflammatory action. Flunixin meglumine† is a relatively new, potent nonsteroidal agent with analgesic, anti-inflammatory, and antipyretic activity. Administration of 1.0 mg per kg once to twice daily intravenously, intramuscularly, or orally is recommended for one to five days. The response to this drug is often dramatic, and administration beyond five days is seldom indicated. Aspirin acts via inhibition of the enzyme involved in prostaglandin synthesis and is a theoretically useful adjunct in the long-term control of uveitis. Dosage requirements make this drug less clinically practical in acute cases, but prolonged administration of aspirin (15 mg per kg twice a day) has been used successfully in preventing exacerbations of chronic uveitis.

Mydriatics. A vital therapeutic agent in the uveitis regimen is the parasympatholytic mydriatic-cycloplegic. By dilating the pupil and decreasing iris-lens contact, the chance of posterior synechia formation is diminished. Ciliary spasm is relieved so that the horse is more comfortable, and the iridociliary vessels return to a more normal state under this drug group's influence.

Topical application of 1 to 4 per cent atropine

---

*Butazolidin, Jensen-Salsbery Labs, Kansas City, MO 64141
†Banamine, Schering Corp., Kenilworth, NJ 07033

solution or ointment is indicated hourly until the pupil is dilated, or at least 6 and preferably 10 times daily for the first 48 hours. Once the pupil is dilated, frequency of administration may be reduced to one to three times daily. In cases refractory to atropine, 10 per cent phenylephrine hydrochloride can be used topically in conjunction with atropine to effect.

Horses on an intense parasympatholytic regimen should be monitored for signs of colic, as systemic effects are occasionally seen associated with topical atropine administered at frequent intervals. Pupillary dilation may persist for one to four weeks following cessation of therapy.

Antibiotics. Topical and systemic antibiotics may be used in instances in which infection cannot be ruled out or in those horses with high leptospiral titers associated with acute uveitis. Topical antibiotic solutions or ointments may discourage opportunistic bacteria during intense corticosteroid therapy of an already vulnerable eye. Broad-spectrum antibiotic ophthalmic preparations, such as chloramphenicol, neomycin-polymyxin B, or gentamicin, are commonly employed topically. Frequency of administration generally parallels that of topical steroid application. Since current evidence suggests an immune rather than an infectious basis for most uveitis, however, antibiotics assume a less prominent role in the therapeutic scheme.

Other Drugs. Oral diethylcarbamazine citrate (4 mg per kg once daily for 21 days, given in the food) has been utilized in cases of equine uveitis believed secondary to *Onchocerca cervicalis* in which dermal and conjunctival biopsies indicate the presence of microfilariae. Present recommendations discourage use of the drug in cases of active uveitis, since the presence of dead larvae may exacerbate the inflammatory condition. The precise role of the parasite in equine uveitis is not yet determined, however, and widespread controversy exists regarding the necessity or benefit of such microfilaricidal therapy even in the quiescent eye.

No therapy is indicated in nonpainful eyes with lesions of chronic uveitis. Should the eye cause the animal discomfort, symptomatic therapy as described for acute uveitis may be instituted. Extremely painful, chronically inflamed eyes are candidates for enucleation.

Equine uveitis presents both a diagnostic and therapeutic challenge to the veterinary practitioner. Recognition of acute and chronic inflammatory lesions is essential both prognostically and in the formulation of a successful medical plan. Symptomatic therapy must be initially aggressive and of sufficient duration for successful resolution of the uveitis. Preservation of ocular function following a successful therapeutic regimen warrants the time and expense involved.

Supplemental Readings

1. Bistner, A., and Shaw, D.: Uveitis in the horse. Compend. Contin. Ed., 2:S35, 1980.
2. Henkind, P., Walsh, J. B., and Berger, A. W.: Physicians' Desk Reference for Ophthalmology. Oradell, NJ, Medical Economics Co., 1979.
3. Rebhun, W. C.: Diagnosis and treatment of equine uveitis. J. Am. Vet. Med. Assoc., 175:803, 1979.
4. Severin, G. A.: Veterinary Ophthalmology Notes, 2nd ed. Ft. Collins, CO, Colorado State University Press, 1976. pp. 37–44, 215–220.

OCULAR DISCHARGE IN YOUNG HORSES

Gay Wiles Senk, GLEN HEAD, NEW YORK

Ocular discharge is common in young horses. The animal's age, environment, and involvement of one individual or a group aids in establishing a probable cause. The character of the discharge, the presence of a unilateral or a bilateral problem, and the presence of systemic signs help to establish an allergic, mechanical, or infectious etiology.

UNILATERAL OCULAR DISCHARGE

Unilateral ocular discharge usually involves one individual and indicates a localized ocular problem. Initially, unilateral discharge is usually serous owing to the overflow of tears caused by hypersecretion or obstruction of the excretory system. The presence of thicker seromucoid or mucopurulent discharges indicates chronic inflammation. Causes of unilateral ocular discharge in the young horse are entropion, more commonly seen in foals less than two weeks of age, blocked nasolacrimal duct, either congenital or acquired, corneal ulcerations, and ocular trauma.

ENTROPION

Entropion is an inversion of the eyelid and eyelashes. Epiphora is a common sign accompanying entropion owing to the irritating effect of the lashes on the cornea. In the neonatal foal, entropion is the most common ocular lesion.[2] The lower lid is more commonly affected, and the condition may be more prevalent in weak or premature foals.[2] This author has seen a number of cases in normal, vibrant foals and routinely checks for this condition during the initial neonatal examination. If entropion is present at birth, it is best to determine if the condition can be corrected manually by gently everting the eyelid. It has been my experience that those lids that can be temporarily corrected by manually everting the eyelid will respond to this type of corrective measure within a 12- to 24-hour period. Instruct the attendant to gently evert the lid several times a day while the newborn foal is lying down in the stall so that minimal stress occurs. Do not advocate immediate corrective manipulation by the attendant until the foal has stood and nursed several times so as to avoid immediate stress on the neonate. Once a regimen of lid manipulation has been instituted, apply a protective ocular ointment such as Lacrilube* or an antibiotic ophthalmic ointment such as Neobacimyx† three times a day.

If the entropic lid cannot be manually everted, it will not respond to this conservative method of therapy, and other corrective steps must be instituted after the foal is over 12 hours of age. An ophthalmic ointment to protect the cornea is applied to the affected eye until correction of the entropion is achieved. If entropion is not detected at birth and the foal has epiphora when first examined, a thorough ophthalmic examination is indicated to be certain that mechanical irritation or ulceration of the cornea has not occurred. Staining the cornea with a Fluorescein Strip‡ allows evaluation of corneal damage.

Once evaluation of the cornea and assessment of the severity of the entropion are complete, a plan for correction can be instituted. In those lids that do not respond to manipulation, good results have been attained by infiltrating procaine penicillin G§ under the skin of the affected lid. The author prefers not to sedate foals at such a young age, and most foals will allow this procedure without sedation. Good restraint is essential to prevent the foal from moving its head during the procedure. In fractious foals, sufficient sedation can be attained by giving a 100 lb foal 0.25 to 0.50 ml (0.5 mg per kg to 1.0 mg per kg) xylazine‖ intravenously. The foal is kept in lateral recumbency with adequate handlers utilized in such a manner as to minimize motion and

resistance by the foal. The ventral bony orbit beneath the lower lid is palpated. A 20-gauge 1-in needle is inserted under the skin of the eyelid at the level of the bony orbit. Follow the same technique as used in applying ophthalmic ointment by resting the hand on the foal's head while inserting the needle caudally to avoid damage to the eye should the foal struggle and raise its head. Procaine penicillin G (0.5 to 1.0 ml) is injected under the skin following aspiration. This creates a bleb, which is milked toward the margin of the eyelid and extended to the length of the eyelid beginning rostrally and traveling caudally. During the administration of penicillin, one can observe the underlying conjunctiva start to swell, which mechanically everts the entropic lid. In most instances, 0.5 ml of penicillin is effective. Within an hour, a local tissue reaction occurs, resulting in further swelling of the affected lid. This aids in eversion of the entropic lid. The swelling gradually decreases over a 24- to 36-hour period. This treatment is very rewarding because when the swelling subsides, the problem is resolved and repeated procedures are unnecessary. For nonresponsive congenital entropion or acquired entropion, surgical intervention, involving imbrication sutures or blepharoplasty, is indicated.[4, 5]

BLOCKED NASOLACRIMAL DUCT

A blocked nasolacrimal duct results from swelling of the duct mucosa, the presence of inflammatory cells and debris, or, more rarely, congenital atresia.[2, 3] The initial complaint is unilateral serous discharge due to interference with normal tear drainage through the nasolacrimal system. Atresia usually occurs at or near the duct exit, which lies at the mucocutaneous junction on the nasal floor near the nostril.[2, 3] The condition may affect one or both nasolacrimal ducts. Affected foals are usually two to six weeks of age before the overflow of tears is present.[3, 4] However, epiphora may become apparent any time from birth through the first year of life. Unilateral serous discharge in the young foal is more commonly due to ocular damage such as corneal abrasion or ulceration. In the early stages, epiphora may be the presenting sign before the onset of a swollen eyelid, mucopurulent discharge, or blepharospasm. A good ophthalmic examination and investigation of the cornea with a Fluorescein Strip not only will evaluate the integrity of the cornea but will also establish patency of the nasolacrimal system if dye exits at the nasal orifice.

When atresia of the nasolacrimal duct is present, surgical correction can usually be performed through the nares.[2, 3] Occlusion of the duct by inflammation or debris is usually not a problem in the young foal but may be seen as a primary condition or as a sequela to conjunctivitis in yearlings and two-

---

*Lacrilube, Allergan Pharmaceuticals, Inc., Irvine, CA 92713
†Neobacimyx, Burns-Biotec Labs, Inc., Omaha, NB 68127
‡Fluorescein Strip, Ayerst Labs, New York, NY 10017
§Procaine penicillin G, Pfizer, Inc., New York, NY 10517
‖Rompun, Haver-Lockhart Labs, Shawnee, KS 66201

year-olds. Flushing of the duct to remove any obstructive debris is usually necessary to regain patency. Most horses tolerate flushing without sedation. However, if the horse resists, 0.2 mg per kg (1 ml per 1000-lb horse) to 0.5 mg per kg (2.5 ml per 1000-lb horse) xylazine intravenously provides adequate sedation. A twitch is applied to the upper lip, twisting it away from the affected nostril in order to facilitate opening the nares for access to the duct orifice. Various sizes of flexible male urinary catheters should be available, as well as a Sovereign Feeding Tube and Urethral Catheter* (16 in long, sizes 3½, 5, 8, and 10). After cleansing the orifice with a moist cotton swab, the catheter is passed up the duct as far as possible until resistance is felt.[1, 5] Isotonic saline solution (10 ml) is flushed through the catheter. It is a good practice to place a hand over the affected eye once flushing begins so that the lid closes, thereby lessening the horse's surprise when the eye is irrigated once patency is regained. If back flushing occurs without resolving the obstruction, digital pressure can be applied over the opening of the duct around the catheter to help occlude it during flushing. Once patency is reestablished, instill 1 ml of Gentocin Durafilm Solution† into the catheter before removing it. Flushing the catheter with a small amount of air will clear the Durafilm Solution from the catheter as it is withdrawn. Durafilm Solution helps to control inflammation and lessens recurrence of the occlusion.

BILATERAL OCULAR DISCHARGE WITHOUT SYSTEMIC SIGNS

Bilateral ocular discharge is commonly seen in young foals and yearlings as a local ocular reaction without signs of systemic illness. Individuals are usually bright, alert, eating, and afebrile with no nasal discharge. Examination should evaluate whether an individual or herd problem exists to help establish a possible cause. Most foals affected manifest conjunctivitis with variable signs depending on the duration and severity of the ocular reaction. Signs may include hyperemia, which will vary in intensity, chemosis, which may give the appearance of puffy eyelids, and ocular discharge varying from serous to mucopurulent. Most probable causes of bilateral ocular discharge are allergy, mechanical irritation, or infection. Allergic conjunctivitis may include more than one foal but in general is not a herd problem. Inquisitive individuals who have checked out every possible crevice in their field or paddock may find themselves with red, puffy eyes accompanied by serous discharge. Initial treatment with 1.0 mg per kg flunixin meglumine* or 1 gm per 500 lb phenylbutazone† intravenously and an antibiotic-steroid ophthalmic ointment such as Ophthocort‡ tends to resolve the problem quickly. If a causative antigen is suspected, it should be removed from the foal's environment.

The number of foals affected by mechanical irritation from dust or flies varies. This is a more profound problem in the summer months, and individual assessment of severity is necessary to determine if therapy is indicated. Daily cleansing and monitoring of affected individuals is carried out where feasible. More severely affected individuals require evaluation to determine if corneal abrasions or ulcerations have occurred owing to rubbing of irritated eyes. If uncomplicated conjunctivitis is the problem, most respond to Ophthocort‡ ophthalmic ointment two to three times a day. Others may require concomitant systemic treatment with a nonsteroidal anti-inflammatory agent such as Banamine* or Butazolidin.† It is a good practice to avoid systemic corticosteroids for an anti-inflammatory effect when dealing with foals and young horses so as not to compromise their immune system.

There is very little published about equine infectious conjunctivitis. This problem is most commonly mentioned as a clinical sign accompanying systemic illness such as viral infections of the upper respiratory tract. Other reports indicate the existence of a bacterial organism similar to *Moraxella bovis*, which may cause conjunctivitis in the horse.[5] On several occasions, the author has observed a group of foals with mild signs of conjunctivitis consisting of puffy eyelids, mild redness, and a serous to mucoid discharge. Foals were monitored, but no systemic signs were detected. In a group of foals 7 to 10 days of age, the spread was rapid but uneventful. A few foals were treated symptomatically with Gentocin ophthalmic ointment§ three times a day and 1.0 mg per kg Banamine solution. There was no significant response in those foals that were treated as opposed to those that were not treated. The treatment was discontinued, and all foals recovered uneventfully within a seven-day period.

Empirically, this situation indicates that a probable viral agent had affected this group of foals. In these instances, it is important to monitor the foals for systemic illness to determine if therapy is indicated. A similar syndrome was seen in a group of recently transported yearlings. Upon arrival, a few

---

*Sovereign Feeding Tube and Urethral Catheter, Sherwood Medical Industries, Inc., St. Louis, MO 63103

†Gentocin Durafilm Solution, Schering Corp., Kenilworth, NJ 07033

*Banamine Solution, Schering Corp., Kenilworth, NJ 07033

†Butazolidin, 200 mg per ml, Jensen-Salsbery Labs., Division of Burroughs-Wellcome Co., Kansas City, MO 64141

‡Ophthocort, Parke-Davis and Co., Detroit, MI 48232

§Gentocin Ophthalmic Ointment, Schering Corp., Kenilworth, NJ 07033

were affected with a mucopurulent discharge. Within one week all were affected. The yearlings had a mild to moderate conjunctivitis, which manifested itself as a local bilateral mucopurulent ocular discharge. The ocular discharge was cleaned once to twice a day as needed. Without further treatment, all yearlings recovered uneventfully. Herd outbreaks of what clinically appears to be an infectious conjunctivitis should be monitored for systemic signs. Treatment, other than nursing care and avoidance of stress, does not seem to be indicated when the condition remains localized. If spontaneous recovery does not occur within a 7- to 10-day period, investigation into the possibility of other etiologic agents through conjunctival scraping and culture should be carried out.

BILATERAL OCULAR DISCHARGE WITH SYSTEMIC SIGNS

There is a high incidence of viral infections of the upper respiratory tract in young horses, many accompanied by varying degrees of bilateral ocular discharge. A complete physical examination should be conducted in all cases of bilateral ocular discharge to determine systemic involvement so that proper treatment can be instituted.

References

1. Bistner, S. I., Aguirre, G., and Batik, G.: Atlas of Veterinary Ophthalmic Surgery. Philadelphia, W. B. Saunders Co., 1977, pp. 122–123.
2. Catcott, E. J., and Smithcors, J. F. (eds.): Equine Medicine and Surgery, 2nd ed. Wheaton, IL, American Veterinary Pub. 1972, pp. 414, 654.
3. Gelatt, K. N., Peiffer, R. L., Jr., Gwin, R. M., and Williams, L. W.: The status of equine ophthalmology. J. Equine Med. *1*:13, 1977.
4. Peiffer, R. L., Jr., and Williams, R.: Correction of congenital entropion in a foal. VM SAC, 72:1219, 1977.
5. Severin, G. A.: Veterinary Ophthalmology Notes, 2nd ed. Ft. Collins, CO, Colorado State University Press, 1976. pp. 94–96, 128–129, 131–132, 144.

CORNEAL OPACITIES

Robert M. Gwin, OKLAHOMA CITY, OKLAHOMA

The cornea represents the anterior portion of the ocular fibrous tunic. In order to function, the cornea must remain clear and must maintain its supportive characteristics. Lack of corneal clarity may or may not be associated with a loss of supportive properties.

The cornea consists of four layers: epithelium, stroma, Descemet's membrane, and endothelium. The epithelium and endothelium are lipophilic and hydrophobic structures, whereas the stroma is hydrophilic. Disruption of the epithelial cell or endothelial cell layers results in imbibition of fluid into the corneal stroma. While the corneal stroma is normally avascular, inflammatory and degenerative processes may stimulate stromal neovascularization and cellular infiltration, both of which result in corneal opacification. This chapter discusses several disease processes in which the mechanisms just stated are responsible for corneal opacification.

CORNEAL OPACITIES IN QUIET EYES

CONGENITAL CORNEAL DISEASES

Congenital corneal disease in the foal is relatively uncommon in comparison to other animal species.

The two processes most commonly observed in corneal opacification are persistent pupillary membranes and dermoids.

Persistent pupillary membranes (PPMs) represent strands of persisting mesodermal tissue that arise from the anterior iridal surface and may attach to the endothelial surface of the cornea, resulting in focal corneal opacification. The areas are observed as multifocal plaquelike opacities deep in the cornea. Frequently, strands of mesodermal tissue may be observed attaching to these areas; however, in some cases, the mesodermal tissue may be absent. Treatment is usually not indicated, and vision in all but the most severe cases is not affected. The strands can be severed surgically, or a penetrating corneal transplant can be performed in selected cases.

Congenital dermoids are focal masses that resemble skin and usually arise at the limbus and extend out onto the cornea. The mass may be pigmented and frequently contains hair, sebaceous glands, and other dermal structures. Dermoids frequently cause irritation and may impair vision. Treatment consists of local excision from the conjunctiva and adjacent cornea by superficial keratectomy. Some corneal scarring may occur after superficial keratectomy.

CORNEAL DYSTROPHY AND DEGENERATION

The term dystrophy implies defective nutrition and is used to describe the deposition of crystalline material, often of a calcium and/or lipid nature, in corneal tissues. These deposits have a characteristic light-colored "reflective" appearance. True corneal dystrophies are not associated with previous disease, are bilateral, may be progressive, and frequently involve the corneal stroma. Similar deposits may follow nonspecific inflammation of the cornea. Treatment depends upon the degree of corneal involvement and the depth of the lesion. A superficial keratectomy is indicated if lesions involve the anterior stroma or epithelium and cause visual or cosmetic deficiencies. Deeper stromal lesions require a corneal transplant.

CORNEAL OPACITIES IN RED EYES

ULCERATIVE KERATITIS

Ulcerative keratitis is a common cause of corneal opacification in the horse and results from trauma, foreign bodies, and bacterial and fungal infections. Signs of ulcerative keratitis include pain, blepharospasm, ocular discharge, anterior uveitis, corneal edema, neovascularization, and prolapse of the third eyelid.

Diagnosis of corneal ulceration is made with topical application of moistened sterile strips of fluorescein-impregnated paper. Fluorescein is retained in areas lacking an epithelial surface, since the stain readily penetrates the corneal stroma. It is of paramount importance to determine the cause of an ulcer, especially in severe or refractory cases. Cultures for bacterial and fungal organisms should be taken prior to instillation of a topical anesthetic. Fungal keratitis is observed commonly following prior antibiotic therapy or corticosteroid therapy or both. A scraping of the tissue at the edge of the ulcer may be smeared directly on a slide for immediate staining and microscopic examination. If possible, a biopsy for histopathology is also helpful in diagnosis of bacterial and fungal keratitis.

The conjunctival fornices and membrana nictitans should be examined for foreign bodies. The presence of foreign bodies is usually associated with severe blepharospasm, pain, and lacrimation. The use of tranquilization and nerve blocks (eighth cranial nerve) (p. 378) is indicated in the majority of cases. Lower lid entropion occasionally occurs in foals and may result in corneal ulceration (p. 385).

Therapy of corneal ulceration depends on the etiology. When bacterial ulceration is suspected, antibiotic therapy may be initiated prior to culture and sensitivity results on the basis of direct corneal smears. In general, both gram-positive and gram-negative bacterial rod organisms are sensitive to gentamicin and tobramycin, whereas gram-positive cocci are sensitive to cephaloridine and cefazolin and gram-negative cocci are sensitive to penicillin G (Table 1). In fungal keratitis, 1 to 2 per cent miconazole* and natamycin,† two broad-spectrum, relatively nontoxic antifungal agents, are useful therapeutic agents.

Initial antimicrobial therapy should ideally include subconjunctival deposition of antibiotics (p. 378) and hourly topical therapy. The majority of equine fungal ulcers are associated with a concomitant anterior uveitis. The uveitis alone may result in a blind eye owing to miosis, posterior synechiae, cataract, and phthisis bulbi. Control of uveitis consists of topical cycloplegic-mydriatic agents, such as 1 to 3 per cent atropine sulfate, and systemic antiprostaglandins (p. 382). Frequency and duration of therapy with these drugs is dependent upon the severity of the inflammatory process.

Following resolution of the infectious process and healing of the corneal ulcer, topical corticosteroids may be added to the medications to reduce corneal scarring and to prevent excessive neovascularization and granulation tissue deposition.

In cases of deep corneal ulceration, there is likelihood of corneal rupture. A descemetocele ulcer represents an ulcer that has penetrated the overlying stroma. In most cases, deep stromal and descemetocele ulcers should be treated surgically. They may be covered with adjacent bulbar conjunctival tissue or filled in with a corneal-scleral transposition. A corneal-scleral transposition[3] involves the transposition of adjacent corneal and scleral tissues and has the advantages of immediately filling in the ulcerative defect with healthy corneal tissue

TABLE 1. SELECTION OF ANTIBIOTICS BASED ON BACTERIAL MORPHOLOGY OBSERVED IN SMEARS

	Topical	Subconjunctival
Gram-positive cocci	Cefazolin (30–50 mg/ml) or cephaloridine	Cefazolin (100 mg) or cephaloridine
Gram-positive rods	Gentamicin (14 mg/ml)	Gentamicin (20 mg)
Gram-negative cocci	Penicillin G (100,000 U/ml)	Penicillin G (500,000 U/ml)
Gram-negative rods	Gentamicin (14 mg/ml)	Gentamicin (20 mg)
Two or more bacteria	Cefazolin and gentamicin	Cefazolin and gentamicin
Fungal elements	Natamycin (50 mg/ml) Miconazole (1–2%)	Miconazole (5 mg)

*1 per cent miconazole, Janssen Pharmaceutica, Belgium
†Natacyn, Alcon Labs, Fort Worth, TX 76101

and results in a clearer cornea with less scarring in the central cornea. This technique is more difficult to perform than a conjunctival flap.

CORNEAL LINEAR STROMAL KERATITIS AND ENDOTHELIALITIS

Active corneal lesions are frequently seen in association with equine recurrent uveitis (periodic ophthalmia) (p. 382). The endothelialitis appears secondary to severe anterior uveitis. Clinically, the endothelium may present with plaquelike lesions, while the overlying stroma is edematous secondary to endothelial dysfunction. The lesions may be focal or diffuse.

Linear stromal opacification is also observed in recurrent uveitis. These roadmap linear opacities are found in the mid to deep corneal stroma, are 2 to 3 mm in diameter, may be multiple, and are associated with variable degrees of vascular and inflammatory cell infiltrate. While the cause of this process is not known, the linear, weaving forms of these lesions may represent paths of migrating parasitic organisms.

Focal areas of cellular infiltrate and stromal necrosis occur concomitantly with uveitis and, like the linear stromal opacities, are of unknown etiology and significance. The overlying epithelium is characteristically intact; corneal neovascularization may be extensive.

In general, stromal keratitis and endothelialitis may be treated with topical antibiotic-corticosteroid preparations when the epithelium is intact. The associated uveitis is treated with additional mydriatics and systemic corticosteroids and antiprostaglandins (p. 382).

References

1. Baum, J. K., and Jones, D. B.: Initial therapy of suspected microbial corneal ulcers. Surv. Ophthalmol., 24:97, 1979.
2. Gelatt, K. N., Peterson, G. E., Myers, V., and McClure, R.: Continuous subpalpebral medication in the horse. J. Am. Anim. Hosp. Assoc., 8:35, 1972.
3. Parshall, C. J.: Lamellar corneal-scleral transposition. J. Am. Anim. Hosp. Assoc., 9:270, 1973.

CATARACTS

Dolores J. Kunze, RALEIGH, NORTH CAROLINA

The initial recognition of cataracts in a horse can occur under a variety of circumstances. The horse owner may make the primary complaint of ocular disease, or the veterinarian may make the diagnosis as an incidental finding during a prepurchase, insurance, or neonatal physical examination. Cataracts in horses can be unilateral or bilateral, primary or secondary. They may or may not progress, and they are usually permanent. They usually fall into one of these major categories: congenital cataracts, cataracts secondary to ocular trauma, cataracts secondary to recurrent uveitis, and senile cataracts. A careful examination and a detailed accurate history are essential for determining the type of cataract, the necessary mode of therapy, and an appropriate prognosis.

The normal lens is clear and colorless, but in older horses it may have a slightly bluish tinge. It is suspended behind the iris and is bounded anteriorly by the aqueous humor and posteriorly by the vitreous. Frequently, the Y sutures can be identified, particularly in young animals; the anterior suture is an upright Y and the posterior suture is an inverted Y. The lens capsule, an acellular basement membrane, envelops the lens, providing a barrier against the aqueous humor and the vitreous. The lens has no direct contact with the vascular system, and both nutrients and metabolic wastes move through it by diffusion. An epithelial cell layer directly below the lens capsule is responsible for the majority of the metabolic activity of the lens. Therefore, an injury to this region can result in changes in the membrane potential with subsequent derangement of its biochemical functions.

The transparency of the normal lens is the result of dense concentric packing of the individual stromal cells with minimal discontinuity. This arrangement is possible because the lens is relatively anhydrous. The anhydrous state is maintained by the continuous active transport of cations and the passive extrusion of water. Failure of this system allows localized accumulations of water to form. The resulting vacuolation and subsequent loss of transparency are referred to as a cataract. A cataract is any opacity of the lens or its capsule.

Other cataracts develop with the formation of crystals or aggregates of protein and other substances. Many of the types of cataracts that occur in humans and dogs, such as sugar and radiation cataracts, have not been documented in horses. An inherent biochemical defect, for example an enzyme deficiency, may be the cause of congenital cataracts.

If such a defect exists in horses, it has not yet been identified.

DIAGNOSIS

During the evaluation of a horse with cataracts, thorough ophthalmic and physical examinations should be performed. If systemic disease exists along with ocular disease, the prognosis and therapy can be greatly affected. Both eyes should be examined carefully. The routine ophthalmic examination can be performed with a focal light source and an ophthalmoscope. After evaluating the orbit, eyelids, conjunctiva, sclera, and cornea, the anterior chamber is examined for any signs of previous inflammation or injury. These would include fibrin deposits, atrophy of the corpora nigra, anterior or posterior synechiae, graying or fading of the iris, and the presence of iridal pigment on the anterior lens capsule. A cataract can develop rapidly following anterior uveitis or a direct injury to the lens.

After evaluating the pupillary light reflexes, the pupils should be dilated to maximally expose the lens and fundus. The pupillary aperture of the adult horse is a horizontal ellipse, while that of the foal is almost round. Also, the immature iris responds poorly to mydriatics. If a cataract is present, its location, size, and shape should be noted. Most lens opacities appear white or gray, but those associated with inflammation are yellow or brown-tinged.

Examination of the vitreous and fundus comes next. A persistent hyaloid artery or remnant may be detected floating in the vitreous of a young animal. When these structures do not involve the lens, they often become less apparent or disappear as the foal matures. A small cataract will not prevent the examination of most or all of the vitreous and fundus. The location of a nuclear cataract will usually permit evaluation of a rim of fundus around the opacity. However, complete mature cataracts and total posterior synechiae make examination of the fundus impossible.

The degree of vision loss must be determined because it profoundly influences the course of therapy and the prognosis. A horse with small axial cataracts, such as hyaloid artery cataracts, may have no discernible loss of vision. The animal with nuclear cataracts may be able to negotiate obstacles better in dim lighting or after mydriasis. A large, eccentrically positioned cataract may obstruct a portion of the visual field so that the horse may compensate by an abnormal head carriage or may be reluctant to turn toward the affected side. Examining the animal in unfamiliar surroundings or observing it moving through an obstacle course may be helpful in determining its visual acuity. The state of the fundus, as previously determined, should correlate with the evaluation of vision. The degree of vision loss will depend on the extent of the lens involvement and any coexisting ocular pathology.

The accurate assessment of a foal's vision is critical and may be difficult. The menace response is not a reliable indicator of vision in many young animals, as this response is reinforced with age and experience. It is absent in very young foals. Because a foal will closely follow its dam, the extent of its visual impairment may not be readily apparent until the foal is observed on its own. The development of normal vision depends on adequate light stimulation of the visual pathways during early life. If little or no light can reach the retina during this period, severe neurophysiologic deficits and subsequent blindness can result. The ensuing functional and morphologic abnormalities in the lateral geniculate nuclei and the visual cortex are irreversible. Therefore, for a foal with complete mature cortical cataracts, early diagnosis and correction are essential if a sighted animal is desired.

CONGENITAL CATARACTS

Congenital cataracts are present at birth, having begun during fetal life. Generally, both eyes are affected, and other anomalies, such as microphthalmia, may also be present. Whenever possible, both the sire and the dam should be examined to detect heritability. However, hereditary cataracts appear to be rare in horses.

Cataracts secondary to persistent hyaloid arteries and Y-type cataracts are congenital cataracts that are generally of minor importance. They are often incidental findings, probably because they are commonly small and have a minimal effect on vision. They are usually nonprogressive and do not require surgical correction. The cataract secondary to a persistent hyaloid artery or a hyaloid artery remnant is usually a small opacity in the posterior lens capsule, but a small portion of the lens cortex may be involved as well. The Y-type cataract can appear in either the anterior or posterior lens cortex as a Y-shaped opacity. Under magnification this opacity can appear vacuolar. Aside from a periodic examination to rule out progression of the cataracts, neither of these types requires further medical attention.

The complete cortical and nuclear congenital cataracts are more serious. These are usually noticed in foals soon after birth. Occasionally, the cataracts are not discovered until the animal is weaned or enters training. Although juvenile cataracts might be suspected with such a history, the condition has been present from birth and becomes apparent only when the dam is removed or when the animal is observed closely. The center of the lens is opaque in nuclear cataracts, but the periphery of the lens remains transparent. This area increases as the pupil dilates. Thus, dim lighting or mydriasis may improve the animal's vision. Nuclear cataracts can be progressive, but a few will regress as the animal matures. The complete cortical cataract renders the entire lens opaque, thereby obscuring the fundus even after maximal pupil dilation. Affected animals are blind. If surgery is feasible, it should be attempted at the earliest possible time.

ACQUIRED CATARACTS

Acquired cataracts in horses are common sequelae to ocular injury or inflammation. While severe blunt trauma can result in cataract formation, a perforating eye wound is the more common type of initiating injury. The lens can be injured directly by a penetrating foreign body or by disruption of the lens capsule by posterior synechiae. The resulting injury to the lens capsule interferes with its ability to regulate water and electrolyte movement. Subsequently, vacuoles form, and an opacity develops. The cataract is permanent and can be progressive. Mydriasis may disrupt the initiating synechiae and slow progression of the cataract. Surgery is not indicated if the animal has partial vision in the affected eye. The presence of extensive synechiae would also make surgery impractical because of the likelihood of postoperative complications.

Secondary cataracts are frequently components of the recurrent uveitis syndrome (p. 382). Both eyes are often affected, but involvement may not be symmetrical. These cataracts are usually progressive. The episodes of uveitis can be months to years apart. Even if the cataract does not progress, however, the concurrent chorioretinitis can result in blindness. In the early stages of recurrent uveitis with iridocyclitis, the initial lens involvement may be minimal. Iridal pigment on the anterior lens capsule or posterior synechiae may precede cataract formation; these findings should be noted as prognostic factors. As these cataracts progress and mature, they commonly develop a yellowish or brownish tinge. In the presence of other severe ocular lesions, cataract surgery is of no benefit.

As the lens ages, a change in its refraction can be observed, which produces a readily identifiable demarcation between the nucleus and the cortex. This is referred to as senile nuclear sclerosis. While not an opacity and therefore not a cataract, it will precede senile cataract formation. The development of senile cataracts is a part of the normal aging process in most domestic animals, including horses. These opacities are slowly progressive, but the advanced age of the animal generally dictates against surgery.

THERAPY

There is no successful medical treatment for cataracts. Surgery, which is the only available therapy for cataracts, is indicated when blindness is the direct result of the lens opacity. However, many factors should be considered if cataract surgery is being contemplated. The retina must be functional. Concurrent ocular disease, as with recurrent uveitis, greatly reduces or eliminates the chances for surgical success. Surgical manipulation of extensive posterior synechiae is likely to result in intraocular hemorrhage, thereby jeopardizing a favorable outcome. The presence of other congenital eye anomalies also limits or obviates surgical treatment. Age and temperament can be important, especially with foals; smaller, more tractable animals often make better surgical candidates owing to the ease of postoperative therapy. If the cataractous lens can be removed with minimal trauma and complications, the odds for surgical success are good. In these cases postoperative vision will allow most horses to return to their original function.

The various surgical techniques used for lens removal in horses are beyond the scope of this text. Discission and aspiration, intracapsular extraction, extracapsular extraction, and phacofragmentation have all been used. Aspiration of the lens after discission of the anterior lens capsule generally can be performed in foals under a year of age. At this stage, the lens is still soft and gelatinous. Postoperative uveitis commonly accompanies aspiration, and it can be more severe in older foals. A firm lens can be removed by either intracapsular or extracapsular extraction. The extracapsular procedure leaves the posterior capsule in place after the lens is removed. The entire lens and both capsules are removed with the intracapsular technique. Vitreous prolapse and related complications can accompany this procedure. Phacofragmentation is a relatively new technique of ultrasonic extraction of the lens. The procedure requires the use of an operating microscope. After anterior lens capsule discission, "bursts" of ultrasound break up the lens, and concurrent aspiration removes the pieces of capsule and lens. The large expense of the required equipment limits its availability. Regardless of the surgical technique employed, vigorous medical therapy is required to control the postoperative inflammation.

Supplemental Readings

1. Bistner, S. I., Aguirre, G., and Batik, G.: Atlas of Veterinary Ophthalmic Surgery. Philadelphia, W. B. Saunders Co., 1977, pp. 180–222.
2. Gelatt, K. N.: The eye. *In* Catcott, E. J., and Smithcors, J. F. (eds.): Equine Medicine and Surgery, 2nd ed. Wheaton, IL, American Veterinary Pub., 1972, pp. 399–432.

3. Gelatt, K. N., Meyers, V. S., and McClure, J.: Aspiration of congenital and soft cataracts in foals and young horses. J. Am. Vet. Med. Assoc., *165*:611, 1974.
4. Rathbun, W. B.: Biochemistry of the lens and cataractogenesis: Current concepts. Vet. Clin. North Am. (Small Anim. Pract.), *10*(2):377, 1980.
5. Ruis, R. C.: Diseases of the lens. *In* Kirk, R. W. (ed.): Current Veterinary Therapy VIII: Small Animal Practice. Philadelphia, W. B. Saunders Co., 1980, pp. 565–570.
6. Van Kruiningen, H. J.: Intracapsular cataract extraction in the horse. J. Am. Vet. Med. Assoc., *145*:773, 1964.

OCULAR FUNDUS AND CENTRAL NERVOUS SYSTEM CAUSES OF BLINDNESS

Thomas J. Kern, ITHACA, NEW YORK

Behavioral manifestations of blindness in horses are determined by (1) onset, duration, and severity of the vision loss; (2) symmetry—unilateral versus bilateral; (3) the horse's function and use; and (4) association with other systemic diseases. Sudden profound vision deficit in one or both eyes causes unusual nervousness, decrease in tractability, shying in familiar surroundings, or accidental self-injury. Gradual but equally profound vision loss may be manifested by similar signs, recurrent traumatic injury, and marked dependence upon the presence of other horses, or it may progress unnoticed. In the absence of ocular inflammation, discomfort, discharge, or opacity, the cause of the blindness may challenge discovery.

Vision testing performed on lead in dim and bright light through an obstacle course of large familiar and unfamiliar objects is a crude but useful diagnostic tool. Hoods or blinders can be used to alternately patch the eyes. Riding or driving vision-impaired horses to demonstrate defective vision must be done with caution, if at all. Menace and pupillary reflex evaluation may help to ultimately localize the visual pathway lesion. If the ocular media and cornea are clear and a pupil is present, careful funduscopic examination may localize the lesion in the retina or optic nerve. Indirect funduscopy utilizing a 20D or 28D aspheric condensing lens and a light source (bright penlight or binocular headlamp) provides a panoramic view of topographic fundus relationships. Direct ophthalmoscopy is performed, with or without pupillary dilatation, to characterize any changes in tapetal color pattern, nontapetal background, optic disc, or the normally sparse equine retinal blood vessels. Except for the retinal pigment epithelium in the nontapetal fundus, the retina is transparent, and pathologic changes must be inferred from vascular and tapetal abnormalities.

RETINAL DYSFUNCTION

CONGENITAL ANOMALIES

The true incidence of equine congenital retinal abnormalities is unknown. In foals, retinal detachment or developmental nonattachment is most often associated with multiple ocular anomalies, including microphthalmia, microphakia, lens luxation, congenital cataract, or hypoplastic optic nerves. Etiology can seldom be determined. Genetic origin is possible, though substantiation is difficult. Multiple anomalies occur sporadically in many breeds. Therapy is ineffectual unless cataracts are the major pathologic feature.

NIGHT BLINDNESS

Equine night blindness is a congenital, reportedly nonprogressive, possibly inherited amaurosis that occurs most frequently but not exclusively in Appaloosa horses. Vision deficit spans a broad spectrum and may also involve significant day blindness. Clinical examination usually reveals minimal pathology. Nystagmus and positional strabismus may be prominent. Fundi are generally of normal appearance. Some affected horses have microphthalmic globes. Historically, the animal's vision problems may go unnoticed except to very observant horse owners and handlers. Individuals may repeatedly injure themselves in familiar surroundings, *especially in darkness.* History and ocular examination incriminate the diagnosis. Electroretinography will document the sensory retinal abnormality. The defect is speculated to be a neuroretinal transmission problem. At present, no treatment is available. Identification of affected horses and their removal from breeding programs is recommended.

Experimental vitamin A deficiency has produced night blindness in horses. Though an infrequent clinical suspicion, hypovitaminosis A may be ruled out by history and serial serum vitamin A determinations. Supplementation with vitamin A or its precursors may reverse the signs.

RETINAL DEGENERATION AND OPTIC NERVE ATROPHY

Acquired retinal degeneration in the horse must be generalized or at least widespread and multifocal before visual impairment may be noted. Substantiation of the specific cause for retinal pathology is frequently difficult. Relatively few factors have been documented to explain the pathogenesis. Undoubtedly many more remain to be discovered.

Head, facial, and direct or indirect ocular trauma may result in extensive chorioretinal and/or optic nerve atrophy. The equine retina depends primarily upon the choroid rather than the sparse retinal vasculature for supply of nutrients by diffusion. Choroidal circulatory embarrassment via orbital ciliary artery damage or direct choroidal insult causes atrophy of the outer layers of overlying retina. Once chorioretinal atrophy becomes visible funduscopically as multifocal pigmentary increase or loss, dysfunction is permanent. To forestall such sequelae, traumatized horses should receive prompt therapy for periocular injuries.

Extensive retinal and optic nerve atrophy has also been reported to occur several months following severe blood loss. Specific pathogenesis is unknown but is presumed to be associated with posterior ocular segment vascular insufficiency. No prophylaxis or treatment has been suggested.

Visually significant peripapillary and generalized chorioretinal degeneration are known to follow posterior uveal tract inflammation, usually as part of the equine recurrent uveitis complex (p. 382). Prevention is directed toward diagnosis and elimination of the inciting agent as well as symptomatic control of inflammatory episodes.

Retinal atrophy due to locoweed (Astragalus sp.) intoxication is not amenable to treatment.

RETINAL DETACHMENT

Acquired retinal detachment or separation must be suspected when the equine fundus cannot be examined in focus ophthalmoscopically or when a gray membrane obscures fundus detail. Factors responsible for normal retinal attachment include normal intraocular pressure, support from formed vitreous body, and absence of free fluid in the subretinal space. The immediate cause of retinal detachment may not be obvious. Sudden intraocular

pressure loss, as occurs during perforating injury to the eye, may precipitate such a catastrophe. Inflammatory choroidal effusion or choroidal hemorrhage disrupts tenuous attachment of neural retina, retinal pigment epithelium, and choriocapillaris to one another. Fibrous vitreal traction bands subsequent to uveitis with exudative vitreitis adhere to the inner retina and detach the retina as they contract. The prognosis for retinal reattachment and return of useful vision, regardless of the cause, is guarded at best. Modifying factors include physical extent and duration of detachment and the presence of retinal tears or traction bands. If peripheral retinal disinsertion from the ora ciliaris retinae occurs, reattachment cannot occur.

Therapy to encourage reattachment, when deemed possible even if unlikely, includes daily tranquilization for several weeks. Diuretic administration (for example, with furosemide*) might encourage subretinal fluid resolution. Subconjunctival or systemic corticosteroids are indicated to control ongoing posterior uveal inflammation. Surgical attempts to correct large detachments are heroic and seldom indicated. Subretinal fluid aspiration can be followed by diathermy to encourage chorioretinal adhesion.

GLAUCOMA

Glaucoma, increased intraocular pressure with associated vision loss, is infrequently reported in the horse. Normal equine intraocular pressure is 24 mm Hg measured by applanation tonometry.† Schiotz tonometry is impractical in the standing horse. Individual horses with chronic glaucoma secondary to chronic intraocular inflammation and fibrosis present with enlarged globes, corneal stromal opacity, cornea striae (ruptured Descemet's membrane), cataract, luxated lens, retinal detachment, or retinal or optic nerve degeneration. Presumably, acute secondary glaucoma due to aqueous outflow obstruction with inflammatory debris may occur in uveitis. Congenital glaucoma may accompany multiple ocular malformations.

Experience with therapeutic regimens for equine glaucoma is limited. Echothiophate‡ (0.06 per cent) has been used topically twice daily with limited success. Patients with painful eyes blinded with absolute secondary glaucoma would benefit from enucleation or evisceration and a silicone intrascleral prosthesis.§

*Lasix, American Hoechst Pharmaceuticals, Inc., Somerville, NJ 08876
†Mackay Marq Model 6P–9037, V. Mueller Co., Chicago, IL
‡Phospholine iodide 0.06 per cent, Ayerst Labs. New York, NY 10017
§Jardon Plastics, Southfield, MI

OPTIC NERVE DYSFUNTION

Optic nerve hypoplasia occurs unilaterally or bilaterally in otherwise normal eyes as well as in combination with multiple ocular malformations. The optic disc is small and pale. The retinal vasculature may appear reduced. The cause is unknown. Pupillary reflexes are slow and incomplete, and vision is poor. No therapy is indicated. Acquired optic atrophy must be distinguished from hypoplasia, in which vision begins and remains poor.

Optic neuritis can be visually devastating at its onset or, quite commonly, a silent cause of reduced vision. Ineffectively controlled, it results in permanent optic atrophy. Clinical signs of fulminating, severe inflammation include demonstrable vision loss with dilated unresponsive pupils. Funduscopic examination may show no changes or peripapillary retinal edema, prepapillary vitreal infiltrates, disc hemorrhage, and occasionally a swollen disc. Recurrent posterior uveitis, optic nerve trauma, orbital extension of guttural pouch or paranasal sinus infections, or tumors may all cause optic neuritis. In addition to specific therapy for the suspected etiology, treatment consists of corticosteroid therapy administered to effect by the subconjunctival, retrobulbar, or oral route and maintained as needed. Improvement in vision and pupillary responses may be used to monitor response to therapy.

Optic atrophy follows uncontrolled inflammation from any cause, traumatic ischemia, sudden blood loss, or increased intraocular pressure. The optic disc appears pale, recessed, and usually avascular. The visual prognosis is determined by the extent of atrophy and ultimate resolution of the primary cause.

BLINDNESS OF CENTRAL NERVOUS SYSTEM ORIGIN

Clinical hallmarks include absent menace response, normal findings on ocular examination, and demonstrable vision loss. If lesions are in the lateral geniculate body or above, pupillary reflexes are normal.

Congenital hydrocephalus often results in irreversible atrophy of the optic radiations and visual cortex.

In cerebral diseases of infectious origin, clinical signs of major neurologic dysfunction usually overshadow vision complaints. Cerebrospinal fluid tap results may incriminate the causative agent (p. 331). Therapy of viral encephalomyelitides (Eastern, Western, Venezuelan, and Borna) is supportive, and the prognosis is poor (p. 350). Infarction due to rhinopneumonitis virus may be palliated with systemic corticosteroids. Bacterial encephalitis (due to *Streptococcus equi* or brain abscess) may be responsive to specific antibiotic treatment. Suspected protozoal encephalitis may respond to folic acid inhibitor therapy, and corticosteroid use may be contraindicated (p. 365). Cerebral nematodiasis, due to aberrant strongyle migration, is difficult to confirm antemortem, and the value of nonspecific corticosteroid treatment is questionable.

Encephalomalacia caused by mycotoxicosis induced by *Fusarium moniliformis* ingestion is evidenced by severe cerebral dysfunction and blindness. Treatment is supportive, though the prognosis is poor. Cerebral infarction following accidental intracarotid injection of medication may be treated symptomatically with systemic corticosteroids.

Traumatic occipital cortex injury may result in transient or permanent visual cortex impairment. High-dose systemic corticosteroid therapy or intravenous mannitol therapy or both (p. 339) may relieve inflammatory swelling with return of function. The prognosis depends upon the extent of injury and promptness of treatment.

Hypoxemic necrosis of the visual cortex following cardiac arrest and resuscitation has a guarded prognosis. Systemic corticosteroid use may be indicated.

Metabolic encephalopathy associated with hepatic failure has a guarded prognosis. Therapy is directed toward improvement of liver function based upon the etiology of the liver disease.

Neoplasms causing central blindness in horses are rare. Pituitary tumors of aged horses have been associated with optic atrophy and have been responsive to treatment (p. 164).

Client education for the owner of a terminally blind or vision-impaired horse must consider the horse's use (pet, breeding, show, working, or pleasure animal), temperament and adjustment to vision loss, husbandry and management practices, potential heritability of serious ocular diseases, and discomfort of the specific ocular problems. Visually handicapped animals pose a greater risk to the owners, grooms, handlers, and riders, though they may be suitable for certain purposes. The clinician is obligated to (1) accurately assess the relative extent of the vision loss and (2) realistically predict long-term useful visual function. Horse owners then may utilize and enjoy their equine eye patients as fully as circumstances allow.

References

1. Catcott, E. J., and Smithcors, J. F.: Equine Medicine and Surgery, 2nd ed. American Veterinary Pub., Wheaton, IL, 1972, pp. 399–432.
2. deLahunta, A.: Diagnosis of equine neurologic problems. Cornell Vet., 68:122, 1978.
3. Gelatt, K., Peiffer, R., Gwin, R., and Williams, L.: The status of equine ophthalmology. J. Equine Med. Surg., 1:13, 1977.
4. Rubin, L. F.: Atlas of Veterinary Ophthalmoscopy. Philadelphia, Lea and Febiger, 1974, pp. 289–326.

THE EFFECTS OF ARTIFICIAL LIGHTING ON REPRODUCTION	399
BEHAVIORAL ANESTRUS	400
PROLONGED DIESTRUS	401
OVULATION INDUCTION	402
CONTROL OF OVULATION	404
PROGESTERONE THERAPY	405
OVARIAN TUMORS	408
DISORDERS OF THE CERVIX	409
BACTERIAL ENDOMETRITIS	410
PYOMETRA	414
CAUSES AND PREVENTION OF ABORTION	415
OBSTETRICS	422
RETAINED PLACENTA	425
POSTPARTUM COMPLICATIONS	428
PARTURIENT PERINEAL AND RECTOVESTIBULAR INJURIES	431
INDUCTION OF PARTURITION	438
EVALUATION OF STALLION FERTILITY	442
DISORDERS AFFECTING STALLION FERTILITY	449
ARTIFICIAL BREEDING OF HORSES	456

THE EFFECTS OF ARTIFICIAL LIGHTING ON REPRODUCTION

Dan C. Sharp, GAINESVILLE, FLORIDA

Of all the environmental factors that influence the reproductive cycle of the mare, changes in photoperiod are probably most important. No other environmental factor is as consistent and predictable in its changes, and an evolutionary system would most likely develop around the most predictable cue. Excluding mares that have not undergone a winter anestrus, the average date of the first annual ovulation (onset of the breeding season) changes little from one year to the next even in the face of marked differences in temperature, rainfall, and forage growth. In a seven-year study, the average date of first ovulation was April 1 (Day 91 $\pm$ 16, $\bar{x} \pm$ S.D.) in Thoroughbred and quarter horse mares and May 6 (Day 127 $\pm$ 21, $\bar{x} \pm$ S.D.) in ponies.

The onset of the breeding season can be accelerated by artificially lengthening the day. Burkhardt[1] exposed many mares to gradually increasing artificial light (1000 watt tungsten bulb) beginning on January 1. He increased day length twice as fast as the naturally occurring increase so that the longest day of the year was achieved in March. Light-exposed mares developed estrus in March as opposed to April for controls. A variety of experimental lighting regimens has been studied since Burkhardt's initial report. All of them seem effective. Day length can be instantly increased and then maintained at maximal length using a 200 watt incandescent bulb, which provides 13 to 40 footcandles.[3, 5] Length of the artificial photoperiod can also be increased gradually at the same rate as the natural photoperiod, but starting considerably earlier in the year (October 17) so that maximal day length is achieved by March.[6]

Application of these techniques in the field has met with success. Loy and his associates[4] used 7 to 15 footcandles, starting the lighting program in late November and increasing the length of day by 15 to 30 minutes per week until May. Thirty-six per cent of the Thoroughbred mares exposed to the artificial lights were bred by March 31, compared with none in a group of mares that was unlighted. Cooper and Wert[2] used one 200 watt incandescent bulb per stall in a lighting regimen used over a six-year period in a band of Standardbred mares. Light treatment was begun in October, and the length of day was increased by 30 minutes per week so that maximal day length (16 hrs) was achieved by January and subsequently maintained. After five years of the program, 50 per cent of the mares were foaling during the period from November to January, compared with 3.8 per cent at the onset of the program.

The preceding reports indicate that lighting can be used to stimulate an early onset of the breeding season. Most schedules employ gradually increasing day length up to a maximal amount of 16 hours. Although minimal light intensity is not yet known, most of the successful studies used 10 to 20 footcandles (approximately one 200 watt incandescent bulb per 12 ft stall). In all of the experiments and field trials there was a lag of 40 to 60 days between the onset of the lighting program and the onset of the breeding season because of an obligatory transition period in which follicles develop in both size and numbers. The majority of mares require 40 to 60 days to go through this transition period, regardless of whether it is a naturally or artificially induced onset of the breeding season. The time lag should be considered in planning a lighting schedule.

Although the mechanisms by which artificial lighting accelerates the onset of the breeding season are not well understood, several clues have recently become available. Exposure to only 2½ hrs of artificial light (average 15 footcandles) in addition to natural daylight can effectively stimulate the onset of the breeding season if applied after sunset rather than before sunrise. This suggests that mares may be sensitive to light at a specific time of day (photosensitive period) and that exposure to light at other times of day is ineffective. The biochemical events that occur during this time involve secretion of a pineal hormone, melatonin, because removal of the pineal gland abolishes the ability of mares to respond to a stimulatory photoperiod.

The significance of these techniques to the breeder is obvious. By stimulating an early onset of the breeding season, the breeder can see that the normal mares are bred early and thus deliver an early foal. More important, the breeder can gain precious time to work with problem breeding mares, thus offering a greater chance of solving some of their problems and getting a greater percentage of them in foal.

References

1. Burkhardt, J.: Transition from anestrus in the mare and the effects of artificial lighting. J. Agric. Sci., Camb., 37:64, 1947.
2. Cooper, W. L., and Wert, N. E.: Wintertime breeding of mares using artificial light and insemination: Six years' experience. Proc. 21st Annu. Meet. Am. Assoc. Eq. Pract., 1975, pp. 245–253.

3. Kooistra, L. H., and Ginther, O. J.: Effect of photoperiod on reproductive activity and hair in mares. Am. J. Vet. Res., 36:1413, 1975.
4. Loy, R. G.: Effects of artificial lighting regimes on reproductive patterns in mares. Proc. 14th Annu. Meet. Am. Assoc. Eq. Pract., 1968, pp. 159–167.
5. Nishikawa, Y.: Studies on reproduction in horses. Japan Racing Association, 1959.
6. Sharp, D. C., and Ginther, O. J.: Stimulation of follicular activity and estrous behaviour in anestrous mares with light and temperature. J. Anim. Sci., 41:1368, 1975.

BEHAVIORAL ANESTRUS

Jeffrey B. Grimmett, GAINESVILLE, FLORIDA

Behavioral anestrus is a psychic disorder of mares characterized by the absence of receptivity to teasing during physiologic estrus.

INCIDENCE

The incidence of behavioral anestrus varies with teasing efficiency but may be as high as 15 per cent even on well-managed breeding farms. Highly nervous mares are most commonly affected, especially foaling mares whose maternal instincts interfere with the teasing procedure. Maiden mares also are prone to silent heats, particularly when being introduced to the teasing routine. It has been suggested that the sex center in the hypothalamus of such mares has reduced sensitivity or is totally unresponsive to normal neurohumoral signals.

MANAGEMENT

The immediate goal in dealing with behavioral anestrus is to identify those mares that are cycling. Rectal palpation of the ovaries, uterus, and cervix together with visual examination of the vagina and cervix on a repeated basis are the most appropriate means of assessing the mare's reproductive status. Periodic progesterone assay, when available, may be used to identify ovarian cyclicity. These examinations should be carried out two or three times a week in concert with regular teasing. After identification, "silent heat" mares should be closely monitored, especially as visual and palpable changes associated with proestrus begin to develop. Some time and precision may be gained if $PGF_{2\alpha}$ or one of its analogues is administered and if reproductive change is closely monitored from the second day postinjection.

The method of teasing can have a profound effect on a mare's behavior. Teasing systems vary considerably between farms, but certain essentials are required for any successful teasing program. A standard teasing procedure should be followed, allowing mares to become accustomed to the routine and thus minimizing nervous suppression of signs. The mare should be calmly presented to a vigorous stallion and her reactions evaluated. A systematic method of recording should be established in addition to accurate observation, preferably by the same person. Intense stimulation and much patience is required when teasing mares with diminished estrous behavior. Techniques such as changing stallions, changing location, flank and vulval palpation, and mounting may be required before mares with prolonged reaction time will exhibit estrus. The operator may need to look for more subtle behavioral changes and should be aware of the individual idiosyncrasies of each mare. In general, unresponsive mares are better teased individually, as group methods tend to identify only the mares that show signs freely. Occasionally a mare may respond better in a more natural situation, unrestrained in the presence of a teaser stallion that has a surgically deviated penis.

Special attention should be given to maiden and foaling mares. Maiden mares should be gently introduced to the teasing system and will often improve after being bred once. Some foaling mares will only show estrus signs when their foal is taken out of sight, while others must have the foal nearby. Obviously some trial and error is in order.

Most mares when intensively teased at full estrus will show some estrous sign to an observant handler and thus pose no further problem to breeding. A few even under optimal conditions will continue to be nonreceptive. The majority of these will stand for natural service when suitably restrained. Appropriate forms of restraint include use of the twitch, kneestrap, breeding hobbles, and tranquilization. Rarely, a mare may resist all attempts at breeding so violently as to pose a threat to safety. In such instances, artificial insemination, if permitted, is the final solution.

Supplemental Readings

1. Allen, W. E.: Abnormalities of oestrous cycle in the mare. Vet. Rec., *104*:166, 1977.
2. Allen, W. E., and Newcombe, J. R.: Anestrous conditions in the mare, their diagnosis and treatment. Vet. Rec., *100*:338, 1977.
3. Ginther, O. J.: Reproductive Biology of the Mare: Basic and Applied Aspects. Ann Arbor, MI, McNaughton and Gunn, 1979.
4. Hughes, J. P., and Stabenfeldt, G. H.: Anestrus in the mare. Proc. 23rd Annu. Conv. Am. Assoc. Eq. Pract., 1977, pp. 89–96.
5. Kenney, R. M., Ganjam, V. K., and Bergman, R. V.: Non-infectious breeding problems in mares. Vet. Scope, *19*(1):16, 1975.

PROLONGED DIESTRUS

Steven D. Van Camp, STARKVILLE, MISSISSIPPI

Because humans have imposed a short breeding season on many breeds of horses, any interruption of the mare's cycle during this season can greatly reduce fertility. Prolonged diestrus is a common cyclic abnormality the causes of which must be recognized in order to manage mares for maximal fertility.

Prolonged diestrus is associated with persistence of the corpus luteum (CL) and is manifested as a failure to return to estrus on schedule. Persistent CL may occur spontaneously, after early embryonic death, in association with pyometra or endometrial degeneration and possibly in association with lactation. The life span of the CL is prolonged owing to failure of prostaglandins (PG) to induce luteolysis. This failure may relate to lack of PG release, to failure of the CL to respond to PG, or to the presence of antagonistic endocrine substances at the time of PG release.

Spontaneous persistence of the CL may occur at any time during the ovulatory portion of the mare's cycle and may extend for up to 90 days. Elevated progesterone levels produced by the CL prevent the return to estrus. Ovulation may occur during the prolonged diestrus.

Spontaneous persistence of the CL is defined as that occurring without known endometrial abnormality that would interfere with PG production. Mechanisms that have been suggested as important in the occurrence of this phenomenon include:

1. Presence of an immature CL at the time of PG release. It is known that the CL is incapable of responding to PG for four to five days after ovulation. If a diestrous ovulation occurs a few days before the normal PG release, the immature CL that results can continue functioning, causing maintenance of progesterone levels too high to allow the resumption of estrus.

2. Insufficient PG release, resulting in failure of luteolysis or incomplete luteolysis. The mare's CL may require a biphasic surge of PG to cause complete lysis. If either part of the surge is inadequate, the function of the CL may continue uninterrupted.

Persistence of the CL may occur as a result of uterine changes or endometrial pathology that blocks PG release. Examples are pyometra and endometrial degeneration. Not all cases of pyometra in mares interfere with the cycle, but if the cervix remains closed and fluid persists in the uterine lumen, release of PG to the circulation is interfered with. Endometrial degeneration may result from a variety of causes. Since PG is produced by the endometrial glands, severe destruction of these tissues will prevent normal PG production. Seasonal endometrial atrophy is a potential cause of lack of PG release.

Early embryonic death after the formation of endometrial cups (38 days) is another cause of mares failing to return to estrus. The presence of high levels of pregnant mare serum gonadotrophin (PMSG) from day 38 to near day 120 has the apparent effect of maintaining luteal function. Whether PMSG prevents luteolysis or induces the formation of new CLs is not completely clear. Current thinking indicates a luteotrophic role for PMSG, rather than a folliculogenic one.

Lactational anestrus is a term that has been used to describe cyclic failure in mares suckling foals. Rarely is true anestrus with ovarian inactivity involved, as with sows and beef cows. Since many mares stop cycling after the so-called "foal heat," a spontaneous persistence of CL is the most likely explanation for these cases.

THERAPY

The basis for treatment of all prolonged diestrus cases except those due to persisting PMSG levels is the induction of luteolysis. This is accomplished directly by administration of exogenous PG or by stimulation of endogenous PG release through uterine irritation.

Prostaglandins are available commercially in several forms that are approved for use in horses: a natural $PGF_{2\alpha}$ compound, dinoprost tromethamine,* and two analogues, prostalene† and fluprostenol.‡ All three are designed for parenteral administration, using the following dosage schedule for luteolysis:

dinoprost tromethamine	10 mg intramuscularly
prostalene	2 mg subcutaneously
fluprostenol	250 µg intramuscularly

Single luteolytic doses are effective in terminating CL life in a high percentage of cases when a mature CL is present. A higher number of responses have been noted by some practitioners when two doses are administered on subsequent days.

Following the administration of dinoprost, some degree of sweating is observed in virtually all mares within 15 to 20 minutes of treatment. Occasionally sweating is profuse and persistent. Mild abdominal discomfort may be evident in a small number of treated mares for a short time after treatment. Rarely, a transient posterior ataxia is noted. The prostaglandin analogues have few noticeable side effects.

The mare is particularly variable in response time from administration of exogenous PG until estrus and ovulation occur. Practitioners should be aware of the variability imposed by follicular status at the time of treatment, and an ovarian examination is indicated whenever PG is administered. Mares that have follicles larger than 40 mm in diameter at the time of treatment have a variable post-treatment ovulatory interval. About two thirds of these mares ovulate within three to seven days after treatment. The remaining one third show regression of the large follicle and replacement with a small one that ruptures in 6 to 12 days after treatment. Some mares that have follicles larger than 40 mm in diameter will ovulate this follicle in one to three days after treatment but fail to show heat during this time.

---

*Prostin, The Upjohn Co., Kalamazoo, MI 49001
†Synchrocept, Diamond Labs, Inc., Des Moines, IA 50303
‡Equimate, Haver-Lockhart Labs, Shawnee, KS 66201

Mares with smaller follicles (less than 35 mm in diameter) tend to be more consistent and ovulate five to nine days after treatment.

Indirect stimulation of endogenous PG is best accomplished by saline infusion of the uterus. The endometrium of mares is highly sensitive to manipulation or mild irritation and readily responds with PG release. Using strict asepsis, the cervix is gently dilated with the gloved finger, and a suitable catheter is directed into the uterine lumen. Warm saline (500 to 1000 ml) is infused by gravity or forced flow. Prophylactic antibiotics may be added to the solution.

Clinical procedures such as invasion of the cervix, endometrial biopsy, or even endometrial culture will also release PG and cause a return to estrus if a mature CL present.

Prostaglandin therapy, either direct or indirect, is ineffective in reestablishing cycles in mares with persisting PMSG levels. Virtually all mares aborting after 38 days will fail to return to estrus until 100 to 120 days for this reason. No therapeutic regimen is helpful in these cases.

Supplemental Readings

1. Hughes, J. P.: Clinical examination and abnormalities in the mare. *In* Morrow, D. (ed.): Current Therapy in Theriogenology. Philadelphia, W. B. Saunders Co., 1980, pp. 706–721.
2. Hughes, J. P., and Loy, R. G.: Variations in ovulatory response associated with the use of prostaglandins to manipulate the lifespan of the normal diestrus corpus luteum or the prolonged corpus luteum of the mare. Proc. 24th Annu. Conv. Am. Assoc. Eq. Pract., 1978, pp. 173–175.
3. Hughes, J. P., and Stabenfeldt, G. H.: Anestrus in the mare. Proc. 23rd Annu. Conv. Am. Assoc. Eq. Pract., 1977, pp. 89–96.
4. Hughes, J. P., Stabenfeldt, G. H., and Kennedy, P. C.: The estrous cycle and selected functional and pathologic ovarian abnormalities in the mare. Vet. Clin. North Am. (Large Anim. Pract.), 2(2):225, 1980.
5. Kenney, R. M.: Cyclic and pathologic changes of the mare endometrium as detected by biopsy, with a note on early embryonic death. J. Am. Vet. Med. Assoc., *172*:241, 1978.
6. Neely, D. P., Kindahl, H., Stabenfeldt, G. H., Edqvist, L.-E., and Hughes, J. P.: Prostaglandin release pattern in the mare: Physiological, pathophysiological and therapeutic responses. J. Reprod. Fertil. Suppl., 27:181, 1979.

OVULATION INDUCTION

Steven M. Hopkins, GAINESVILLE, FLORIDA

The induction of ovulation by exogenous hormones is utilized in brood mare management primarily to limit the number of breedings per conception. Inducing ovulation conserves a heavily used stallion and decreases the potential for bacterial contamination and physical trauma possible with each natural cover. There is, however, little merit in using hormones in a mare that has an established regular ovulation pattern.

Mares that are candidates for ovulation induction fall into two categories. First are those mares bred during the seasonal ovulatory period at the optimal time of their estrous cycle who fail to ovulate within 48 hours. These mares are clinically normal but may have variable estrous lengths due to individual idio-syncrasies. Management errors can be a factor, since teasing observations are subjective and may be incorrectly interpreted. The history of these mares indicates that they foal annually but require multiple covers before conception. The second class of mares are those bred during the transitional phase of their reproductive cycle. This transitional period is variable in length depending on the individual horse but in most instances occurs during the increasing photoperiod in early spring. These are often barren mares, and an attempt is made to settle them early in the season. Transitional mares frequently show strong estrous signs, but insufficient luteinizing hormone (LH) release from the pituitary gland impedes ovulation.[1]

A complete anamnesis and examination of the genital tract is necessary before considering ovulation induction. The transitional stage mare with endometrial gland atrophy from insufficient estrogen-progesterone priming or a mare in persistent diestrus are not candidates for ovulation induction. Each mare must meet the following criteria. There should be a palpable follicle, generally between 30 and 80 mm in diameter. The uterine horns should be symmetrical and should have an edematous consistency, and the borders of the cervix should be short and indistinct owing to relaxation. In cases of suspected uterine infection, negative bacterial culture and biopsy should precede any breeding attempts. A biopsy is particularly important in assessing transitional mares' uterine gland maturation.

Once ovulation induction is undertaken, most mares can be expected to ovulate within 24 to 48 hours.[2] This interval coincides with the average viability of capacitated spermatozoa of 48 hours.

There are three types of hormones available for ovulation induction: chorionic gonadotrophin, anterior pituitary extracts, and releasing hormones.

Human chorionic gonadotrophin* (HCG) has LH activity as its principal function and is obtained from the urine of pregnant women. A dose of 2000 to 3000 USP units injected intravenously gives consistent results, although 10,000 USP units intramuscularly or subcutaneously can be used. The chorionic gonadotrophins are purified proteins and are potentially antigenic. On serial HCG injections in a controlled study[3] some mares formed antibodies sufficient to neutralize a therapeutic dose; however, they exhibited no ovulatory refractoriness to the HCG. Anaphylactic reactions are possible but are rare. Unused portions of the drug may be refrigerated but should be used within 30 days or discarded.

The second group of hormones are those of anterior pituitary origin. These hormones, depending on the manufacturer, are isolated from the pituitaries of horses or other domestic animals. Pituitary extracts give erratic results in the horse[3] compared to HCG and have the disadvantage that unused portions must be refrozen to maintain potency.

The final group are gonadotrophic releasing hormones (GnRH). They are small proteins (10 amino acids) and are not highly antigenic. GnRH causes endogenous LH release from the anterior pituitary and appears to be as efficacious as HCG. The main drawback with GnRH is that there may not be adequate quantities of LH stored within the pituitary to cause ovulation. More studies need to be done in this area, especially in the transitional stage mare.

Because multiple ovulations may be caused by induction, accurate assessment of the ovaries by rectal palpation is essential prior to treatment. There are several alternatives to consider with the presence of two potentially ovulatory follicles: (1) If the breeding season is flexible, it is best to wait and cover the mare on an estrus with only one mature follicle. (2) If the mare has a "split" ovulatory pattern in which one follicle ovulates several hours prior to the other, breeding is attempted 12 hours after the first ovulation. This allows the initial ovum to degenerate while the second is still viable. (3) Breed after ovulation induction. Both follicles may simultaneously rupture, but clinical evidence indicates that the number of double ovulations exceeds the actual number of twin pregnancies.[5]

Mares that have multiple follicles and are covered should be examined at day 30 of gestation for two vesicles. In the event of twin pregnancy, abortion is indicated and should be undertaken before the development of the endometrial cups (p. 438).

Failure of HCG to cause ovulation occurs most often during the transitional period. Some follicles seem to be refractory to HCG irrespective of the dose used, and repeat injections are not indicated. Ovulatory failure may be due to a deficiency or immaturity of the LH receptors.

Ovulation induction is also used in estrus synchronization for embryo transfers. A successful transfer requires that the donor and recipient mares have an ovulatory synchrony of ±12 hours. HCG may be used on a few mares rather than maintaining a large band of recipients.

References

1. Ginther, O. J.: Regulation of reproductive seasonality in mares. Proc. Soc. Theriogenol., September, 1978, pp. 1–9.
2. Loy, R. G., and Hughes, J. P.: The effects of human chorionic gonadotrophin on ovulation, length of estrus and fertility in the mare. Cornell Vet., 56:41, 1966.
3. Loy, R. G.: Exogenous hormone therapy in mares. Proc. Soc. Theriogenol., September, 1976, pp. 8–13.
4. Roberts, S. J.: Gestation and pregnancy diagnosis in the mare. In Morrow, D. A. (ed.): Current Therapy in Theriogenology. Philadelphia, W. B. Saunders Co., 1980, pp. 736–746.
5. Roser, J. F., Kiefer, B. L., Evans, J. W., Neely, D. P., and Pacheco, C. A.: The development of antibodies to human chorionic gonadotrophin following its repeated injection in the cyclic mare. J. Reprod. Fertil., Suppl., 27:173, 1979.

*Chorisol T.M., Burns-Biotec, Omaha, NB 68127

CONTROL OF OVULATION

Robert G. Loy, LEXINGTON, KENTUCKY

In spite of the advent of newer agents and methods of control of estrus and ovulation in mammalian species, the precise control of ovulation time in mares is still difficult. The major reason for this difficulty is the lesser role of the luteal phase of the estrous cycle, and the correspondingly greater role of the follicular phase in governing total cycle length. Most of the methods used to control ovulation in other livestock species modify the luteal phase. The use of prostaglandin (PG) $F_{2\alpha}$ to shorten and the progestogens to prolong the luteal phase have relatively little direct effect on patterns of follicular development. Neither do combinations of these agents precisely control ovulation in mares because they fail to control certain aspects of follicular development. The inclusion of human chorionic gonadotrophin (HCG) along with either of the preceding agents or combinations of them adds little to the precision of control, since HCG can modify the follicular phase only by shortening it slightly.

Some general comments will be made before discussing the methods and limitations of ovulation control in mares. First, it is extremely difficult to consistently induce a useful ovulation by any hormonal treatment in deeply acyclic mares, such as those in seasonally induced anestrus and those deeply acyclic following foaling. Second, in spite of several reports suggesting advancement of first ovulations following seasonal acyclicity by means of progestogen treatments late in the period of transition from anestrus into the cyclic state, the evidence that such advancement actually can be accomplished is very tenuous. In order to allow any useful control over ovulation time, mares must be cyclic or so near the first ovulation of the season as to be considered essentially cyclic.[5, 7]

Given these circumstances, a range of degrees of control of ovulation time is possible using various agents presently available to the veterinarian.

ADVANCING OVULATION WITHIN AN ESTROUS PERIOD

Human chorionic gonadotrophin (HCG) reliably advances the time of ovulation of a potentially competent follicle. HCG permits a precise knowledge of ovulation time with respect to time of administration, provided it is given relatively early in estrus when a palpable follicle is present. Refractoriness to the ovulatory stimulus does not develop with repeated use of HCG.[6]

ADVANCING ESTRUS AND THE ASSOCIATED OVULATION

This entails the use of PG to shorten the luteal phase and thereby the entire estrous cycle. Precise targeting of ovulation is not possible. Following treatment on any given day postovulation, the distribution of intervals from treatment to ovulation is quite broad. This precludes the possibility of closely grouping ovulations in a large group of mares by either a single dose or any time-spaced series of doses of PG.

The average time saved by PG given in diestrus is about a week. HCG can be incorporated in this scheme to shave a little time off the follicular phase, again provided it is given relatively early in the postprostaglandin estrus.

Variability of response intervals after PG treatment is a characteristic of premature luteal regression and not of differences among proprietary brands or analogues of PG.[3]

GROUP OVULATIONS WITHIN A TIME PERIOD SHORTER THAN A NORMAL ESTROUS CYCLE

Progestogens alone administered for about 18 days may be used for this kind of ovulation control in mares. Progesterone in fairly high doses (200 mg per day in oil) and other progestogens do not inhibit follicular development uniformly. Thus, when progesterone given to block ovulation and allow regression of the corpus luteum is withdrawn from a group of mares, follicles in a wide range of developmental stages exist. This results in ovulation of the most mature follicles in a short time with a much longer interval to ovulation of the least mature follicles. The resulting range of time during which ovulations occur can be as long as one half a normal cycle length, and ovulations are uniformly, rather than normally, distributed during this interval.[2]

Two doses of PG spaced 10 days to two weeks apart can provide a similar or slightly lesser degree of control. A treatment regimen in which PG is given on the last day of a 10-day progestogen treatment provides about the same precision of control as progestogen alone but does allow reduction of the treatment period by about 50 per cent.

SYNCHRONIZING OR TARGETING OVULATION

The relatively long, variable period of follicular development in mares makes precise control of ovulation time much more difficult than in females of other livestock species. It is extremely important to exert a high degree of control over follicular development during the treatment period. While ovulations have been confined to a fairly short time span in small groups of mares using an oral progestogen followed by HCG, it is likely that the full range of variability that is possible following progestogen treatment was not experienced in this study.[5]

A treatment regimen of combined ovarian steroids (150 mg progesterone, 10 mg estradiol-17β) provides quite uniform inhibition of earlier stages of follicular development. When mares were given this treatment for 10 days, 20 mares having no luteal function at the end of treatment ovulated during a five-day period (days 9 to 13 after the last injection), with 18 of the 20 ovulating 10 to 12 days after treatment. For reasons covered in detail in the original report, it is necessary to give a luteolytic injection of PG on the last day of steroid treatment for maximal precision of control.[4]

More recent unpublished studies (Pemstein, Taylor and Loy) have indicated that the combined steroid-prostaglandin treatment may be used to obtain acceptably precise control of ovulation time in the early breeding season but only if mares have been adequately stimulated by an artificially increased photoperiod prior to beginning the treatment (p. 399). This agrees with the results of Palmer[5] and Squires et al.[7] In our experience, however, it appears that the individuality of a mare's response to a given lighting regimen is more critical than a specific interval of increased photoperiod. Since the response to light is quite variable, we suggest that for precise control of ovulation, mares in the central

Kentucky area (probably wherever seasonal changes in day length occur) should be subjected to an increased photoperiod for at least 70 days prior to the start of the steroid treatment. Additional cautions regarding the use of this method may be found in the original report.[4]

References

1. Ginther, O. J.: Reproductive Biology of the Mare: Basic and Applied Aspects. Ann Arbor, Michigan, McNaughton and Gunn, Inc., 1979.
2. Holtan, D. W., Douglas, R. H., and Ginther, O. J.: Estrus, ovulation and conception following synchronization with progesterone, prostaglandin F$_{2\alpha}$ and human chorionic gonadotrophin in pony mares. J. Anim. Sci., 44:431, 1977.
3. Loy, R. G., Buell, J. R., Stevenson, W., and Hamm, D.: Sources of variation in response intervals after prostaglandin treatment in mares with functional corpora lutea. J. Reprod. Fertil. Suppl., 27:229, 1979.
4. Loy, R. G., Pemstein, R., O'Canna, D., and Douglas, R. H.: Control of ovulation in cycling mares with ovarian steroids and prostaglandin. Theriogenology, 15:191, 1981.
5. Palmer, E.: Reproductive management of mares without detection of oestrus. J. Reprod. Fertil. Suppl., 27:263, 1979.
6. Roser, J. F., Kiefer, B. L., Evans, J. W., Neely, D. P., and Pacheco, C. A.: The development of antibodies to human chorionic gonadotrophin following its repeated injection in the cyclic mare. J. Reprod. Fertil. Suppl., 27:173, 1979.
7. Squires, E. L., Stevens, W. B., McGlothlin, D. E., and Pickett, B. W.: Effect of an oral progestin on the estrous cycle and fertility of mares. J. Anim. Sci., 49:729, 1977.

PROGESTERONE THERAPY

Dan L. Hawkins, LEXINGTON, KENTUCKY

Progesterone affects the mare in several ways. Plasma progesterone concentrations greater than 1.0 ng per ml cause rejection of advances by a stallion; disappearance of edema from tissues of the reproductive tract and closing of the cervix; increase in the development, tortuosity, and activity of endometrial glands; and inhibition of secretion of luteinizing hormone but little if any effect on follicle stimulating hormone.

Various metabolites of progesterone, collectively termed progestins, are functional in maintenance of pregnancy and are present in concentrations of 1 to 2 ng per ml plasma or greater at all stages of pregnancy in the mare. In addition to the effects of progestins listed earlier, they may cause the increased uterine tone of early pregnancy in the mare and have a "quieting" effect on the myometrium during pregnancy. They are also important in the production of endometrial secretions during pregnancy and in the hormonal function of the fetoplacental unit. In early pregnancy, progestins are of ovarian origin, but as early as 60 to 90 days, the placenta begins

producing progesterone, and by 150 to 180 days, it is the principal source of progestins.

The practicing veterinarian can obtain progesterone in propylene glycol,* oil,† or aqueous‡ vehicles. Using ovariectomized mares, studies of plasma progesterone concentration following intramuscular administration of progesterone have correlated plasma concentrations with dosages of progesterone in each of these vehicles. In one study, repositol progesterone (in propylene glycol) was administered intramuscularly on Days one and seven at doses of 500 mg, 1000 mg, and 2000 mg.[4] After 500 mg progesterone, concentrations peaked in six hours but returned to near 1.0 ng per ml in two days. At 1000 mg and 2000 mg, plasma progesterone was maintained at approximately 2.0 and 4.0 ng per ml, re-

---

*Repogest (50 mg per ml), Burns-Biotec Division, Chromalloy Pharmaceutical, Inc., Omaha, NB 68127

†Progesterone Injection (100 mg per ml), Carter-Glogan Labs, Inc., Glendale, AZ

‡Progesterone Suspension (50 mg per ml), N.F. (aqueous), Lannet Co., Inc., Philadelphia, PA

spectively, for seven days after injection and was 1.5 and 3.5 ng per ml, respectively, 11 days after injection. In the same study, progesterone in oil was administered in seven daily intramuscular injections at dosages of 50 mg, 100 mg, and 200 mg each day. Plasma progesterone concentrations were not maintained greater than 1.0 ng per ml for 24 hours with 50 mg per day. However, they remained at approximately 1.5 ng per ml during the last four days of 100 mg per day dosage and at approximately 3.5 ng per ml throughout the injection sequence of 200 mg per day. Ganjam et al.[3] administered intramuscular progesterone in an aqueous vehicle to mares at 150 mg and 300 mg daily. They observed that 150 mg per day for 21 days or 300 mg per day for 14 days was required to produce progesterone concentrations of 5 to 7 ng per ml plasma. The data from each of these investigations suggest the occurrence of an "accumulative effect" on plasma progesterone concentrations with repeated daily injections.

There are several oral synthetic progestogen products for use in other domestic species, but the most promising product for use in the horse is allyl trenbolone (17α-allyl-estratriene 4-9-11, 17β-ol-3-one).* There have been several studies of potential clinical applications,[1, 6, 7, 9] but it is not yet available to the equine practitioner.

Plasma progestins are assayed with sensitive competitive protein-binding assays (CPBA) and radioimmunoassays (RIA). The latter method is more specific for progesterone by utilizing an antiserum raised against antigens such as 11α-hydroxyprogesteronehemisuccinate. Reliable progestin values on field cases can be obtained if frozen plasma samples are sent to a university or diagnostic laboratory equipped to run assays for the horse.

CLINICAL USES OF PROGESTERONE

ESTRUS SUPPRESSION

Progesterone may be used to suppress estrous behavior in mares used for racing, rodeo, showing, or other competitive events. Daily intramuscular administration of 50 mg progesterone in oil beginning prior to the onset of estrus prevents estrous behavior but not ovulation, while 100 mg blocks estrus and ovulation.[5] When treatment is initiated on the first day of estrus, neither dosage is effective. A dose of 200 mg per day progesterone in oil is necessary to block estrous behavior in a normal, cycling mare that is in estrus at the start of treatment. For a mare showing estrus during the transitional or anovulatory season or a mare in diestrus, a smaller

*Regumate, Roussel Uclaf, France

dose of 50 to 100 mg per day should block estrous behavior. The propylene glycol vehicle should not be used, as it is readily picked up on drug testing programs.

Not infrequently, a trainer may request progesterone for a mare showing exaggerated psychic manifestations of estrus so that she will "go out of heat." Very few of these mares are actually showing acceptance of the stallion. They generally do not have any ovarian, uterine, or cervical changes associated with physiologic estrus, and their behavior is more that of agitation in which the tail is swished about and thrown up and urine forcefully expelled. In my experience, progesterone has not been a satisfactory treatment for a mare showing this behavior.

UTERINE INVOLUTION

Progesterone can be used to aid involution of the uterus in the postpartum mare. In mares in which fetal membranes are retained long enough that the uterus becomes refractory to oxytocin, daily intramuscular injections of 100 mg progesterone in oil and 1 mg estradiol 17-β will cause additional uterine response. The same dosage scheme carried out for five days will enhance uterine involution and tone in the mare that has a flaccid uterus and minimal involution at six to nine days postpartum.

IRREGULAR ESTRUS

Disruption of irregular estrous behavior that occurs during the early part of the breeding season may be accomplished with intramuscular treatment with 100 mg per day progesterone in oil for seven days. Van Niekerk et al.[8] found that behavioral estrus was blocked within two days of the first injection and that most mares were in an ovulatory estrus within three days following the last treatment. Mares during this period that were not showing estrus but had active ovaries responded similarly. The status of ovarian activity has an effect on the success of this treatment regimen. Mares with abundant follicular activity at the time of the first injection may give a positive response most consistently, while mares with slight to moderate ovarian activity are frequently disappointing. More recently, Squires et al.[7] and Allen et al.[1] have reported success using the synthetic oral progestin allyl trenbolone to treat mares in the transitional phase of the breeding season.

PREVENTION OF ABORTION

The major use of progesterone has been to prevent fetal death in abortion-prone mares. Although evidence is lacking to support the thesis that early fetal death or abortion is commonly due to a progesterone deficiency, there are no reported adverse effects resulting from progesterone therapy during pregnancy, and some mares with a history of repeated abortions will deliver a live foal while on a program of progesterone administration. Progesterone in a propylene glycol vehicle (repositol progesterone) is the form most frequently used by practitioners to support pregnancy. Treatment regimens employed once pregnancy is diagnosed range from 250 to 500 mg administered at intervals of 7 to 30 days. Recent work[4] indicates that such regimens of repositol progesterone probably do not significantly elevate plasma progesterone concentrations in the pregnant mare.

Determining which mare should receive progesterone therapy is difficult. By far the most common indication is a history of one or more incidences of fetal loss, especially during early pregnancy. A second indication is detection of poor uterine tone during early pregnancy examinations. However, recent evidence suggests that the enhanced uterine tone of early pregnancy may be partly due to estrogens, possibly produced by the developing conceptus.[2] An additional indication for progesterone therapy is low plasma progesterone concentrations either during a previous pregnancy that failed or during a current pregnancy.

There are two progesterone therapy regimens that elevate plasma progesterone in pregnant mares. In the first regimen, the mare is given 100 to 150 mg per day progesterone in oil intramuscularly when she is approximately 21 days postovulation and has shown no cervical relaxation. This dose is continued until she is either diagnosed not in foal or is 45 to 50 days pregnant. At this time, a more convenient schedule of 1000 mg per week repositol progesterone may be employed until 150 to 180 days of pregnancy. If the owner or manager prefers to continue therapy, the mare can be placed on 500 mg per week repositol progesterone until near term. In the second regimen, intramuscular administration of 1000 mg per week repositol progesterone is initiated when the mare is diagnosed pregnant.

MANAGEMENT OF TWIN PREGNANCY

Exogenous progesterone may be employed as part of a protocol for destruction of one vesicle in a twin pregnancy. The procedure is generally more successful if destruction of the vesicle is completed by 34 to 36 days of pregnancy. Phenylbutazone (4 gm daily orally) and progesterone in oil (200 mg per day intramuscularly) are given to the mare for two days before the vesicle is destroyed by rectal manipulation. Afterward she is maintained on phenylbutazone (2 gm per day) and progesterone in oil (200 mg per day intramuscularly) for 14 days unless she is diagnosed not in foal. Once a single pregnancy is confirmed, the phenylbutazone therapy is stopped, and the mare may be maintained on the dosage schedule described previously for maintenance of pregnancy.

References

1. Allen, W. R., Urwin, V., Simpson, D. J., Greenwood, R. E. S., Crowhurst, R. C., Ellis, D. R., Rickets, S. W., Hunt, M. D. N., and Digby, N. J.: Preliminary studies on the use of an oral progestogen to induce oestrus and ovulation in seasonally anoestrous Thoroughbred mares. Equine Vet. J., 12:141, 1980.
2. Berg, S. L., and Ginther, O. J.: Effect of estrogens on uterine tone and life span of the corpus luteum in mares. J. Anim. Sci., 47:203, 1978.
3. Ganjam, V. K., Kenney, R. M., and Flickinger, G.: Effect of exogenous progesterone on its endogenous levels: Biological half-life of progesterone and lack of progesterone binding in mares. J. Reprod. Fertil. Suppl., 23:183, 1975.
4. Hawkins, D. L., Neely, D. P., and Stabenfeldt, G. H.: Plasma progesterone concentrations derived from the administration of exogenous progesterone to ovariectomized mares. J. Reprod. Fertil. Suppl., 27:211, 1979.
5. Loy, R. G., and Swan, S. M.: Effects of exogenous progestogens on reproductive phenomena in mares. J. Anim. Sci., 25:821, 1966.
6. Palmer, E.: Reproductive management of mares without detection of oestrus. J. Reprod. Fertil. Suppl., 27:?^^, 1979.
7. Squires, E. L., Stevens, W. B., McGlothlin, D. E., and Pickett, B. W.: Effect of an oral progestin on the estrous cycle and fertility of mares. J. Anim. Sci., 49:729, 1979.
8. van Niekerk, C. H., Coubrough, R. I., and Doms, H. W. H.: Progesterone treatment of mares with abnormal oestrus cycles early in the breeding season. J. S. Afr. Vet. Med. Assoc., 44:37, 1973.
9. Webel, S. K.: Oestrus control in horses with a progestin. J. Anim. Sci., 41:385 (Abstr.), 1975.

OVARIAN TUMORS

Irwin K. M. Liu, DAVIS, CALIFORNIA

A number of types of equine ovarian tumors have been reported. These include teratomas, melanomas, epitheliomas, cystadenomas, dysgerminomas, hemangiomas, adenocarcinomas, arrhenoblastomas, hemoblastomas, and granulosa-theca cell tumors (granulosa cell tumors). Of all ovarian tumors reported in the horse, granulosa-theca cell tumors and teratomas are most often encountered, with granulosa-theca cell tumors being by far the most common.

Teratomas are composed of misplaced embryonic structures and include tissues such as bone, skin, teeth, cartilage, nerves, vessels, and hair. Granulosa-theca cell tumors are composed predominantly of neoplastic granulosa cells with frequent thecal cell involvement.

There is no apparent age or breed predilection for all types of tumors, and metastasis is rare. A presumptive diagnosis of ovarian neoplasia is made via rectal palpation of a large ovarian mass. The ovarian mass is usually unilateral, firm in consistency, and may range in size from 6 to 40 cm in diameter.

Other than in granulosa-theca cell tumors, the contralateral ovary is usually normal in size and consistency and remains functional. Clinical confirmation of neoplasia is based on persistence of the large ovarian mass, and definitive diagnosis is based on gross and microscopic examination of the mass following surgical removal.

Hormonal patterns and clinical signs for tumors other than granulosa-theca cell tumors and arrhenoblastomas have not been documented. A recent report on an arrhenoblastoma in a mare revealed significantly elevated testosterone levels with stallion-like behavior and a small, firm, and inactive contralateral ovary.

GRANULOSA-THECA CELL TUMORS

Clinical signs include nymphomania, anestrus, and stallion-like behavior. Abdominal discomfort and physical change with development of a heavy crested neck and increased muscling through the forelegs and chest have been reported.

Preliminary diagnosis of granulosa-theca cell tumor is based on (1) a persistent, large, and often multicystic ovarian mass affecting one ovary that may increase in size after several months, (2) abnormally elevated levels of testosterone, (3) clinical signs noted before, and (4) a small, firm, and inactive contralateral ovary. Estrogen levels have not been diagnostically useful.

Differential diagnoses include hematomas, teratomas, cystadenomas, and other tumors if a large ovarian mass is felt on rectal palpation. Hematomas of the ovary are generally presented as large masses on the ovary, often indistinguishable in texture from neoplasia, and are generally unilateral. Within weeks, however, the hematoma will subside. Teratomas, cystadenomas, and other tumors must be differentiated following surgical removal, with gross and microscopic examinations of the mass. Before diagnosing a granulosa-theca cell tumor in mares exhibiting stallion-like behavior, excessive use of anabolic steroids and XY testicular feminization must be ruled out. In the latter cases, there is no ovarian mass.

Mares that develop granulosa-theca cell tumors are generally infertile owing to hormonal imbalance, resulting in the suppression of the unaffected ovary. Granulosa-theca cell tumors may be diagnosed in pregnant mares; however, it is believed that conception occurs prior to active development of the tumor and subsequent hormonal imbalances.

HORMONAL PATTERNS

Testosterone levels are generally elevated in mares with granulosa-theca cell tumors, regardless of clinical behavioral patterns. In most instances, mares exhibiting stallion-like behavior have significantly elevated testosterone levels with Leydig cell involvement.

TREATMENT

Surgical removal of the tumor is the only satisfactory method of management, regardless of the type of tumor. Vaginal, abdominal, and flank approaches are generally utilized in removal of the tumor. The selected approach is dependent upon the size, age, and disposition of the mare. Regardless of surgical approach, all mares are withheld from feed 24 hours prior to surgery. Postsurgically, the majority of mares with granulosa-theca cell tumors will return to normal estrus, provided the neoplasm is unilateral. Return to cyclic ovarian activity usually occurs during the following reproductive season. Some mares fail to return to estrus as long as 1½ years following surgical removal of the affected ovary. Most mares will return to normal reproductive function and are capable of conceiving and delivering a live foal, provided there are no other causes for infertility.

Supplemental Readings

1. Clark, T. L.: Clinical management of equine ovarian neoplasms. J. Reprod. Fertil. Suppl., 23:331, 1975.
2. Meagher, D. M., Wheat J. D., Hughes, J. P., Stabenfeldt, G. H., and Harris, B. A.: Granulosa cell tumors in mares:

A review of 78 cases. Proc. 23rd Annu. Conv. Am. Assoc. Eq. Pract., 1977, pp. 133–143.
3. Stabenfeldt, G. H., Hughes, J. P., Kennedy, P. C., Meagher, D. M., and Neely, D. P.: Clinical findings, pathological changes and endocrinological secretory patterns in mares with ovarian tumors. J. Reprod. Fertil. Suppl., 27:277, 1979.

DISORDERS OF THE CERVIX

George K. Haibel, GAINESVILLE, FLORIDA

The equine cervix is a dynamic structure that must be capable of both estrous relaxation to allow escape of postbreeding contaminants and diestrous closure for maintenance of uterine integrity during pregnancy. Any abnormality that reduces the efficiency of these functions will result in lowered fertility. The tendency of the equine cervix to react to trauma or inflammation with fibrosis is the main source of serious lesions.

The mare's cervix is sphincterlike and simple when compared to that of other domestic animals. The cervical canal lacks annular rings and is essentially a continuation of the longitudinal folds of endometrium. Its luminal mucosa is highly folded and lined by columnar epithelium that contains many mucus-producing goblet cells. The intravaginal portion of the cervix (portio vaginalis) protrudes from the surrounding vaginal fornix. A sagittal frenulum is generally present. Palpable shape and the mechanical basis for closure are provided by the tubular tunica muscularis, which consists of several smooth muscle layers interposed by abundant, collagen-rich connective tissue.

The cervix alters its structure under hormonal control to perform divergent functions. Apposition of the glans penis and relaxed cervix during copulation results in intrauterine deposition of semen. The open cervix of estrus allows the free outward flow of uterine secretions and exudates, which clears the uterus of contaminants. Diestral closure renders the cervical lumen virtually impenetrable by debris and bacteria, ensuring uterine integrity for the establishment and maintenance of pregnancy. The fully effaced cervix at parturition gives the impression of vaginal-uterine continuity and allows unimpeded expulsion of the fetus.

Cervical lesions cause infertility by obstructing the lumen or by preventing adequate closure. Foaling trauma is a prime cause of cervical damage. Malformations and neoplasia are uncommon. Transluminal cervical adhesions are the result of deep inflammation or laceration of the luminal mucosa.

Intrauterine irrigation with irritating solutions such as iodine may lead to a chemical cervicitis. An indolent cervicitis may also follow acute puerperal metritis. Cervical bruising or penetrating laceration of the vaginal fornix can occur at breeding. Laceration or avulsion may follow uncomplicated delivery but is more commonly due to forced extraction. Manipulation necessary for correction of posture or fetotomy can easily cause cervical trauma. Rupture or excessive stretching of the muscular tunic at parturition without tearing of the mucosa can result in an incompetent cervix.

EXAMINATION OF THE CERVIX

Evaluation of the cervix occurs at several points in the routine genital examination. The size, shape, and consistency of the cervix are readily palpable per rectum. Vaginoscopic examination of the intravaginal cervix should not confuse variations in normal structures with lesions. The cervical lumen should be evaluated with a finger in every nonpregnant mare and is easily accomplished during uterine culture or endometrial biopsy. Examination for intraluminal lesions is best done during estrus or following administration of exogenous estrogen. If present, the possibility of concurrent intrauterine adhesions should be considered. The integrity of the muscular tunic in suspected cervical incompetence must be evaluated during diestrus.

THERAPY

Adhesions involving the intravaginal cervix and vaginal fornix can be ignored, circumvented by artificial insemination or reinforced breeding, or surgically corrected, depending on their severity. General surgical considerations for cervical surgery are similar to those described elsewhere (p. 431). Excision is generally successful. Traction applied to the cervix to enhance accessibility alters the relationships of the vaginal fornix. Proposed lines of excision should be well identified prior to traction and the anatomic effects of excision verified during the procedure. Transluminal adhesions are less amenable to repair and have a tendency to recur. Excision or digital breakdown may be followed by stenting the lumen with an indwelling urinary catheter, daily manual probing, or placement of bland pessaries.

Reconstructive repair of cervical lacerations requires careful dissection and tissue identification. Surgery is best performed at least 30 days postpartum with the mare in diestrus to enhance muscularis recognition and to minimize mucosal edema. Dissection of the defect and adhesions should reestablish the layers of the cervix, which are then sutured separately. The luminal mucosa is everted with No. 1 chromic catgut in a continuous horizontal mattress suture. The muscularis is closed with a simple continuous pattern of the same material, and the vaginal mucosa is closed with an everting pattern. Well-defined defects in the muscular tunic may be repaired by suturing in a similar fashion to a full-thickness laceration, after incising the overlying intact mucosa. Additional support in the form of a buried retention suture involves placing a nonabsorbable suture submucosally around the muscular tunic of the intravaginal portion of the cervix. Repair of lacerations frequently results in new adhesions. Prognosis for fertility is always guarded. Lacerations tend to recur at subsequent foalings.

The diagnosis of cervical conditions results from thorough examination of the genital tract. Iatrogenic contributions to many lesions should be remembered. The cervix should not be incriminated as a cause of infertility, nor should restorative procedures be contemplated without evaluation of the uterus by endometrial biopsy. Surgical results are frequently frustrating, and the prognosis for fertility is therefore guarded for all but the simplest problems.

Supplemental Readings

1. Evans, L. J., Tate, L. P., Cooper, W. L., and Robertson, J. T.: Surgical repair of cervical lacerations and the incompetent cervix. Proc. 25th Annu. Conv. Am. Assoc. Eq. Pract., 483–486, 1979.
2. Ginther, O. J.: Reproductive Biology of the Mare. Ann Arbor, MI, McNaughton and Gunn, 1979.
3. Walker, D. F., and Vaughan, J. T.: Bovine and Equine Urogenital Surgery. Philadelphia, Lea and Febiger, 1980.

BACTERIAL ENDOMETRITIS

A. C. Asbury, GAINESVILLE, FLORIDA

The economic impact of uterine infections on equine fertility is enormous. Bacterial endometritis was the most important cause of infertility in a large survey of mares more than 50 years ago. In spite of the development of sophisticated antimicrobial agents during the ensuing half century, the same statement can be made today. Thus, the availability of a wide spectrum of specific antibiotics has not solved what would appear to be a simple cause-effect relationship of etiologic agent to disease.

The reasons for this failure are complex and not completely understood. Endometritis is a disorder perpetuated by anatomic, physiologic, and immunologic failures in the mare. The presence of bacteria in the uterus is only one part of the complex. In order to manage endometritis successfully, it is necessary to understand the predisposing factors, develop an efficient diagnostic routine, and employ a therapeutic regimen that takes the complexities of the disorder into account.

PATHOGENESIS

Bacterial contamination of the reproductive tract is inevitable for all brood mares. Countless organisms gain access to the vagina and uterus during breeding and foaling. The fertile mare responds to this bacterial invasion with a highly efficient defense system that rapidly eliminates the organisms from the uterus, allowing survival of the embryo. When this system fails, the contaminating bacteria become established, producing inflammation that persists long enough to produce an environment that is incompatible with pregnancy.

Stallion semen contains millions of potentially pathogenic bacteria that are deposited directly into the uterus during coitus. The organisms originate from the surface of the penis and prepuce, urethral diverticulum, and the urethra itself. Prebreeding washing may reduce contamination, but no technique, including collection of semen by artificial vagina, will eliminate bacteria from the ejaculate. It is impossible, then, to breed mares by any method that will totally prevent contamination of the uterus.

Parturition is another event in which bacteria gain entrance to the mare's reproductive tract. In normal foaling, it is logical that most contaminants are expelled by rapid delivery of the placental membranes and uterine involution. Nevertheless, uterine cultures of these mares during the immediate postpartum period will yield a wide array of organisms with the potential to produce endometritis. Any variation from normal parturition, even retention of the placenta for a few hours, will dramatically increase the numbers of bacteria.

Additional sources of uterine contamination include perineal conformation defects that predispose to pneumovagina and fecal aspiration and iatrogenic causes. Irritants such as urine pooling in the cranial vagina may contribute to the problem.

The evidence for a competent uterine defense system is the number of mares that conceive, maintain pregnancy, and deliver healthy foals annually. The uterine environment must be essentially free from bacteria and inflammatory byproducts by the fourth day postovulation, when the embryo descends into the uterus.

The anatomy of the tubular genitalia of normal mares is a key component of the defense mechanism. During estrus, when the entire tract is relaxed and dilatable, three structures act as valves, allowing uterine contents to be expelled while external contaminants are excluded. These are the cervix, the vestibular sphincter, and the vulvar sphincter. Mucus produced by uterine glands and cervical epithelium provides the medium to literally flush uterine contents to the outside.

Another important component of the system is the mobilization of polymorphonuclear leukocytes (PMNs) into the uterine lumen. Phagocytosis of bacteria by these cells is critical in inactivation of the organisms before they can multiply. In the normal mare, PMNs can be detected in the uterus within a few hours of the contamination, and bacteria, PMNs, and inflammatory byproducts begin to flow through the open cervix soon thereafter.

Failure of the defense mechanism may result from anatomic causes (inability of the uterus to contract, failure of the cervix to open) or immunologic causes (inability of PMN to mobilize, ingest, and kill bacteria). Failure may also relate to chronic, low-level contamination through anatomic defects that perpetually bathe the uterus with organisms that can never totally be eliminated.

DIAGNOSIS

The dilemma in treating bacterial endometritis lies in the problems of accurately identifying the disorder as much as employing specific therapy. Since indiscriminate antibiotic treatment in mares that are not actually infected may be detrimental and since failure to recognize and treat low-grade inflammation may result in persistent infertility, an accurate diagnosis is imperative. History, physical examination, and laboratory aids are all part of the diagnostic regimen.

Endometritis is by definition an inflammation. Determination that an inflammatory process is involved is the key to accurate diagnosis. Cultural findings are meaningless without knowledge of the inflammatory status of the uterus.

The physical examination of the reproductive tract should be the primary diagnostic procedure. Changes in the tubular system as detected by palpation and vaginoscopy can provide immediate evidence of inflammation. Fluid accumulation in the uterine lumen, hyperemia of the cervix or vagina, and exudates are examples.

Supportive evidence of inflammation can be obtained by endometrial cytology and endometrial biopsy. Staining endometrial smears and examining them for the presence of PMNs provides a rapid, simple screening test. In the mare there are few neutrophils in normal uterine secretions, so their presence in significant numbers is a valid sign of active endometritis.

Uterine biopsy is the most definitive technique for confirming inflammatory changes in the endometrium. Superficial, diffuse, moderate infiltrations of lymphocytes, plasma cells, and occasionally PMNs correlate well with clinical endometritis. Isolated circumscribed foci of lymphocytes, when widely scattered, are less significant. There is increasing acceptance by practitioners of the endometrial biopsy as a diagnostic tool. Its value in assessing the efficacy of therapy is an additional factor.

Uterine culture does not by itself establish the presence or degree of inflammation. Recovery of infectious agents from the uterus merely indicates the probable etiology of the inflammatory process. Cultures should be representative of the uterus only and should be made with instruments and techniques that avoid contamination by organisms residing in the vaginal tract or by outside contaminants. Since the principal uterine pathogens are opportunistic bacteria that are commonly present on skin, in the caudal vagina, and in the environment, the interpretation of a contaminated culture becomes difficult.

Laboratory technique for handling uterine cultures should provide both qualitative and quantitative information. Direct streaking of swabs on plates without intermediate holding in nutrient media is essential for both types of information.

The principal bacterial pathogens causing endometritis are *Streptococcus zooepidemicus, Escherichia coli, Pseudomonas aeruginosa,* and *Klebsiella pneumoniae.* These four organisms are found in over 80 per cent of confirmed cases of uterine infection. In the presence of convincing evidence of inflammation, Corynebacterium sp, Proteus sp, and rarely Staphylococcus sp should be considered pathogenic. Most isolates of alpha-hemolytic Streptococci, Enterobacter sp, and *Staphylococcus epidermidis* cannot be correlated with inflammatory changes and are viewed as contaminants.

Yeasts, particularly Candida sp and rarely fungi such as Aspergillus sp, may be isolated from mares with concurrent signs of inflammation. These organisms should be recoverable repeatedly to be significant. Most cases of yeast or fungal infections are secondary to antibiotic therapy and may prove to be more stubborn to manage than the original bacterial problem. Severe, prolonged Candida infections have resulted in permanent changes in the tubular genitalia, such as intraluminal, cervical, or vaginal adhesions.

THERAPY

Once a reliable diagnosis of bacterial endometritis has been established, management of the disorder must include (1) correction of anatomic defects when indicated, (2) reduction of bacterial numbers in the endometrium and uterine lumen, and (3) prevention of recurrence of the inflammation.

The mare with poor vulvar conformation may need nothing more than a Caslick's operation to accomplish all three therapeutic objectives. In fact, this simple labial suturing survives as the most effective tool in managing infertility of infectious origin. More complex anatomic defects such as perineal body damage or rectovestibular injuries are discussed on p. 431.

Antibiotic therapy is currently the logical approach to achieving the second objective, reducing bacterial numbers in the uterus. Differences of opinion exist about almost every aspect of the use of antibiotics in the treatment of uterine infections in mares. The questions involve such issues as local versus systemic administration, choice of drug, type and volume of the vehicle, and frequency of treatment.

The basis for most of these opinions is experience. Experimental evidence is lacking to form a sound basis for making the necessary decisions. Current research on minimum inhibitory concentrations of drugs in endometrial tissue will provide some guidelines, but until a reliable experimental model for endometritis is available, these facts may be difficult to translate into therapeutic efficacy.

Majority opinion today supports topical treatment of the uterus by infusion of antibiotics through the cervix in a volume of vehicle adequate to distribute the drug uniformly throughout the organ. The use of large volumes of vehicle to stretch the uterus and provide contact with all of its surface area is also logical. The problem with this regimen is the escape of a portion of the drug through the cervix when the infusion is completed. Forcing antibiotic solutions into the uterine lumen under pressure is an interesting concept that merits further appraisal.

A treatment regimen that represents the author's opinion is based on the following guidelines: (1) Select as specific an antibiotic as possible based on culture results and in vitro antibiotic sensitivity testing; (2) select a drug and vehicle that are relatively nonirritating to the endometrium; (3) administer by intrauterine infusion using aseptic technique daily during estrus for at least three days and longer if time and economics permit; (4) use a minimal volume of 200 ml, an amount that will be retained in the uterus of most mares without flowback through the cervix.

There are variations to these guidelines that should be observed. Antibiotic sensitivity testing does not always correlate with in vivo efficacy when applied to the equine uterus. As an example, polymyxin B, which is invariably impressive in the laboratory against Pseudomonas and Klebsiella cultures, is seldom, if ever, of value in treating endometritis. Nitrofurazone and related compounds are similarly inconsistent. Drugs from the tetracycline family should be avoided for intrauterine infusion owing to questions relating to their irritant qualities. Antibiotics with a primary antibacterial action should not be used for treatment of yeasts or fungi.

Table 1 lists antibiotics that may be used for intrauterine infusion in mares. Not all of these drugs have been officially approved for this purpose, and appropriate discretion is advised.

A particularly perplexing problem encountered in managing specific bacterial infections is the so-called superinfection. In these cases, the primary organism is eliminated from cultural findings, but another, usually more stubborn one, takes over. This situation may be noted when treatment for streptococci results in a pure recovery of Pseudomonas at the next subsequent estrus. Occasionally Pseudomonas and Klebsiella are involved in the same interaction. The phenomenon of superinfection has been noted to occur spontaneously in experimentally infected mares in which no antibiotic therapy has been employed. This observation suggests that both organisms are involved initially, but one is masked by the other. Changes in the uterine environment may predispose to the reduction in numbers of one agent and favor multiplication of the other. Superinfection, if noted often, may be an indication for use of

TABLE 1. SUGGESTED ANTIBIOTICS FOR UTERINE INFUSION

Drug	Dose Per Infusion	Comments*
Amikacin†	2 gm	Gram-negative spectrum
Ampicillin‡	3 gm	Use only soluble products
Carbenicillin§	6 gm	At this dose is effective in some Pseudomonas cases
Chloramphenicol‖	2–3 gm	If oral solution used, may precipitate in saline
Gentamicin sulfate**	2 gm	Buffer with $NaHCO_3$ when using small volumes (less than 200 ml)
Kanamycin sulfate††	1–2 gm	Most *E. coli* are sensitive
Neomycin sulfate	4 gm	*E. coli*, some Klebsiella, but seldom Pseudomonas
Potassium penicillin G‡‡	5 million units	Preferred for Streptococci
Ticarcillin§§	3–6 gm	Most endometritis pathogens are susceptible. Higher dose recommended for Pseudomonas
Amphotericin B‖	50 mg	Use the IV preparation. Dilute in water, *not* saline. For Candida sp and fungi

*Except where indicated, sterile saline is the appropriate vehicle.
†Amikacin sulfate, Bristol Labs, Syracuse, NY 13057
‡Amp-Equine, Beecham Labs, Bristol, TN 37620
§Pyopen, Beecham Labs, Bristol, TN 37620
‖Chloramphenicol Oral Solution, Pitman-Moore, Washington Crossing, NJ 08560
**Gentocin, Schering Corp., Kenilworth, NJ 07033
††Kantrim, Bristol Labs, Syracuse, NY 13057
‡‡Pencillin G Potassium for injection, E.R. Squibb & Sons, Princeton, NJ 08540
§§Ticar, Beecham Labs, Bristol, TN 37620
‖Fungizone, E.R. Squibb & Sons, Princeton, NJ 08540

broad-spectrum antibiotics or combinations of narrower spectrum drugs.

Many endometritis cases, particularly the more chronic, fail to yield specific bacteria on culture, yet the endometrium is known to be inflamed. A decision must be made in these instances whether to use antibiotic therapy without knowledge of the etiologic agent or to use a less specific, nonantibiotic approach. Previous cultural history may aid in the decision.

The use of irritating disinfectant solutions in the mare's uterus should be approached cautiously. The mare is extremely sensitive to irritant substances introduced into the reproductive tract and may respond with necrosis and subsequent fibrotic changes of the endometrium, cervix, and vagina. Strong iodine solutions and chlorhexidine diacetate* are contraindicated for this reason.

One nonantibiotic regimen that has been used with some success in chronic and culturally negative cases is infusions with dilute povidone-iodine solutions. A variety of these compounds are marketed, and the available or titratable iodine content of each should be noted to calculate the appropriate dilution. The maximal strength of the infused solution

should not exceed one part of a stock solution containing 1 per cent available iodine in 10 parts of final solution.

Even at these concentrations, the solutions are irritating to some mares. Discomfort and straining following infusion may be noted. Prior to each subsequent treatment, evaluation of the degree of irritation caused by the previous infusion should be made. Any cervical or vaginal edema or hyperemia is grounds for discontinuation of therapy. Failure to monitor the irritation carefully may result in severe and, rarely, permanent changes in the reproductive tract.

Ideally, the povidone-iodine infusions, using 250 to 500 ml of solution, should continue for five or six days. Histologic evidence for an improvement in the endometrium has been observed with this treatment, and fertility has been restored in a number of difficult mares.

Evaluation of therapy for endometritis is based on the disappearance of inflammatory signs and demonstration of negative uterine cultures during subsequent estrous periods. Endometrial biopsy is the ideal method for assessing the efficacy of treatment.

Once the uterus has been returned to an acceptable state, careful management is indicated to prevent recurrence of the infection, since the uterine defense mechanisms are as important as the initial

*Nolvasan, Fort Dodge Labs, Fort Dodge, IA 50501

therapy. Indiscriminate breeding or failure to maintain anatomic integrity will usually cause an immediate recurrence of the problem.

Artificial insemination (AI), using antibiotic extenders, is the best management tool for these susceptible mares. Where AI is not permitted, mares should be managed for minimal contamination at breeding. The infusion of antibiotic semen extenders into the uterus just prior to natural service is helpful (p. 453). Limitation of the number of natural breedings is also indicated. Postbreeding infusion with antibiotics may be used for 48 hours after ovulation without compromising embryo survival.

Supplemental Readings

1. Baker, C. V., and Kenney, R. M.: Systematic approach to the diagnosis of the infertile or subfertile mare. *In* Morrow, D. A. (ed.): Current Therapy in Theriogenology. Philadelphia, W. B. Saunders Co., 1980.
2. Blanchard, T. L., Garcia, M. C., Hurtgen, J. P., and Kenney, R. M.: Comparison of two techniques for obtaining endometrial bacteriologic cultures in the mare. Theriogenology, *16*: 85, 1981.
3. Conboy, H. C.: Diagnosis and therapy of equine endometritis. Proc. 24th Annu. Con. Am. Assoc. Eq. Pract., 1978, pp.165–171.
4. Garg, R. C., and Powers, T. E.: Some interactions, incompatiblties and adverse effects of antimicrobrial drugs. *In* Morrow, D. A. (ed.): Current Therapy in Theriogenology. Philadelphia, W. B. Saunders Co., 1980.
5. Hughes, J. P.: Clinical examination and abnormalities in the mare. *In* Morrow, D. A. (ed.): Current Therapy in Theriogenology. Philadelphia, W. B. Saunders Co., 1980.
6. Kenney, R. M.: Cyclic and pathologic changes of the mare endometrium as detected by biopsy, with a note on early embryonic death. J. Am. Vet. Med. Assoc., 3:241, 1978.
7. Woolcock, J. B.: Equine bacterial endometritis: Diagnosis, interpretation and treatment. Vet. Clin. North Am. (Large Anim. Pract.), 2(2):241, 1980.

PYOMETRA

Irwin K. M. Liu, DAVIS, CALIFORNIA

Pyometra is an accumulation of abnormal fluids in the uterus accompanied by distention of the organ. Interference with the patency of the cervix and with natural drainage of fluids from the uterus is often considered a causative factor. Cervical adhesions or irregular, tortuous, and abnormally tight cervices, particularly during the follicular phase of the estrous cycle, may be predisposing factors. Pyometra can be found, however, in mares with apparently normal cervices.

CLINICAL SIGNS

Clinical signs include discharge from the vulva, which may vary from watery to creamlike in consistency, occurring particularly during estrus. In some instances in which the condition is prolonged, the discharge may become caseous, and cottage cheese–like material may be observed. The discharge may range in volume from 1 to 60 l. Isolation of bacteria of various species from the discharge, although common, is not the rule.

Systemic complications of pyometra are rare but when present may result in weight loss, depression, and anorexia. Hematologic findings in systemically normal mares include a mild depression anemia and a mild leukopenia. Those exhibiting clinical signs of systemic involvement usually do not show any marked changes in the blood picture; however, toxicity of the granulocytic series may be apparent.

The estrous cycles of affected mares may vary considerably and may range from failure to cycle to shorter estrous cycles. Hormonal concentrations remain unaffected.

Diagnosis of pyometra is based upon rectal palpation of a fluid-filled uterus with or without the observation of excessive discharge from the external os of the cervix or the vulva. It is imperative that pregnancy, particularly during the gestational period of 80 to 120 days, be included in the differential diagnosis if purulent discharge from the vulva or cervix is not noticeable. A tentative diagnosis of pregnancy can be obtained through the use of the Mare Immunological Pregnancy (MIP) Test if a fetus is not palpable. Ballottement of the fetus is conclusive evidence of pregnancy.

GENERAL CONSIDERATIONS FOR TREATMENT

Treatment of chronic pyometra in mares is usually not indicated unless there is unsightly discharge of pus or signs of systemic disease. If treatment is elected, the uterus generally returns to a reasonable size and consistency if drainage is performed during the early stages of the disease. In most instances, a mare with pyometra is brought to the attention of the practitioner during the advanced stages of the disease, and treatment is usually followed by a return of the condition after a few weeks. If left untreated, accumulated fluid may inspissate within the uterus or may be expelled during the follicular phases of the estrous cycle. Expulsion and inspissation of the fluid may require months to years. Where severe systemic signs are noted, an attempt should be made to treat the condition. Severe endometrial damage is inevitable, and the prognosis for future maintenance of a full-term foal is poor.

If the mare is likely to be used as a donor for embryo transfer, treatment of pyometra is essential to avoid possible involvement of the oviducts. If treatment is successful, the mare still may not enter a follicular phase of the estrous cycle and may not ovulate. This is due to unpredictable release of prostaglandin (PG)$F_{2\alpha}$ by the damaged endometrium. Exogenous $PGF_{2\alpha}$ should be utilized to ensure complete luteolysis and subsequent ovulation.

TREATMENT

Repeated lavage of the uterus with povidone-iodine, diluted to 1 part in 10 parts of warm water, is necessary to remove the accumulated exudate. A nasogastric tube or similar apparatus is useful for this purpose. Care must be exercised not to overfill an already distended uterus and not to excessively manipulate and traumatize the compromised uterus. Fluid is siphoned off through the tube, and the flow may be enhanced by gently massaging the uterus by palpation per rectum. Injection of estradiol propionate (5 to 10 mg) intramuscularly to aid in softening and relaxation of the cervix may be useful. The administration of estrogen will also condition the uterus to respond to a subsequent injection of oxytocin intramuscularly (5 to 20 units), which will help expel the contents from its lumen. $PGF_{2\alpha}$ is indicated to bring about the regression of active corpus luteum and subsequent relaxation of the cervix to facilitate drainage of fluid from the uterus during the induced follicular phase.

The presence of cervical adhesions will prevent drainage of exudate from the uterus. If present, they should be manually separated utilizing one or more well-lubricated gloved fingers. Adhesions will reform unless a pessary is utilized or unless frequent manual manipulation is performed to maintain patency.

When mares become systemically ill and when drainage is followed by recurrence of pyometra, hysterectomy is indicated. Hysterectomy can be performed within several days following complete removal of exudate from the uterus, provided systemic signs have regressed. It is during this period that the uterus will have contracted to its minimal size thereby facilitating surgical extirpation.

ANTIMICROBIAL THERAPY

Supportive systemic therapy is usually not indicated. There is no evidence for its usefulness in treating infections of the uterus.

In situations in which mares become systemically ill, systemic administration of antimicrobials may be useful; however, evacuation of uterine contents in most instances will alleviate the condition.

Supplemental Reading

1. Hughes, J. P., Stabenfeldt, G. H., Kindahl, H., Kennedy, P. C., Edqvist, L. E., Neely, D. P., and Schalm, O. W.: Pyometra in the mare. J. Reprod. Fertil. Suppl., 27:321, 1979.

CAUSES AND PREVENTION OF ABORTION

Dean P. Neely, EAST LANSING, MICHIGAN

Abortion is the termination of a pregnancy and expulsion of the fetus during the period between the completion of embryonic organogenesis and term gestation. Fetal abortion should be considered separately from embryonic loss, which occurs prior to organogenesis.

EMBRYONIC LOSS

The embryonic stage, from fertilization of the ovum to the end of organogenesis, ends between 30 and 60 days of gestation. Embryonic loss within this period can result in absorption (resorption) of the embryonic tissues and fluid without expulsion of tissue through the cervical canal. Only if the luteal influence is removed, such as by prostaglandin therapy, so that the cervical canal opens, may products of this early embryonic stage be observed.

Early embryonic losses can occur in 10 to 20 per cent of pregnancies, with the greatest incidence in lactating mares and mares bred in "foal heat."[10] If the conceptus is lost prior to 35 or 36 days of gestation, the primary corpus luteum can persist for up to 30 to 60 days before undergoing luteolysis and returning the mare to estrus.

Should conceptus loss occur after the formation of the endometrial cups and their production of pregnant mare serum gonadotrophin (PMSG) around 35 to 38 days of gestation, the mare generally will not return to estrus until the endometrial cups have been rejected from the endometrium approximately 90 to 150 days from the date of conception. The presence of PMSG in the circulation appears to inhibit estrous behavior even if the corpora lutea are lysed by prostaglandin therapy.

Few causes of early embryonic death have been accurately identified. Moderate to severe generalized endometrial fibrosis, determined by histopathologic evaluations of endometrial biopsies,[8] is one of the best documented etiologies. It is recommended that mares with mild to moderate endometrial fibrosis be bred by minimal contamination techniques utilizing semen extenders (p. 453). Progesterone supplementation has also been utilized by the author during the first two to three months of pregnancy. With severe generalized endometrial fibrosis, embryo transfer techniques can be utilized to maintain the mare's genetics within the progeny.

Nutritional deficiencies (energy and protein) and stress are often incriminated in embryonic deaths. Embryonic resorption has occurred with mares placed on negative protein rations. The greater incidence observed in lactating mares may relate to nutritional stress from the nutrient drain of lactation or to incomplete uterine endometrial involution following parturition.

Chromosomal abnormalities are associated with at least one third of early conceptus losses in the human. The difficulty in obtaining embryonic tissue and the limited number of equine cytogenetic laboratories have delayed demonstration of this phenomenon in the horse. Other causes of embryonic deaths suggested include progesterone deficiency (p. 405), hormonal imbalance, immunologic rejection, toxins, drugs, and bacterial or viral agents. These generally lack diagnostic evidence, though iatrogenic administration of luteolytic drugs or ingestion of estrogenic toxins could result in loss.

FETAL ABORTION

The fetal abortion rate in mares is 4 to 14 per cent, with the higher incidence in mares over 15 years of age and in mares bred in "foal heat." Fetal abortions can be early, generally occurring prior to six months' gestation, or late, occurring from six months to term. This separation is based on the premise that equine fetuses less than five to seven months' gestational age are usually aborted in an autolytic state because they lack the maturity to respond to the abortive agent. Death is often sudden, and the fetus remains in utero and becomes autolysed prior to abortion. In this autolysed state, a generalized bacterial invasion can often result; thus, a bacterial etiology is often attached to early fetal losses.

Equine fetuses approximately six months' gestational age and older have developed a degree of hypothalamic-pituitary-adrenal maturity as well as immunologic abilities. Thus, when these older fetuses are challenged by an abortive agent, they respond with stress hormones and some immune responses. Such responses often elicit a rapid relaxation of the cervix and uterine contractions, resulting in the fetus being expelled fresh or only slightly autolysed.

SUBMISSION OF SPECIMENS FOR DIAGNOSIS

Only 40 to 65 per cent of abortions are currently diagnosed with available laboratory facilities. To improve these percentages, coordination and cooperation between owners, practitioners, and diagnostic laboratories are needed.

Practitioners should establish a protocol to follow with each abortion. This protocol should be arranged with the diagnostic laboratory so that proper transport methods, tissue preservatives, and selected culture media are readily available when the need occurs.

Most diagnostic laboratories prefer that the complete fetus and its placenta be submitted with minimal delay in a chilled, not frozen, condition. The submission of the placenta is of prime importance, since placental lesions are associated with approximately 30 to 40 per cent of abortions.

Should delivery of the entire fetus to the laboratory be impossible, it is advisable to collect selected organ tissue specimens in a sterile manner and to individually package these in sterile containers. Such packaging avoids cross-contamination for microbiologic and immunofluorescent staining procedures.

Similar tissues should be obtained for histopathologic examination. Sections of placental tissue should also be included for histopathologic examination. Tissues should be sectioned in 5 mm thick specimens, with sections extending across the boundary zone to include normal and abnormal tissue. Adequate volumes of fixative are required. Each diagnostic laboratory usually has a protocol of the tissue specimens it prefers.

NONINFECTIOUS EQUINE ABORTIONS

TWINNING

Twinning accounts for 20 to 30 per cent of all diagnosed abortions. Twin losses may occur throughout gestation but primarily as twin fetal abortions during the eighth to tenth month of gestation. In mares conceiving twins, approximately 65 to 75 per cent abort, and only about 15 per cent deliver both twins alive. Of these, nearly half of the foals die soon after birth.[6] The breed incidence of twin abortions is as follows: Thoroughbreds, 1 to 5 per cent; draft horses, 0.2 to 3.2 per cent; Arabians, 0.2 to 0.5 per cent; and pony breeds, rarely.

The general picture of twin abortions is that of a mare in late gestation that has premature mammary development followed by abortion. One twin is usually small with some autolysis, while the larger twin is emaciated but in a fresh condition.

Examination of the placentae of twin abortions reveals an area of avillous contact between the two chorionic surfaces. Should the mare be on pasture and only a single placenta found, with only one fetus or even no fetus recovered, the diagnosis could subjectively be made by the presence of a well-demarcated avillous chorionic surface area free of infectious lesions.

Twin abortion is associated with placental insufficiency due to the lack of adequate chorionic attachment to the uterine endometrium. Immunologic rejection between the two fetuses has also been proposed as an etiology of twin deaths.[15] Support for this is derived from the presence of plasma cells in tissue bridges where the two chorions contact.

Two approaches have been utilized to decrease the losses associated with twin abortions: prevention and elimination. Prevention of twin conceptions is based on the knowledge that nearly all equine twins are dizygotic, arising from two separate ovulations.

Prevention of Twin Conceptions

1. Avoid breeding the mare when two mature follicles are present as determined by rectal palpation or ultrasound scanning of the ovaries.

2. Delay breeding the mare until 12 to 24 hours after one follicle has ovulated but before the second mature follicle ovulates. This protocol is based on the assumption that an ovum from the first follicle has a fertilizable life span of only 6 to 12 hours.

3. Aspirate one follicle with a needle in an attempt to prevent its ovulation, then breed to fertilize the remaining mature follicle.

4. Surgically occlude one oviduct, with the assumption that a follicle will form on each ovary. This assumption is correct only 50 to 60 per cent of the time.

This author does not agree with the surgical removal of one ovary in an attempt to prevent double ovulations. If only one ovary remains, it will then produce two follicles with the same regularity as occurred when two ovaries were present. The sensitivity to hypothalamic-pituitary hormones, not the presence of two ovaries, appears to control the number of follicles produced.

Elimination of Twin Conceptuses

Therapy to eliminate twin conceptions is based on early diagnosis. Twin pregnancies can be diagnosed by rectal examination at 25 to 45 days or by ultrasound scanning of the uterus per rectum at 18 to 23 days. Should the twin pregnancy advance beyond 50 to 60 days, it becomes progressively more difficult to distinguish the two separate chorionic vesicles.

Methods to eliminate twin conceptions include the following.

1. Abortion of both twins using prostaglandins or intrauterine irrigation. If an attempt is to be made at rebreeding during the same season, abortion should be performed prior to 35 days before endometrial cups form and PMSG is produced.

2. Needle aspiration of one of the twin embryonic vesicles via a vaginopericervical approach. Success has been minimal for this author.

3. Attempting the manual crushing of one of the twin embryonic vesicles per rectum. This is rarely successful without loss of both embryos.

4. Repeated regular massage and gentle movement of one twin embryonic vesicle to disrupt its endometrial contact. R. Pascoe of Australia has reported success with this technique.[12]

5. Severely limiting the nutritional supply to the mare that has twin embryonic vesicles. H. Merkt[10] of West Germany reports approximately a 60 per cent success rate in resorption of one twin embryo, but occasionally both embryos are resorbed.

With the manipulative techniques, various dosages of antiprostaglandin drugs and/or exogenous progesterone have been used. There is no evidence these drugs are beneficial.[12]

ANOMALIES

Anomalies are responsible for 2 to 10 per cent of diagnosed fetal abortions. The majority of anomalies result in abortion between 6 and 10 months of gestation and can be classified as placental, umbilical cord, or fetal anomalies.

Placental Anomalies

Placental anomalies associated with abortion include body pregnancies, hydroallantois, chorionic surface deficiencies, and premature chorioallantois separation. Body pregnancy is rare. The conceptus develops within the body of the uterus, and the placenta fails to extend into the uterine horns. The placental chorionic horns are underdeveloped with obliteration of their lumens and deep irregular folds on their surface. The fetus eventually dies and has the retarded growth and emaciation associated with placental insufficiency. Body pregnancies do not generally recur. Some practitioners have suggested initiating early abortion when the initial pregnancy examination indicates that the embryo is located in the body of the uterus. The validity of rectal diagnosis of body pregnancy is dubious. Possibly with the advent of ultrasound scanning techniques, such developmental anomalies could be verified.

Hydroallantois is also rare. Signs include rapid distention of the abdomen over a two-week interval during the sixth to tenth month of gestation. This abdominal distention is the result of an increased quantity of allantoic fluid, often associated with vascular anomalies of the allantois. The abdominal distention can result in dyspnea and difficult locomotion. Approximately half of the mares spontaneously abort. The remaining mares are examined for the dyspnea and discomfort signs. On rectal examination, a large, fluid-distended uterus is noted, but the fetus is generally not ballotted. Rupture of the chorioallantois through a manually dilated cervix releases the allantoic fluid and initiates abortion. With the rapid loss of fluid from the uterus, systemic shock may occur, requiring fluid administration and corticosteroids. The abortion may require manual extraction of the fetus because the uterus is often refractile to oxytocic drugs.

Chorionic surface deficiencies of the placenta result in a lack of placental chorionic villi. Surface deficiencies include chorionic hypoplasia or atrophy and large chorioallantoic cysts or similar space-occupying lesions of the chorion. These are very rare conditions resulting in placental insufficiency signs and abortion in late gestation.

Premature chorioallantoic separation occurs at parturition. As the mare enters the second stage of labor, the chorioallantois fails to rupture at the cervical star, and a bulging, red, villus-surfaced chorion is presented at the vulva. Treatment requires immediate diagnosis and manual rupture of the chorioallantois if the fetus is to be born alive without anoxic damage. The cause of the unyielding cervical star is not known, but the incidence of premature separation of the placenta is much greater with hormonally induced parturition.

Umbilical Cord Anomalies

Umbilical cord anomalies resulting in fetal abortion are primarily torsion and premature rupture of the cord. Torsion has been overdiagnosed in the past owing to the normal twists present in the equine umbilical cord. Signs of vascular obstruction are essential for the diagnosis of umbilical cord torsion. Cords with torsion are usually excessively long (greater than 80 cm) and tightly twisted, obstruction being associated with edema and hemorrhage into the cord vessel walls. Alternate dilation and constrictions in both the urachus and vessels occur. The fetus is generally somewhat autolysed when aborted at six to eight months of gestation.

Premature rupture of the umbilical cord usually occurs during parturition. These umbilical cords are usually short (less than 35 cm) and rupture prematurely near the abdomen, causing blood to pool within the amniotic cavity.

Urachal cysts, allantoic cysts, and calcified cysts on the umbilical cord are remnants of the early yolk sac placentation and should not be incriminated as a cause of fetal loss unless they are associated with vascular obstruction.

Fetal Developmental Anomalies

Fetal developmental anomalies may result in abortion from three months' gestation to term. The contracted foal syndrome may occur with as great as 3 to 4 per cent of diagnosed equine abortions. These fetuses have contracted forelimbs and occasionally torticollis, scoliosis, and/or skull deformities. There has been a suggestion of an increasing incidence of this diagnosis in Kentucky over the past decade related to an increased use of drugs in pregnant mares. There is no research to support this suggestion.

Other fetal anomalies, such as hydrocephalus and schistosomus reflexus, occur rarely. The etiology of these gross anatomic deformities is unknown, but most are not considered genetic.

HORMONAL IMBALANCE AND STRESS

Hormonal imbalance or stress as a cause of embryonic or fetal loss has probably been overemphasized. Progesterone deficiency, PMSG deficiency, estrogen excess or deficiency, glucocorticoid excess (stress), and thyroxin deficiency have all been incriminated as causing abortion.

Progesterone deficiency has received much attention as a cause of conceptus loss and is discussed elsewhere (p. 405).

Estrogens increase rapidly in the mare's system after approximately 60 to 90 days of gestation owing to production from the fetal-placental unit. Insufficient estrogens have been suggested as a cause of fetal abortion, and stilbestrol was recommended for abortion prevention. Studies have since indicated that stilbestrol does not aid in pregnancy maintenance and that implants of 50 mg of stilbestrol can cause abortion.

Prolonged periods of stress during the last few months of gestation have been associated with abortion in mares. Severe laminitis, chronic peritoneal pain, and chronic obstructive pulmonary disease have all been recorded as etiologies of stress-induced abortions. The therapy for these conditions may include prolonged corticosteroid therapy, which may contribute to factors initiating the abortion.

Two forms of therapy appear to aid in helping to prevent some late term "stress-induced" abortions. One is antiprostaglandin therapy in the form of phenylbutazone, flunixin meglumine,* or meclofenamic acid.† Prostaglandins increase in association with uterine contraction and cervical relaxation, so therapy to suppress these effects may prevent expulsion of the fetus. The second line of therapy is progesterone administration if the mare is in her last month of gestation. This therapy is suggested only to simulate the normal increase in progesterone seen in the mare's serum during the last month of gestation.

The suggestion that decreased thyroid hormone levels may be associated with abortion is difficult to justify based on experiments demonstrating that thyroidectomized mares can conceive and deliver normal foals.

NUTRITIONAL, TOXIC, AND DRUG-RELATED CAUSES OF ABORTION

With undiagnosed late gestation abortions, nutritional deficiencies and ingestion of toxic agents or therapeutic agents are often considered as causes. Low energy intake and negative protein balance may cause maternal weight loss and may be involved with stress-related abortion. Selenium deficiencies have been suggested to cause early embryonic deaths and abortion, but definitive evidence is lacking. Blood selenium levels should be determined in suspected cases, but it is the author's experience that other mares on the same farms with similar low blood selenium levels will foal normally. Selenium may be given by injection of vitamin E and selenium,‡ 25 mg selenium and 680 IU vitamin E every two weeks, or by providing oral supplementation,§

1 mg selenium and 200 IU vitamin E daily. Selenium toxicosis is possible with oversupplementation.

Iodide deficiency can cause term gestation abortions of goitrous foals that have poor muscular development, long hair, and occasionally contracted tendons. The condition is no longer reported with present diets. Therapy would include the feeding of iodized salt or sodium iodide. Application of tincture of iodine to the skin also results in rapid absorption of iodide.

Iodide excess in the diet has been reported as a cause of congenital goiters in foals from mares on diets of dried seaweed (kelp) or mixed concentrates containing high iodides. These mares have occasionally aborted goitrous fetuses in late gestation.

Late gestation abortions have been reported in the central eastern United States associated with abnormally thick placentae, agalactia, and occasionally prolonged gestation. The University of Missouri has related these problems to fescue pastures. Mycotoxins that are related to fescue abortions in cattle have not been identified, but selenium deficiency on these pastures is suspected. It is recommended that mares be removed from fescue pasture 60 days before foaling or that a good-quality alfalfa hay be provided on pasture to decrease fescue intake.

Pastures have also been related to unidentified abortions occurring during the spring months in central Kentucky. These abortions occur between two and four months of gestation, and a 5 to 12 per cent incidence has occurred on affected farms. Abortions have occurred in late May and early June with a relation to only certain pastures. One considered etiology is a toxicosis related to climatic changes affecting certain plants on the pastures. An opposing etiologic viewpoint is that mares bred during the early breeding season have a greater incidence of estrous signs occurring during pregnancy, which can cause cervical relaxation and an ascending bacterial placental infection resulting in abortions. The recommendation at present is to avoid putting mares on pastures that have been incriminated in previous abortions.

Administration of corticosteroids, estrogens, prostaglandins, and oxytocin can cause abortion. Anthelmintics such as organophosphates, carbon tetrachloride, and phenothiazines have also been incriminated in abortions. Avoiding use of these anthelmintics during late gestation is recommended.

INFECTIOUS ABORTION

Infectious equine abortion can be divided into bacterial, mycotic, or viral etiologies. There is insufficient evidence to incriminate protozoal and mycoplasma organisms as causing equine abortion other than through maternal stress.

---

*Banamine, Schering Corp., Kenilworth, NJ 07033
†Arquel, Parke-Davis Co., Detroit, MI 48232
‡E-Se, Burns-Biotec, Omaha, NB 68127
§Vit. E plus Selenium, Vita Vet Lab, Marion, IN 46952

BACTERIAL CAUSES OF ABORTION

Bacterial etiologies are associated with 7 to 13 per cent of diagnosed equine abortions. Bacteria enter the fetal-placental unit either via hematogenous spread from systemic infection or by ascending the vagina and cervical canal to cause a chorionitis.

Ascending placentitis can be caused by *Streptococcus zooepidemicus, Escherichia coli, Pseudomonas aeruginosa, Staphylococcus aureus, Klebsiella pneumoniae*, and other, rarely reported bacteria. The majority of these abortions are reported during the fifth to tenth month of gestation, with placental lesions observed. Bacteria have also been incriminated in early gestation abortions based only on bacterial isolation from uterine cultures after the abortion. This is indirect evidence at best.

Lesions in ascending placentitis include a thickened, edematous placenta with a tenacious tan-brown exudate over the affected chorionic surface. The diseased portion spreads from the cervical star of the allantochorion and ascends forward onto the body of the placenta. A distinct, well-demarcated line often separates the normal velvety chorionic villi from the tenacious exudative surface. Factors predisposing mares to ascending placentitis can be pneumovagina and damage to the mucosal surface of the cervical canal.

Therapeutic measures involve episioplasty (Caslick operation) in mares with defective vulva closure and cervical canal repair if required (p. 409). The use of artificial insemination or semen extenders containing antibiotics can aid in preventing bacterial contamination at the time of breeding (p. 453).

Bacterial abortion from hematogenous infection has occurred infrequently since the eradication of *Salmonella abortus equi*. Most reported cases now involve mares with severe or prolonged systemic infections.

Corynebacterium pseudotuberculosis has resulted in 6 to 10 months' gestation abortions in mares previously undergoing prolonged treatment for multiple abscesses caused by this organism. Often no lesions occur in the placenta, but the fetus may have abscesses in its liver, lungs, kidneys, and other organs.

Systemic *Streptococcus zooepidemicus* or *Escherichia coli* infections in mares can result in abortion during late gestation. The placentae of these infected mares may have a multifocal chorionitis over the entire surface. The fetus is usually in a fresh state with stress findings.

Leptospira pomona has been reported to cause 8 to 10 months' gestation abortions. The organism enters the uterus approximately one to three weeks after systemic illness in the mare. The fetus is usually autolysed, and efforts to demonstrate the organism by culture or fluorescent antibody staining are often unsuccessful. Rising antibody titers and blood inoculation tests have been used in some diagnoses. No treatment or vaccinations have been used owing to the rarity of Leptospira abortion.

Salmonella abortus equi has been extinct from the United States since 1932. In the early 1900s, it was associated with 5 to 10 months' gestation abortion with a 10 to 90 per cent incidence in reported outbreaks. The organism was ingested in contaminated feed or water and entered the pregnant uterus via the hematogenous route. After a 14- to 28-day incubation period, the fetus was aborted in an autolysed condition with an edematous, necrotic, and hemorrhagic placenta. Diagnosis was based on culture of the organism. A bacterin administered at four and nine months of gestation aided in eliminating the disease.

MYCOTIC CAUSES OF ABORTION

Fungal organisms are responsible for 3 to 10 per cent of diagnosed equine abortions. Abortions are sporadic and can occur between 5 and 10 months of gestation, with the later gestational stages most common. *Aspergillus fumigatus* is the most commonly identified organism, followed by Mucor sp and rarely *Absidia corymbifera* and *Allescheria boydii*.

Mycotic abortions are generally due to an ascending placentitis with the predisposing factors described earlier. The lesions of a bacterial and mycotic chorioplacentitis cannot be differentiated grossly, though mycotic placentitis may occasionally be a drier leather-textured chorionitis. Diagnosis of mycotic abortion is derived from impression smears or histologic examination of the chorion demonstrating the hyphae. Cultures verify the specific organism.

Prevention involves decreasing vaginal-cervical exposure to fungi by utilizing an episioplasty. Therapy after a mycotic abortion is generally not required. These mares generally rebreed without problem.

VIRAL CAUSES OF ABORTION

Viruses are responsible for 3 to 15 per cent of equine abortions. Equine herpesvirus 1 represents the majority of these diagnoses.

EQUINE HERPESVIRUS 1

Equine herpesvirus 1 (EHV-1) infection is also called rhinopneumonitis because of the respiratory syndrome occurring in young horses with this virus. Abortions due to EHV-1 have been diagnosed between four months' gestation and term, with the majority occurring between 8 and 10 months. The abortions are sporadic, with 1 to 90 per cent of the mares losing their fetuses.

Abortions generally occur one to four months after an outbreak of EHV-1 respiratory disease in the weanlings on the farm. Usually there are no impending signs of abortion, and the mare rapidly expels the fetus and its membrane without signs of maternal illness. Fetuses aborted after the seventh month of gestation are generally in a fresh condition and may be contained within intact placental membranes. Fetuses aborted prior to six months' gestation may be autolysed, and it may be extremely difficult to identify a viral etiology. Doll et al.[3] reported causing abortions in mares exposed to the virus at 70 to 80 days of gestation, so early abortions of EHV-1 etiology should not be excluded from consideration. Equine herpesvirus 1 abortions do not generally affect later fertility.

The majority of EHV-1 abortions result in a fresh fetus that may be slightly jaundiced and have petechiation of mucous membranes, subcutaneous edema, excessive pleural-peritoneal fluid, pulmonary edema, and spleen enlargement. A more definitive sign is the presence of pinpoint white foci on the liver surface, indicative of necrotic sites. These signs are variable and may be present in only 25 per cent of the cases.

Histopathologic lesions identified in EHV-1 aborted fetuses include bronchitis, pneumonitis, necrosis of splenic lymphoid follicles, and focal liver necrosis. The presence of intranuclear inclusion bodies in hepatic, adrenal cortex, bronchiole, and/or splenic cells is considered pathognomonic of EHV-1. Immunofluorescent staining of the viral antigen and/or viral isolation represent a positive diagnosis.

Vaccines for EHV-1 are available, but the level of immune protection against abortion is frequently questioned. Antibody titers to EHV-1 are short-lived with both natural exposure and vaccination. These titers remain elevated only three to four months after a challenge.[11] Much of the poor response from vaccines can be related directly to the failure to maintain a three- to four-month revaccination schedule.

Presently two EHV-1 vaccines are commercially available: Rhinomune* and Pneumabort-K.† Rhinomune is an attenuated live virus vaccine marketed only for the prevention of respiratory EHV-1. Prior to 1977 it was marketed for EHV-1 abortion protection also, but this recommendation was removed when reports of EHV-1 abortions occurred after immunization.[4] Evaluation of one report[4] reveals that mares were last vaccinated three to five months

prior to abortion and that stress may have been involved. The manufacturer was recommending vaccination only every six months with Rhinomune, so it is quite possible that the vaccine failed to produce immunity of sufficient duration. Protection may have been sufficient if the vaccine had been utilized every three months. From personal experience, this author has successfully utilized the Rhinomune vaccine given at two, five, and eight months of gestation in over 400 mares when a positive diagnosis of EHV-1 respiratory infection occurred in weanlings on the same farms. Maintenance of a serum neutralization titer greater than 1:64 appears to protect mares from natural EHV-1 exposure.[11]

Pneumabort-K is a killed EHV-1 vaccine marketed since 1979 for the prevention of both respiratory and abortion forms of the disease. Protection against abortion appears good and may be related to the manufacturer's recommendation to administer the vaccine on a bimonthly schedule between the fifth and ninth months of pregnancy.

It is the author's opinion that mares should also be vaccinated during early gestation. Owing to the difficulty in observing early abortions, let alone identifying an etiologic agent from an autolytic fetus, it is quite possible that EHV-1 could cause early fetal loss as noted in the few mares that Doll et al.[3] experimentally exposed to the virus at 70 to 80 days of gestation.

Diagnosed cases of EHV-1 abortions in Kentucky have decreased from approximately 25 per cent in the 1950s to near 10 per cent in the 1970s. Bryans[2] related this decreased incidence in Kentucky to the increased use of EHV-1 vaccines.

Equine herpesvirus-1 has also been implicated as a cause of posterior paresis in horses. The paresis generally occurs approximately one week after mild respiratory signs of the disease. This neurologic form of the disease appears to be related to an intense immune response following exposure to EHV-1.

EQUINE VIRAL ARTERITIS

Equine viral arteritis (EVA) has been associated with abortions between 5 and 10 months of gestation. In the 1950s it occurred with a 1 to 80 per cent incidence on certain eastern United States farms but currently is of rare occurrence as an abortive agent. Reasons for the near extinction of abortive forms of this disease are unknown.

Equine viral arteritis is characterized by an incubation period of 2 to 10 days before horses show systemic illness. Signs of the disease include depression, fever, leukopenia, keratitis, palpebral edema, lacrimation, photophobia, and edematous swelling of the extremities and ventral abdomen. Histopathologically, these lesions are the result of necrosis of the media of small arteries.

---

*Rhinomune, Norden Labs, Lincoln NB 68521
†Pneumabort-K, Ft. Dodge Labs, Ft. Dodge, IA 50501

After the onset of illness, mares can abort in 1 to 14 days. The aborted fetuses are generally autolysed, and diagnosis is made by immunofluorescent antigen staining and viral isolation of fetal tissues. Recovered horses tend to have prolonged immunity to reinfection.

Serologic titers of the equine population indicate that the virus is still present, but the abortigenic form of the disease has nearly disappeared. The Standardbred breed tends to maintain a greater incidence of EVA titers for unknown reasons. A vaccine has been developed but is not utilized owing to the low incidence of disease.

OTHER VIRUSES

The equine infectious anemia (EIA) virus may cause abortion in the last half of gestation, but at a very low incidence. Kemen and Coggins[7] have demonstrated in utero transmission of EIA virus to the fetus in one of 52 pregnant mares seropositive to EIA. This mare had lost weight for several months prior to aborting an eight-month-old live fetus. Diagnosis of transmission was made by inoculating a susceptible pony with a spleen emulsion from the fetus. The mare may have aborted from the stress of illness, or the viral infection in the fetus may have caused the foal to initiate its own stress-related delivery. Foals of seropositive mares generally are born seronegative but can become infected by colostral or milk transmission of the virus.

The equine influenza viruses have not been shown to cause abortions. It is possible that severe stress and associated secondary bacterial infections may lead to abortion. The equine herpesvirus-3, which causes equine coital exanthema with formation of vesicular and ulcerative lesions on the external genitalia of stallions and mares, has no reported abortigenic effects.

References

1. Allen, W. R.: Hormonal control of early pregnancy in the mare. Vet. Clin. North Am. (Large Anim. Pract.), 2:291, 1980.
2. Bryans, J. T.: Application of management procedures and prophylactic immunization to the control of equine rhinopneumonitis. Proc. Am. Assoc. Eq. Pract., 26th Annu. Conv. 1980, p. 259.
3. Doll, E. R., Crowe, M. E. W., Bryans, J. T., and McCollum, W. H.: Infection immunity in equine virus abortion. Cornell Vet., 45:387, 1955.
4. Eaglesome, M. D., Mitchell, D., and Henry, J. N. R.: Control and prevention of equine herpesvirus 1 abortion. J. Reprod. Fertil. Suppl., 27:607, 1979.
5. Hawkins, D. L., Neely, D. P., and Stabenfeldt, G. H.: Plasma progesterone concentrations derived from the administration of exogenous progesterone to ovariectomized mares. J. Reprod. Fertil. Suppl., 27:211, 1979.
6. Jeffcott, L. B., and Whitwell, K. E.: Twinning as a cause of foetal and neonatal loss in the Thoroughbred mare. J. Comp. Pathol., 83:91, 1973.
7. Kemen, M. J., and Coggins, L.: Equine infectious anemia: Transmission from infected mares to foals. J. Am. Vet. Med. Assoc., 161:496, 1972.
8. Kenny, R. M.: Cyclic and pathological changes of the mare endometrium as detected by biopsy with a note on early embryonic death. J. Am. Vet. Med. Assoc., 172:241, 1978.
9. Mahaffey, L. W.: Abortion in mares. Vet. Rec., 82:681, 1968.
10. Merkt, H., and Günzel, A. R.: A survey of early pregnancy losses in West German Thoroughbred mares. Equine Vet. J., 11:256, 1979.
11. Neely, D. P., and Hawkins, D. L.: A two-year study of the clinical and serologic responses of horses to a modified live-virus equine rhinopneumonitis vaccine. J. Equine Med. Surg., 2:532, 1978.
12. Pascoe, R. R.: A possible new treatment for twin pregnancy in the mare. Equine Vet. J., 11:64, 1979.
13. Platt, H.: Aetiological aspects of abortion in the Thoroughbred mare. J. Comp. Pathol., 83:199, 1973.
14. Prickett, M. E.: Abortion and placental lesions in the mare. J. Am. Vet. Med. Assoc., 157:1465, 1970.
15. Whitwell, K. E.: Investigations into fetal and neonatal losses in the horse. Vet. Clin. North Am. (Large Anim. Pract.), 2:313, 1980.

OBSTETRICS

Maarten Drost, GAINESVILLE, FLORIDA
A. C. Asbury, GAINESVILLE, FLORIDA

NORMAL PARTURITION

The length of gestation in the mare is extremely variable and may range all the way from 305 to 365 days and still be considered normal. The mare has some degree of voluntary control over the time of onset of parturition and has been known to delay the onset for a number of days as she waits for an undisturbed time, generally during the quiet hours of the night.

The fetus is an active participant in the birth process, as it rotates from a dorsopubic to a dorsosacral position during the last 24 hours of gestation. Signs of impending parturition are not obvious in the mare. Relaxation of the pelvic ligaments may be obscured by the well-developed croup muscles. Vulvar changes are limited to a lengthening of the labia. The flank region will appear sunken in. The udder of the mare, which has gradually become distended over a period of several days, will show some dried precolostral secretions (waxing) at the ends of the teats 24 to 48 hours prepartum.

During the first stage of labor, the mare will be restless, will walk around with a raised tail, and will urinate frequent small amounts. She will show signs of colic as she alternately lies down and gets up, while slight sweating becomes noticeable in the flank region and behind the elbows. It takes approximately two hours for the cervix to completely dilate and to become effaced.

The second stage of parturition is normally heralded by rupture of the chorioallantois. This is the stage of true labor, and it is rapid and forceful. The fetus may be expelled in less than five minutes, but on the average it requires 20 minutes. If not completed in 40 minutes, complications may have arisen, and a clinical examination of the fetus and the birth canal is indicated.

The third and final stage is that of delivery of the placenta and involution of the uterus. The fetal membranes are expelled 15 to 90 minutes after the birth of the foal, and the uterus frequently returns to its normal nongravid dimension in 10 to 14 days.

RESTRAINT AND EXAMINATION OF THE MARE IN LABOR

Examination of parturient mares must be made in a manner that offers maximal safety to both the examiner and the mare. While the ideal location for foaling may be a clean, grassy field, most mares are presented to the veterinarian in a box stall. The use of the door frame as partial protection for the examiner is common practice, but in fact mares may be more relaxed and the examiner may be provided more flexibility if the examination is made in the center of the stall. Stocks should be avoided for obstetrical procedures, as rapid changes of position by the mare may injure her and the operator.

Some restraint is advisable in all cases. Even the most placid mare may become excited and dangerous during parturition. A twitch or lip chain will often suffice. A sideline, applied on the side most suitable to the veterinarian, will restrict kicking and still allow a four-point stance.

Chemical sedation of the mare may be indicated, but drugs that might depress the fetus should be used with discretion. Light sedation with acepromazine (5 to 6 mg per 100 kg intravenously) has a minimal effect on the foal. Chloral hydrate in sedative doses (7 to 10 gm intravenously) has been found useful in relaxing anxious mares. Xylazine

alone is a poor choice to sedate the parturient mare, as some individuals become hypersensitive in the rear quarters following its administration.

When the disposition of the dam or the difficulty of the procedure indicates, short-term general anesthesia is helpful. Xylazine (1 mg per kg intravenously) followed by ketamine (2 mg per kg intravenously) after full xylazine effect provides an ideal restraint for rapid procedures. Muscular relaxation and analgesia persist for 10 to 12 minutes, enough for a careful examination and some corrective manipulation.

An alternative and longer general anesthetic approach is achieved with glyceryl guaiacolate (1 l, 5 per cent, in 5 per cent dextrose) with a thiobarbiturate (thiamylal sodium, 1 to 2 gm) administered rapidly intravenously. The barbiturates should be used only when the foal is dead.

When an apparently serious dystocia or major obstetrical procedure is anticipated, induction, intubation, and inhalation anesthesia should be used. The degree of muscular relaxation provided by halothane is often enough to permit vaginal delivery that is otherwise impossible. Should vaginal delivery fail, the mare is properly anesthetized for cesarean section, which may be resorted to without further delay.

The keys to successful obstetrical examination are cleanliness and ample lubrication. Prior to the genital examination the tail should be wrapped and the perineal area thoroughly scrubbed with a nonirritating surgical scrub (povidone scrub). Repeated cleansing during the procedures is usually necessitated by frequent defecation. The operator's hands and arms should be scrubbed meticulously. Lubrication should be ample and constantly renewed. Petrolatum is an excellent obstetrical lubricant. Sterile methylcellulose preparations are adequate but need more frequent replenishment. Soaps and particularly detergents are poor lubricants, as they defat the tissues and actually reduce lubrication.

The examination itself should be rapid but thorough, determining presentation, position, and posture of the fetus. In addition, the size and viability of the fetus are determined as well as the degree of freshness of the tissues and the adequacy of pelvic size. Never overlook the possibility of more than one fetus.

The expulsive efforts of the mare are induced by the introduction of the arms in the birth canal and may be so forceful as to necessitate more drastic restraint and relaxation.

CAUSES OF DYSTOCIA

Postural abnormalities are the most common fetal cause of dystocia. Ninety-nine per cent of the foals are delivered in an anterior longitudinal presentation. Left lateral retention of the head and, less frequently, ventral retention of the head between the forelimbs are more likely to occur when the foal fails to participate in its delivery because it is weak or dead. For the same reasons, one or both forelimbs may be retained at the carpus. When the foal is in posterior presentation, the hindlimbs may be retained at the hocks or at the hips (true breech). Transverse presentations are extremely rare, as are monsters, and these foals are best delivered by cesarean section. An exception is the hydrocephalic foal in which the soft skull may be collapsed with the aid of a guarded knife or the fetotome. The absolute oversized fetus also occurs rarely and is again best delivered by cesarean section. As in other species, it does not always follow that a longer gestation period results in a larger foal.

Of the maternal causes of dystocia, the tight vestibulovaginal sphincter, particularly of the primiparous mare, may delay parturition and predisposes to lacerations and rectovaginal tears. The small vulva or the vulvar opening that has been reduced by a Caslick operation may further stagnate the delivery process. Torsion of the uterus can be an insidious cause of dystocia. Reduction of the diameter of the birth canal may be the result of previous trauma such as old healed pelvic fractures, sacroiliac luxation, tumors, or hematomas. Premature separation of the chorioallantois constitutes a very serious cause of dystocia. While the foal is threatened by hypoxia, the presence of the membranes themselves diminishes the diameter of the birth canal.

OBSTETRICAL PROCEDURES

MUTATION

The success of mutation, or correction of abnormalities of presentation, position, and posture, is dependent on restraint, lubrication, and room to maneuver. Repulsion of the fetus to gain room is best accomplished manually. Instruments for repulsion, such as rods and crutches, easily inflict damage because of rigidity and are not recommended. The reproductive efficiency of mares is greatly reduced by trauma during parturition.

Postural corrections, as in returning a retained forelimb to its normal posture, may require both arms in the birth canal, one to repel and one to correct. The fetal foot should be cupped in the hand to protect the birth canal during the correction.

Mutation of a laterally deviated head can be extremely taxing owing to the length of the foal's neck. An obstetrical chain over the poll and through the mouth may be of value; blunt eye hooks are helpful in some cases. Repulsion is an essential portion of this type of mutation.

EXTRACTION

Once the fetus is aligned, traction should be applied by no more than two adults. Efforts should be in synchrony with the expulsive efforts of the mare. Obstetrical chains should be placed around the pastern only, with the eye on the dorsal aspect of the limb. Fetal extractors are contraindicated for equine obstetrics.

Rotation of the foal is not helpful because the pelvic canal has a circular cross-section. Should a hip-lock be encountered, it may be overcome by placing a halter on the foal and applying traction along the spinal column instead of along the forelimbs.

PARTIAL FETOTOMY

In cases in which vaginal delivery of a dead foal is prevented by a simple postural abnormality, a partial fetotomy, limited to one or two cuts, may be indicated. Since the vaginal and cervical mucosa of the mare is highly sensitive to prolonged or traumatic procedures, partial fetotomy must be undertaken carefully and quickly.

Relaxation, ample lubrication, and excellent instrumentation are all key ingredients for this procedure. Removal of one limb or a head should be the extent of the operation. Extreme care should be taken to protect the mucosa when placing wires and fetotomes. Epidural anesthesia is helpful.

The sequelae to any protracted obstetrical manipulation, including fetotomy, are multiple and irreversible adhesions of the cervix or vagina or both. These often are equated with sterility in future years. Total fetotomy is contraindicated in equine obstetrics.

CESAREAN SECTION

If the initial examination indicates or if preliminary obstetrical procedures are unrewarding, the decision to perform a cesarean section should be made promptly. Modern inhalation anesthesia and improved surgical techniques have made this procedure a logical alternative. Much is gained by proceeding without delay.

As long as the foal is alive, induction should be made without barbiturates. Glyceryl guaiacolate alone or the xylazine-ketamine combination will allow for intubation. The general anesthetic agent of choice is halothane.

After anesthetizing the mare and while preparation of the surgical site is in progress, one last valiant attempt at vaginal delivery should be made.

The surgical approach is either via the midline or the lower left flank. Midline incision is preferred when gross uterine contamination is present, owing to better chances of exteriorization of the uterus. After removal of the fetus, the placenta should be dissected back from the wound edges to prevent its accidental inclusion in the uterine suture line. The placenta should be left in the uterine lumen.

Postpartum care of the mare should include regular rectal palpation of the uterus to detect and reduce any adhesions as they form. This process should begin within a day or two following surgery. Prognosis for future productivity of the mare is excellent in cases attended to promptly and in which peritonitis is controlled.

When elective cesarean section is contemplated owing to known problems, such as pelvic abnormalities, particular attention must be paid to fetal maturity. The same criteria as those for induction of labor apply (p. 438). The safest approach, when supervision is adequate, is to actually allow the mare to begin labor before starting the surgery. Fetal viability is optimal when all the maturation processes are complete.

Supplemental Readings

1. Richter, J. and Götze, R.: Tiergeburtshilfe, 3rd. ed. Berlin, Verlag Paul Parey, 1980.
2. Roberts, S. J.: Veterinary Obstetrics and Genital Diseases, 2nd ed. Ithaca, NY, published by author, 1971.
3. Vandeplassche, M.: Obstetrician's view of the physiology of equine parturition and dystocia. Equine Vet. J, *12*:45, 1980.

RETAINED PLACENTA

J. Pierre Held, KNOXVILLE, TENNESSEE

A review of equine placentation is helpful in understanding the physiologic process involved in the normal expulsion of fetal membranes and in the etiology of retained placenta. Placentation in the mare is epitheliochorial, which means that the fetal membranes do not invade the uterine tissue, except in the endometrial cup area, where trophoblast cells break through the uterine epithelium.[3] The fully developed organ of nutrient exchange, the microcotyledon, is an interdigitation of chorionic and endometrial epithelium. After the microcotyledons are fully formed (approximately 150 days), the placental barrier is confined to the villi and crypts of the microplacentomes. Several areas of the chorion are devoid of villi.[5] These are (1) the cervical star, located at the internal os of the cervix; during parturition the allantochorion breaks at this location; (2) the tip of both horns opposite the fallopian tube opening; (3) the endometrial cup site; and (4) invaginated placental folds; these folds usually occur over major allantoic vessels. At most of the avillous spots, glandular secretions accumulate between the chorion and endometrial epithelium.

Retained placenta has long been thought to be due to placental edema, preventing normal release of the membranes. This belief led to the rule of thumb that any placenta weighing more than 6.3 kg (14 lbs) had some degree of pathology. In a study involving over 200 normal foalings,[5] it has been shown, however, that the normal weight for an equine Thoroughbred placenta varies between 4 and 8 kg (8.8 and 17.6 lbs). It has been further shown that placentae are mostly retained in the nonpregnant horn even though the incidence of edema is higher in the pregnant horn.[4] Clinical experience indicates that delayed separation of the allantochorion seems to be a fairly localized phenomenon. If manual separation is attempted, areas of loose placenta alternate with areas where the fetal membranes remain firmly attached.

Factors predisposing to retained placenta include (1) induction of parturition before all signs of impending foaling are present (cervical dilation, a minimum of 330 days' pregnancy, and a full udder with distended teats); (2) cesarean section; delayed uterine involution following surgical removal of the fetus will often cause prolonged retention if no treatment is instituted. Defective separation of the allantochorion should not be confused with the inability to release the membranes due to inadvertent suturing of membranes to the uterine wall; (3) any obstetrical work, including fetotomy, will delay uterine involution and, therefore, normal separation of the placenta; (4) after prolonged delivery, uterine involution is delayed, especially on the nonpregnant horn. This might be the reason why membranes are usually retained in the nonpregnant rather than the pregnant uterine horn.

MANAGEMENT OF RETAINED PLACENTA

REMOVAL OF THE FETAL MEMBRANES

Several different approaches are advocated for removal of fetal membranes. Advantages and disadvantages are listed in Table 1.

TABLE 1. ADVANTAGES AND DISADVANTAGES OF VARIOUS METHODS FOR REMOVAL OF RETAINED FETAL MEMBRANES

Method	Advantage	Disadvantage
Oxytocin; repeated bolus injections	Easy to apply No special equipment needed Might be given by owner	Possibility of uterine cramps Might cause excessive discomfort to the mare
Oxytocin; as a drip	Can be given to effect Method giving the most reliable results	Time involved to place catheter and set up infusion equipment
Povidone-iodine solution; infusion into allantoic space	Most physiologic method, as it stimulates endogenous oxytocin release	Time involvement Possiblity of membrane rupture before expulsion Difficulty to perform clean and leakless application, especially on restless mares
Manual separation	None	Danger of excessive bleeding Several attempts might be needed Increased uterine contamination

Oxytocin Bolus. Bolus injection of oxytocin gives satisfactory results in most cases. Large doses of oxytocin (over 60 IU) might cause a spasmodic contraction of the whole myometrium, and are therefore of little value. If bolus injections are used, no more than 30 to 40 IU should be given intravenously at intervals of 15 to 20 minutes.

Oxytocin Infusion. Intravenous oxytocin infusion is in my opinion the method of choice. Eighty to 100 IU of oxytocin is prepared in 500 ml saline. The speed of infusion is adjusted according to the mare's reactions, the flow rate being slowed if excessive abdominal pain is present. With this method, which might be time-consuming, most of the retained membranes are expelled within one half hour. Gentle traction on the placenta will speed up expulsion.

Uterine Infusion. Infusion of a large volume of a povidone-iodine solution is another way to stimulate uterine contraction. Povidone-iodine solution diluted 1:10 (10 to 12 liters) is infused into the allantochorionic space using a stomach tube.[2] At the end of the infusion, the stomach tube is withdrawn, and the opening in the fetal membranes is tied with umbilical tape. At this point, the membranes may be squeezed to force the fluid into the uterus. The pressure of the fluid expanding the uterus, vagina, and the cervix will stimulate endogenous oxytocin release. Membranes are usually expelled within 30 minutes. The main advantage of this method is that the uterus is not invaded and, therefore, the risk of contamination is reduced.

Manual Removal. Manual separation of the allantochorion is still used, especially in some European countries. The risk of hemorrhage and infection is very high with this traumatic method. Manual separation has also been used in cesarean sections at the time of surgery to prevent postsurgical retention. The membranes are at this time usually too firmly attached to be removed without excessive trauma.

After the removal, the placenta should be carefully examined to make sure that all the membranes have been expelled. In some instances, especially if the membranes have been forcibly extracted, the placenta may break close to the tip of the horn. The best treatment for this partial retention is either oxytocin or manual removal if the membranes are not too firmly attached. Antimicrobial therapy, as described later, might also be instituted. Repeated oxytocin injection 12 to 24 hours apart is indicated in any case in which delayed uterine involution is diagnosed. Rectal examination is, therefore, an important clinical tool to monitor a patient's progress.

CHEMOTHERAPY

In addition to removal of all fetal membranes from the uterus, antibiotics and anti-inflammmatory drugs are often indicated in the treatment of retained placenta, especially in protracted cases or cases in which severe uterine contamination is suspected (Table 2). During the first six to eight hours after foaling, bacterial growth remains in an acceptable range. If the placenta is retained for more than eight hours, bacteria multiply rapidly, and antimicrobial therapy should be started.

1. Intrauterine medication should be used only if the uterus has been invaded manually or if it contains large amounts of fluid. Repeated intrauterine medication should be used very selectively, as every time the uterus is invaded, more contaminants are introduced. Strict asepsis must be observed. The

TABLE 2. SUPPORTIVE THERAPY FOLLOWING REMOVAL OF RETAINED PLACENTA

	Intrauterine Treatment	Parenteral Antimicrobial Therapy	Phenylbutazone	Oxytocin
Placenta removed in less than 8 hrs postpartum without invading uterus	None	None	None	None
Placenta removed in less than 8 hrs after obstetrical work; minimal contamination	One treatment after placenta has been removed	None	None	One IV infusion after delivery of the foal
Placenta removed in less than 8 hrs after obstetrical work; marked contamination	One treatment after placenta has been removed	3–4 days	None	Two IV infusions 12 hrs apart
Membranes removed after more than 8 hrs	One treatment or as needed, if delayed uterine involution with fluid pooling is present	3–4 days or as needed	3–4 days or as needed	Daily IV infusion for 2–3 days or as needed

two antibiotics of choice for intrauterine application are tetracycline hydrochloride capsules (2 gm) or nitrofurazone-urea boluses (six to eight boluses at 180 mg each).

2. Parenteral antibiotic therapy—according to some work done in the bovine species, intramuscular injections of sodium penicillin (22,000 IU per kg twice a day) provide effective levels in the uterus.[1] Parenteral antibiotic medication is preferred over intrauterine infusion in order to avoid unnecessary contamination of an already damaged uterus.

3. Anti-inflammatory medication—especially in protracted cases of retained placenta, phenylbutazone (2 gm orally twice a day) might be helpful in preventing the metritis-laminitis syndrome (p. 428). The analgesic properties of phenylbutazone might also help eliminate excessive abdominal pain caused by the rapid uterine involution.

REFRACTORY CASES

On occasion, routine therapeutic procedures fail to cause delivery of the membranes, and a tightly adhered area of chorion is palpable. The danger of forcibly stripping these membranes away from the endometrium should be recognized. Permanent endometrial damage may occur, resulting in compromise of the mare's future productivity.

In these protracted cases, chemotherapy combining local and systemic antibiotics and oxytocin as well as phenylbutazone should be instituted. Each

time the uterus is medicated, the site of placental attachment might be explored for release of the chorion. Usually no more than three or four days of treatment are needed even in the most stubborn cases. Careful client education is generally a necessary part of the therapeutic regimen.

CONCLUSIONS

The importance of limiting uterine contamination cannot be stressed enough. Every time the uterus is manipulated, even if strict aseptic conditions are used, additional contaminants are introduced, increasing the danger of the metritis-laminitis complex. The key to successful treatment of retained placenta is rapid uterine involution combined with antimicrobial therapy when indicated.

References

1. Ayliffe, R. R., and Noakes, D. E.: Some preliminary studies on the uptake of sodium benzylpenicillin by the endometrium of the cow. Vet. Rec., *102*:215, 1978.
2. Burns, S. J., Judge, N. G., Martin, F. E., and Adams, L. G.: Management of retained placenta in mares. Proc. 23rd Annu. Meet. Am. Assoc. Eq. Pract., 1977, pp. 381–390.
3. Samuel, C. A., Allen, W. R., and Steven, D. H.: Studies on the equine placenta. II. Ultrastructure of the placental barrier. J. Reprod. Fertil., *48*:257, 1976.
4. Vandeplassche, M., Spincemaille, J., and Bouters, R.: Etiology, pathogenesis and treatment of retained placenta in the mare. Eq. Vet. J., *3*:144, 1971.
5. Whitwell, K. E., and Jeffcott, L. B.: Morphological studies on the fetal membranes of the normal singleton foal at term. Res. Vet. Sci., *19*:44, 1975.

POSTPARTUM COMPLICATIONS

Walter W. Zent, LEXINGTON, KENTUCKY

During foaling and in the immediate postpartum period, a variety of injuries and disorders develop that can have serious consequences for the mare. The age and breed of the dam have some influence on the incidence of these complications, but many are purely accidents associated with the rapid and often violent birth process. The clinician must quickly diagnose the cause of postpartum disorders, since early recognition of the problem may improve the success of treatment. Frequently diagnosis is made difficult because the clinical signs of many postpartum problems are nonspecific.

PROLAPSED UTERUS

The mare's uterus, composed of a body and two horns, is suspended cranially and laterally by the broad ligaments. The cranial attachment of the broad ligaments makes uterine prolapse less likely than in the cow. Uterine prolapse can occur after normal delivery but is more common following dystocia or retention of the placental membranes. It is my opinion that uterine prolapse is more common in Standardbreds than in Thoroughbreds.

Occasionally the tip of one uterine horn may partially prolapse after foaling, causing pain and straining that frequently result in a total eversion of the organ. Mares that have a history of uterine prolapse are more likely to repeat after subsequent foalings and should be observed closely in the early postpartum period. The principles in treating uterine prolapse are (1) control of straining, (2) cleaning and replacing the uterus, and (3) preventing recurrence. Straining is best controlled by first sedating the mare with moderate doses of xylazine* and pentazocine,† followed by epidural anesthesia with 8 to 10 ml of 2 per cent lidocaine.‡

The uterus should be carefully and thoroughly washed with a dilute solution of a mild disinfectant such as povidone-iodine solution.§ If the placenta can be easily removed, it is advantageous to do so before replacing the uterus. The uterus is examined for lacerations and is carefully replaced, attempting to straighten out the horns as completely as possible. Antibiotic boluses are placed into the uterine lumen, and the vulva is sutured with a heavy material such as umbilical tape to prevent reprolapse.

Systemic antibiotics are indicated to control in-fection. Kanamycin* at 5 mg per kg twice a day and procaine penicillin,† 10 million units twice a day, make a satisfactory broad-spectrum combination. If the mare's vital signs remain normal, no attempt should be made to medicate the uterus for several days. If there are signs of toxemia or an elevated temperature, the uterus should be examined, and treatment for metritis should be instituted if necessary.

UTERINE RUPTURE

Uterine rupture may occur during dystocia or in normal delivery. If the rupture is large, the mare will rapidly show signs of hemorrhagic shock. Death of the mare is inevitable in these cases. If the serosa remains intact, there are signs of hemorrhage and colic, but the mare will usually survive.

Smaller uterine ruptures, such as those produced by perforation during dystocia, may not produce signs for several hours. Signs of peritonitis gradually become evident after this time. Heroic antibiotic therapy may control some of these infections, but the prognosis is grave. Gentamicin,‡ 2 mg per kg four times a day, and sodium penicillin,§ 10 million units twice a day, is my choice of an antibiotic combination. The rent in the uterus is difficult to find, but if antibiotics fail to bring about improvement, surgical repair of the uterus may be indicated. This is usually done through a midline laparotomy.

HEMORRHAGE

Hemorrhage from a uterine artery is most common in older mares and is a significant cause of death in aged brood mares. Multiparous mares over 11 years of age are the prime candidates, but rarely a postpartum hemorrhage will occur in a younger animal.

These hemorrhages are not always fatal. If the broad ligament that surrounds the artery remains intact, the ligament may contain the hemorrhage. The result is a large hematoma that dissects between the myometrium and the serosa of the uterus. The resulting clot is capable of controlling the arterial bleeding, and survival of the mare depends on the quantity of blood lost. If the broad ligament rup-

*Rompun, Haver-Lockhart Labs, Shawnee, KS 66201
†Talwin, Winthrop Labs, New York, NY 10017
‡Xylocaine, Astra Pharmaceutical Products, Inc., Worcester, MA 01606
§Betadine, Purdue Frederick Co., Norwalk, CN 06856

*Kantrim, Bristol Labs, Syracuse, NY 13201
†Cristicillin, E. R. Squibb & Sons, Princeton, NJ 08540
‡Gentocin, Schering Corp., Kenilworth, NJ 07033
§Sodium Penicillin G, E. R. Squibb & Sons, Princeton, NJ 08540

tures with the artery or if the uterine serosa ruptures during hematoma formation, the blood quickly moves out into the peritoneal cavity.

Clinical signs of postpartum hemorrhage include mild to severe colic, sweating, pale mucous membanes, and elevated pulse rate. Shock and death may be the ultimate fates. The only possible treatment is to keep the mare as quiet as possible, including mild sedation if necessary. Blood transfusions, plasma expanders, or fluid therapy do not seem to alter the course of these cases and may even be contraindicated if the mare becomes excited by the treatment procedures.

Postpartum hemorrhages can occur before, during, or after foaling. Dystocia does not seem to be important in the incidence. Some management practices are logical to minimize the chances for arterial rupture in older mares during the periparturient period. It is prudent to minimize handling of older mares at this time. Shipping, deworming, foot care, and minor surgery should be scheduled during a safer time period. Even the routine Caslick's operation after foaling should be delayed a few days to minimize excitement and stress.

CERVICAL LACERATION

Laceration of the mare's cervix can occur during parturition and is commonly associated with dystocia. The injury may be produced by an oversized fetus, by obstetrical chains, or by fetotomy wire. Small cervical lacerations that do not interfere with closure of the os during diestrus are of no consequence, but serious trauma can have a profound effect on future reproductive performance.

I favor attempting to repair cervical lacerations during estrus when exposure and retraction are easier. When attempting repair of these injuries, it is important to free all of the adhesions between the cervix and the vaginal wall. The integrity of the lumen of the cervical canal must be maintained.

Many cervical lacerations can be prevented. Sufficient time should be allowed for maximal dilation to occur before attempting to deliver a foal. Cutting instruments that might predispose to cervical trauma should not be passed through the cervix. In difficult cases of dystocia, cesarean section should be considered if excessive manipulation or fetotomy is needed for vaginal delivery. The reproductive potential following cesarean section is greater than following cervical damage.

VAGINAL RUPTURE

Vaginal rupture can occur by perforation of the foal's foot through the vaginal wall or as a result of obstetrical procedures. The dorsal vaginal wall is most susceptible when the feet of the foal are the cause. The vagina may rupture at any point from the cervix caudally. Cranial vaginal ruptures communicate directly with the peritoneal cavity. Concurrent damage to the colon or rectum need not occur.

In mares in which a dorsal vaginal injury is not discovered at the time of foaling, the presenting signs are those of peritonitis, appearing as early as a few hours postpartum. There is seldom a prolapse of bowel through a laceration in this location.

Repair of a dorsal vaginal rupture is most easily accomplished in the standing animal. The mare should be restrained in stocks and sedated as was described earlier. Epidural anesthesia with 10 ml of 2 per cent lidocaine is indicated. Intraperitoneal administration of an antibiotic solution such as 10 million units sodium penicillin and 500 mg of gentamicin, buffered with sodium bicarbonate* (1 ml 7.5 per cent $NaHCO_3$ per 50 mg gentamicin), is easily accomplished through the rent in the vagina prior to repair. The volume of the infusion should be at least 500 ml. Stay sutures placed adjacent to the cervix may permit some retraction of the wound to a more accessible area, but the heavy postpartum uterus may make retraction difficult.

The edges of the laceration should be apposed with resorbable sutures. Completely sealing the wound is not necessary if the major portions of the edges are apposed. Following repair, a Caslick's operation will reduce the chances of air aspiration into the peritoneal cavity.

When laceration of the ventral wall of the vagina occurs, a frequent sequela is herniation of portions of the viscera, usually small intestine. If this prolapse occurs before delivery of the foal, it may complicate the dystocia. Vigorous attempts to deliver the foal vaginally can lead to serious trauma and contamination of the gut. Immediate cesarean section is therefore indicated. It is helpful to completely suture the labia prior to anesthesia induction to protect the herniating intestine.

If the prolapsed gut has been badly damaged prior to the clinician's arrival, the only choice may be euthanasia of the mare and salvage of the foal. The ideal approach to this problem is to shoot the mare and to immediately remove the foal through a slash incision. Chemical euthanasia greatly reduces foal survival.

RECTOVESTIBULAR INJURIES

Rectovestibular injuries occur during foaling when a foot fails to pass the vaginovestibular sphinc-

---

*Sodium Bicarbonate Sterile Solution 7.5%, Med Tech, Inc., Elwood, KS 66024

ter and the abdominal contractions of the mare force the foot dorsally and caudally. The resulting injury is a perforation of the vestibular roof and the rectum. If the situation is detected at this time and the foal is repelled and delivered vaginally, the more serious third-degree perineal laceration can be prevented.

In the case of either injury, repair should not be attempted for several weeks to allow resolution of edema and inflammation. Some rectovestibular fistulas will heal without surgery. Details on repair of these perineal and rectovestibular problems appear elsewhere (p. 431).

VULVAR LACERATION

Vulvar lacerations are common aftermaths of foaling. One of the frequent causes is failure to adequately open the previous year's Caslick's operation. If the laceration is severe, time must be allowed for resolution of inflammation before repair is attempted.

Extensive pressure on the labia during delivery can disrupt the circulation, resulting in vulvar necrosis. The resulting damage may reduce the amount of tissue remaining and may require a deeper closure than the simple Caslick's procedure. In the worst of these cases, it is often prudent to delay repair until after breeding the mare, thus allowing more healing time.

GASTROINTESTINAL COMPLICATIONS OF FOALING

A variety of intestinal complications can follow parturition in the mare, ranging from simple constipation to a ruptured viscus. The signs observed are often confusing and make the differential diagnosis challenging.

Constipation is a frequent occurrence following delivery of the first foal. Bruising of the vagina and perineal area cause pain, which makes the mare reluctant to defecate. The resulting constipation is generally mild and will usually respond to mineral oil, 1 gal orally, and a little time.

A more serious intestinal problem follows bruising of the small colon when this organ is compressed between the uterus and pelvis during delivery. These mares will show signs of constipation soon after foaling. By the second day postpartum, signs of mild colic appear, and temperature may be elevated. At about 72 hours, signs of peritonitis are evident, such as fever, congested mucous membranes, elevated white blood cell count, and colic of increasing severity. Rectal examination at this time will usually reveal a large sausage-shaped mass involving the small colon.

Immediate surgical intervention to resect the damaged bowel is indicated. Any delay will increase the possibility of further breakdown of the colon wall with resulting irreversible peritonitis.

The most serious intestinal problem related to parturition is rupture of the rectum, small colon, or cecum. Rectal and small colon rupture follows entrapment of the organs and compression during delivery. Cecal rupture, usually at the base of the cecum, occurs because of distention of the organ at the time of delivery. Abdominal compression is apparently forceful enough to cause the rupture. These mares develop peritonitis within a few hours with fatal results.

One management technique that may reduce the incidence of cecal rupture is the reduction of roughage intake by mares in the last few days prepartum. Most mares voluntarily eat less hay as parturition nears, but individual animals, especially in groups that compete for feed, may lose this natural instinct.

Rectal prolapse is occasionally an aftermath of foaling (p. 254). Immediate replacement of the prolapse may appear to be a satisfactory solution, but the short mesentery of the rectum may have been damaged in the process with compromise in the blood supply as a sequela. These mares follow the same pattern as the cases with bruised colon, with necrosis of the avascular portion of the rectal wall leading to leakage and peritonitis.

Surgical correction of rectal damage is difficult owing to the limited access to the area. One approach is to reprolapse the rectum and anastomose the healthy ends outside of the anus. It may help to have a second operator, working through a ventral midline incision. This allows delineation of the damaged area of the rectum and can provide extra stretching of the mesentery to make it more accessible.

METRITIS-LAMINITIS-TOXEMIA SYNDROME

Postpartum metritis, while not common, is extremely serious owing to the rapid development of laminitis, septicemia, and toxemia.

Acute metritis may result from dystocia, retained placenta, or any massive contamination of the uterine lumen. The mare is usually depressed and anorectic 24 to 36 hours after foaling. The rectal temperature may range from 101 to 106° F. The mucous membranes become congested, then muddy or purple. Depression progresses rapidly. There may be an increase in the digital pulse at any time, signifying the onset of laminitis.

The uterus usually contains several gallons of a chocolate-colored, fetid fluid, which distends the organ and pulls it over the pelvic brim. A small piece of placenta is frequently found in one horn. This membrane should be removed if it is readily lifted out without tearing. If the placenta is tightly adherent to the endometrium, it is best left until complete separation has occurred.

Treatment should be directed at evacuation of the uterus to eliminate toxins. Large volumes of dilute povidone-iodine solution are pumped into the uterus using a stomach tube, pump, and a 5-gal bucket. The contents are then siphoned off. This washing procedure is repeated until the character of the fluid drained off is similar to that being pumped in. The entire procedure should be repeated at least twice a day.

When the uterus is emptied, antibiotic boluses should be introduced into the lumen. Systemic antibiotic therapy is imperative. Sodium penicillin (10 million units intravenously twice a day) and kanamycin (10 mg per kg twice a day) or gentamicin (2 mg per kg four times a day) offer broad-spectrum coverage.

When acute metritis is treated vigorously from the onset, laminitis is an infrequent sequela. When laminitis does occur, however, it may develop very quickly and with dire consequences. Puerperal laminitis often results in sloughing of the feet, necessitating euthanasia. The laminitis should be treated with anti-inflammatory drugs such as phenylbutazone* (4 gm daily) or dexamethasone† (20 mg daily).

If the mare can be kept on a 3- to 4-in bedding of sand, uniform sole pressure is maintained, which reduces the chance of coffin bone rotation. Ice is helpful in reducing the inflammation in the feet, and forced exercise, where possible, will improve blood flow from the feet and help prevent rotation. It must be remembered that the laminitis in these cases is secondary to the metritis, so prompt and diligent treatment of the uterus is essential to correct the entire problem. Metritis-laminitis-toxemia syndrome is highly fatal in mares that do not receive adequate care.

Supplemental Readings

1. Richter, J., and Gotze, R.: Tiergeburtshilfe, 3rd. ed. Berlin, Verlag Paul Parey, 1980.
2. Roberts, S. J.: Veterinary Obstetrics and Genital Diseases, 2nd ed. Ithaca, NY, published by author, 1971.
3. Vadeplassche, M.: Obstetrician's view of the physiology of equine parturition and dystocia. Equine Vet. J., *12*:45, 1980.

---

*Butazolidin, Jensen-Salsbery Labs, Kansas City, MO 64141
†Azium, Schering Corp., Kenilworth, NJ 07033

PARTURIENT PERINEAL AND RECTOVESTIBULAR INJURIES

Rolf M. Embertson, GAINESVILLE, FLORIDA

Several types of injuries may be associated with parturition in the mare. These include vaginal and cervical contusions and lacerations, uterine rupture or prolapse, urinary bladder eversion or prolapse, perineal lacerations, and rectovestibular fistulas.[5] The perineal and rectovestibular injuries are the most common type that require surgical repair. These injuries are usually the result of malpositioning of the fetus with the forefeet traumatizing the vestibule or perineum during delivery. Damage can also occur as the result of delivery of an oversized fetus or from overzealous assistance during foaling.

Perineal and rectovestibular injuries are classified by type and severity. First-degree perineal lacerations involve the mucosa of the vestibule and dermis of the dorsal commissure of the vulva. Second-degree lacerations involve the vestibular mucosa and submucosa, the dermis of the dorsal commissure of the vulva, and the perineal body musculature, including the constrictor vulvae. Third-degree lacerations involve the walls of the rectum and vestibule, the perineal septum and musculature, and the anal sphincter. Rectovestibular fistulas involve the dorsal wall of the vestibule, the perineal septum, and the ventral wall of the rectum.[3] When applied to the condition that usually occurs in the mare, rectovestibular is the proper terminology rather than the commonly used rectovaginal or rectovulvar.[4]

Third-degree lacerations are more commonly seen in the primiparous mare, when the forefoot of the fetus may catch on the low annular fold of the hymen at the vaginovestibular junction.[6] Continued expulsion drives the foot up through the dorsum of the vestibule and into the rectum. If this situation

---

Special thanks to Dr. A. C. Asbury, Dr. P. T. Colahan, and Dr. James T. Robertson for their assistance.

is corrected by manual assistance or by natural means, the result is a rectovestibular fistula; if not corrected, the expulsive efforts of delivery will result in a third-degree laceration.

Surgical repair of these injuries in the acute state is generally not recommended, as the vast majority of attempts are unsuccessful. Bacterial contamination, tissue inflammation, and devitalization create a poor environment for successful surgery. Vaginal lacerations that reach the peritoneal reflection are rare and require immediate attention, including suturing the vaginal rent to prevent evisceration and severe peritonitis. A minimum of three to four weeks' delay in repair is necessary to allow for resolution of the inflammation, wound margin epithelialization, and wound contracture.[4-6] The dimensions of the wound will decrease significantly by this time. In rare cases, some rectovestibular fistulas may heal without surgical assistance. Following the acute injury, little treatment is necessary until surgery is performed. However, daily cleansing of the wound may be of benefit, and current tetanus prophylaxis is mandatory.

If parturition results in a rectovestibular fistula or third-degree laceration and the foal lives, under most circumstances it is advisable to wait until weaning before operative repair of the mare is performed. This is especially true if the mare and foal are subjected to a hospital environment, exposing the foal to hospital diseases and hazards. Also, the special postoperative diet required of the mare may adversely affect her lactation. Even if the dystocia results in a dead fetus, it is unlikely that the mare can be bred during the same breeding season. Breeding should be delayed two to three months to allow for adequate tissue healing. Another time factor is that more than one surgical attempt is sometimes necessary to complete the repair.

FIRST-DEGREE PERINEAL LACERATIONS

The laceration can be repaired with a Caslick procedure, using nonabsorbable monofilament suture material in an interrupted or continuous pattern.[6] No special dietary considerations are necessary in repair of this type of wound.

SECOND-DEGREE PERINEAL LACERATIONS

Because of the damage to the perineal body and vestibular sphincter, repair of a second-degree laceration by a Caslick procedure is usually inadequate. A simple Caslick suture leaves a sunken perineum, which predisposes to pneumovagina and its associated problems. Perineal body reconstruction

is necessary. No special dietary considerations are required in preparation for surgery. The repair can be done under local anesthesia or an epidural block.

A triangular section of mucous membrane is removed from the dorsal and dorsolateral aspect of the vestibule. The base of this triangle is the mucocutaneous junction of the vulva with the apex located in the vestibule. The incised edges of vestibular mucosa are sutured together, as are the raw submucosal surfaces and the edges of cutaneous perineum. Sexual rest is mandatory for four to eight weeks to allow adequate time for healing.[3, 6]

THIRD-DEGREE PERINEAL LACERATIONS

PREPARATION AND ANESTHESIA

Preoperative preparation is extremely important in the success of third-degree laceration repair. Soft feces are necessary before the surgery is performed. To accomplish this, several different feeding and laxative regimens have been used, including lush green grass pasture, pelleted rations, wet bran mashes, danthron, magnesium sulfate, mineral oil, and dioctyl sodium sulfosuccinate (DSS), all with reported success. Abrupt changes in feeding should be avoided by adjusting the diet gradually over a three- to five-day period. Prolonged fasting to empty the intestinal tract has been advocated by some. However, this is not necessary and may predispose the mare to enteritis and diarrhea.[3]

Although individual mares will vary in treatment regimens necessary to produce and maintain soft feces, the following program has worked well. Place the mare on lush green grass pasture (if available) supplemented with a pelleted ration. No hay is fed. Assuming she weighs 450 kg, administer 1 lb of magnesium sulfate in 2 gal of water once daily via a nasogastric tube. On alternate days, 400 ml of DSS are added until the feces are soft, at which time the surgery is performed. Fasting the mare 24 hours prior to surgery is desirable to reduce the amount of feces in the operative and immediate postoperative period.

Phenylbutazone (4 mg per kg intravenously) and procaine penicillin G (20,000 IU per kg intramuscularly) are administered three to four hours preoperatively, ensuring effective blood levels during surgery. Phenylbutazone may help decrease postoperative inflammation and swelling and lessen the mare's tendency to strain. Although no definite advantage for using antibiotics has been proved, the inevitable contamination of the surgery site and the large anaerobic bacterial population in the feces justify the use of penicillin. Intraoperative wound irrigation with either sterile saline or potassium penicillin G in saline may also be beneficial. Tetanus prophylaxis is mandatory.[3]

The mare is placed in the stocks and tranquilized. Acepromazine HCl* (0.05 mg per kg intravenously) with xylazine† (0.55 mg per kg intravenously) or acepromazine HCl (0.05 mg per kg intravenously) with 30 per cent chloral hydrate and 25 per cent magnesium sulfate‡ (60 to 100 ml per 450 kg intravenously) can be used. The diuretic effect of xylazine may cause micturition intraoperatively.

The tail is wrapped, and the tail head is clipped and prepared for epidural anesthesia. Seven to 10 ml of 2 per cent lidocaine or mepivacaine HCl§ will adequately anesthetize the intended operative field. More than 10 ml of anesthetic solution may partially anesthetize the mare's rear legs, causing posterior ataxia or even recumbency. General anesthesia is indicated in those mares that go down and become very frightened and thrash about. Although positioning becomes a problem, the procedure can be completed under general anesthesia or postponed. Quiet mares should be kept comfortable until they can stand.

While waiting for the epidural to take effect, the rectum is manually evacuated as far cranial as possible. The rectum, vestibule, and perineum are cleansed with a nonirritating antiseptic solution diluted in water, preferably povidone-iodine. The surgical field is then sprayed with povidone-iodine solution.

PRINCIPLES OF REPAIR

Many different variations of rectovestibular surgery are found in the literature. Success of the surgery depends on the careful observation of basic surgical principles and proper preparation of the patient. The feces must be soft before the surgery is performed and maintained soft for an additional two weeks. Postoperative pain combined with firm feces may lead to rectal impaction and subsequent repair dehiscence. Suture material needs to be strong and must cause minimal tissue reaction. Chromic gut has been used successfully but is not the ideal suture material owing to the inflammatory reaction it may produce. Sutures should be placed 1.0 to 1.5 cm apart using hand ties and surgeon's knots and should be checked for adequate tension. Loose sutures lead to poor tissue apposition, fistulation, and possible dehiscence of the repair. Maximal tissue apposition with minimal suture tension is accomplished by adequate dissection, creating

generous flaps of rectal wall and vestibular wall. Suturing these flaps will leave a thick, strong rectovestibular septum when healed. Hemorrhage excessive enough to require vessel ligation is usually not encountered. However, severe hemorrhage should be controlled, as hematomas in the repair are undesirable.[3, 4, 6]

OPERATIVE TECHNIQUES

The surgical techniques described involve two phases. The first phase consists of dissection and reconstruction of the rectovestibular septum. The second phase consists of dissection and reconstruction of the perineal body.[6] Some authors recommend that the surgery be performed in one stage, with both phases of repair completed in one procedure. The advantages of single-stage over two-stage repair, where the second phase is done about two weeks later, include less preoperative and postoperative care, less hospitalization, and one surgical procedure. The advantage of a two-stage repair is that during the healing period of the rectovestibular septum, the mare can defecate more easily because of the larger anal orifice. There is less chance of the rectum becoming impacted and of straining to defecate, which may lead to dehiscence or fistulation of the repair.

For adequate visualization of the surgical field, Balfour retractors or stay sutures placed through the labia and perineal tissue can be used. Either can be sutured to the skin or held by an assistant. A surgical light or a head lamp worn by the surgeon or both provide illumination.

The techniques that will be described include the six-bite vertical suture pattern, the four-bite knot-in-the-rectum pattern, the three-layer closure, and the rectal pull-back technique. The dissection is similar for all the techniques, but the rectal pull-back technique requires a more generous cranial dissection. The intact rectovestibular shelf is incised cranially 2 to 3 cm in a horizontal plane. Dissection is then directed caudally on each side along the junction of the rectal and vestibular mucosa and is continued to the cutaneous perineum. If a six-bite vertical pattern is used, the flaps created should be thicker on the rectal side than the vestibular side. In the four-bite knot-in-the-rectum and rectal pullback techniques, the vestibular flaps should be made thicker. Flaps of equal thickness are created for the three-layer closure.[3]

The six-bite vertical suture pattern repair (Fig. 1) uses heavy nonabsorbable polyester suture material*† and a large half-circle cutting edge needle.

*Acepromazine, Ayerst Labs, Inc., New York, NY 10017
†Rompun, Haver-Lockhart, Shawnee, KS 66201
‡Chloral-Thesia, Med-Tech, Inc., Elwood, KS 66024
§Carbocaine, Winthrop Labs, New York, NY 10016

*Ethibond, Ethicon, Inc., Somerville, NJ 08876
†Mersilene, Ethicon, Inc., Somerville, NJ 08876

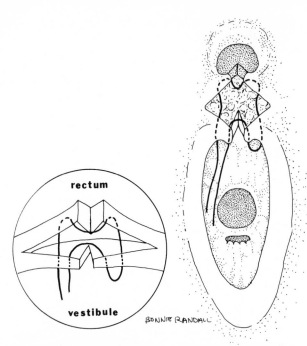

Figure 1. The six-bite vertical suture pattern used in repair of third-degree perineal lacerations; suture placement. (Adapted from Colahan, P. T.: Equine Medicine and Surgery. Santa Barbara, CA, American Veterinary Pub., 1982, and Walker, D. F., and Vaughan, J. T.: Urogenital Surgery. Philadelphia, Lea and Febiger, 1980.)

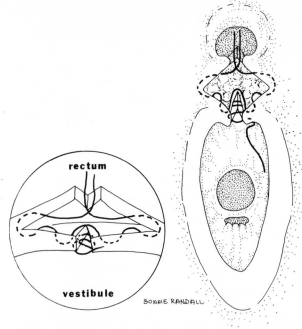

Figure 2. The four-bite knot-in-the-rectum technique used in repair of third-degree perineal lacerations; suture placement. (Adapted from Colahan, P. T.: Equine Medicine and Surgery. Santa Barbara, CA, American Veterinary Pub., 1982, and Walker, D. F., and Vaughan, J. T.: Urogenital Surgery. Philadelphia, Lea and Febiger, 1980.)

Each suture is knotted in the vestibule, leaving long (10 cm) ends for easy removal in 14 days. In Phase 1 of the repair, the first bite is placed deep through the left vestibular flap starting in the vestibule. The second bite is placed through the left rectal flap, emerging just below the rectal mucosa. The third bite is placed in the right rectal flap, emerging in the plane of dissection. The fourth bite is placed deep through the right vestibular flap, emerging in the vestibule. The fifth bite is placed up through the right vestibular flap near its edge, and the sixth bite is placed down through the left vestibular flap near its edge, emerging in the vestibule. The suture is then tied under tension, which will appose the rectal flaps and invert the vestibular flaps into the vestibule. This pattern is started in the cranial pocket created in the rectovestibular septum by dissection and is continued caudally 4 to 6 cm from the cutaneous perineum. No suture can be allowed to penetrate the rectal mucosa.[6]

The second phase of this repair is similar to the perineal body reconstruction procedure previously described.

The four-bite knot-in-the-rectum technique (Fig. 2) begins by placing a continuous horizontal mattress pattern using No. 1 chromic gut in the edges of the vestibular flaps. The suture is run from the cranial aspect of the laceration caudally one third of

the length of the laceration, where it is tied. This suture inverts the vestibular mucosa into the vestibule and will be continued later in the procedure. The pocket created in the intact rectovestibular septum is obliterated with pursestring sutures of No. 2 chromic gut. A four-bite modified Lembert pattern is then begun using No. 5 polyester.* The first bite is placed in the perivestibular tissue of the right vestibular flap. The second bite is placed in the submucosa of the right vestibular flap closer to its edge. The third bite is placed in the submucosa of the left vestibular flap, and the fourth bite is placed in the perivestibular tissue of the left flap further from its edge. The suture is then tied under tension, inverting the vestibular tissues into the vestibule and pulling the rectal mucosa closer together. The ends of the suture are left long to facilitate removal in 14 days. This suture pattern and the continuous horizontal suture pattern are continued alternately, caudally to the cutaneous perineum.

The rectal submucosa is not sutured in this method. As the tissues heal, the rectal mucosa will heal over the granulating bed. The second phase of this technique is done two weeks later. The repair of the perineal body is done in a slightly different fashion than previously explained.[2, 3]

---

*Mersilene, Ethicon, Inc., Somerville, NJ 08876

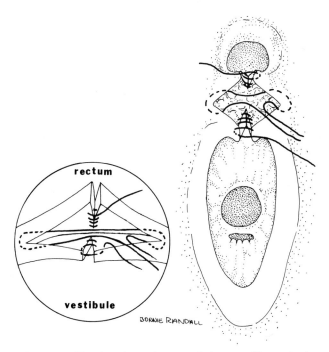

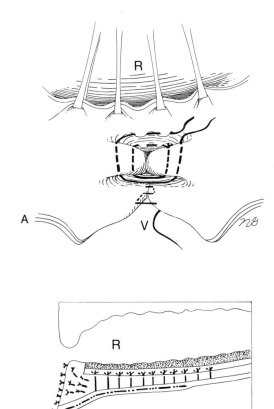

Figure 3. The three-layer closure technique used in repair of third-degree perineal lacerations; suture placement. (Adapted from Colahan, P. T.: Equine Medicine and Surgery. Santa Barbara, CA, American Veterinary Pub., 1982, and Walker, D. F., and Vaughan, J. T.: Urogenital Surgery. Philadelphia, Lea and Febiger, 1980.)

The three-layer closure (Fig. 3) uses monofilament nonabsorbable suture material with all internal sutures buried. First, continuous Lembert suture of No. 0 polypropylene* is placed in the vestibular submucosa. Then, simple interrupted sutures of No. 2 nylon are placed in the connective tissue shelf between the rectal and vestibular walls. The most cranial sutures are preplaced, then tied in sequence. The rectal submucosa is then apposed in the same manner as the vestibular submucosa. Suture lines are placed alternately because of the limited working space. The sutures do not penetrate the mucosa of either the rectum or vestibule. Simple interrupted sutures are then placed in the cutaneous perineum, and the perineal body is reconstructed to complete the procedure.[4]

The rectal pull-back technique (Fig. 4) is commenced by pulling the rectal floor caudally to the anal sphincter with three long Allis tissue forceps. These are placed in the submucosa along the caudal margin of the intact rectal shelf. The pocket created in the intact rectovestibular septum is obliterated with pursestring sutures of No. 2 chromic gut. A four-bite pattern using No. 3 chromic gut is then started. The first bite is large and is placed in the

Figure 4. *A,* The rectal pull-back technique used in repair of third-degree perineal lacerations; suture placement and Allis tissue forceps grasping the rectal floor. R, rectum; V, vestibule. *B,* The rectal pull-back technique depicting a sagittal view of the finished surgery. R, rectum; V, vestibule. (Courtesy of Dr. James T. Robinson.)

right vestibular flap; the second bite is also large and is placed in the left vestibular flap; the third bite is small and is placed in the rectal submucosa on the left side; the fourth bite is also small and is placed in the rectal submucosa on the right side. This suture is then tied under tension on the right side of the dissected plane. With each suture placement, the rectal floor is retracted caudally before the rectal submucosal bites are taken. The suture does not penetrate the rectal mucosa or the vestibular mucosa. The four-bite pattern is continued caudally about one fourth the length of the laceration. Then a continuous horizontal mattress pattern placed in the edges of the vestibular flaps using No. 0 chromic gut is begun. This pattern is continued

*Prolene, Ethicon, Inc., Somerville, NJ 08876

to the point where the four-bite suture ended, then is tied, and the remainder is left in the vestibule until it is needed again. In this manner, the two suture patterns are alternated to the perineum. If the rectal floor cannot be pulled back to the anal sphincter, the four-bite pattern is continued, incorporating the rectal flaps and apposing the rectal mucosa. Simple interrupted sutures in the cutaneous perineum and a routine vulvoplasty complete this procedure. In this technique, an intact rectal floor is secured to the repaired rectovestibular septum (Robertson, J. T., personal communication, 1981).

POSTOPERATIVE MANAGEMENT

Soft feces must be maintained for 14 days postoperatively. The mare should remain on the same diet and should receive laxatives as needed. Phenylbutazone and penicillin therapy are continued for 48 to 72 hours postoperatively. Excessive examination of the surgical site may disrupt the repair and should be avoided. Only in the case of rectal impactions should the rectum be manually evacuated or should enemas be administered. Sutures are removed in 12 to 14 days. The reproductive tract is examined in four to six weeks, and artificial insemination is possible in six to eight weeks; however, natural breeding should be delayed for at least three months.[3]

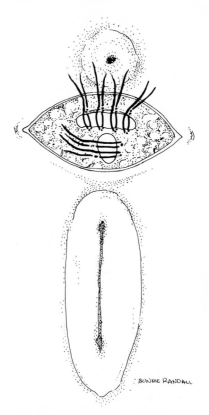

Figure 5. The horizontal perineal approach to repair of a rectovestibular fistula; suture placement. (Adapted from Colahan, P. T.: Equine Medicine and Surgery. Santa Barbara, CA, American Veterinary Pub., 1982.)

RECTOVESTIBULAR FISTULAS

The surgical preparation, anesthesia, principles of repair, and postoperative management for rectovestibular fistulas are the same as discussed for third-degree perineal lacerations. As with third-degree lacerations, different techniques have been used successfully to repair rectovestibular fistulas. Essentially four techniques with individual variations have been used. These include the creation and subsequent repair of a third-degree laceration, a horizontal perineal approach, a vestibular approach, and a rectal approach. Repair of the fistula through creation of a third-degree laceration or by a rectal approach is generally not recommended.

The horizontal perineal approach (Fig. 5) consists of incising the perineum in a horizontal plane midway between the anus and vulva. Dissection through the rectovestibular septum is done carefully so that no perforations are made into the rectum or vagina. The dissection is continued 3 to 4 cm cranial to the fistula, incising the edges of the fistula along the rectal and vestibular mucosal junction.

The principal lines of stress in the rectal wall occur at right angles to its longitudinal axis. Distract-

ing forces applied to a fistula closed along these lines of stress (transversely) would be less than fistulas closed against these lines of stress (longitudinally). Sutures of No. 1 chromic gut, polyglactin 910,* or polypropylene directed longitudinally are preplaced in the rectal submucosa using a Lembert pattern. Tying these sutures converts the fistula to a transverse closure, inverting the rectal mucosa into the rectum. Sutures perforating the rectal mucosa are not acceptable. The vestibular fistula is closed in a similar manner, except the sutures are placed transversely, creating a longitudinal closure.[6] Some surgeons prefer to close the rectal fistula in a longitudinal direction, as the sutures are easier to place. This type of closure can be successful if the sutures are placed accurately and if adequate bites of submucosa are taken.[3] The space created by dissection is then closed with simple interrupted sutures, and the cutaneous perineum is sutured with No. 00 nylon.[3, 6] Alternatively, the dead space can be packed with gauze, which is gradually removed over four to five days as the wound fills with granulation tis-

---

*Vicryl, Ethicon, Inc., Somerville, NJ 08876

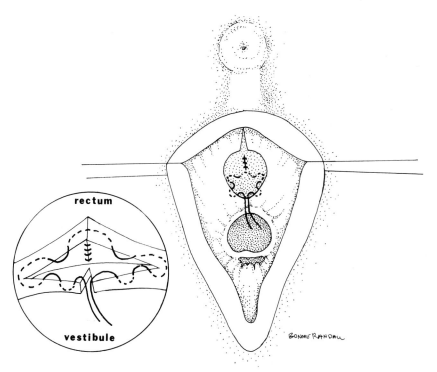

rectum

vestibule

BONNIE RANDALL

Figure 6. The vestibular approach to repair of a rectovestibular fistula; suture placement. (Adapted from Colahan, P. T.: Equine Medicine and Surgery. Santa Barbara, CA, American Veterinary Pub., 1982, and Walker, D. F., and Vaughan, J. T.: Urogenital Surgery. Philadelphia, Lea and Febiger, 1980.)

sue. (Robertson, J. T., personal communication, 1981).

In the vestibular approach (Fig. 6), the entire surgical procedure is performed through the vestibule. The cranial half of the circumference of the fistula is incised along the rectal and vestibular mucosal junction. To facilitate dissection of the caudal half of the fistula, a 3 to 4 cm longitudinal incision is made through the vestibular mucosa and submucosa from the caudal edge posteriorly. A continuous Lembert pattern using No. 0 polypropylene is placed in the rectal submucosa, inverting the rectal mucosa into the rectum. A five-bite suture is then placed in an interrupted pattern to close the vestibular fistula. Placement is as follows: Starting at the cranial aspect in the plane of dissection, a bite is taken in the right vestibular submucosa, right perivestibular tissue, right and left rectal submucosa, left perivestibular tissue, and left vestibular submucosa. The suture is tied in the plane of dissection, obliterating any dead space and inverting the vestibular mucosa into the vestibule. This pattern is continued caudad to completely close the fistula. (Brown, M. P., personal communication, 1981).

PROGNOSIS FOR FUTURE FERTILITY

The conception and foaling rates of mares with repaired perineal lacerations and rectovestibular fis-

tulas are not significantly reduced. Once repaired, concurrent vaginitis or endometritis usually resolves during the first postoperative estrus, with appropriate therapy employed as necessary. With attendance and proper care at subsequent foalings, additional severe perineal injuries occur infrequently. The prognosis for future fertility is very good (Asbury, A. C., personal communication, 1981).

References

1. Aanes, W. A.: Surgical repair of third-degree perineal laceration and rectovaginal fistula in the mare. J. Am. Vet. Med. Assoc., *144*:485, 1964.
2. Aanes, W. A.: Progress in recto-vaginal surgery. Proc. 19th Annu. Con. Am. Assoc. Eq. Pract., 1973, p. 225.
3. Colahan, P. T.: Female urogenital surgery. *In* Mansmann R. A., and McAllister, E. S. (eds.): Equine Medicine and Surgery, 3rd ed. Santa Barbara, CA, American Veterinary Pub., 1982.
4. Stickle, R. L., Fessler, J. F., and Adams, S. B.: A single-stage technique for repair of rectovestibular lacerations in the mare. Vet. Surg., 8:25, 1979.
5. Vaughan, J. T.: The genital system; horse. *In* Oehme, F. W., and Prier, J. E. (eds.): Textbook of Large Animal Surgery. Baltimore, Williams and Wilkins, 1971, pp. 498–505.
6. Walker, D. F., and Vaughan, J. T.: Perineal lacerations and rectovaginal fistulas. *In* Bovine and Equine Urogenital Surgery. Philadelphia, Lea and Febiger, 1980, pp. 197–213.

INDUCTION OF PARTURITION

Robert B. Hillman, ITHACA, NEW YORK

Over the past decade, induced parturition has become an integral part of many brood mare practices throughout the world. While this technique ensures the presence of professional assistance at foaling and is of particular advantage when employed on mares that have experienced previous foaling difficulties, it is not without hazards. Each situation should be carefully evaluated, and full consideration must be given to the risks involved before a decision is made to begin an induction. Once a successful induction has been performed on a farm, it is often difficult to curb the owners' enthusiasm, as they then want all foalings induced and often want them induced at their convenience rather than waiting until the mare is ready. To succumb to this enthusiasm is to invite disaster. Induction of parturition is a critical procedure, and strict adherence to rigid guidelines is essential to ensure success. It is necessary to understand the limitations of this technique, to carefully select the cases in which it is to be employed, and, once started, to continually monitor the foaling through its completion.

INDUCTION SITE

Mares should be placed in the area to be used for foaling at least a month prior to the estimated due date. This allows the mare to become familiar with and relaxed in this environment, but more important, it allows her enough time to develop antibodies against any pathogens present so that the colostrum will provide specific protection for the newborn foal. The foaling area and pregnant mares should be isolated from any transient populations entering the breeding farm. The pregnant mare should receive a tetanus toxoid booster upon arrival at the foaling area. Other vaccinations deemed necessary by past farm experience can also be administered at this time to ensure maximal colostral protection for the foal.

The foaling stall should be of ample size (12 ft × 12 ft), should be dry, warm, and well-bedded, and should be provided with good ventilation but should be free of drafts. It should allow observation without disturbing the mare.

INDICATIONS

Induction of parturition in the mare has been recommended for many clinical conditions as well as for managerial, teaching, and research purposes.

CLINICAL CONDITIONS

1. Delayed parturition due to uterine atony, that is, a mare that has reached term, appears ready to foal with colostrum in the udder, relaxed vulva, and sacrosciatic ligaments and cervix, but that does not go into labor.

2. Mares with a history of having produced dead or severely hypoxic foals owing to premature placental separation associated with delayed parturition should be considered as candidates.

3. Mares that have suffered injuries or tears at previous foalings should have professional assistance to prevent or minimize trauma at foaling.

4. Gestations prolonged beyond 365 days and associated with a very large fetus require careful supervision. (Note: Many mares that carry beyond 365 days will produce a foal of normal or even small size, and these mares usually do not require veterinary assistance.)

5. Impending rupture of the prepubic tendon due to prolonged, excessive ventral edema or hydrops of the amnion.

6. Mares that have produced icteric foals (neonatal isoerythrolysis) can be induced at term to prevent ingestion of colostrum prior to checking it for compatibility with the newborn foal's blood.

7. Loss of colostrum (this is better handled by milking the mare and freezing the colostrum).

8. Injuries, arthritis, or other painful skeletal diseases that may become aggravated in late pregnancy.

9. Induced parturition can also be used to provide a nurse mare for a valuable orphan foal, a foal whose dam fails to lactate, or a foal rejected by its dam.

MANAGERIAL INDICATIONS

Convenience. When a mare has a history of foaling problems and it is anticipated that veterinary assistance will be necessary, it is desirable to schedule the foaling during the day at a time convenient for the veterinarian and the farm management.

Economic Considerations. Most mares foal at night, so scheduling an induced foaling during the day, in addition to being more convenient, eliminates the expense of emergency night calls and false alarms. It also reduces the need and expense of prolonged night watches.

438

TEACHING

Scheduling an induced foaling enables a large group of veterinary or animal husbandry students to observe the entire procedure from examination and preparation of the mare through the actual stages of foaling, including postpartum care of the mare and foal.

RESEARCH

Induction of parturition enables researchers to obtain colostrum-deprived foals when studying the effects of various diseases and vaccines.

Induced parturition has assisted in behavioral studies of the mare and foal during and immediately after foaling, in studies of neonatal physiology, and in the evaluation of hormonal changes in the mare and foal at parturition.

INDUCTION CRITERIA

The criteria used to select the proper time for induction include (1) length of gestation, (2) udder enlargement with the presence of milk, (3) relaxation of the sacrosciatic ligaments, and (4) cervical softening.

Length of Gestation. It is essential that induction take place only after a gestation period of sufficient length (a minimum of 330 days) to ensure the necessary fetal maturity for successful adaptation to the extrauterine environment. Normal gestation in the mare covers a wide range from 320 to 360 days or more. Experienced equine practitioners and researchers recommend a minimum of 330 days' gestation to ensure adequate fetal maturity at the time of induction.

Udder Enlargement with the Presence of Milk. Mammary development begins approximately four weeks prior to parturition and gradually increases to reach a maximal size at the time of foaling. The teats become distended just a few hours prior to foaling. The udder secretion at first is scant, thick, sticky, and of amber color. As foaling becomes imminent, the quantity increases, the viscosity decreases, and the color changes to gray or yellow-white. The udder is judged acceptable for induction to begin when it is enlarged and the teats are distended with an ample supply of smokey gray to yellow-white colostrum. The presence of a sufficient supply of colostrum in the udder is the most important indication of sufficient fetal maturity for induction to be carried out.

Relaxation of the Sacrosciatic Ligaments. Sufficient relaxation of the sacrosciatic ligaments is indicated by a softening on either side of the tail-head. Maximal relaxation at foaling is accompanied by relaxation and lengthening of the vulva just prior to foaling.

Cervical Relaxation. The degree of cervical relaxation is determined by gentle vaginal examination after the previously listed criteria have been carefully checked. After wrapping the tail and thoroughly cleaning the vulva with a disinfectant soap, a well-lubricated, gloved hand is inserted into the vagina to locate the cervix and determine the degree of relaxation. A mare that is eligible for induction must have a soft, easily compressed cervix or a cervix that is starting to dilate. It is not necessary to penetrate the cervix to determine the extent of relaxation. Careful palpation through the vaginal wall will enable the clinician to determine the position of the fetus.

METHODS OF INDUCTION

OXYTOCIN

Oxytocin was the agent used in the first report of induced parturition in mares and is still used by more practitioners than other agents. Many trials and extensive use by brood mare veterinarians have confirmed that this agent, when used on properly evaluated mares, is rapid and safe to both the mare and the foal. The oxytocin has been administered intramuscularly in doses ranging from 20 to 150 IU. Our trials indicate a direct relationship between the dose and the time of appearance and degree of expression of foaling signs. The 20 IU dose results in a slower, quieter foaling, whereas doses of greater than 100 IU result in the rapid completion of a more active foaling. Trials using graded doses revealed that 40 to 60 IU of oxytocin given intramuscularly will result in a quiet, safe foaling that will be completed in less than one hour. Recently published data indicate that smaller doses (2.5 to 10 IU) administered intravenously either over a 15-minute infusion or as a bolus are sufficient to induce foaling in pony mares. It was proposed that the smaller doses were more physiologic, but an intravenous dose for full-sized horses has not been worked out.

Approximately 10 minutes after the intramuscular injection of 40 to 60 IU of oxytocin, the signs of parturition commence with frequent passage of small amounts of feces. At 15 minutes postinjection, sweating appears on the neck and gradually spreads over the shoulders. By 20 minutes the mare appears slightly anxious, switches her tail, drips milk, and begins to quietly walk around the stall. Usually by

20 to 25 minutes, the mare lies down and straining begins. If the fetal membranes are not observed at the vulva by 30 minutes, a clean, careful vaginal examination is performed to confirm the proper position of the fetus. Correction of any malpresentation is easily accomplished at this time. Should the red, velvetlike chorioallantois with the cervical star be presented at the vulva, it is opened within the vagina to allow passage of the amnion and foal. Failure to do this will allow premature placental separation and can result in a mildly to severely hypoxic foal. This progression of events at induced foaling precisely mimics natural foalings. Retention of the fetal membranes beyond three hours after foaling has not been observed in most trials, and fertility following oxytocin inductions is not impaired.

Aftercare of the mare and foal has a vital role in ensuring the successful outcome of any foaling, but it takes on extra importance following induction, since any problems that develop are invariably attributed to this technique. With this in mind, the entire induction process should be accomplished in as quiet and unobstrusive a manner as possible. After the second stage of labor is completed and a check has made to ensure that the foal is breathing normally and that its head is free of the amnion, the mare and foal are allowed to lie quietly with the umbilical vessels intact for several minutes. This minimizes loss of placental-fetal blood and results in stronger, more vigorous foals. Once the mare stands and the umbilical cord has separated, the foal's navel should be dipped in mild iodine solution, or an antibiotic powder is applied. A warm, gentle enema should be administered to enhance passage of the meconium. Whenever a foaling is induced, we make it a practice to milk 300 to 500 ml of colostrum from the mare and administer it to the foal using a well-lubricated soft rubber stallion catheter passed through the nose into the stomach. This ensures the presence of an ample supply of colostrum in the foal's digestive tract at the time of maximal immunoglobulin absorption. We have not found it necessary to administer prophylactic antibiotics following most inductions, but do not hesitate to do so if there is any indication of infection (weak, listless foal; evidence of fetal diarrhea; or passage of a heavy, inflamed placenta). Problems with weak, immature foals have been reported when parturition is induced prior to meeting the preinduction criteria and serve to emphasize the need for strict adherence to these guidelines.

Early studies occasionally utilized estrogen to relax the cervix prior to induction with oxytocin. The dose of diethylstilbestrol varied from 12 to 30 mg and was administered 8 to 12 hours prior to the oxytocin injection. Further trials have shown that the exogenous estrogen is not indicated, as relaxation of the cervix is a valuable guide to the proper time for induction.

CORTICOSTEROIDS

While glucocorticoids have been shown to induce parturition in the ewe, sow, cow, and rabbit when administered late in pregnancy, initial trials with horses were uniformly unsuccessful. Later trials using massive doses of dexamethasone (100 mg per day) starting at 321 days of pregnancy for a four-day treatment schedule have resulted in induced foalings from 6½ to 7 days after starting the injections. Resulting foals were small and weak but were healthy and grew at a normal rate. The necessity of repeated dosing and the delay in completion of foaling have combined to deter acceptance of this technique by clinicians.

PROSTAGLANDINS

Prostaglandin has been successfully used to induce foaling in mares prior to development of signs of imminent parturition. The gestation length of these mares ranged from 325 to 367 days, but vaginal examination revealed pale, dry mucous membranes with contracted cervices containing thick tenacious mucous plugs. These mares were treated with flumethasone (10 to 15 mg) and stilbestrol (30 mg) 24 hours prior to receiving the prostaglandin (10 mg). Several mares received an additional 5 mg flumethasone 12 hours after the initial treatment. All mares receiving the two doses of flumethasone foaled within three hours of treatment with prostaglandin. Of five mares receiving a single dose of flumethasone, two foaled within three hours of the administration of the prostaglandin, and the remaining three foaled within three hours of a second injection of prostaglandin (7.5 mg) given three hours after the first one. In all cases, foaling was uneventful, and placental expulsion occurred within an hour.

Fluprostenol, a synthetic prostaglandin analogue, has also been used to induce foaling in mares not showing signs of imminent foaling. Pony mares received 250 μg, while full-sized mares received 1000 μg intramuscularly. All the mares showed first-stage labor (uneasiness, sweating, and mild abdominal discomfort) within 30 minutes. The onset of second-stage labor varied from ½ hour to 3 hours and lasted for 5 to 33 minutes. All foals but one were presented in a normal position. The one dystocia was due to inadequate cervical dilatation. The fetal membranes were expelled within two hours in each case. Of 17 foals from fluprostenol inductions, 13 were judged to be normal and healthy during the adaptive period. One foal was weak initially but improved and developed normally. Two foals suffered fractured ribs; one responded to establish normal behavior at four days of age, whereas one had to be destroyed because of resultant cardiac damage. One foal died during delivery by cesarean section, which was necessary because of failure of the cervix to dilate. These workers described two patterns of response to the fluprostenol injection. In mares that foaled within 90 minutes, prostaglandin levels rose soon after injection and peaked during the maximal expulsive stage of labor, resembling events during natural foaling. In mares that took more than 90 minutes to foal, prostaglandin levels rose at various times after injections and peaked well before the onset of the expulsive stage of labor. They suggested that these differences reflected the hormonal readiness of the mares to foal.

The published reports of fluprostenol inductions utilized mares with varying degrees of mammary development prior to cervical relaxation. While it would be convenient to be able to induce parturition without waiting for mares to meet all the preinduction criteria, it is important for the survival of the foals that they not be induced prematurely. Inasmuch as successful inductions have been accomplished in most cases prior to meeting all the criteria, fluprostenol injections might even be more successful once these criteria were satisfied. Further studies are required before routine applications of this technique can be recommended.

ELECTIVE ABORTION

INDICATIONS

The indications for elective abortion are (1) mismating, (2) purchase of a supposedly open performance mare that is discovered to be pregnant, and (3) twin pregnancy.

TECHNIQUES

Intrauterine Infusions. Intrauterine infusion with saline, antibiotic solution, or a mild iodine solution has been utilized very successfully for many years. The technique involves carefully cleaning the mare, performing a vaginal examination, and, by gentle digital pressure, dilating the cervix. A catheter is then passed into the uterus, and 500 to 1000 ml of solution is infused. Abortion usually occurs within 48 hours. It is best to wait at least one week after breeding to ensure the presence of the embryo within the uterus. If the mare is to be rebred in the same season, it is equally important that the intra-uterine flush be accomplished before 35 days to prevent the formation of the endometrial cups. Once these structures form, even if the embryo is removed, the mare usually does not return to estrus until the cups are rejected by the uterine tissue at about 120 days.

Treatment with Prostaglandins. If prostaglandin is administered after formation of a mature corpus luteum (five days after ovulation) and before the formation of endometrial cups (35 days), a single injection of prostaglandin or its analogue will cause lysis of the CL, loss of the pregnancy, and a return of the mare to estrus. If prostaglandin is used after the formation of the endometrial cups, it must be administered repeatedly to ensure success in terminating pregnancy. Treatment with prostaglandin at daily intervals for four days starting on day 70 produced abortion in all mares tested, whereas a single dose at day 70 and one repeated on day 77 did not produce abortion in any mares tested. The time of abortion following daily treatment did not differ significantly from the time of abortion following injections given every 12 hours, and fewer treatments were required. Mares aborted after 40 days did not return to estrus until the endometrial cups ceased functioning. This emphasizes the fact that if one hopes to rebreed a mare in the same year as the mismating occurred, the abortion should be performed prior to the formation of endometrial cups between days 35 and 40, or return to estrus may be delayed beyond 120 days.

Twin Pregnancy. Mares carrying twins usually abort from mid to late pregnancy when rebreeding is no longer feasible. The few mares that carry twins to term usually produce small, weak foals that fail to grow or perform well and therefore cannot be marketed profitably. For these reasons, when twin pregnancies are diagnosed early, many people elect to induce abortion in an effort to get the mare rebred and pregnant with a single fetus. Either of the previously described techniques can be used to terminate the pregnancy. Another option practiced by some brood mare veterinarians is to crush one embryonic vesicle in hopes that the remaining vesicle will survive and produce a single healthy foal. In this technique, a rectal examination is performed, the portion of the uterus containing one vesicle is cupped in the hand, and gentle pressure is applied by closing the fingers until the vesicle is felt to "pop." Some practitioners report this technique to be successful about 50 per cent of the time. Again, this technique is best applied prior to 35 days of gestation so that in case both pregnancies are lost, the mare will begin to cycle and can be rebred.

Elective abortion of mares after four months of gestation is usually contraindicated owing to complications that may arise due to the large size of the fetus. Once the placenta has taken over the role of supplying the hormones necessary to maintain pregnancy, prostaglandins have been ineffective in precipitating abortion. In one instance, daily dosing with prostaglandin for 10 consecutive days failed to abort two mares that were $6\frac{1}{2}$ months pregnant.

Supplemental Readings

1. Adams, W. M., and Wagner, W. C.: The role of corticosteroids in parturition. Biol. Reprod., 3:223, 1970.
2. Alm, C. C., Sullivan, J. J., and First, N. L.: Induction of premature parturition by parenteral administration of dexamethasone in the mare. J. Am. Vet. Med. Assoc., 165:721. 1974.
3. Burns, S. J.: Clinical safety of dexamethasone in mares during pregnancy. Equine Vet. J., 5:91, 1973.
4. Cooper, W. L.: Clinical aspects of prostaglandins in equine reproduction. Proc. Second Equine Pharmacology Symposium, 1978, p. 225.
5. Douglas, R. H., Squires, E. L., and Ginther, O. J.: Induction of abortion in mares with prostaglandin $F_{2\alpha}$. J. Anim. Sci., 39:404, 1974.
6. First, N. L., and Alm, C. C.: Dexamathasone-induced parturition in pony mares. J. Anim. Sci., 44:1072, 1977.
7. Hillman, R. B.: Induction of parturition in mares. J. Reprod. Fertil. Suppl., 23:641, 1975.
8. Hillman, R. B., and Ganjam, V. K.: Hormonal changes in the mare and foal associated with oxytocin induction of parturition. J. Reprod. Fertil. Suppl., 27:541, 1979.
9. Jeffcott, L. B., and Rossdale, P. D.: A critical review of current methods of induction of parturition in the mare. Equine Vet. J., 9:208, 1977.
10. Kooistra, L. H., and Ginther, O. J.: Termination of pseudopregnancy by administration of prostaglandin $F_{2\alpha}$ and termination of early pregnancy by administration of prostaglandin $F_{2\alpha}$ or colchicine or by removal of the embryo in mares. Am. J. Vet. Res., 37:35, 1976.
11. Lovell, J. D., Stabenfeldt, G. H., Hughes, J. P., and Evans, J. W.: Endocrine patterns of the mare at term. J. Reprod. Fertil. Suppl., 23:449, 1975.
12. Nathanielsz, P. W., Rossdale, P. D., Silver, M., and Comline, R. S.: Studies on fetal neonatal and maternal cortisol metabolism in the mare. J. Reprod. Fertil. Suppl., 23:625, 1975.
13. Pashen, R. L.: Low doses of oxytocin can induce foaling at term. Equine Vet. J., 12:85, 1980.
14. Purvis, A. D.: Elective induction of labor and parturition in the mare. Proc. 18th Annu. Conv. Am. Assoc. Eq. Pract., 1972, p. 113.
15. Purvis, A. D.: The induction of labor in mares as a routine breeding farm procedure. Proc. 23rd Annu. Conv. Am. Assoc. Eq. Pract., 1977, p. 145.
16. Rossdale, P. D., and Jeffcott, L. B.: Problems encountered during induced foaling in pony mares. Vet. Rec., 97:371, 1975.
17. Rossdale, P. D., Jeffcott, L. B., and Allen, W. R.: Foaling induced by a synthetic prostaglandin analogue (fluprostenol). Vet. Rec., 99:26, 1976.
18. Rossdale, P. D., and Mahaffey, L. W.: Parturition in the Thoroughbred mare with particular reference to blood deprivation in the new-born. Vet. Rec., 70:142, 1958.
19. Rossdale, P. D., Pashen, R. L., and Jeffcott, L. B.: The use of synthetic prostaglandin analogue (fluprostenol) to induce foaling. J. Reprod. Fertil. Suppl., 27:521, 1979.
20. Squires, E. L., Hillman, R. B., Pickett, B. W., and Nett, T. M.: Induction of abortion in mares with equimate: Effects on secretion of progesterone, PMSG and reproductive performance. J. Anim. Sci., 50:490, 1980.
21. Van Niekerk, C. H., and Morgenthal, J. C.: Plasma progesterone and oestrogen concentrations during induction of parturition in mares with flumethasone and prostaglandin. Proc. International Congress for Animal Reproduction and Artificial Insemination, 3:386, 1976.

EVALUATION OF STALLION FERTILITY

John P. Hurtgen, KENNETT SQUARE, PENNSYLVANIA

The purpose of a fertility evaluation of a stallion is to assess his libido, mating ability, and the quality of ejaculated semen. Fertility evaluation may be indicated before or after the purchase of a proven or unproven stallion or in the stallion with known or suspected infertility.

The best measure of a horse's fertility is the foaling rate achieved when bred to a large number of mares managed and serviced under recommended conditions. However, it is advisable to evaluate stallions before the onset of their first breeding season. No single test of semen quality or physical characteristic of the horse is highly correlated with stallion fertility. Therefore, a series of observations and tests on the stallion's libido, mating behavior, genitalia, and semen are used to arrive at a best estimate of prospective fertility or to diagnose a case of known infertility.

THE EXAMINATION

Identification. The horse to be evaluated should be identified by name, color and markings, and tattoo number. Identification becomes an important aspect of the examination if the horse is to be examined at a later date.

History. A complete history should be obtained, including the animal's age, prior usage such as breeding, racing, or performance showing, and frequency of ejaculation. A detailed history of services during the week prior to evaluation should be recorded. Severity and duration of prior illness or injury, prior medication history with particular reference to adrenal and anabolic steroids and gonadotropins, vaccinations, present or prior level of fertility, and previous fertility evaluation findings should be noted. Many of the preceding factors have a marked influence on libido and semen quality.

Physical Examination. General body health and condition are noted, as they may be reflective of management conditions. Breeding stallions should not be blind, severely lame, or have conditions known or suspected of being heritable such as wobbler syndrome, umbilical hernia, cryptorchidism, parrot mouth, and others. A known history of these diseases along with evidence of combined immunodeficiency syndrome or other defects in offspring of the stallion should also be recorded.

SEMEN COLLECTION

A suitable mount is the first consideration in the collection of semen. A mare in estrus that is receptive to the stallion is most satisfactory. Some stallions will ejaculate while mounted on a phantom or "dummy" mare. However, most young stallions require training to readily or predictably mount the phantom. An ovariectomized mare may also be used as a mount animal. Injection of the ovariectomized mare with 1 to 2 mg of estradiol one to two days prior to use usually induces a receptive state.

The tail of the mount mare is then wrapped with gauze or placed in a clean plastic bag or sleeve and fastened with tape. The perineal region of the mare is prepared by washing the area with a mild soap or disinfectant, followed by thorough rinsing. The mare is restrained with a twitch or is hobbled.

The Artificial Vagina. The use of an artificial vagina (AV) is the most common method of semen collection from the stallion. Numerous models of equine artificial vaginas are available. The three most common types used are the Missouri,* Japanese,† and Colorado‡ models. The Missouri model AV is the most commonly used in the United States. It consists of a double rubber liner and single rubber collection cone to which a collection vessel can be attached. Internal temperature and pressure of the AV are adjusted by adding warm water between the double liner via a valve stem. The AV is held by leather casing. The Japanese model AV consists of an outer aluminum casing and inner rubber liner.

A sponge rubber ring can be placed inside the AV casing to assist in applying pressure to the glans penis during ejaculation. A solid handle is mounted on the aluminum casing. A collection bag is attached to one end of the AV. Warm water is added to the space between the aluminum casing and rubber liner via a valve opening. The Colorado model AV is larger in diameter and longer than the previous two AVs. It consists of a plastic outer casing to which two inner rubber liners are attached. The innermost liner has a tapered end to which a collection vessel is attached. Warm water is placed between the plastic casing and the outermost rubber liner. It takes longer for the internal temperature to equilibrate in this AV than in the Missouri or Japanese models, but the Colorado model AV tends to maintain internal heat longer than the other two models. It is also much heavier when completely assembled and is held by an outer leather casing. With any AV, the collection vessel should be covered with an insulating hood when semen is collected in an adverse environment.

At the time of semen collection, the internal temperature of the AV should be 44 to 48° C, although many stallions will ejaculate over a wider range of AV temperatures. Warm water at 50° C or above, depending on the type of AV used, is added to the AV water jacket. A dial thermometer is placed inside the AV until the artificial vagina has equilibrated at the desired temperature. If the internal temperature of the AV is above 50° C, damage to sperm may result.

Just before usage, a small amount of a sterile lubricating jelly*† is placed on a plastic disposable sleeve or glass rod and is used to lubricate the rubber liner. Lubricants containing disinfectants or substances that are detrimental to spermatozoa should not be used. The plastic sleeve can be draped over the end of the AV to prevent entry of dust or drying of the jelly prior to semen collection. The semen collection vessel is prewarmed prior to semen collection.

The Condom. Although a representative ejaculate can be collected using a condom‡ or breeder's bag, it is not commonly used. Problems encountered with the use of a condom for semen collection from the stallion may include loss of semen from the condom, the need for the stallion to enter the mare, difficulty of intromission by some stallions, and loss of the condom from the penis before or after semen collection. However, the use of a condom to collect semen from stallions with certain mating or ejaculatory disturbances has been invaluable (p. 449).

---

*Equine Artificial Vagina, NASCO, Fort Atkinson, WI
†Japanese Aluminum Vagina, Scott Medical Supply, Hayward, CA
‡Colorado Artificial Vagina, Lane Manufacturing Co., Denver, CO

*K-Y Lubricating Jelly (sterile), Johnson and Johnson Co., New Brunswick, NJ
†Vaseline Pure Petroleum Jelly, Cheesebrough Ponds, Inc., Greenwich, CT
‡Equine Condom, Jorgenson Labs, Loveland, CO

The Dismount Sample. Collection of a dismount sample for the evaluation of stallion fertility is not recommended. This practice always results in the collection of a sample that is not representative of the whole ejaculate and requires intromission to occur. The dismount sample is obtained by collecting the seminal drippings from the urethra following ejaculation. This practice, however, is commonly performed on farms to determine that ejaculation of spermatozoa has occurred or to monitor the presence or absence of blood in an ejaculate. The absence of blood cells in the dismount sample does not ensure the clinician that hemospermia has not occurred.

Preparation of the Stallion. Clean, warm (40 to 42° C) water should be used for washing the stallion. Disposable plastic bags may be used as liners for buckets. Clean paper towels or cotton are used along with a mild disinfectant or nonirritating, nonresidual soap.

The stallion is allowed to tease an estrous mare at a tease rail or in a chute until an erection is attained. The penis is then grasped and washed until the smegma and dirt have been removed. Particular attention is given to cleansing the fossa glandis that surrounds the urethra. The penis is rinsed with copious amounts of clean, warm water and is then dried with a towel.

Manipulation of the glans penis usually causes the stallion to emit preejaculatory fluid, which will cleanse the urethra. A sterile swab is then inserted into the urethra of the stallion's erect penis. The swab is used to inoculate culture media to determine the bacteriologic status of the urethra and internal genitalia. A second urethral swabbing will be taken following ejaculation. The prepuce, penis, and urethral process are closely observed for evidence of injury or abnormalities during the teasing and washing procedures.

Semen Collection. Semen should be collected in an open area to provide safety to all individuals involved and solid footing to the mare, stallion, and collector. After the mount mare has been adequately prepared and restrained for semen collection, the stallion is exposed to the mare. The stallion is allowed to mount the mare from the rear or slightly to the left side of the mare after attaining full penile erection. The mare handler, stallion handler, and collector are on the left side of the mount to provide optimal movement and safety to each of the individuals involved in the procedure. After the stallion has mounted, the penis is deflected away from the buttocks of the mare to prevent contamination of the penis and to allow some of the preejaculatory secretions to wash out the urethra. The penis is directed into the AV. The AV is held at about a 30° angle above the horizontal. The AV can be stabilized against the mare's flank to maintain its proper positioning. When intromission occurs and the stallion begins thrusting, the collector should place one or two fingers on the ventral base of the penis to feel the urethral pulsations that usually accompany ejaculation. Usually, three to nine strong, rhythmic pulsations accompany ejaculation. After the onset of ejaculation, the anterior end of the AV is lowered to allow semen to enter the collection vessel. After ejaculation, the stallion dismounts. The artificial vagina should be handed to an assistant. The base of the penis is immediately grasped and held with an encircling grip. This will keep the glans penis engorged. A sterile swab is inserted into the dilated urethra. Again, suitable culture media is inoculated using this swab specimen. The penis, urethral process, distal urethra, and fossa glandis are again observed for evidence of injury, irritation, or other abnormalities.

The artificial vagina is taken to the laboratory. About 50 per cent of the water is poured out of the AV liner so that any remaining semen can flow into the collection vessel. The collection vessel is removed and is placed in an incubator or under a warmed hood. If the AV is equipped with a gel filter, it should be removed immediately, as gel will tend to migrate through the filter. If the semen was not filtered during collection and the sample contains gel, it should be aspirated from the semen using a syringe. With this technique, the tip of a syringe is touched to the coagulated gel that can be visualized through the collection vessel. Once aspiration of the gel has commenced, the syringe is raised out of the semen and aspiration is continued. Only if gel or large particles of dirt or debris remain in the semen should it be filtered again at this point. Filtration removes a significant number of sperm cells from the semen sample.

Evaluation of Semen. Because no single test of semen or sperm quality is highly correlated with intrinsic fertility, a series of tests is performed. Although the correlation of some parameters of semen quality with fertility has not been well documented, most appear to have some relationship to fertility. Certain examination procedures are conducted routinely on all stallions presented for fertility or breeding soundness examination. However, the clinician should be aware of additional tests of semen quality that may be performed when presented with stallions with special problems.

It is important that the laboratory be properly prepared before semen is collected. This means that a warming plate or incubator is adjusted to 35 to 37° C and that sufficient glass slides, coverslips, stain, calibrated glass or plastic ware, and seminal extender are available and warm. All materials that contact semen should be warm and chemically clean. A light or phase contrast microscope should be available and equipped with $4\times$ or $10\times$, $40\times$, and oil immersion ($100\times$) objectives.

MOTILITY. The motility of spermatozoa in raw

semen should be estimated promptly after semen collection. It is usually recommended that the total percentage of motile sperm and the incidence of progressively motile spermatozoa be estimated and recorded. Motility estimates are made after a drop of semen has been placed on a warm glass slide. The drop is then covered with a coverslip and is viewed under 40, 100, or 400× magnification. While viewing the raw semen sample for motility, special notes should be made of the presence of white blood cells, red blood cells, and spermatocytes. These cell types may not be visible when semen smears are made with certain stains.

Motility may be adversely affected by the presence of gel, debris, soap, water, urine, bacterial toxins, or blood. Additionally, sperm cells tend to adhere to the glass surfaces of the slide or coverslip. Rapid changes in temperature are also detrimental to sperm cell motility. This is especially apparent if the small drop is exposed to a cold slide. Some stallions occasionally, or even consistently, produce semen that is characterized by agglutination of sperm cells. The correlation of sperm cell agglutination to stallion fertility is not clear. Because many factors may aid in the agglutination of sperm cells, such as the presence of gel, debris, or blood, these potential causes should be eliminated. Dilution of semen with an extender usually decreases the degree of agglutination.

The longevity of motility in raw and extended semen samples is also a useful test in evaluating semen quality, particularly in some infertile stallions. Aliquots of semen are placed in plastic tubes that are capped and free of air. Semen is incubated at 22° C in a dark and draft-free area. Motility is estimated at one- to two-hour intervals until progressive motility falls to less than 10 per cent. The results of this test can be influenced by the use of seminal extenders which may enhance or adversely affect sperm cell motility. Additionally, the spermatozoa of individual stallions may respond differently to a seemingly "acceptable" extender.

pH. If the pH of semen is to be measured, it should be measured using a pH meter immediately after collection. The use of pH paper is too inaccurate to be of value. The pH of normal semen is 7.35 to 7.7. Seminal pH may be elevated in semen from stallions in which the ampullae fail to empty. Presence of urine in semen or inflammation of the internal genitalia will also usually elevate seminal pH. Seminal color and odor or determination of seminal plasma creatinine or urea nitrogen concentrations are also useful in determining whether there is urine in semen.

SPERM CELL MORPHOLOGY. Though many stains can be used for stallion sperm (hematoxylin and eosin [H & E], Williams', eosin nigrosin, Cassarett's, India ink, and others), all have limitations. The Williams', Cassarett's and H & E stains require

special laboratory assistance for staining, and there is a delay in receiving the finished smears for interpretation. Smears made with India ink are of poor quality and should not be used for stallion spermatozoa. Eosin nigrosin–stained smears are quickly prepared and can be interpreted immediately. However, white blood cells and spermatocytes cannot be identified using the eosin nigrosin background stain. It is suggested that eosin nigrosin be used to prepare two or three smears from each ejaculate. An additional one or two unstained smears of raw semen are made for subsequent staining with H & E, if indicated. Be sure to identify each slide with the animal's name, ejaculate number, and date of collection. Cells are viewed at 1000× magnification using an oil immersion objective.

The eosin nigrosin–stained smear is prepared by placing a very small drop of stain on a warm slide. A small drop of semen is then added to the stain and gently mixed with it. The edge of a second warm slide is used to draw the stain-semen droplet across the slide to form a film. The smear should be quickly dried on a warm surface. A smear of raw semen is prepared in the same manner but without addition of stain.

Preparation of smears on slides incubated at less than 35° C, delay in preparation of smears, and staining itself will cause varying degrees of damage to spermatozoa. Damage to the sperm cell acrosome, including complete loss of the acrosome, and damage to the midpiece segment are the most commonly induced artifacts of sperm on stained smears. In order to obtain more repeatable and accurate sperm cell morphology counts that are virtually free of the artifacts observed in stained smears, four to six drops of raw semen may be fixed in 2 ml of buffered formol saline or buffered glutaraldehyde. These samples are usually viewed as a wet mount preparation using phase contrast microscopy. This appears to be a superior method of evaluating acrosomal integrity and differentiating among proximal droplets, abnormal midpiece segments, and artifactual midpiece alterations.

CONCENTRATION. The concentration of spermatozoa is usually determined using a spectrophotometer after a standard curve has been developed or with a hemocytometer. In the spectrophotometric method, the percentage transmittance of formol saline–diluted stallion semen is usually performed at dilutions of 1:10 or 1:20 and a wavelength of 525 mμ. The hemocytometer should be used for samples with very low concentrations of spermatozoa or in samples containing a high incidence of non–sperm cells or debris.

The hemocytometer method of determining sperm concentration is done using formol saline–diluted raw semen at a dilution ratio ranging from 1:20 to 1:100. A red blood cell dilution pipette is most commonly used. Commercially available diluting systems used for determining white or red blood cell concentrations in blood are also useful for dilution of semen.* Final concentration of spermatozoa in semen is calculated by accounting for dilution factors and volume of the sample over the hemocytometer grid that is counted. The concentration of spermatozoa in semen should be recorded in units of spermatozoa per milliliter of semen.

VOLUME. The volume of gel-free semen is recorded. The presence and volume of the gel fraction in semen should also be recorded.

TOTAL NUMBER OF SPERM CELLS PER EJACULATE. The total number of sperm cells in the ejaculate is determined by multiplying the volume of gel-free semen by the concentration of spermatozoa.

COLOR. Seminal color should be noted and recorded. The color of normal stallion semen ranges from opalescent to slightly milky. This color range is reflective of sperm cell concentration. Even in very concentrated samples, stallion semen should not have a granular appearance. Gel-free semen that is watery, pink, red, amber, or brown in color or granular in appearance should be viewed with suspicion. The cause of these qualitative changes in semen should be determined.

The color of the gel fraction of semen should also be noted. The color and physical characteristics of the gel are occasionally altered in stallions with inflammation of the internal genitalia.

Examination of the Genitalia. Though examination of the external and internal genitalia may be performed prior to semen collection, most stallions are more tractable after semen collection, and the physical examination is less likely to interfere with breeding performance of inexperienced stallions or stallions with behavioral problems.

The stallion's penis, prepuce, urethral process and fossa glandis have been carefully examined during washing of the stallion and semen collection. The testicles and epididymides are palpated for their presence, location, size, consistency, and shape. The length, width, and height of each testicle is measured using calipers. When the testes are held in the ventral aspect of the scrotal sac, the total width of the scrotum and testicles is determined. The head, body, and tail of each epididymis is examined as thoroughly as is practical. Specific measurements of these parts is usually not made.

The internal genitalia are examined per rectum. Using the pelvic urethra as a landmark, the vesicular glands and ampullae are located. The presence, size, and consistency of these internal genital organs are noted. The bulbourethral glands cannot be identified per rectum. The vasa deferentia are often difficult to examine in their entirety from the ampullae to the internal inguinal rings. The degree of patency of the internal inguinal rings is noted. Examination of the internal genitalia has been of great diagnostic value in selected cases of stallion infertility. The internal genitalia of stallions should not be examined unless adequate restraint facilities are available.

INTERPRETATION OF EXAMINATION FINDINGS

Although lower foaling rates are frequently accepted in the horse breeding industry, highly fertile stallions repeatedly achieve foaling rates of 80 per cent or more when bred to reproductively healthy mares under good management conditions. Because foaling rates are determined by the percentage of mares that deliver foals following service during an entire breeding season, it is obvious that a given stallion's fertility may be highly influenced by management factors such as the number of cycles in which mares are serviced. Additionally, stallions with a large book may be limited to servicing each mare too infrequently for maximal fertility. Management factors relating to breeding mares must be considered in any potential stallion fertility assessment. In this respect, a stallion's libido toward estrous mares, behavior toward handlers and mares, mounting ability, and efficiency of ejaculation become very important aspects of the breeding soundness evaluation of stallions. These components of stallion fertility are difficult to assess on a single examination of the stallion in a given environment. However, obvious deviations from normal should be considered. It may be necessary to evaluate a horse repeatedly over a period of time and under a variety of circumstances to arrive at an accurate assessment of the problem. If stallions are evaluated sufficiently in advance of the breeding season, these behavioral or mating problems can usually be overcome so that the ensuing breeding season is not partially or totally lost.

Tests of Semen Quality. Ideally, it is hoped that tests of semen quality would reflect the intrinsic fertility of a stallion or the effects of reproductive tract disease and, therefore, would be good predictors of fertility. However, many factors influence the results of semen quality tests. Factors influencing these test results include age of the stallion, use of exogenous hormones and drugs, frequency of ejaculation, and such semen handling factors as method of staining, interval from semen collection to evaluation, type of extender used, method of semen collection, and experience of the examiner.

The relationship between tests of semen quality and fertility is further complicated by intended frequency of stallion use, method of breeding, time lag

---

*Unopette Test 5851 or Unopette Test 5855, Becton-Dickinson, Rutherford, NJ

between stallion evaluation and the actual breeding season, breeding hygiene, reproductive health of mares bred to the stallion, and others. It is for these reasons that the evaluation of stallions must be performed in a systematic and thorough manner.

TOTAL SPERM NUMBER PER EJACULATE AND TESTICULAR SIZE. Daily sperm output for normal stallions averages 4×10^9 sperm cells in young stallions and 6×10^9 sperm cells in mature stallions. There is a direct correlation between testicular size and daily sperm cell output. The dimensions of the testes of normal stallions are approximately 9 to 10 cm in length, 5 to 6 cm in width, and 5 to 6.5 cm in height. Total scrotal width should be greater than 10 cm in mature stallions. To accurately estimate daily sperm cell output by a stallion, it is probably necessary to collect one ejaculate per day for seven days. Daily sperm cell output is then determined during the subsequent seven-day period. This becomes impractical under most circumstances.

Stallions in regular usage (three to seven ejaculates per week) that ejaculate fewer than 3×10^9 spermatozoa per day should be viewed with suspicion. In other words, a reason for the below average number of sperm cells should be determined. Common causes of low numbers of sperm cells per ejaculate include small testes, testicular degeneration, overuse, incomplete ejaculation, and administration of exogenous hormones or other drugs to stallions. If inadequate numbers of spermatozoa are collected during the nonbreeding season, it is suggested that the horse be reevaluated during the breeding season.

Of special note is the number of spermatozoa ejaculated by stallions recently retired from racing or performance training and presented for prepurchase or breeding soundness evaluation. The effects of racing or performance and their associated stresses of transportation, housing, and training on semen quality is unknown. However, the administration of oral and systemic compounds, including hormones, is common. It is known that exogenously administered testosterone, estrogen, and certain anabolic steroids decrease sperm output and testicular size in stallions. The effects of the majority of compounds administered to racehorses on semen quality and prospective fertility are unknown. The effects of dosage and frequency of administration of these compounds on semen quality are likewise unknown. Clinical experience suggests that the interval from withdrawal of these compounds to the onset of normal semen quality varies tremendously among stallions. This effect is probably related to the drug or combination of drugs administered, sequence of drug combinations, dosage, frequency of administration, age at which use of these compounds was initiated, and innate stallion differences. The clinician needs to be extremely cautious in the evalua-

tion of these horses because conditions such as testicular hypoplasia or chronic degenerative atrophy present a similar semen quality.

MOTILITY. Using the suggested method of evaluating sperm motility, it is important to remember that the motility value recorded is an estimate. Motility is frequently lower in sexually rested stallions compared to the same stallions in regular breeding usage. The spermatozoa of some stallions have a tendency to agglutinate. The cause of this phenomenon or its influence on fertility is not known. However, estimates of progressive motility are likely to be decreased. In general, temperature shock of semen will depress sperm motility. As the incidence of sperm tail defects increases, progressive motility decreases. There is considerable variation in motility estimates from one examiner to another and with the same examiner. Therefore, it should not be surprising that the correlation between sperm motility and fertility would be low. The motility of spermatozoa in second ejaculates is usually the same or higher than in first ejaculates.

Fertile stallions should ejaculate semen in which 50 per cent or more of spermatozoa are progressively motile. It is also expected that at least 10 per cent of spermatozoa from stallions in regular usage should remain progressively motile for six or more hours after collection when stored in a dark, draft-free environment at room temperature. Stallions whose sperm exhibit less than 50 per cent progressive motility in raw semen or that have less than 10 per cent progressively motile sperm two hours after semen collection should be suspected of having potential infertility problems.

pH. The pH of normal stallion semen ranges from 7.35 to 7.7 A pH value above 7.7 may be suggestive of ejaculatory failure, incomplete ejaculation, or the presence of urine in the ejaculate. The pH of presperm fluid is usually 7.8 to 8.2. pH is usually the same or slghtly elevated in second ejaculates compared to first ejaculates. Inflammatory conditions of the internal genitalia may also result in elevated pH.

SPERM CELL MORPHOLOGY. Morphologically abnormal spermatozoa are found in the semen of all stallions. Abaxial attachment of the midpiece segment to the sperm head is normal. The sperm head is not symmetrical but has a less convex surface on the side of midpiece attachment compared to the opposite side. The normal sperm cell does not contain a proximal or distal cytoplasmic droplet. The midpiece and sperm tail are straight.

The etiology of many sperm abnormalities has not been determined. Morphologic abnormalities of sperm may originate in the testis or epididymis or may be induced artifacts due to semen storage or handling methods. An upper limit for sperm abnormalities in prospectively fertile horses has not been established. However, it is reasonable to assume that as the incidence of abnormal sperm forms increases, fertility will be adversely affected. Whether the presence of morphologically abnormal spermatozoa alters the viability or fertilizing ability of normal spermatozoa has not been established in the horse.

Abnormalities of the acrosome and head shape, proximal cytoplasmic droplets, tightly coiled tails, detached heads, and midpiece abnormalities are most commonly associated with impaired spermatogenesis and infertility. The significance of the distal cytoplasmic droplet defect on fertility is not fully known, but it appears to be of little consequence. As the frequency of ejaculation is increased, the incidence of sperm with distal droplets usually decreases. This effect is most dramatic in sexually rested stallions. A similar effect may also be observed in the incidence of bent tails and detached heads.

The examiner should be extremely aware of artifactual changes in sperm morphology that result from temperature shock, storage of raw semen, and staining. Commonly observed artifacts of spermatozoa include complete loss of the acrosome, fraying or thickening of the midpiece segment, slight bending of the tail, and, occasionally, detachment of sperm heads. On occasion, these same defects are associated with impaired spermatogenesis or sperm maturation. To avoid many of the problems associated with artifactual changes in spermatozoa, fixation immediately after collection in buffered formol saline or buffered glutaraldehyde has been recommended. Cells are then viewed under a phase contrast microscope using a wet mount preparation.

Though a wide range may be acceptable for normal stallions, most stallions in regular usage have less than a 10 to 15 per cent incidence of any single morphologic defect and have more than 60 per cent morphologically normal sperm cells. Abnormalities of the acrosome and midpiece segment are usually less than 5 per cent.

It is commonly recommended that mares be inseminated using 100 to 500 $\times$ 10^6 normal spermatozoa or progressively motile, morphologically normal sperm for the artificial insemination. The number of sperm cells necessary to achieve acceptable fertility using natural service is unknown.

ADDITIONAL TESTS OF SEMEN QUALITY. In selected stallions or under certain mating management conditions, additional tests of semen quality may be indicated. Some of these tests have been termed "stress" tests. Longevity of sperm motility or ability to withstand freezing are examples of these tests. Resuspension of the centrifuged sperm pellet in an artificial extender in a stallion of low fertility may be attempted. This has been of value in a limited number of infertile stallions. Determination of osmotic pressure, oxygen consumption, or chemical constituents of seminal plasma may also be helpful. Wright's or H & E staining is frequently helpful in differentiating spermatocytes from red or white blood cells.

OVERALL INTERPRETATION OF SEMEN QUALITY TESTS. Because no single test of semen quality is well correlated with fertility, many parameters of semen quality are assessed. If tests result in below normal ranges for stallion semen, an effort should be made to determine the cause. Particular effort should be made to eliminate errors in laboratory technique or semen handling. The evaluation of breeding potential of stallions requires that the examination be performed in a systematic and thorough manner. In cases of doubt, reexamination is rcommended.

The fertility of a given stallion can be dramatically influenced by frequency of use, breeding potential of mated females, timing of service, method of breeding, stallion behavior, and other factors. Under certain management conditions, subfertile stallions may achieve a very acceptable foaling rate. On the other hand, stallions of apparently normal fertility potential may perform poorly. Many of the steps in the evaluation of an infertile stallion may provide clues to assist in optimizing the fertility of an otherwise infertile horse.

Supplemental Readings

1. Bielanski, W.: The evaluation of stallion semen in aspects of fertility control and its use for artificial insemination. J. Reprod. Fertil. Suppl., 23:19, 1975.
2. Cooper, W. l.; Artificial breeding of horses. Vet. Clin. North Am. (Large Anim. Pract.), 2:267, 1980.
3. Gebauer, M. R., Pickett, B. W., Voss, J. L., and Swierstra, E. E.: Reproductive physiology of the stallion: Daily sperm output and testicular measurements. J. Am. Vet. Med. Assoc., *165*:711, 1974.
4. Kenney R. M.: Clinical fertility evaluation of the stallion. Proc. 21st Annu. Conv. Am. Assoc. Eq. Pract., 1975, pp. 336–355.
5. Swierstra, E. E., Gebauer, M. R., and Pickett, B. W.: Reproductive physiology of the stallion. I. Spermatogenesis and testis composition. J. Reprod. Fertil., 40:113, 1974.

DISORDERS AFFECTING STALLION FERTILITY

John P. Hurtgen, KENNETT SQUARE, PENNSYLVANIA

Many conditions may affect stallion fertility even though tests of semen quality are acceptable. These conditions include behavioral or mating disorders, traumatic injuries, lesions of the penis or urethral process, and contamination of semen.

BEHAVIORAL OR MATING DISORDERS

Libido is probably a heritable trait but is also a learned experience highly influenced by enviromental factors. Young stallions used for racing or performance are discouraged from demonstrating sexual interest in mares by application of a stallion "ring" to the penis to prevent erection or by discipline to discourage vocalization in the presence of a mare. Such training may lead to aberrant breeding behavior such as lack of interest in an estrous mare, failure to attain penile erection, repeated "drop" and retraction of the penis, mounting without erection, abnormal mounting position, excessive biting, repeated intromission without ejaculation, premature "belling" or enlargement of the glans penis, abrupt dismount during ejaculation, and apparent loss of body balance during ejaculation. These conditions are most commonly observed and are most easily corrected in young, inexperienced stallions but may also occur in sexually experienced horses.

Although the cause of behavioral abnormality can rarely be determined, a thorough history of the horse's use, prior treatment, management, and behavior can be helpful in removing factors associated with abnormal breeding behavior and encouraging acceptable breeding patterns. Factors discouraging normal breeding patterns include excessive discipline of the shy or low libido stallion, muzzling, stallion "rings," lack of variation in mount animals, noisy surroundings, and confined breeding areas. Though washing the penis is stimulatory for most horses, it can cause distraction and anxiety in others. In these cases, the horse should gain confidence in the breeding procedure before routine cleansing of the penis or culturing of the urethra is initiated. Excessive biting of the mount mare can be controlled by discipline or by muzzling the stallion.

Premature "belling" of the glans penis, which makes intromission difficult, is usually associated with prolonged teasing or a prolonged interval from mounting to intromission. These procedures increase the volume of semen but have no effect on the number of sperm cells ejaculated. The condition is also observed when stallions breed mares that have been tightly sutured or have poor perineal conformation. Stallions that "bell" prematurely should be encouraged to mount quickly after the penis has been cleansed. Manual guidance of the penis into the vagina and lubrication of the tips of the vulva are also helpful.

Although a stallion should not normally mount the mare until erection has occurred, mounting without erection may be tolerated and even encouraged in the training of stallions with very low libido so that the stallion learns that mounting is acceptable behavior.

Probably the most challenging behavioral problem is failure to ejaculate despite repeated mounting and intromission. In natural service, this behavior increases contamination of the mare's reproductive tract, the risk of vaginal lacerations, and the risk of stallion injury. Many of these stallions are thought to have ejaculated based on "flagging" of the tail or pulsation of the urethra, but emission of 20 to 60 ml of seminal fluid with few sperm cells is common. Because such horses may require up to four or more hours to ejaculate and thus tie up the breeding shed, farm managers and veterinarians may avoid using such a stallion for an initial or repeat service of a mare. This attitude by personnel may lead to less frequent stallion usage and thus may exaggerate the infertility problem.

Though the ultimate goal for therapy in the horse that has an increased number of mounts per ejaculate may be one mount per ejaculate, establishing a predictable pattern for the horse and handlers may be just as important. Initially, semen should be collected using an artificial vagina so that the ejaculatory pattern of the horse becomes known. The temperature, pressure, and degree of lubrication of the artificial vagina should be noted. Personnel used for handling the stallion and semen collection should be the same for each attempted collection. Once the behavioral pattern has been determined, single factors can be varied until a favorable response is elicited. In our experience, one of the most beneficial factors is use of a phantom. When it is necessary to obtain a semen sample from young, inexperienced stallions that repeatedly mount and enter the artificial vagina without ejaculation, use of a condom for semen collection is very helpful. Once horses become accustomed to ejaculating in the condom, they readily adapt to collection using an artificial vagina. Testosterone, human chorionic gonadotrophin, oxytocin, ephedrine, and prostaglandin are not helpful. Certain of these compounds have undesirable side effects in stallions, such as reduced spermatogenesis following use of testosterone and temporary incoordination following prostaglandin administration.

Stallions being used for two or three services per day may develop abnormal mating behavior patterns such as excessive mounts per ejaculate, biting, premature dismounting, or lack of libido. Semen collection in an artificial vagina and insemination of mares on an every-other-day basis are obvious solutions to the problem. Other alternatives include limitation of a stallion's book, limiting stallion usage to once per day or less frequently if needed, more careful selection of mares to be bred through the practice of ovarian and cervical palpation, and judicious use of human chorionic gonadotrophin (HCG) to induce ovulation at a more predictable time (p. 402). Mares usually ovulate 24 to 28 hours after administration of HCG during early estrus. Therefore, mares should be bred the day following treatment. If stallion usage is limited to one mating per day and a mare passes out of estrus without being served, she may be returned to estrus by administration of prostaglandin five or more days after ovulation (p. 401).

There appears to be a seasonal influence on mating desire in stallions. During periods of short daylight, libido may be somewhat depressed, and number of mounts per ejaculate may be increased. Exposure to 15 hours of light per day begining 60 or more days prior to the onset of the breeding season may be beneficial in stallions breeding a significant number of mares early in the breeding season.

Stallions that readily achieve erection of the penis but are reluctant to mount, those that have an increased number of mounts per ejaculate, or those that prematurely dismount with or without ejaculation may do so in response to pain resulting from foot, pastern, hock, stifle, or back problems or from abdominal visceral adhesions. Inadequate diameter of the artificial vagina or painful lesions affecting the penis should also be considered. The chronic or short-term use of analgesic or anti-inflammatory agents such as phenylbutazone, flunixin meglumine, or aspirin may be beneficial. Owing to the possibly heritable nature of such locomotor problems as cerebellar hypoplasia and wobbler syndrome and owing to the danger that affected horses impose on the handlers and the horse, affected animals should not be used for breeding.

TRAUMATIC INJURIES TO THE GENITALIA

The Penis and Prepuce. Traumatic injuries of the penis, prepuce, or testicles are frequently the result of kicking by a mare during breeding, improperly fitted stallion "rings," and breeding "stitches." Proper restraint of mares cannot be overemphasized. Most mares are serviced after a twitch has been applied to the upper lip. If a mare begins kicking during breeding, her head should be pulled toward the side of the stallion handler so that her buttocks move away from the stallion. Individual mares may require more restraint, including tranquilization.

Other less commonly encountered injuries to the penis may result from an improperly fitted, cracked, or wrinkled covering over the phantom. In artificial vaginas (AV) in which the rubber liner is held over the outer casing with rubber bands, the bands may on rare occasion slip off the AV during thrusting and encircle the penis. If the rubber band is quickly stripped from the erect penis, a seroma will result. To remove the band, an encircling grip of the penis is made proximal to the rubber band, which is then cut and removed from the penis. Stallions may also traumatize the genitalia when attempting to breed estrous mares across a fence. Stallion pastures and paddocks should be separated from mare paddocks by double fencing at least 10 feet apart.

The response of the penis and prepuce to trauma is edema or, occasionally, hemorrhage. Preputial edema is usually generalized, whereas edema of the penis may be localized. Traumatic injury frequently results in prolapse of the penis from the preputial sheath, the penis usually bowing in a posterior direction. The edematous penis or prepuce must be elevated and supported to aid fluid return from the damaged tissues. Support can be applied by a stallion "supporter" or by use of bandaging material to encircle the abdomen and include the penis and prepuce. If only the penis has been traumatized, it can be maintained in the preputial cavity using retention sutures to close the preputial orifice. If the injured penis or preputial membranes are being maintained within the preputial cavity, the penis can be manually withdrawn from the prepuce for cleansing. Pressure bandaging of the penis is also beneficial to prevent further swelling and to reduce existing edema. Applying ointment to the penis prevents drying of the penile skin. If the penis will not return to the prepuce (paraphimosis), exercise should be limited to prevent further bruising or abrasion of the edematous penis. Cold water hydrotherapy and massage (two to four times per day for 15 to 30 minutes per treatment) are indicated to prevent further fluid accumulation. After the threat of further edema or hemorrhage has ceased, warm water hydrotherapy may be indicated to aid in movement of fluid out of the affected tissues.

If superficial lacerations or abrasions accompany seroma or hematoma of the penis or preputial edema, antibiotics should be incorporated into the ointment applied to the skin surface. Systemic antibiotics are indicated when deeper lacerations of the tissues have occurred. Phenylbutazone, aspirin, or flunixin meglumine are helpful for their anti-inflammatory and analgesic actions. Treatment may be necessary for as little as two to three days to as long as two to three months.

Tranquilizers are contraindicated in horses with paraphimosis or penile injuries. These agents tend to cause further prolapse and accumulation of fluid in the penis. Stallions should be kept free from sexual stimulation to avoid further hemorrhage or edema, which could result from increased blood pressure during erection.

In addition to being a sequela to injury, paraphimosis may also be associated with equine infectious anemia, purpura hemorrhagica, rhinopneumonitis, exhaustion, starvation, or penile paralysis. To prevent secondary traumatic injury, the prolapsed penis must be elevated and moistened with ointments.

PENILE PARALYSIS

Penile paralysis may result from local neurologic damage, rabies, and use of phenothiazine tranquilizers. Tranquilizer-induced paralysis of the penis, which has been observed following the use of propiopromazine and acepromazine but not xylazine, results in a seemingly partial erection of the penis. The corpus cavernosum penis is uniformly filled, and there is no edema. However, the corpus cavernosum penis contains a blood clot. The penis is painful on deep palpation for about two weeks after the onset of paralysis. The condition is usually observed in stallions but also in geldings receiving exogenous testosterone therapy. In most circumstances, amputation of the penis is necessary after the acute inflammation of the corpus cavernosum penis has subsided. If superficial abrasions, lacerations, or hematoma of the penis have not occurred and to avoid some of the complications associated with amputation of the penis, a penis retraction operation may be performed. One such penile retraction operation is the Bolz technique.

In valuable breeding stallions, two possible methods of therapy may be attempted. The stallion can be trained to ejaculate into an artificial vagina in spite of paralysis of the penis. Owing to reduced sensitivity of the majority of the penis, the water temperature and pressure in the vagina may need to be increased. Alternatively, the organized hematoma in the corpus cavernosum can be encouraged to recanalize by sexually stimulating the stallion three times per day for 15 to 30 minutes per session.

URETHRAL TRAUMA

Trauma of the urethra that causes inflammation or stricture formation may result from direct trauma to the penis, urethral calculi, repeated catheterization, improper use of the endoscope in the stallion's urethra, constricting stallion rings, and irritating chemicals. When minor lacerations of the urethral process are cauterized with agents such as silver nitrate, care must be taken so that the silver nitrate does not gain access to the urethra proper.

TESTICULAR TRAUMA

Occasionally, trauma to the testicles and epididymes may occur owing to a kick from a mare during service. Trauma to the testicles usually results in scrotal edema, elevated scrotal temperature, pain, hematocele, and, uncommonly, enlargement of the affected testis. Acute orchitis usually results in temporary or permanent degenerative atrophy of the affected testis, which becomes small and fibrotic.

Treatment of acute orchitis and epididymitis consists of support of the stallion's scrotum and testes, cold water hydrotherapy, systemic treatment to alleviate pain and inflammation, and prophylactic use of antibiotics.

Success is largely dependent on immediate initiation of treatment. Unilateral castration may be indicated to prevent inflammation and degenerative changes in the opposite testis.

On rare occasions, traumatic injury to the scrotal contents may result in a blockage of the epididymal duct system. Obstruction of the duct system of the stallion is suspected when the stallion ejaculates semen devoid of sperm. True obstruction or aplasia of the duct system in the stallion is exceedingly rare. Some stallions fail to ejaculate sperm cells in the first ejaculate even though a normal volume of semen is produced. Repeated attempts to collect semen result in clumps of dead sperm cells before motile sperm cells are finally collected. These ejaculates are also characterized by a high incidence of detached sperm heads. This syndrome is thought to be due to a unilateral or bilateral stasis of sperm cells in the ampullae. Vigorous massage of the enlarged ampullae and vasa deferentia and prolonged sexual stimulation of the stallion are thought to be helpful. The condition may or may not recur in the same individual. Regular semen collection or natural service are logical prophylactic measures even during the nonbreeding season.

TUMORLIKE LESIONS OF THE GENITALIA

PENILE NEOPLASMS

Squamous cell carcinomas of the penis and prepuce are common tumors in the stallion. This tumor, which tends to affect nonpigmented areas, is locally invasive and granulomatous in appearance. Metastasis to regional lymph nodes has been reported. If the lesion is localized, cryosurgical excision is recommended. More extensive lesions are alleviated by surgical excision of the granulomatous nodules, although amputation of the penis may be necessary. Other tumors of the penis and prepuce include the melanoma, sarcoid, hemangioma, and fibropapilloma. Tumors of the penis may interfere with intromission and frequently result in hemospermia. Stallions with fibropapilloma (warts) should not be used for natural mating during the period of infectivity. Although fibropapillomas usually regress spontaneously, surgical excision may be indicated to reduce the period of recovery. Autogenous vaccines can also be used in the treatment of warts, but the efficacy of autogenous vaccination has not been tested (p. 536). Melanomas on the prepuce or scrotum are rather common in gray horses. They do not affect fertility and are only rarely removed surgically.

HABRONEMIASIS

Neoplasms of the penis or prepuce may readily be confused with the advanced lesions of habronemiasis, affecting the skin of the prepuce, penis, or mucous membranes of the urethra (p. 196). *Habronema muscae* eggs are deposited on the moist surfaces of the urethral process or prepuce. The eggs hatch, and resulting larvae invade tissues in the area. Lacerations or breaks in the skin or mucous membranes probably facilitate larval migration. The tissue responds to the larvae with edema, inflammation, and granuloma formation. The initial lesion on the urethral process may be localized edema of the urethral mucosa and may result in sporadic hemospermia. More chronic cases appear granulomatous and are frequently ulcerated. If lesions are on the urethral process, hemospermia is common. Although the lesion is at the end of the urethra, blood is invariably ejaculated only at the end of ejaculation unless the lesions are extensive. Hematuria is rarely encountered. Because the larvae themselves are usually dead, it is unlikely that systemic administration of organophosphates would be efficacious. Topical and systemic treatment with anti-inflammatory agents offers temporary cessation of granuloma formation. When therapy is discontinued, lesions frequently proliferate again. Surgical amputation of the urethral process has been performed in a number of stallions with habronemiasis of the distal urethral process. Local cautery of unhealed areas of the sutured mucocutaneous junction may be necessary. Sexual stimulation of the horse should be avoided for at least two weeks. Surgically corrected lesions of the urethral process are susceptible to bleeding following trauma of the penis during natural mating or semen collection because the urethral mucosa tends to be slightly everted following surgery. The lesions of habronemiasis may completely or partially regress during cold months of the year. *Collitroga hominivorax* (screwworm fly) larvae have also been incriminated in such lesions of the penis and prepuce.

TESTICULAR NEOPLASMS

Testicular tumors include seminomas, lipomas, teratomas, and interstitial cell tumors. Sertoli cell tumor of the equine testis has not been reported. Testicular tumors are rare in the horse but may be seen in older horses, the seminoma being most frequently described. Testicular tumors, which are usually unilateral, result in swelling, which may be fluctuant and somewhat painful. Metastasis is rare. Testicular tumors need to be differentiated from abscesses or hematomas, which may also cause a localized, firm, space-occupying mass. Because tumors cause testicular degeneration, a decreased number of sperm and an increased incidence of abnormal sperm cells and spermatocytes may be present in the ejaculate. As these lesions are usually not painful, the libido of affected stallions is not altered. The onset of testicular enlargement is not usually noticed by the owner. Unilateral castration of stallions is recommended. Palpation of the inguinal lymph nodes and histologic evaluation of the excised testis and spermatic cord are helpful in determining if metastasis has occurred.

TESTICULAR TORSION

Acute 360° torsion of the stallion's testis, though rare, must also be differentiated from tumors. The very acute onset of the condition, signs of colic, and the young age of affected horses are helpful in establishing a diagnosis. A more common form of testicular rotation is a transient 180° rotation of the testis often encountered during the breeding soundness evaluation of stallions. Invariably, a single testis is involved. Libido and semen quality of affected horses appear unaltered. In cases of 180° rotation of the testis, the tail of the epididymis is directed anteriorly. The malposition of the testis is thought to occur during descent of the testicle into the scrotum.

HEMOSPERMIA

Blood in semen, hemospermia, lowers fertility, the degree of infertility being related to the amount of blood in the semen. Hemospermia, which may be intermittent or a consistent problem, is always secondary to some disease or abnormality of the penis, urethra, or internal genitalia that often results in painful ejaculation. The correction of hemospermia in stallions is, therefore, aimed at correction of the underlying cause of bleeding.

Hemospermia is best diagnosed by collection of semen using an artificial vagina. Depending on the amount of blood in the ejaculate, semen may be faint pink to red in color, hemospermia becoming more severe as the frequency of ejaculation increases. The incidence of progressively motile sperm cells is decreased, primarily because of the increased agglutination of sperm cells to red cells. The presence of red blood cells can also be determined using Wright's or H & E staining of air-dried semen smears. Laboratory tests for the presence of occult blood may also be useful in monitoring the occurrence of hemospermia, although stallion semen free of red blood cells will yield a slightly positive reaction.

Many times the source of bleeding can be readily identified. Traumatic lacerations or viral papillomatosis of the penis and cutaneous habronemiasis of the distal urethral process are easily diagnosed common causes of persistent or sporadic hemospermia. These conditions must be differentiated from tumors. Bacterial urethritis, urethral ulceration, or rupture of urethral subepithelial vessels is also a potential cause of hemospermia, which can be diagnosed by examining the penile and pelvic urethra with a small-diameter, flexible fiberscope at least 100 cm long. With this instrument, a subischial urethrostomy is not necessary. Inflammation of the internal genitalia is also a cause of hemospermia. In stallions used for natural service, caution must be exercised in diagnosing hemospermia if blood is observed on the stallion's penis or at the mare's vulva following service. Rupture or stretching of the hymenal ring, vaginal lacerations or bruising, rupture of the vagina, or tearing of a sutured vulva should also be considered as a source of blood.

Sexual rest is indicated in horses with hemospermia. Specific therapy should then be initiated based on the cause of bleeding. Antibiotic ointments should be applied to superficial lacerations of the urethral process, glans penis, or shaft of the penis. Systemic anti-inflammatory agents and topical corticoteroids applied to early lesions of Habronema may allow an affected stallion to remain in limited service until lesions regress or can be surgically excised. Proliferative lesions of Habronema are best corrected by surgical removal. If the distal end of the urethral process is amputated, care must be taken to ensure that the incision line is well healed before reinitiating service. In most cases, some degree of focal cautery of the amputated urethral pro-

cess is necessary. If local cautery is done using silver nitrate, care must be taken so that the chemical does not gain access to the urethra. This will result in irritation and necrosis of the mucosa and further problems with hemospermia. Lesions of fibropapillomatosis usually regress spontaneously. If they do not, surgical removal is recommended. An open-ended or Polish model artificial vagina can be used to collect blood-free ejaculates from stallions with early lesions of Habronema or with irritation to the distal urethra. The blood-free jets of semen are caught and used for the artificial insemination of mares.

In cases of bacterial urethritis or inflammation of the internal genitalia, the causative organism should be identified and antibiotic sensitivity determined. Systemic and local treatment of these conditions is recommended, but success is limited. In the case of stallions with persistent genital infections, semen in an extender containing an appropriate antibiotic can be used to inseminate mares. For natural service, the extender (Table 1) containing the appropriate antibiotic is infused into the mare's uterus just prior to intromission by the stallion. Endometritis has not been a problem in mares bred using either of these schemes. These stallions achieve normal fertility when matings are managed in this manner.

UROSPERMIA

Urine in semen or urination during ejaculation is referred to as urospermia. Ejaculates containing urine usually have an elevated pH, decreased sperm cell motility, elevated osmotic pressure, are a light yellow to amber in color, and may also smell of urine and contain much sediment. The elevation of pH is dependent on how much urine enters the seminal collection vessel. Some ejaculates, therefore, have a pH value within the normal range for stallions. Determination of creatinine or urea nitrogen concentration of semen appears to be the most definitive test for urine contamination of semen. Creatinine concentrations above 2.0 mg per dl or urea nitrogen concentrations above 30 mg per dl are observed in urine-contaminated ejaculates. The fertil-

TABLE 1. FORMULA FOR A SEMEN EXTENDER SUITABLE FOR ARTIFICIAL INSEMINATION AND FOR INTRAUTERINE INFUSION FOLLOWING NATURAL SERVICE

Instant nonfat dry milk	2.4 gm
Glucose	4.9 gm
Gentamicin	100.0 mg
7.5% sodium bicarbonate	2.0 ml
Distilled water to	100.0 ml

ity of ejaculates containing urine is probably reduced owing to the effect of urine on sperm cell quality and the effect of urine on the mare's endometrium. The cause of urospermia is unknown. The condition is intermittent, and in the majority of cases, urine is ejaculated near the end of ejaculation. During natural service, urination during ejaculation is rarely suspected. Reduced fertility is the usual presenting complaint.

Owing to the unpredictable occurrence of urospermia from one ejaculate to the next within the same horse, it is difficult to assess the efficacy of treatments. If possible, semen from affected horses should be collected with an artificial vagina so that contaminated ejaculates can be discarded. To reduce the frequency of urination during ejaculation, it may be beneficial to use the horse for breeding only after urination has occurred. Urination frequently occurs following exercise, after exposure to fecal matter from another horse, and after feeding and fresh bedding of the stall. Many studs will urinate in response to whistling. Some stallions will still urinate during ejaculation even though urination has occurred prior to semen collection. Diuretic administration to induce urination prior to semen collection is not beneficial, nor is administration of ephedrine sulfate. Because urine is usually passed near the end of the ejaculatory process, an open-ended artificial vagina may be used to separate uncontaminated and contaminated semen.

INFECTION OF THE GENITALIA

Contamination of semen by bacteria almost always occurs even though semen is collected in as clean a manner as possible. Extreme caution must be exercised in diagnosing a bacterial infection of the genitalia. The prepuce, surface of the penis, fossa glandis, and distal urethra are heavily contaminated with bacteria, including organisms strongly suspected of being pathogenic to the stallion's and mare's reproductive organs. These surface contaminants, which include nonpathogenic environmental bacteria and such potential pathogens as Pseudomonas sp, *Klebsiella pneumoniae, Streptococcus zooepidemicus, Escherichia coli,* and *Staphylococcus aureus,* gain entry into semen during natural service or semen collection. Though these organisms may be potentially pathogenic to the stallion's reproductive tract, inflammation of the genitalia and active shedding of these organisms during breeding are uncommon. Similarly, most young or reproductively healthy mares are unaffected by the contamination of the mare's reproductive tract during natural service, but mares with reduced uterine resistance may be susceptible to infection.

In the evaluation of breeding soundness in stal-

lions, a urethral swabbing is made of the washed, rinsed, and dried penis before and after first ejaculation. The stallion is considered free of infection if the type of bacteria recovered is inconsistent in the two swab specimens, the number of organisms is sharply reduced in postejaculate urethral swabbings compared to preejaculate swab cultures, inflammatory cells are absent in semen, and a pure growth of a pathogen is not obtained when culturing the postejaculate swab specimen. If one or more of the preceding criteria is not met, the stallion is considered potentially infected, and further efforts are made to confirm the presence of the bacteria and their source. In many cases, it is difficult to differentiate inflammatory cells from germinal cells of the seminiferous tubules. The presence of the latter type of cell is suspected when round cells are observed in the slide prepared for motility estimation. With certain stains, white blood cells and spermatocytes are not visible. Therefore, air-dried smears should be stained with Wright's or H & E stain. If excessive numbers of white blood cells are present in semen, the sample may appear flocculent or granular, or the purulent material may be grossly visible.

Genital infection of the stallion is also suspected if mares served by the stallion repeatedly develop endometritis that is caused by an organism recovered from the stallion or his semen. Because the environment or genital instruments could be sources of bacteria causing endometritis, the stallion is considered only a potential source of the offending organism.

Stallions should not harbor *Hemophilus equigenitalis,* the organism of contagious equine metritis (CEM), on their genitalia. Because the stallion is frequently involved in the transmission of the organism to mares, affected stallions should not be considered sound breeders.

The fertility of mares bred by artificial insemination using raw semen is comparable to fertility following use of semen diluted in extender containing antibiotics. However, the incidence of postbreeding uterine infections seems markedly decreased in mares bred using antibiotic-extended semen. With the appropriate selection of antibiotics, semen diluted in extender usually fails to yield bacteria when cultured on blood agar. In an artificial insemination program, the pH and osmotic pressure of the extender should be monitored if fertility rates are below normal because some extenders have an adverse effect on semen quality and stallion fertility, and individual stallion spermatozoa may be adversely affected by an otherwise acceptable extender. The pH of extender should be 7.2 to 7.4 and osmotic pressure should be 300 to 330 mOsm.

Though raw semen may contain numerous bacteria, endometritis following natural service is not common because of the natural resistance mechanisms of the mare's endometrium and the bacteriostatic properties of seminal plasma. In mares that become infected following natural service, the infusion of the uterus with an extender (Table 1) containing antibiotics immediately prior to service is helpful. Infusion of the uterus with an appropriate antibiotic 2 to 24 hours (preferably 6 hours) following natural cover is also used successfully in stallions known to consistently infect mares with Pseudomonas or Klebsiella..

In stallions that shed pathogenic bacteria in their semen, an attempt should be made to locate the source of the bacteria. Bacterial urethritis, frequently associated with cystitis, is probably the most commonly diagnosed inflammatory condition of the stallion's genital tract. Hemospermia and an increased number of mounts per ejaculate are frequently associated with urethritis. Systemic antibiotic treatment may be helpful in such cases, but limited vascular supply to the urethra and failure of many drugs to be excreted via the urinary system limit the success of this route of therapy. Local irrigation of the urethra with nonirritating antibacterials is also used. Sexual rest is indicated. Seminal vesiculitis and ampullitis are rare in the horse. During the acute phase of inflammation, such organs are likely to be enlarged and painful to palpation. In more chronic cases, the organs tend to be nonpainful, and enlargement or induration of areas of the organs may be evident on palpation. Inflammation of the prostate and bulbourethral glands has not been reported in the stallion.

Fiberscopic examination of the penile and pelvic urethra with particular attention to the ducts of the accessory sex glands and opening to the bladder should be part of the diagnostic work-up. Additionally, fluid can be collected directly from the vesicular glands by passing a sterile, flexible catheter into the pelvic urethra following sexual stimulation of the stallion. Following sexual stimulation of the stallion, the vesicular glands fill with fluid. With the catheter in position within the pelvic urethra, the contents of the vesicular glands are expressed by manual decompression of each gland per rectum. The fluid can then be biochemically or bacteriologically analyzed.

Because the preejaculatory dripping of fluid from the urethra is thought to originate primarily from the bulbourethral glands, analysis of this fluid may indirectly allow the clinician to evaluate this organ.

At present, palpation per rectum appears to be the only method of evaluating the ampullae. Though bacterial epididymitis may occur in stallions, palpation is the only method of evaluating this organ without direct invasion of the epididymis, which is likely to result in the formation of adhesions and duct blockage.

Orchitis, inflammation of the testis of bacterial origin, may occur following trauma, strangles, or other systemic infections. Acutely, the testes are enlarged, painful, and warm to palpation. The scrotum may also be edematous, and injury to the epididymal ducts is common. Therapy, including systemic antibiotics and local cold water hydrotherapy, must be initiated promptly. Elevation of the enlarged and painful testicles is also indicated. Hydrotherapy should be applied four or more times per day for 15 to 30-minute periods for at least one week. Chronic orchitis or unsuccessful treatment of acute orchitis usually results in the affected testis becoming small, firm, and frequently nodular in consistency. Sperm cell production is below normal, and there is an increased incidence of abnormal sperm cells.

References

1. Cooper, W. L.: Artificial breeding of horses. Vet. Clin. North Am. (Large Anim. Pract.); 2:267; 1980.
2. Kenney, R. M.: Clinical fertility evaluation of the stallion. Proc. 21st Annu. Conv. Am. Asso. Eq. Pract., 1975, pp. 336–355.
3. Pickett, B. W., and Voss, J. L.: Abnormalities of mating behavior in domestic stallions. J. Reprod. Fertil. Suppl., 23:129, 1975.
4. Rasbech, N. O.: Ejaculatory disorders of the stallion. J. Reprod. Fertil. Suppl., 23:123; 1975.
5. Voss, J. L., and Pickett, B. W.: Diagnosis and treatment of haemospermia in the stallion. J. Reprod. Fertil. Suppl., 23:151, 1975.
6. Walker, D. F., and Vaughan, J. T.: Bovine and Equine Urogenital Surgery. Philadelphia, Lea and Febiger, 1980, pp. 125–169.

ARTIFICIAL BREEDING OF HORSES*

Wendell L. Cooper, KENNETT SQUARE, PENNSYLVANIA

Artificial breeding programs should be aimed at (1) achieving efficient use of stallions, people, and facilities, (2) ensuring safety to stallion, mares, and people, and (3) preventing uterine infections in the mare and spread of pathogens to the stallion's genital tract. Effective management is the key to carrying out such programs, and success or failure depends largely on the total management of each individual establishment.[13] On well-managed operations, conception rates of 80 per cent or above with sizeable bookings are expected. Live-foal rates and registered-foal rates are the best reflection of total management. Live-foal rates of 76 to 80 per cent are being achieved by some of the best operations using artificial breeding, even when rigorous selection against mares of reduced fertility is not exercised.

THE STALLION

The fertility potential of each individual stallion should be estimated as precisely as possible and utilized in management decisions such as limiting the stallion's book of mares to a given number, how close to ovulation one must breed in order to optimize the opportunity for conception, as well as how to determine the number of mares one can inseminate with the number of normal, motile sperm in a given ejaculate. Stallions must be treated as individuals in this respect because there are high variations in fertility potential between stallions. The best way to prove a stallion's fertility is in actual use when problems will quickly become apparent. However, this trial and error method can be very costly during the first one or two seasons in which the stallion is introduced to service if problems are present. Problems such as low sperm numbers, high percentage of primary sperm abnormalities, and basic sperm defects leading to poor progressive motility can be detected and allowed for if an evaluation of potential fertility is made prior to use. Other problems such as strong seasonal effects and short longevity of sperm in the mare tract may be more difficult to define by the usual one-time stallion fertility evaluation but often do show up when in vitro longevity tests are performed.

SEMEN COLLECTION

Having used all the stallion semen collection devices available, our experience shows that a properly constructed and prepared artificial vagina will yield the best results in stallion performance, ejaculate quality, and maximum sperm harvest. Each operator will have to choose the artificial vagina that best suits his needs. I would suggest choosing one that is least complicated, easy to sterilize, and lightweight. Stallions of average or higher libido can be trained to use any kind of artificial vagina. However, most artificial vaginas are longer than necessary, since stallions will work well in an artificial vagina that is only 20 inches in length. The diameter should be only 1 in greater than the diameter of the erect glans penis (about 5 in). The smaller and less complicated artificial vaginas will have less sperm loss in the collection system, since sperm loss is dependent upon sperm concentration and the area of the collection system wetted by the ejaculate.

Preparation of the artificial vagina includes filling it with the proper amount of water at the proper temperature, lubricating the liner, and placing the semen receptacle onto the artificial vagina. Preparation of the artificial vagina should be timed closely with stallion teasing and preparation to prevent excessive cooling prior to collection. This timing can be quite precise when experience tells you the time required to stimulate and wash the penis of a given stallion. Knowing the stallion's penis size and filling the artificial vagina with the proper amount of water to give the desired internal pressure are important. Using the same volume of water each time provides consistency, which is important for stallion performance. The internal temperature is important and should be between 45 and 48° C. This temperature, which is above that of the body, is stimulating to the stallion but not high enough to be uncomfortable. Again, consistent temperature will yield consistent stallion performance.

Consistency of stallion performance and efficiency in collection of semen have been greatly augmented with the use of the dummy or phantom mare. Such devices had been used for bulls and were first reported being used for stallions by Polish workers.[14] We first implemented it for therapeutic use in a stallion with tarsitis in 1970 and quickly realized its value for routine semen collection. The popularity of the phantom mare has spread rapidly and now it is widely used throughout the United States and

*(Reprinted with permission from Cooper, W. L.: Artificial breeding of horses. Vet. Clin. North Am. (Large Anim. Pract.), 2:267, 1980.)

Canada. A phantom mare essentially is a padded tubular structure of such height to accommodate the stallion for which it is to be used. It can be made adjustable for height when more than one stallion will be using it. The width (including 4 in of foam padding) should be no greater than 22 in.

Stallions accept the phantom as a sexual object very readily. Some may accept it on first introduction and mount it immediately, whereas others may require a short training period (one to three days, rarely extending to as long as two weeks). Training involves use of an estrual mare beside the phantom placed in such a manner as to have her rear quarter one to two feet anterior to the posterior end of the phantom. The stallion is brought to the mare's rear quarter at an angle with his head and neck extending over the rear end of the phantom. Do not allow the stallion to attempt mounting until he is well aroused. When the stallion attempts to mount across the end of the phantom, pull his head to the near side and he will land astride the phantom. Once astride the phantom with the artificial vagina placed over the penis, the stallion will begin thrusting, ending in ejaculation. After repeating this process a few times the stallion will be conditioned. When trained, most stallions do not require a tease mare beside the phantom, although a few do. Some stallions with high libido do not require a mare at all and will respond to the phantom alone.

In addition to routine and therapeutic use in stallions with physical problems, phantoms can help stallions with some behavioral problems such as mare shyness, delayed ejaculation (several mounts prior to ejaculation), vicious biting while breeding, and violent thrusting, which can cause mare injury. Using the dummy, we have obtained dramatic improvement in the ease and efficiency with which the semen of such stallions can be collected. When a stallion's semen is collected by use of an artificial vagina mounted on a phantom mare, one should not switch back to natural service even if only one mare is to be bred that day. Consistency of use gives better stallion performance.

THE EJACULATE

Variation in semen volume is due primarily to individual variation in size of the accessory glands. Semen volume is also influenced by the amount of premount sexual stimulation, by consistency in preparation of the artificial vagina, as well as by seasonal variation in gel content.[12] In a given season, one can obtain rather consistent semen volumes by holding premount sexual stimulation to a minimum and being absolutely consistent in preparation of the artificial vagina. Many breeders are unjustly concerned about semen volume and consider it a pri-

mary criterion of ejaculate quality. Rather, total sperm number (that is, concentration × volume) is vitally important.

"Sperm count" (sperm concentration) is another term often referred to which, in itself, is meaningless. When concerned with semen quality, one should think in terms of total numbers and morphologically normal sperm. Each ejaculate should be evaluated on its own merits prior to use in insemination because there are times when individual ejaculates from stallions of known high fertility are of lowered sperm quality. This is usually seen as reduced progressive motility or increased morphologic abnormalities, or both. There also can be incomplete ejaculation at times, which leads to ejaculates with drastically lowered sperm numbers. This makes clear the necessity for sperm counting in each ejaculate. Sperm counting is usually unnecessary when only one or two mares are to be inseminated with the ejaculate of a stallion of average fertility. Visualization of the ejaculate by an experienced person plus viewing undiluted samples under the microscope can be used to estimate sperm concentration with enough accuracy for dividing ejaculates for insemination for a few mares. When stallions with low sperm output are used or if many mares must be inseminated on a given day, sperm counting becomes critical. This leads us to the question of how many sperm must be used to inseminate mares in order to ensure good fertility.

Controlled work by Pickett et al. indicates that between 100 and 500 million sperm need to be inseminated to have a reasonable chance of conception.[10] In our experience, this is a fair estimate if one includes a factor for morphologic normalcy. These numbers provide a base to begin working with a given stallion. We believe that, on the average, 100 million morphologically normal, progressively motile sperm is an adequate number to begin breeding, while realizing that there are individual stallions from which more or fewer sperm will be needed. For example, exceptional stallions can be used with much less than 100 million normal motile sperm per insemination, whereas others will require more than 500 million to achieve acceptable conception rates. Such variation probably reflects intrinsic sperm characteristics, which we currently have no practical means of identifying. Working with individual stallions for one or more seasons will allow one to learn what sperm numbers and quality are necessary for insemination. This requires the keeping of a daily log book in which is recorded information pertaining to the collection and evaluation of each ejaculate. This includes the number of mounts per ejaculation, ejaculate volume, gel volume, initial progressive motility, sperm concentration, any abnormalities seen, names of mares inseminated with each ejaculate, and numbers of sperm each received. Such information can be important when problems arise or for routine evaluation of a given stallion's performance.

METHODS OF SPERM COUNTING

Two methods are available for counting sperm: with a hemocytometer (the basic method) and with a spectrophotometer calibrated by hemocytometer counting. Hemocytometer counting is the most accurate method but is limited by the skill of the person using it. Inaccuracy arises mainly in use of the blood cell pipette. We have overcome this somewhat by using 5 or 10 microliter Eppindorf pipettes to replace the blood cell pipette. These can be used by the inexperienced person with less chance for inaccuracy. When several stallions are used daily, the spectrophotometric method of sperm counting can be used to reduce the time involved in sperm counting. The spectrophotometer measures light transmission through a solution and is nonselective as regards sperm. This means that inaccuracy develops when nonsperm, particulate matter such as epithelial cells, blood cells, or foreign material is in the ejaculate. The spectrophotometer is also no more accurate than the hemocytometer counting that was done to calibrate it. A further inaccuracy can occur when the glass cuvettes become scratched with use.

USE OF STORED STALLION SEMEN

Semen can be stored either in the frozen or unfrozen state. Attempts have been made to develop successful methods of freezing stallion semen,[5, 8] yet none developed to date will provide conception rates approximating those attained by use of fresh semen. Most attempts toward further development of frozen semen in the United States have been abandoned. In addition, little incentive has been given by horse breeding associations toward this end. Discouragement is the rule rather than the exception.

In regard to low temperature nonfreezing storage, work by Nishikawa et al. tends to show that stallion semen does not withstand storage well at 5° C for 24 to 48 hours and that fertility suffers.[6] Again, individual stallion variations exist. In general, one should limit use of stallion semen to use in the fresh state, and insemination should be made within two hours of collection.

SEMEN EXTENDERS

After 15 years of intensive experience in breeding mares (five years using raw semen and ten years using extended, fresh semen with the extender containing antibiotics), there is no difference in overall conception rates between raw and extended semen. However, there is a lowered uterine infection rate when antibiotic-treated semen is used. For that reason alone, I would no longer consider use of raw semen for insemination because all raw semen is highly contaminated with bacteria when collected with the artificial vagina. Laymen tend to expect too much from semen extenders by expecting an extender to improve quality of sperm and provide greatly prolonged viability. A semen extender should provide some cryoprotective activity as well as substrates, which sperm can utilize as an exogenous energy source. Most important are the antibiotics to reduce bacterial contamination. Other additives may be used in attempts to maintain sperm cell membrane integrity. Ideally, an extender should be as simple as possible and should not be difficult to make or store.

Cryoprotectives for Semen Extenders. Egg yolk provides cryoprotective activity by virtue of its lipoproteins. It has been used successfully for years in bull semen extenders with no problems insofar as fertility is concerned but is not suitable for stallion semen. I found in one brief period of use in 1970 that it was disastrous to fertility of stallion semen; Kenney et al. found that longevity of motility of sperm was twice as long in skim milk extender as compared to egg yolk extender.[4] Skim milk has cryoprotective activity also but without harmful effects on fertility. Our controlled work in 1979 showed that when extended with skim milk, stallion sperm could withstand rapid temperature drops to 0° C for 10 minutes without affecting sperm motility or respiration irreversibly.[1] The cryoprotective agent in skim milk has not been identified, but it apparently binds to sperm cell membranes because sperm exposed to skim milk exhibit their cryoprotection through at least two washings. Glycerol is a common additive for its cryoprotective activity in freezing sperm of many species but has been shown to be detrimental to stallion sperm fertility.

Energy Source. Energy sources that can be broken down by the enzymes contained in spermatozoa must be chosen. Glucose is such a source for stallion sperm and performs very well in stallion semen extenders. Other workers have used lactose and raffinose with some success.

Buffers. We have tried a few zwitterion buffers and found Trisma hydrochloride to be the most successful, but all have the deficiency of raising the osmolarity to above 400 mOsm. We have found that sodium bicarbonate is best suited to extenders for stallion semen. When allowed to stand for two or more hours, the bicarbonate will cause the pH to rise but apparently causes no problem to sperm. We have adopted one semen extender, which has now been used successfully for 10 years. The following is its formula:

Dry skim milk (Sanalac)	2.4 gm
Glucose	4.9 gm
Water (deionized or distilled)	96 ml
Sodium bicarbonate (8.4%)	1.6 ml
Gentocin solution	2.0 ml
(Gentamicin sulfate, 50 mg/ml)	

The extender can be made up in large batches (one liter or more). The batches can be divided into 50 or 100 ml aliquots, placed in sterile plastic bags (Whirl Pak), and frozen for future use. We recommend semen-to-extender ratios of 1:1 to 1:3, depending on the sperm concentration of the ejaculate and the number of mares to be bred.

PRACTICAL CONSIDERATIONS CONCERNING THE TIMING OF ARTIFICIAL INSEMINATION

The ideal time to inseminate mares would be just prior to ovulation. In a practical sense this is not necessary when a stallion of average or better fertility is mated to a mare of equal fertility. Stallion sperm can be expected to be fertile for at least 48 hours in the mare tract and, with some stallions, for much longer. We have three documented cases of insemination taking place six days prior to ovulation with conception and live foals following. We have adopted a three-days-a-week system of semen collection and insemination. This divides the week into two 48-hour periods between inseminations and one 72-hour period. In two seasons of use involving close to 2000 mares, we cannot find any statistical difference between mares' conception rates when bred prior to a 48-hour interinsemination period or a 72-hour interinsemination period.

There are a few stallions that produce sperm of short viability in the mare tract. They identify themselves quickly and must be managed so that insemination is performed close to ovulation.

POSTOVULATION INSEMINATION

Postovulation insemination can be successful when carried out before 12 hours have elapsed.[11] The condition of the cervix is used to determine whether or not the mare should be inseminated. The cervix is useful for this purpose because progesterone levels rise with ovulation and cause the cervix to be closed 24 hours after ovulation. Therefore, if the mare has ovulated without prior insemination and the cervix is still wide open, she should be inseminated. If it is closed or nearly so, she

should not be inseminated because conception rate will be essentially nil.

MEANS OF INSEMINATION

Nothing but chemically clean, sterile, disposable equipment for collection, processing, and deposition of semen into the mare is used. This not only saves much labor but, in contrast to washed glassware or plastics, ensures freedom from residues that harm sperm. For insemination, we prefer to use a 30 ml disposable syringe attached to a plastic disposable infusion pipette.

SITE OF SEMEN DEPOSITION IN THE MARE

The semen is deposited in the body of the uterus. We have no experience in deposition of sperm into the ipsilateral uterine horn and have not been stimulated to try because of the high conception and foaling rates obtained by insemination into the uterine body.

EVALUATION OF PROGRAM SUCCESS AND INDIVIDUAL STALLION FERTILITY IN AN ARTIFICIAL BREEDING PROGRAM

Two main criteria should be used to evaluate stallion fertility and breeding success: quality of mares bred and total management of those mares. To be able to accurately assess these criteria, one must be closely associated with both procedures. The veterinarian doing the mare examination, semen collection, evaluation, and insemination should have an accurate picture of both the mares and their overall management. A properly managed group of maiden mares under six years of age is the best indicator of breeding success. In this group, one should expect 90 to 100 per cent conception rates. If much lower, there is usually a management or fertility problem; usually, it is the former.

A veterinarian for a large breeding farm recently indicated that he was thinking of abandoning the use of semen extender because he could get no better than 70 per cent conception rates. When asked to break down the fertility rates by stallion, he found that his best two stallions got 90 and 92 per cent of their mares in foal under the insemination program that was yielding 70 per cent overall. Furthermore, neither the insemination program nor the fertility of the other stallions was at fault. The truth was that the best stallions were receiving the best quality of mares for breeding and the overall problem was that the farm retained too many mares with severe fertility problems.

In summary, inseminating mares with properly extended semen containing a broad-spectrum antibiotic has been rewarding in the past 15 years when combined with total mare management for fertility, since it provides high conception and live-foal rates as well as reduced infection rates.

References

1. Cooper, W. L.: The effect of rapid temperature changes on oxygen uptake by and motility of stallion spermatozoa. Conference of the Society of Theriogenology, 13–14, Sept. 1979.
2. Hughes, J. P., and Loy, R. G.: Artificial insemination in the equine. Cornell Vet., *60*:463, 1970.
3. Kenney, R. M., and Cooper, W. L.: Therapeutic use of a phantom for semen collection from a stallion. J. Am. Vet. Med. Assoc., *165*:706, 1974.
4. Kenney, R. M., Kingston, R. S., Rajamannon, A. H., and Ranberg, C. F.: Stallion semen characteristics for predicting fertility. Proc. Seventeenth Annu. Conv. Am. Assoc. Eq. Pract., 1971, pp. 53–67.
5. Krause, D., and Grove, D.: Deep freezing of jackass and stallion semen in concentrated pellet form. J. Reprod. Fertil., *14*:139, 1967.
6. Nishikawa, Y.: Studies on the preservation of raw and frozen horse semen. J. Reprod. Fertil. Suppl., 23:99, 1975.
7. Nishikawa, Y.: Studies on the protective effects of eggyolk and glycerol on the freezability of horse sperm. Proceedings of the Seventh International Congress on Animal Reproduction and Artificial Insemination, 2:1545, 1972.
8. Pace, M. M., and Sullivan, J. J.: Effect of timing of insemination numbers of spermatozoa and extender components on the pregnancy rate in mares inseminated with frozen stallion semen. J. Reprod. Fertil. Suppl. 23:115, 1975.
9. Pickett, B. W.: Impotence and abnormal sexual behavior in the stallion. Theriogenology, 8:329, 1977.
10. Pickett, B. W., and Voss, J. L.: The effect of semen extenders and sperm number on mare fertility. J. Reprod. Fertil. Suppl. 23:95, 1975.
11. Saltzman, A. A.: Inseminations of mares after ovulation. Sovetsk. Zootech., No. 4:77, 1939 (Anim. Breed. Abs. 8, 16, 1940).
12. Thompson, D. L., Jr., Pickett, B. W., Berndtson, W. E., Voss, J. L., and Nett, J. M.: Reproductive physiology of the stallion. VIII: Artificial photoperiod, collection interval and seminal characteristics, sexual behavior and concentration of LH and testosterone in serum. J. Anim. Sci., *44*:656, 1977.
13. Von Lepel, J. FRHR: Maintenance of fertility in the horse including artificial insemination, Equine Vet. J., 7:97, 1975.
14. Wierzbowski, S.: Odruchy plciowe ogierow. [The sexual reflexes of stallions.] Roczn. Nauk Roln. [B], *73*:753, 1959.

Section 10

RESPIRATORY DISEASES

Edited by N. E. Robinson

THE DIAGNOSIS AND TREATMENT OF COUGHING 463

ANTIMICROBIAL TREATMENT OF RESPIRATORY DISEASE 467

EMERGENCY VENTILATION 475

OXYGEN THERAPY 478

SINUSITIS 481

GUTTURAL POUCH DISEASE 485

PHARYNGITIS 490

SOFT PALATE DISPLACEMENT 493

DISEASES OF THE EPIGLOTTIS 494

LARYNGEAL HEMIPLEGIA 496

FOAL PNEUMONIA AND LUNG ABSCESSES 501

CHRONIC AIRWAY DISEASE 505

SUMMER PASTURE–ASSOCIATED OBSTRUCTIVE PULMONARY DISEASE 512

EXERCISE-INDUCED PULMONARY HEMORRHAGE 516

LUNG PARASITES 520

PLEURITIS 523

THE DIAGNOSIS AND TREATMENT OF COUGHING

Gregory L. Ferraro, ARCADIA, CALIFORNIA

The causes of coughing can be many and varied. Therefore, any attempt by the practitioner to use a blanket cure for this common complaint will produce unsatisfactory results. In every case, the abnormalities that cause the persistent cough must be determined prior to treatment. Most often, one will find a single cause, but multiple causes are possible. The veterinarian must piece together facts obtained from a careful history, a thorough clinical examination, and laboratory data into a meaningful picture of the causal relationship between the abnormalities discovered and the complaint of coughing. Once the suspected cause is discovered, a reasonable and ideally successful program of therapy can be instituted. One must be prepared for prolonged therapy in many cases and for therapeutic failure in some. To avoid serious misunderstandings or unhappiness on the part of the client, these possibilities should always be discussed with the owner before long, arduous, and expensive treatment programs are embarked upon. Many patients presenting with a chronic cough have a history of several courses of unsuccessful treatment. The reasons for failure of previous treatment regimens should be investigated, with the hope of providing information useful in determining the cause of the cough. This knowledge will also keep the clinician from repeating ineffective therapy.

THE HISTORY OF THE COMPLAINT

The history of the coughing horse must be taken very carefully. One must determine exactly when and how often animals cough and what type of cough is heard. Very often, the client who complains that the horse is coughing "all the time" will reveal upon further questioning that the animal coughs only in relationship to certain definite events, such as feeding, exercise, or the return to the stall. This specificity of time and place can be quite helpful in determining the cause. Animals that cough in association with exercise do so because the exercise is aggravating to the condition or because the abnormality does not manifest itself unless the respiratory tract is stressed by work. If coughing is related to exercise, the veterinarian should try to determine if it occurs throughout the exercise period or only at the beginning or end. Horses with guttural pouch disease, for example, often cough toward the end of exercise because the exertion stimulates drainage of the pouches into the pharynx,

thereby stimulating the cough reflex. Coughing that occurs throughout the exercise period or only in the first minute or two immediately after the completion of the workout is often related to pharyngeal problems such as an entrapped epiglottis or upward displacement of the soft palate.

If coughing is unrelated to exercise, the veterinarian should determine what other events are associated. Some animals cough only while eating, because of a sensitivity to hay or dust pollens, or because of a mechanical defect of the pharynx or larynx that prevents the proper sealing of the rima glottidis. An arytenoepiglottic fold or a chondroma of the arytenoid cartilage can cause this latter type of cough. Many animals cough only while in their stalls, which may indicate an environmental cause such as poor ventilation, dusty stalls, or poor-quality bedding. Animals with allergic-type bronchial disease may also present with this type of complaint.

THE CLINICAL EXAMINATION

Once a thorough and accurate history is obtained, the veterinarian begins the clinical examination, being guided by facts obtained from the history and eliminating those causes of coughing that do not coincide with that history. The single most important determination made in the clinical examination is whether the cough originates in the upper or lower respiratory tract. Treatment for chronic lung disease will have disappointing results if a problem of the larynx or pharynx is the source of the cough. The clinical examination is initially conducted at rest but should be repeated immediately postexercise, because many respiratory conditions become more obvious or manifest themselves only after exercise.

The examination should begin with observation of the head and throat area. The veterinarian should examine the nares for any signs of discharge, and the sinus area should be visually examined and percussed. One should inspect for signs of asymmetry of the face, which could indicate diseased sinuses. Palpation of the submandibular and parotid glands, guttural pouches, and larynx should always be included in the examination of the head and neck.

The clinical examination must always include a thorough auscultation and percussion of the chest. Auscultation should be conducted in a quiet environment and is aided by temporarily holding a large plastic bag over the nose of the patient to cause deeper and more rapid respiration. Percussion must

463

be very thorough and should be conducted while observing the patient's response as well as listening to the sounds elicited, since animals with pleuritic lesions often show resentment or pain on percussion of their chests. An upper thrust at the base of the sternum may also elicit a grunt or cough in animals with chronic pleuritic adhesions.

The next phase in the clinical examination is conducted with the flexible fiberoptic endoscope. This part of the examination is conducted at rest and, if necessary, is repeated after exercise. Conditions such as guttural pouch drainage or mucopurulent discharge within the trachea as a result of chronic tracheobronchial disease are often seen only after exercise. All parts of the pharynx and larynx must be examined, and the endoscope should always be passed through the larynx and into the proximal trachea to search for inflammation, exudate, or foreign material.

During the physical examination, the veterinarian should also try to elicit a cough by the patient in order to determine its character. Sometimes this can be done by manipulation of the pharynx and larynx, but very often the veterinarian may have to watch the animal at exercise or in the stall and wait for coughing to occur naturally.

The clinical examination may also include any laboratory tests the veterinarian feels necessary. A complete blood count (CBC) and fecal examination are usually performed, and a transtracheal wash and culture or a pharyngeal culture and biopsy may also be desirable.

The clinical examination must include observation of the patient's housing and environment. A significant number of animals presenting as chronic coughers are helped more by a change of environment than by the use of specific therapeutic agents. Poor housing and dusty environments cannot be overcome by chemotherapy.

Upon the completion of history-taking and the clinical examination, the veterinarian should then be able, based upon evaluation of the facts, to determine the probable cause of the cough. If that is not the case, the examination should be repeated or the patient referred to someone with more sophisticated diagnostic tools.

VIRAL INFECTIONS OF THE RESPIRATORY TRACT

Viral respiratory infections such as equine influenza (p. 31) and rhinopneumonitis (p. 41) are very common in horses and are almost always accompanied by coughing. The cough, which usually follows the onset of the disease by one or two days, is due to damage of the respiratory mucosa by the infecting virus and generally persists until the integ-

rity of this tissue is restored. In uncomplicated viral respiratory infections, clinical improvement is seen in five to seven days, but complete healing of the respiratory mucosa requires approximately 21 days. Coughing may persist at least that long. Many commercially available cough preparations are helpful in reducing the severity of coughing. Those containing expectorants are preferred by the author.

UPPER RESPIRATORY CAUSES OF COUGHING

Pharyngitis. Pharyngitis is a commonly recognized problem in performance horses. Coughing is not a sign of uncomplicated pharyngitis. The treatment of pharyngitis is discussed on page 491.

Acute Guttural Pouch Disease. Acute guttural pouch infection and inflammation produce different clinical signs than the classical empyema of the pouches (p. 485). Acute inflammation does not result in large amounts of purulent exudate at the nostrils when the animal lowers its head. Rather, it is often subclinical, with the only complaint being a cough toward the end of the exercise period. The diagnosis is made by endoscopic examination immediately after exercise and observation of a discharge, which is usually mucopurulent in character, from one or both pouch openings. Since this discharge may only be visible a short time after exercise, the examination must be conducted immediately after exercise.

A definitive diagnosis of a guttural pouch infection can only be made by passing the endoscope into the pouch and observing inflamed mucosa and an exudate. Since this can be time-consuming and rather difficult, most clinicians are content to assume a diagnosis based on the observation of exudate at the pouch openings and a response to therapy.

Treatment of acute guttural pouch inflammation requires flushing of the pouch, which can be accomplished in one of two ways. A metal Chambers mare catheter* can be blindly passed up the nostril and into the pouch opening once or twice daily for approximately five days. This procedure takes practice, but with reasonable experience, most clinicians can master it easily.

The catheter is passed up the floor of the ventral meatus. Upon reaching the pharynx, the catheter tip is turned laterally and somewhat dorsally. The instrument is slid gently along the wall of the pharynx until it slides through the pouch openings and into the pouch. It is easy to tell when the catheter is placed correctly, for it will slide to the hub of the instrument only when it is within the pouch. If the

*Chambers mare catheter (metal), Jen-Sal Labs, Burroughs Wellcome Co., Kansas City, MO

pouch opening has been missed, the catheter will stop short of the hub when it strikes the dorsal pharynx.

Alternatively, an indwelling catheter is placed in the pouch with the aid of an endoscope. The end of the catheter projects out of the nostril and is sutured in place for a period of a few days, and the desired solution is flushed up the catheter several times daily. Several types of catheters are suitable. Two commonly used are the Foley catheter* or the indwelling intrauterine infuser made by Fort Dodge Labs.† If the latter is used, the clinician should suture the ram's horn–like end to the catheter. This procedure ensures that the endpiece will not come loose and be retained in the pouch. Most clinicians feel that the self-retaining catheters should not be left in the animal for more than three or four days, as the catheters themselves become a source of inflammation.

There has been considerable debate as to which infusion solutions are the most effective for treatment (p. 486). Some antibiotics are suitable if culture and sensitivity tests have been obtained. If not, it is probably better to use mild, nonirritating antiseptic agents such as a 5 to 10 per cent solution of povidone-iodine‡ in physiologic saline. There are major nerve branches running through or close to the guttural pouch, and the instillation of irritating or heat-producing compounds such as hydrogen peroxide or hydrogen peroxide–organic iodine combinations may cause pharyngeal paralysis. If the diagnosis has been correct, a response to therapy should occur, and coughing should subside in a few days. In animals treated with indwelling catheters, a discharge may continue throughout treatment and for up to three days after the removal of the catheters.

Pharyngeal Ulcers. Pharyngeal ulcers can cause irritation sufficient to cause coughing if they are large or located in particularly sensitive areas such as the free border of the soft palate. Coughing associated with these lesions is frequently noticed during exercise and also when the animal is eating. They are readily diagnosed with the use of the fiberoptic endoscope. These ulcers are amenable to treatment by chemical cautery with a mild agent such as Harter's iodine (Table 1). Cautery may have to be repeated several times. Depending on the location of the lesion, cautery may be accomplished using a shielded uterine culture swab or by passing a catheter through the endoscope and infusing the cauterizing agent directly onto the ulcerated area.

Laryngitis and Tracheitis. These conditions

---

*Foley catheter, Bickford, Inc., East Aurora, NY
†Indwelling intrauterine infuser, Fort Dodge Labs, Fort Dodge, IA
‡Betadine solution, Purdue Frederick Co., Norwalk, CT

TABLE 1. HARTER'S IODINE

Phenol	400 ml
Belladonna extract	800 ml
Tincture of iodine #70	1200 ml
Glycerine	1600 ml
	4000 ml

cause coughing at any time during the animal's daily routine, but if the tracheal inflammation is due to failure of the rima glottidis to seal during swallowing, coughing will be most noticeable when the animal eats or drinks. When tracheitis is diagnosed with the fiberoptic endoscope, the clinician should try to determine if there is a failure of closure of the rima glottidis. The two common causes of this are abnormalities of the epiglottis and postsurgical complications of laryngoplasty because either the arytenoid cartilage has been retracted too severely or the retracting sutures have been placed improperly. The endoscope should be passed through the opening of the larynx to examine the luminal surface of the cricoid cartilage and to determine if the laryngoplastic suture has invaded the mucosa, causing the tracheitis and an associated chondritis. Abnormalities of this type are very serious and often require surgical correction. If failure of sealing of the rima glottidis is suspected, the lungs should also be examined for evidence of an inhalation pneumonia. If the tracheitis is not complicated by a failure of the rima glottidic seal, treatment is usually simple. Systemic antibiotic therapy or a combination of antibiotic and anti-inflammatory therapy is usually sufficient. Culture and sensitivity tests may be helpful in selecting the appropriate antibiotic.

Arytenoepiglottic Folds. Entrapment of the epiglottis by an arytenoepiglottic fold can be a cause of coughing, particularly if the fold was adhered to the dorsal surface of the epiglottis or has become severely inflamed and ulcerated. Because this condition interferes with swallowing, the cough in these animals occurs during eating and also periodically throughout the exercise period when the animal attempts to swallow the respiratory secretions that develop during the gallop. Correction of this problem is surgical (p. 494), and if coughing is a sign, it will persist despite medical treatment until surgical correction is accomplished. Coughing may not be associated with this condition, however, especially if the entrapment is intermittent. Other causes of coughing must be eliminated before the diagnosis of coughing due to entrapment of the epiglottis is made. Also, it should be noted that some animals can perform quite well in spite of an entrapment, and, therefore, if an intermittent cough is the only complaint, surgical correction may be postponed until such time as the condition affects performance.

al Displacement of the Soft Palate. Horses
...isplace the soft palate dorsal to the epiglottis
/ swallowing or during exercise frequently cough
... eral times until the palate returns to the correct
position. Animals with chronic dorsal displacement
of the soft palate frequently have a persistent intermittent cough in addition to exercise intolerance
and an expiratory gurgle during exercise. While dorsal displacement of the soft palate can be readily
observed with the endoscope, it should not be designated as the cause of coughing unless associated
respiratory signs can also be demonstrated, because
many normal animals displace the soft palate with
the endoscope in the pharynx.

The clinician should not confuse chronic dorsal
displacement of the soft palate with soft palate paresis. True soft palate paresis, either complete or
partial, is associated with problems of deglutition
and is usually accompanied by extrusion of food from
the nostrils. Animals suffering from soft palate paresis eventually succumb to inhalation pneumonia.

While many treatments are currently proposed
for the correction of dorsal displacement of the soft
palate (p. 493), it is the opinion of this author that
none is effective. An attempt should be made to
manage the problem with training aids (such as bits,
nose bands, and tongue ties), and if these are ineffective, retirement from athletic competition is advised.

Chondromas of the Arytenoid Cartilages.
Infection of the arytenoid cartilage that results in
the formation of a chondroma can result in coughing
as well as other clinical signs. Chondromas most
often protrude through the mucosal surface on the
medial or intraluminal surface of the arytenoid cartilage. While they generally first appear unilaterally,
they often form a kissing lesion on the opposite arytenoid cartilage, leading to bilateral chondroma
formation. Coughing is often one of the earliest complaints. Clinical signs progress as the chondroma
enlarges and leads to an abnormal sound during exercise. This sound is very similar to that heard with
laryngeal hemiplegia, except that the noise is heard
on both inspiration and expiration. Advanced cases
of chondritis of the arytenoids exhibit severe dyspnea even at rest. The diagnosis is made by examining the larynx via the fiberoptic endoscope. The
only effective treatment is surgical removal of the
affected cartilage (p. 499). The prognosis for a return
to pasture soundness is quite good, but the likelihood of a return to athletic competition has yet to
be determined.

Suprapharyngeal Swellings. Space-occupying
lesions such as abscesses or tumors located in close
proximity to the larynx or pharynx are a further
cause of coughing. Severe phlebitis of the jugular
vein with thrombosis is also sometimes associated
with coughing. Coughing in cases such as these is
a secondary problem, and adequate treatment of the

primary problem should result in cessation of the
cough.

TREATMENT OF PULMONARY SOURCES OF COUGHING

Pulmonary causes of chronic coughing include
parasitism, chronic obstructive pulmonary disease,
and pleuritis.

Parasitism. Coughing in the horse as a result of
parasitic infestation is usually due to infection with
Parascaris equorum or *Dictyocaulus arnfieldi.*
Coughing is a common sign of heavy infestations of
both of these parasites, and so any horse, especially
a younger animal, suspected of having pulmonary
disease should be examined for infestations of these
parasites. The diagnosis of *Parascaris equorum* infestation is easily made via a fecal examination. If
heavy infestation is found, coughing may be a result
of larval migration of this parasite through the lung
parenchyma. Treatment of this condition is administration of thiabendazole* via a stomach tube at a
dose of 440 mg per kg. At this level, thiabendazole
is considered to be larvicidal. The diagnosis and
treatment of *Dictyocaulus arnfieldi* infestation is described in detail elsewhere (p. 520). In this author's
opinion, the most effective treatment for this parasite is two doses of thiabendazole at a level of 440
mg per kg administered orally at 24 hour intervals.

Chronic Obstructive Pulmonary Disease. Animals suspected of having chronic obstructive lung
disease or chronic bronchiolitis (p. 505) require a
thorough clinical examination and evaluation. Careful auscultation and percussion of the chest both at
rest and after exercise are the first steps in this examination, even though they are often totally un-
revealing. An endoscopic examination should be
conducted immediately after exercise to determine
if a mucopurulent exudate is present in the distal
trachea. This material may only be evident for one
to two hours after the exercise period, and its presence in the trachea is good presumptive evidence
that chronic bronchiolitis exists. Radiographic examination of the chest is not available to all practicing veterinarians but can be very useful in protracted cases for determining both the severity of
the disease and the possible prognosis for recovery.
Therapy of chronic obstructive pulmonary disease
is described in detail elsewhere (p. 507). Medical
therapy will always be prolonged and should be accompanied by improvement of the horse's environment. The prognosis should always be guarded.

Chronic Pleuritis. While not a common cause
of coughing, chronic pleuritic lesions such as abscesses or adhesions can often be associated with a
chronic cough, which can often be elicited by ex-

---

*Thiabendazole, Merck and Co., Inc., Rahway, NJ 07065

erting an upward pressure at the base of the sternum or by leaning against the right or left side of the animal's chest and forcing sideways movement. A complete blood count should be taken to determine if the hemogram is consistent with the presence of an abscess. Several blood samples may be necessary, taken at different times, with at least one taken a day or two after strenuous exercise. Serum protein fractionation may also be helpful to determine the presence of a chronic inflammatory process. One should expect to see a decrease in albumin levels and an increase in the α1, α2, and possibly also the gamma globulin levels in these cases. A positive diagnosis may only be possible, however, with a radiographic examination of the chest. If chronic pleuritic adhesions or abscesses are present, treatment may often prove to be extremely difficult. Protracted antibiotic therapy is almost always indicated, however (for example, 2.5 gm kanamycin sulfate twice a day for two to three weeks, followed by a rest period of two weeks and a repeat treatment period of two to three weeks). While this may prove helpful in minimizing signs, complete recovery, if possible, will probably require an extended rest period of several months (p. 523).

CONCLUSION

The successful treatment of the coughing horse is dependent upon several factors. The most important of these is proper identification of the cause of the cough. Only after that determination has been made can successful treatment be accomplished. Treatment of these patients generally requires an extended period of time and involves several important elements. These include chemotherapy, patient management, environmental control, and sometimes surgical intervention. Horse owners should be informed of these procedures and of the often guarded nature of the prognosis to avoid misunderstandings in protracted cases. Shotgun treatment, or therapy instituted without a thorough knowledge of the causative factors of the cough, should always be avoided.

Supplemental Readings

1. Exercise-induced pulmonary hemorrhage in the racing horse. Proc. 26th Annu. Conv. Am. Assoc. Eq. Pract., 1980.
2. Illinois Veterinary Respiratory Symposium, University of Illinois at Urbana, November 13–15, 1978.
3. Pearce, H. G.: Aspects of lower respiratory tract disease in the horse. NZ Vet. J., 27:1, 1979.
4. Proc. Equine Respiratory Disease Symposium, Ohio State University, May 19–20, 1980. Am. Assoc. Eq. Pract. Newsletter, No. 2, June, 1980.
5. Round, M. C.: Lungworm infection (Dictyocaulus arnfieldi) of horses and donkeys. Vet. Rec., 99:393, 1976.
6. Symposium on Equine Respiratory Disease. Vet. Clin. North Am. (Large Anim. Pract.), 1(1), 1979.

ANTIMICROBIAL TREATMENT OF RESPIRATORY DISEASE

Jill Beech, KENNETT SQUARE, PENNSYLVANIA

A wide range of antibiotics is used to treat respiratory infection in horses. The choice of antibiotics is often based on the veterinarian's clinical experience, especially when bacterial cultures are not done or are negative. In addition to the sensitivity patterns of the various microbes, other factors are important in determining the therapeutic outcome (p. 43).

DOSAGES AND ROUTES OF ADMINISTRATION

The tissue concentration of an antibiotic can be affected by the dose and the route and rate of administration. If it is given in too low a dose or in a site with poor blood flow, effective tissue levels may not be reached. Rate of intravenous infusion is important. Bolus injection usually results in a higher tissue level, as the highest local concentrations are associated with the highest peak serum values. However, the minimum inhibitory concentration (MIC) for the particular pathogen must be considered when deciding which method is optimal. If it is high, a high-dose intravenous bolus may be best, but if the MIC is low, intramuscular injection would be preferable because it would maximize the time period when the drug level in bronchial fluids exceeds the MIC. Serum protein binding inhibits antibiotic penetration of tissues, but for most antibiotics, the active free portion of the drug is not significantly reduced until this exceeds 80 per cent (Table 1).

TABLE 1. SERUM PROTEIN BINDING OF ANTIBIOTICS*

Extensive (>80%)	Moderately High (50–80%)	Low (<50%)
Penicillin V	Penicillin G	Ampicillin (4–10)
Erythromycin (5)	Cephalothin	Chloramphenicol
Sulfadimethoxine	Trimethoprim	Oxytetracycline (10–30)
	Sulfamethoxazole	Aminoglycosides Gentamicin (20–40)
		Amikacin (25)
		Cephaloridine
		Cephalexin
		Spectinomycin

*Percentage of peak serum levels reached in bronchi or sputum is in parentheses.[18, 25] (Adapted from Baggott, J. D.: Distribution of antimicrobial agents in normal and diseased animals. J. Am. Vet. Med. Assoc., *176*:1085, 1980.)

PRESENCE OF INFLAMMATION AND EXUDATE

Pus and a low pH can slow bacterial growth and decrease the efficacy of cell wall synthesis inhibitors such as the penicillins. Despite its penetrating ability, penicillin may be ineffective for these reasons in abscesses. Cell breakdown products in pus may bind drugs, such as gentamicin and polymyxin B, and decrease their activity. Changes in pH may also affect diffusion of the antibiotic through the bacterial cell membrane and can decrease the effectiveness of drugs, such as the aminoglycosides and sulfas. Weak acids, such as tetracycline and nitrofurantoin, are more effective, whereas weak bases, such as erythromycin and aminoglycosides, have decreased activity in the lower pH ranges. The effect of pH must always be taken into account when adding antibiotics to infusing solutions. Fibrin may alter drug penetration. For example, penicillin G penetrates it better than sulfonamides.[2]

Antibiotic penetration of the blood-bronchus barrier varies. Local inflammation of airways increases bronchial penetration, but when this subsides and sputum production falls, levels of many antibiotics, such as ampicillin and cephalexin, decrease. This does not occur with gentamicin or tetracycline. Patients with chronic bronchitis may also have slower clearance of intrabronchial antibiotics. Intrabronchial bleeding from any cause increases secretion levels. For intraparenchymal lung damage without significant purulent tracheobronchitis, alveolar and interstitial fluid antibiotic concentrations closely approximate serum levels. Certain gram-negative organisms (but not gram-negative bacilli) do not need continuous exposure to antibiotics to be inhibited; for example, the inhibitory effects of macrolides, tetracyclines, and beta lactamase–resistant penicillins persist for several hours after drug levels disappear from the area.

HOST FACTORS

Host factors, such as phagocytosis and intracellular killing of bacteria, are also essential to recovery, and these can be affected by antibiotic dosing. After periods of treatment with antibiotic concentrations above the MIC, postantibiotic leukocyte enhancement or enhanced bacterial susceptibility to phagocytosis and killing occurs. Other host influences on phagocytosis and bacterial killing also play a role, and immunocompromised horses cannot respond optimally to antimicrobial treatment.

DRUG INTERACTIONS (p. 43)

Certain antibiotics may inactivate others when mixed prior to injection, even though they may be synergistic when given simultaneously yet separately. An example is the combination of gentamicin and carbenicillin.

Cost of the drug and frequency, ease, and route of administration are all very important and may prevent use of the ideal antibiotic in some patients. Clinical experience often is a major influence. For example, in our area, oxytetracycline is commonly used and in general is thought to be very efficacious, yet clinicians elsewhere do not use oxytetracycline because of side effects. A review of 58 cases of foal pneumonia in our clinic revealed that oxytetracycline, penicillin, and chloramphenicol appeared to give the best clinical responses despite evaluation of the sensitivities of the various organisms cultured suggesting that chloramphenicol, gentamicin, and erythromycin would be the best. Ampicillin and aminoglycosides were used less frequently, and erythromycin was not used at this time. Regardless of the antibiotic chosen, the disease must be treated for an appropriate length of time. For very severe pneumonia and pleuritis, treatment may need to be continued for 6 to 10 weeks. When chronic treatment is needed, it is often necessary to change the antibiotic after several weeks; for example, oxytetracycline treatment is usually not continued for more than two weeks and aminoglycosides rarely beyond two to three weeks. Drugs such as penicillin, ampicillin, and chloramphenicol have been used continuously for long periods. Myositis and phlebitis may dictate the need for change to an oral drug. To date we have not had any undesirable side effects from long-term use of oral chloramphenicol, trimethoprim-sulfa, isoniazid, ampicillin, or cephalexin.

Different antibiotics available for use and commonly used in treating respiratory disease will be briefly discussed. The previously mentioned factors, as well as possible toxicity, must be considered when choosing a drug. Unfortunately, most data on dosages are for mature horses, and there is no information specific for foals. Therefore, doses used are usually the same as for mature horses. Many of the drugs we use have not been approved by the FDA for systemic administration in horses.

PENICILLIN G

Penicillin is effective against many gram-positive and gram-negative cocci and most anaerobes except *Bacillus fragilus*. However, anaerobes are not thought to be of great clinical importance in most equine respiratory infections.[9] Penicillin is moderately highly protein-bound (52 to 54 per cent), and, therefore, serum levels do not reflect the biologically available drug. The sodium and potassium salts are used intravenously and more rarely intramuscularly. Procaine penicillin G and benzathine penicillin salts are given intramuscularly. The latter is rarely used because blood levels, although persistent, are very low. Doses commonly used are in Table 2.

Drug combinations such as Combiotic,* Azimycin,† and Longicil S‡ are not good choices because in order to give the preferred dose of penicillin, an

---

*Combiotic, Pfizer, Inc., New York NY 10017
†Azimycin, Schering Corp., Kenilworth, NJ 07033
‡Longicil S, Ft. Dodge Labs, Inc., Ft. Dodge, IA 50501

TABLE 2. DOSES OF ANTIBIOTICS COMMONLY USED IN TREATMENT OF RESPIRATORY DISEASE AND CONCENTRATIONS IN HORSE SERUM

Antibiotic	Dose/kg	Route	Times/Day	Peak Concentration Time (hr)	Peak Concentration µg/ml	Concentration End of Period Time (hr)	Concentration End of Period µg/ml	Reference
K penicillin G	20×10^3 U	IM	4	1	0.5	6	0.3	8
	40×10^3 U	IM	4	1	2.2	6	1.6	8
	20×10^3 U	IV	4	1/2	2.7–4.4	6	0.0	8
	200×10^3 U	PO		1/2	1.4	12	0.12	8
Na penicillin G	30×10^6 U	IM	4	1/4	6.1	6	0.65	8
		IV	4					
Procaine penicillin G	22×10^3 U	IM	2	2	1.8	12	0.5	8
Ampicillin Na	11 mg	IM	4	1/2	5.3–16.0	6	4.4–5.6	4
Ampicillin trihydrate	11 mg	IM	2	2	1.0–2.1	8	0.18–2.1	4
	22 mg	IM	2	2	2.4–3.2	8	2.4–3.0	4
Amikacin	6.6 mg	IM	3–4?	1/2	15.1	6	0.9	11
	6.6 mg	IV	?	1/2	89.1	3	0.4	11
Gentamicin	1.7 mg	IM	4	1	5.2–16.0	8	0.5–0.7	3
	4.4 mg	IM	4	1/2	15–21	8	1.2–1.5	3
Kanamycin	5 mg	IM	3	1	17.6–21.4	8	~1.5	8
Oxytetracycline	5 mg	IV	2	1/2	5–8	7	1.0	8
	4.4 mg	IV	2	1/2	5.6	12	2.27	18
Sulfamethazine	220 mg on day 1	IV	1					Package insert
	110 mg on day 2	IV	1					
Chloramphenicol succinate	22 mg	IV	4–6	≤1/2	21.5	4	~1.0	5
	22 mg	IM	4	1/4–1/2	11–12	5	~2.0	5
	50 mg	IM	3	1	32.9	8	6.5	10
Chloramphenicol palmitate	50 mg	PO	4	1	46.4 ± 6.3	6	10.6 ± 1	10
Trimethoprim sulfadiazine	5.5 mg	PO	2–3	1/3	~3.2	6–7	<0.5	1
	5.5 mg	IV	2–3	1/2	7.5	6–7	~1.0	1
Isoniazid	5–15 mg	PO	2					14

Note: These dose regimens may not be FDA approved. Consult medication label on each drug for FDA recommendation or approval.

excessively high dose of dihydrostreptomycin would be injected. Also, the inclusion of a steroid with antibiotics is contraindicated in treatment of infectious respiratory disease. Combiotic contains 200,000 units of procaine penicillin G per ml and 250 mg of dihydrostreptomycin per ml. In a 500 kg horse, a dose of 22,000 units per kg (10,000 units per lb) of penicillin would be approximately 55 ml, which would contain 13.75 gm of dihydrostreptomycin (DSM), a dose higher than that usually recommended. It would also be an excessively large volume for frequent injection even if it were divided at multiple sites. If the usual dose of 5.5 mg per kg of DSM were used, the dose of penicillin would be only 4400 units per kg (2×10^3 units per lb); this would result in very low serum levels and presumably even lower tissue levels. Rollins et al.[16] found that this dose of penicillin (4400 units per kg) given as either Combiotic or Azimycin yielded peak blood levels that would generally be inadequate, as they were less than the desired minimum range of 0.5 to 1.0 μg per ml.

The MIC for most susceptible microorganisms generally ranges from 0.5 to 1.0 μg per ml (0.75 to 1.5 units per ml).[8] This includes the usual respiratory pathogens such as beta-hemolytic streptococci and nonpenicillinase-producing staphylococci but not Pasteurella. Penetration into pleural fluid and bronchial secretions is fairly good. If one accepts the general rule of the necessity to maintain an in vivo concentration at the infection site of at least two to four times the MIC, the use of intramuscular benzyl penicillin salts would not be advised, except for the most susceptible microorganisms.[8] The inactivation by pus further decreases the efficacy. When high levels are needed, frequent (at least four times daily) intravenous bolus administration of large doses is necessary. Intramuscular doses of potassium or sodium penicillin salts will achieve neither high nor persistent levels; however, when the microorganism is quite sensitive, then twice daily dosing of procaine penicillin G is usually adequate. Occasionally procaine penicillin may elicit signs of rapid forced expiration, hyperesthesia, excitability, incoordination, and muscle tremors; care must be taken not to inject the drug into a blood vessel.

AMPICILLIN

Ampicillin has a broader spectrum than penicillin (Table 3), is relatively nontoxic, and penetrates most tissues well. As it is less protein-bound than penicillin, more is biologically available. Aqueous and suspension forms are available. Doses commonly used are in Table 2.

Oral ampicillin has been used clinically in several foals with streptococcal respiratory infection with good results after the intramuscular use was stopped. However, when concentrations were measured in two mature horses receiving 22 mg per kg (10 mg per lb) orally four times daily, serum levels were low, never exceeding 2 μg per ml in one horse and never more than 0.9 μg per ml in the other, although they persisted over an eight-hour period. In humans, oral bacampicillin reaches higher and earlier peaks than ampicillin, and it might have the same advantages in horses. Ampicillin penetrates the pleural cavity like penicillin; however, as less is protein bound and elimination is less rapid, levels may be higher. Except for a few microorganisms, susceptibility patterns would suggest little advantage to its use compared to penicillin. However, it causes very little tissue reaction, and its intramuscular use results in higher and more consistent serum levels that intramuscular penicillin G.

CHLORAMPHENICOL

Chloramphenicol has a wide antibacterial spectrum, including most anaerobes (Table 3). In our clinic, except for *Corynebacterium equi*, Proteus, *Klebsiella pneumoniae*, Pseudomonas, and *Escherichia coli*, more than 95 per cent of all respiratory pathogen isolates are sensitive to it. It penetrates most tissues and secretions well and is one of the few antibiotics that penetrates well intracellularly. It is safe when used orally for several months. Although it is usually not a drug routinely chosen for use or to initiate treatment, we have used it successfully in horses with pneumonia or pleuritis, especially where it is impossible to inject drugs or where the owners are unable to administer drugs by injection. The increase in resistance of salmonella to chloramphenicol has raised questions about its use in animals. Certainly its use should be selective. In our clinic, in vitro susceptibility patterns showed an increase in resistance by *C. equi* and *E. coli*. Data on serum levels and doses used clinically have varied widely.[5, 8, 10, 13, 15, 17] One study showed that 15 mg per kg (7 mg per lb) of chloramphenicol orally gave adequate levels for only three to four hours; Davis found that 22 mg per kg (10 mg per lb) orally resulted in blood levels less than 4 μg per ml, but Oh-Ishi reported that 50 mg per kg (23 mg per lb) could give a peak of 46 μg per ml.[5, 10, 13, 17] Davis also suggested, contrary to the package insert, that intramuscular Chloromycetin* may produce greater concentrations than intravenous use.[5] The oral tablets or capsules (Anacetin†) are easier to administer than the liquid; as the taste is very bitter, they must be mixed with something to disguise the taste.

---

*Chloromycetin, Parke-Davis, Morris Plains, NJ 07950
†Anacetin, Bioceutic Laboratories, St. Joseph, MO 64502

TABLE 3. ANTIBIOTIC SENSITIVITY TEST RESULTS

	Beta-hemolytic Streptococci		E. coli		Hemolytic Staphylococci		Pasteurella sp		Proteus vulgaris		Pseudomonas sp		Enterobacter sp		Corynebacterium sp		Bordetella bronchiseptica	Klebsiella pneumoniae
No. of isolates	65*	49†	72*	87†	43*	16†	21*	27†	19*	6†	44*	13†	13*	11†	22*	8†	4†	7†
Amikacin	95	ND		100	37	ND	81	100	21	100	0	100	8	100	73	ND	100	100
Ampicillin	99	100	36	60	93	19	95	55	42	0	5	0	92	22 (0–67)	100	63	50	0
Chloromycetin	95	98	85	72	100	94	95	98	26	50	2	0	46	70	86	75	100	43
Cephalosporin	95	100	33	35	77	100	95	95	0	0	2	0	15	64	91	0	50	71
Erythromycin	92	98	5	ND	81	94	95	ND	5	ND	5	ND	46	ND	82	100	ND	ND
Furadantin	86	100	64	93	100	100	91	100	95	17	86	0	85	41	95	50	0	86
Gentamicin	83	100	97	90	77	69	71	100	26	83	7	92	62	75	68	100	100	86
Kanamycin	5	ND	40	43	72	ND	62	100	47	67	25	8	54	70	50	ND	100	43
Neomycin	3	ND	38	45	33	ND	76	93	5	67	0	8	15	70	68	ND	100	43
Penicillin	91	100	3	ND	42	19	24	40	16	ND	2	ND	38	ND	50	0	ND	ND
Streptomycin	9	ND	11	20	77	ND	76	43	5	34	9	0	62	33	50	ND	0	43
Tetracycline	31	8	25	28		81		50		0		ND		80	55	100	100	43

*From University of Pennsylvania Microbiology Laboratory, 1978
†From University of Pennsylvania Microbiology Laboratory, January 1–June 30, 1981
Numbers indicate the percentage of isolates sensitive to a given antibiotic.
ND = not done

When the oral liquid form has been used intravenously, hemolysis results but is not usually of clinical significance. Intravenous administration results in such rapid clearance that its use by this route, except in certain instances when a rapid serum rise is needed, is probably less desirable than frequent oral administration.

GENTAMICIN

Gentamicin is a broad-spectrum antibiotic but is primarily active against gram-negative organisms (Table 3). It is not active against anaerobes because its intracellular uptake depends on oxygen. As there is potential for nephrotoxicity, one should monitor the creatinine level at least once a week. Foals and mature horses have been kept on the antibiotic (2.2 mg per kg or 1.0 mg per lb intramuscularly four times daily) for three weeks without problems. Some clinicians have reported nephrotoxicity in young foals. In human infants, levels can be extremely variable, and clearance rates for foals are unknown. Levels measured in the urine of mature horses have been highly variable.[3] Unless absolutely essential, aminoglycosides, including gentamicin, should not be used in animals with impaired renal function. If they must be used in those cases, dosing frequency should be decreased because of the decreased clearance. Peripheral neuromuscular blockade can occur after aminoglycosides, and this may be enhanced by general anesthesia.

Although one study in humans showed that protein binding could be as high as 20 to 25 per cent, protein binding generally is thought to be almost nil, and aminoglycosides penetrate well into pleural fluid. There has been controversy over levels obtained in bronchial secretions, and they may be inadequate for certain bacteria; the drug is cleared more slowly from bronchial secretions than from serum. Inflammation does not appear to significantly increase the penetration into bronchial fluids. Levels are highest after rapid intravenous administration, which yields a maximal gradient between serum and bronchial fluid. Therefore, when high levels are needed in bronchial secretions, bolus injection, not long-term infusion, is probably most advisable. High doses may produce nephrotoxic serum levels, although these rapidly decline. Because of aminoglycosides' poor penetration, endotracheal administration in addition to systemic medication has been advocated in treating severe gram-negative bronchopneumonia in humans. The former yields high and sustained levels within bronchial secretions with low levels in the blood. The drug is given multiple times daily with the patient in different positions to encourage wide deposition. This is different from the method commonly used in horses in which isolated intratracheal injection of varying amounts, sometimes in combination with steroids, has been popularized. Uneven drug distribution must be tremendous with this method, and the effects have never been carefully evaluated or compared with a placebo; it is possible that the mechanical effect on bronchial clearance may be the reason for its reported efficacy. The inclusion of steroids is ill advised in the presence of infectious disease. Widely indiscriminate use of the drug could lead to an increase in resistance of bacteria, and in humans this has become a major problem necessitating development of more expensive aminoglycosides and semisynthetic penicillins. Doses suggested for use are in Table 2. We commonly use 2.2 mg per kg (1 mg per lb) intramuscularly four times daily.

KANAMYCIN

Pharmacokinetics of kanamycin are similar to those of gentamicin; however, its antimicrobial spectrum is much less and in our clinic is similar to that of neomycin (Table 3). When used for treating respiratory infections, it is frequently used in combination with penicillin. This use might be questioned, as it would not appear to significantly broaden the spectrum of activity and except where specifically indicated probably is less effective than use of a single broad-spectrum drug such as chloramphenicol. Unlike gentamicin, it has very low activity against beta-hemolytic streptococci. After the commonly used dose of 5 mg per kg (2.3 mg per lb) intramuscularly, a peak serum level of 18 μg per ml is reached in about an hour; this rapidly declines to 3 μg per ml at six hours and is about 2 μg per ml by eight hours.[8]

AMIKACIN

Amikacin is a broad-spectrum aminoglycoside. Initial data showed that 6.6 mg per kg (3 mg per lb), either intramuscularly or intravenously, resulted in levels above 4 μg per ml in serum for four to six hours. This was the concentration that inhibited growth of Klebsiella, *E. coli*, and several Pseudomonas and Serratia species.[11] Intravenous dosing yielded much higher initial peak levels for one hour; if a wide serum–bronchial secretion gradient enhances penetration of the latter as it does for gentamicin, then intravenous dosing would be preferable when treating pneumonia. Its use should be restricted to specific gram-negative infections, as indiscriminate use could result in development of resistant strains. It has been used clinically and appears to be safe.

DIHYDROSTREPTOMYCIN AND STREPTOMYCIN

These drugs are rarely used now except for their common use in combination with penicillin. For reasons stated earlier, use of combination antibiotic mixtures is ill-advised. Because of the resistance patterns and rather poor penetration into bronchial fluid, at the present time there is little reason to recommend its use in treating equine respiratory infections. However, a dose frequency used has been 5 to 7 mg per kg (2.3 to 3.2 mg per lb) intramuscularly three times daily.[8, 16] This dose gives serum levels that persist above 4.5 μg per ml for at least six hours.

OXYTETRACYCLINE

This bacteriostatic drug is very commonly and successfully used in treating equine respiratory tract infections. Despite its rather limited spectrum of activity and the wide range of bacterial sensitivity patterns, clinical response of horses with pneumonia has often been excellent. Serum protein binding is low, and it penetrates bronchial secretions quite well (Table 1). It may be combined with sulfonamides for the first week of use. Its use is not advisable in a very stressed animal or one with a gastrointestinal problem, as diarrhea may result. Large doses or use in severely stressed animals has been associated with colitis and death.[15] In our clinic, no gastrointestinal problems have been seen, except it mildly exacerbated diarrhea in a foal with Salmonella infection and has sometimes been associated with transient soft feces. MacKellar suggested that large doses of vitamin B complex controlled oxytetracycline-induced diarrhea.[15] It is irritating and can cause phlebitis and also a severe local reaction if injected perivascularly. Rapid administration can cause collapse. After a dose of 4.4 mg per kg (2 mg per lb), a peak level of 5.6 μg per ml occurs at 30 minutes, and concentrations exceed 2 μg per ml for 12 hours. Occasionally 11 mg per kg (5 mg per lb) is given intravenously once daily, but more frequently 4.4 to 5.5 mg per kg is administered twice daily.[18] It should not be given intramuscularly because of local reaction and low blood levels.

NEOMYCIN

This aminoglycoside has a narrower spectrum than gentamicin, but it is somewhat similar to or only slightly narrower than that of kanamycin. The oral form of neomycin* (200 mg per ml concentration) has been used intravenously and intramuscularly, although it is not approved for this use. A dose of 4.4 mg per kg intramuscularly two or three times a day yields fairly high blood and pleural fluid levels. Intramuscular use does cause myositis, and local reactions may be sufficient to cause one to discontinue its use. Reactions are usually transient and subside when it is discontinued. Like other aminoglycosides, it may not penetrate bronchial secretions very well.

ERYTHROMYCIN

This bacteriostatic drug is becoming used more frequently, as it is effective against a wide spectrum of microorganisms (Table 3), including many anaerobes. Although it has been reported to cause diarrhea after three to four days of use,[8] other clinicians have seen no ill effects or only transient mild diarrhea. The pediatric syrup is apparently well accepted by foals for oral use. It has been successfully used in treating a few foals with *Corynebacterium equi* pneumonia and lung abscesses. The dose is usually 10 mg per kg (4.4 mg per lb) intravenously in three to four doses.[8] It is commonly used orally in foals in a dose 1⅓ to 2 times this. After intramuscular administration of 4 mg per kg, Knight was unable to obtain a serum level above 1 μg per ml.[8] It diffuses into pleural fluids and has a high lung tissue–serum concentration ratio. Levels in bronchial fluids are lower.

TRIMETHOPRIM-SULFA

This broad-spectrum antimicrobial combination is often used in human pneumonias and has been used to less extent in horses. Knight reported that it is useful in upper respiratory infections, especially those caused by *Bordetella bronchiseptica*.[8] As the intravenous form is not available in the United States, the oral drug is used. The dose of trimethoprim should be at least 5.5 mg per kg (2.5 mg per lb) two or three times a day. For a 400 kg horse, this would be 29 tablets of Tribrissen 480† (containing a total of 11.2 gm of sulfadiazine) two to three times daily. Alexander reported that at this oral dose, concentrations in serum never exceeded 3 μg per ml and were about 0.5 μg per ml by 400 minutes.[1] Intravenous dosing yielded peak levels of 8

*Biosol, The Upjohn Co., Kalamazoo, MI 49001
†Tribrissen, Burroughs Wellcome Co., Research Triangle Park, NC 27709

μg per ml, and by 400 minutes the concentration was 1 μg per ml.

SPECTINOMYCIN

This aminocyclitol is effective against many gram-negative organisms and has a high lung-serum concentration ratio. It is sometimes used to treat equine respiratory infections, although in humans its use is limited to treatment of acute gonorrhea. In the horse, a dose of 20 mg per kg (9.9 mg per lb) intramuscularly three times a day has been suggested. However, it may be irritating by this route.

TYLOSIN

This macrolide is mainly effective against mycoplasma and some gram-positive microorganisms. It is rarely used for treating equine respiratory infections. A dose of 10 mg per kg (4.6 mg per lb) intramuscularly twice daily has been suggested; at this dose, a serum concentration of 1 μg per ml has been measured at four hours.

ISONIAZID

The antimicrobial spectrum of this drug appears to be limited to mycobacteria or similar organisms. Its small size allows it to penetrate granulation tissue and abscesses. There have been anecdotal reports of its efficacy in chronic infections, but convincing evidence of its value has not yet been presented.[8, 9, 14] The usual dose used is 5 to 15 mg per kg (2.3 to 6.7 mg per lb) orally twice daily.[14]

SULFONAMIDES

These drugs have wide antimicrobial activity against many gram-positive and gram-negative organisms, and they are well distributed throughout all body tissues and pleural fluid. Rapid intravenous administration may result in trembling, excitement, and increased heart rate. Intravenous administration should always be slow and should be discontinued if undesirable side effects occur. Doses used vary with each drug. Sulfamethazine has been used at a single daily dose of 60 to 150 mg per kg, either intramuscularly or orally.[15] Commonly we use 220 mg per kg (100 mg per lb) intravenously once the first day followed by 110 mg per kg (50 mg per lb) intravenously once each subsequent treatment day.

CEPHALOSPORINS

This group of antibiotics is highly effective against Pasteurella, beta-hemolytic streptococci, and hemolytic Staphylococci. Oral cephalexin has been used at a dose of 22 to 33 mg per kg (10 to 15 mg per lb) four times daily for four weeks with no undesirable side effects in one mature horse. Serum levels in that horse ranged from 10 to 31 μg per ml. The drug is expensive, and except in specific infections in which an oral drug is needed, it would not be a primary drug of choice in respiratory infections.

NEBULIZATION

Nebulization as a method of antibiotic administration has not been mentioned because of lack of information. There is controversy over its use in other species, and one suspects that in most cases it would not be a good means of treating horses with lower respiratory tract infections. Certain antibiotics can cause bronchoconstriction when nebulized, and this could worsen a respiratory disease. Nebulizers also have the potential for spreading disease, and most nebulized material never penetrates the lower respiratory tract.

This review of antibiotics, while serving as a source of available information upon which the practitioner can superimpose his or her clinical experience and individual patient and client factors, reveals our need for data on epidemiology and bacteriology in equine respiratory diseases and on drug dosages and drug disposition.

References

1. Alexander, F., and Collett, R. A.: Trimethoprim in the horse. Equine Vet. J., 7:203, 1975.
2. Aronson, A. L.: The use, misuse and abuse of antibacterial agents. Mod. Vet. Pract., 56:383, 1975.
3. Beech, J., Kohn, C., Leitch, M., Weinstein, A., and Gallagher, M.: Therapeutic use of gentamicin in horses: Concentrations in serum, urine and synovial fluid and evaluation of renal function. Am. J. Vet. Res., 38:1085, 1977.
4. Beech, J., Kohn, C., Leitch, M., Weinstein, A., and Gallagher, M.: Serum and synovial fluid levels of sodium ampicillin (Totacillin) and ampicillin trihydrate (Polyflex) in horses. J. Equine Med. Surg., 3:350, 1979.
5. Davis, L. E., Neff, C. A., Baggot, J. D., and Powers, T. E.: Pharmacokinetics of chloramphenicol in domesticated animals. Am. J. Vet. Res., 33:2259, 1972.
6. Doll, E. R., Wallace, M. E., and McCollum, W. H.: Serum levels of horses following intramuscular injection of aqueous suspension of procaine penicillin. Vet. Med., 45:309, 1950.
7. English, P. B.: The therapeutic serum concentrations of penicillin: The relationship between dose rate and plasma concentration after parenteral administration of benzyl penicillin (Penicillin G). Vet. Rec., 77:810, 1965.

8. Knight, H. D.: Antimicrobial agents used in the horse. Proc. 21st Annu. Conv. Am. Assoc. Eq. Pract. 1975, pp. 131–144 (and preparatory data).
9. Knight, H. D., Hietala, S. K., and Jang, S.: Antibacterial treatment of abscesses. J. Am. Vet. Med. Assoc., *176*:1095, 1980.
10. Oh-Ishi, S.: Blood concentration of chloramphenicol in horses after intramuscular or oral administration. Jap. J. Vet. Sci., *30*:25, 1968.
11. Orsini, J.: Serum, synovial and peritoneal levels of Amikacin SO$_4$ in the horse after IM and IV injection. Unpublished data, 1980.
12. Pedersoli, W. M., Belmonte, A. A., Purohit, R. C., and Ravis, W. R.: Pharmacokinetics of gentamicin in the horse. Am. J. Vet. Res., *41*:351, 1980.
13. Pilloud, M.: Pharmacokinetics, plasma protein binding and dosage of chloramphenicol in cattle and horses. Res. Vet. Sci., *15*:231, 1973.
14. Roberts, W. D.: Isoniazid in equine therapy. Proc 17th Annu. Conv. Am. Assoc. Eq. Pract. 1971, pp. 33–34.
15. Roberts, M. C., and English, P. B.: Antimicrobial chemotherapy in the horse. II. The application of antimicrobial therapy. J. Eq. Med. Surg., 3:308, 1979.
16. Rollins, L. D., Teske, R. H., Condon, R. J., and Carter, G. G.: Serum penicillin and dihydrostreptomycin concentrations in horses after intramuscular administration of selected preparations containing these antibiotics. J. Am. Vet. Med. Assoc., *161*:490, 1972.
17. Sisodia, C. S., Kramer, L. L., Gupta, V. S., Lerner, D. J. and Taksas, L.: A pharmacologic study of chloramphenicol in horses. Can. J. Comp. Med., *39*:216, 1975.
18. Teske, R. H., Rollins, L. D., Condon, R. J., and Carter, G. G.: Serum oxytetracycline concentrations after intravenous and intramuscular administration in horses. J. Am. Vet. Med. Assoc., *162*:119, 1973.

EMERGENCY VENTILATION

Thomas W. Riebold, CORVALLIS, OREGON

Emergency ventilation is indicated when apnea or hypoventilation occurs in horses. Common causes of apnea and hypoventilation are overdosage with anesthetic agents or muscle relaxants, anaphylaxis, airway obstruction, central nervous system injury, and chest trauma. Clinical signs indicating the need for emergency ventilation include lack of respiratory movements, accentuated respiratory efforts with little gas flow from the nostrils, and cyanosis. In some cases, usually horses that have received an overdose of succinylcholine, chest movements and flaring of the nostrils are present, causing one to believe that gas exchange is occurring. However, on closer inspection, one will note asynchrony of the chest movements and nasal flaring and will be unable to detect passage of little more than small puffs of expired gas from the nostrils. While cyanosis can be due to hypoventilation, it is also observed in horses with lung disease in which ventilation is adequate as well as in shock when peripheral blood flow is reduced.

Although apnea and hypoventilation can result from a variety of causes, the pathophysiologic sequence of events is similar in all cases. For example, following acute airway obstruction, arterial oxygen tension falls from a normal 90 torr to 35 torr within two minutes. This hypoxemia contributes to cellular hypoxia, acidosis, cardiac arrhythmias, and ultimately death. Carbon dioxide retention also contributes to acidosis and cardiac arrhythmias. To avoid this series of events, symptomatic therapy must be promptly initiated while the cause of the apnea is determined, after which specific therapy may be instituted. Ventilation is increased either by the use of pharmacologic agents or by endotracheal intubation and mechanical ventilation with oxygen or air.

RESPIRATORY STIMULANTS

The older analeptic agents (pentylenetetrazol, nikethamide, amphetamine, and picrotoxin) are obsolete because they do not stimulate a hypoxic respiratory center and may cause convulsions. Doxopram* is the agent of choice for relief of respiratory depression. It increases ventilation by stimulating the peripheral chemoreceptors rather than the respiratory center. Doxopram is given at a dose rate of 0.5 mg per kg intravenously. The respiratory rate usually increases within one minute, and the increase in rate usually lasts for 5 to 10 minutes. One must closely observe the horse for a recurrence of apnea as the effect of the drug dissipates. With repeated administration, doxopram becomes less effective, so the cause of the apnea must be determined and corrected.

NARCOTIC ANTAGONISTS

If the cause of the apnea or respiratory depression is an overdose of a narcotic, one of the narcotic an-

---

*Dopram-V, A. H. Robins, Inc., Richmond, VA 23770

tagonists should be administered. The three antagonists available are levallorphan,* nalorphine,† and naloxone.‡ Naloxone is the preferred agent, as overdosage will not produce sedation and respiratory depression. This is in contrast to overdosage of levallorphan or nalorphine. Levallorphan is given at a dose rate of 0.02 to 0.04 mg per kg (0.83 to 1.9 mg per 100 lbs), nalorphine at 0.01 mg per kg (0.4 mg per 100 lbs), and naloxone at 0.01 mg per kg (0.4 mg per 100 lbs). All are administered intravenously. The sedative effects of the narcotics may outlast the arousal effects of the antagonist, and, therefore, the horse must be closely observed for recurrence of respiratory depression. If respiratory depression does recur, additional antagonist should be administered.

VENTILATION

The best treatment for respiratory depression, apnea, and hypoventilation is endotracheal intubation and mechanical ventilation with oxygen. Mechanical ventilation eliminates hypoxia and respiratory acidosis and provides time for the veterinarian to determine the cause of the respiratory depression or apnea and institute specific therapy. If oxygen is unavailable, compressed air will usually provide adequate arterial oxygen tension. Intubation is preferred to use of a mask for ventilation. If a mask is used, it must fit tightly around the horse's muzzle to avoid leakage during the inspiratory phase of the respiratory cycle. Masks provide a less efficient method of ventilation and are not effective if the underlying cause of hypoventilation is upper airway obstruction.

Intermittent positive pressure ventilation consists of two phases. During the inspiratory phase, positive airway pressure causes gas to flow into the lungs but also reduces venous return to the heart. During expiration, airway pressure rapidly returns to 0 cm H_2O, allowing adequate cardiac filling. To avoid the untoward cardiovascular effects of mechanical ventilation, the inspiratory phase of the respiratory cycle must last no more than 2.0 to 3.0 sec. In order to deliver the tidal volume to an adult horse in this period of time, the equipment must generate gas flows of 250 l per min.

Endotracheal intubation of the horse is performed blindly. The head and neck are extended to make the orotracheal axis approach 180°. The endotracheal tube§‖ is inserted, advanced, and manipulated

until it enters the larynx. If resistance or an obstruction is encountered, the tube is redirected to avoid injury to the epiglottis and laryngeal and pharyngeal tissues and is advanced again until it enters the larynx. If an obstruction impairs passage of the endotracheal tube, a tracheostomy is indicated. In this article, different techniques of emergency ventilation are described for use with an endotracheal tube. If intubation is not possible, the same techniques can be used with a tracheostomy tube. The optimal sizes of the endotracheal or tracheostomy tube for use with horses of differing sizes are shown in Table 1. Because the tracheostomy tube is placed between two tracheal rings, it must have a smaller diameter than the endotracheal tube used for the same size horse.

If the respiratory emergency occurs in the hospital setting and an anesthetic machine is available, the horse should be intubated and connected to the anesthetic machine.*†‡ The rebreathing bag is filled with oxygen, and ventilation is provided by manual compression and release of the bag. A respiratory rate of six to eight breaths per min with a 2.0- to 3.0-sec inspiratory time and tidal volume of 15 to 22 ml per kg usually provides adequate ventilation. In the absence of equipment to measure the tidal volume, an inspiratory pressure of 25 to 30 cm H_2O coupled with visual observation of adequate thoracic expansion during inflation provides a good indication of an adequate tidal volume.

If anesthetic overdosage is the cause of apnea, the anesthetic plane should be decreased. If a horse will not ventilate adequately under minimal levels of surgical anesthesia, one has the choice of supporting ventilation either by manual compression of the rebreathing bag or with mechanical ventilation.§‖** For extended periods of anesthesia, mechanical ventilation is more efficient and consistent. Ventilators are adjusted to provide a respiratory rate of six to eight breaths per min with a 2.0-sec inspiratory time and 25 to 30 cm H_2O inspiratory pressure and tidal volume of 15 to 22 ml per kg.

If the horse is under intravenous anesthesia, "Bird" ventilators†† can be connected directly to the endotracheal tube of the horse. When this method is utilized, either 100 per cent oxygen or an oxygen-air mixture can be delivered to the horse. Usually an oxygen-air mixture is utilized, as it allows higher gas flows to be generated by the ventilator,

---

*Lorfan, Roche Labs, Nutley, NJ 07110
†Nalline, Merck and Co., Rahway, NJ 07065
‡Naloxone, Pitman-Moore, Washington Crossing, NJ 08560
§Cole Equine Tube, Lane Manufacturing, Inc., Denver, CO
‖Silicone Endotracheal Tube, Bivona Surgical Instruments, Inc., Hammond, IN

*Narkovet-E, North American Drager, Telford, PA 18969
†VML, Fraser Harlake, Inc., Lancaster, NY 14086
‡Vet-Tec LAVC-2000, JD Medical Distributing Co., Phoenix, AZ
§Model M7, Mallard Medical, Inc., Plymouth, MI
‖Narkovet-E Anesthesia Control Center, North American Drager, Telford, PA 18969
**Vet-Tec LAVC-3000, JD Medical Distributing Co., Phoenix, AZ
††Bird Corp., Palm Springs, CA

TABLE 1. SIZE OF ENDOTRACHEAL AND TRACHEOSTOMY TUBES FOR HORSES

Weight of Horse (lbs)	Cuffed Endo-tracheal Tube (mm i.d.)	Cole Equine Tube	Tracheos-tomy Tube (mm o.d.)
70–300	11–16	Foal, weanling	8–13
300–500	16–20	Weanling	13–18
500–750	20–25	Weanling, adult	20–22
750–1000	25–30	Adult	22–25
>1000	30–40	Adult	25–

thereby providing efficient ventilation and adequate oxygenation. The previously mentioned ventilatory guidelines are used when adjusting the ventilator.

For field use, methods of emergency ventilation include use of a demand valve, the Vetaspirator,* and insufflation of the lungs with a nasogastric tube. Each of these methods involves the use of easily transported equipment and an oxygen source, usually an "E" cylinder equipped with a regulator, preferably one providing adjustable line pressure.

The demand valve,† when connected to an endotracheal tube, enables a horse to spontaneously ventilate on oxygen or allows administration of oxygen by intermittent positive pressure ventilation. Following intubation, the endotracheal tube is connected to the demand valve. Oxygen flow is controlled by a button on the valve. Inspiration occurs while the button is compressed and continues until an adequate tidal volume (as assessed by thoracic expansion) is delivered. The button is then released by the operator, and passive exhalation occurs. If the button is not released, oxygen flow will cease when the pressure within the airway of the horse reaches 54 cm H_2O. Usually an inspiratory pressure of 25 to 30 cm H_2O is sufficient to deliver an adequate tidal volume to an apneic horse unless respiratory compliance is altered by disease or abdominal tympany. In individuals with decreased compliance, higher inspiratory pressures are required to deliver an adequate tidal volume. However, one rarely requires the maximal inspiratory pressure provided by the demand valve even in these individuals, and its use in normal horses may cause ruptured alveoli. No manipulations of the demand valve are required for spontaneous ventilation to occur. The negative pressure created by the horse's inspiratory effort causes the demand valve to open and oxygen flow to begin. Flow continues until the horse begins to exhale, causing the valve to close, oxygen flow to cease, and exhalation to occur. By its design, the demand valve prevents rebreathing of exhaled gases.

A two-stage regulator is used with the demand valve because it permits increases in gas supply line pressure, enabling the demand valve to deliver higher oxygen flows. When the supply line pressure is 80 psi, the demand valve can generate an oxygen flow of 275 l per min, enough to efficiently ventilate a 1200 lb horse. In larger horses, the demand valve's flow capability is exceeded, and inspiratory time is longer than optimal (greater than 3.0 sec). In these cases, the gas supply line pressure must be increased to allow higher oxygen flow rates and more efficient ventilation.

The same criteria are used as guidelines for ventilation with this method as with other methods. Using these guidelines, an "E" cylinder of oxygen lasts about 15 min, depending upon the size of the horse. As the cylinder empties, the inspiratory time becomes progressively longer and ventilation more inefficient.

The Vetaspirator is a portable unit capable of supplying intermittent positive pressure ventilation. Other required equipment includes either an endotracheal tube or mask and an oxygen source and regulator. The Vetaspirator can generate flows of 130 l per min and, therefore, provides progressively less efficient ventilation as the size of the horse increases. The unit is connected to the endotracheal tube of the apneic horse. Oxygen flow is governed by alternately opening and closing a valve on the unit. The same guidelines for mechanical ventilation in horses are used with this method. Ideally, one wishes to obtain an inspiratory time of 2 to 3 sec. However, when this mode of ventilation is used in larger horses, this inspiratory time probably will not be obtained.

The third method of ventilation for use in the field is insufflation. This method requires the least equipment but is an inefficient method of intermittent positive pressure ventilation, especially in larger horses. Equipment required includes a large nasogastric tube and an oxygen source and regulator. The nasogastric tube is connected to the oxygen regulator, and the cylinder is opened slightly until oxygen flow is felt about 15 to 18 inches from the tube tip. This corresponds to a flow rate of about 80 l per min. The nasogastric tube is inserted nasally through the ventral meatus into the trachea. Entrance into the larynx is made easier if the horse's head and neck are extended. Following placement of the tube, occlusion of the nostrils causes lung inflation, and release allows exhalation. Routine guidelines are followed for the respiratory rate and tidal volume. This method is more efficient if used with endotracheal intubation. Following intubation, the nasogastric tube is inserted into the endotracheal tube, and alternate occlusion and release of the endotracheal tube orifice provide ventilation.

---

*Vetaspirator, Veterinarian's Specialties, Cedar Rapids, IA

†Model 5040, Hudson Oxygen Therapy Sales Co., Wadsworth, OH 44281

Supplemental Readings

1. Riebold, T. W., Evans, A. T., and Robinson, N. E.: Evaluation of the demand valve for resuscitation of horses. J. Am. Vet. Med. Assoc., *176*:623, 1980.
2. Riebold, T. W., Evans, A. T., and Robinson, N. E.: Emergency ventilation in the horse. Proc. 25th Annu. Conv. Am. Assoc. Eq. Pract. 1979, p. 113.
3. Steffey, E. P.: Anesthetic management of the horse with respiratory disease. Vet. Clin. North Am. (Large Anim. Pract.), *1*:113, 1979.
4. Steffey, E. P., and Berry, J. D.: Flow rates from an intermittent positive pressure breathing-anesthetic delivery apparatus for horses. Am. J. Vet. Res., *38*:685, 1977.
5. Thurman, J. C., Trim, C. M., and Hartsfield, S. M.: Mechanical ventilation of the anesthetized horse. Proc. 22nd Annu. Conv. Am. Assoc. Eq. Pract. 1976, pp. 341–345.

OXYGEN THERAPY

Thomas W. Riebold, CORVALLIS, OREGON

This section deals primarily with oxygen supplementation in horses capable of spontaneous ventilation. Oxygen therapy and mechanical ventilation for apneic horses is covered elsewhere (p. 475).

Oxygen therapy increases alveolar oxygen tension in a ventilating horse and thereby increases blood oxygen tension. It will not correct the acidosis and carbon dioxide retention that result from inadequate alveolar ventilation, nor will the provision of oxygen via a face mask increase blood oxygen content in an apneic animal. For example, a horse that has a severe upper airway obstruction that hinders air flow and increases the work of breathing is better treated with a tracheostomy than by oxygen therapy, because if the lungs are healthy, gas exchange will be normal if air can be delivered to the alveoli. Oxygen therapy will not compensate for a lack of hemoglobin because the amount of oxygen that is carried in solution in plasma is minimal in comparison to the amount transported on hemoglobin. If a horse is anemic enough to be hypoxic, it must receive additional erythrocytes to improve oxygen delivery to the tissues.

Oxygen therapy is indicated when gas exchange is impaired by pulmonary or cardiovascular disease. Horses with decreased tissue blood flow, such as horses with gastrointestinal obstruction resulting in shock, may also benefit from supplemental oxygen prior to induction and during recovery from anesthesia. In addition, healthy horses may need supplemental oxygen when lung function is impaired by anesthesia and/or recumbency. For example, horses undergoing elective surgery with intravenous anesthesia are frequently hypoxemic, as are horses recovering from inhalation anesthesia.

Clinical signs indicating a need for oxygen therapy include tachypnea, tachycardia, cyanosis, and prolonged gingival perfusion time. Cyanosis is evident only in severe hypoxemia when blood contains at least 1 gm per dl of reduced hemoglobin. Arterial oxygen tension may be reduced considerably below normal in many anesthetized horses that show no outward signs of hypoxemia. It is, therefore, a wise practice to provide supplemental oxygen to all anesthetized horses. Because of a lack of hemoglobin, anemic horses may not show cyanosis even with severe hypoxemia. While prolonged gingival perfusion time is indicative of poor tissue perfusion, many horses with this sign may benefit from oxygen therapy because pulmonary gas exchange may also be impaired by reduced pulmonary blood flow or vascular pressures.

The goal of oxygen therapy is to return arterial oxygen content to normal. In most situations, an arterial oxygen tension of greater than 85 torr is sufficient. Even with extensive pulmonary disease, it is rarely necessary to use pure oxygen to achieve normal oxygen content, and in most cases 40 to 60 per cent inspired oxygen concentrations will suffice. This is fortunate because oxygen delivery systems are rarely adequate to deliver pure oxygen.

Before a decision is made to administer supplemental oxygen to a horse, the adequacy of alveolar ventilation must be determined either subjectively by correlating the amount of effort used to breathe with air flow at the nares or objectively by measuring arterial oxygen and carbon dioxide tensions. Also, the benefits of oxygen therapy must be weighed against the risks. If the restraint involved with oxygen therapy increases struggling by the horse, more oxygen may be consumed than is administered. Another consideration is the cost of the equipment and personnel which may prohibit prolonged oxygen therapy in an animal of limited value.

There are several methods of administering higher than atmospheric concentrations of oxygen to horses. In standing horses, they include oxygen masks and insufflation. In small foals, the Kirschner Oxygen Therapy Unit* can be used. In anesthetized horses, techniques involving insufflation and a demand valve can be utilized.

---

*Intensive Care Oxygen Therapy Unit, Kirschner, Aberdeen, MD 21001

OXYGEN CAGES

The Kirschner Oxygen Therapy Unit is an excellent method of providing an environment with controlled temperature, humidity, and oxygen and carbon dioxide levels. Unfortunately, the largest model is designed for use with large dogs. While the cage works well with small calves, it does not lend itself well to use with foals. Most foals are too tall to stand or lie comfortably in the cage. Until a similar cage is produced in a larger model, its use is limited to small neonatal foals. Product literature describes its use with these foals.

Although a homemade oxygen cage of suitable size can be lined with plastic to make it airtight, several problems are associated with this method. Leaks make it difficult to attain predictable oxygen concentrations, and unless some provision is made for carbon dioxide removal, it may accumulate in the system. Heat accumulation may be a problem, as the unit is most often not equipped to maintain a constant ambient temperature. Unless some method of prompt removal of feces and urine is available, ammonia fumes can be an added insult to the respiratory tract.

At this point in time, oxygen cages are of little value in foals because of the small size of the commercially available unit and the problems associated with the home-built units. In addition, the feeding schedule of newborn foals necessitates opening the oxygen cage at frequent intervals, causing loss of the oxygen-enriched atmosphere. Because foals have a small tidal volume, it is easier to supplement the inspired oxygen concentration using nasotracheal insufflation or a face mask than with an oxygen therapy unit.

FACE MASK

A face mask* can be used to administer oxygen to horses. Most commonly, a face mask is used to increase inspired oxygen concentrations and not to replace all of the horse's inspired air with pure oxygen. Masks that completely replace room air with pure oxygen have a nonrebreathing valve in the system that causes all exhaled gases to be vented to the atmosphere. High oxygen flows must be used to meet the animal's minute volume, and the mask must fit tightly around the horse's muzzle to prevent leakage or dilution of the oxygen with room air. The mask should contain minimal exhaled gas between breaths, as this gas contains carbon dioxide, which contributes to hypercarbia.

Most horses do not require the administration of pure oxygen, and supplementation with a mask is

_____

*Equine Inhalation Apparatus, Snyder Veterinary Products Co., Taos, NM 87571

usually sufficient. In this instance, the system need not be sophisticated because a leakproof system with a nonrebreathing valve is not required. Instead of purchasing a commercial mask, one can be made from a plastic 1 gal jug, 1 l. bottle, or other plastic container appropriate for the size of the horse. This type of mask is disposable after the need for oxygen therapy has passed, minimizing cross-infection between horses from contaminated masks. The mask should be slightly larger than the horse's muzzle. The bottom is removed from the container, and a hole is made in either side to allow a piece of twine to be tied to one side, passed over the horse's poll, and tied to the other side, holding the mask in place. The mask should fit loosely and comfortably around the horse's muzzle to allow elimination of expired gases and dilution of the oxygen with room air during inspiration. The continuous flow of oxygen into the mask between breaths forces expired gas out of the mask, and since the gas in the mask is the first inhaled by the horse, the resultant inspired gas has an oxygen concentration exceeding that of room air.

An appropriate length of tubing is used to connect the mask to a flowmeter and regulator mounted on an oxygen cylinder. Usually the horses are restrained either by an assistant or in stocks, cross-ties, or other devices when this method of oxygen therapy is used. Some horses, when confined to their stall without being restrained by an assistant, will try to remove the mask by rubbing it against the wall or may get the mask caught in the hay manger or feed box. Oxygen is introduced into the mask at a flow rate of about 15 l per min in an adult horse. With this system, the final inspired oxygen concentration is a function of the oxygen flow rate into the mask and the minute volume of the horse. As the minute volume of the horse increases, at a given oxygen flow rate the inspired oxygen concentration declines and approaches that of room air.

The advantage of this system is its simplicity; little equipment and technical skill are required to administer oxygen therapy to the horse. The disadvantages of this method are the need for restraint of most horses and, in horses with a large minute volume, the final inspired oxygen concentration does not greatly exceed that of room air. In the latter group of horses, the oxygen flow rate should be increased to improve the inspired oxygen concentration.

INSUFFLATION

Insufflation is similar to using a mask in that an oxygen reservoir is created by displacing expired gas from the dead space. In this instance, the reservoir is the horse's own conducting airway rather than an externally applied mask. Depending upon placement of the insufflation tube, the reservoir consists of the nasal passages, nasopharynx, and cranial trachea. The simplest method of insufflation involves placement of a small nasogastric tube in the nasopharynx.

When nasopharyngeal insufflation is used, the horse should be monitored for signs of abdominal discomfort due to gastric dilation caused by swallowing large volumes of oxygen and air. The tube tip should not be allowed to contact the esophageal orifice during nasopharyngeal insufflation, as this could encourage the horse to swallow the gas mixture.

Nasotracheal insufflation allows administration of higher oxygen concentrations than nasopharyngeal insufflation when using the same oxygen flow rate. To place the tube in the trachea, the horse's head and neck should be extended after the tube tip has reached the level of the nasopharynx, and the tube should be manipulated and advanced until it enters the trachea. Correct placement of the tube is confirmed by lack of resistance to advancement of the tube and the inability to obtain a vacuum in the tube during aspiration. The tube should be advanced so that the tip lies about 12 in. into the trachea. If the tube tip remains in the larynx, it may cause coughing. The tube also should not be advanced to contact the carina, as this also causes severe coughing.

The advantages to insufflation are its simplicity in terms of equipment and technical skill that are required and the lack of restraint needed. A nasogastric tube is used for insufflation because it is readily available and because, in addition to the orifice at the end of the tube, there are two others in the wall of the tube. This tends to reduce jetting of the gas as it leaves the tube and helps to prevent mechanical trauma to the tracheal mucosa. In foals, a stallion urinary catheter or a piece of an intravenous administration set is substituted for the nasogastric tube.

The nasotracheal tube is taped to the horse's halter, although on occasion, it may be sutured to the nares. From there, the insufflation tube passes through a braid in the horse's mane and is connected with additional tubing to a point above the horse's head on the stall wall or ceiling and then to the oxygen cylinder and regulator-flowmeter.* By having the tube pass through a braid in the horse's mane, it is able to slide back and forth as the horse turns its head. The tubing should be long enough to allow the horse enough freedom to walk around its stall, yet should be short enough not to get tangled in the legs. For adult horses, oxygen flow rates of 10 to 15 l per min are sufficient. Using this method, arterial oxygen tensions in healthy standing horses can be increased from a normal value of 90 torr to 210 torr. If the oxygen is to be administered for periods of time exceeding a few hours, a humidifier* should be included in the system to prevent drying of the respiratory tract.

Most horses tolerate insufflation very well. Some horses object to the presence of the nasotracheal tube and continually cough and sneeze. In certain cases, nasotracheal insufflation is contraindicated. In horses with an upper airway obstruction, the lumen of the airway must not only be large enough to allow passage of the nasotracheal tube but also must be large enough to allow escape of the insufflated oxygen and expired gases in order to avoid abnormal airway pressure and ruptured alveoli. In those cases or in horses that will not tolerate a nasotracheal tube, oxygen may be insufflated through a tracheostomy tube. The tracheostomy is usually performed in the midcervical area unless the airway obstruction is more caudal, necessitating that the tracheostomy be performed closer to the thoracic inlet. Following placement of the tracheostomy tube, a catheter or length of small tubing is passed through the tracheostomy tube and into the trachea. Again, it should not be advanced to the point where it contacts the carina. If there is an upper airway obstruction, one must be sure that the size of the insufflation tube does not compromise the lumen of the tracheostomy tube to the point where ventilation is hindered. The insufflation tube is attached to the horse in much the same manner as the nasotracheal tube and is connected to the oxygen source. Humidifiers are recommended if the oxygen therapy is prolonged. The advantages of this method are similar to those of nasotracheal insufflation. The primary disadvantage to this method is the need for a tracheostomy and the resultant aftercare, but in cases with airway obstruction, there is no alternative. One potential complication of this method is subcutaneous emphysema if the insufflation tube becomes dislodged.

In emergency situations, oxygen can be insufflated through a large (10- to 12-gauge) catheter, or a needle can be percutaneously placed in the midcervical trachea. Care should be taken to avoid contact with a tracheal ring during catheter placement. The catheter is either sutured or securely taped in place and connected to the oxygen source in routine fashion. The catheter should be long enough (3 to 5 in) that it does not back out of the trachea and cause severe subcutaneous emphysema. Oxygen flow rates of 10 l per min are used.

Often no provision is made to increase the inspired oxygen concentration of horses under intravenous anesthesia. Oxygen can be administered by nasotracheal insufflation, or if the horse is intubated, the insufflation tube can be passed into the endotracheal tube. In horses recovering from anesthesia, nasotracheal insufflation with oxygen is advisable to prevent hypoxia resulting from anesthesia and/or recumbency.

DEMAND VALVE

Another method of administering oxygen to these horses is with a demand valve (p. 477).* Following intubation, the horse is connected to a demand valve, allowing it to spontaneously ventilate on oxygen. In addition, the valve allows intermittent positive pressure ventilation, permitting the operator to "sigh" the horse once or twice every five minutes. That is, every five minutes a button on the demand valve is compressed to force oxygen into the horse until adequate thoracic expansion occurs and then is released to allow exhalation. This maneuver helps to prevent atelectasis and improves oxygenation in the horse.

Oxygen toxicity is a possibility in animals that are administered high oxygen concentrations for prolonged periods of time. Dogs allowed to breathe 100 per cent oxygen at sea level died in three days,

---

*Demand valve, Model 5040, Hudson Oxygen Therapy Sales Co., Wadsworth, OH 44281

while those breathing 50 per cent oxygen did not show signs of toxicity. Toxic signs include pulmonary edema, decreased pulmonary compliance, and tracheobronchitis. In addition, the administration of unhumidified oxygen causes drying of the respiratory tract, making elimination of pulmonary secretions more difficult. In equine oxygen therapy, administration of oxygen in concentrations exceeding 50 per cent of the inspired gas is unlikely. It is more likely that complications would be due to the administration of unhumidified gases.

Supplemental Readings

1. Garner, H. E., Moore, J. N., Auer, J. A., Traver, D. S., Johnson, J. H., Coffman, J. R., and Tritschler, L. G.: Postoperative care of equine abdominal crisis. Vet. Anesth., 4:40, 1977.
2. Moore, J. N., Garner, H. E., Johnson, J. H., and Huesgen, J. G.: Continuous administration of oxygen during the immediate post-anesthetic period. VM SAC, 73:1397, 1978.
3. Riebold, T. W., Evans, A. T., and Robinson, N. E.: Evaluation of the demand valve for resuscitation of horses. J. Am. Vet. Med. Assoc., 176:626, 1980.
4. Steffey, E. P.: Anesthetic management of the horse with respiratory disease. Vet. Clin. North Am. (Large Anim. Pract.), 1:113, 1979.
5. Thurmon, J. C.: Oxygen therapy—a review. Proc. Illinois Veterinary Respiratory Symposium, 1978, p. 188.

SINUSITIS

Dallas O. Goble, KNOXVILLE, TENNESSEE

ANATOMY

Sinusitis, a condition recognized for centuries, still presents a challenging diagnostic and therapeutic problem to the equine practitioner. Because examination of the paranasal sinuses is limited by the bones of the skull, familiarity with the anatomy of the sinuses is mandatory for proper clinical evaluation (Figs. 1 and 2). The sphenopalatine, ethmoidal, and frontal sinuses communicate through the posterior maxillary sinus, which opens into the nasal cavity via the nasomaxillary opening, located in the posterior portion of the middle meatus. The anterior maxillary sinus, which may or may not communicate with the posterior maxillary sinus, depending on the completeness of the osseous septum, drains to the nasal cavity through a separate orifice, also in the middle meatus. The maxillary sinuses are divided into medial and lateral compartments by the nasolacrimal duct.

The frontal sinus is divided into frontal and turbinate portions (Figs. 2 and 3), both of which communicate with the posterior maxillary sinus through the large frontomaxillary opening. The small sphenopalatine and ethmoid sinuses, which are of less clinical importance, also drain into the posterior maxillary sinus.

ETIOLOGY

Dental problems, such as patent infundibulum, cement necrosis, alveolar periostitis, or a fractured tooth, are the most frequent causes of sinusitis. The fourth upper cheek tooth (first molar), the root of which is usually located in the anterior maxillary sinus, is by far the most common tooth associated with sinusitis. Infections from dental problems are usually mixed with numerous organisms present. Sinusitis is observed with greater frequency in four-,

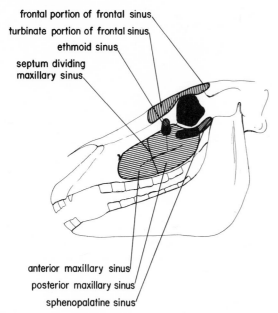

frontal portion of frontal sinus
turbinate portion of frontal sinus
ethmoid sinus
septum dividing
maxillary sinus

anterior maxillary sinus
posterior maxillary sinus
sphenopalatine sinus

Figure 1. The lateral view of the paranasal sinuses in the horse.

five-, and six-year-old horses than in any other age range. The improper shedding of deciduous teeth and dental crowding may be factors relating to frequent occurrence in this age group.

The second most common cause of sinusitis is a bacterial infection following a systemic viral or bacterial respiratory infection, not infrequently strangles. Strangles complications are less frequent than previously, owing in part to better management, treatment, and in some instances vaccination programs on endemic farms. Streptococcus and Staphylococcus are the organisms most frequently isolated from sinusitis secondary to respiratory infection. Many times a mixed infection includes Pseudomonas species.

Less frequent causes of sinusitis include trauma from puncture wounds, kicks, or other accidents. Tumors must also be considered when there is deformity of the facial bones or a blood-tinged nasal discharge. Maxillary cysts are sometimes misdiagnosed as tumors. Mycotic infections of the paranasal sinuses are infrequent. Allergic sinusitis as recognized in humans is difficult to document in the horse but may predispose to secondary bacterial infections.

Atresia of the nasomaxillary opening, seen primarily in horses less than one year old, is a further cause of facial distortion that may be confused with sinusitis. Diagnosis prior to severe facial distortion and surgical intervention to produce a nasomaxillary fistula may allow for correction. The prognosis for complete recovery is guarded.

DIAGNOSIS AND CLINICAL SIGNS

A complete physical examination is the single most important feature in the diagnostic protocol.

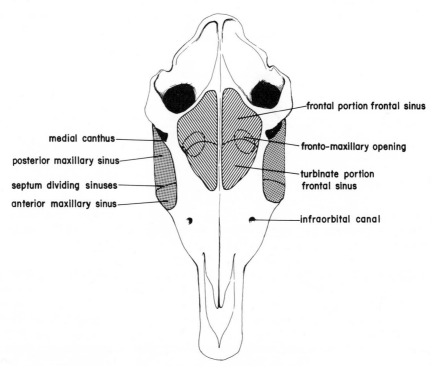

medial canthus
posterior maxillary sinus
septum dividing sinuses
anterior maxillary sinus

frontal portion frontal sinus
fronto-maxillary opening
turbinate portion frontal sinus
infraorbital canal

Figure 2. Frontal view of the paranasal sinuses in the horse.

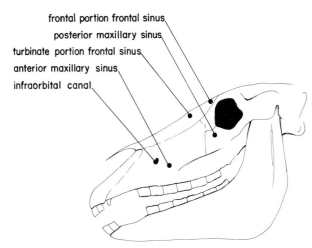

frontal portion frontal sinus
posterior maxillary sinus
turbinate portion frontal sinus
anterior maxillary sinus
infraorbital canal

Figure 3. The common sites of diagnostic trephines.

An accurate history is beneficial but is often difficult to obtain because horses frequently change trainers, owners, or caretakers. After the physical examination and history have been completed, it may be necessary to utilize special diagnostic procedures to arrive at a definitive diagnosis.

The history should attempt to answer the following questions:

1. How long has the problem been present?
2. Is the discharge unilateral or bilateral?
3. Was the discharge the first indication of illness, or were there concurrently other signs of disease?
4. What has been the character of the discharge, and has it contained blood?
5. Does the horse make increased respiratory sound on exercise?
6. Does the exudate appear spontaneously, or is it more profuse when the head is down?
7. Does the horse hold its head sideways when eating, or does it have abnormal mastication?
8. Has any trauma occurred to the patient prior to occurrence of discharge?
9. Are other horses on the farm affected, and what are their ages?
10. What was the duration, nature, and effect of previous treatments (if any)?

Questions related to allergies should be pursued if the case does not fit any other reasonable diagnostic pattern. Added significance is given to allergy if the problem is more severe in association with a change of surroundings, feed, or bedding.

Physical examination is difficult because the paranasal sinuses are encased in the bones of the skull. Facial symmetry must be carefully observed and any assymetry of the skull examined in detail. Alopecia or elevation of the hair over a particular area may indicate chronic infection. Percussion of the sinuses is often a useful diagnostic technique. Placing the thumb in the interdental space to open the mouth during percussion will improve resonance when healthy sinuses are percussed and will emphasize the lack of resonance in fluid-filled sinuses.

The color, consistency, and odor of the nasal discharge should be noted. A thick yellow tenacious exudate is commonly observed with streptococcal infections but is not accompanied by a distinct odor. Exudates with a greenish tint and fruitlike odor are characteristic of Pseudomonas infections. Staphylococcal infections tend to produce a white exudate of a more fluid consistency than do streptococcal infections. When blood or a blood-tinged nasal discharge is observed or reported in the history, a tumor must be placed high on the differential diagnosis. Hemangiosarcoma will sometimes produce profuse epistaxis prior to the horse developing obvious facial swelling. This is unusual, however, and more frequently a chronic blood-tinged nasal discharge will be found on examination. It should be recalled that sinusitis is associated with dental problems in over 50 per cent of the cases and that the bacterial infections will be mixed.

A mouth speculum, flashlight, and infundibulum pick are essential to examine the teeth. The horse should be sedated and the oral cavity thoroughly rinsed prior to examination. Loose or fractured teeth and gingival problems are identified by palpation of each tooth. Placement of the infundibulum pick ⅜ inch past the table surface within any of the infundibula is suggestive of a patent opening into the sinus. When teeth are involved in sinusitis, there is often an obvious fetid odor.

Epiphora is often present on the side of the head affected by sinusitis owing to inflammation of the nasolacrimal duct. In addition, the horse will sometimes have snoring or increased respiratory sounds at exercise.

If the examination as described is inconclusive, special diagnostic techniques may be necessary to obtain a definitive diagnosis and to make a more accurate prognosis.

SPECIAL DIAGNOSTIC TECHNIQUES

Radiology. A 14 × 17 in film is most desirable for radiographic examination of the paranasal sinuses. Smaller films (10 × 12 in) can be used but make identification of structures difficult. The lateral view of the sinuses can easily be taken in the standing horse tranquilized with xylazine. The dorsoventral view can usually also be obtained in the standing horse. The film should be evaluated for fluid lines in the sinuses, bone lysis, or soft tissue masses. Alveolar disease and fluid lines are most easily observed on the lateral views, while soft tissue masses are best observed on the dorsoventral view.

Optimal radiographs are obtained with a high-output radiographic machine, but in practice situations with a cooperative patient, a portable unit can yield diagnostic radiographs.

Endoscopy. Endoscopic equipment, either a rigid boroscope or a flexible fiberoptic unit, is of limited value in the evaluation of sinusitis. With the flexible endoscope, the nasomaxillary opening in the middle meatus can be examined for the presence of a discharge. Bulging of the turbinate portion of the maxillary and frontal sinuses may also be observed but is difficult to recognize unless severe.

Diagnostic Trephine. Trephining the sinus or sinuses is a most useful technique for both diagnosis and treatment of sinusitis. The anatomic locations of trephine sites are shown in Figure 3. The technique can be accomplished in the standing horse. For diagnosis, it is most useful to trephine the posterior maxillary sinus because infection in the frontal, sphenopalatine, and ethmoidal sinuses drains to the nares via the posterior maxillary sinus. The anterior maxillary sinus should also be trephined if nothing is obtained from the posterior sinus, since these two sinuses do not always communicate. Sedation and a small amount of local anesthetic allow penetration of the sinus with a $\frac{1}{8}$ to $\frac{3}{16}$ in diameter Stienmann pin. A hand chuck allows control of the depth of penetration, in which 1 to $1\frac{1}{2}$ in is usually satisfactory. A polyethylene catheter can be introduced through the hole produced with the Stienmann pin, and aspiration of the sinus can be attempted. The catheter should be sufficient in size to tightly fit the hole, which facilitates both aspiration and flushing. Exudates should be sent to the laboratory for culture, sensitivity, and cytology. The polyethylene tube can be sutured in place and utilized for repeated flushing of the sinus if need be.

THERAPY

The treatment of sinusitis depends on the etiology. The owner must be made well aware that the period of treatment may be long (two to five weeks), the cost usually high, and the results of treatment not always successful. The more chronic the infection, the more guarded the prognosis, and this is usually true regardless of the infectious agent present. If severe facial distortion has occurred, the prognosis for complete recovery is more unfavorable.

CHRONIC SINUSITIS

The most successful treatment of chronic sinusitis is surgical trephining and volume flushing of the affected sinus. When the primary cause of sinusitis is dental problems, the affected tooth or teeth must be extracted or repelled. This surgical procedure is well documented in the literature and will not be described in detail.[1-3] Particular care must be exercised that all bone or tooth fragments are removed at the time of surgery.

Bacterial culture, sensitivity, and cytology results are necessary for successful treatment. The samples for laboratory evaluation should be taken immediately upon opening the sinus to prevent contamination that would give misleading bacteriologic results.

The most frequent organisms found in association with chronic sinusitis are beta-hemolytic Streptococcus and Staphylococcus. In those cases in which dental problems are the primary etiology, infections are usually mixed. When Pseudomonas is the primary pathogen, the prognosis for recovery is unfavorable.

The lining membranes of the sinuses are often thickened and inflamed from chronic infection. Unless the major portion of this tissue is surgically removed, the sinusitis will remain even with intensive treatment. The bone flap technique offers the best approach for surgical excision of the inflammatory tissue.[4] If the nasomaxillary duct is obstructed, the bone flap approach allows creation of a new opening through the turbinate portion of the maxillary sinus. A gauze seton can be placed through the nostril and tied over the sinus to maintain patency but may be unnecessary with twice daily volume flushing.

Once drainage has been established, antibiotics should be used concurrently with local flushing. Antibiotic therapy should begin immediately following recovery from anesthesia. The author uses penicillin G at a rate of 20,000 to 40,000 units per kg of body weight per day divided into twice daily injections or ampicillin at a dose rate of 20 mg per kg twice daily. Ampicillin is preferable to penicillin because of its wider spectrum of action but has the disadvantage of being more expensive and is irritating to tissue. An excellent combination of antibiotics utilizes procaine penicillin G at the preceding dosage plus kanamycin at 5 mg per kg twice a day. Once the culture and sensitivity results are received, the antibiotic can be changed if necessary.

Within six hours after surgery, the sinus should be flushed the first time. At least 1 l. of warm normal saline should be used to flush blood from the sinus because blood is an ideal medium for bacterial growth. The sinus should then be flushed every 12 hours. Beginning on the third postsurgical day, hydrogen peroxide should be utilized once a day to loosen debris. A 1:1000 solution of potassium permanganate may also be used as a flush solution of 300 to 500 ml twice daily, or the appropriate antibiotic can be added to the saline flushes. As soon as the saline flushes stop bringing exudate from the sinus, they should be stopped. A prolonged flushing period or an irritating solution itself can produce a continuance of an exudate after the infection is controlled. It is desirable to flush for only five to six days, but with chronic sinusitis the flush period will usually last 10 to 14 days and sometimes longer. Clinical judgment must be used regarding the time to terminate the flushing protocol.

Fungal sinusitis is uncommon. Amphotericin B intravenously at the rate of 0.3 mg per kg in 1 l. of 5 per cent dextrose is the treatment of choice. The amphotericin B dosage should be increased over a five-day period to a daily dose of 0.5 mg per kg body weight. Because amphotericin B is nephrotoxic, careful monitoring of the BUN is mandatory.

Careful observation of appetite and general attitude of the patient must also be maintained during the treatment period. Treatment usually needs to be 15 to 20 days in duration. If the BUN increases rapidly or goes above 40 mg per 100 ml, treatment is discontinued for three days or until the BUN returns to 25 mg per 100 ml or less. Retreatment can begin, but the dosage should be maintained at 0.3 to 0.4 mg per kg of body weight. The prognosis in cases of fungal sinusitis is unfavorable.

Chronic sinusitis associated with neoplasia has an unfavorable prognosis because the disease is often well advanced before clinical signs are recognized. Surgical excision and radiation therapy offer the greatest hope of prolonging the patient's life. Careful examination of the external lymph nodes, endoscopic examination of the pharynx, and thoracic radiographs should be performed prior to expensive surgical and radiation therapy. These procedures could determine if metastasis has already occurred, making surgery unjustified.

ACUTE SINUSITIS

Systemic respiratory infections are frequently accompanied by sinusitis. These cases are generally self-limiting and clear spontaneously as recovery from the initial infection occurs. If the discharge persists for two weeks or longer after recovery from the systemic infection, the condition should be considered chronic and should be treated by trephining as described earlier. Systemic antibiotics alone will seldom be an effective treatment unless administered in the very early stages of the disease. The exudate will frequently decrease or even disappear while on treatment but often reappears after treatment is stopped.

References

1. Baker, G. J.: Surgery of the head and neck. *In* Catcott, E. J., and Smithcors, J. F. (eds.): Equine Medicine and Surgery, 2nd ed. Wheaton, IL, American Veterinary Pub., 1972, pp. 752–758.
2. Milne, D. W., and Turner, A. S.: An Atlas of Surgical Approaches to the Bones of the Horse. Philadelphia, W. B. Saunders Co., 1979, pp. 178–185.
3. Schneider, J. E. *In* Oehme, F. W., and Prier, J. E. (eds.): Textbook of Large Animal Surgery. Baltimore, Williams and Wilkins, 1974, pp. 348–350.
4. Wheat, J. D.: Sinus drainage and tooth repulsion in the horse. Proc. 19th Annu. Conv. Assoc. Eq. Pract., 1973. pp. 171–176.

GUTTURAL POUCH DISEASE

David E. Freeman, KENNETT SQUARE, PENNSYLVANIA

EMPYEMA

Empyema of the guttural pouches usually develops as a chronic sequela to upper respiratory tract infections, especially those caused by Streptococcus sp., or as a complication of guttural pouch tympany. Although the incidence of guttural pouch catarrh or empyema or both is low, there is a tendency to overdiagnose these conditions in horses with vague upper respiratory tract problems.

CLINICAL SIGNS AND DIAGNOSIS

The clinical signs of guttural pouch empyema include intermittent nasal discharge, swelling of adjacent lymph nodes, parotid swelling and pain, and interference with breathing. These signs are not pathognomonic, so endoscopic and radiographic examinations of the guttural pouch are necessary to make the diagnosis and to establish the severity and nature of the disease,

On endoscopic examination, opaque mucopurulent material is seen at the pharyngeal orifice on the affected side and adhering to the lining of the guttural pouch. An accumulation of exudate within the guttural pouch is evident on standing lateral radiographs as a fluid line or as a partial obliteration of the normal guttural pouch contour. Radiopaque foreign bodies may also be demonstrated on radiographs.

Bacterial cultures and sensitivity testing of fluid aspirates or saline washings should be interpreted in the light of clinical findings because bacteria and fungi can be retrieved from normal guttural pouches and other parts of the horse's upper respiratory tract.

TOPICAL TREATMENT

Repeated infusion of the affected guttural pouch is a safe and often effective method for treating empyema and should be the first line of treatment in all but the most severe cases.

METHODS OF GUTTURAL POUCH INFUSION

Guttural pouches are treated topically by infusing medicated solutions through an indwelling catheter introduced along the nasal passages and into the pharyngeal opening of the guttural pouch. A self-retaining uterine catheter* can be inserted through its introducer, which has been bent at the distal tip and guided into the guttural pouch under endoscopic observation. The introducer is then removed, and a butterfly bandage of adhesive tape is applied to the catheter shaft and is sutured to the nostril.

The commercially available uterine catheter suffers from the disadvantage that its coiled plastic grapple can become secured to the inflamed mucosa and detaches when the catheter is removed. A more satisfactory indwelling catheter can be made from a length of PE240 polyethylene tubing† that has a number of coils formed at one end by heating it with hot water and wrapping it around the barrel of a 50 ml syringe. This tubing can also be inserted by the method described before and is advanced until all its coils lie within the cavity of the guttural pouch. The guttural pouch can also be catheterized at Viborg's triangle with a $5\frac{1}{4}$ in, 14-gauge intravenous catheter‡ or with a length of PE240 polyethylene tubing inserted percutaneously through a large-bore

needle. A disadvantage of the latter methods is that the percutaneous catheter provides a tract that allows the infection to spread into tissues outside the guttural pouch.

An intravenous infusion set can be used to connect the catheter to a bottle containing the required volume of medication, and pressure can be generated in the bottle by injecting air into it. The bottle is then inverted, and approximately 200 ml of solution is infused rapidly. Toward the end of the infusion, the horse's head is lowered to allow free drainage of the guttural pouch contents. A sample of the contents, obtained by infusing an antibiotic-free solution prior to treatment with antibiotics, should be used for culture and sensitivity tests. Infusions should be repeated twice daily until the infection has resolved, and the horse should be fed from the ground at all times to allow drainage of exudate from the guttural pouch. After 7 to 10 days, treatment should be interrupted briefly to assess the response.

INFUSION SOLUTIONS

Infusion solutions improve the environment within the guttural pouch by dislodging and removing dead cells, debris, particles of food material, and mediators of the inflammatory response. They should be inexpensive, stable, and easily administered by the owner or lay personnel.

Irritating solutions should not be infused because they can induce neuritis of the cranial nerves over the guttural pouch, resulting in coughing and dysphagia. They can also modify the nature of and increase the amount of nasal discharge, thereby masking the outward signs of response to treatment. Mixtures of antibiotics or antibiotics and other drugs should be avoided because possible interactions in solution can interfere with antimicrobial activity.[10] The pH and ionic composition of the infusion solution should also be close to optimal for any antimicrobial agent that it contains.[1]

Antibiotics are rarely infused into the guttural pouch because they are unable to penetrate tissues or kill organisms within the brief contact period achieved, and many are inactivated by the products of inflammation.[1] In addition, the amounts of antibiotic required to reach effective concentrations over the infected tissues lead to considerable waste and expense.

The most popular antiseptic for guttural pouch infusion is a 10 per cent (v/v) solution of the iodophor povidone-iodine* in physiologic saline. The free iodine liberated from this solution accounts for its low to intermediate germicidal properties.[5] Pov-

---

*Indwelling Uterine Infuser, Fort Dodge Labs, Fort Dodge, IA 50501

†Intramedic, Clay-Adams, Division of Becton-Dickinson and Co., Rutherford, NJ 07070

‡Angiocath, The Deseret Co., Sandy, UT 84070

---

*Betadine, The Purdue Frederick Co., Norwalk, CT 06856

idone-iodine exerts its bactericidal effects over a wide pH range but is more effective in an acid environment than at a neutral or higher pH.[5] Numerous organic and inorganic agents neutralize the effects of iodine, and this may be a disadvantage in the presence of exudates. However, iodine solutions are superior to other antiseptics because they kill immediately on contact and achieve excellent penetration.[5]

If large volumes of necrotic tissue and exudate have accumulated in the guttural pouch, it should be lavaged as often as necessary by rapid infusion of 1 l. of warmed physiologic saline. The horse should be allowed to lower its head during this procedure to prevent aspiration of fluid draining into the pharynx.

SYSTEMIC TREATMENT

Some antibiotics given systemically reach the infected tissues in higher concentrations and for longer intervals than can be achieved with topical application. However, systemic treatment of guttural pouch empyema is rarely indicated unless there is evidence that the infection is spreading and involving other tissues. In these cases, penicillin is often the drug of choice because streptococci, the most common causes of guttural pouch and upper respiratory tract infections in the horse, are uniformly sensitive to it.[1] Penicillin can also achieve excellent penetration into infected and necrotic tissue.[1] However, it is less effective against bacteria that are not actively growing and multiplying, as in the late stages of infection[10] or in suppurative processes contained in cavities[1] like the guttural pouch. This underscores the need for drainage, either through surgery or local irrigation, rather than total reliance on systemic antibiotics.

SURGERY

If medical treatment is unsuccessful and drainage through the pharyngeal orifice is insufficient to cope with the volume of exudate produced, the guttural pouch can be drained surgically through a Whitehouse approach or through a hyovertebrotomy combined with an opening through Viborg's triangle.[3] Irrespective of the surgical approach, the ventral incision is always left open to allow egress of purulent contents. Surgery is always indicated when the purulent material in the guttural pouch has become inspissated or molded into ovoid masses called *chondroids*.

After surgery, the guttural pouch is flushed twice daily through an indwelling rubber tube that has been placed through the ventral incision. Systemic

antibiotics can also be given for the first five days after surgery, and local infusions are discontinued when the ventral incision heals usually in two to three weeks. Although surgical treatment is frequently successful, it should be approached with care to avoid the potential risk of intraoperative nerve damage.

GUTTURAL POUCH MYCOSIS

Guttural pouch mycosis is a localized or diffuse fungal invasion on the roof of the medial compartment of the guttural pouch, caudal to the articulation of the stylohyoid bone. The wide variety of clinical signs that arise from this disease can be explained by the close proximity of the predilection site to a number of important structures in the wall of the medial compartment.[2] Diagnosis can be confirmed by identifying the diphtheritic membrane on endoscopic examination of the affected guttural pouch.

Fungal erosion of the wall of the internal carotid artery causes profuse spontaneous hemorrhage, and this is the most common clinical manifestation of guttural pouch mycosis. Management of this hemorrhage is difficult because it is unpredictable and can recur with little if any warning. The second most common clinical sign is dysphagia caused by neuritis of the pharyngeal and laryngeal branches of the vagus nerve and the pharyngeal branch of the glossopharyngeal nerve. Horses that develop dysphagia may eventually recover their ability to swallow, but a small number develop aspiration pneumonia.

TOPICAL TREATMENT

Guttural pouch mycosis can be treated by topical infusions applying the same principles and with the same methods described in the topical treatment of empyema. The response to treatment is slow, so infusions should be continued for four to six weeks.

METHODS

It is difficult to apply topical infusions directly to the infection site because it is usually confined to the roof of the guttural pouch where the organisms are well protected within a superficial layer of necrotic tissue and fibrin. This problem can be circumvented by nebulizing fungicidal and fungistatic agents through a catheter placed in the guttural pouch, or the horse can be anesthetized and placed in dorsal recumbency so that infusion solutions can bathe the roof of the medial compartment.[2] Solutions can also be infused directly beneath the diphtheritic membrane and against the infected mucosal surface by injecting them through stiff polyethylene tubing passed along the biopsy channel of the fiberoptic endoscope. Vigorous flushing of the lesion may serve to macerate, undermine, and detach the necrotic debris and fungal mat.

INFUSION SOLUTIONS

The true etiology of guttural pouch mycosis is unknown, so treatment must often be directed against a presumptive pathogen such as *Aspergillus nidulans*. This and other saprophytic fungi are often found in the superficial layers of the lesion and in lesser numbers in the underlying tissues. A 10 per cent solution of povidone-iodine is both fungicidal and fungistatic and can be used topically against these organisms.[5] Although the clinical response is often slow and disappointing, there are few, if any, inexpensive, safe, and effective alternatives to this agent.

Daily infusions of 1 per cent gentian violet have been used,[4] but this dye is only effective against Candida sp, a genus that is rarely involved. A 4 per cent solution of formaldehyde was infused in one horse,[2] but this agent is slow-acting, is inactivated by organic matter, and is irritating to mucosal surfaces when applied in effective concentrations.[5]

A number of antibiotics such as amphotericin B, nystatin, and clotrimazole have been considered for topical application in cases of guttural pouch mycosis but are not recommended. Amphotericin B is unstable, especially in an acid environment, and binding to tissue constituents only limits its diffusion to the infected areas.[10] Nystatin is mainly effective against *C. albicans* and appears to have little activity against Aspergillus sp,[10] the organisms most frequently involved. Clotrimazole is not available in a liquid preparation suitable for application to mucous membranes. Pimaricin* as a 5 per cent suspension and miconazole† at a concentration of 1 mg per ml warrant consideration for treatment of guttural pouch mycosis, but neither has been evaluated for this purpose. Because these antibiotics are expensive, they should only be administered topically by a method that allows controlled application to the infected tissues. They must also be administered over a long period, and the expense of such treatment may preclude their use.

Enzymes have been applied topically to the diphtheritic membrane[2] in an attempt to remove clotted blood, mucus, and fibrinous and purulent exudate.[9] This treatment is not recommended because enzymes have specific pH requirements and

must have prolonged and intimate contact with their substrates.[9] They can also induce a local inflammatory response, remove tissue barriers that limit spread of infection, and interfere with blood clotting.[9] Dimethylsulfoxide has been used as a vehicle to enhance drug penetration to infected tissues but is too expensive and irritating to infuse into the guttural pouch over a prolonged period.

SYSTEMIC AND ORAL TREATMENT

Care should be taken when choosing a drug for treatment of guttural pouch mycosis because many antifungal agents are only active against dermatophytes. For example, griseofulvin has no place in the treatment of guttural pouch mycosis because it is not effective against the organisms that cause systemic mycotic infections.[10] In addition, it attains low levels in serum and tissues and is deposited mainly in the stratum corneum,[10] a cell layer that is not present in the mucosal lining of the guttural pouch.

Although there are no reports of the use of amphotericin B in the treatment of guttural pouch mycosis, it has been used systemically and topically for the treatment of other fungal infections in the horse.[7] Horses appear to tolerate the drug, although it can cause phlebitis, depression, kidney damage, fever, hypokalemia, and weight loss.[7, 10] Prolonged therapy can also cause anemia, and although it is usually mild,[7] this can be a grave complication in a horse that is prone to hemorrhage. Although a number of treatment regimens have been used in attempts to minimize adverse side effects,[1, 10] amphotericin B is generally not recommended for treatment of guttural pouch mycosis. Unfortunately, there are no reports on the use of flucytosine in the horse, although the combination of this drug and amphotericin B can act synergistically on susceptible organisms and amphotericin B can prevent the emergence of strains resistant to flucytosine.[10]

Potassium iodide has been given orally and sodium iodide has been infused intravenously to treat mycotic infections in animals. However, there is little critical assessment of these forms of treatment, and there is no clinical evidence in favor of using these drugs against guttural pouch mycosis.

Corticosteroids or phenylbutazone may be administered in certain cases to alleviate the inflammatory response to mycotic infection and to reduce neuritis and fibrosis in the infected tissue.[2] However, prolonged corticosteroid therapy is not recommended because it may exacerbate the mycotic invasion by reducing local tissue defenses against it.

Thiabendazole* has been used in an insufficient number of horses with guttural pouch mycosis to

---

*Natamycin, Alcon Labs, Inc., Fort Worth, TX 76101
†Monistat IV, Janssen Pharmaceuticals, Inc., New Brunswick, NJ 08903

---

*Equizole, Merck and Co., Inc., Rahway, NJ 07065

allow critical assessment of its value in treating this disease. It is a potent, broad-spectrum fungicidal and fungistatic agent[8] that has been used successfully in the treatment of aspergillosis in animals.[6] It is readily taken in the feed and can be given at a dose rate of 10 to 20 mg per kg twice a day for four weeks. Although oral thiabendazole is readily absorbed, a large part of the absorbed drug is converted into metabolic products that are less fungicidal than the parent compound.[8] Agents such as levamisole that stimulate the immune system may also prove to be valuable in the treatment of guttural pouch mycosis, but the immune status of affected horses is unknown at present.

It is common practice to administer tranquilizers, such as acepromazine, as an emergency measure to horses that are bleeding from guttural pouch mycosis on the basis that these drugs cause a drop in blood pressure and thereby reduce the severity of hemorrhage. However, agents that induce a hypotensive effect should be avoided because they can worsen the hypovolemic shock caused by severe blood loss.

Although transfused red blood cells have a short life span in horses, whole blood (see p. 325) should be administered to cases that have suffered acute and massive hemorrhage. Treatment of severe hemorrhage should also include polyionic solutions* or lactated Ringer's solutions. These solutions should be given to supplement blood transfusions or as the sole means of fluid replacement if blood is not available.

In summary, few drugs are available for safe and effective treatment of guttural pouch mycosis. Even under optimal conditions, the response to medical treatment is too slow to remove the risk of complications such as fatal hemorrhage. Some cases resolve spontaneously, and this must be considered when evaluating a treatment method. Another problem often encountered in treating this disease is that there are few if any outward signs that can be used to monitor the response to treatment.

SURGICAL TREATMENT

Proximal ligation of the affected internal carotid artery may fail to prevent hemorrhage from guttural pouch mycosis because the circle of Willis maintains blood pressure at the infection site. To overcome this problem, the artery can be ligated close to its origin, and a balloon catheter can be inserted distal

*Normosol-R, Abbott Labs, North Chicago, IL 60064

to the ligature.[4] The balloon is advanced beyond the mycotic lesion, as determined by measurement and endoscopy, and is inflated so that the infected segment of artery is isolated from the cerebrovascular system.[4] In severe cases, the mycotic lesion can be removed surgically, or parts of it can be detached in a piecemeal fashion with the biopsy attachment of the fiberoptic endoscope. To prevent intraoperative hemorrhage, surgical removal of the diphtheritic membrane should be combined with occlusion of the internal carotid artery, even in horses that have no previous history of hemorrhage from the guttural pouch. In some horses, the external carotid artery or the maxillary artery is affected. In these cases, a balloon catheter should be introduced into the external carotid artery distal to the origin of the linguofacial trunk, and the balloon should be inflated beyond the roof of the guttural pouch.

References

1. Aronson, A. L., and Kirk, R. W.: Antimicrobial drugs. *In* Ettinger, S. J. (ed.): Textbook of Veterinary Internal Medicine, Vol. 1. Philadelphia, W. B. Saunders Co., 1975, pp. 153–180.
2. Cook, W. R.: Diseases of the ear, nose and throat in the horse. Part 1. The ear. *In* Grunsell, C. S. G. (ed.): The Veterinary Annual. Bristol, England, John Wright and Sons, Ltd., 1971, pp. 12–43.
3. Freeman, D. E.: Diagnosis and treatment of diseases of the guttural pouch (Part II). Compend. Contin. Educ. Pract. Vet., 2(2):525, 1980.
4. Freeman, D. E., and Donawick, W. J.; Occlusion of internal carotid artery in the horse by means of a balloon-tipped catheter: Clinical use of a method to prevent epistaxis caused by guttural pouch mycosis. J. Am. Vet. Med. Assoc., 176:236, 1980.
5. Harvey, S. C.: Antiseptics and disinfectants; fungicides; ectoparasiticides. *In* Goodman, L. S., and Gilman, A. (eds.): The Pharmacological Basis of Therapeutics, 5th ed. New York, Macmillan Co., 1975, pp. 987–1017.
6. Lane, J. G., Clayton-Jones, D. G., Thoday, K. L., and Thomsett, L. R.: The diagnosis and successful treatment of *Asperigillus fumigatus* infection of the frontal sinuses and nasal chambers of the dog. J. Small Anim. Pract., 15:79, 1974.
7. McCullan, W. C., Joyce, J. R., Hanselka, D. V., and Heitmann, J. M.: Amphotericin B for the treatment of localized subcutaneous phycomycosis in the horse. J. Am. Vet. Med. Assoc., 170:1293, 1977.
8. Robinson, H. J., Phares, H. F., and Graessle, O. E.: Antimycotic properties of thiabendazole. J. Invest. Dermatol., 42:479, 1964.
9. Swinyard, E. A.: Surface-acting drugs. *In* Goodman, L. S., and Gilman, A. (eds.): The Pharmacological Basis of Therapeutics, 5th ed. New York, Macmillan Co., 1975, pp. 946–959.
10. Weinstein, L.: Antimicrobial agents. *In* Goodman L. S., and Gilman, A. (eds.): The Pharmacological Basis of Therapeutics, 5th ed. New York, Macmillan Co., 1975, pp. 1090–1247.

PHARYNGITIS

Warwick M. Bayly, PULLMAN, WASHINGTON

Pharyngitis in the horse is more accurately described as pharyngeal lymphoid hyperplasia (PLH) or lymphoid follicular hyperplasia. In its chronic form, it has traditionally been regarded as one of the more common causes of decreased athletic performance in young racehorses (two- and three-year-olds).

ETIOLOGY

A number of possible causes of PLH have been suggested. One widely held opinion is that it most frequently develops in response to an equine viral respiratory infection. Attempts to isolate equine influenza (EI) or equine herpesvirus 1 (EHV-1) from pharyngeal cultures are, however, generally unsuccessful. Equine herpesvirus 2 (EHV-2) has been reported as a possible cause of pharyngitis and is a relatively common isolate from swabs of the pharynx.[1] This organism, however, is ubiquitous and can survive for long periods of time in equine lymphocytes. Consequently, its importance in the development of severe or clinical PLH has been questioned. Bacteria that may be cultured from the pharynx of a horse with PLH are usually incidental findings or else represent a secondary infection following initial viral invasion or the effect of another noxious agent. The author has been able to produce a grade 4 PLH by repeatedly spraying irritant chemicals onto the pharyngeal mucous membranes, and it is possible that under certain circumstances, chemical trauma could be primarily responsible for the development of clinical lesions. It is relatively common for a racehorse to be exposed to environmental pollutants from industry or poorly ventilated barns. These physical factors are more likely to combine with stresses such as those due to training and racing to aggravate or worsen existing PLH, rather than acting as primary causes of the syndrome.

Horses do not possess compact masses of lymphoid tissue or tonsils as found in other species. Instead, small follicles of lymphoid tissue are spread diffusely over the dorsal and lateral surfaces of the nasopharynx and pharynx, extending from the dorsal pharyngeal recess caudal to the posterior pillars of the soft palate. The presence of these follicles results in the large number of small nodular areas that are seen in the normal equine pharynx. This lymphoid tissue is capable of mounting a nonspecific inflammatory response to any noxious stimulus, be it viral, bacterial, chemical, or physical. The extent of this response varies with the age of the horse, the nature of the inciting agent, the duration of exposure to it, and the presence of any other stressful factors in the animal's environment.

Existing opinion concerning PLH is based largely on the interpretation of the clinical observations of a number of equine practitioners. Hypotheses advanced to explain poor performance of horses with PLH include (1) obstruction of air flow by follicles, (2) the release of mediators from irritated or inflamed pharyngeal tissue that stimulate bronchoconstriction either directly or by nervous reflex, and (3) the existence of concurrent lower respiratory tract disease caused by EI or EHV-1. The last theory is supported by the observation that exercise intolerance is more common in horses with PLH and a cough than those with the pharyngeal lesions alone. In-depth investigation is needed to clarify the pathophysiology of this disease.

CLINICAL SIGNS

Clinical signs are variable and include harsh inspiratory and/or expiratory sounds during exercise, dysphagia, cough, serous or purulent nasal exudate, and pain on deep palpation of the larynx and pharynx. Exercise intolerance and abnormal respiratory sounds are the most consistent of these signs. The diagnosis may be suggested by a history of loss of form and the clinical signs and is confirmed by endoscopic examination of the upper respiratory tract.

So variable are the degrees of PLH that may occur in a horse that a four-point grading system has been developed to assist in assessing the severity of the pharyngeal lesions seen endoscopically.[6] Grade 1 PLH is considered normal in a young horse. There are a number of small white follicles on the dorsal pharyngeal wall. They appear relatively inactive with no sign of associated edema or hyperemia. In each of the subsequent grades, the area covered by follicles, their size, and the amount of hyperemia and edema increase until in grade 4 all the visible surfaces of the pharyngeal mucous membranes are involved. There are many large pink and white follicles seen, which appear to coalesce and frequently form polyps. Grades 3 and 4 are most commonly associated with loss of athletic performance.

It is noteworthy, however, that grades 3 and 4 PLH can be found in horses of all breeds, and many two- and three-year-olds that are training and racing well can be found to have PLH equally as severe as that in other horses displaying exercise intolerance. It is the author's belief that if a horse is showing signs of decreased performance and is found to have PLH, attempts should be made to determine whether there is concomitant disease of the lower airways. These horses are usually afebrile, with a total white blood cell count within the normal range and lungs that are normal on auscultation. A tracheal wash, however, may show cytologic changes compatible with a low-grade infectious or inflammatory process, and culture may reveal the presence of a common pathogenic organism such as Streptococcus.

THERAPY

Because pharyngitis represents a nonspecific inflammation and because definite information concerning its etiology and pathogenesis is unavailable, therapeutic regimens for the syndrome are very diverse. Many approaches and medications have been tried with varying success. The common factor in most of these treatments is rest, and it is unanimously agreed that rest is essential for satisfactory recovery.

Grade 1 PLH should not be considered abnormal, and the cause of any exercise intolerance in these cases should be sought elsewhere. Grade 2 PLH must also be considered a mild abnormality unless no other possible cause of poor performance can be detected. Animals with grade 2 PLH respond well to a rest period of 30 to 45 days. They do not usually require any additional therapy. This is also the period needed for reepithelialization of the mucous membranes of the lower respiratory tract following infection with equine influenza. Grades 3 and 4 PLH also improve greatly with rest alone but often also require surgical intervention to obtain a "satisfactory" result. (This means either that the pharynx is free of all follicles or that only a grade 1 PLH remains.)

CAUTERY

The surgery requires general anesthesia and a standard laryngotomy approach on the ventral midline in the space between the thyroid and cricoid cartilages. The affected regions of the pharynx and nasopharynx are then electrically or chemically cauterized. The most popular cautery agent is a 50 per cent solution of trichloroacetic acid (TCA),* which is introduced on a cotton pledget on the end of a plastic rod. An ideal instrument is a commercially available uterine culture swab. Chemical cauterizing agents are extremely irritating and can cause adverse reactions such as ulceration and scarring if applied to structures such as the arytenoid cartilages

or the epiglottis. For this reason, the plastic rod and cotton tip are ensheathed in an outer protective guard for introduction into the pharynx. The guard may be a large catheter or simply the outer cover of a uterine culture rod.

The best results are obtained with the patient anesthetized. An assistant views the cautery process via an endoscope inserted up a nostril. This is helpful owing to the limited view afforded the surgeon via the approach site and because of the rostral spread of the lymphoid follicles, particularly in cases of grade 3 or 4 PLH. The observer is able to tell the surgeon when to advance the cotton tip and in which direction to move it.

The rod does not have to be sterile and is swept back and forth across the affected area. In cases of grades 3 and 4 PLH, insufficient TCA might be carried on the tip to cauterize the affected area at once. Instead, the rod and guard must be withdrawn and reintroduced many times before the whole area is covered. If anesthesia is being maintained via gas, the plane must be sufficiently deep to allow the endotracheal tube to be withdrawn into the mouth while the application of the TCA proceeds.

Postsurgical care consists of daily cleaning of the laryngotomy site, which is left to heal by secondary intention. The patient usually develops a bilateral nasal discharge about 24 to 36 hours after surgery, and this may continue for up to a week. Endoscopic examination two to three days after surgery generally reveals hyperemia with some gray or purplish discoloration of the cauterized area. The swelling can be severe, and it is advisable to have a tracheotomy tube beside the horse's stall for the first 72 postoperative hours, although it is rarely needed. Provided the incision site is kept clean, postsurgical antibiotic therapy is not indicated. Rest for 30 to 60 days is recommended, after which the horses are put back into training.

Electrocautery is performed in the same way as chemical cautery, except that a guard is not needed to protect the arytenoids and the epiglottis. Other chemical agents such as Lugol's iodine* and vinegar (5 per cent acetic acid) have been tried. Chemical cautery can be performed in the standing, heavily sedated horse by passing an endoscope up one nostril and the plastic rod and guard up the other. This author feels that better results are obtained when the procedure is performed with the aid of general anesthesia.

Recently a cryosurgical approach has been developed for use in treating PLH. The aim of this technique is the same as that of chemical or electrocautery, namely, to induce necrosis and subsequent sloughing of the nasopharyngeal mucosa. The pro-

---

*Mallinckrodt Chemical Works, St. Louis, MO 63147

*Med-Tech, Inc, Elwood, KS 66024

cedure is performed with the animal anesthetized, and an endoscope is passed up one nostril. A 60-cm-long insulated probe with a valve at the tip is passed up the other nostril and is placed in close proximity to the affected area. The tissue is sprayed with a refrigerant such as Freon 22* for about two minutes. The area covered with each application varies with the closeness of the tip to the pharyngeal mucosa. The procedure may take longer than 20 minutes, and for this reason, general anesthesia is needed for best results.

THROAT SPRAYS

A number of throat sprays have been tried in horses suffering from PLH. These usually involve a combination of drugs and are administered in repeated doses via a catheter inserted up the nose. An ideal implement can be made by taking a plastic artificial insemination pipette, heating one end and sealing it, and then blowing a small bubble in the plastic at the closed end. A 22-gauge needle is heated and used to poke numerous holes in the bubble from all sides. This catheter can be easily passed up the nose and is of such a length that the bubble sits at the entrance to the nasopharynx. Because passage is done blindly, it is possible for the end to lodge in the dorsal pharyngeal recess rather than the nasopharynx, with the result that the effect of the spray is lost. Pharyngeal sprays have been concocted from many agents, which generally fall into one of two classes: anti-inflammatory or antimicrobial. Two of the more popular combinations are 150 ml dimethyl sulfoxide,† 350 ml nitrofurazone solution,‡ and 1000 mg prednisolone.§ [7] Twenty-five ml of this solution is sprayed on the pharynx twice daily until the desired result is achieved or until another approach is tried. Another popular combination is equal parts of DMSO and organic iodide.‖ The rationale behind the choice of agents in the second formula is puzzling, as the former decreases inflammation and the latter stimulates it. Results using this mixture have been variable.

Pharyngeal sprays should not be considered viable alternatives to rest or surgery. Sprays are indicated when it is believed that the degree of PLH is sufficiently mild that a rest from competition is not indicated or when it is desirable to enable a horse to remain in training to allow it to start in a chosen race or event. In such cases, the idea behind the use of the spray is to reduce the severity of the PLH (for example, from grade 3 to grade 2) in the hope of reducing the degree of any existing exercise intolerance. In such situations, the veterinarian must be sure that the horse has no concomitant pulmonary disease that may be exacerbated by continued stress, and the horse should be empirically treated systemically in case such a condition does exist. With the exception of these instances, the author sees no indication for, or value in, treating PLH with antibiotics. Similarly, cough syrups and large doses of vitamins B and C appear to have little direct beneficial effect.

PREVENTION

Finally, mention should be made of prophylaxis, or rather, attempted prophylaxis. The level of immunity of athletic horses against EI and EHV-1 varies greatly among stables. It is this author's opinion that horses on a regular vaccination program display grade 3 or 4 lesions and exercise intolerance less frequently than those that are not being immunized as frequently. "Regular" in this context means vaccinating at least every 60 days against EI and EHV-1. This program should begin prior to the time the young horse is exposed to field viruses. The most frequent source of such exposure is older horses, which act as carriers of the viruses. In many cases, the horse should be first vaccinated at two months of age and should receive regular injections every 60 days while in a "high-risk" habitat until it is at least four years of age. In other instances, the animal may be vaccinated less frequently in its early life if it is kept isolated from older horses, especially those coming and going from the racetrack. Under such circumstances, regular 60-day interval vaccination should begin about two months before the horse is introduced to a high-risk environment such as a sale ring or a training farm.

In summary, whether PLH is a clinical entity capable of hampering athletic performance remains to be determined scientifically. No specific etiologic agents have been positively identified, although there is a strong clinical impression that EI and EHV-1 play a role in its pathogenesis. With this in mind, there is reason to believe that the observed exercise intolerance associated with some cases of PLH may be due to coexisting lower airway disease. This also remains to be proved. Until the pathophysiologic aspects of PLH can be elucidated, the best approach to handling the syndrome consists of rest for 30 to 45 days. This rest period may or may not follow pharyngeal cautery, depending on the severity of the lesions. Pharyngeal sprays are indicated when it is wished to keep the horse in regular training and competition.

---

*Freon 22, Virginia Chemicals, Inc., Portsmouth, VA
†Domoso, Diamond Labs, Inc., Des Moines, IA 50304
‡Clay-Park Labs, Inc., Bronx, NY 10456
§Interstate Drug Exchange, Plainview, NY 11803
‖Povidone-iodine solution, Clay-Park Labs, Inc., Bronx, NY 10456

References

1. Blakeslee, J. R., Olsen, R. G., McAllister, E. S., Fassbender, J., and Dennis, R.: Evidence of respiratory tract infection induced by equine herpesvirus, type 2, in the horse. Can. J. Microbiol., *21*:1940, 1975.
2. Boles, C. L.: Abnormalities of the upper respiratory tract. Vet. Clin. North Am. (Large Anim. Pract.), *1*(1):102, 1979.
3. Boles, C. L.: Treatment of upper airway abnormalities. Vet. Clin. North Am. (Large Anim. Pract.), *1*(1):135, 1979.
4. McAllister, E. S., and Blakeslee, J. R.: Clinical observations of pharyngitis in the horse. J. Am. Vet. Med. Assoc., *170*:739, 1977.
5. Montgomery, T.: A clinical consideration of the causes of chronic pharyngitis in the equine. Equine Pract., *3*(1):26, 1981.
6. Raker, C. W.: Diseases of the pharynx. Mod. Vet. Pract., *57*:396, 1976.
7. Raker, C. W., and Boles, C. L.: Pharyngeal lymphoid hyperplasia in the horse. J. Equine Med. Surg., *2*:202, 1978.

SOFT PALATE DISPLACEMENT

Dennis R. Geiser, KNOXVILLE, TENNESSEE

ETIOLOGY AND PATHOPHYSIOLOGY

Soft palate paresis, soft palate elongation, and dorsal displacement of the soft palate are terms that have been used to describe this syndrome in the horse. The etiology of soft palate displacement is unknown, but the following causes have been suggested: (1) edema or swelling of the palate due to irritation, pharyngitis, or turbulent air flow; (2) a congenital abnormality; (3) cranial nerve damage; (4) hypoplasia of the epiglottis; and (5) asynchronous action of the palate, pharynx, epiglottis, and strap muscles.

Dorsal displacement of the soft palate causes airway obstruction due to displacement of the caudal free border of the palate above the epiglottis. This allows the palate to be pulled into the rima glottidis on inspiration. Vibration or fluttering of the palate occurs on expiration. The end result is obstructed air flow into the lungs and exercise intolerance.

CLINICAL SIGNS AND DIAGNOSIS

The primary complaint is exercise intolerance, especially choking during the last quarter of a race or at the end of a workout. The racehorse may actually stop at the end of the race. Other signs include a fluttering respiratory noise, a missed breathing effort because of swallowing to reposition the palate, and mouth breathing.

The diagnosis is made by endoscopic examination and observation of clinical signs during exercise. The introduction of the endoscope into the pharynx may elicit the swallowing reflex and cause the palate to be displaced above the epiglottis. The normal horse will usually swallow again in a few minutes, repositioning the palate below the epiglottis. In ab-normal horses, the palate may remain above the epiglottis despite swallowing. This finding, along with a fluttering respiratory noise, mouth breathing, and swallowing during exercise, would be good evidence for abnormal dorsal displacement of the soft palate. A horse with abnormal displacement of the soft palate will eventually breathe through the mouth when the nostrils are occluded. Normal horses will fight until the nostrils are uncovered.

There is a predisposition for abnormal displacement of the soft palate in horses 16 hands and over, horses with narrow heads, and horses four to six years old.

TREATMENT

When the cause of dorsal displacement of the soft palate is thought to be edema or inflammation, medical treatment should be attempted. Surgical resection should not be attempted until appropriate rest or medical therapy has reduced the swelling to a minimal amount. This is essential because resection of the edematous soft palate produces excessive shortening when postoperative rest reduces the inflammation.

Conservative therapy may include (1) anti-inflammatory agents such as phenylbutazone* (4 mg per kg orally daily) or dexamethasone† (declining dosage starting at 0.02 to 0.05 mg per kg) given systemically; (2) diuretics such as furosemide‡ (0.5 to 1.0 mg per kg twice a day for two or three days) or trichlormethiazide§ (0.4 to 0.8 mg per kg once a day

---

*Phenylbutazone, Butler Co., Columbus, OH 43228
†Dexamethasone, Beecham Co., Bristol, TN 37620
‡Lasix, National Labs, Somerville, NJ 08876
§Naquasone, Schering Corp., Kenilworth, NJ 07033

for three to four days); (3) throat sprays, which are usually a combination of antibiotics, prednisolone,* or dexamethasone, and DMSO† (a popular mixture contains 1 oz DMSO, 2 oz Predef 2x,‡ and 5 oz Furacin solution sprayed via nasal catheter twice a day); (4) paddock or pasture rest for a minimum of four to six months; and (5) tying the tongue during exercise. The duration of therapy ranges from 7 to 14 days with additional rest up to 6 months. Diuretics should be used carefully to avoid excessive dehydration. In my opinion, the palate requires an extended rest period before surgical intervention is attempted. A product that is used frequently is Naquasone,§ which contains a combination of dexamethasone (5 mg) and trichlormethiazide (200 mg). One to two boluses are crushed and given orally every day for three to five days.

Surgical shortening of the palate is attempted when a positive diagnosis of dorsal displacement is made and after adequate time is allowed for any edema or inflammation to subside. The laryngotomy approach is used as in epiglottic entrapment and ventriculectomy. After entering the larynx, the V-shaped caudal border of the palate is visualized. An Allis tissue forceps is placed on either side of the apex of the V. A $\frac{1}{4}$-in incision is made extending straight forward from the apex. Using a Metzenbaum curved scissors, the caudal margin is removed from the end of the small incision at the apex back to the pharyngeal wall. Traction may be placed on the palate with the Allis forceps. The same procedure is repeated for the other half of the palate. This will remove approximately $\frac{1}{4}$ to $\frac{1}{2}$ in from the center and lesser amounts toward the pharyngeal wall, preserving the V shape of the caudal border. No attempt is made to suture the caudal border, and hemorrhage is usually minimal.

The exact amount of tissue to resect is difficult to estimate. It is better to be conservative. It may be necessary to repeat the procedure if enough tissue is not removed the first time. The owner should be informed of this possibility.

An extended rest period (four to six months) is necessary between procedures because swelling from the first attempt may still be present. Postoperative care includes placement of a laryngotomy tube in the larynx for 24 to 36 hours, anti-inflammatory drugs (phenylbutazone 4 mg per kg orally daily), and tetanus prophylaxis.* Food should be withheld for 24 hours immediately postoperatively. A bran mash is fed for four to five days after surgery. Hay is then introduced gradually. The horse should rest in a stall for three weeks with a total rest period of 90 to 120 days before resuming training.

The major postoperative complication is dysphagia and regurgitation of food and water through the nose owing to excessive shortening of the palate. This problem cannot be alleviated once it occurs.

References

1. Cook, W. R.: Some observations on disease of the ear, nose, and throat in the horse and endoscopy using a flexible fiberoptic endoscope. Vet. Rec., *94*:533, 1974.
2. Schneider, J. E.: The Respiratory System. *In* Oehme, F. W., and Prier, J. E. (eds.): Textbook of Large Animal Surgery. Baltimore, Williams and Wilkins, 1974, p. 340.

*Deltasone, Upjohn Co., Kalamazoo, MI 49001
†Domoso, Diamond Labs, Des Moines, IA 50304
‡Predef 2x, Upjohn Co., Kalamazoo, MI 49001
§Naquasone, Schering Corp., Kenilworth NJ 07033

*Tetanus toxoid, Super Tet, Haver-Lockhart Labs, Shawnee, KS 66201

DISEASES OF THE EPIGLOTTIS

Dennis R. Geiser, KNOXVILLE, TENNESSEE

ARYTENOEPIGLOTTIC ENTRAPMENT

ETIOLOGY AND PATHOPHYSIOLOGY

Epiglottic entrapment is either an acquired or congenital condition, but the exact cause is unknown. Arytenoepiglottic entrapment can be associated with hypoplasia of the epiglottis, pathologic dorsal displacement of the soft palate, and an excessive amount or length of the arytenoepiglottic folds that occurs as a congenital abnormality. The fact that entrapment appears in older horses that have been normal suggests that the condition can be acquired.

Obstruction to air flow, turbulence, and improper functioning of the epiglottis probably occur because the epiglottis is engulfed, to varying degrees, in folds of mucous membrane running from the ventral free border of the epiglottis to the mucous membrane of the arytenoid cartilage. Entrapment, complete or partial, may occur after swallowing and during exercise.

HISTORY AND DIAGNOSIS

The horse with epiglottic entrapment is usually presented with a history of varying degrees of exercise intolerance, abnormal respiratory fluttering, rattling or gurgling, and excessive coughing, especially when eating. The diagnosis is made from the history, clinical signs, and endoscopic examination. The criteria used to determine the presence of an entrapped epiglottis are (1) the presence of the gross outline of the epiglottis without serration of the free margins and typical branching vascular patterns on the epiglottis, (2) excessive elevation of the tip of the epiglottis above the soft palate, and (3) occasionally what appears to be ulceration of the tip of the epiglottis but is in fact ulceration of the arytenoepiglottic fold covering the epiglottis.

TREATMENT

The treatment of epiglottic entrapment is the surgical excision of the excessive amount of the arytenoepiglottic fold through a laryngotomy. The horse is placed under general anesthesia and in dorsal recumbency. A 10 cm midline incision is made directly over the ventral aspect of the larynx. The paired sternothyroideus muscle is divided on the midline by blunt dissection. The fat layer immediately ventral to the larynx is dissected free. The triangular cricothyroid membrane is identified, and a stab incision is made in it with a scalpel. The incision is extended forward to the apex and caudal to the cricoid cartilage. The lumen of the larynx is now visible. Additional exposure may be gained by splitting the thyroid cartilage at the cranial end of the cricothyroid membrane. At this time, the endotracheal tube must be removed to visualize the soft palate and arytenoepiglottic folds. The V-shaped free caudal margin of the soft palate can be seen with the transverse arytenoepiglottic folds dorsal to it (below it as you view the area with the horse in dorsal recumbency). The fold may be retracted into the laryngeal lumen with an Allis tissue forceps. The excess fold is then resected with a scissors. Time is allowed for hemostasis. A tracheostomy tube ("J" tube) is inserted into the lumen via the laryngotomy incision. It is left in place for 36 to 48 hours and then removed. The incision is left to heal by secondary intention. This requires approximately three weeks.

Postoperative care includes the following: (1) tetanus prophylaxis with tetanus toxoid* intramuscu-

larly; (2) antibiotics (procaine penicillin G, 10,000 units per lb twice a day for three to five days); (3) nonsteroidal anti-inflammatory agents (phenylbutazone* (4 mg per kg intravenously for one day, then 4 mg per kg orally for five days); (4) no food for 24 hours postoperatively, with use of a muzzle or cross tie; and (5) daily cleansing of the incision area with saline to remove discharges.

Three to four weeks of stall rest after surgery is recommended. An additional 45 to 60 days of turnout is also recommended.

The procedure can also be accomplished through an oral approach. This requires a general anesthetic, mouth speculum (McAllen type), and long-handled instruments (scissors or biopsy forceps). Excision of the arytenoepiglottic fold is accomplished blindly by palpation.

The prognosis for return to function is good in 90 per cent of the cases. Those with a hypoplastic epiglottis carry a poor prognosis.

HYPOPLASIA OF THE EPIGLOTTIS

ETIOLOGY AND PATHOPHYSIOLOGY

Hypoplasia of the epiglottis is considered a congenital anomaly. Because of the extremely small size and short length of the epiglottis, it cannot function properly in relation to the palate and arytenoids. There may also be an asynchronization between the palate and epiglottis during swallowing. Hypoplasia of the epiglottis is usually accompanied by dorsal displacement of the soft palate and may predispose an animal to arytenoepiglottic entrapment. The small epiglottis allows the palate to displace dorsally and creates a poor seal with the arytenoids and pharynx during deglutition.

CLINICAL SIGNS AND DIAGNOSIS

Epiglottic hypoplasia produces abnormal respiratory noise because of the dorsal displacement of the soft palate. Decreased exercise tolerance, increased swallowing during exercise, and coughing while eating may also be described. The definitive diagnosis can only be made on endoscopic examination.

TREATMENT

There is no specific therapy for hypoplasia of the epiglottis. The prognosis for function as an athlete is poor.

*Tetanus toxoid, Super-Tet, Haver-Lockhart Labs, Shawnee, KS 66201

*Phenylbutazone, Butler Co., Columbus, OH 43228

SUBEPIGLOTTAL CYSTS

ETIOLOGY AND PATHOPHYSIOLOGY

Subepiglottal cysts are congenital problems involving dilatation of the remnant of the embryonic thyroglossal duct. Cysts formed from Rathke's pouch and subepiglottal cysts may also be classified as pharyngeal cysts.

The subepiglottal cyst produces airway obstruction by elevating the epiglottis above the soft palate and into the rima glottidis. Large cysts also prevent proper functioning of the epiglottis during deglutition.

CLINICAL SIGNS AND DIAGNOSIS

The subepiglottal cyst may be present at birth, but clinical signs are not manifested until the horse is placed in training or is forced to exercise. Choking, coughing, and occasionally severe respiratory distress may be noticed when exercise begins. The severity of clinical signs depends on the size and location of the cyst. Abnormal respiratory sounds may also be heard on expiration and inspiration.

A definitive diagnosis is made by endoscopic examination.

TREATMENT

Subepiglottal cysts are removed surgically. The laryngotomy approach is used to enter the pharynx.

The epiglottis is everted into the larynx for better visualization. If necessary, the thyroid cartilage may be split. If possible, the cyst should be dissected from the epiglottis without rupture. If the cyst ruptures or the entire secretory membrane cannot be removed, cautery of the area should be attempted with Lugol's iodine or another strong cautery agent. Care must be taken not to injure the adjacent mucous membrane and free border of the epiglottis either by cautery or dissection. If the total cyst is removed by dissection, the mucous membrane can be sutured with absorbable suture material (size 00). A laryngotomy tube is placed into the larynx. The tube is removed in two to three days, and the incision is left to granulate. Swelling due to cautery may be a problem, and the surgical area should be examined endoscopically prior to removal of the laryngotomy tube.

The prognosis for return to function after successful removal of the cyst is favorable. The major long-term postoperative complication is adhesions of the epiglottis to the soft palate or adjacent pharyngeal wall.

References

1. Boles, C. L.: Epiglottic entrapment and follicular pharyngitis: Diagnosis and treatment. Proc. 21st Annu. Meet. Am. Assoc. Eq. Pract., 1975, p. 29.
2. Boles, C. L., Raker, C. W., and Wheat, J. D.: Epiglottic entrapment by arytenoepiglottic folds in the horse. J. Am. Vet. Med. Assoc., 172:338, 1978.
3. Spiers, V. C.: Entrapment of the epiglottis in horses. Equine Vet. J. 1:267, 1977.

LARYNGEAL HEMIPLEGIA

Gordon J. Baker, URBANA, ILLINOIS

For more than two centuries, veterinarians have recognized laryngeal hemiplegia in the horse. Inspiratory stridor during exercise and the characteristic roaring or whistling noises are the key clinical signs. With the introduction of the rhinolaryngoscope, at first a rigid optical telescope, and, in the past 15 years, flexible fiberoptic endoscopes, a greater understanding of idiopathic laryngeal hemiplegia (ILH) has been achieved. Endoscopic observations, together with studies of laryngeal muscle and recurrent nerve pathology and electrophysiology, have expanded our knowledge of the function and malfunction of the larynx of the horse.

Since the mid-19th century, veterinary surgeons have developed a series of surgical techniques to relieve the laryngeal obstruction caused by recurrent nerve paralysis. Unfortunately, few critical studies have evaluated the effectiveness of these procedures, and consequently, the literature on the subject of the surgical treatment of ILH is an extremely misleading field to explore. The key question is still unresolved; that is, how do we assess the surgical result? Is elimination of noise at exercise the answer? All too often the literature compares the poor performance of an *unfit* laryngeal hemiplegic to that of the same horse postsurgically and *fit*. It is, therefore, hardly surprising that claims of 80 per cent surgical success rates have been made.

Haynes[11] has recently suggested that failures in the surgical treatment of upper respiratory disease may be divided into four general categories: (1) failure to diagnose (incorrect diagnosis), (2) failure in client communication, (3) failure in surgical technique, and (4) failure to avoid complications. To these categories we should perhaps add a fifth, namely, failure to evaluate and record results effectively.

ETIOLOGY AND PATHOGENESIS

If either recurrent laryngeal nerve (RLN) is damaged, there is loss of motor function on the corresponding side of the larynx. The duration and degree of motor loss depends upon the severity of the neuropathy and may be permanent, such as following jugular phlebitis, strangles, abscessation, or auditory tube diverticulum disease. The majority of cases of laryngeal hemiplegias, however, do not result from such diseases and are designated as idiopathic (hence, idiopathic laryngeal hemiplegia, or ILH). Such clinical cases are seen in larger horses and are universally left-sided. Horses of all sizes with endoscopically normal larynges have histochemical evidence of bilateral neurogenic atrophy of the intralaryngeal muscles supplied by the RLN,[6, 9, 15] and both RLNs exhibit evidence of distal demyelination and also regeneration.[7] The factors that express the clinical disease of hemiplegia on the left side are unknown but may interfere with regeneration. Whether these factors are simple compression or stretching is unproved, but such etiologies have been suggested. Observations of fetal neurogenic atrophy and neonatal hemiplegia[10] lend strength to Cook's suggestion that the disease is inherited as a simple recessive factor.[5]

DIAGNOSIS

Horses with laryngeal hemiplegia are noisy when exercised, but not all noisy horses have ILH, although the rasping roar (le cheval qui scie du bois) may be very suggestive.[2] Because noise at exercise can be produced by any nasal, pharyngeal, or tracheal obstruction (for example, pharyngeal lymphoid hyperplasia), a full history should determine the degree of fitness (or lack of fitness) and the pace and conditions under which the noise is heard. While training and racing times can be used to assess the performance of race horses, a quantitative measurement of the effect of ILH on the performance of hunters, show jumpers, eventers, and pleasure horses is not available.

A complete physical examination should rule out intercurrent disease that may also affect the animal's performance, such as lower airway disease, musculoskeletal problems, or heart disease.

The larynx should be palpated for scar tissue (indicating previous surgery) and for ossification. Atrophy of the cricoarytenoideus dorsalis (CAD) muscle is assessed by hooking a finger over the top of the larynx on either side and using a sweeping movement to compare the prominence of the muscular processes of the arytenoid cartilages. With practice, atrophy of the CAD can be detected. Pressure on the *right* arytenoid or on the cricothyroid ligament will reduce the glottis, and if the *left* side is paralyzed, the horse may well make an inspiratory noise.

A preliminary diagnosis can be made by endoscopic examination at rest. If the horse resists examination at this stage, it is best to proceed to the exercise test and to try endoscopy again after the horse has been worked hard, rather than to tranquilize the animal. The exercise test should demonstrate the noise or the nature of the poor performance or exercise intolerance that is the basis for the consultation. The endoscopic examination should then be repeated.

LARYNGOSCOPIC DIAGNOSIS

Cook[2-4] and Johnson et al.[13] have described the endoscopic appearance of the normal and hemiplegic larynx. There is agreement as to the endoscopic appearance of the normal resting, the fully adducted (i.e., closed), and the fully abducted (i.e., dilated) larynx.

The normal larynx is bilaterally symmetrical both at rest and when fully abducted and adducted. Care should be taken in assessing asymmetry, and the endoscopic examination should be carried out through each nostril successively. Many horses react to the endoscope, and very little glottal movement is seen, giving a narrow rima glottidis in quiet horses and a fixed, dilated rima glottidis in excitable individuals. Full closure and full dilation can be stimulated by slapping the chest on alternate sides, by stimulating a swallowing movement, or by blocking the external nares. Only 40 per cent of horses exhibit rhythmic laryngeal movement at rest, and frequently movements of the two sides of the larynx are asynchronous. Observations of a group of horses in training over a four-year period failed to show any progression of asynchrony to left hemiplegia (Baker, unpublished data). Similarly, asynchronous movement has been seen in horses and ponies of all ages and sizes, and in the author's opinion such movement is normal.

In most cases of laryngeal hemiplegia, there is some compensatory, partial abduction of the right arytenoid and vocal ligament as well as the obvious medial displacement of the paralyzed side.

Failure to fully dilate the rima glottidis is confirmed by the postexercise endoscopic examination when the asymmetry of the hemiplegic larynx is exaggerated.

In summary, horses with ILH demonstrate noise at exercise, some impairment of athletic ability, and paralysis of the left vocal ligament as seen on endoscopic examination.

THERAPY

The only satisfactory treatment of ILH is surgical, but a critical analysis should be made of each case before laryngeal surgery is advised. It could be argued that those horses required to perform in short races and under conditions of less than maximal exertion, such as jumpers, dressage horses, and hunters, can perform such tasks quite effectively despite their laryngeal obstruction. Perhaps the future will bring techniques to assist in evaluating such horses.

Horses with acquired ILH should be evaluated monthly for up to six months before surgical treatment is undertaken. Normal RLN function may return in horses with iatrogenic neuritis (edema or phlebitis) at times varying from five days to five months after injury.

The ideal surgical technique should enlarge and streamline the rima glottidis and should have neither short-term nor long-term complications. This has been recognized since the mid-19th century, when Gunther, at first alone and later with his son, carried out the first partial laryngectomy procedures. It is not the object of this section to give a review of the evolution of laryngeal surgery in the horse from that time (see Johnson and Garner, 1975)[12] but to present a personal opinion of those techniques that are used currently.

SURGICAL TECHNIQUES

VENTRICULECTOMY

The larynx may be opened with the horse standing after sedation and local anesthesia, but general anesthesia and the use of a cuffed endotracheal tube are preferred. The horse is positioned on its back, and after suitable surgical preparation and nose support, a 10 to 12 cm ventral midline skin incision is made on either side of a line joining the caudal borders of the mandibles. The cricothyroid ligament is divided, and a self-retaining retractor is used to expose the vocal ligaments. Ventriculectomy is facilitated by everting the lateral ventricle on the paralyzed side using a bur. The bur is inserted deeply into the ventricle, and by rotating and lifting, the mucous membrane is drawn out. The bur may then

be removed, and further traction and sharp dissection complete the excision. Some surgeons routinely strip both ventricles, but this is considered to be unnecessary. Others excise part of the vocal ligament and, using chromic catgut, suture the excision site.

A Papes or "J" tube is inserted through the laryngotomy wound to protect from asphyxia as a result of postoperative edema. This tube is removed after 24 to 48 hours, and the horse is stall-rested until the laryngotomy incision has closed (three to four weeks). After a further month's rest, the training program can be resumed.

LARYNGOPLASTY

Under general anesthesia, the horse is positioned with the affected side uppermost and the neck extended. The chin is raised, and the surgical site is prepared. A 12 cm skin incision is made immediately below the linguofacial vein cranial to its junction with the jugular vein. Simple, blunt dissection elevates the linguofacial vein, and digital manipulation deepens the dissection through the fascial tissue to expose the lateral surface of the larynx and the overlying pharyngeal muscles. Dissection of the larynx is made easier by having the animal's neck extended and slightly rotated by a wedge or sandbag beneath the chin and ramus of the mandible. The caudal lamina of the cricoid cartilage is exposed, carefully avoiding damage to the cranial thyroid artery and vein. The fascial plane between the thyropharyngeus and cricopharyngeus muscles is divided to expose the muscular process of the arytenoid cartilage. The cricopharyngeus muscle is elevated from the dorsal aspect of the atrophied cricoarytenoideus dorsalis muscle. The laryngeal suture or prosthesis (nonabsorbable polyester—Mersilene No. 1—or polypropylene—Prolene—on a 30 mm half-circle trochar point needle) must be positioned as close to the midline as possible. The needle is inserted beneath the caudal margin of the cricoid lamina to emerge cranially on the midline, encompassing a 1.5 to 2 cm bite of the lamina. The needle and the free end are then retrieved using curved forceps beneath the elevated cricopharyngeus muscle. The suture is manipulated to slide smoothly in this position, and the needle is then directed in a cranial direction through the muscular process of the arytenoid cartilage. Its position can be checked by laryngoscopy and suture manipulation or by palpation of the arytenoid cartilage as the suture is tightened and tied. In this way, the rima glottidis is dilated by the induced outward rotation of the arytenoid cartilage about the cricoarytenoid joint.

The fascial plane between the cricopharyngeus and thyropharyngeus muscles is apposed over the suture, and the surgical incision is closed in a routine manner. The horse is then positioned for a left ventriculectomy. No drainage materials are used routinely, but a Penrose drain may be indicated in repeat operations in which the degree of surgical trauma is magnified by the scar tissue or other factors.

The postoperative treatment consists of tetanus prophylaxis, antibiotic therapy, and daily wound cleansing. The horse can resume training four weeks after closure of the ventriculectomy incision.

ARYTENOIDECTOMY

In the face of laryngeal chondritis, abscessation, chondroma formation, ossification with laryngeal obstruction, or failed laryngoplasty, surgeons are re-evaluating forms of partial or submucosal arytenoidectomy as a salvage procedure.[16]

A ventral midline laryngotomy is used, and the incision should be extended cranially through the junction of the laminae of the thyroid cartilage if exposure through the cricothyroid ligament is inadequate. Anesthesia is maintained using a cuffed endotracheal tube inserted through a midcervical tracheostomy incision.

An incision is made along the cranial edge of the vocal ligament, and the lateral ventricle is everted. The arytenoid cartilage is dissected after injection of 1:10,000 epinephrine both submucosally and lateral and dorsal to the cartilage itself. A curved periosteal elevator is used to lift the mucosa from the vocal process of the arytenoid, and this dissection is continued as far as possible onto the rostral margin of the arytenoid cartilage (corniculate process). Care must be taken in the deeper lateral and dorsal dissection of the cartilage to keep close to the cartilage itself and so avoid severe hemorrhage. This procedure may not be easy in the presence of advanced cartilage inflammation, necrosis, or abscessation. The arytenoidectomy site is then sutured with interrupted sutures of 2–0 chromic gut or polypropylene.

The laryngotomy incision is treated as for a ventriculectomy. Postoperative care should include antibiotics, analgesics, and diuretics as indicated. If intraoperative hemorrhage is severe, laryngeal packing and a tracheostomy tube are essential.

RESULTS OF SURGICAL PROCEDURES

Table 1 presents a summary of 326 horses operated upon by the author for the treatment of laryngeal obstruction (310 with ILH, 6 with acquired hemiplegia, and 10 with "chondritis" syndrome). This study represents an attempt to critically assess the surgical treatment of ILH. The value of personal

TABLE 1. RESULTS OF SURGICAL CORRECTION OF LARYNGEAL HEMIPLEGIA

1. Time surveyed		1965–1979
2. Number of surgical corrections of laryngeal hemiplegia		326
3. Follow-up numbers (Follow-up = 6 months postoperatively and includes preoperative and postoperative exercise test and laryngoscopy)		165
4. *Techniques used in 3*		
Permanent tracheostomy tube	16	
Unilateral ventriculectomy	67	
Laryngoplasty (includes unilateral ventriculectomy)	96	
Arytenoidectomy	2	
5. *Postoperative noise*	*Ventriculectomy*	*Laryngoplasty*
No change	45%	10%
Slightly reduced	27	32
Greatly reduced	28	28
Absent	0	30

Note: Total 4 exceeds Total 3 because 16 horses had more than one procedure on separate occasions.

reexamination was emphasized when owner-trainer questionnaire returns were compared with the follow-up examination results. Owners-trainers of ventriculectomized horses reported that they were satisfied in 60 per cent of cases, whereas personal examination produced only 28 per cent in which the noise was greatly reduced. Obviously the quality of noise assessment is subjective and, therefore, is subject to major error and bias. The application of radiostethoscope recordings and analysis of amplitude envelopes[1] would perhaps overcome such errors in future surveys, or as indicated earlier, the development of methods to measure tracheal air flows telemetrically could be invaluable.

After excision of the lateral ventricle, 28 per cent of horses were deemed satisfactory, but none was regarded as silent to the rider's ear. Endoscopic examination refuted earlier claims that scar tissue can retract the paralyzed vocal ligament and arytenoid. In no case was rima glottidis enlargement detected. This suggests that effective (nonturbulent) air flow is influenced not only by the size of the airway but also by the nature of its wall. If the ventriculectomy results in the laryngeal vestibule becoming streamlined, then effective (relatively silent) air flow will result. It appears, however, that this result is only achieved in less than one third of cases and cannot be forecast preoperatively.

The laryngoplasty results are much better than the results of a ventriculectomy in that 58 per cent were much improved. In earlier reports of up to 80 per cent satisfactory results from laryngoplasties, the methods of assessment were not defined.[14]

Very few complications were recorded in the ventriculectomy series, confirming the opinion that

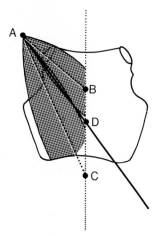

Figure 1. Diagram of the dorsal surface of the cricoid cartilage with vectors of cricoarytenoideus dorsalis action. AB, cranial belly; AC, caudal belly; AD, combined. AD represents the ideal suture position. A, muscular process of arytenoid.

ventriculectomy or the Williams-Hobday operation is a safe procedure. Only one case resulted in chondroma formation and laryngeal obstruction; this horse was subsequently destroyed.

A number of authors have reviewed laryngoplasty complications.[8] Suture sinus formation, separation of the suture, esophageal obstruction, and acute and chronic coughing have been described. Care must be taken to ensure the correct placement of the suture to effect not only outward rotation of the rostral margin of the arytenoid cartilage but also good abduction of the vocal process and vocal ligament. The vector of the suture should be from a point as close to the median crest of the cricoid as possible (Fig. 1).

The choice of suture material has also been reviewed, and although elastic (Lycra) material is the choice of some surgeons, the majority are satisfied with the results of inelastic nonabsorbable materials.

In this series, no serious wound problems or suture sinuses occurred. Surgical edema was minimal, and wound healing was very good. In eight cases, good early abduction was replaced by collapse (at five weeks to five months after operations), and in six cases, at reoperation the knot in the suture was intact, but it had cut through the muscular process of the arytenoid. In three of these cases, it proved impossible to reanchor the suture to the muscular process. Great care should be taken if the needle technique is used rather than the drilling technique of Marks et al.[14] to avoid stress fractures of the muscular process, which may result in subsequent failure of the prosthesis.

A more serious problem appears to result from the induced failure of the glottal closure mechanisms and changes in pharyngeal function.[8] Nearly 40 per cent of laryngoplasty horses show coughing as they feed during the first month after the laryngoplasty, and 20 per cent remain as intermittent, chronic, feeding-induced coughers. In this series, there was no apparent relationship between the chronicity and severity of coughing and the degree of rima abduction.

At the present time, the results of surgical treatment of ILH can be summarized by saying that ventriculectomy is a safe operation but is only effective in less than 30 per cent of cases, whereas laryngoplasty is effective in nearly 60 per cent of cases but is not without problems.

References

1. Attenburrow, D. P.: Respiratory sounds recorded by radio stethoscope from normal horses at exercise. Equine Vet. J., *10*:176, 1978.
2. Cook, W. R.: The diagnosis of respiratory unsoundness in the horse. Vet. Rec., 77:516, 1965.
3. Cook, W. R.: A comparison of idiopathic laryngeal paralysis in man and horse. J. Laryngol. Otol., 84:819, 1970.
4. Cook, W. S.: Some observations on diseases of the ear, nose and throat in the horse and endoscopy using a flexible fiberoptic endoscope. Vet. Rec., 94:533, 1974.
5. Cook, W. R.: Hereditary roaring in the horse. Am. Assoc. Eq. Pract. Newsletter, June, 1978, p. 33.
6. Duncan, I. D., Griffiths, I. R., McQueen, A., and Baker, G. J.: The pathology of equine laryngeal hemiplegia. Acta Neuropathol., 27:337, 1974.
7. Duncan, I. D., Griffiths, I. R. and Madrid, R. E.: A light and electron microscope study of the neuropathy of equine idiopathic laryngeal hemiplegia. Neuropathol. Appl. Neurobiol., 4:483, 1978.
8. Greet, T. R. C., Baker, G. J., and Lee, R.: The effect of laryngoplasty on pharyngeal function in the horse. Equine Vet. J., *11*:153, 1979.
9. Gunn, H. M.: Histochemical observations on laryngeal skeletal muscle fibres in "normal" horses. Equine Vet. J., 4:144, 1972.
10. Gunn, H. M.: Further observations on laryngeal skeletal muscle in the horse. Equine Vet. J., 5:77, 1973.
11. Haynes, P. F.: Surgical failures in upper respiratory surgery. Proc. 24th Annu. Conv. Am. Assoc. Eq. Pract., 1978, pp. 223–249.
12. Johnson, J. H., and Garner, H. E.: Complications in equine laryngeal surgery. Archives, 4(2):57, 1975.
13. Johnson, J. H., Moore, J. N., Garner, H. E., Coffman, J. R., Tritschler, L. G., and Traver, D. S.: Clinical characterization of the larynx in laryngeal hemiplegia. Proc. 23rd Annu. Conv. Am. Assoc. Eq. Pract., 1977, p. 259.
14. Marks, D., Mackay-Smith, M. P., Cushing, L. S. and Leslie, J. A.: Etiology and diagnosis of laryngeal hemiplegia in horses. J. Am. Vet. Med. Assoc., 157:429, 1970.
15. Quinlan, T., Goulden, B. E., and Davies, A. S.: Bilateral asymmetry of equine laryngeal muscle. NZ Vet. J., 23:145, 1975.
16. White, N. A., and Blackwell, R. B.: Partial arytenoidectomy in the horse. Vet. Surg., 9(1):5, 1980.

FOAL PNEUMONIA AND LUNG ABSCESSES

W. L. Scrutchfield, COLLEGE STATION, TEXAS

R. J. Martens, COLLEGE STATION, TEXAS

Pneumonia is an important economic problem in foals. In a survey conducted by the American Association of Equine Practitioners covering the years 1976 and 1977, it was estimated that approximately 9 per cent of foals are affected by the pneumonia syndrome. Approximately 12 per cent of the affected foals died (more than 1 per cent of the total).[3]

Several management factors contribute to foal pneumonia, including overcrowding, poor ventilation, and contaminated feed, bedding, and water supply. Rough and excessive handling as well as hauling are stressful.

An effective parasite control program is very important in the prevention of pneumonia. Ascarid migration through the lungs increases the stress on foals.

The failure of passive transfer of immunity via colostrum greatly increases the foal's chances of developing infections, including foal pneumonia. It has been estimated that 10 per cent of foals have failure of passive transfer (colostral immunity). Arabian foals affected with combined immunodeficiency develop fatal respiratory tract infections within the first six months of life.

ETIOLOGY

INFECTIOUS AGENTS

VIRAL AGENTS

Viral respiratory agents in the horse include equine influenza virus (myxovirus influenza A-equi-1 and A-equi-2) (p. 3); rhinopneumonitis virus (herpesvirus type 1) (p. 4); equine rhinovirus (p. 6); and adenovirus (p. 5). While these are generally considered upper respiratory infections, concurrent aerogenous and hematogenous spread of the virus may cause disease of the lungs. Viral infections of the lower respiratory tract result in interstitial pneumonia, bronchitis, and secondary bacterial pneumonia. The viruses increase the susceptibility of the respiratory tract to secondary infection with bacteria due to epithelial cell necrosis, accumulation of inflammatory exudates, disruption of mucociliary transport, and interference with macrophage activity.

BACTERIA

Many different species of bacteria have been isolated from foal pneumonia cases. More than one species may infect the same foal. *Streptococcus zooepidemicus* and *S. equi* are the most common bacteria isolated in equine respiratory infections. These are often associated with upper respiratory tract infections (strangles); however, both may be involved in foal pneumonia and infrequently lung abscesses.

The most severe foal pneumonia is caused by *Corynebacterium equi*. Clinical signs are usually not evident until a large amount of the foal's lung tissue is involved. Frequently there are multiple abscesses throughout the lungs. Enteritis and arthritis may also be seen in affected foals. Certain farms have *C. equi* infections each year with high death losses.

Actinobacillus equuli can cause acute respiratory infections accompanied by septicemia or arthritis or both in very young foals. Older foals (three to six months) with acute or chronic pneumonia that has failed to respond to antibiotic therapy may have an Actinobacillus infection. Actinobacillus infections in foals have become very important in certain areas of the country.[6]

While *Klebsiella pneumoniae* can be a primary pathogen, usually it is a secondary pathogen in equine respiratory infections. When found, it is resistant to many antibiotics. *Bordetella bronchiseptica* has been recoverd from upper respiratory infections and pneumonia in foals. Generally it is an individual animal problem and is treated as such. Salmonella sp can produce septicemia, diarrhea, and septic arthritis in foals two to eight weeks old. Approximately 30 per cent of these foals have pneumonia associated with this disease complex.

OTHER AGENTS PREDISPOSING FOALS TO PNEUMONIA

Pneumocystis carinii, a ubiquitous protozoan, should be considered in foals with chronic illness, debilitation, and long-term antibiotic or anti-inflammatory therapy. While the diagnosis is usually made at necropsy, transtracheal washings stained with Gomori methenamine silver may reveal the organisms.[5]

Skin testing indicates that coccidioidomycosis may be common in horses in the Southwest. The few cases in the literature are described as a chronic, febrile, wasting disease with respiratory signs.

Dictyocaulus arnfieldi may cause respiratory disease signs in horses, as may the migration of immature *Parascaris equorum* through the lungs. Both parasites may predispose the foal to pneumonia (p. 520).

HISTORY

A history of previous respiratory problems on the farm should be obtained in any suspected case of foal pneumonia. The results of previous culture and sensitivity testing and response to therapy are often helpful in diagnosis of a current problem. The age of the foal is important, as failure of passive transfer of colostral immunity may be involved in the development of respiratory infections in the very young foal. Infections start to appear in Arabian foals with combined immunodeficiency around 40 to 60 days of age. Determine if and when the foal has had previous treatment, as it may alter the clinical picture and laboratory examinations.

CLINICAL SIGNS

The first sign of foal pneumonia is often an increased respiratory rate with some difficulty in breathing. The attitude of the foal varies from alert to very depressed. The mare's udder may be distended owing to lack of nursing. Often a mucopurulent nasal discharge and elevated temperature are present. Coughing may or may not be present.

A complete physical examination should be done to be sure the respiratory signs are primary and not secondary to some other condition. The rate and character of respiration should be determined before catching and handling the foal. Observe the presence or absence of nasal discharge. A serous nasal discharge suggests viral infection or the presence of some irritating agent such as dust. A mucopurulent discharge indicates bacterial infection. Frequently, foals with *C. equi* pneumonia do not have a nasal discharge. Observe and palpate the intermandibular and retropharyngeal areas for the presence of enlarged lymph nodes.

Auscultate both sides of the thorax, over the trachea, and the upper airway. Auscultation should be done at rest with a bag over the foal's nose to increase the depth of respiration. Exaggerated and harsh vesicular sounds indicate interstitial pneumonia. Moist rales and dry rhonchi indicate the presence of airway fluid and airway inflammation, respectively. Crepitant adventitious sounds are often heard early in pneumonia. Harsh inspiratory sounds may be the only abnormal sounds heard, although pulmonary abscessation is present. This is especially true in cases of *C. equi* pneumonia. Differentiate between referred sounds from the upper airway and abnormal lung sounds to help determine if true lower airway disease is present.

Endoscopy of the upper respiratory tract is indicated in chronic or nonresponsive pneumonia cases, especially if there are inspiratory "rattling" and indications of an upper airway obstruction. In one report, three foals with nonresponsive pneumonia were found to have subepiglottic cysts as the inciting cause.[7]

LABORATORY EXAMINATION

A blood sample for complete blood count should be obtained early in the examination before the foal becomes excited. The results are somewhat variable, but the following are general guidelines. A mild lymphopenia indicates a viral infection. Lymphocyte counts under 1000 per mm^3 may indicate an immunodeficiency, especially in Arabian foals. Most foals with bacterial pneumonia will have a mild to moderate neutrophilic leukocytosis (10,000 to 20,000 WBC per mm^3). The WBC count may be much higher in severe cases. Usually the elevated WBC count returns toward normal with clinical improvement. It would be desirable to check foals under 10 days of age for failure of passive transfer of immunity via colostrum. This can be done by the zinc sulfate turbidity test or by single radial immunodiffusion (p. 323).

TRANSTRACHEAL ASPIRATION

While evaluation of tracheal aspirates has been controversial, it is still the best technique to obtain cultures and determine susceptibilities of the etiologic agent or agents. Gram stain of direct smears may indicate appropriate initial antibiotic therapy. The technique and evaluation of transtracheal aspiration are discussed elsewhere (p. 513).

RADIOGRAPHY

Many portable radiograph machines can be used to assess the thorax in standing foals. Radiographs are especially helpful in diagnosing lung abscesses and in following the progression or resolution of pneumonia. Regular-speed intensifying screens can be used in very young foals, but to obtain good-quality thoracic radiographs in older foals, rare-earth screens* should be used.[1] Rare-earth screens are six times "faster" than regular-speed screens, so the milliampere seconds (MAS) can be divided by six, thus reducing the length of exposure, which

---

*Quanta-3, E.I. du Pont de Nemours and Co., Wilmington, DE 19898

TABLE 1. TECHNIQUE CHART FOR RADIOGRAPHY OF THE FOAL THORAX
(MIDTHORACIC MEASUREMENT: 24 CM)

Machine	FFD*	Air-Gap	Film	Screens	MA‡	Time (secs)	MAS§	KVP†
Min X-Ray (30 MA)	32"	Yes	X-L 1 Kodak	Regular Speed	10	0.3	3.3	100
Min X-Ray (30 MA)	32"	Yes	X-L 1 Kodak	Q-3	10	0.05	0.5	100
Bowie (20 MA, 80 kv)	32"	Yes	X-L 1 Kodak	Q-3	20	0.1	2.0	80

*Focal film distance
†Kilovolt peak
‡Milliamperes
§Milliampere seconds.

decreases the amount of motion and minimizes radiation exposure. An exposure that would normally require 12 MAS with regular-speed screens will only need 2 MAS with rare-earth screens.

An air-gap of 3 to 4 in. between the foal's thorax and the x-ray cassette replaces a grid and minimizes scattered radiation. The cassette can be taped to a wall and the foal positioned to maintain the required air-gap.

A technique chart (Table 1), currently in use at Texas A & M University, indicates the exposure requirements for thoracic radiographs of foals with a midthoracic width of 11 in (24 cm). This chart indicates the techniques for two readily available portable radiographic machines; however, similar techniques may be used for any machine with an equivalent capacity. The highest possible kilovolt peak should always be used to minimize radiation exposure. When examining larger or smaller foals, it will be necessary to increase or decrease the MAS accordingly.

TREATMENT

The choice of antibiotics for treatment of a case of pneumonia should be guided by previous experience on the farm, identification of the etiologic agent and its susceptibility, the dose and frequency of administration, possible side effects, and cost. An article by Knight[2] is very helpful for determining dosages, routes, and frequency of administration of antibiotics in horses (also see pp. 43 and 467).

Since a high percentage of foal pneumonia is due to penicillin-sensitive organisms, penicillin is often used for initial therapy. Penicillin is relatively inexpensive and nontoxic, except in the small percentage of individuals that have hypersensitivity reactions. Procaine penicillin G at 5000 to 10,000 units per lb (10,000 to 20,000 units per kg) intramuscularly twice a day is often effective, especially against beta-hemolytic streptococci. Procaine and benzathine penicillin may not produce high enough blood levels to be effective against more resistant organisms. Much higher blood levels can be obtained by the use of penicillin salts (potassium penicillin G or sodium penicillin G) at 6000 to 50,000 units per lb (12,000 to 100,000 units per kg) intravenously or intramuscularly four times a day. The simultaneous use of procaine penicillin G and penicillin salts will give both high and sustained blood levels. This combination should be considered in the foal that is severely affected.

Aminoglycosides are often combined with penicillin for their effect against gram-negative organisms and their synergism with penicillin. Kanamycin sulfate* at 5 mg per lb (10 mg per kg) twice a day can be effective. Gentamicin sulfate† is expensive but may be economical in foals because of the low total dosage required. A dosage of 0.8 mg per lb (1.8 mg per kg) three times a day or 1 mg per lb (2.2 mg per kg) two times a day should not be exceeded because of the danger of nephrotoxicity. After five days of treatment or if the patient is not adequately hydrated, serial monitoring of urine for protein, blood, and casts is indicated. These changes appear earlier than elevated blood urea nitrogen (BUN) and serum creatinine in nephrotoxicity due to gentamicin.[4] Dihydrostreptomycin is less useful than either kanamycin or gentamicin because many organisms are resistant to it.

The trimethoprim-sulfonamide combination products‡§ appear to be useful in the treatment of pneumonia. This combination has bactericidal rather than bacteriostatic activity. The dosage suggested is 14 mg per lb per day (30 mg per kg per day) orally. More work needs to be done to define effective dosages for horses.

Other antibiotics that can be used to treat foal pneumonia include ampicillin, chloramphenicol, erythromycin, and tetracycline.

*Kantrim, Bristol Labs, Des Moines, IA 50317
†Gentocin, Schering Corp., Kenilworth, NJ 07033
‡Di-Trim, Diamond Labs, Des Moines, IA 50317
§Tribrissen, Jensen-Salsbery Labs, Kansas City, MO 64141

Bronchodilator-expectorant products, such as Quibron* or Slo-Phyllin Syrup,† are helpful in foals with labored breathing. These contain theophylline for a bronchodilator and guaifenesin as an expectorant. Ten ml three or four times a day orally (100 mg theophylline, 60 mg guaifenesin per 10 ml) appears to be effective. Excessive theophylline doses may be associated with toxicity such as seizures or ventricular arrhythmias. As there is improvement in breathing, the dosage should be decreased or stopped.

If the foal's temperature is elevated excessively and the foal is depressed, nonsteroidal anti-inflammatory drugs, such as phenylbutazone, flunixin meglumine,‡ or dipyrone, are indicated. Their use will improve the foal's attitude and appetite but will eliminate the value of body temperature as an indicator of response to treatment. Antipyretic therapy should be stopped when the foal feels better so that body temperature can be used as an indicator of response to therapy.

It would be the rare foal pneumonia case that would benefit from corticosteroids. The foal's pulmonary defense mechanisms have already been compromised. Corticosteroids contribute to the impairment of the immune system, especially when used repeatedly.

NEBULIZATION

The benefits of nebulization in the treatment of foal pneumonia are questionable. The possible benefits include mobilization of secretions that have increased viscosity and decreased elasticity. Pharmacologic agents, including bronchodilators, mucolytics, and antibiotics may be delivered by this route. Bronchodilators are necessary if using any other agents, since the latter are irritants and cause some degree of bronchoconstriction.

Ultrasonic nebulizors should be used to deliver the correct particle size. Sterile physiologic saline may be used alone, or many different combinations may be used in nebulization.

One example is: 10 ml of gentamicin (50 mg per ml), 10 ml aminophylline (250 mg total), and 80 ml physiologic sterile saline.

Hazards of aerosol therapy include (1) contamination of equipment, resulting in spread of infection; (2) precipitation of bronchospasm; (3) fluid overload of the lungs if the patient has moist secretions; and (4) swelling of dried retained secretions, which may obstruct airways.

TRANSFUSION

If there are indications of failure of passive transfer of immunity via colostrum, a plasma transfusion from a suitable donor is indicated (p. 324).

LUNG ABSCESSES

Lung abscesses may be caused by nearly all the bacteria involved with foal pneumonia. Abscesses are present in a high percentage of foals infected with *C. equi*. Careful auscultation and percussion may reveal dull areas, suggesting the possibility of abscesses, but a more definite diagnosis is made by radiology. An abscess or abscesses may be present and may not be seen on radiographs because of the heart shadow.

Treatment of lung abscesses must include intensive long-term antimicrobial therapy. Empirically, 20 per cent sodium iodide given intravenously in a dosage of 10 to 20 ml per day for five to seven days followed by organic iodide orally seems to be beneficial. Levamisole*† at a dosage of 1 mg per lb (2 mg per kg) orally every other day for three weeks may help stimulate a compromised immune system. All forms of stress should be avoided.

References

1. King, G. K., Martens, R. J., and McCall, V. H.: Equine thoracic radiography. Part I. Air-gap rare-earth radiography of the normal equine thorax. Part II. Radiographic patterns of equine pulmonary and pleural disease using air-gap rare-earth radiography. Comp. Cont. Ed., 3:278, 1981.
2. Knight, H. D.: Antimicrobial agents used in the horse. Proc. 21st Annu. Conv. Am. Assoc. Eq. Pract., 1975, pp. 131–144.
3. Morris Animal Foundation: Report of Foal Pneumonia Panel, Denver, CO, May 8–9, 1978. J. Equine Med. Surg., September 1978, p. 400, and October 1978, p. 428.
4. Riviere, J. E., Traver, D. S., and Coppoc, G. L.: Gentamicin toxic nephropathy in horses with disseminated bacterial infection. J. Am. Vet. Med. Assoc., 180:648, 1982.
5. Shively, J. N., Dellers, R. W., Byergelt, C. D., Hsu, F. S., Kabelac, L. P., Moe, K. K., Tennant, B., and Vaughan, J. T.: Pneumocystis carinii pneumonia in two foals. J. Am. Vet. Med. Assoc., 162:648, 1973.
6. Simpson, R. B., and Rideout, M. I.: Bacterial respiratory infections in Texas foals: Causal agents and management procedures. Southwest. Vet., 33:145, 1980.
7. Stick, J. A., and Boles, C.: Subepiglottic cyst in three foals. J. Am. Vet. Med. Assoc., 177:62, 1980.

---

*Quibron, Mead Johnson Pharmaceutical Division, Evansville, IN 47721

†Slo-Phyllin Syrup, Dooner Labs, Inc., Fort Washington, PA 19034

‡Banamine, Schering Corp., Kenilworth, NJ 07033

---

*Ripercol, American Cyanamid Co., Princeton, NJ 08540
†Levasole, Pitman-Moore, Washington Crossing, NJ 08560

CHRONIC AIRWAY DISEASE

Frederik J. Derksen, EAST LANSING, MICHIGAN

The practitioner commonly encounters horses with a history of exercise intolerance and clinical signs of mild airway disease, including abnormal secretions in the trachea and, to the astute clinician, increased bronchial tones. These animals are in contrast to horses with complete exercise intolerance, chronic mucopurulent nasal discharge, hypoxemia, cyanosis, chronic cough, and inspiratory and expiratory dyspnea. The latter horses are often referred to as "heavy" or suffering from heaves. Between these two extremes, a wide spectrum of clinical signs is recognized. This chapter will discuss the disease syndrome exemplified by these two cases.

Attempts to categorize the variety of clinical manifestations of this disease syndrome into pathophysiologic entities have met with failure and have resulted in a confusing nomenclature. Names such as chronic bronchitis, chronic bronchiolitis, chronic asthmoid bronchitis. allergic bronchitis, alveolar emphysema, and emphysema are pathologic diagnoses that the clinician, at the present state of the art, cannot establish with certainty. In any event, it may be that these pathologic changes are closely related and represent different stages of the same disease process. This does not imply that chronic airway disease (CAD) has only one pathogenesis. It is more likely that a variety of etiologies lead to common pathologic and functional alterations. Presently it appears that subdivision of CAD on clinical grounds is unwarranted.

INCIDENCE

Chronic airway disease is in large part a disease of domestication. The condition is uncommon in warm countries, where horses are kept on grass and spend most of their time in the fresh air. In temperate climates where most horses are kept in barns and fed hay for long periods, the disease is common. Mild forms of the disease are most evident in performance horses and occur in mature animals of all ages. The more severe forms with dyspnea at rest are uncommon in horses under five years of age. Horses of all breeds and both sexes are affected.[6]

HISTORY AND CLINICAL SIGNS

Mildly affected horses may show no signs at rest or during light exercise but are unable to perform to capacity. Some horses cough when exposed to dust or cold air. They may work well in warm weather but perform poorly in winter months. Animals may have suffered from viral respiratory tract infection and may have never completely recovered. The more severely affected animal usually presents with a history of progressive deterioration from mild exercise intolerance to dyspnea and coughing. Persistent bouts of coughing may be elicited when horses are exposed to dust or cold air. Often the owners indicate that animals improve on pasture but that exacerbations occur after indoor housing or work. In a few instances, horses are presented with severe dyspnea of acute onset. Careful questioning as to changes in management often reveals recent exposure to "new" antigenic material such as dust from chickens or molds. Animals may show an increased abdominal effort at end-expiration or during the entire expiratory phase. A line of hypertrophy of the abdominal muscles often develops along the ventrocaudal edge of the rib cage (heave line). Nasal discharge may be slight and serous in nature or copious and mucopurulent. In the later stages, inspiratory dyspnea with flaring of the nostrils may also be observed. The disease may result in anorexia, weight loss, depression, and inability to perform even the smallest task.[1]

PATHOLOGY

The primary pathologic lesion present in horses with clinical signs of CAD is bronchiolitis. In addition, mucus plugging of bronchioles, peribronchiolar fibrosis, bronchitis with diffuse epithelial hyperplasia and metaplasia, acinar overinflation (also called alveolar emphysema), emphysema with destruction of the alveolar walls, and right ventricular hypertrophy may also be present.[2]

PATHOGENESIS

Although several hypotheses concerning the pathogenesis of CAD in the horse have been advanced, insufficient scientific data exist to confirm or refute their validity. It is likely that the syndrome describes several disease entities, and, therefore, more than one mechanism may be involved in the generation of CAD. Possible etiologic factors include specific and nonspecific airway hypersensitivities, viral and bacterial infections, and diet.

Common management practices expose the respiratory system of the horse to large loads of organic and inorganic pollutants ranging from straw, hay, and racetrack dust to molds, ammonia, ozone, and sulfur dioxide from air pollution. Because a close correlation exists between exposure to organic dust and incidence of CAD, it has been postulated that animals mount an inappropriate immune response to one or more antigens in the environment, resulting in a specific hypersensitivity. Little is known about the immunopathology of this phenomenon, but studies in which horses with CAD were challenged with organic dust, *Micropolyspora faeni*, and *Asperigillus fumigatus* antigens support this hypothesis.[9] Recent investigations in our laboratory have implicated the parasympathetic nervous system in the production of clinical signs in experimentally induced pulmonary hypersensitivity in horses. Vagal blockade reversed the hyperpnea and reduced airway obstruction in horses sensitized to ovalbumin and challenged with homologous antigen. It was concluded that stimulation of pulmonary receptors by the allergic reaction initiated a vagal reflex, resulting in hyperpnea and bronchoconstriction.

In experimental animals and humans, viral infections or chronic exposure to air pollutants may render airways hypersensitive to otherwise innocuous stimuli, such as cold or mechanical stimulation by rapid air flow. The hypersensitivity is nonspecific in that many different stimulants are effective in triggering bronchoconstriction. Clinical observations of exacerbation of signs of dyspnea after exposure of some horses to dust, cold air, or exercise suggest that this mechanism may also be important in the pathogenesis of CAD in horses.

Many authors report that CAD commonly follows viral and bacterial respiratory tract infections. A similar correlation exists between infectious respiratory diseases and asthma in humans. The significance of this correlation and the mechanisms whereby airway infections lead to CAD are presently unknown.

Dietary factors have been incriminated in the pathogenesis of CAD for centuries. Recently Breeze et al. showed that the oral administation of 3-methylindole causes chronic bronchiolitis and obstructive pulmonary disease in the horse.[3] Three-methylindole is a metabolite of the aminoacid L-tryptophan and is present in the feces of domestic mammals.

DIAGNOSIS

AUSCULTATION AND PERCUSSION

Auscultatory findings vary with the extent of lung disease. Mild cases may be asymptomatic, but when the animal is forced to breathe deeply by occluding the nostrils for about 30 sec after exercise, bronchial tones and vesicular sounds are more evident than normal. Occasionally a wheeze is heard at the end of exhalation, suggesting the presence of exudate in small airways. Percussion findings are normal in these cases. In more severely affected animals, auscultation may reveal a spectrum of abnormal lung sounds, including harsh bronchial tones and vesicular sounds, rales, wheezes, and crepitant sounds in various lung areas. Sounds associated with large bronchi are best heard at the beginning of exhalation when air flow rates are greatest, and sounds associated with small airways are most evident at the end of expiration, as in that part of the respiratory cycle, small airways are compressed. Percussion may be normal or may suggest a caudal extension of the lung field beyond normal limits.

ENDOSCOPY

With the advent of the fiberoptic endoscope in veterinary medicine, endoscopy has become a valuable tool in the assessment of chronic airway disease. This diagnostic technique may be especially helpful in mildly affected cases in which diagnosis is a challenge. The upper respiratory system is assessed on the way to the trachea and mainstem bronchi. With the 180 cm scope now available, the entire trachea up to the carina can be observed in most 500 kg horses. Because of their poor cough reflex, most horses will allow passage of the fiberoptic scope without tranquilization. An occasional cough is normal, but when passage of the scope into the trachea results in paroxysmal bouts of coughing, a hyperirritable airway is suspected. In horses suffering from CAD, variable amounts of yellow, viscous exudate are present in the trachea, either in the form of tags along the wall or pooled on the floor of the trachea, most commonly near the thoracic inlet. Most if not all horses with CAD have accumulations of yellow, viscous material in the trachea, but the amount does not seem to correlate well with the severity of clinical signs.

TRANSTRACHEAL WASH

Transtracheal washing (p. 513) may be helpful to distinguish horses with CAD from animals with chronic pneumonia or other chronic lung diseases. Cultures of transtracheal washings of horses with CAD usually fail to grow pathogenic bacteria, and cytologic examination characterizes the fluid as a nonseptic exudate or modified transudate. A normal cytology excludes bronchitis and bronchiolitis, but airway obstruction may still be present owing to functional bronchoconstriction. Transtracheal washings are not helpful in assessing the extent of lung damage in horses with CAD.

RADIOGRAPHY

Most practitioners do not have the radiographic equipment necessary to take diagnostic chest radiographs of mature horses. Even with the best equipment presently available, radiographic detail is poor, and variables, such as the point in the respiratory cycle where the film is taken, are difficult to control. Generally, radiography reveals increased density of the lung field with accentuation of the bronchial pattern. Thoracic radiographs are helpful in detecting focal or miliary lesions in the lung and in distinguishing these cases from animals with CAD. Thoracic radiographs have not been helpful in assessing the severity of CAD for therapeutic and prognostic purposes.

DIAGNOSTIC USE OF BRONCHODILATORS

The clinician may wish to determine the role of airway narrowing due to bronchospasm in the production of dyspnea. Isoproterenol,* a beta-adrenergic agonist, may be used to achieve airway smooth muscle relaxation. The drug (0.2 mg) is diluted in 50 cc of saline and administered intravenously until the heart rate doubles. Alternatively, atropine,† a parasympatholytic agent, at a dose of 4.0 μg per kg may be administered intravenously. Reversion of clinical signs of dyspnea and lung sounds toward normal constitutes a positive response. This test does not distinguish between reversible and nonreversible lung disease, as has been proposed in the past. For example, in cases with bronchiolitis and mucous plugging of airways, atropine or isoproterenol may have no clinical effect, while the disease may be reversible if treated properly.

LUNG FUNCTION TESTS

Presently lung function tests are utilized in equine medicine on an experimental basis. With one exception, equipment necessary is generally not available to the practicing veterinarian. The simplest and so far perhaps the most sensitive test of lung function is measurement of the arterial blood oxygen tension. Arterial blood is most easily collected from the common carotid artery. Determinations of PaO_2 can be made up to five hours after collection if blood is kept in a sealed glass syringe on ice, but if blood is stored in a plastic syringe, determinations must be made within one hour. At sea level, PaO_2 less than 83 mm Hg^2 is considered

abnormal. Arterial oxygen tension decreases with altitude, so that at higher altitudes, a lower PaO_2 may be normal.

THERAPY

ALTERATION OF THE ENVIRONMENT

The most important factor in the development of chronic airway disease in the majority of cases appears to be exposure of the respiratory system to organic dust. Established management practices are so ingrained that despite this fact, the main thrust of therapy is often directed toward drug administration with inevitably poor results. No therapeutic effort can succeed unless the horse's environment is altered and the exposure to dust or allergens is drastically reduced. This fact needs to be stressed to owners who otherwise may not be willing to follow recommendations. Damp, dusty barns with poor ventilation tend to exacerbate clinical signs of CAD, whereas the environment least likely to stress the respiratory system is a pasture with a modest shelter against inclement weather. If a pasture is not available, horses with CAD should be housed in well-ventilated areas with as little dust as possible. Animals may be bedded on moist wood shavings or clay. Pelleted feed should be substituted for hay, and all feed should be moistened.

In mild cases of CAD in which bronchitis and bronchiolitis are the predominant lesions, rest is an important part of the therapeutic regimen. Animals are rested for 30 to 90 days, depending upon the severity of the condition, and even moderate exercise to keep the animal in racing shape is not recommended. Although there is no scientific evidence to support this notion in the horse, it is my clinical impression that exercise resulting in large degrees of air flow through diseased airways is responsible for perpetuating airway irritation.

BRONCHODILATOR THERAPY

Since narrowing of airways by excess mucus secretion, inflammation, or bronchospasm is characteristic of CAD in the horse, bronchodilators are potentially useful therapeutic agents (Table 1). Bronchodilator drugs act by inducing airway smooth muscle relaxation through a variety of mechanisms (Fig. 1).

ANTICHOLINERGIC DRUGS

Some of the earliest remedies used in the treatment of heaves in horses contained anticholinergic drugs related to atropine. Atropine is an important

*Isuprel, Breon Labs, New York, NY 10017
†Atropine, Fort Dodge Labs, Fort Dodge, IA 50501

TABLE 1. BRONCHODILATOR DRUGS

Generic Name	Mechanism of Action	Dose	Route
Atropine	Parasympatholytic: prevents formation of cGMP	4.0 μg/kg	IV
Isoproterenol	Sympathomimetic β_2 agonist; increases cAMP production	0.4 μg/kg	IV
Ephedrine	Sympathomimetic norepinephrine release and β_2 agonist	0.7 mg/kg BID	Oral
Clenbuterol*	Sympathomimetic β_2 agonist; increases cAMP production	0.8 μg/kg BID	IV Oral
Theophylline*	Phosphodiesterase inhibitor; prevents breakdown of cAMP	1.0 mg/kg QID	Oral

*Not approved for use in horses in North America

parasympatholytic drug that is particularly effective as a muscarinic blocker of neurotransmission by acetylcholine to smooth muscle. Thus, bronchodilation is one of the main effects of systemic administration. In addition, parasympathetic blockade results in decreased secretion by submucosal glands and drying of the respiratory mucosa. The effect of atropine as a pulmonary parasympatholytic drug illustrates two important and discrete functions of the vagal supply to the lung, namely the maintenance of bronchial tone and stimulation of airway secretions.

Atropine at a dose of 4.0 μg per kg will decrease work of breathing and airway secretions in normal horses as well as in horses with CAD. The decreased

work of breathing is not clinically evident in normal horses but can be demonstrated with pulmonary function tests. In horses with CAD, especially those in which vagally mediated bronchoconstriction plays a prominent role in the pathogenesis of dyspnea, clinical improvement is evident 20 minutes after treatment and persists for up to 12 hours. Drying of airway secretions may be advantageous in cases in which excessive secretion is observed but undesirable when expectoration is a goal of therapy. Side effects of atropine treatment include mydriasis, tachycardia, central nervous system excitation, and bowel stasis. Its potentially serious side effects preclude its use as a useful therapeutic agent in the horse. Potentially, this class of drugs has great use-

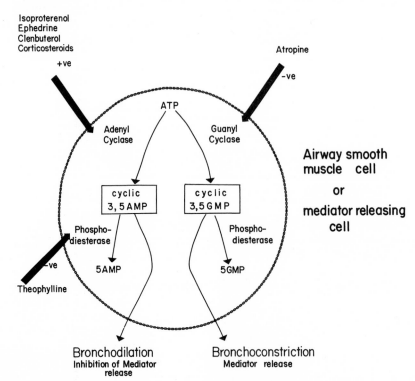

Figure 1. Schematic representation of the effect of therapeutic agents on airway smooth muscle tone and release of mediators.

fulness in the treatment of CAD, and new anticholinergic agents with more potent bronchodilator effects and fewer side effects are presently being evaluated in bronchodilator therapy in humans.

SYMPATHOMIMETIC AGENTS

Sympathomimetic agents, including epinephrine, isoproterenol, ephedrine,* and clenbuterol,† cause bronchodilation by stimulation of beta$_2$-adrenergic receptors in large and small airways. Airway smooth muscle relaxation is brought about by increased cyclic AMP production in the smooth muscle cell and mast cell. Bronchodilation occurs naturally by this mechanism when animals are stressed and when sympathetic nervous system activity increases, but other receptors (alpha, beta$_1$) are then also stimulated in a variety of organ systems. Sympathomimetic bronchodilators were developed for their specific effect on beta$_2$ receptors present in the bronchi, vascular beds, and uterus, thereby minimizing undesirable side effects on other organ systems such as the heart and the gastrointestinal tract. In addition, a prolonged action is desirable. In some instances, prolonged action is achieved by the preparation of slow release formulations.

Ephedrine is a moderately active beta$_2$ stimulator, but its main mechanism of action is through the release of stored norepinephrine. Consequently, it has both alpha- and beta-adrenergic properties. Therapeutic doses tend to cause depletion of the stored norepinephrine, resulting in tolerance, so that progressively more of the drug is needed to achieve the same degree of bronchodilation. Few controlled studies as to its efficacy are available, but clinically the drug appears effective in some cases. The recommended dosage is 0.7 mg per kg twice a day per os for seven days.

Isoproterenol is a catecholamine with potent beta$_2$ activity. It has virtually no alpha-adrenergic properties, but it has marked beta$_1$ effects. The drug is one of the most powerful bronchodilators and has a rapid onset of action. However, its bronchodilator effects may last as little as one hour. When given intravenously, 0.2 mg of the drug should be diluted in 50 ml of saline and the heart rate should be monitored continuously. The recommended dose is 0.4 μg per kg but infusion should be discontinued when the heart rate doubles. In humans, aerosol is more effective and achieves bronchodilation with fewer side effects, but in horses this route of administration is not practical for long-term therapy because of the need for frequent treatments. Isoproterenol should not be administered orally, as absorption is erratic.[12] Undesirable side effects are mainly due to its beta$_1$-adrenergic properties and include tachycardia, nervousness, tremors, and sweating. Isoproterenol may be useful in the treatment of acute exacerbations of bronchospasm, but because of its short duration of action and side effects, it is undesirable for long-term therapy in the horse.

Clenbuterol is a specific beta$_2$ agonist as well as an expectorant. Its depressant effects on the airway smooth musculature have been demonstrated in a series of studies in various animal species, including the horse. In the therapeutic dose range, the drug has little effect on the muscle of the gastrointestinal tract and the heart, and, therefore, side effects are minimal. Clenbuterol is well absorbed after oral administration and has a long duration of action. The drug can be administered orally or intravenously at a dose of 0.8 μg per kg twice a day. In Europe, the drug has been on the market for several years, but on the North American continent, it is available only for clinical trials. Curti[5] and Sasse and Hajer[10] report that clenbuterol is very efficacious in the treatment of CAD.

PHOSPHODIESTERASE INHIBITORS

Phosphodiesterase inhibitors, of which the commonest member is theophylline,* act by inhibiting the breakdown of cyclic AMP, thereby promoting smooth muscle relaxation and interfering with the liberation of mediators that cause bronchospasm (Fig. 1). Presently theophylline is not available for use in the horse, but experience in this clinic indicates its effectiveness in most cases of CAD with a history of acute exacerbations when exposed to dust inside a barn. Empirically, the drug is given orally four times a day at a dose of 1.0 mg per kg. Expense and the frequency of administration are the major deterrents. Scientific study of proper dose levels, absorption, excretion, and efficacy of the drug is needed before usage can be recommended.

EXPECTORANT THERAPY

Expectorant therapy is controversial in the treatment of pulmonary disorders in humans and animals, and although it is commonly used to facilitate movement of respiratory tract secretions, few scientific reports confirm its efficacy. Since mucous plugging of airways is a common finding in horses with CAD, improved mucokinesis is a reasonable objective of therapy. Expectoration can be promoted by systemic administration of expectorants or by nebulization (Table 2).

---

*Ephedrine, Breon Labs, New York, NY 10017
†Ventipulmin, Boehringer Ingelheim, Ridgefield, CT 06877

---

*Theo-dur, Key Pharmaceuticals, Miami, FL 33169

TABLE 2. EXPECTORANT DRUGS

Generic Name	Mechanism of Action	Dose	Route
Water saline	Hydration and dilution	0.1 ml/kg QID	Nebulization
Propylene glycol	Wetting action	2% solution 0.1 ml/kg	Nebulization
Acetylcysteine (Mucomyst)	Splits disulfide bonds		Nebulization
Iodides	Gastropulmonary mucokinetic reflex; stimulation of bronchial glands	0.5 mg/kg twice a week	IV
Glyceryl guaiacolate	Gastropulmonary mucokinetic reflex	3.0 mg/kg	Oral
Bromhexine	Gastropulmonary mucokinetic reflex; stimulation of bronchial glands	30 mg/kg	Oral

NEBULIZATION

The process of nebulization produces a particulate liquid suspension, which, depending on particle size, electrical charge, and other characteristics, is deposited at various sites in the respiratory tract. Larger particles are trapped in the upper airway and trachea, while particles smaller than 5 μ may reach the lower respiratory system. Few nebulizers presently in use for treatment of respiratory diseases in horses are capable of producing particles that are sufficiently‡ small to reach the lower respiratory system in significant quantities. Water and saline are the most commonly used solutions and serve to hydrate airway secretions, thereby promoting their removal. Water is more irritating than saline and may evoke coughing. Propylene glycol,* a hygroscopic agent, may be added to the solution in order to promote particle stability and penetration. A 2 per cent solution of propylene glycol is isotonic and nonirritating.

Volatile oils are common ingredients in nebulization solutions. Although the scented fumes may have an aesthetic appeal, no evidence for their effectiveness is forthcoming.

Acetylcysteine† is a true mucolytic agent that may be administered via nebulization. The drug ruptures the disulfide bridges of mucoprotein, thereby breaking the complex protein network into less viscous strands. The drug is not available for use in horses, and I have had no experience with it.

MUCOKINETIC AGENTS

Iodides‡ are popular mucokinetic agents that can be administered either orally or intravenously. Iodides are thought to act by direct stimulation of bronchial glands to increase secretion, thus liquefying the existing sputum. They may also stimulate secretion via a gastropulmonary reflex mediated through the vagus nerve and also increase cilioexcitation. Adverse side effects include edema of the face and neck with laryngeal edema severe enough to cause dyspnea. Iodides appear clinically useful in some cases of CAD and are in common use, although no controlled studies as to their efficacy are available.

Bromhexine* is a mucokinetic agent with a mechanism of action similar to the iodides. In Europe, the drug has been marketed for several years, and clinical studies have shown its efficacy.[8]

Glyceryl guaiacolate† in combination with various salts such as ammonium chloride, ammonium carbonate, and potassium citrate is a commonly used expectorant. The mechanism of action of this combination is mainly through the gastropulmonary mucokinetic reflex, mediated via the vagus nerve, although glyceryl guaiacolate is also thought to increase mucociliary clearance directly. Scientific evidence for its effectiveness in any species is scant, and clinical experience suggests that the compounds are not helpful in the treatment of CAD.

CORTICOSTEROIDS

Corticosteroids have a beneficial effect on most cases of CAD. It is presently thought that steroids stabilize the membranes of lysosomes, thereby preventing the release of their content of hydrolytic enzymes that would destroy the cell and cause an inflammatory response in the tissues. Although good evidence exists that this occurs in laboratory experiments, it is much less certain that this mechanism is of importance in vivo.[12] Steroids may also inhibit cellular migration, potentiate the actions of beta$_2$ receptor stimulants, and inhibit the enzyme catechol-0-methyl transferase, which breaks down

---

*Propylene glycol, Burroughs Wellcome Co., Research Triangle Park, NC 27708

†Mucomyst, Mead Johnson and Co., Evansville, IN 47721
‡Sodium iodide, Haver-Lockhart Labs, Shawnee, KS 66201

---

*Bisolvon, Boehringer Ingelheim, Ridgefield, CT 06877
†Glycom, Bio-Ceutic Labs, St. Joseph, MO 64502

catecholamines and increases the availability of the enzyme cyclic AMP. The latter enzyme promotes airway smooth muscle relaxation and inhibits mediator release from lysosomes.

The undesirable side effects of steroid therapy are potentially serious and may develop weeks after initiation of treatment. Therefore, these drugs should be used with caution. Prolonged use of high dosages may lead to Cushingoid signs such as depression, muscle wasting, a long, dry hair coat, hyperglycemia, polydipsia, and polyuria. More commonly, the immunologic status is impaired, resulting in the flareup or establishment of respiratory or other infections. Exogenous steroids depress the release of ACTH from the posterior pituitary, resulting in adrenocortical atrophy. Clinical signs of adrenal insufficiency may be evident after withdrawal of only two weeks of steroid therapy. Signs include depression, anorexia, electrolyte loss, polyuria, and dehydration. Despite possible serious complications, steroid therapy has proved useful in the treatment of horses with CAD. In order to prevent steroid dependence, prednisolone* is administered orally every other day in the morning at a dose of 0.5 mg per kg. Endogenous blood steroid levels peak in the morning and decline to reach the lowest level in the early evening. By giving the drug every 48 hours in the morning, sufficient stimulation of the adrenal cortex occurs to prevent steroid dependence. After two weeks of steroid therapy, the response to treatment is evaluated, and the dose level is gradually reduced until a minimal effective dose is reached. The use of longer-acting steroids such as dexamethasone is not recommended because of the increased risk of adrenocortical depression. Steroid therapy should not be initiated if concurrent infections are suspected.[11]

Antibiotics

In animals affected with CAD, clearance of potential pathogens from the lung is likely to be impaired. Therefore, animals may be more susceptible to challenges by environmental pathogens resulting in the common concurrence of CAD and infectious bronchitis, bronchiolitis, and pneumonia.

Culture of transtracheal washings (p. 513) is an important tool in the detection of these cases. In vitro antibiotic sensitivity testing should be done on isolates to determine the most effective and least expensive antibiotic. Cultures from tracheal washes often produce gram-positive cocci, which are sensitive to procaine penicillin G† at a dose of 20,000 IU per kg administered intramuscularly twice a day for at least two weeks. In all cases, adequate dosage

and duration of the treatment regimen are important in order to maximize therapeutic response and minimize development of resistance. Antibiotic therapy is dealt with in more detail on pp. 43 and 467.

ISONIAZID

Isoniazid* is an antimicrobial agent commonly used in the treatment of CAD in horses. Its reported efficacy is surprising, as in vitro the agent has only antimycobacterial properties without any effect against pathogens commonly encountered in the horse. Presently, no in vivo studies supporting the efficacy of isoniazid in the treatment of CAD are available. A commonly used oral dose is 2 mg per kg for 30 to 90 days, but undesirable side effects, including anorexia, ataxia, incoordination, and apparent blindness, have been observed at doses as low as 4 mg per kg. In view of its doubtful efficacy and its small safety margin, the use of isoniazid in the treatment of CAD cannot be recommended.

Miscellaneous Therapy

ANTIHISTAMINES

Antihistamines† alone or in combination with other drugs have been used extensively in the treatment of CAD. Few scientific studies exist to evaluate the efficacy of antihistamines in the treatment of CAD in the horse, and in my experience, these drugs are ineffective. Histamine may be only one of many mediators released in the lung, and, therefore, antihistamines cannot be expected to produce significant improvement. Most commonly used antihistamines are used in combination with ephedrine in oral preparations,‡ and the efficacy of this combination may be attributed to the beta agonist.

ANTHELMINTICS

Two anthelmintic drugs, levamisole and diethylcarbamazine, have been commonly used in the treatment of CAD in horses. Levamisole§ is a known stimulator of cell-mediated immunity, and the efficacy of this drug in the treatment of CAD in the horse is attributed to this mechanism. Therefore, when using the drug, the clinician should consider the relevance of immunomodulation in the disease process. It is not at all clear that cell-mediated immunity is important in the pathogenesis of CAD, and although successful treatment of advanced cases of CAD has been reported in the lit-

---

*Prednisolone, Butler Co., Columbus, OH 43228
†Procaine Penicillin G, Pfizer, New York, NY 10017

*Isoniazid, Eli Lilly and Co., Indianapolis, IN 46225
†A-H Solution, Jensen-Salsbery Labs, Kansas City, MO 64141
‡Equi-Hist, Equine Products of Maryland, Pikesville, MD 21208
§Levasole, Pitman-Moore, Washington Crossing, NJ 08560

erature,[4] levamisole's ineffectiveness in most cases may be related to the irrelevance of immunomodulation. The treatment regimen most commonly used is 5.5 mg per kg intramuscularly. The treatment may be repeated.

Diethylcarbamazine* is known to inhibit release of mediators such as slow-reacting substance of anaphylaxis (SRS-A), and it also has been found to inhibit prostaglandin $F_{2\alpha}$–induced bronchospasm in some species. This action is dose-dependent, because at high doses, mediator release may be stimulated rather than suppressed. Presently, the effect of diethylcarbamazine on mediator release in the equid is unknown, and in addition, the role of SRS-A and $PGF_{2\alpha}$ in the pathogenesis of CAD in the horse is unclear. Clinical experience with the drug suggests limited efficacy in a few cases when used at a dose of 6.5 mg per kg orally for 14 days.

References

1. Beech, J.: Diseases of the lung. Vet. Clin. North Am. *1*:149, 1979.
2. Breeze, R. G.: Heaves. Vet. Clin. North Am., *1*:219, 1979.
3. Breeze, R. G., Lee, H. A., and Grant, B. D.: Toxic lung disease. Mod. Vet. Pract., *59*:301, 1978.
4. Calverley, A. H.: Levamisole phosphate as a treatment for heaves. Proc. 23rd Annu. Conv. Am. Assoc. Eq. Pract., 1977, pp. 353–365.
5. Curti, P. C.: Untersuchungen zur klinischen pharmakoligie eines neuen spezifisch adrenergischen β_2 bronchodilatators. Int. J. Clin. Pharmacol., *9*:305, 1974.
6. Cook, W. R.: Chronic bronchitis and alveolar emphysema in the horse. Vet. Rec., *99*:448, 1976.
7. Derksen, F. J., and Robinson, N. E.: The effect of reversible vagal blockade on normal conscious ponies and ponies with induced allergic lung disease. Proc. 26th Annu. Conv. Am. Assoc. Eq. Pract., 1980, p. 477.
8. Geide, H.: Moderne therapie von erkrankungen der atmungsorgane des pferdes. Tierarzl. Umschau, *22*:478, 1967.
9. McPherson, E. A., Lawson, G. H. K., Murphy, T. R., Nicholson, J. M., Breeze, R. G., and Pirie, A. M.: Chronic obstructive pulmonary disease in horses: Aetiological studies: Response to intradermal and inhalation antigenic challenge. Equine Vet. J., *11*(3):159, 1979.
10. Sasse, H. H. L., and Hajer, R: Enkele veterinair-klinische ervaringen met het gebruike van een β_2-receptoren stimulerend sympaticomymeticum by paarden met longaandoeningen. Tijdschr. Diergeneeskd., *102*:1232, 1977.
11. Willoughby, R. A.: Corticosteroids in the management of respiratory disorders in horses. Proc. American College of Veterinary Internal Medicine, Dallas, 1978, pp. 48–60.
12. Ziment, I.: Respiratory Pharmacology and Therapeutics, Philadelphia, W.B. Saunders Co., 1978, pp. 147–180.

*Caricide, American Cyanamid Co., Princeton, NJ 08540

SUMMER PASTURE–ASSOCIATED OBSTRUCTIVE PULMONARY DISEASE

Ralph E. Beadle, BATON ROUGE, LOUISIANA

Chronic obstructive pulmonary disease in horses (COPD or heaves) is a condition that occurs in all parts of the United States. This condition is observed predominantly in horses exposed to stables and their associated moldy hay or bedding and dust. A major component of the therapy for such cases is minimizing exposure to causative factors by turning the animals out to pasture when possible.

A syndrome with similar clinical signs, but occurring under differing conditions, exists in horses in the southeastern region of the United States. Significant numbers of horses in this region that graze pasture land in the summer develop an obstructive pulmonary disease. Because this syndrome is not seen in pastured horses in the winter, it has been called summer pasture–associated obstructive pulmonary disease (SPAOPD). States where horses are known to be affected include Florida, Georgia, Louisiana, and Mississippi. Horses in neighboring states may be affected as well.

The onset of the condition in susceptible horses is variable with respect to the month of the year. In some years, horses may experience problems in late May, whereas in other years, they may experience respiratory difficulties beginning in late July or early August. A triad of environmental factors that seem to be associated with the full expression of the syndrome is a hot and humid climate and high soil moisture content.

There does not seem to be a sex or breed predilection for this condition. Most horses affected with this condition are at least three years of age. Affected horses are remarkably improved during the cooler winter months whether eating hay or grazing rye grass pasture. They will, however, show signs again the following summer.

ETIOLOGY

Specific investigations into the etiology of SPAOPD have not been undertaken. Factors that may be responsible for the condition include allergy and diet. The immunologic mechanisms thought to be involved are type I and type III allergic reactions. Indeed, there are cases in the literature in which the offending antigen was identified with the use of allergen skin testing, and hyposensitization was achieved.[4] The history of these cases suggests that these horses may have been affected with SPAOPD. However, the paucity of these reports suggests that another cause may be responsible for a significant number of these cases. The possibility exists that some of the horses are ingesting a pulmonary phytotoxin or a precursor to such a toxin in the grass.[3]

PATHOGENESIS

The pathogenesis of this condition is not well understood because of the equivocal nature of the etiology. There does seem to be a stimulation of the parasympathetic nervous system to the lungs with an accompanying bronchoconstriction and increased mucus production. Another important feature of the pathogenesis is the migration of large numbers of neutrophils into the airways of these horses. Type I and type III allergic reactions could account for these aspects of the condition.

The chemical structure of indolic compounds could allow them to serve as direct mediators for parasympathetic stimulation. Lush native grasses that contain such indolic compounds or their precursors, such as tryptophan, might be ingested by horses in quantities sufficient to produce reversible bronchoconstriction. Acute bovine pulmonary emphysema is such a condition reported to occur in cattle at pasture.[5] A similar condition may exist in horses, as 3-methylindole has produced an obstructive pulmonary disease syndrome experimentally in horses.[3]

A bacterial infection is present in the airways of some of the horses, especially those that are not treated early in the condition. This is probably the result of decreased phagocytic function in macrophages receiving inadequate oxygen owing to constricted and mucus-plugged airways.

CLINICAL FINDINGS

Horses with this condition show varying degrees of exercise intolerance. In the most severe cases, even a short walk in the pasture can be an exhausting experience for the animal. Severely affected horses will also show a pronounced abdominal lift (heave line) at the end of exhalation. In addition, these animals will show varying degrees of anorexia and weight loss. The respiratory rate and heart rate may be increased and the depth of respiration diminished. Coughing is almost always a clinical sign described by the owner. Auscultation of the lungs reveals sibilant rhonchi in all areas of the lungs, and percussion reveals moderately to grossly enlarged lung fields. The rhonchi are heard at the end of exhalation in early cases but may be heard earlier in exhalation or even during inhalation if the severity of the condition has progressed sufficiently. Rales may also be auscultated during inspiration in the severely affected cases. Fever is not a feature of this condition even though a concomitant bacterial bronchitis and bronchiolitis may be present as described earlier.

Radiographic examination of the thorax will confirm the enlargement of the lung field. Radiographic signs associated with other lung diseases are not commonly seen.

CLINICAL PATHOLOGY

No consistent changes are seen in the hemograms of these patients. Blood gas analyses reveal a decreased arterial oxygen tension and a normal arterial carbon dioxide tension.

The cytology of tracheobronchial aspirates is abnormal and will be discussed later.

SPECIAL DIAGNOSTIC PROCEDURES

Additional diagnostic procedures used to confirm a diagnosis of SPAOPD include tracheobronchial aspiration, allergen skin testing, and the intravenous atropine response test.

Tracheobronchial Aspiration

Tracheobronchial aspiration of sterile saline injected into the airway provides a sample that can give information about events occurring in the airways of these animals. Sterile technique should be used in performing this procedure. Hair is clipped from a 10 cm square area of skin over the junction of the middle and lower thirds of the cervical trachea. The area is then thoroughly scrubbed and disinfected. Analgesia is achieved by injecting 1 to 2 ml of local anesthetic subcutaneously at the intended aspiration site. A 1 cm incision is made in the skin and subcutaneous tissue over the trachea at the site of the local block. An Oschner trocar and cannula* are slipped between two adjacent tracheal rings and are directed down the trachea. The trocar is removed, and a No. 8 French polypropylene catheter† is inserted through the cannula. Use of such a stiff catheter prevents the horse from coughing the tip of the catheter into the laryngeal or pharyngeal area. Thirty ml of sterile physiologic saline solution are injected into the catheter and are aspirated as quickly as possible. Usually 10 to 15 ml of aspirate are recovered. The recovered sample is divided into two portions and is used for cytologic and bacterial analyses. Once the aspiration is complete, the catheter and cannula are removed from the horse, and the incision is closed with two or three simple interrupted sutures. A tetanus toxoid booster is administered if the vaccination history warrants it (p. 29).

Massive numbers of neutrophils are present in the aspirate along with copious amounts of mucus. Lymphocytes, eosinophils, and ciliated epithelial cells are an uncommon finding. Small numbers of macrophages are occasionally seen, especially in the recovering patient. Bacteria may be present in the aspirate in either the free or phagocytized form.

Bacterial examinations routinely performed on the aspirate should include Gram staining, culturing on equine blood agar, and antibiotic sensitivity testing.

ALLERGEN SKIN TESTING

The antigens used for allergen skin testing are obtained commercially. Center Labs, Inc.,‡ and Dome Labs§ are two companies that provide such antigens. The antigens used in any particular case are chosen with the aid of a thorough and complete history of the animal in question. A human or veterinary allergist in the same geographic area can be helpful in recommending appropriate antigens. Mixed antigens can be used in a screening procedure to decrease the number of injections needed. Subsequent injections of individual antigens are used to differentiate between the antigens causing a positive reaction when using mixed antigens. The volume of antigen used is determined by the manufacturer's recommendations. Injections are made intradermally with a tuberculin syringe and a 25-gauge needle. A positive control of 1:100,000 histamine phosphate and a negative diluent control are used. The injections are usually made on the side of the neck after it has been clipped. Results of the

test are read at 30 minutes, 4 hours, and 24 hours after injection and are categorized according to the following criteria: (1) negative—the swelling is less than 5 mm greater than the diameter of the negative control; (2) 1+—the swelling is 5 to 9 mm greater than the diameter of the negative control; (3) 2+—the swelling is 10 to 14 mm greater than the diameter of the negative control; (4) 3+—the swelling is 15 to 19 mm greater than the diameter of the negative control; (5) 4+—the swelling is 20 mm or more greater than the diameter of the negative control. Positive reactions occurring within 30 minutes are called type I allergic reactions. Type III and type IV allergic reactions are positive at 4 and 24 hours, respectively, after antigen injection.

INTRAVENOUS ATROPINE TEST

A further diagnostic procedure is the use of an atropine test. An intravenous dose of 0.022 mg per kg will cause a marked reduction in the end-expiratory lift and adventitial lung sounds within five minutes postinjection. A favorable response to atropine gives a more favorable prognosis for response to treatment. Larger doses of atropine should not be used in order to avoid side effects such as decreased intestinal motility and colic.

NECROPSY

Necropsy specimens are not usually obtained from these cases because the disease is not fatal. Limited histologic examinations of tissues from these animals have revealed increased numbers of goblet cells in the bronchi with some hyperplasia of the epithelial lining. Also, many bronchioles and occasionally bronchi appear to be plugged with mucus.

DIAGNOSIS

Diagnosis of SPAOPD is made on the basis of history, clinical signs, and results of the specialized diagnostic procedures. Diagnosis of a secondary bacterial infection accompanying the primary condition is more difficult. The cytology and bacterial findings associated with the tracheobronchial aspirate are very useful in this regard. The occasional presence of bacteria in the aspirate is not sufficient evidence to make this diagnosis, as some bacteria are normal inhabitants of the airways.

When an accompanying bacterial infection is present, there will be moderate to large numbers of bacteria in the aspirate, and the neutrophils will show signs of degeneration with karyolysis. Contam-

---

*MX13-62, Miltex Instrument Co., Lake Success, NY 11042
†Sherwood Medical Supplies, Inc., St. Louis, MO 63103
‡Center Labs, Inc., Div. of Alcon Labs, Inc., Port Washington, NY 11050
§Dome Labs, Div. of Miles Labs, Inc., West Haven CT 06502

inating bacteria and commensal organisms will not be present in such large numbers, and the neutrophils associated with them will appear well preserved. In some cases, repeated tracheobronchial aspirates may be needed to confirm an organism as a true pathogen and not a contaminant.

TREATMENT

The objectives of the treatment are to dilate the airways and to prevent further stimulation for bronchoconstriction and mucus secretion. Therefore, the pillars of the treatment regimen are to remove the animal from the offending pasture and to achieve effective bronchodilation.

ENVIRONMENTAL MANAGEMENT

The most critical aspect of therapy is an environmental change. The horse should be removed from pasture and placed in a stall on a diet of hay or pelleted feed and water free choice. This therapy by itself may be sufficient to alleviate clinical signs if a patient is treated early. In such cases, clinical signs will regress in 7 to 10 days after being taken off pasture. Patients not responding to environmental changes usually have an accompanying infection. Appropriate antibacterial drugs, selected on the basis of culture and sensitivity testing, should be used to treat the infection.

BRONCHODILATORS

Bronchodilation is beneficial in letting the horse exchange gases more efficiently in the lungs. It also provides a more healthful environment for the phagocytic cells of the airways. Phagocytosis is thereby enhanced, and infections can be more readily controlled.

The theory of bronchodilation as it is presently understood involves pharmacologic manipulation of the ratio of $3',5'$ cyclic adenosine monophosphate (cAMP) to $3',5'$ cyclic guanyl monophosphate (cGMP) in the smooth muscle cells of the airways. The desired result is to obtain a cAMP:cGMP ratio with a high value, which is associated with the relaxation of airway smooth muscle cells.

β_2 STIMULATORS

The cAMP level in the airway smooth muscle cells can be increased by increasing the rate of formation of cAMP from adenosine triphosphate (ATP). β_2-stimulating drugs are able to activate the enzyme adenyl cyclase in the airway smooth muscle cell

membranes. This, in turn, stimulates the preceding reaction. No β_2 stimulators are presently cleared for use in horses in the United States. Clenbuterol may become available soon. The recommended dosage is 0.8 μg per kg of body weight both orally and parenterally. Terbutaline sulfate is a β_2 stimulator available from manufacturers of drugs for use in humans, but the dosage for repeated administration in horses is not known. On a single injection basis, a dosage of 3.3 μg per kg intravenously will be effective as a bronchodilator. The primary sign of overdosage of β_2 stimulators in horses is sweating, which lasts for 30 to 60 minutes.

METHYLXANTHINES

Theophylline and its water-soluble congener aminophylline are able to increase cAMP levels in various body cells by inhibiting the enzyme phosphodiesterase, which is responsible for the breakdown of cAMP. Therapeutic dosages for theophylline in the horse are unavailable in the literature. At present, there is disagreement about the half-life of theophylline in equine plasma, and until this question is resolved, it is not possible to recommend an appropriate dosage regimen for this drug in the horse. An oral dose of 4 to 7 mg per kg of aminophylline has been recommended for use in horses,[2] but because theophylline is the active drug contained in aminophylline, no information is available for use of this drug on a repeated basis in horses either. If repeated dosages are attempted, the patient should be observed for signs of toxicity, especially cardiac arrhythmias.

COMBINATION THERAPY

Because the methylxanthines and the β_2-stimulating drugs act by different means to increase the levels of cAMP in cells, a combination of these two drug types should effect a better degree of bronchodilation than the use of either one alone.

PARASYMPATHOLYTIC AGENTS

Parasympatholytic drugs are quite effective as bronchodilators for this condition. Their mechanism of action is to decrease the cGMP levels in appropriate cells by competitively inhibiting the stimulation of guanyl cyclase by parasympathomimetic agents. As mentioned previously, a 0.022 mg per kg dose of atropine sulfate is particularly effective in treating this condition. Continuous administration of atropine is not recommended, since such a procedure increases the viscosity of the mucus in the airways and inhibits the effectiveness of the mucociliary escalator in clearing inhaled material such as bacteria from the lungs. The chance of an infection developing in the airways under such conditions is greatly enhanced. Therefore, atropine should be used only in those cases in which bronchoconstriction is extremely advanced and in which aggressive short-term therapy is needed to effect immediate improvement in pulmonary gas exchange.

GLUCOCORTICOIDS

Glucocorticoids, such as dexamethasone, are also effective in alleviating the signs associated with this condition. Animals will respond to an oral or parenteral dose of 20 mg of dexamethasone in about 12 hours. Response to such a dose will usually last about 48 hours. Because dexamethasone may cause adrenocortical suppression, it should not be administered on a continuous basis. Prednisolone may be given orally at a dosage of 4 to 7 mg per kg on an alternate-day basis to avoid this adrenocortical suppression.[1]

The mechanism of action of glucocorticoids in this syndrome is not well understood. They inhibit any inflammatory response occurring in the airways. They may also inhibit antibody formation, may prevent the release of lysozymes from neutrophils by membrane stabilization, and may increase the sensitivity of adenyl cyclase to β_2-stimulating drugs.

MISCELLANEOUS DRUGS

Other drugs that have been tried but do not seem to be effective for this condition include the antihistamines, diethylcarbamazine, levamisole, orgotein, and the nonsteroidal anti-inflammatory agents such as phenylbutazone, meclofenamic acid, and flunixin meglumine. Diuretics such as furosemide are not recommended, as they tend to decrease the hydration of the mucus and make it more viscous.

HYPOSENSITIZATION

Hyposensitization may be attempted with the aid of knowledge gained from allergen skin testing in affected horses. The amount of allergen used and the frequency of administration of allergen for the hyposensitization procedure should be done according to the recommendations of the manufacturer of the allergen. Two of these manufacturers were listed earlier. It should be remembered that hyposensitization will only be effective in those cases that have a type I allergy. The results reported so far for this procedure have been variable, and the procedure is still being evaluated in horses.

PREVENTION

SPAOPD can be controlled somewhat by observing the animals closely in the summer for the first signs of the condition. Removal from pasture for a period of time sufficient to alleviate the signs is recommended. The horse can then be put back to pasture until signs recur. Such an alternating procedure will control the condition early in the summer, but as the season progresses, the animals may have to be removed from pasture completely until the onset of cooler weather in November and December.

References

1. Beech, J.: Diseases of the lung. Vet. Clin. North Am. (Large Anim. Pract.) *1*(1):149, 1979.
2. Beech, J.: Principles of therapy. Vet. Clin. North Am. (Large Anim. Pract.) *1*(1):73, 1979.
3. Breeze, R. G., Lee, H. H., and Grant, B. D.: Toxic lung disease. Mod. Vet. Pract., 59:301, 1978.
4. Carr, S. H.: Hyposensitization of horses with heaves by injectable allergens: A field report. J. Equine Med. Surg., 2:101, 1978.
5. Hammond, A. C., Bradley, B. J., Yokoyama, M. T., Carlson, J. R., and Dickinson, E. O.: 3-Methylindole and naturally occurring acute bovine pulmonary edema and emphysema. Am. J. Vet. Res., 40:1398, 1979.

EXERCISE-INDUCED PULMONARY HEMORRHAGE

John R. Pascoe, DAVIS, CALIFORNIA

Exercise-induced pulmonary hemorrhage (EIPH) is characterized by the presence of blood in the tracheobronchial tree following periods of competitive exercise.[8] Horses with blood present at one or both nostrils following training or racing have been recognized for at least 300 years, and the syndrome has been described by a variety of terms, including "broken blood vessels," "bleeding," "epistaxis," and, more recently, "pulmonary hemorrhage." The incidence of bleeding was believed to be low, and based on observations of blood at the nostrils, was reported to vary between 0.5 and 2.5 per cent.[3]

The introduction of the flexible fiberoptic endoscope has facilitated examination of the equine upper respiratory tract and has allowed improved understanding of the EIPH syndrome. Recent surveys have shown that the blood occasionally observed at the nostrils originates from the lung and not from the nasal vasculature. Endoscopic examination of 1180 Thoroughbred horses after racing showed that 42 per cent had blood present in the tracheobronchial tree.[7] Only 15 (3 per cent) of these horses had blood present at the nostrils at the time of examination. A survey of 249 Standardbred horses yielded similar results.[7] EIPH also occurs in quarter horses and horses used for jumping, steeple chasing, and eventing, but prevalence data are not available.

No association has been demonstrated between racing finishing position and the frequency of EIPH in Thoroughbreds and Standardbreds. There is no sex predisposition. The higher frequency of pulmonary hemorrhage in older horses is believed to be due to the persistence of pulmonary lesion(s) and possibly reflects an inability of the lung to adequately repair damaged regions in the face of continued training.

The effect of EIPH on performance is variable; some horses finish strongly, others cannot sustain their drive to the finish, while others reduce speed significantly and may stop during the race. Many of these latter horses have a distressed or anxious facial expression, "cool out" slowly, cough occasionally, and swallow often. Repeated swallowing is often one of the first signs noted by astute horseowners and handlers and is an indication that blood is being cleared from the respiratory tract into the gastrointestinal tract.

Diagnosis of EIPH can be readily established by endoscopic examination of the upper respiratory tract and, if this is not possible, by cytologic examination of a tracheobronchial aspirate. The optimal time for endoscopic examination is 30 to 120 minutes after exercise. Examination should not be restricted to the postracing period, as EIPH can often be detected following training. The presence of macrophages containing intracytoplasmic droplets of hemosiderin in a tracheobronchial aspirate (p. 513) is strongly suggestive of recent pulmonary hemorrhage. Microbiologic culture of the aspirate may provide additional information on the disease status of the lungs.

Each case of EIPH should be individually evaluated to determine if respiratory disease predisposed to pulmonary hemorrhage. Obtaining an adequate history of previous respiratory infection is often difficult because of the continual movement of horses among trainers and the lack of individual patient records. Auscultation and percussion of the thorax should be performed carefully. Although a consistent radiographic pattern diagnostic for EIPH has not been recognized, thoracic radiographs often provide additional information that is useful in directing therapy. Abnormal radiographic patterns, such as the presence of circumscribed pulmonary densities, cavitary lesions, or pleural effusion, suggest previous or concurrent pulmonary disease, which demands closer evaluation and appropriate treatment. Cytology and bacterial culture of a tracheobronchial aspirate and hematologic examination provide additional guidelines for rational therapy. Although assay of fecal samples for occult blood has been suggested as an aid to the diagnosis of EIPH, this is not reliable, and a positive result should not be viewed as definitive evidence of EIPH.

THERAPY

The variety of current treatment modalities and management procedures underscores the limited understanding of the pathophysiology of EIPH. Treatment is largely empiric and is usually directed at prophylaxis. In addition, reports of the efficacy of various preparations have been mostly anecdotal and unsupported by clinical trials.

Supportive treatment is usually not required. In most horses, hemorrhage ceases soon after racing, and blood is usually cleared from the airways within six hours. Massive fatal episodes of pulmonary hemorrhage occur following rupture of major pulmonary vessels, erosion of vessel walls intimately associated with focal pneumonic lesions or pulmonary abscesses, and following pleural tearing, which disrupts the pulmonary architecture. Therapy in these cases is usually supportive and of limited value.

A small number of horses continue to bleed into the airways for several days to weeks following racing. These horses are often afebrile, listless, and dull and eat poorly. Hematologic examination usually indicates developing anemia. These horses should be carefully evaluated for concurrent pulmonary disease and should be treated accordingly. In addition, rest and supportive therapy with hematinics are indicated (p. 297).

COAGULANTS

Historically, preparations used in the treatment of EIPH have been coagulants or drugs intended to correct specific deficiencies in the coagulation process. Since coagulation screening tests have failed to demonstrate any defects in hemostasis (Pascoe, J., unpublished data, 1980; Bayley, W., personal communication, 1980), it is difficult to justify the continued use of vitamin K or related preparations, tranexamic acid,* or mixtures of oxalic and malonic acid.

ESTROGENS

Conjugated estrogens have been widely used in the management of EIPH. The rationale for their use has not been documented, and testimonials of their effectiveness alone or in combination with furosemide vary considerably and are unsupported by clinical trials. The commonly used preparations are a mixture of sodium estrone sulfate and sodium equilin sulfate† and potassium estrone sulfate.‡§ By convention, these preparations are usually administered within one hour of racing at dose rates of 0.05 to 0.25 mg per kg intravenously and 0.05 to 0.1 mg per kg intravenously, respectively.

FUROSEMIDE

For at least 15 years, furosemide‖ has been the most popular drug for the control of EIPH. It was probably introduced because EIPH was thought to result from pulmonary edema. Although furosemide is approved for the treatment of pulmonary edema in horses, there is no clinical evidence that horses experience pulmonary edema either during or while recovering from racing. Like the conjugated estrogens, furosemide seems firmly entrenched as a racing medication despite the lack of clinical trials to support its effectiveness in controlling EIPH.

Without racing board restrictions, the conventional dose of furosemide is 0.3 to 0.6 mg per kg intravenously given 60 to 90 minutes prior to racing. At most racetracks where furosemide is permitted as a raceday medication for the control of EIPH, it usually cannot be legally administered within 180 minutes of racing. With this restriction, the dose is slightly higher (0.3 to 0.8 mg per kg intravenously or intramuscularly). For horses in which EIPH is refractory and is believed to seriously impair performance, 0.6 to 1.1 mg per kg of furosemide divided into two doses is given, the initial dose at five to six hours and the remainder at three hours prior to racing.

Furosemide (1 mg per kg intravenously) decreases pulmonary vascular pressures and increases pulmonary vascular capacitance in standing resting horses and tethered swimming horses.[5,6] These hemodynamic effects are transient (less than 120 min-

utes) and presumably result from furosemide's ability to reduce plasma volume via diuresis. Reductions in plasma volume by diuresis are dose-dependent, and since lower furosemide dosages (less than 1.0 mg per kg intravenously) are commonly used to control EIPH, the alterations in hemodynamic parameters would presumably be lower and of shorter duration. If, in fact, such changes in cardiopulmonary vascular dynamics could reduce the amount of hemorrhage in exercising horses with EIPH, then current time restrictions further limit the effective use of furosemide.

The continued use of furosemide as a permitted race medication is a contentious issue. Its diuretic action decreases the urinary concentrations of drugs and, using current techniques, makes the detection of prohibited medications more difficult. It is also purported to improve racing performance, although performance trials in Standardbred horses have not substantiated this.[12] The effect of furosemide on the performance of horses known to experience EIPH has not been evaluated. Additionally, surveys have shown that at least 50 per cent of horses treated with furosemide to control EIPH still had endoscopic evidence of hemorrhage in the tracheobronchial tree. Since these were single observations, it is not known whether furosemide treatment decreased the amount of hemorrhage that may have otherwise occurred.[8]

DISODIUM CROMOGLYCATE

Disodium cromoglycate (cromolyn sodium)* stabilizes mast cells, preventing the release of vasoactive amines and slow reacting substance of anaphylaxis (SRS-A). It is used prophylactically to prevent allergy- and exercise-induced bronchoconstriction (EIB) in humans. Both allergic pulmonary disease and EIB may occur in horses and may be predisposing factors to EIPH. Recently, a synergistic relationship between the combination of cold air breathing, exercise, and bronchoconstriction has been shown in some human patients with bronchial asthma.[11] Additionally, during viral upper respiratory tract infections, a transient airway hyperreactivity may occur in response to cold, dry air.[1]

Bronchoconstriction may be especially important in some horses exercising or racing in cold weather. It is likely that such horses would show impaired performance and may be predisposed to EIPH. Concurrent viral upper respiratory tract infections could exacerbate the bronchoconstriction. Limited experience with disodium cromoglycate in horses has shown that pharyngeal insufflation of 200 or 300

---

*Vasolamin S 10 per cent, Ilium Labs, Smithfield, Australia
†Premarin, Ayerst Labs, New York, NY 10017
‡Estro IV, Western Serum, Tempe, AZ 86514
§Tri-Estro, Triple Crown, Ft. Collins, CO 80521
‖Lasix, American Hoechst Co., Somerville, NJ 08876

*Intal, Fisons Corp, Bedford, MA 01730

mg about 45 minutes prior to exercise or exposure to allergens prevents bronchoconstriction for three to four hours.[2] Its efficacy in the treatment of EIPH is unknown.

CLENBUTEROL

Clenbuterol is a long-acting β_2- adrenergic receptor stimulant that causes bronchodilation, enhances the activity of ciliated bronchial epithelial cells, and is secretolytic.[10] Although European trials have shown that the drug is effective in horses with chronic obstructive pulmonary disease, clenbuterol is still being investigated in the United States. Should clenbuterol become commercially available for use in horses, it may provide a useful adjunct to therapy in horses with EIPH and concurrent obstructive airway disease.

FEED SUPPLEMENTS

A variety of feed supplements that claim to prevent "bleeding" are commercially available and usually contain some combination of vitamin K, ascorbic acid, and bioflavinoids. The efficacy of these supplements in preventing EIPH has not been tested, and manufacturers' testimonials should be evaluated accordingly.

As stated earlier, the difficulty in providing reasonable therapeutic guidelines for the management of EIPH arises because of our limited understanding of this clinical syndrome. Each case should be thoroughly evaluated for subclinical or clinical respiratory disease and treated accordingly. In the absence of other clinical abnormalities, horses that experience EIPH should be monitored for subsequent infectious respiratory disease. Free blood in the respiratory tract provides an excellent medium for bacterial growth, and in some cases, particularly in the face of continued training, fulminant respiratory disease may occur. Although the effectiveness of rest in controlling EIPH is unknown, three months of enforced rest is an amount arbitrarily recommended prior to the resumption of training. Unfortunately, the economics of racing dictate that many of these horses continue racing, and rest is not possible until a period of orthopedic convalescence ensues or until severe respiratory infection limits the performance ability of the horse. Unfortunately, the

degree of pulmonary damage is often severe enough by this stage that it is unlikely that the horse will return to and continue racing without further episodes of pulmonary hemorrhage, despite therapy and rest.

Should a specific syndrome be recognized that is characterized by EIPH without concurrent pulmonary pathology and associated with mechanisms in exercise physiology, then specific prophylactic therapy may be possible. This would then provide the framework for a more rational approach to therapy, clinical management, and training procedures and for the subsequent evaluation of the efficacy of these procedures.

References

1. Aquilina, A. T., Hall, W. J., Douglas, R. G., Jr., and Vtell, M.: Airway reactivity in subjects with upper viral respiratory tract infections: The effects of exercise and cold air. Am. Rev. Respir. Dis., 122:3, 1980.
2. Beech, J.: Principles of therapy. Vet. Clin. North Am. (Large Anim. Pract.), 1(1):73, 1979.
3. Cook, W.R.: Epistaxis in the racehorse. Equine Vet. J., 6:45, 1974.
4. Fregin, G. F., and Deem, D. A.: Epistaxis in horses with atrial fibrillation. Proc. 26th Annu. Conv. Am. Assoc. Eq. Pract. 1980, pp. 431–433.
5. Milne, D. W., Muir, W. W., Skarda, R. T., Fregin, G. F., and Nicholl, J. K.: The hemodynamic response of the horse to swimming with and without furosemide. J. Equine Med. Surg., 1:331, 1977.
6. Muir, W. W., Milne, D. W., and Skarda, R. T.: Acute hemodynamic effects of furosemide administered intravenously in the horse. Am. J. Vet. Res., 37:117, 1976.
7. Pascoe, J. R.: Exercise-induced pulmonary hemorrhage: Current status. Am. Assoc. Eq. Pract. Newsletter, June 1970, p. 87.
8. Pascoe, J. R., Ferraro, G. L., Cannon, J. H., Arthur, R. M., and Wheat, J. D.: Exercise-induced pulmonary hemorrhage in racing thoroughbreds: A preliminary survey. Am. J. Vet. Res., 42:703, 1981.
9. Robinson, N. E.: Functional abnormalities caused by upper-airway obstruction and heaves: Their relationship to the etiology of epistaxis. Vet. Clin. North Am. (Large Anim. Pract.,) 1(1):17, 1979.
10. Sasse, H. H. L., and Hajer, R.: Veterinary and clinical experience with the use of a beta 2-receptor stimulating sympathicomimetic agent (NAB-365) in horses with respiratory diseases. Tijdschr. Diergeneesk., 102:31, 1977.
11. Strauss, R. H., McFadden, E. R., Jr., Ingram, R. H., Jr., and Jaeger, J. J.: Enhancement of exercise-induced asthma by cold air. N. Engl. J. Med., 297:743, 1977.
12. Tobin, T., Roberts, B. C., Swerczek, T. W., and Crisman, M.: The pharmacology of furosemide in the horse. III. Dose and time relationships, effects of repeated dosing and performance effects. J. Equine Med. Surg., 2:216, 1978.

LUNG PARASITES

Hilary M. Clayton, GLASGOW, SCOTLAND

Horses may cough for a variety of reasons, and it is in cases of chronic coughing (of several months' duration) that lungworm infection should be considered in the differential diagnosis. Although it is closely related to the lungworms of cattle and sheep, comparatively little is known about the equine lungworm, *Dictyocaulus arnfieldi*. One reason for this lack of information is that the parasite is particularly difficult to culture in the laboratory, and this has limited the number of experimental studies. In addition, *D. arnfieldi* usually arises as a problem in an individual or a small group of horses, in contrast to the situation in ruminants, in which outbreaks of clinical disease resulting in considerable economic loss have stimulated extensive research activity.

PATHOGENESIS

Lungworm infection in horses and donkeys was reviewed by Round.[4] All equidae are susceptible to infection, but the donkey appears to be the natural host and is seldom affected clinically. On the other hand, respiratory disease is a problem in infected horses and ponies, which seem to be less well-adapted hosts. It is necessary to understand the behavior of the parasite in the donkey population before considering the acquisition of infection by other species.

Most donkeys are infected early in life during grazing. The larvae migrate through the gut wall and are carried to the lungs, where they mature in the bronchi toward the periphery of the lobes. The adults are threadlike worms, up to 10 cm in length, and have a prepatent period of two to three months. Eggs laid in the bronchi are carried by the mucociliary blanket toward the larynx and then are swallowed. They hatch within a few hours after being passed in the feces, so for diagnostic purposes, feces should be examined for the presence of larvae using a Baermann technique rather than using one of the egg counting methods.

Surveys throughout the world indicate that *D. arnfieldi* is widespread in donkeys with a prevalence of 50 to 70 per cent. Contributing to the high infection rate is the fact that the parasite is not susceptible to routine anthelmintic treatment, and owners are not stimulated to seek specific therapy, since most donkeys show no obvious effects. Despite the absence of overt clinical signs, the parasite causes pathologic changes in the lungs.[3] At necropsy, the presence of pale, raised areas of overinflated pulmonary tissue is characteristic of *D. arnfieldi* infection. These circumscribed lesions often form distinct wedge-shaped areas around the lung periphery.

They are most numerous in the caudal lobes, which is consistent with the distribution of an agent arriving in the lungs via the hematogenous route. The small bronchi supplying the overinflated areas are often occluded by a mucous exudate and coiled worms. Histopathologic examination reveals epithelial hyperplasia with an increase in size and number of the goblet cells. The presence of adult worms in the bronchi stimulates little exudation, whereas any hatched first-stage larvae are surrounded by an intense mucopurulent reaction consisting of mucus, polymorphonuclear leukocytes, and eosinophils. These pathologic changes may predispose to other pulmonary diseases, such as allergic conditions and respiratory viruses.

In the donkey, patent lungworm infections persist for many years without seasonal variation in the magnitude of the fecal egg output. In temperate areas, the larvae are unable to winter on pasture, and development to the infective stage occurs only during the summer months. This seasonal availability of larvae is reflected by the fact that donkey foals develop patent infections in the late summer or autumn regardless of the month of birth.

Pastures contaminated by donkeys are the usual source of infection for horses and ponies, and the response to infection in these animals depends largely upon age. For example, a pony foal will develop a patent lungworm infection in the absence of overt clinical signs, although the duration of patency is usually shorter than in donkeys. In older horses and ponies, larval development in the lungs is retarded. As a result, the worms remain small and immature, and the infection does not become patent and cannot, therefore, be diagnosed by fecal examination. It is in these nonpatent infections that clinical signs develop, predominantly coughing and sometimes also an increase in respiratory rate and adventitious lung sounds. Affected animals will cough not only during exercise but also at rest, and the cough persists for many months. Even at necropsy it is difficult to confirm the presence of *D. arnfieldi*, since the larvae are small (less than 1 cm long) and are difficult to recover from the lungs. However, the pathologic changes resembling those described in the donkey are characteristic of *D. arnfieldi* infection.

DIAGNOSIS

The diagnosis of equine lungworm infections is based upon the history and clinical signs, microscopic examination of feces and tracheal washings, and, in some cases, necropsy examination.

The majority of donkeys have patent infections in the absence of overt clinical signs, and larvae can be recovered from the feces using a Baermann technique. The first-stage *D. arnfieldi* larva is recognized by its sluggish movements and the presence of a small spike on the end of the tail, which can be brought into focus after killing the larva with a drop of iodine or alcohol. The problems of larval differentiation can be minimized by taking feces directly from the rectum to avoid contamination, but in some low-level excretors, feces may have to be examined on more than one occasion before the larvae are detected.

In horses and ponies, fecal examination is of limited value, since the infection is usually nonpatent. When Baermann examination is negative, the clinical signs, predominantly a chronic cough, present problems in differential diagnosis from other conditions such as chronic obstructive pulmonary disease (COPD) (p. 505). An accurate history can be of value, particularly if there has been mixed grazing with donkeys, but it is very difficult either to confirm that lungworm is the etiologic agent or to eliminate this parasite as a possible cause.

One useful diagnostic aid in differentiating parasitic lung disease from COPD is cytologic examination of bronchial washings. In normal horses, few cells are present. Horses affected with COPD usually have excess mucus production with an increased number of inflammatory cells, mainly neutrophils but also macrophages. Parasitic infections also give rise to excess mucus, neutrophils, and macrophages, but characteristically, eosinophils are often seen. In the future, the rapidly expanding field of immunoparasitology may provide a serologic test for the diagnosis of lungworm in horses.

THERAPY

When we consider therapy of *D. arnfieldi* infection, one of the biggest problems is the method of evaluation of the response to treatment. Three criteria are used. The first of these is the clinical response, which assumes that if a horse stops coughing after treatment, this not only proves the efficacy of the anthelmintic against lungworm but also confirms the diagnosis. In many cases, these assumptions may be correct, but it is also possible that recovery was either coincidental or dependent upon some unrelated property of the drug. A second method of evaluating the effect of the anthelmintic is to determine the post-treatment depression of fecal larval counts. The drawbacks are that some anthelmintics cause only a temporary suppression of egg production of female worms, while others kill the most mature parasites but are ineffective against the earlier stages. In either case, there will be a marked

TABLE 1. *D. ARNFIELDI* LARVAL COUNTS AND NECROPSY RECOVERIES FROM DONKEYS TREATED WITH MEBENDAZOLE AND UNTREATED CONTROLS*

| Treatment Group | Fecal Larval Count (larvae/gm) | | No. Worms Recovered at Necropsy |
	Pre-treatment	Post-treatment	
Control	212 (25–584)	315 (10–1100)	143 (16–408)
Mebendazole 15–20 mg/kg/day for 5 days	208 (13–630)	0	2 (0–4)

*Each group comprised four donkeys, and results show average values and ranges for each group.

effect on larval output, but patency will be reestablished in a relatively short period of time. The third test, the controlled trial, gives a more accurate assessment of anthelmintic efficacy by comparing the worm burdens of treated animals with untreated controls at necropsy. In the case of *D. arnfieldi*, the only controlled trial used mebendazole* at two dosage rates.[1] The lower dosage rate proved ineffective, but when given at a rate of 15 to 20 mg per kg per day for five days, the worm burdens of the donkeys in the treated group were decreased by 75 to 100 per cent compared with the control group, and post-treatment fecal larval counts were reduced to zero in every animal. No adverse effects were seen. The results are summarized in Table 1.

As a follow-up to this study, Clayton and Trawford[2] treated 140 donkeys with mebendazole as described before. The number of animals with patent lungworm infections fell from 66 per cent before treatment to 23 per cent one month post-treatment. After grazing heavily contaminated pastures for six months, only 38 per cent of the treated donkeys were passing larvae. In contrast, in the control group, the number of animals with patent infections rose from 80 per cent in April to over 90 per cent in October. In addition, the fecal larval counts of individual donkeys in the control group were significantly higher than those of the treated group. The results are illustrated in Figure 1.

Veterinarians have reported a remission of clinical signs in horses suffering from a chronic cough of unknown etiology following treatment with fenbendazole† at a dose rate of 15 mg per kg. On the contrary, in naturally infected donkeys, doses of fenbendazole as high as 60 mg per kg resulted in only a temporary (three to four weeks) depression of fecal larval counts.

---

*Telmin, Pitman-Moore, Washington Crossing, NJ 08560
†Panacur, American Hoechst Co., Somerville, NJ 08876

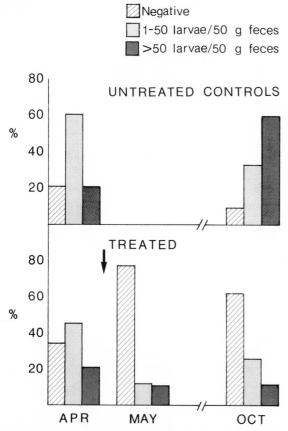

Figure 1. *D. arnfieldi* fecal larval counts of donkeys treated with 3.5g mebendazole daily for 5 days and untreated controls.
☐ Negative
☐ 1–50 larvae/50g feces
■ >50 larvae/50g feces

Before the newer benzimidazole derivatives became available, Round[4] used thiabendazole* at 440 mg per kg given twice with a 24-hour interval between treatments. In donkeys, the fecal larval counts were negative 28 days later. This treatment regimen has not been evaluated in a critical trial, however, and some animals have shown depression and anorexia after therapy. Other drugs that have been used include diethylcarbamazine and cyanacethydrazide, neither of which had a lasting effect on fecal larval output.

*Equizole, Merck and Co., Rahway, NJ 07065

Levamisole* has also been reported to produce a good clinical response when used at 7.5 to 15 mg per kg, but this drug has a low safety margin in equidae. Signs of toxicity have been seen after treatment with 20 mg per kg, and some horses develop a severe local reaction following injection of levamisole.

At the present time, the only anthelmintic with proven efficacy against equine lungworms is mebendazole at a dosage rate of 15 to 20 mg per kg per day for five days. Donkeys that graze with horses or ponies should be evaluated annually and retreated as necessary. It is anticipated that other benzimidazole derivatives might be effective against *D. arnfieldi*, but until critical trials have been conducted to determine the optimal dosage rate for each compound, mebendazole remains the treatment of choice.

D. arnfieldi is not the only parasite found in equine lungs. In foals, the intestinal nematode *Parascaris equorum* undergoes a hepatic-tracheal migration. Larvae arrive in the lungs by the hematogenous route, then migrate along the airways toward the trachea and larynx. Their presence stimulates excess mucus production, and in heavy infections, coughing and a mucoid or purulent nasal discharge may be seen. The effect of anthelmintics on the tissue stages of *P. equorum* has not been investigated, and therapy at this stage is not usually necessary, since the respiratory signs are transient. However, if treatment is being considered, high doses of the benzimidazoles would probably offer the best chance of success.

References

1. Clayton, H. M., and Neave, R. M. S.: Efficacy of mebendazole against *Dictyocaulus arnfieldi* in the donkey. Vet. Rec., *104*:571, 1979.
2. Clayton, H. M., and Trawford, A. F.: Anthelmintic control of lungworm in donkeys. Equine Vet. J. *13*(3):192, 1981.
3. Nicholls, J. M., Clayton, H. M., Duncan, J. L., and Buntain, B.: Lungworm (*Dictyocaulus arnfieldi*) infection in donkeys. Vet. Rec., *104*:567, 1979.
4. Round, M. C.: Lungworm infection (*Dictyocaulus arnfieldi*) of horses and donkeys. Vet. Rec., *99*:393, 1976.

*Ripercol, American Cyanamid Co., Princeton, NJ 08540

PLEURITIS

Stephen M. Reed, PULLMAN, WASHINGTON

Pleural effusion, the presence of an abnormally large amount of fluid within the pleural space, can be a primary disease or a complication of cardiac disease, hepatic disorders, neoplasia, or respiratory infections. Pleural effusions may also accompany diseases that result in protein loss from the gastrointestinal tract or kidney. In one study, idiopathic pleural effusion was recognized in approximately 38 per cent of the cases.[11]

The pleura consists of visceral and parietal layers. The former covers the lungs, and the latter lines the chest wall, mediastinum, and diaphragm. The mediastinum of the horse is incomplete, being fenestrated in the caudal ventral portion. One important anatomic feature differentiating the horse from other species is that both the visceral and parietal pleura receive their blood supply from the systemic circulation, while in most species, the visceral layer is supplied from the pulmonary circulation.

The parietal pleura is well supplied with pain receptors from the intercostal and phrenic nerves, whereas the visceral pleura has no pain receptors but does receive innervation from autonomic fibers. The lymphatic drainage from the visceral pleura is into the tracheobronchial lymph nodes, and the parietal pleura drains into the sternal nodes, with the exception of the mediastinal and diaphragmatic sections of the parietal pleura, which drain into the mediastinal nodes.

The fluid within the pleural space is constantly being formed and removed. Its production and resorption are controlled by the plasma oncotic pressure, pleural capillary hydrostatic pressure, capillary permeability, and lymphatic drainage. In most species, protein-free fluid is constantly entering the pleural space from the parietal side and leaving via the visceral pleura, while protein enters from both the visceral and parietal surfaces and exits through the lymphatics. In the horse, because the parietal and visceral pleura receive their blood supply from the systemic circulation, it is possible that the net driving force for protein-free fluid filtration is greater than in species such as the dog.

The initial question when a pleural effusion is identified is whether that effusion is a transudate or an exudate. If the effusion is a transudate, an underlying cause of congestive heart failure, renal failure, hepatic failure, or protein-losing gastroenteropathy is sought and, if found, is treated. If, on the other hand, an exudate is identified, further diagnostic procedures are required to help determine the cause of pleural disease.

A transudate is noninflammatory in origin and results from causes such as hypoproteinemia or venous stasis. Transudates are nonclotting, clear, or yellow fluids that contain few cells and no bacteria and that have a specific gravity of less than 1.017 and a total protein of less than 3 gm per dl.[3] The usual cells that may be present include small lymphocytes and erythrocytes with an occasional endothelial or mesothelial cell.

An exudate is inflammatory in origin and results from infections, trauma, neoplasia, or inflammation due to a foreign body. Exudates clot rapidly, are clear or cloudy, and contain numerous cells and often bacteria. The specific gravity is greater than 1.017, and the total protein is greater than 3 gm per dl.[3] In this type of effusion, one may expect to find neutrophils, lymphocytes, and erythrocytes, although a large number of reactive mesothelial or neoplastic cells is not an uncommon finding. The presence of intracellular or extracellular bacteria often indicates a septic process.

Most commonly in equine medicine, pleural effusions are modified transudates or exudates indicating inflammation of the pleural surfaces. A modified transudate is a transudate that has been altered by addition of protein and cells. This type of effusion is often serosanguineous, contains a protein level greater than 2.5 gm per dl, and has a variable number of macrophages, lymphocytes, erythrocytes, neutrophils, and mesothelial cells. It is often seen in association with neoplasia.

The minimal examination of a fluid removed from a serous body cavity should include appearance, coagulation, measurement of total protein, and cytologic examination as well as direct examination for bacteria and bacterial culture.

HISTORY AND CLINICAL SIGNS

The evaluation of a horse suspected to be suffering from pleural effusion or pleuritis is aided by an accurate history. This disease may follow a recent stressful event such as a prolonged trip or exposure to a large number of new horses. Because pleuritis is often associated with respiratory infection, knowledge of the patient's vaccination status as well as the health and vaccination status of other horses with which it has been in recent contact is important. The previous geographic location can be important because fungal agents such as *Coccidiodes immitis* and *Nocardia*[4] sp, as well as other systemic fungi that may cause pleuritis, are common in the southwestern United States.

The clinical signs of pleural effusion in the horse are dependent upon the amount of fluid within the pleural space as well as the underlying cause. It is not uncommon for horses to be febrile, depressed, thin, and have pitting edema of subcutaneous tissue in the pectoral region. If only a small amount of fluid is present within the pleural cavity, no abnormal signs may be detected. If several liters of fluid are present, the patient is usually dyspneic at rest or following slight exertion. One report suggests that 10 l of fluid or greater often results in dyspnea.[11]

When the parietal pleura is inflamed, the horse may show signs of pain when moving or when pressure is applied over the ribs; however, the longer the fluid is present within the pleural space, the less commonly is pain a feature of the disease. This may result from formation of firm fibrous adhesions or a cushion created by large volumes of intrapleural fluid. Respiration is often shallow and guarded, and close examination may reveal asymmetric movements of the chest wall. Nasal discharge and cough are common if the pleural effusion is associated with pneumonia.

Airway sounds are absent in the ventral thorax below the pleural fluid level, while in the dorsal lung regions, airway sounds may be normal or abnormal depending upon the amount of pulmonary disease. Fluid within the trachea may be detected if pneumonia accompanies a pleural effusion. The cardiac sounds generally radiate over a wider region than normal, unless there is an accompanying pericarditis, in which case they may be difficult to detect. Pleural friction rubs are not always a consistent feature; however, their presence is highly suggestive of pleuritis.

A fluid line may not always be detected by auscultation unless ventilation is increased by temporarily occluding or placing a bag over the nares. The increased ventilation results in increased sounds above the fluid line, making absence of sounds ventrally more easily detected. Percussion will also help identify the presence of a fluid line. This is performed by use of a plexor and pleximeter. I feel most comfortable when assisted by another person to judge the change in resonance. The normal limits of pleural reflection are the 17th intercostal (IC) space at the level of the tuber coxae, the 15th IC space at the level of the tuber ischii, the 13th IC space at the midchest, the 11th IC space at the point of the shoulder, and ending at the point of the elbow.[7]

THORACENTESIS

Thoracentesis is essential for physical, chemical, cytologic, and bacteriologic examinations of pleural fluid.[9] It is also of therapeutic benefit in most cases. The most common locations for thoracentesis are the seventh intercostal space on the right side and the eighth or ninth intercostal space on the left side. The site is dependent upon the fluid level, which has been identified on physical examination or by use of other diagnostic aids such as radiography or ultrasonography. The procedure must be performed with aseptic technique and is conducted with the animal restrained in a stall or stocks. A 14- to 18-gauge, 3- to 4-in needle or catheter, a 3-in teat cannula, or a bitch catheter may be utilized. A three-way stopcock and syringe should be available to avoid developing pneumothorax. Local anesthesia of the skin and underlying muscle is important to alleviate pain. A small stab incision is made through the skin using a No. 10 or No. 15 scalpel blade. The cannula or catheter, attached to the stopcock and syringe, is pushed into the chest cavity along the anterior border of the rib in order to avoid the intercostal vessels.

The aspirate that is collected should be examined for color, turbidity, odor, and presence of coagulation. Measurement of specific gravity, total protein, and cytologic composition are also important diagnostic aids. All samples collected should be submitted for a direct examination to determine whether bacteria are present and should be cultured both aerobically and anaerobically.

OTHER DIAGNOSTIC AIDS

Other diagnostic aids to evaluate a patient with a pleural effusion include hematology, radiography, ultrasonography, transtracheal aspiration for bacterial culture and viral isolation as well as serologic titers against common viral respiratory pathogens. B-mode ultrasonography is often helpful in locating a sequestered fluid-filled area. The transtracheal aspiration for bacterial culture is most beneficial when pleural effusion is associated with pneumonia, especially if aspiration or bacterial pneumonia has occurred. The hematologic parameters alone may reveal only nonspecific changes of stress, infection, or chronic disease. If the process has been long-standing, one may recognize an elevated total protein often associated with an increased fibrinogen and globulin fraction with a lower than normal serum albumin level.

THERAPY

Treatment of a pleural effusion in the horse has four objectives: (1) the establishment of drainage; (2) administration of appropriate antibiotic or antimicrobial therapy; (3) use of drugs for alleviation of pain and inflammation; and (4) nursing care, which may include rest, hand feeding, and sometimes intravenous fluid therapy. Beyond these it may also be helpful to administer diuretics, such as furosemide, as well as agents that activate plasminogen to break down fibrin such as streptokinase. Each of these therapies will be discussed in more detail emphasizing its importance and describing the technique.

DRAINAGE

Drainage of a pleural effusion can be accomplished with a syringe and needle, although a permanent drain is often more convenient. The technique for applying such a drain involves making a stab wound at the 9th or 10th intercostal space on the left in order to tunnel a fenestrated polyethylene catheter* beneath the skin in a craniad direction for 1 to 2 intercostal spaces (Fig. 1*A*). The drain is then stabbed or pushed through the chest wall into the pleural space. Once the drain is in place, a sterile, one-way chest drain valve† should be attached to prevent leakage of air into the thorax. This drain may be permanently fixed in place by use of suture and bandage material (Fig. 1*B*). Drains may be allowed to drain continuously or may be elevated to a level at which drainage no longer occurs and may be fixed there with an adhesive dressing. The drains may then be periodically lowered to remove accumulated fluid. When a permanent drain is applied in this fashion, caution must be used to keep the chest wound, drainage tube, and one-way valve aseptic. Since fluid often accumulates to a different degree on each side of the thorax and may even be of a different character on each side, a drain in both the right and left sides is usually necessary.

Continuous drainage appears to be the most efficacious treatment. However, it can be hazardous, as it provides a route of entry for infectious agents and so may compound rather than improve the condition. In addition, if not adequately sealed, the drain may act as a portal of entry for air, causing pneumothorax and atelectasis. The removal of the restrictive forces (air or fluid) followed by reexpansion of the pulmonary tissue relieves dyspnea and pain and often decreases the patient's anxiety associated with difficult breathing. In addition, the removal of inflammatory products can be very helpful in decreasing the generalized toxemia and pyrexia that may accompany pleural effusion.

When treating a pleural effusion that is a transudate, attention must be directed toward identifying and correcting the underlying case. If the effusion is a result of elevated hydrostatic pressure, as with

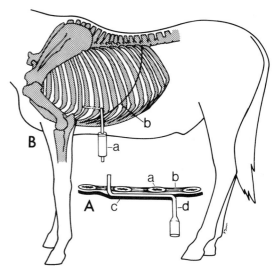

Figure 1. Technique for placement of a drain in the pleural cavity. *A.* The drain tube (d) is tunneled beneath the skin (c) before puncturing the intercostal muscles (b) between the ribs (a). *B.* Anatomical location of drain. Pleural reflection is shown (b), as is the one-way valve on the drain tube.

right- or left-sided congestive heart failure, there is likely very little one can do for the animal, although use of drugs such as digitalis combined with diuretics may be helpful (p. 140). If the transudate is a result of decreased plasma oncotic pressure, it is usually secondary to hypoalbuminemia. The causes of hypoalbuminemia include starvation, parasitism, intestinal malabsorption, hepatic failure, and renal failure. Treatment of this type of effusion may involve use of furosemide* at a dosage of 250 to 500 mg per 450 kg once or twice a day. This treatment is only symptomatic and may help alleviate the clinical signs of dyspnea but does not correct the underlying disease.

Treatment of a modified transudate should involve chronic drainage, along with antimicrobial therapy to combat secondary bacterial infections, and nursing care. If the diagnosis of a neoplastic condition is confirmed, further treatment is not realistic.

INTRAVENOUS FLUIDS

In many instances, the administration of intravenous polyionic isotonic fluids such as saline or lactated Ringer's for circulatory support may be helpful. These should be given at a dose of 10 to 20 ml per 1b of body weight during or following the period of fluid removal. I have, on occasion, seen horses that collapse during removal of fluid from the

---

*Argyle trocar catheter, 20 or 28 French, Sherwood Medical Industries, Inc., St. Louis, MO
†Heimlick, Bard-Parker, Rutherford, NJ

*Lasix, American Hoescht Co., Somerville, NJ 08876

pleural space. The cause of this is unknown but may be related to increase in venous capacitance following removal of the space-occupying lesion.[10]

ANTIMICROBIAL THERAPY

The use of systemic antimicrobial therapy is important and should be performed according to results of sensitivity testing of aerobic and anaerobic bacterial cultures.[1] The culture and sensitivity tests should be performed on both the transtracheal wash and thoracentesis fluids. The usual organisms isolated from pleural effusion are Streptococcus sp and coliforms. I have found *S. zooepidemicus* to be the most frequent pathogen isolated, followed by *Escherichia coli*. Other less common isolates include Pasteurella sp, Klebsiella sp, Bordetella, Actinobacillus, and Nocardia. The significance of these agents, especially Actinobacillus as a primary pathogen of the respiratory tract in adult horses, is debatable;[6] however, if they are recovered as the sole pathogenic organism on initial transtracheal aspiration or thoracentesis, it is important to initiate treatment. The usual antibiotic of choice is penicillin (10,000 U per lb, 22,000 U per kg twice a day). However, aminoglycosides such as gentamicin* at 0.8 mg per lb (1.8 mg per kg) intramuscularly three times a day and kanamycin† at 5 mg per lb (11 mg per kg) intramuscularly twice a day are effective against most gram-negative organisms. Other agents that may be beneficial include combinations of trimethoprim and sulfamethoxazole‡ and chloramphenicol, 20 mg per lb (50 mg per kg) four times a day, which may be given orally, as well as sodium ampicillin, 5 mg per lb (11 mg per kg) three times a day. Further information on antimicrobial therapy is available elsewhere in this text (p. 43). The best route of administration for antimicrobial therapy is intramuscular or intravenous. Other routes that have been described include intratracheal injections and local infusions into the pleural space; however, in this author's hands, the latter methods have given poor results.

ANTI-INFLAMMATORY AGENTS

Anti-inflammatory agents help reduce pain and may aid in decreasing the production of pleural ef-

*Gentocin, Schering Corp., Kenilworth, NJ 07033
†Kantrim, Bristol Labs, Syracuse, NY 13201
‡Bactrim DS, Roche, Nutley, NJ 07110

fusions. Phenylbutazone at a dose of 4 gm (0.008 mg per kg) divided twice a day is the usual drug choice, although other nonsteroidal anti-inflammatory agents such as flunixin meglumine* may also be helpful (1.1 mg per kg). The use of corticosteroids such as dexamethasone at 0.1 to 0.2 mg per kg once a day and prednisone at 1.0 mg per kg orally has been described by other authors to reduce fluid reaccumulation.[12] These drugs appear to provide a euphoric effect in the patient; however, some causes of pleural effusion in the horse, such as lymphosarcoma, may be associated with significant immunosuppression.[5] Therefore, drugs that may further promote this should be used cautiously.

NURSING CARE

The fourth essential component of treatment of pleural effusions is rest with adequate nursing care. These patients are very ill and have toxic byproducts within the pleural space. Pleural fluid restricts lung expansion and limits the activity of the animal. Additional stress must be avoided at all costs.

References

1. Bartlett, J. G.: Diagnostic accuracy of transtracheal aspiration bacteriologic studies. Am. Rev. Respir. Dis., *115*:777, 1977.
2. Beech, J.: Principles of therapy, Vet. Clin. North Am. (Large Anim. Pract)., *1*(1):73, 1979.
3. Benjamin, M. M.: Outline of Veterinary Clinical Pathology, 2nd ed. Ames, IA, The Iowa State University Press, 1972, pp. 149–152.
4. Deem, D., and Harrington, D. D.: *Nocardia brasiliensis* in a horse with pneumonia and pleuritis. Cornell Vet., *70*:321, 1980.
5. Dopson, L., Reed, S., and Perryman, L.: Immunosuppression associated with lymphosarcoma in three horses, submitted for publication, 1982.
6. Jubb, K. V. F., and Kennedy, P. C.: Pathology of Domestic Animals, Vol. 1. New York, Academic Press, 1963, p. 431.
7. Kohn, C. N.: Recognition and management of equine viral respiratory disease. Compend. Contin. Ed., *3*(3):S101, 1981.
8. Knight, H. D.: Antimicrobial agents used in the horse. Proc. 21st Ann. Conv. Am. Assoc. Eq. Pract., 1975, pp. 131–144.
9. Moore, J. N., Johnson, J. H., Traver, D. S., Garner, H. E., and Coffman, J. R.: Thoracentesis. Vet. Surg., *6*(1):38, 1977.
10. Ross, J. N.: Shock. Proc. Am. Coll. Vet. Intern. Med., July, 1980.
11. Smith, B. P.: Pleuritis and pleural effusion in the horse: A study of 37 cases. J. Am. Vet. Med. Assoc., *170*:208, 1977.
12. Smith, B. P.: Diseases of the pleura. Vet. Clin. North Am. (Large Anim. Pract), *1*(1):197, 1979.

*Banamine, Schering Corp., Kenilworth, NJ 07033

Section 11

SKIN DISEASES

Edited by A. A. Stannard

COMMON ECTOPARASITES AND THEIR CONTROL 529

URTICARIA AND ANGIOEDEMA 535

PAPILLOMATOSIS (WARTS) 536

SURGICAL TREATMENT OF EQUINE SARCOID 537

BCG THERAPY FOR EQUINE SARCOID 539

PEMPHIGUS FOLIACEUS 541

FOLLICULITIS AND FURUNCULOSIS 542

NODULAR COLLAGENOLYTIC GRANULOMA (NODULAR NECROBIOSIS) 545

DISEASES OF ABNORMAL KERATINIZATION (SEBORRHEA) 546

CONTACT DERMATITIS 547

SCRATCHES 549

PHYCOMYCOSIS 550

HABRONEMIASIS 551

DERMATOPHILOSIS 553

SPOROTRICHOSIS 555

ONCHOCERCIASIS 557

SWEET OR QUEENSLAND ITCH (CULICOIDES HYPERSENSITIVITY) 558

COMMON ECTOPARASITES AND THEIR CONTROL

Edmond C. Loomis, DAVIS, CALIFORNIA

Ectoparasites and pests of horses include mites, ticks, lice, flies, gnats, and mosquitoes. Dense populations of some species may cause anemia, anorexia, colic, dermatitis, emaciation, hair loss, tail rubbing, unthriftiness, weakness, and, if left untreated, death. Some species also carry serious diseases of animals and humans.

PREVENTION

The horse owner is responsible for applying good methods of sanitation and management to prevent parasites and pests on or in horses. Recommendations are included under certain species that may minimize or eliminate problems and thereby provide more effective chemical control.

Pesticides listed alphabetically in Table 1 include chemicals named in the Federal Register for horses (nonfood use), and all are effective when used at the proper concentration, dosage, and application method. Dermal application of emulsifiable concentrate spray solutions, aerosols, or ready-to-use smears should be tested on a small area with some breeds (for example, Arabians and palominos) because of possible skin sensitivity to petroleum derivatives used in different formulations. Some pesticides may not be found in every state if separate registration is required or if distributorship is not available. Also, all manufacturers' names are not included for each pesticide because of the many different formulators who obtain basic compounds and prepare mixtures under a variety of trade names.

MITES

Mites are microscopic, permanent parasites that cause a variety of skin conditions called mange. Two species, *Psoroptes equi* and *Chorioptes bovis* (var. *equi*) live on the skin surface. *P. equi* is more common on the poll, mane, and tail, while *C. bovis* is found below the hock and knees. Both produce skin lesions, loss of hair, with scabs appearing over the thickened skin. *Sarcoptes scabiei* forms tunnels by burrowing under the skin of the neck, shoulders, head, chest, flank, and abdomen. Small nodules form around the burrows with eventual loss of hair and scab development.

Life cycles of these mites are similar. Daily oviposition occurs in the skin (under scabs) or in the burrow during an adult life span of 12 to 15 days.

Eggs hatch in about four days, and mites reach maturity in 10 to 14 days. Transmission is by contact with infested horses, blankets, curry combs, and other common gear. It is important to isolate infested horses and to keep all equipment separate until the disease is controlled.

Skin scabs and scrapings should be taken for differential diagnosis of mange mites, ringworm, or dermal habronemiasis. Treatment requires thorough dipping or use of high-powered sprays (100 psi) for sarcoptic mange. A stiff brush–wash method (to dislodge scabs) is recommended to kill psoroptic and chorioptic mites. Two treatments seven days apart are necessary for all types of mange (℞ 1 and 13, Table 1).

Chiggers (red bugs) are larvae of trombiculid mites, which normally infest reptiles, birds, and rodents. In the absence of their normal hosts, the mites may attack horses. A massive infestation of larvae may cause intense itching, rubbing of affected parts, and severe dermatitis. Mangelike lesions may be found over the entire body but appear more frequently on the legs, neck, and head. Chiggers can be controlled by application of a pesticide wash (℞ 1,4,6, or 13, Table 1). One application is sufficient, and affected horses should not be repastured in mite-infested areas for one month. Area control for chiggers is not feasible.

TICKS

Of the many species that attack livestock, only a few are found on horses. Infestations are more common during spring and fall months, when ticks actively seek their hosts. Ticks go unnoticed in the long winter hair coat until large numbers appear on the head, neck, mane, flanks, chest, and abdomen. Animals begin to rub, scratch, or bite the affected body areas, and dense tick populations may cause weakness, ascites, anorexia, anemia, paralysis, and death.

All ticks have four stages: egg, larvae (six-legged), nymph, and adult (the last two are eight-legged). Most species use a variety of small rodents and larger wildlife on which larvae (seed ticks) and nymphs feed before the adults attach to horses. These species use two or more hosts to complete their life cycle, which requires a period of two to three years. However, ticks commonly found on horses are one host species, of which the larva, nymph, and adult remain in place to feed and mate

TABLE 1. RECOMMENDED PESTICIDES FOR EXTERNAL PARASITE CONTROL ON HORSES

Parasite(s)	Guides for Treatment	Pesticide and Manufacturer[1]	Formulations[2]	Concentration and Application[3]
Black fly Face fly Gnats Horn fly Stable fly Mosquitoes Lice Mites Ticks (on body)	For most flies, gnats, and mosquitoes, hand wash with sponge or direct mist spray and low-pressure sprays (30 psi) to head, neck, chest, withers, and abdomen. For biting stable fly, direct treatments to lower body areas and legs. For lice, mites, and ticks on body areas, use high-pressure spray (80–100 psi) to penetrate long hair coat and thoroughly wet skin. Retreatment necessary in 7 days for mites, in 14 days for lice. For black flies and gnats attacking ears, apply thin smear of jelly or dust well on inside edges of both ears. Resmethrin and tetramethrin are repellents; brush on lightly, but do not wet skin—for flies, gnats, and mosquitoes. For dusts, half-fill a sock and tap lightly to head areas for face fly, to withers for horn fly, or to ears for gnats and black fly.	1. Coumaphos (Co-Ral)—BV 2. Dichlorvos (Vapona)—DS 3. Dichlorvos (Vapona) + crotoxyphos (Ciodrin)—BV 4. Dioxathion (Conav)—TH 5. Dioxathion (Conav) + dichlorvos (Vapona)—TH 6. Malathion—AC, CC 7. Methoxychlor—TC, DP 8. Petroleum jelly 9. Pyrethrins + piperonyl butoxide 10. Resmethrin + cyclopropane carboxylate—F 11. Stirofos (Rabon)—DS 12. Tetramethrin—F 13. Toxaphene—HI	EC or dust EC EC EC EC or dust EC EC EC or gel EC	0.06% HW, SP, 1% HD; for flies, lice, ticks 0.93% prepared solution HW, MSP 1% + 0.25% MSP for flies; 0.15% + 0.05% SP for lice; 0.02% + 0.3% SP for ticks 0.15% HW, SP 0.12% + 0.005% HW, SP 0.5% HW, SP; 4–5% HD 0.5% HW, SP Ready to use 0.1% + 1% MSP 10% + 0.5% prepared solution WO 1% HW, SP; 2% WO 0.4% prepared solution WO 0.5% HW, SP for flies, mites, ticks; 0.25% SP for lice
Blow flies and screwworms (in wounds)	Apply thoroughly into and around wounds once weekly until healed.	14. Coumaphos (Co-Ral)—BV 15. Lindane—BW 16. Ronnel (Korlan)—FL	EC or dust Aerosol solution Aerosol solution or smear	0.25% HW; 5% HD 3% SP 2.5% SP; 5% smear
Bot flies (bots in stomach)	Orally in feed 1 month after first frost. Do not treat colts under 4 months of age or mares in last month of pregnancy. Withhold water for 4–6 hours before treatment and 3–4 hours after. Do not treat more often than every 30 days. Orally by syringe before first frost. Contraindications as for powder, but withhold food overnight before treatment and 3–4 hours after. Orally in feed 1 month after first frost. Contraindications as for dichlorvos.	17. Dichlorvos (Vapona)—DS 18. Trichlorfon (Neguvon)–BV	Powder Paste Powder	20% powder, 14–18 mg/lb or half this amount given twice 8–12 hours apart. 32 cc/1200 lbs 90% powder; 1 packet of 5 gm/250 lbs

Table continued on the opposite page

TABLE 1. RECOMMENDED PESTICIDES FOR EXTERNAL PARASITE CONTROL ON HORSES *(Continued)*

Parasite(s)	Guides for Treatment	Pesticide and Manufacturer[1]	Formulations[2]	Concentration and Application[3]
Bot flies (eggs on hairs)	Use in lukewarm water over areas where eggs are attached, and repeat once weekly until after first frost.	19. Coumaphos (Co-Ral)—BV	EC	0.06% HW, MSP
		20. Dioxathion (Conav)—TH	EC	0.15% HW, MSP
		21. Malathion—AC	EC	0.5% HW, MSP
		22. Stirofos (Rabon)—DS	EC	0.5% HW, MSP
		23. Toxaphene—HI	EC	0.25% HW, MSP
Ear ticks	Spray or dust into deep recesses of both ears. Apply 1 oz into recesses of each ear.	24. Coumaphos (Co-Ral)—BV	Aerosol or dust	3% aerosol SP; 5% HD
		25. Lindane—BW	Aerosol	3% SP
		26. Ronnel (Korlan)—FL	Aerosol or smear	2.5% SP; 5% smear
		27. Dioxathion (Conav) + dichlorvos (Vapona)—TH	EC	0.12% + 0.005% solution in rubber-tipped oil can

[1]AC = American Cyanamid Co.; BV = Bayvet-Cutter; BW = Burroughs Wellcome, Cooper Div.; CC = Chevron Chemical Co.; DC = Dow Chemical; DP = duPont de Nemours & Co.; DS = Diamond Shamrock; F = Farnum Co.; FL = Franklin Labs; HI = Hercules Incorporated; TC = Techne Corp.; TH = Thompson-Hayward Chemical Co.

[2]EC = Emulsifiable concentrate

[3]HD = hand dust; HW = hand wash; MSP = mist spray; SP = spray; WO = wipe-on

and need less than one year for complete development. These include *Anocentor nitens* (tropical horse tick) in Texas, Georgia, and Florida; *Boophilus annulatus* (cattle tick) along the Texas-Mexico border; *Dermacentor albipictus* (winter tick) in northern states from Washington to Maine and in western states south to Texas; and *Otobius megnini* (spinous ear tick) in warm, arid regions of southwestern states.

A. nitens, though mainly in the ears, also attacks the nasal diverticula, mane, abdomen, and anal and inguinal areas. The tick carries equine piroplasmosis, and tick bites predispose horses to screwworm attack. *D. albipictus* may occur over all body areas but prefers the abdomen and areas between the legs. This tick carries anaplasmosis to livestock. *O. megnini* larvae and nymphs feed deep inside the ear (also on livestock, pets, and wildlife), drop to the ground, and crawl into cracks in corral posts, feed troughs, and barn sidings and even hide under the bark of trees. Here they molt to adults, mate, and die after the females lay eggs. Severe ear infestations cause pain and irritation, and blood wounds invite screwworm attacks or secondary infection. Perforation of the eardrum (deafness) and death from meningitis may result. *B. annulatus*, chiefly found on cattle, may occur on any body area and is the vector of babesiosis (Texas cattle fever).

There are seven multihost species of which adults may occur on horses. *Amblyomma americanum* (Lone Star tick) is found in the Plains states north to Missouri and eastward to the Atlantic coast and carries Rocky Mountain spotted fever and tularemia. *A. cajennense* (Cayenne tick) occurs in southern Texas and, on horses, prefers the ears and other natural cavities. *A. maculatum* (Gulf coast tick) is found in areas of high temperature, rainfall, and humidity and in states along the Gulf of Mexico and

invades primarily the concave portion of the outer ears of horses and cattle, providing sites for screwworm attacks. *Dermacentor andersoni* (Rocky Mountain tick) is distributed throughout the north central and western states, where it transmits Rocky Mountain spotted fever, Colorado tick fever, Powassan encephalitis virus, tularemia, anaplasmosis, and tick-bite paralysis. *D. occidentalis* (Pacific Coast tick) occurs in Oregon and California, where it transmits tularemia, anaplasmosis, and tick-bite paralysis. *Ixodes scapularis* (black-legged tick) is widespread along the east coast and in the Plains states from Iowa to Texas, while *I. pacificus* is common in the Pacific coast states; adults of both *Ixodes* cause intense irritation because of their long mouth parts but to date are not vectors of any disease.

Horses should be examined particularly from fall to spring months and especially after trail rides, exercise in grasslands, and brush-covered "tick country," after movement of stock from brushy rangeland to paddocks, and after horses are transported intrastate and interstate following shows, rides, and other events. Reexamination of stock should be made in five to seven days to detect engorged ticks overlooked in the first inspection. Both ears should be routinely inspected, and a pesticide application should be made into each ear when ticks are found (Rx 24–27, Table 1).

Mechanical clearing or burning of brush and shrubs and pastures used for grazing will reduce tick habitat and animal infestation by multihost ticks. For one-host ticks, rotation of horses between blocks of pastures for several months will cause high mortality of larval ticks and will help prevent reinfestation.

Many pesticides are available, and to date, ticks have not acquired resistance to these compounds (Rx 1,3, or 13, Table 1). Chemical application methods follow closely those recommended for louse control. If ticks are not discovered until late winter, chemical sprays to the ground surface of paddocks and stalls (between bedding removal) will help prevent reinfestation (R 6,11, or 13, Table 1).

LICE

Three species of lice are common on horses: the blood-sucking *Haematopinus asini* and biting lice, *Trichodectes pilosus* and *T. equi*. These lice do not transfer to cattle, nor can species peculiar to cattle live on horses. Louse infestations are commonly seen in winter when the horse's hair coat is long or when animals are overstocked on poor pasture.

Lice occur on all body areas, but owing to self-grooming by the horse, they are usually first seen on the head, neck, mane, and tail. Lice depend mainly on animal contact to transfer from an infested horse to a clean one. Some horses are highly susceptible to lice and are termed "louse carriers." These animals should be routinely inspected and treated. Hair parts should be made in areas where horses scratch, rub, or bite to detect lice at an early stage before scabbed lesions develop. Left untreated, blood-sucking lice in particular cause anemia, weakness, and contribute to stunted growth in young stock and to the loss of condition and weight in older animals.

The life cycles of these lice are similar in time needed to develop from egg (nit) to nymph to adult. Eggs incubate for 5 to 14 days, whereupon the nymphs emerge and feed for about two weeks before becoming adults. Mating occurs one week later, and female lice lay from 50 to 100 eggs in a life span of four to five weeks.

Numerous pesticides are available for louse control, and all are effective if horses are thoroughly treated and retreated two weeks later to kill young lice hatching from eggs not affected by the first treatment (R 1,3–6, 11, or 13, Table 1). Horses may be sprayed with high-pressure sprays (100 psi), but some animals are difficult to control, and these individuals are commonly treated by thorough brushing of the pesticide solution onto louse-infected body areas. Blankets, brushes, and rope halters should be soaked in boiling water, and leather articles, including saddles, can be rubbed with the pesticide solution; retreat articles in two weeks.

FLIES, GNATS, AND MOSQUITOES

This group contains the largest and most diversified number of pests and parasites of horses, with all species passing through four stages of development: egg, larva (maggot), pupa (resting stage), and adult. The life cycle from egg to adult may be as short as eight days (house fly, face fly, and mosquitoes) or may require as long as one year (horse flies, bot flies, and certain gnats). Adults include blood-feeders (biting stable fly, horn fly, horse flies, black flies, gnats, and mosquitoes), those that feed on liquid secretions from animals, from manure, or from plant debris (house fly, face fly, and blow flies), and those that do not feed because they lack suitable mouth parts (bot flies). With few exceptions, the numerous species in each subgroup are cosmopolitan in distribution.

HOUSE FLY AND STABLE FLY

In summer, the house fly (*Musca domestica*) and biting stable fly (*Stomoxys calcitrans*) commonly take 8 and 21 days, respectively, to reproduce. They breed in manure piles commonly found inside stalls, in paddock areas, or in piles of mixed manure and bedding, wet feed, decomposed plant debris, piles of rotted fruit or vegetables, garbage, and pet droppings. These species transmit many disease agents to animals and humans. Those diseases commonly found in horses and livestock include equine infectious anemia, vesicular stomatitis, anthrax, brucellosis, leptospirosis, anaplasmosis, the stomach worm, *Habronema muscae*, and dermal myiasis, or "summer sore."

Basic farm management practices will reduce natural attractors and will eliminate breeding areas of these flies. Manure and soiled bedding should be removed from stalls at least twice a week in summer and less often in cooler weather. Stable wastes should not be stockpiled but should be immediately spread thinly in the arena as a cushion or delivered elsewhere for fertilizer use. All troughs, bowls, and other water devices should have nonleak or automatic valves for water control. Sanitation around barns, tack sheds, and the residence is as important as manure and water management.

Chemical control with any pesticides listed in Table 2 may assist in fly reduction. Spray application can be made to surfaces where flies rest and may be effective for two to four weeks (R 28–32, Table 2). Space sprays or fogs are most valuable to quickly kill large numbers of flies (R 33–35, Table 2). Bait compounds are useful to help support good sanitation but must be located in places where flies congregate (R 36–38, Table 2).

HORN FLY

The horn fly, *Haematobia irritans*, sucks blood. Horses are attacked when they are pastured with cattle, ridden into rangeland, or kept in paddocks

TABLE 2. RECOMMENDED INSECTICIDES FOR FLY CONTROL IN HORSE STABLES AND BARNS
(not for use on horses)

Insecticide and Manufacturer[1]	Concentration and Formulation[2]	Spray Mixture (%)	Remarks
Residual Surface Sprays (Long-Term Kill)			
28. Dimethoate (Cygon)—AC	23% EC	4 gal/100 gal water (1%)	Spray interior and exterior surfaces where flies rest. Apply to point of runoff (drip). Do not contaminate feed or water. Remove horses from buildings before spraying, and do not return them until spray has dried. Do not spray animals.
29. Fenthion (Baytex)	45% EC	3 gal/100 gal water (1%)	
30. Permethrin (Atroban)—BW	25% WP	1 pkg (189 gm)/5 gal water (0.25%)	
(Ectiban)—ICI	25% WP	6 oz/11 gal water (.125%)	
31. Stirofos (Rabon)—DS	24.3% EC	4 gal/100 gal water (1%)	
32. Stirofos (Rabon) + dichlorvos (Vapona)—DS "Ravap"	23% + 6% EC	1 gal/75 gal water (0.35% + 0.1%)	
Space Spray (Quick Knockdown)			
33. Dichlorvos (Vapona)—DS	23% EC	0.5 gal/25 gal water (0.5%)	Spray directly on resting flies or mist spray or fog in air where flies are numerous. Time applications to coincide with daily pattern of fly activity.
34. Naled (Dibrom)—CC	58% EC	20 oz/25 gal water (0.5%)	
35. Pyrethrins + piperonyl butoxide	0.1% solution	Ready to use	
Fly Baits			
36. Dichlorvos—BW	0.46% granules	Use as dry bait or liquid spray by mixing 1 lb/gal water.	Sprinkle dry on ground or on wet sacking. May use liquid applied to surfaces where flies rest.
37. Dichlorvos (Vapona) + ronnel (Korlan)—ZC	0.9% dichlorvos + 0.25% ronnel granules	Use as dry bait or liquid spray by mixing 1 lb/gal water.	
38. Methomyl (Lannate) + (z)-9-Triosene (Muscalure)—ZC	1% methomyl + 0.025% muscalure	Use as dry bait.	Sprinkle on ground at 0.25 lb/500 ft².

[1]AC = American Cyanamid Co.; BW = Burroughs Wellcome, Cooper Div.; CC = Chevron Chemical Co.; DS = Diamond Shamrock Corp.; ICI = Imperial Chemicals Industry, Ltd.; ZC = Zoecon Corp.
[2]EC = emulsifiable concentrate; WP = wettable powder

near cattle on pastures. This fly breeds in fresh cow feces, and the cycle from egg to adult takes 10 days in summer and 30 days in cool weather. Horn flies are easy to control with any pesticide. A light spray or sponge wash to the withers is sufficient rather than treatment of entire body areas (℞ 1,5–7, 11 or 13, Table 1).

FACE FLY

The face fly, *Musca autumnalis,* attacks horses that are pastured with cattle, kept near cattle on pasture, or ridden into rangeland areas. They breed only in fresh cow feces found on rangeland or pasture, and the life cycle takes eight days in summer and two to three weeks in cooler weather. This pest occurs in all states except those in the southwest and Alaska and Hawaii. The flies cause intense irritation when they feed on mucous secretions from the horse's mouth, nostrils, eyes, or from fresh

wounds caused by blood-sucking horse flies, gnats, horn flies, and ticks. The fly is a vector of eye worms, Thelazia sp, in eastern states. Face flies are difficult to control because they visit only for brief feeding periods. Stringy masks fixed to halters prevent flies from landing on the face. Chemical control requires daily application of pesticide wipe-ons, smears, or dusts to the face, muzzle, and around the eyes (℞ 1, 6, 9, 10, or 12, Table 1).

HORSE FLY

Horse flies are vicious biters because of their intermittent blood-feeding habits. Horses become nervous and are often unmanageable, and blood spots invite further attack by screwworm flies. Horse flies transmit equine infectious anemia and, because of their intermittent feeding habits, can physically transmit other blood diseases if the right circumstances exist. Horse flies lay eggs on plant leaves and moist soil around the edges of ponds and ditches. Larvae winter in muddy soil, and adults appear in summer to regenerate the next one-year cycle. Control of breeding sources is impractical. Individual animal treatments with repellent-type pesticides may protect horses for one to two days (℞ 10 or 12, Table 1).

BLOW FLIES

Blow flies lay eggs in necrotic tissue of wounds (castration, navels of newborns, afterbirths, or animal carcasses) and in garbage containing meat scraps. The black blow fly, *Phormia regina*, is more abundant during spring and fall and takes two to four weeks to cycle from egg to adult. Green blow flies, Phaenicia sp, are more prevalent during the summer and require one to two weeks for development from egg to adult. The adults may attack old wounds, but eggs also are deposited in dead carcasses, garbage, dead snails, pet droppings, and decayed fruit and vegetable wastes. Control of blow fly attack on animals is best achieved by repetitive treatment until wounds are thoroughly healed (℞ 14–16, Table 1). Collection and disposal of animal offal and carcasses and general ranch sanitation will help prevent breeding sources of these flies.

SCREWWORM FLY

The primary screwworm fly, *Cochliomyia hominivorax,* lays eggs in fresh wounds (navels of newborns, vulva, or cuts from nails, wire, or other objects). The Southwest Screwworm Eradication program, using mass releases of sterilized flies, has greatly reduced the damaging effects of this fly, and occasional attacks on domestic animals and wildlife are restricted to areas bordering Mexico. Fresh wounds should be treated with pesticide smears, aerosol sprays, or dusts to guard against fly attacks (℞ 14–16, Table 1).

BOT FLY

Bot flies include three species in North America, and most widespread is the common bot, *Gasterophilus intestinalis*. Adults are nearly the size of bees and have no functional mouth parts, and so they do not bite as is commonly believed. Adults are active from midsummer until the first frost. The activity of adults laying eggs on the hairs of horses causes animals to bunch, seek protection in dense shrubbery or in water, or to run in an erratic manner. Larval migration causes irritation in oral tissues and pus pockets in the gums. In the stomach, bots cause colic, occasional blockage of the pyloric valve, and, in rare instances, rupture of the stomach wall resulting in peritonitis. Eggs of *G. intestinalis* are glued to hairs on the lower body areas and legs, those of the nose bot, *G. hemorrhoidalis*, on the lips, and those of the throat bot fly, *G. nasalis*, under the jaw and throat. Moisture, warmth, and friction from licking eggs of the common bot stimulate larval hatch and subsequent ingestion, whereas larvae of the other two bot flies hatch without any stimulation and crawl into the mouth. All bot larvae spend from three to six weeks in the mucous membranes of gums and then migrate to the stomach. After 8 to 10 months, the older larvae move through the intestines and pass out in the droppings. They spend from one to two months on the ground before emerging in the summer or autumn. For external treatment of bot eggs, a warm water wash that contains a pesticide will stimulate hatching and kill the larvae (℞ 19–23, Table 1). For internal treatment, pesticide powders added to grain supplement are available, but if palatability is a factor with some horses, then paste formulations for injection into the oral cavity may be used (℞ 17 and 18, Table 1) (p. 283).

GNATS

Gnats belong to many different groups, but the more common blood-sucking types are the black flies (buffalo gnats or Simuliidae), biting midges (Leptoconops), and "no-see-ums" (Culicoides). These may be distributed from coastal plains to high mountainous areas. Adults attack various body areas, including the ears. Horses react by restless movement around paddocks, head tossing, ear flicking, tail switching, skin twitching, or by moving indoors, into water, into shrubbery, or under trees. Lesions caused by blood-sucking gnats ooze serum and form papules or blisters. Repeated attacks may cause a high level of sensitivity; intense skin wheals develop that later emit a discharge. On some animals, severe dermatitis with subsequent irritation results in hair loss from constant rubbing or biting of affected areas. Breeding sources include slow-moving water in streams, creeks, irrigation supplies, and drainage ditches (Simuliidae), muddy soil margins of ponds, ground pools (including hoof prints), tree holes, or liquid manure (*Culicoides*), and in dry cracks of adobe-like soil (*Leptoconops*). Control of these sources is difficult and not economically feasible. Daily application of repellents as sprays, wipe-ons, or smears offers some protection (℞ 8, 9, 10, or 12, Table 1). Keeping animals inside stables during the day or evening whenever certain gnats become more active is often effective, as is the application of ear nets.

MOSQUITOES

Mosquitoes are particularly important because they transmit viruses causing Western equine encephalomyelitis, Eastern equine encephalomyelitis, and Venezuelan equine encephalomyelitis (WEE, EEE, and VEE). Some species also cause papular skin reaction and severe dermatitis as a result of individual horse sensitivity to the bites. These disease vectors are widely distributed from sea level to 8000 ft elevation. Eggs are laid directly on water or on dry surfaces—on the ground, inside tree holes, or in man-made containers (cans, buckets, or rubber tires); eggs hatch when water later covers eggs laid in these dry areas. The cycle from egg to adult may require only one week during warm weather. Common breeding sources around horse stables are low spots in corrals and paddocks, large, infrequently used water troughs, irrigated pastures, drain ditches, flooded meadows, creeks, tree holes, containers, leaf-choked rain gutters, and poorly covered septic tanks and drains. Mosquito control largely depends on elimination of standing water; container disposal, rain gutter maintenance each spring, water troughs stocked with minnows (mosquito-fish), filling of low spots in corrals or paddocks, and weed control along ditch banks are some of the methods that help reduce mosquito breeding. Vaccines are available for all three viral diseases, and yearly vaccination is advised, depending on ranch location and the extent of interstate travel (p. 40). Daily application of repellent as sprays, wipe-ons, or smears offers some protection against mosquito attacks (℞ 9, 10, or 12, Table 1).

Supplemental Readings

1. Harwood, R. F., and James, M. T.: Entomology in Human and Animal Health. New York, Macmillan, 1979, 548 pp.
2. Loomis, E. C., Hughes, J. P., and Bramhall, E. L.: The Common Parasites of Horses. University of California Division of Agricultural Science, Bulletin 4006, 1975, 35 pp.

URTICARIA AND ANGIOEDEMA

Richard E. Halliwell, GAINESVILLE, FLORIDA

Both urticaria and angioedema result from release of histamine and other pharmacologic agents from blood basophils and tissue mast cells. The difference between the two conditions is merely the site and extent of the pathologic event. The conditions can affect horses of all ages, and no breed or sex incidence has been documented.

This condition most commonly arises from a type I allergic reaction but may also arise through a type III reaction or from the direct histamine-like activity or histamine-releasing activity of some insect saliva and snake venoms.

CLINICAL SIGNS

The classical clinical sign of both of these conditions is edema. In the case of urticaria, wheals of varying size are distributed randomly over the body surface. The degree of pruritus is variable.

Angioedema may also arise at any part of the body, but the edema fluid will gravitate ventrally. The head is most commonly affected.

DIAGNOSIS

The most important factor in establishing the diagnosis is that the edematous lesions pit on pressure. This is easily documented in the early stages, but in the more chronic cases, a cellular infiltrate follows, and the pitting edema is less apparent.

Dermatophytosis can mimic urticaria and can have an equally sudden onset. Edema is not a feature of the latter condition, and the hair readily epilates, leaving a circular area of crusty alopecia.

THERAPY

Nonspecific therapy is directed toward preventing further release of and combating the effects of histamine. Corticosteroids are the drugs of choice. In the acute case, dexamethasone may be given intravenously in a dosage of 10 to 20 mg. Alternatively, prednisone or prednisolone may be given orally at an initial dose of up to 600 mg daily.

All nonspecific therapy should be accompanied by a diligent search for the etiology. On the first occurence, this may be unrewarding, but in the recurrent case, a pattern may become established, which should facilitate in identification of the offending allergen(s). Despite the most diligent searches, a specific cause is only found in about 50 per cent of cases of recurrent urticaria or angioedema.

Attention should be given to any changes in hay

or concentrates or dietary supplements. Because it may take months or years to become sensitized to a dietary component, an allergic reaction need not necessarily be the result of a recent introduction. A sensible initial approach is to take the horse off all sweet feed and supplements. If the condition resolves, the diagnosis must be confirmed by exacerbation upon reintroduction of the offending item.

Drug allergy is also often implicated in the etiology of urticaria and angioedema. The potential exists for almost any drug to induce allergic reactions, and carrier vehicles may also do so. The most common offender is penicillin.

A search should also be made for concurrent internal disease, as urticaria is sometimes encountered in humans in association with infections and malignancies. The condition has been associated with a case of lymphosarcoma in the horse.

Snake bites ordinarily cause angioedema and may lead to tissue necrosis. The head and feet are the most commonly affected sites. If a snake bite is suspected, long-term therapy with corticosteroids is necessary, and other supportive therapy may be indicated.

Insect bites are uncommon causes of urticaria, although type I hypersensitivity is often readily demonstrable upon intradermal skin testing. This may be because the amount of histamine released upon the bite of an insect is insufficient to cause a visible wheal, although it may be sufficient to cause pruritus. Infestation with the straw itch mite (Pyemotes sp) can cause urticaria.

PAPILLOMATOSIS (WARTS)

Gordon H. Theilen, DAVIS, CALIFORNIA

Warts usually occur on the lips, muzzle, external nares, and legs of one- to three-year-old horses. There may be a few or as many as 100 or more. Growth occurs for four to eight weeks, and then in most horses, warts spontaneously regress.[9] Endemics have been described on some large breeding farms. Congenital cutaneous papillomatosis has been reported in foals ranging in age at the time of biopsy from one hour to five days.[1, 4, 6, 8] Congenital warts are not restricted to the muzzle. Most breeds and both sexes are involved in both traditional and congenital warts. Warts are caused by the equine papilloma virus (EPV).[2, 3]

CLINICOPATHOLOGIC ASPECTS

Following exposure to EPV under experimental conditions, the incubation period is about 60 days, with growth and regression of papillomas taking another 60 days. After the lesions mature, they become necrotic and usually disappear within one to two weeks. Warts probably persist and present a medical problem only in immune-deficient individuals. In such horses, however, warts may occur on parts other than the muzzle and often persist for one to two years or longer. Persistent warts are often multiple lesions of the ear or the legs. These locations are atypical for equine warts and may result from transfer of virus by brushes and combs or by rubbing the infected muzzle on the legs. Atypical warts may also be found in non–immune-suppressed horses.

When several papillomas of the muzzle exist together, they are small, measuring 2 to 10 mm in diameter. Occasionally, when only a few warts develop, they reach a diameter of 15 to 20 mm or larger. Equine warts rarely cause an economic problem or alter body function. Grossly, lesions are elevated, circumscribed, horny masses having fronds similar in appearance to a small cauliflower.

DIFFERENTIAL DIAGNOSIS

Verrucous-type sarcoids may be mistaken for warts.[9] These sarcoids begin as nonpigmented lesions, appear pinkish, and have a smooth surface. As they age, the epithelium becomes more pigmented and wartlike. They occur most frequently on the ears, eyelids, other areas of the head, and on the legs. Histologically, verrucous sarcoids are mainly fibroblastic cells and are fibromatous tumors. Sarcoids are seen at any age in the horse, but in the United States they are seen more frequently in saddle-type and not so frequently in running horses. Experimentally, bovine papilloma virus (BPV) injected into the equine epidermis will induce sarcoid-like lesions.[5, 7]

PREVENTION AND CONTROL

Theoretically, susceptible horses could be vaccinated against warts using a vaccine similar to that for cattle but prepared from equine wart material. An equine wart vaccine is unnecessary because of the few endemic situations and rapid regression of most warts. There is little health problem associated with equine papillomas; hence, control measures have rarely been attempted. Contaminated fomites such as curry combs, brushes, and surgical instruments are believed to be a main source of spread.

THERAPY

Cryosurgery by freezing the warts to −20°C or hyperthermia, heating the warts to 42 to 44°C for 20 minutes or to 50°C for 30 seconds, is usually curative. An autogenous vaccine can be made to treat horses with persistently active warts. A homogenate of tissue is diluted 1:10 in saline and is filtered through gauze. The final solution is centrifuged at 300 rpm for 5 minutes. Formaldehyde is added to the supernatant fluid to a final concentration of 0.5 per cent formaldehyde. The vaccine can be stored for up to two to four weeks at 4°C until used. Two ml is injected intradermally at 14-day intervals for three to four injections.

References

1. Atwell, R. B., and Summers, P. M.: Congenital papilloma in a foal. Aust. Vet. J., 53:299, 1977.
2. Cook, R. H., and Olson, C.: Experimental transmission of cutaneous papilloma of the horse. Am. J. Pathol., 27:1087, 1951.
3. Fulton, R. E., Doane, F. W., and MacPherson, L. W.: The fine structure of equine papillomas and the equine papilloma virus. J. Ultrastruct. Res., 30:328, 1970.
4. Garma-Avina, A., Valli, V. E., and Lumsden, J. H.: Equine congenital cutaneous papillomatosis: A report of 5 cases. Equine Vet. J., 13:59, 1981.
5. Lancaster, W. D., Theilen, G. H., and Olson, C.: Equine sarcoid: Evidence for a bovine papilloma virus etiology. Intervirology, 11:227, 1979.
6. Njoko, C. O., and Burwash, W. A.: Congenital cutaneous papilloma in a foal. Cornell Vet., 62:54, 1972.
7. Olson, C., Jr., and Cook, R. H.: Cutaneous sarcoma-like lesions of the horse caused by the agent of bovine papilloma. Proc. Soc. Exp. Biol. Med., 77:281, 1951.
8. Schueler, R. L.: Congenital equine papillomatosis. J. Am. Vet. Med. Assoc., 162:640, 1977.
9. Theilen, G. H., and Madewell, B. R.: Equine papillomatosis. *In* Theilen, G. H., and Madewell, B. R. (eds.): Veterinary Cancer Medicine. Philadelphia, Lea and Febiger, 1979, p. 151.

SURGICAL TREATMENT OF EQUINE SARCOID

Murray P. Brown, GAINESVILLE, FLORIDA

Sarcoids are the most common skin tumors occurring in horses, donkeys, and mules.[5] There is no apparent disease predilection for sex, age, breed, coat color, or season.[8] The most common sites are the head (ears, eyelids, and commissures of the mouth), legs, and ventral abdomen. The tumors may be single or multiple.

Sarcoids are classified as either verrucous (warty) or fibroblastic (proud flesh) or a combination of the two types. They may be broad-based (sessile) or pedunculated.[5]

Verrucous sarcoids have a dry, horny, cauliflower-like surface and are usually less than 6 cm in diameter. Some are very flat and consist of a sharply bordered area of slightly thickened skin with a mildly roughened surface and are partially or completely devoid of hair. Verrucous sarcoids that have been traumatized frequently transform into the fibroblastic type.

The fibroblastic type is a firm, fibrous nodule within the dermis. The overlying epidermis is usually ulcerated. It is sessile or pedunculated and may exceed 20 cm in diameter.

Sarcoids are thought to be viral in origin. The relationship between bovine papilloma virus (BPV) and equine sarcoids is still uncertain. Growth rates of sarcoids are highly variable. After its initial appearance, a sarcoid may remain static for years and then suddenly may exhibit very rapid growth. In other cases, particularly with the fibroblastic type, growth may be rapid and aggressive from the beginning.

Sarcoids are locally invasive, and it may be impossible to identify the junction of the sarcoid with the surrounding tissues. This presents a surgical problem in that it is difficult to know if the tumor has been completely resected. Incomplete resection may possibly account for the high rate of recurrence, which may approach 50 per cent following surgery. Sarcoids do not metastasize, but the animal may possibly autotransplant the tumor in other areas of normal skin by biting or rubbing the lesion. Although spontaneous regression may occur, this is not frequently observed.

Other skin lesions that must be differentiated from fibroblastic sarcoids are granulation tissue, cutaneous habronemiasis, squamous cell carcinoma, phycomycosis, and fibroma. Small sessile verrucous sarcoids on the nose or lips may be mistaken for equine papillomas. The very flat verrucous type with partial or complete hair loss and a roughened surface must be distinguished from dermatophytosis. Neurofibromas (schwannomas) involving the eyelids closely resemble sarcoids but usually have a lower incidence of recurrence following excision.

Histologic examination is necessary for a definitive diagnosis. Nevertheless, efforts to obtain biopsy material, short of complete excision of the tumor, are not recommended because such an insult may increase the growth rate and aggressiveness of an inactive sarcoid.

THERAPY

Many forms of treatment have been described for equine sarcoids. Unfortunately, it is very difficult to compare the efficacy of different therapeutic regimens because well-controlled studies have not been done. In my experience, consistent results have not been obtained with any form of treatment. Two factors may account for this: (1) variability in technique and (2) aggressiveness of the tumor being treated.

SURGICAL RESECTION

Wide surgical resection of the sarcoid, including a 0.5 to 1.0 cm margin of normal tissue, is occasionally successful in cases in which the limits of the tumor are well defined and in which there is an abundance of normal tissue to allow liberal dissection. Closure of the wound in such cases may result in primary healing. However, the tendency for sarcoids to develop in areas lacking surplus skin does not often provide the opportunity for this form of management. Since autotransplantation may occur, it must be remembered that instruments that contact the tumor should not be used on the normal adjacent skin.

At present, surgical treatment is usually combined with other forms of therapy. Resection by electroscalpel, followed by electrocautery of the tumor bed, usually gives better results than scalpel dissection alone. The topical application of cytotoxic agents, such as 5-fluorouracil* or podophyllin,† can be combined with surgery. In cases in which surgery is not feasible for anatomic or economic reasons and the sarcoid is relatively small, the application of one of these agents to the sarcoid may cause regression. My experience, however, has not shown either one of these drugs to be a reliable means of treatment.

There are no good controlled studies to indicate that autogenous sarcoid vaccines are effective. If improperly prepared, the vaccine may produce tumor growth at each vaccination site.

HYPERTHERMIA

The application of hyperthermia to very small sarcoids and to sarcoid beds following surgical resection has been moderately successful. Hyperthermia of large tumor beds can become a relatively long procedure because of the small surface area covered ($1 \text{ cm}^2 \times 3$ to 4 mm deep) by each application of the hyperthermia electrode.* The need for many tedious systematic applications of the electrode to cover large beds also presents the possibility that some portions of the bed may be inadequately treated or missed completely.

RADIATION

Gamma radiation in the form of cesium or iridium implants has yielded good results in sarcoids located in the eyelids. For best results, the tumor should be surgically debulked before the radiation source is implanted. Although this form of treatment usually results in fewer lid deformities than cryosurgery, fibrous thickening of the eyelids following iridium therapy has been observed. The irradiation hazard to the therapist in this form of treatment must always be weighed against the potential therapeutic benefits to the patient. Irradiation therapy must be performed by a qualified radiologist.

CRYOSURGERY

Cryosurgery has produced the most consistent results in sarcoid therapy.[1-3] The mechanisms of cryonecrosis are well documented[7] and should be understood before cryosurgery is performed. This procedure can be done using xylazine tranquilization (local anesthesia is usually unnecessary) or general anesthesia, depending on the size and location of the sarcoid and temperament of the animal. Prior to freezing the tumor, hair and debris should be removed from the area to reduce contamination and to increase coolant contact with the sarcoid. Liquid nitrogen is the most commonly used cryogen and is applied as a spray or with a cryoprobe.† If spray application is used, it may be necessary to protect adjacent structures from freezing by placing styro-

---

*Efudex, Roche Labs, Nutley, NJ 07110
†Verrex, C&M Pharmacal, Hazel Park, MI 48030

*Model RF-22A Thermoprobe, Hach Chemical Co., Loveland, CO 80537
†CS-76, Frigitronics of Connecticut, Inc., Shelton, CT 06484

foam, dense cardboard, or petrolatum-coated gauze around the sarcoid. Some prefer not to use such insulators because the cryogen may run under the insulator and cause unwanted freezing of the surrounding skin without the operator's awareness.[1] It is recommended that the lesion be frozen at least twice to a temperature of $-20°$ C for adequate cellular destruction and tissue necrosis. Freezing three times to $-30°$ C has been reported to increase the rate of success.[1] After each freezing, the tissue should be allowed to thaw at room temperature without additional warming aids.

It is strongly recommended that tissue temperatures attained during cryosurgery be monitored by inserting thermocouple needles 0.5 cm from the tumor margin and 0.5 cm below the base of the tumor. Such monitoring is extremely critical when freezing around such structures as the eyes, tendons, and ligaments. Eyelid deformities and corneal damage may result from overzealous freezing of periocular tumors. Chronic lameness and draining tracts have been observed following cryonecrosis of collateral ligaments.

Sarcoids larger than 5 cm in diameter are usually more effectively managed by surgical resection followed by freezing of the tumor bed. If surgical resection is done prior to freezing, some hemorrhage should be expected after thawing occurs.

Following cryosurgery, the lesion will become edematous with some serosanguineous discharge. Within a few days, lesions located in the skin become encrusted and may have a leathery appearance. As the mass begins to separate from the surrounding tissue, there may be some discharge. Cryonecrosis at a mucocutaneous junction often results in considerable purulent discharge. Clients should be warned that the sloughing tissue may have a bad odor. Sloughing and secondary intention healing may require three to eight weeks, depending on the size of the lesion. Self-mutilation is not usually a problem. Although bandaging is not recommended following cryosurgery, fly protection should be provided when necessary. Following healing, depigmentation of hair at the site of cryosurgery should be expected.

References

1. Fretz, P. B., and Barber, S.: Prospective analysis of cryosurgery as the sole treatment for equine sarcoids. Vet. Clin. North Am. (Small Anim. Pract.), *10*:847, 1980.
2. Joyce, J. R.: Cryosurgical treatment of tumors of horses and cattle. J. Am. Vet. Med. Assoc., *168*:226, 1976.
3. Lane, J. G.: The treatment of equine sarcoids by cryosurgery. Equine Vet. J., *9*:127, 1977.
4. Murray, D. E., Ladds, P. W., and Campbell, R. S. F.: Granulomatous and neoplastic diseases of the skin of horses. Aust. Vet. J., *54*:338, 1978.
5. Ragland, W. L., Keown, G. H., and Spencer, G. R.: Equine sarcoid. Equine Vet. J., *2*:2, 1970.
6. Roberts, W. D.: Experimental treatment of equine sarcoid. VM SAC., *65*:67, 1970.
7. Seim, H. B.: Mechanisms of cold-induced cellular death. Vet. Clin. North Am. (Small Anim. Pract.), *10*:755, 1980.
8. Stannard, A. J., and Pulley, L. T.: Equine sarcoid. *In* Moulton, J. E. (ed.): Tumors in Domestic Animals, 2nd ed. Berkeley, University of California Press, 1978, pp. 18–22.

BCG THERAPY FOR EQUINE SARCOID

Donald D. Flemming, DAVIS, CALIFORNIA

Bacillus Calmette-Guérin (BCG) is an attenuated strain of *Mycobacterium bovis* used as a vaccine against tuberculosis. BCG is a potent reticuloendothelial stimulant that has been used extensively in cancer chemotherapy. Both reconstituted commercial BCG vaccine[5] and a modified cell wall preparation in oil[2] have been used successfully in the treatment of equine sarcoid.

Several factors affect the success of BCG as an anticancer agent:[1] (1) Tumor size is a primary factor, BCG therapy being most effective against small, well-localized primary tumors, such as equine sarcoids. (2) Adequate dose is important, but this has not been established in horses. (3) Close association between the BCG vaccine and the tumor cells is a factor ensured by injecting BCG into the lesion. (4) The ability of the patient to react by generating an immune response to the BCG antigens is a factor that has not been investigated in horses, but in humans, the ability to react is shown by a positive tuberculin test. (5) The ability of the host to generate an immune response to tumor-specific antigens may constitute a major factor in the success of BCG anticancer therapy. Tumor-specific antigens have been demonstrated in equine sarcoid.[3]

The upper limit in the size of lesions that can be expected to respond to BCG treatment has not been determined, but lesions up to 6 cm have been treated successfully. Lesions of any size, but especially those greater than 6 cm in any one dimension, should, if possible, be reduced in mass by surgical excision to the level of the surrounding normal skin. When using the cell wall BCG preparation, vigorous cleansing of the area with materials such as povidone-iodine is not recommended prior to the injection of the vaccine, as this may cause disruption of the cell wall emulsion.

When using the reconstituted vaccine,* multiple injections should be made into the base of the tumor until a total of 1 ml (4.9 × 10⁶ viable bacilli) of vaccine has been administered. These injections should be repeated every two weeks if needed for regression of the tumor. The greatest number of treatments so far reported has been four. Treatments in excess of this number may or may not be necessary and should be used with caution.

The dosage of the modified cell wall preparation† is based on the surface area of the tumor remaining after surgical debulking. The vaccine is administered by multiple injections into the lesion until 0.0090 ml per mm^2 surface area has been given. This is repeated after one week. Subsequent injections are determined by the tissue reaction. If the reaction is mild, then the dates of injection are determined by adding one week to the number of the most recent injection. For example, if the most recent injection was the second, the next injection would be in three weeks. If the reaction is severe, treatments should be given a minimum of four weeks apart. As with the reconstituted vaccine, a maximum of four treatments has been reported sufficient for remissions. Treatments beyond this number should be performed with caution.

General anesthesia is not usually required for the administration of BCG vaccine. Sedation with xylazine‡ is generally all that is necessary. Local anesthetic blocks are not required. The vaccine should be given slowly and carefully, as there are frequently channels within necrotic tissue that will allow easy passage to the surface, resulting in loss of the vaccine.

---

*BCG vaccine, N. F. Glaxo Labs, Ltd., Greenford, Middlesex, England; distributed by Eli Lilly and Co., Indianapolis, IN 46225

†BCG vaccine, Elars Bioresearch Labs, Fort Collins, CO 80526

‡Rompun, Bayvet-Cutter Labs, Shawnee, KS 66201

Inflammatory reactions are common with intralesional BCG therapy. These are most often seen between 3 and 10 days post-treatment but may occur almost immediately. The tissue reaction may lead to edema, necrosis, and copious discharge. The horse's owner should be forewarned that the lesions will generally look much worse before improvement occurs. Complete remission may not occur for several months after treatment ceases.

Adverse reactions to the modified cell wall preparation have not been reported. There is, however, one report of two anaphylactic deaths in horses following the second treatment with the reconstituted commercial BCG vaccine.[4] If this product is used, pretreatment 30 minutes prior to the injection with antiprostaglandins (flunixin meglumine, 1 mg per kg intravenously)* and steroids (prednisolone, 2 mg per kg intramuscularly)† is recommended. It is suggested that horses be observed for 30 minutes post-injection, and drugs for treatment of anaphylaxis should be readily available.

Treatments with either of the currently available BCG vaccines are complex and require multiple visits but will result in generally high rates of remission with no recurrences for up to 18 months in successful cases. Time spent on client education relating to equine sarcoid and its treatment and prognosis is usually time well spent.

References

1. Bast, R. C., Zbar, B., Borsos, T., and Rapp, H. J.: BCG and cancer. N. Eng. J. Med., *290*:1413, 1974.
2. Murphy, J. M., Severin, G. A., Lavach, J. D., Helper, D. I., and Leuker, D. C.: Immunotherapy in ocular equine sarcoid. J. Am. Vet. Med. Assoc., *174*:269, 1979.
3. Watson, R. E., and Larson, K. A.: Detection of tumor-specific antigens in an equine sarcoid cell line. Am. J. Vet. Res., *34*:1601, 1973.
4. Winston, T., Rings, M., and Wyman, M.: Treatment of equine sarcoids (letter). J. Am. Vet. Med. Assoc., *174*:775, 1979.
5. Wyman, M., Rings, M. D., Tarr, M. J., and Alden, C. L.: Immunotherapy in equine sarcoid: A report of two cases. J. Am. Vet. Med. Assoc., *171*:449, 1977.

---

*Banamine, Schering Corp., Kenilworth, NJ 07033

†Solu-Delta-Cortef, The Upjohn Co., Kalamazoo, MI 49001

PEMPHIGUS FOLIACEUS

Thomas O. Manning, ITHACA, NEW YORK

Pemphigus foliaceus is an autoimmune bullous skin disorder. The age of onset varies widely, and the condition may occur in horses as young as six months. The disease often begins on the ventral half of the body and gradually extends to the entire body surface; acute generalized eruptions are seen. Pemphigus foliaceus is characterized by flaccid bullae, epidermal collarettes, erosions, oozing, and crusting. In advanced stages, bullae are few and may be absent, so that the resemblance to a generalized exfoliative dermatitis is great. Pain, occasional pruritus, depression, ventral pitting edema, and pyrexia may be reported. Oral lesions are extremely rare.

The diagnosis of pemphigus foliaceus is made on the basis of physical examination, histopathologic examination of skin biopsy specimens, and immunofluorescence studies of skin and sera. The earliest histopathologic change is acantholysis within the upper epidermis, leading to cleft formation in the superficial epidermis. Immunofluorescence tests on patient skin (direct) or serum (indirect) may demonstrate the presence of an autoantibody (usually IgG), with or without complement, directed against an intercellular antigen of the epidermis.

THERAPY

Prior to the initiation of therapy, a complete physical examination and clinical pathology work-up are important in assessing the patient's present state of health, prognosis, and baseline information to determine future responses to medication.

Therapy of pemphigus foliaceus consists of large doses of glucocorticoids and the concurrent use of other immunosuppressive drugs when glucocorticoids are ineffective or intolerable. Initially, cases should be treated with oral prednisolone, 2 mg per kg per day. Improvement should be noted within 10 days. Daily medication should be continued until all signs of active disease disappear. Once the active lesions have subsided, full body clipping and shampooing will dramatically improve the appearance and general attitude of the horse. Once the disease is in remission, the dose of corticosteroids is gradually reduced until the minimal daily maintenance dose is established. This should be followed by alternate-morning steroid therapy with prednisolone or prednisone, the goal of maintenance therapy being control of the disease with alternate-day therapy using as low a dose of steroid as possible. After two to three months, the dose of steroids can be further reduced by 5 mg every other day until the maintenance dose of 0.5 mg per kg on alternate days is reached.

There are no objective criteria to determine when treatment can be stopped or reduced. Immunofluorescence studies, direct or indirect, are not consistent with the horse's therapeutic response and, therefore, are not applicable to the therapeutic management of the disease. The incidence of naturally occurring remission of equine pemphigus foliaceus is not known. In human cases of pemphigus foliaceus, steroid-induced drug-free remissions are reported to occur infrequently. Thus, steroid therapy is continued for life.

It is the opinion of this author that a combination of corticosteroids and gold may be the preferred method of control for pemphigus foliaceus in the horse. Clinical experience in the use of immunosuppressive drugs to treat autoimmune diseases in the horse, however, is limited. Gold (aurothioglucose)* may be given from the initiation of steroid therapy or may be added after two to four weeks when alternate-day steroid treatment begins. Aurothioglucose should be administered intramuscularly (1 mg per kg) at weekly intervals. Prior to therapy, test doses of 20 and 50 mg are given at weekly intervals. It is strongly recommended that therapy be monitored by weekly physical examination, hemogram, urinalysis, and measurements of blood urea nitrogen, creatinine, serum glutamic oxaloacetic transaminase, and sorbitol dehydrogenase. When remission of signs has been achieved, after approximately six to eight weeks, all steroids are stopped. The therapeutic dose of aurothioglucose is decreased in frequency to bimonthly and then monthly injections. It may be advisable to inject the large therapeutic doses of aurothioglucose in multiple intramuscular sites.

Complications of gold therapy have been reported in humans but not in the horse. Toxicity most frequently develops during the initial course of gold therapy. Toxic reactions developing during maintenance therapy are rare. The toxic side effects of gold compounds are listed on all package inserts, the most common being stomatitis and dermatitis. Complications are not usually severe and may not recur if gold therapy is cautiously resumed after the adverse reaction has subsided. One must remember, however, that this is an experimental treatment in the horse and is not an approved therapy.

As in corticosteroid therapy, there are no objective criteria for cessation of treatment. Response to treatment varies with each patient. Currently, the only reliable way of assessing disease activity is routine observation of clinical signs.

---

*Solganol, Aurothioglucose, Schering Corp., Kenilworth, NJ 07033

Supplemental Readings

1. Johnson, M. E., Scott, D. W., Smith, V. A., Smith, C. A., and Lewis, R. M.: Pemphigus foliaceus in the horse. Equine Pract., 3(2):40, 1981.
2. Manning, T. O., Scott, D. W., Kruth, S. A., Sozanski, M., and Lewis, R. M.: Three cases of canine pemphigus foli-
3. aceus and observations on chrysotherapy. J.A.A.H.A., 16(2): 189, 1980.
4. Manning, T. O., Scott, D. W., Rebhun, W. C., Smith, C. A., and Lewis, R. M.: Pemphigus–bullous pemphigoid in a horse. Equine Pract., 3(5):38, 1981.
5. Power, H. T., McEvoy, E. O., and Manning, T. O.: Use of a gold compound for treatment of pemphigus foliaceus in a foal. J. Am. Vet. Med. Assoc., 180:400, 1982.

FOLLICULITIS AND FURUNCULOSIS

Danny W. Scott, ITHACA, NEW YORK

Folliculitis is inflammation of hair follicles. When the inflammatory process breaks through the hair follicles and extends into the surrounding dermis and subcutis, the process is called furunculosis. When multiple areas of furunculosis coalesce, the resultant focal area of induration and fistulous tracts is called a carbuncle ("boil").

Inflammatory disease of the hair follicles is common in the horse and is multifactorial in etiology. Etiologic agents associated with equine folliculitis and furunculosis include bacteria (especially *Staphylococcus aureus* and *Dermatophilus congolensis*), fungi (especially Trichophyton and Microsporum sp), and parasites (*Demodex equi* and *Pelodera strongyloides*). Important predisposing factors include mechanical trauma from tack and biting insects; heat and moisture (hot, humid weather; rain; heavy work and exercise); and poor sanitation.

The primary skin lesion of equine folliculitis is a follicular papule. Pustules are rarely seen. Frequently, one first notices erect hairs over a 2 to 3 mm papule that is more easily felt than seen. These lesions occasionally will spontaneously regress but usually progressively enlarge. Some lesions will enlarge to 6 to 10 mm in diameter, develop a central ulcer that may discharge a serosanguineous material, then become encrusted. The chronic or healing phase is characterized by progressive flattening of the lesion and a static or gradually expanding circular area of alopecia and scaling. Hairs at the periphery of these lesions are often easily epilated.

Some lesions will progress to furunculosis. This stage is characterized by varying combinations of nodules, draining tracts, ulcers, and crusts. Large lesions are often associated with severe inflammatory edema and may assume an edematous plaque or urticarial appearance. Scarring, leukoderma, and leukotrichia may follow. Uncommonly, an urticarial eruption will precede the follicular dermatosis by 24 to 48 hours. This may be seen with dermatophytosis and staphylococcosis.

Although folliculitis and furunculosis can affect any and all hairy areas of skin, the predisposed areas are those under the saddle and tack, the neck, the dorsal lumbosacral region, and the posterior aspect of the pastern. Pruritus and pain are variable. Pruritus is more commonly seen with dermatophytosis, while pain is more commonly associated with staphylococcosis and dermatophilosis.

The diagnosis of equine folliculitis and furunculosis is usually made on the basis of some combination of history, physical examination, skin scrapings, direct smears of exudative material or macerated crusts, KOH preparations, fungal culture, bacterial culture, and skin biopsy. Staphylococcosis often begins in spring and early summer, dermatophytosis in fall and winter, and dermatophilosis in the rainy season. Evidence of contagion may suggest dermatophytosis or dermatophilosis.

Physical examination may assist in the differential diagnosis, as staphylococcosis and dermatophytosis tend to involve the saddle and tack areas first, while dermatophilosis tends to involve the dorsal lumbosacral region. However, "atypical" forms of each disease are not uncommon, so physical examination never excludes any of the etiologic possibilities. It is extremely important to remember that in the chronic or healing stage, all of these disorders are often characterized by circular areas of alopecia and scaling (so-called classic ringworm lesions).

Microscopic examination of crusts is extremely helpful in equine dermatoses. Crusts may be macerated in sterile water or saline, stained and examined, or fixed in 10 per cent formalin and processed for histologic examination. Dermatophytosis and dermatophilosis are often diagnosed in this manner. Other laboratory tests are discussed later.

BACTERIAL SKIN INFECTION

Bacterial infection (acne, heat rash, summer rash, summer scab, sweating eczema of the saddle region, saddle scab, and saddle boils) accounts for about one third of the cases of equine folliculitis and furunculosis. No age, breed, or sex predilections are evident. About 90 per cent of the cases begin in spring and early summer. This period coincides with shedding, heavy riding and work schedules, higher environmental temperature and humidity, and increased insect population densities. Poorly groomed horses may be at risk.

Skin lesions initially affect the saddle and tack areas in about 90 per cent of the cases. The lesions are painful in up to 70 per cent of the cases, rendering the horse unfit for riding or work, but are rarely pruritic. No evidence of contagion to humans or other animals has been seen. Whether or not immunity develops is unclear, but cases of chronically recurrent lesions are well known.

Very little information is available concerning the normal cutaneous bacterial flora of the horse. Micrococcus sp, coagulase-negative Staphylococcus sp, nonhemolytic streptococci, Bacillus sp, Corynebacterium sp, Flavobacterium sp, and Nocardia sp appear to be common isolates from normal horse skin (Table 1). Bacteriophage typing on 68 strains of coagulase-positive *Staphylococcus aureus* isolated from the nostrils, tonsils, and intestinal contents of healthy horses and from pathogenic materials (suppurative lesions) revealed that 31 strains (45.6 per cent) were biotype E, 27 strains (39.7 per cent) were biotype C, 8 strains (11.8 per cent) were biotype B, and 2 strains (2.9 per cent) were biotype A.

The most common bacterial agent (excluding *Dermatophilus congolensis*) isolated from cases of folliculitis is *Staphylococcus aureus*, with *Corynebacterium pseudotuberculosis* (Canadian horsepox) and streptococci being rare. As pustules are rarely seen, bacterial culture involves surgical preparation and removal of an intact follicular papule and culture of the tissue. To date, all *S. aureus* isolates have showed in vitro sensitivity to penicillin, tetracycline, chloramphenicol, ampicillin, erythromycin, lincomycin, kanamycin, and gentamicin. Skin biopsy reveals varying degrees of folliculitis and furunculosis, with extensive tissue eosinophilia and collagenolysis often accompanying furunculosis, and bacteria visible within the tissue reaction in 30 per cent of the specimens.

THERAPY

Therapy of bacterial skin infection varies with the severity and stage of the disease. Mild cases of folliculitis may resolve spontaneously. More severe

TABLE 1. BACTERIA AND FUNGI ISOLATED FROM THE SKIN OF NORMAL HORSES

Bacteria	Fungi
Micrococcus	Alternaria
Bacillus	Aspergillus
Corynebacterium	Hormodendrum
Coagulase-negative Staphylococcus	Penicillium
Nonhemolytic Streptococcus	Fusarium
Flavobacterium	Monotospora
Nocardia	Diplosporium
	Paecilomyces
	Scopulariopsis

From a qualitative study conducted by D. W. Scott and J. Bentinck-Smith at the New York State College of Veterinary Medicine. Cultures performed on hair and skin scrapings from three different areas (neck, thorax, and rump) from each of four normal horses.

cases of folliculitis require topical antibacterial therapy. Iodophors*† or chlorhexidine‡ are applied daily for five to seven days, then twice weekly until the dermatosis is resolved. Cases progressing to furunculosis require systemic antibiotics (such as procaine penicillin G, 22,000 IU per kg intramuscularly twice daily for 7 to 10 days) in addition to topical therapy. Resting the horse until the dermatosis is resolved is advised. Healing is usually complete within two to four weeks. It has been reported that daily iodophor shampoos, before and after work, are an effective preventive measure in horses with recurrent staphylococcosis.

DERMATOPHYTOSIS

Dermatophytosis (dermatomycosis, ringworm, tinea, girth itch, or jockey itch) is common in horses and accounts for about one third of the cases of equine folliculitis and furunculosis. No breed or sex predilections are known. Young animals are more susceptible, but any age group may be affected. The increased susceptibility of the young horse is probably not due to age per se, but reflects a lack of previous exposure. Adult horses can be reinfected, but reinfections are usually less severe and are of shorter duration.

The incubation period for experimental and naturally occurring equine dermatophytosis is 4 to 30 days. About 70 per cent of the cases begin in fall and winter. This period coincides with close housing, a paucity of sunshine, and resultant crowded, dark, damp, and dirty environments. Some authors have noticed an increased incidence of equine der-

*Betadine, Purdue Frederick, Norwalk, CT 06856
†Weladol, Pitman-Moore, Washington Crossing, NJ 08560
‡Nolvasan, Fort Dodge Labs, Fort Dodge, IA 50501

matophytosis with wet, warm weather and a resultant increased insect population.

Skin lesions initially affect the saddle and tack areas in about 90 per cent of the cases. Lesions may be limited to the pastern region (scratches or grease heel) and may wax and wane (analogous to "athlete's foot" in humans) with stress, local irritation, moisture, and filth. Dermatophytosis may also present as multifocal or generalized scaling (seborrhea sicca) without significant alopecia. The lesions are pruritic in about 33 per cent of the cases and may be painful in up to 20 per cent of the cases. The zoonotic importance of equine dermatophytosis is disputed.

The most common fungi associated with equine dermatophytosis are *Trichophyton equinum, T. mentagrophytes, T. verrucosum, Microsporum gypseum,* and *M. canis.* Other rarely isolated dermatophytes include *Keratinomyces ajelloi, T. terrestre, T. schoenleini, T. tonsurans, M. equinum,* and *M. cookei.*

DIAGNOSIS

Wood's light examination is rarely positive in the horse. Potassium hydroxide preparations may be quite useful in the hands of experienced personnel but are less than rewarding for the average clinician. Fungal culture is the most reliable method for definitive diagnosis but is difficult to perform and interpret. It is extremely important to adequately prepare equine skin before attempting to culture for fungi. An area of stubbled hairs and crusts should be gently cleansed with a nonantiseptic soap and water and should be rinsed and allowed to air dry. This is done to reduce the tremendous numbers of saprophytic fungi that populate normal equine skin (Table 1) and that tend to overgrow both the culture plates and any pathogen that may be present. When using Dermatophyte Testing Medium (DTM), pathogenic fungi will cause the red color change to occur at the same time that their initial white colony growth is seen (usually three to seven days). It has been recommended that one to two drops of a sterile, injectable B complex vitamin preparation be added to culture plates, as one strain of *T. equinum (T. equinum,* var. *equinum)* has a unique nicotinic acid requirement. Skin biopsy reveals varying degrees of folliculitis and furunculosis, with fungi demonstrable in 67 per cent of the culturally positive cases.

THERAPY

Dermatophytosis is usually a self-limiting disease, with spontaneous remission occurring in one to three months even without therapy. Thus, treat-

ment is usually directed at shortening the course and severity of the disease, preventing contagion to other animals and humans, and reducing environmental contamination. To this end, topical fungicides are all that is indicated in the specific therapy of equine dermatophytosis. Topical fungicides of choice include 3 per cent captan*, 2 to 5 per cent lime sulfur†, iodophors, and 0.5 per cent sodium hypochlorite.‡ Captan is the least irritating but must be applied while wearing protective gloves, as it is a contact sensitizer in humans. Lime sulfur is drying, rarely irritating, and smelly, and stains skin, the hair coat, and jewelry. Iodophors are expensive, staining, and may be irritating. Topical fungicides should be applied as total body dips once daily for five to seven days, then twice weekly until the dermatosis is resolved (two to four weeks). Good nutrition and plenty of fresh air and sunshine are beneficial.

Although oral griseofulvin§ has been recommended for the treatment of equine dermatophytosis (10 mg per kg once daily for 7 to 10 days; 6.25 to 12.5 gm in a quart of milk via a stomach tube; repeat in 7 to 10 days), there is no evidence that this product is effective, nor is there any indication that vitamin and mineral preparations are of any benefit.

As viable fungal elements may persist on fomites and in the environment for over a year, fungicidal treatment of tack, blankets, grooming utensils, and stalls is indicated. Formaldehyde and lime sulfur are most effective.

DEMODICOSIS

Demodicosis (demodectic mange, follicular mange) is an extremely rare dermatosis in the horse. No age, breed, or sex predilections have been reported. Although some authors have suggested that poor nutrition and other stresses are predisposing factors, most reported cases have involved healthy, well-cared-for horses. Most cases have occurred during the warm weather.

Two species of demodicid mites occur in normal equine skin. *Demodex folliculorum,* var. *equi,* inhabits the pilosebaceous apparatus of the eyelids and muzzle, and *D. equi* inhabits the rest of the body skin. Only *D. equi* has been linked with skin disease.

Skin lesions most commonly occur over the withers, thorax, and neck but may involve the face and

*Orthocide, Ortho Products, Div. of Chevron Chemical Co., San Francisco, CA 94119
†Orthorix, Ortho Products, Div. of Chevron Chemical Co., San Francisco, CA 94119
‡Clorox, Clorox Co., Oakland, CA 94612
§Fulvicin, Schering Corp., Kenilworth, NJ 07033

ears and any other area of the body. Pruritus and secondary pyoderma may occur. Demodicosis is not contagious.

Diagnosis is based on skin scrapings or skin biopsy or both. As with any other animal species, the demodicid mites should be demonstrated in large numbers before they are credited with a disease process.

To date, no therapeutic agents have been shown to have any clearly beneficial effect in equine demodicosis. Anecdotal successes have been obtained with topical lime sulfur, rotenone, lindane, and organophosphates. Some cases have been reported to undergo spontaneous remission.

Supplemental Readings

1. Bennison, J. C.: Demodicosis of horses with particular reference to equine members of the genus Demodex. J. R. Army Vet. Corps, *14*:34, 66, 1943.

2. Blood, D. C., and Henderson, J. A.: Veterinary Medicine IV. Baltimore, Williams & Wilkins Co., 1974.
3. Hutyra, F., and Marek, J.: Special Pathology and Therapeutics of the Diseases of Domestic Animals III. Chicago, Alexander Eger, 1926.
4. Jungerman, P. F., and Schwartzman, R. M.: Veterinary Medical Mycology. Philadelphia, Lea & Febiger, 1972.
5. Pascoe, R. R.: The nature and treatment of skin conditions observed in horses in Queensland. Aust. Vet. J., *49*:35, 1973.
6. Pascoe, R. R.: Equine dermatoses. Vet. Rev., No. 14. University of Sydney Post-Graduate Foundation in Veterinary Science, Sydney, Australia, 1974.
7. Pascoe, R. R.: The epidemiology of ringworm in racehorses caused by *Trichophyton equinum var autotrophicum*. Aust. Vet. J., *55*:403, 1979.
8. Scott, D. W., and Manning, T. O.: Equine folliculitis and furunculosis. Equine Pract., *2*(6):20, 1980.
9. Shimizu, A., and Kato, E.: Bacteriophage typing of *Staphylococcus aureus* isolated from horses in Japan. Jap. J. Vet. Sci., *41*:409, 1979.
10. Stannard, A. A.: Equine dermatology. Proc. 22nd Annu. Conv. Am. Assoc. Eq. Pract., 1976, p. 273.

NODULAR COLLAGENOLYTIC GRANULOMA
(Nodular Necrobiosis)

Craig E. Griffin, SAN DIEGO, CALIFORNIA

Nodular collagenolytic granuloma is a common skin disease of the horse. Although the etiology and pathogenesis are unknown, a hypersensitivity reaction is thought to be involved. Histopathologic examination reveals focal microscopic areas of collagen degeneration surrounded by an infiltrate of eosinophils. Some nodules, especially older ones, may become mineralized.

CLINICAL SIGNS

No age, breed, or sex predilections have been noted. The characteristic lesions are multiple intradermal nodules. The nodules vary from 0.5 to several centimeters in diameter and remain freely movable from the underlying fascia. Alopecia and ulcerations are usually not present unless the nodule is subjected to trauma. Pain and pruritus are absent. The distribution most commonly includes the back, withers, and neck. Clinically, nodular collagenolytic granuloma is distinguished from hypoderma by the absence of a breathing pore. Definitive diagnosis is based on characteristic histopathologic findings.

THERAPY

Treatment includes systemic corticosteroids, corticosteroids injected into the lesion, or surgical excision. The treatment of choice depends on the number and type of lesions. When just a few nodules are present, injection of triamcinolone acetonide, 3 to 5 mg per nodule, is sufficient. The total dose of triamcinolone should not exceed 20 mg. Besides the usual side effects that have been attributed to corticosteroid therapy, laminitis should also be considered when treating any equine species. When the number of nodules exceeds four to six per horse, prednisone, 400 to 600 mg per day for two to three weeks, is the treatment of choice. When only one or two nodules are present, surgical excision may be indicated. In other cases, surgical excision may be necessary to remove mineralized lesions, which may be refractory to systemic or local corticosteroid therapy.

The prognosis is good, especially if the lesions are relatively new and not mineralized. However, the client must also be warned that recurrences are possible and that retreatment may be required.

DISEASES OF ABNORMAL KERATINIZATION (SEBORRHEA)

Peter J. Ihrke, DAVIS, CALIFORNIA

The term *seborrhea* is used in both humans and domestic animals to describe various poorly understood diseases characterized clinically by scaling and crust formation. Regardless of etiology, an abnormal keratinization process seems to be a common link in these diseases. Although no evidence exists that excess sebum production is important in the pathogenesis of equine seborrhea or the other equine keratinization defect diseases, the term *equine seborrheic diseases* is still useful as a general classification term for a group of diseases with probable similar underlying etiologies and similar recommended treatment regimens. In contrast to canine seborrheic diseases, there is no evidence that hypothyroidism can cause equine seborrhea.

LOCALIZED SEBORRHEA

Mane and Tail Seborrhea

Mane and tail seborrhea is the most common seborrheic disease. No age, breed, or sex predilection has been noted. Moderate to heavy scaling is seen in the mane or tail regions or both. Keratinous crusts may be present. Both dry and oily forms of the disease may be seen. There is little or no inflammation, pruritus, or alopecia. If significant pruritus is present, differential diagnoses of culicoides hypersensitivity, pediculosis, and cutaneous onchocerciasis should be considered. Although a skin biopsy may be occasionally useful in ruling out other diseases, no specific laboratory tests are indicated.

Since equine mane and tail seborrhea is an idiopathic disease, no specific curative therapy is available. It is important for the owner to understand that, similar to dandruff in humans, control rather than cure is the goal of therapy. As equine seborrhea is essentially a cosmetic disease, many owners elect not to treat their horses.

Substantial benefit is seen with the regular use of human or canine antiseborrheic shampoos. Veterinary products such as Lytar,* Mycodex Tar and Sulfur,† Sebafon,‡ and Oxydex,§ as well as products for humans such as Polytar,‖ have been used suc-

cessfully. The shampoo is lathered well, allowed to remain on the affected area for 10 minutes, and then rinsed thoroughly. Usually, shampooing of the affected areas is recommended twice weekly during the first week followed by weekly administration. A dilute solution of Alpha-Keri bath oil* (1 capful per quart of water) in a spray bottle has been beneficial occasionally for very dry seborrhea in show horses.

Poor-quality food has been implicated in some cases of equine seborrhea. The addition of extra concentrates or corn oil (up to 1 cup daily) or both to the ration may be beneficial.

Cannon Keratosis

A moderately well-demarcated seborrhea may be seen on the anterior surface of the rear cannon bones. Both scaling and crusting are usually present. Hairs may be easily epilated when adherent crusts are removed. Ringworm may be considered as a differential diagnosis, but usually the distribution and character of the lesions are diagnostic. A dermatophyte culture should be considered in atypical cases.

Antiseborrheic shampoos applied in a similar manner as mentioned before may be effective palliatively. In severe cases, topical corticosteroid creams or ointments applied twice daily are beneficial. For economic reasons, generic 1 per cent hydrocortisone products are most frequently used.

Linear Keratosis

Linear keratosis is a characteristic seborrheic disease that primarily affects quarter horses. No sex predilection has been noted. The condition usually develops between one and five years of age. A similar linear exfoliative disease, lichen striatus, is documented in humans. In horses, the striking predilection for quarter horses and the occurrence of the disease in closely related animals indicate that hereditary factors may be involved.

Clinically, this condition consists of one or more linear, usually vertically oriented bands of alopecia and keratinous crusting. Lesions vary from about 0.25 to 0.75 cm in width and 5 to 50 cm in length.

*Lytar, D.V.M., Inc., Miami, FL 33143
†Mycodex Tar and Sulfur Pet Shampoo, Beecham Labs, Bristol, TN 37620
‡Sebafon, Winthrop Labs, New York, NY 10016
§Oxydex, D.V.M., Inc., Miami, FL 33143
‖Polytar, Stiefel Labs, Coral Gables, FL 33134

*Alpha Keri Bath Oil, Westwood Pharmaceuticals, Buffalo, NY 14213

The neck and lateral aspect of the thorax are the most common sites. Pruritus is uncommon. Generally this condition persists throughout the horse's life.

The diagnosis of this disease does not usually present a problem. The linear configuration usually readily differentiates it from dermatophytosis. Scars resulting from linear trauma such as scratches or whip marks must be differentiated.

The owner should be advised that this is a cosmetic disorder but that it is probably incurable. Antiseborrheic shampoos such as those mentioned earlier may be somewhat palliative, but regular use every three or four days is often necessary even for partial control. Topical corticosteroid creams or ointments may be beneficial in reducing scaling.

Owing to the unanswered questions as to the possible heritability of this condition, owners should be advised of the potential problem of using affected animals for breeding purposes.

GENERALIZED SEBORRHEA

Occasionally, a generalized form of seborrhea is seen. Before a diagnosis of idiopathic equine generalized seborrhea is made, several important differential diagnoses must be ruled out.

Equine pemphigus foliaceus presents as a generalized exfoliative disease. The lesions most frequently begin on the face and lower extremities. However, in addition to a generalized scaling, crusting, and alopecia, other signs such as depression, dependent edema, and pruritus are often seen. Conventional formalin-fixed biopsies of new lesions are recommmended, and immunofluorescence is advisable if available (p. 541).

An unusual generalized granulomatous disease greatly resembling equine pemphigus foliaceus is also seen occasionally in the horse. Skin biopsy reveals a granulomatous inflammation of the dermis. Many internal organs are also involved, as determined at necropsy.

If both of these causes of chronic exfoliative dermatitis are satisfactorily ruled out and if no other explanation for the scaling is available, the animal may be considered to have idiopathic generalized equine seborrhea. Current recommendations are to manage these horses as described in the section on mane and tail seborrhea. Obviously, the cost of shampoo becomes more of a factor in treating generalized seborrhea, and products such as Sebafon and Lytar that are available in gallon jugs are usually recommended.

Supplemental Reading

Stannard, A. A.: Equine dermatology. Proc. 22nd Annu. Conv. Am. Assoc. Eq. Pract., 1976, p. 273.

CONTACT DERMATITIS

Peter J. Ihrke, DAVIS, CALIFORNIA

Contact dermatitis may be either allergic or irritant in origin, but the majority of cases are believed to be due to irritants. In most instances, it is extremely difficult to determine the cause of contact dermatitis, but since the diagnosis and therapy of irritant and allergic contact dermatitis are essentially the same, differentiation is not mandatory.

ETIOLOGY AND PATHOGENESIS

Irritant contact dermatitis is a reaction of the skin to an irritating concentration of an offending agent. Since the substances damage the skin by direct toxic action, no immune mechanism is responsible. Allergic contact dermatitis is a delayed hypersensitivity reaction (type IV) in which a sensitive animal reacts to a nonirritating concentration of an offending agent. The offending agents are usually simple chemicals acting as haptenes that become antigenic upon union with epidermal proteins.

PREDISPOSING FACTORS

Moisture is an important predisposing factor in contact dermatitis, since it decreases the effectiveness of the normal skin barrier and increases the intimacy of contact between the agent and the skin surface. For example, a sweating horse is an ideal circumstance for contact dermatitis to occur in association with riding tack. Horses kept in a wet or muddy environment may develop contact dermatitis of their distal extremities (so-called mud fever). The concentration of the offending agent, the duration of contact time, and any preexisting skin irritation are also important factors. Many topical medications used in the treatment of skin diseases can potentially produce a contact dermatitis that exacerbates the lesions rather than contributing to healing.

CLINICAL SIGNS

Contact dermatitis in horses is seen most commonly around the muzzle, lower extremities, and in the areas of contact with riding tack. The increased frequency of the problem around the muzzle and distal extremities correlates well with the fact that these areas may have less protective hair and have a greater chance of contacting an offending substance.

Lesions caused by medications obviously have a distribution similar to the distribution of the product on the skin. Horses with diarrhea may exhibit a severe perianal irritant contact dermatitis.

Acute contact dermatitis lesions may show erythema, exudation, pruritus, and alopecia. Primary lesions such as papules or vesicles, if present at all, are usually transient in nature. While many species of domestic animals commonly show hyperpigmentation of the skin as a sequela to contact reactions, horses may depigment at the site of contact. Leukoderma (depigmentation of the skin) and leukotrichia (depigmentation of the hair) may both be permanent sequelae.

DIAGNOSIS

Substantial detective work by both the veterinarian and the owner may be necessary to determine the cause of many cases of contact dermatitis.

Dyes and preservatives are most commonly suspected in association with tack. Rubber bits have also been known to cause reactions around the mouth. Creosote and other wood preservatives applied to fencing may cause lesions on the muzzle. Occasionally, the bedding material of a horse has been responsible for more generalized lesions.

Iatrogenic lesions may be caused by both home remedies and veterinary products. Blisters or leg sweats may produce severe contact reactions, and insecticidal products mixed either properly or improperly can produce generalized lesions. Various fly sprays have also been implicated.

In order to make a tentative diagnosis of contact dermatitis, the lesions must be compatible with this type of skin disease, and the lesion localization should be compatible with the potential distribution of contact dermatitis. The onset of clinical signs may be quite rapid in cases of irritant contact dermatitis in comparison to a usually more gradual onset in cases of allergic contact dermatitis. It should be stressed that in humans, many if not most cases of allergic contact dermatitis occur in association with substances that are not particularly new in the environment. The same probably is true in the horse.

In most cases, the clinician must rely on historic data and clinical signs in making a tentative diagnosis of contact dermatitis. No specific laboratory test is available to establish this diagnosis in veterinary medicine. Although patch testing is the method of choice in diagnosing allergic contact dermatitis in humans, it is impractical in veterinary medicine and frequently unrewarding, since most cases are probably irritant in nature. Skin biopsy is infrequently helpful, since few specific changes are seen. An acute to chronic nonspecific dermatitis is usually seen.

THERAPY

The most effective therapy in the treatment of any contact dermatitis is the avoidance of the offending substance. As has been mentioned previously, the identification of the offending substance or substances may be quite difficult. An attempt should always be made to eliminate various potential causes in a sequential manner. In most cases, some improvement should be noted between three and seven days after the substance has been eliminated from the environment.

Even if a positive identification of the offending substance is not made, the animal may be treated palliatively with either systemic or topical corticosteroids. In mild localized cases, a 1 per cent hydrocortisone cream may be sufficient. In severe cases, systemic corticosteroids (400 to 600 mg prednisolone daily per average 450 kg horse for five to seven days) may be beneficial. If any of the offending substance is still thought to be in contact with the horse's skin, a gentle shampoo should be used.

SCRATCHES

William C. McMullan, COLLEGE STATION, TEXAS

Scratches (grease heel, mud fever, cracked heels) is an eczematous dermatitis of the heel and palmar pastern. It is not contagious, but several affected horses may be seen at one stable. Breeds with "feathers" are especially prone to the condition if grooming is inadequate or if stabling facilities are unsanitary, muddy, or otherwise neglected. When draft horses are confined to a stanchion at night, the rear feet are more often affected owing to urine and fecal scalding. Field stubble, grit from track surfaces, lime dust, irritant plants and chemicals, heel bug mites, fire ants, and a number of other agents can initially irritate the skin. This irritated or "chapped" stage when the heels are reddened, dry, and scurfy constitutes "scratches." With continued irritation and exercise, inflammation becomes more severe, exudation becomes apparent (grease heel), and the hair is matted. Lameness and/or edema of the limb may be present, and some horses show a stringhalt-type gait. This damaged skin allows a variety of organisms to gain entry and perpetuate the problem. In chronic cases, fissures develop in the skin (cracked heels), and a fetid discharge is present. Occasionally, and probably dependent upon the particular agent (Staphylococcus, for instance), vegetative granulomatous lesions (grapes) are seen. Some of these masses become heavily cornified.

TREATMENT

Development of the more serious later stages of this disease may be prevented if treatment is instituted early. In the "chapped" stage, the lesions should be cleaned with a mild soap and warm water, dried, and then clipped. Relatively clean heels may be clipped without washing. The simplest cases may then be medicated with a soothing ointment such as udder ointment or zinc oxide.* Leg wraps extending to ground level offer protection against secondary infection. More severely irritated but still nonexudative noninfected lesions respond more rapidly to a corticosteroid ointment.† In this stage as well as the others, lasting success of therapy is directly dependent upon the ability to identify and eliminate predisposing factors or etiologic agents.

If the disease has progressed to the exudative stage, soaking in a mild cleansing soap will be necessary to remove exudate, scabs, and accumulated debris. Clip after drying. Astringent lotions, such as white lotion (zinc sulfate and lead acetate) or calamine lotion, should be applied several times a day in the form of a soak bandage: Cover the heels and pastern with several layers of flexible gauze and pour on the lotion, saturating the gauze. After eight hours, remove and discard the gauze dressing and repeat the process. Once the lesions are no longer exudative, the area should be treated with an antibiotic-corticosteroid ointment* under a bandage for several more days. Recurrence of the problem can be prevented by keeping the hair clipped and by daily application of soothing ointment before exercise.

Grossly contaminated lesions (severe grease or cracked heels) are cleaned and clipped as before but with more effort. Then a poultice, linseed meal, or poultice powder† should be applied twice a day for two days, each time preceded by a povidone-iodine wash; then astringent lotions and finally ointments should be started. In these cases, appropriate chemotherapeutic agents are of benefit both topically and systemically if the invading microbe can be identified. For bacteria, penicillin or sulfapyridine are most often used. Fungicidal ointments may be used if a mycosis is suspected. On an empirical basis, an effective topical mixture is 30 ml DMSO,‡ 30 gm thiabendazole (TBZ) powder, and 0.5 kg sulfa cream.§ If the infection extends into the coronary band or frog, the loose horn tissue must be removed to permit effective medication.

Granulomatous masses (grapes) must be removed surgically, electrocautery being the preferred method. Postoperative care consists of basic wound care.

Supplemental Readings

1. Lundvall, R.L.: *In* Catcott, E. J., and Smithcors, J. F. (eds.): Equine Medicine and Surgery. Wheaton, IL, American Veterinary Pub., 1963, p. 299.
2. Stannard, A. A.: *In* Catcott, E. J., and Smithcors, J. F. (eds.): Equine Medicine and Surgery, 2nd ed. Wheaton, IL, American Veterinary Pub., 1972, p. 386.

---

*Desitin, Leeming/Pacquin, Division of Pfizer, New York, NY 10017

†Vetalog Ointment, E. R. Squibb and Sons, Princeton, NJ 08540

*Panalog Ointment, E. R. Squibb and Sons, Princeton, NJ 08540

†Poltis Powder, Jensen-Salsbery Labs, Kansas City, MO 64141

‡Domoso, Diamond Labs, Des Moines, IA 50303

§Vermorsal or Morumide. Beecham Labs, Bristol, TN 37620

PHYCOMYCOSIS

William C. McMullan, COLLEGE STATION, TEXAS

Phycomycosis is an extremely pruritic, granulomatous fungal disease of the skin and subcutaneous tissue of the legs, ventral abdomen, and head. Necrotic tracts containing gritty, grey-white masses of hyphae and surrounding reactive tissue ("leeches") are found in exuberant granulation tissue. Ninety per cent of the cases are from Gulf Coast areas.

Hyphomyces destruens and *Entomophthora coronata* are the fungi most frequently isolated.[1]

HISTORY

At the site of an apparently insignificant wound, there is, in just a few days, an explosion of granulation tissue, much of which is partially necrotic. The horse chews at it frequently. Various wound medications are of no benefit. Bandages have a foul odor.

CLINICAL SIGNS

The distal extremities are most commonly involved, especially the pastern and fetlock. The granulation mass may encircle the limb and extend vertically up to 30 cm. It has a nasty appearance and a foul odor. Exudation, necrosis, and pruritus are prime characteristics of the disease, but the presence of "leeches" in draining tracts and/or deep within the granulation and fibrous tissue is diagnostic. Proximal swelling or lymph node involvement or both may be present. Internal spread is rare.

DIAGNOSIS

The presence of firm, rough-textured, gray to yellow-white, branching cores "leeches" within an exudative, pruritic, granulomatous lesion is sufficient for field diagnosis. Histologic examination of several deep biopsy specimens and examination of "leeches" for fungal hyphae confirm the field diagnosis.

TREATMENT

Immediate, radical, surgical removal of all infected tissue is essential. Do not wait for the biopsy report. General anesthesia and tourniquet application are essential if the lesion is larger than 3 cm in diameter. Start in normal tissue at a proximal perimeter and cut as deeply as possible perpendicular to the skin. Extend the cut distal and ventral to the granulation mass. Be sure "leeches" are not left in tracts going into the normal tissue. Remove all granulation and fibrous connective tissue. A light freeze of the surgical site seems to be helpful in reducing recurrence of infection. A tight, thick pressure wrap is applied to control postsurgical hemorrhage. Recurrence is to be expected, and repeat surgery is indicated if new foci of infection are observed at daily bandage changes. These are first apparent as dark red to black hemorrhagic patches 1 to 5 mm in diameter in the new granulation bed. A full-depth excision of this spot plus 5 mm into normal granulation tissue should be done without waiting for leeches to appear. One major surgical procedure and two to three minor "retrims" are customary in the average case.

Lesions close to the bulbs of the heel or coronary band should be inspected carefully for evidence of infection. If present, one should not hesitate to remove with hoof nippers any portion of the frog or wall that will allow access to a fungal focus.

In cases with small wounds, a gauze dressing pad soaked in amphotericin B solution* (50 gm amphotericin B in 10 ml sterile H_2O) and 10 ml of DMSO† may be applied to the site daily for one week. As this is impractical in large wounds, they should simply be cleansed daily. New foci that appear may be thoroughly infiltrated with amphotericin B solution by injection with a 22-gauge needle and syringe.

Topical fungicides or griseofulvin or both have not been beneficial. Systemic treatment with amphotericin B is effective but should in all cases be combined with surgical removal.[2] The starting dose is 150 mg amphotericin B solution per 450 kg added to 1 l 5 per cent dextrose given intravenously with a 16-gauge 5 cm needle to prevent perivascular injection. Every third day, the dose is increased by 50 mg until a maximum of 350 to 400 mg per day is reached at day 15 to 18 and then is continued on a daily or alternate-day schedule until day 30. Response to therapy will in part govern the intensity of treatment. The blood urea nitrogen (BUN) and hematocrit should be monitored weekly. If the patient becomes severely depressed or anorectic or if the BUN exceeds 40 mg per 100 ml, systemic therapy should be temporarily discontinued or reduced. Expense is an important factor with systemic treatment; a 30-day treatment for a 450 kg horse costs $600 to $900 (1981 prices) for amphotericin B alone.

A phenolized vaccine has been reported to be ef-

---

*Fungizone, E. R. Squibb and Sons, Princeton, NJ 08540
†Domoso, Diamond Labs, Des Moines, IA 50303

fective when used alone or, preferably, with surgery.[3] Three doses of 2 ml each are given subcutaneously a week apart, with improvement noted within seven days. Oral potassium iodide 20 g *sid* is also recommended.

Cryotherapy (double freeze-thaw to −20° C) is effective on early lesions that are less than 1 cm in thickness. Failures result with thicker lesions because leeches are frequently found at the very depth of a lesion and are unaffected.

References

1. Bridges, C. H.: Mycotic Diseases. *In* Catcott, E. J., and Smithcors, J. F. (eds.): Equine Medicine and Surgery, 2nd ed. Wheaton, IL, American Veterinary Pub., 1972, p. 124.
2. McMullan, W. C., Joyce, J. R., Hanselka, D. V., and Heitmann, J. M.: Amphotericin B for the treatment of localized subcutaneous phycomycosis in the horse. J. Am Vet Med. Assoc., *170*:1293, 1977.
3. Miller, R. I.: Tropical Veterinary Science. James Cook University, N. Queensland, Australia, personal communication.

HABRONEMIASIS

William C. McMullan, COLLEGE STATION, TEXAS

Habronemiasis ("summer sore") is a seasonal, granulomatous, occasionally mildly pruritic disease that occurs at the site of minor wounds or natural body moisture (sheath, eyes) in sensitized horses. Habronema sp larvae deposited there by the house fly and stable fly are the sources of irritation.[1]

CLINICAL SIGNS

Hemorrhagic reddish-brown exuberant granulation tissue covered with a greasy coagulated exudate is typical at wound sites and on lesions of the penis, sheath, and urethral process. A few lesions become quite massive. Conjunctival lesions at the medial canthus are more strawberry-like in texture and up to 5 mm in size. Lesions 1 to 2 cm nasal to the medial canthus are usually small, about 1 to 5 mm in diameter, with openings that lead to small subcutaneous sinuses containing larvae and exudate.

Caseocalcareous granules are sometimes found in conjunctival lesions, on the underside of scabs covering wounds, or in granulation tissue. They seldom become larger than a grain of rice and do not branch like "leeches" found in lesions of phycomycosis.

DIAGNOSIS

A symptomatic diagnosis can be confirmed by biopsy or by identifying larvae in a scraping or minced tissue suspension.

TREATMENT

A combination of local and systemic therapy is most effective.

Local. Any of several paste mixtures are about equal in efficacy. The main ingredients include an organophosphate, usually 30 ml fenthion* or 1 oz trichlorfon powder.† The organophosphate is added to ¾ lb heated petrolatum or nitrofurazone ointment.‡ An anti-inflammatory agent is also added, such as 10 mg triamcinolone acetonide powder,§ dexamethasone powder,‖ and/or 90 ml DMSO.** Thiabendazole†† has anti-inflammatory and larvicidal properties and can be added to any of the preceding mixtures advantageously. The resultant paste should be applied daily, and the site should be bandaged to prevent reinfection.

Systemic. Trichlorfon‡‡ at 22 mg per kg is given intravenously in 1 l of 5 per cent dextrose or saline by means of a 5 cm, 16-gauge needle, being careful to avoid perivascular injection. The solution is preferably autoclaved before use. Precautions ordinarily observed with organophosphate use should be followed. This intravenous treatment may be repeated in two weeks if necessary. Pretreatment with atropine is unnecessary and may cause ileus and flatulent colic.

Systemic corticosteroid therapy minimizes the hypersensitivity tissue reaction and has been used successfully as the only systemic treatment.[4] Prednisolone orally at 800 mg per 450 kg mixed in sweet feed each morning for one week followed by 400 mg per 450 kg each morning for a second week is effective, as is triamcinolone acetonide oral power,§§ 10 mg each morning for four days followed by 10 mg every other day for four doses.

---

*Spotton, Cutter Labs, Shawnee, KS 66201
†Dylox, Mobay Chemical Corp., Kansas City, MO 64120
‡Furacin dressing, Norden Labs, Lincoln, NB 68521
§Vetalog, E. R. Squibb and Sons, Princeton, NJ 08540
‖Azium, Schering Corp., Kenilworth, NJ 07033
**Domoso, Diamond Labs, Des Moines, IA 50303
††Equizole Powder, Merck & Co., Rahway, NJ 07065
‡‡Combot, Haver-Lockhart Labs, Shawnee, KS 66201
§§Vetalog Powder, E. R. Squibb and Sons, Princeton, NJ 08540

Diethylcarbamazine liquid or tablets* added to sweet feed at 6.6 mg per kg twice a day for two to three weeks is effective on early lesions. It is not effective in those horses with massive lesions or a lesion recurring in the same location as a year previously. Apparently, excessive fibrous tissue impairs the distribution of the drug.

Subcutaneous or intralesion injection of fenthion and/or short-acting corticosteroids is effective. Five ml of each is injected for a 5 cm lesion.

Avermectin is an experimental injectable anthelmintic with good activity against summer sores following a single intramuscular injection of 0.2 mg per kg. Improvement occurs in seven days.[2]

Conjunctival habronemiasis can be treated by instilling two drops of fenthion† in the eye once a day along with a corticosteroid-antibiotic ophthalmic preparation three times a day. If granules are embedded in the mucous membrane or granulation tissue, they should be washed out with saline or removed with forceps after anesthetizing the tissues with proparacaine hydrochloride‡ or topical lidocaine.§

Lesions of a thickness within the capability of a cryotherapy unit have been treated successfully, using a double freeze-thaw cycle.[3] Massive lesions are removed surgically and treated both systemically and locally.

Horses with recurrent infection in the same location the same year or the next year are sometimes medically unresponsive and must be treated surgically. A technique for excision of chronic urethral process lesions has been described.[5]

For the average case, my choice of therapy is intravenous trichlorfon, daily application of summer sore paste under a bandage, and systemic corticosteroids. Regardless of the chosen therapy, the granulating wound must still be attended in the usual manner, with excision, pressure bandages, corticosteroid ointments, copper sulfate, and so forth.

Fly control, though admittedly difficult, will reduce the incidence of the disease. Prompt and proper removal and disposal of droppings and soiled bedding are vital. Residual sprays on the walls, a barn mist system or individual stall misters, repellents applied to the horses, and cattle insecticide ear tags‖ affixed to the mane and tail are all helpful. Consult your county agent or university entomologist as to selection of products that work best in your area (p. 529).

Elimination of adult Habronema sp from the stomach is another logical point of attack, but unfortunately, many of the wormers in use are ineffective against Habronema sp, a fact leading to an increased incidence of this disease in the last 20 years. Products with known efficacy are dichlorvos* and carbon disulfide. All horses on the premises should be treated. Predosing by 30 minutes with 8 qt 2 per cent $NaHCO_3$ will increase anthelmintic efficacy by helping to dissolve the mucus plugs of a *Habronema (Draschia) megastoma* nodule. This species is by far the most resistant to treatment and also is the one most often involved in summer sores. Therefore, this phase of treatment, while well intended, is likely to be only partially successful.

PROPHYLAXIS

Fly control and elimination of adults of the species, as indicated, constitute the principal prophylactic measures. These are especially recommended on farms that have an annual problem or "repeaters." Prompt treatment of fresh wounds with a summer sore paste or insecticidal wound medication is indicated.

Breeding stallions with an anticipated recurrent infection of the urethral process or penis may as a last resort be maintained on a long-term, low-level, alternate-day corticosteroid schedule beginning with the onset of fly season. With oral prednisolone, after a week at 400 mg per 450 kg once a day, continue through the hot weather at a dose of 350 mg per 450 kg every other morning. With triamcinolone acetonide oral powder, after 10 mg each day for two doses and 10 mg every other day for four doses, continue with 10 mg twice a week. With any long-term corticosteroid therapy, be sure the handler is alerted for signs of iatrogenic Cushing's disease (hyperadrenalism), such as polydipsia, polyuria, muscle wasting, poor wound healing, and decreased resistance to infection. Upon arrival of cool weather, corticosteroid therapy should be terminated gradually, and stress should be avoided during this time.

References

1. Georgi, J. R.: Parasitology for Veterinarians, 2nd ed. Philadelphia, W. B. Saunders Co., 1974.
2. Herd, R. P., and Donham, J. C.: Efficacy of ivermectin against "summer sores" due to *Draschia* and *Habronema* infection in horses. Proc. 26th Annu. Meet. Am. Assoc. Vet. Parasitol., 1981, p. 8.
3. Migiola, S., Blanton, A. B., and Davenport, J. W.: Cryosurgical treatment of equine cutaneous habronemiasis. VM SAC, 73:1073, 1978.
4. Stannard, A. A.: Personal communication, Davis, California, 1979.
5. Stick, J. A.: Amputation of the equine urethral process affected with habronemiasis. VM SAC, 74:1453, 1979.

---

*Caricide, American Cyanamid, Princeton, NJ 08540
†Tiguvon, Cutter Labs, Shawnee, KS 66201
‡Opthaine, E. R. Squibb and Sons, Princeton, NJ 08540
§Xylocaine, Astra Pharmaceutical Products, Worcester, MA 01606
‖Ectrin, Diamond Shamrock, Dallas, TX 75201

---

*Equigard, E. R. Squibb and Sons, Princeton, NJ 08540

DERMATOPHILOSIS

Reginald R. R. Pascoe, OAKEY, QUEENSLAND, AUSTRALIA

Dermatophilosis is a dermatitis caused by *Dermatophilus congolensis*. The disease is characterized by exudation, matting of the hair at skin level, loss of hair without pruritus, and excessive scab formation.

The disease occurs worldwide but is most common in Africa and Australia. *D. congolensis* is also the etiologic agent of dermatophilosis of cattle (cutaneous streptotrichosis) and mycotic dermatitis and strawberry footrot in sheep. Equine dermatophilosis is not contagious to humans.

EPIDEMIOLOGY

Horses of all ages are susceptible. In foals, the infection is usually observed on the face and back only, except under severe wet conditions, when it may extend to all parts of the body as a moist, eczematous type of dermatitis. The disease appears at any time of the year but is always associated with periods of heavy rain or prolonged light rain with overcast, humid weather conditions. Warm, moist weather favors rapid spread, the longer, wetter periods being associated with generalized infection of the whole horse. Contact with infected animals leads to the spread of the disease. While the origin of infection is still obscure, the organism has only once been isolated from soil samples; it must, therefore, be suspected that the skin and hair of previously infected horses act as reservoirs of the disease.

The method of transmission is unclear; stable flies (*Stomoxys calcitrans*) and house flies (*Musca domestica*) transmit the disease mechanically, the flies remaining contaminated for up to 24 hours after original contact. Once the disease has occurred on a horse establishment, it becomes enzootic, and when favorable weather conditions occur, fresh cases of the disease appear.

The organism invades cutaneous abrasions and creates a bacterial dermatitis. Even minor abrasions can be a source of infection if excessive wetting of the skin occurs either from rain or continual wetting of the nose and legs by grass. In race horses, the abrasions can be caused by cinders striking the hind legs from the hocks downward.

PATHOGENESIS

In horses with longer hair (during the winter months), the exudate, epithelial debris, and mycetial forms of the organism cause matting of the hairs not unlike ringworm in the horse. In shorter-haired horses, the lesions are smaller and drier, and as the disease follows the natural water drainage patterns on the horse, so the areas of "scald" lines appear on the horse's skin.

White-skinned areas are more sensitive to infection and exhibit erythema, especially on the nose, often leading to an erroneous diagnosis of sunburn. The characteristic scald appearance is followed by cracking and exudation from the skin, with accumulation of scab, exudate, and fine hairs matted together.

The areas around the pastern, fetlocks, and bulb of the heels crack, fissure, and scab, leading to lameness. Edema of the fetlock extending up the cannon bone is fairly common, as is exudation and secondary infection; healing is slow, and repeated wetting leads to a chronic dermatitis associated with secondary infections.

DIAGNOSIS

In acute early cases, *D. congolensis* may be readily isolated from fresh lesions by culture on blood agar plates. Isolation from chronic or healing lesions is difficult and may be misleading owing to overgrowth of contaminants. A different method of culture is necessary for old chronic lesions; this involves placing small pieces of scabs in 5 ml bijou bottles, moistening with 1 ml distilled water, and allowing the bottles to stand open for 3½ hours on the bench, then incubating in 20 per cent carbon dioxide for 15 minutes. The bottles are then carefully removed, and with a bacteriologic loop, samples are taken from the water surface, are plated on 5 per cent ox blood agar, and are incubated at 37° C in 20 per cent carbon dioxide for 24 to 48 hours. Abundant, small, embedding, hemolytic, rough, fimbriated colonies typical of *D. congolensis* are obtained, usually in relatively pure culture. Stained smears from the colonies confirm the diagnosis.

Impression smears taken directly from the underside of freshly removed scabs and stained with either methylene blue or Giemsa stain show the presence of typical branching mycelia-like organisms. Invasion of lesions with secondary organisms such as staphylococci can increase the amount of purulent exudation between the hair mat and the skin. The disease in most horses is self-limiting if conditions favorable for its spread or maintenance are removed.

CLINICAL SIGNS

With long-haired horses, removal of the matted hairs leaves a moist, gray to pink, slightly raised skin; the lesions are slightly ovoid in shape, hence, the resemblance to ringworm. With short-haired horses, the matted hair scab is much smaller and is often palpated more easily than it is seen. Early in the disease, it occurs as small 1 to 2 mm hard, shot-like lesions that may be plucked by fingernail from among the normal hair. It is still the characteristic scab as seen in long-haired horses, that is, hairs embedded in the scab with the roots visible under the lower surface of the scab.

Generalized lesions show a definite pattern of distribution on the back-line of the horse. The most severely affected areas are the head, loins, and croup. The neck and chest are affected less severely owing to a more angular slope, which allows better rain run-off. The infection follows natural drainage lines on the horse's body.

Where paddock horses graze in wet pasture conditions, the lesions are confined to the nose and lower legs, usually as high as the fetlock. Racehorses working on long grass or cinder tracks tend to have leg lesions only, with an extension of infection up the front of the hind cannon bone to the hock caused by flying debris cast by the front hooves while the horse is working.

TREATMENT AND CONTROL

When large groups of horses become infected, treatment with local medication can be difficult; it has been observed over many years that the disease is usually self-limiting and requires minimal treatment. Paddocked horses are most commonly affected by generalized infection of the head and back, and provided that prolonged wet weather is not a factor, treatment is only given to horses showing the secondary signs of loss of condition, pain, and swelling of affected legs. Untreated horses show regression of signs and healing of lesions in three to four weeks. Horses that show more severe infection are treated individually.

General Treatment. Remove all horses from unfavorable environmental conditions; stable to keep them out of the rain or away from boggy ground; keep stable floors dry, and ensure that bedding is dry and nonirritating.

Skin lesions should be cleaned with a surgical scrub of povidone-iodine* and thoroughly dried to loosen and remove all scabs and debris from the skin. In uncomplicated mild cases, this is usually

*Betadine, Purdue Frederick, Norwalk, CT 06856

sufficient. The lesions form smaller, looser scabs and soon heal. In more severe cases, the horse is treated as before, and then 0.25 per cent chloramphenicol is washed over the infected area and allowed to dry. This is repeated for three days; healing occurs in most horses.

Local Treatment. In more severe cases where cracks or fissures of the skin have occurred around the legs, nose, and even occasionally on the body, the area becomes extremely painful. The area should be gently cleaned, 0.25 per cent chloramphenicol should be applied, and if improvement is not rapidly effected, the area should be treated with emollient creams containing both antibiotics and corticosteroids. One such compound available in Australia contains 2 mg nitrofurazone, 5 mg neomycin sulfate, 2.5 mg prednisolone, 20 mg chlorophyll, 100 mg cod liver oil, and 450 mg propylene glycol per gram of ointment. Another contains 0.5 per cent neomycin sulfate and 0.5 per cent hydrocortisone. Astringents such as white lotion (20 gm zinc sulfate and 30 gm lead acetate in 500 ml water) applied to the leg lesions daily for five days also reduce swelling and inflammation.

Protective bandages must be used with caution, as chafing, which occasionally exacerbates the condition of the pastern and fetlock, often occurs.

Systemic Treatment. Where lesions are severe or widespread, systemic antibiotics are necessary and, in most instances, work extremely well. Good response is obtained with both streptomycin and penicillin, and usually both are combined and given intramuscularly for three to five days at a dose rate of 10 mg per kg penicillin and 10 mg per kg streptomycin.

Supplemental Readings

1. Haalstra, R. T.: Isolation of *Dermatophilus congolensis* from skin lesions in the diagnosis of streptotrichosis. Vet. Rec., 77:824, 1965.
2. Kaplan, W.: *Dermatophilus*—a recently recognized disease in the United States. S. West. Vet., 20:14, 1966.
3. Kaplan, W., and Johnston, W. J.: Equine Dermatophilus (cutaneous streptotrichosis) in Georgia. J. Am. Vet. Med. Assoc., 149:1162, 1966.
4. Pascoe, R. R.: An outbreak of mycotic dermatitis in horses in southeastern Queensland. Aust. Vet. J., 47:112, 1971.
5. Pascoe, R. R.: Further observations on *Dermatophilus* infections in horses. Aust. Vet. J., 48:32, 1972.
6. Pier, A. C., Richards, J. L., and Farrell, E. F.: Fluorescent antibody and cultural techniques in cutaneous streptotrichosis. Am. J. Vet. Res., 25:1014, 1964.
7. Richards, J. L., and Pier, A. C.: Transmission of *Dermatophilus congolensis* by *Stomoxys calcitrans* and *Musca domestica*. Am. J. Vet. Res., 27:419, 1966.

SPOROTRICHOSIS

Paul Morris, MANHATTAN, KANSAS

ETIOLOGY

Sporotrichosis, a nodular, granulomatous disease seen occasionally in the horse, is caused by the dimorphic fungus *Sporothrix (Sporotrichum) schenckii*. The organism is a ubiquitous saprophyte found worldwide but more often in areas with a temperate or tropical climate and high humidity. Its natural habitat is the external surface of various plants, the most common of which include thorns of rose or barberry bushes, sphagnum moss, and salt marsh grasses. Infections develop after injury and inoculation of the skin.[4]

CLINICAL SIGNS

Sporotrichosis occurs in cutaneous, cutaneolymphatic, and disseminated forms. In the horse, the cutaneolymphatic type is the most common. After inoculation into the skin, a primary lesion occurs on the exposed part of the body, usually a limb and less often an upper part of the body, such as the shoulder, hip, or perineal region. Progressively, subcutaneous nodules from 1 to 5 cm in diameter develop along the lymphatics draining the region. The lymphatics may become corded, and the nodules, particularly the larger ones, may ulcerate, discharge a small amount of creamy exudate, and later become encrusted. Extension of infection typically follows the lymphatics and consistently involves only one side of the body or one limb. History and careful observation of an affected limb will often reveal a distal wound at which the infection developed initially.[1, 2, 4]

The disseminated form, although not reported in the horse, has occurred in other species as a sequela to the cutaneolymphatic form. Rarely, pulmonary infections have resulted from inhalation of the fungus.

DIFFERENTIAL DIAGNOSIS

Differential diagnoses include both bacterial and fungal diseases that cause granulomatous skin lesions. Some of the fungal diseases may have coexisting pulmonary lesions (blastomycosis, coccidioidomycosis, cryptococcosis, or histoplasmosis). The likelihood of any of the differentials is based in part on the horse's geographic history.

Bacterial diseases such as *Corynebacterium pseu-*
dotuberculosis and *Staphylococcus aureus* infection can easily be confirmed or ruled out by culture. *Corynebacterium pseudotuberculosis* infection is seen mainly in California, although cases have been reported elsewhere in the United States. Verification of *Staphylococcus aureus* pyogranulomas requires multiple, consistent isolations. *Actinomyces* sp have been isolated by culture from enlarged, firm lymph nodes or fistulous tracts in the mandibular, pharyngeal, and cervical regions. Cutaneous glanders caused by *Pseudomonas mallei* has not been reported in the United States in recent years but is seen in Europe, Asia, and Africa. The diagnosis of glanders is confirmed by finding the organism in smears, a positive complement fixation serology test, or a positive reaction to the mallein test.

Systemic and subcutaneous mycoses resulting in cutaneous or cutaneolymphatic granulomatous skin lesions may need to be considered, depending on geographic location, and are described elsewhere (p. 32).

Cutaneous mastocytosis, a nodular disease with larger ulcerating lesions, is seen more often on the upper body, especially the head, neck, and back, than on the lower limbs. Biopsy provides a definitive diagnosis.

DIAGNOSIS

The most reliable way to confirm a diagnosis of sporotrichosis is to culture an aspirate of exudate using Saboraud-dextrose slants, brain-heart infusion glucose blood agar, or Francis glucose-cystine blood agar plates. Chloramphenicol (0.05 mg per ml) and cycloheximide (0.5 mg per ml) can be added to reduce the number of bacterial and mold contaminants. Growth usually occurs in two to seven days. If a mycelial phase is demonstrated at room temperature and "cigar bodies" at 37°C, the diagnosis is made.

S. schenckii can also be identified by submitting an aspirate of exudate or a piece of tissue to the Center for Disease Control (CDC) laboratory in Atlanta, Georgia, for a fluorescent antibody (FA) test. The test is rapid and very sensitive. Cases have been detected by FA that were negative on culture.[5]

Although cytology of exudates or histopathology of biopsies is generally unrewarding, it occasionally reveals the organism and provides a quick diagnosis. Biopsies are taken only when there are no nodules to aspirate or when there are other differential diagnoses that would be confirmed by biopsy. Special fungal stains (periodic acid–Schiff, Grocott's or Gomori's methenamine silver, or Goodpasture's) can be utilized to demonstrate the pleomorphic (oval, rounded, or cigar-shaped) yeast organisms in granulomatous tissue.

Serologic tests using latex agglutination and tube agglutination can also be helpful in the diagnosis.[4]

TREATMENT

The cutaneolymphatic form of sporotrichosis responds well to iodide therapy. The inorganic iodides, sodium or potassium iodide, or the organic iodide, ethylene diamine dihydroiodide (EDDI), can be utilized. Sodium iodide, which is available in a 20 per cent solution,* can be given intravenously; the other two are administered orally. Some veterinarians start with intravenous sodium iodide, but it is not necessary, since oral iodides are absorbed rapidly.[7] Less cost is incurred in the treatment if oral iodides alone are used.

EDDI may offer some advantage over the inorganic iodides because the iodine in EDDI may be retained in tissues longer than iodine from sodium iodide.[6] EDDI† has been used at a dosage of 1 to 2 mg per kg (active ingredient) once or twice daily for one week, then reduced to 0.5 to 1 mg per kg once daily for the remainder of the treatment. Alternatively, potassium iodide‡ can be used at a similar dosage, although dosages up to 40 mg per kg have been used for short periods. Care should be exercised in storing potassium iodide, since iodine in this form is unstable in the presence of moisture, sunlight, and high temperatures. Potassium iodate§ is not subject to these problems and may be used in place of potassium iodide. The oral iodides are usually administered with sweet feed but when necessary can be mixed with molasses and administered with a plastic syringe. The iodine content of each iodide is listed in Table 1.

With treatment, the lesions should regress in three to four weeks. Therapy should be continued for three to four weeks after the lesions disappear, or relapses will occur. In these cases, reinstitution

*20 per cent Sodium iodide, Med Tech, Elwood, KS 66024
†EDDI can be purchased as pure chemical in 100 lb drums from West Design Chemical Group, P.O. Box 1386, Shawnee Mission, KS 66222; or Whitmoyer Labs, Inc., 19 N. Railroad St., P.O. Box 288, Myerstown, PA 17067. EDDI blended mixtures are usually preferred: GEN-I (8.8 per cent EDDI, soybean meal carrier) 40#, West Design; Biodin (9.2 per cent EDDI, salt carrier) 25# or 100# Whitmoyer Labs. Soybean carrier is better, as EDDI may separate from salt carrier.
‡Potassium iodide, Fisher Scientific, Pittsburgh, PA 15219
§Potassium iodate, Mallincrodt, Paris, KY 40361

TABLE 1. IODINE CONTENT OF VARIOUS MEDICATIONS USED IN TREATMENT OF SPOROTRICHOSIS[7]

Iodide	Iodine %
Ethylene diamine dihydroiodide	80.0
Potassium iodide	76.45
Potassium iodate	59.3
Sodium iodide	84.7

of iodide therapy at the same or higher dosage will generally allow recovery.

Tolerance to iodine therapy varies, and some horses may show signs of iodism, such as scaly dermatitis, depression, anorexia, fever, coughing, lacrimation, serous nasal discharge, salivation, nervousness, or cardiovascular abnormalities. In such cases, the dosage may be reduced or therapy temporarily discontinued.[7, 9]

For rare cases not responding to iodide therapy, griseofulvin has been used. Response to therapy has been variable. Amphotericin B has been used in the disseminated form of sporotrichosis in other species.

PUBLIC HEALTH SIGNIFICANCE

It is important to remember that any person coming in contact with an animal with sporotrichosis and exposed to lesions, exudates, or infected material can become infected by the accidental inoculation or contamination of broken skin.[4]

References

1. Bridges, C.: Mycotic diseases. *In* Catcott, E. J., and Smithcors, J. F. (eds.): Equine Medicine and Surgery. Wheaton, IL, American Veterinary Pub., 1972, pp. 119–136.
2. Fishburn, F., and Kelley D. C.: Sporotrichosis in a horse. J. Am. Vet. Med Assoc., 151:45, 1967.
3. Huber, W.: Antifungal and antiviral agents. *In* Jones, L. M., Booth, N. H., and McDonald, L. E. (eds.): Veterinary Pharmacology and Therapeutics. Ames, IA, Iowa State University Press, 1977, pp. 974–978.
4. Kaplan, W., and Ajello, L.: Subcutaneous mycoses. *In* Steele, J. H. (ed.): CRC Handbook Series in Zoonoses. Vol. II. Boca Raton, FL, CRC Press, 1980, pp. 459–468.
5. Kaplan, W., and Ochoa, A. G.: Application of the fluorescent antibody technique to the rapid diagnosis of sporotrichosis. J. Lab. Clin. Med., 62:835, 1963.
6. Miller, J. K., and Swanson, E. W.: Metabolism of EDDI and sodium or potassium iodide by dairy cows. J. Dairy Sci., 56:378, 1973.
7. Rossoff, I. S.: Handbook of Veterinary Drugs. New York, Springer Verlag, 1974, pp. 475–476, 541.
8. Scott, D. W.: Sporotrichosis. *In* Kirk, R. W. (ed.): Current Veterinary Therapy VI. Philadelphia, W. B. Saunders Co., 1977, pp. 557–558.
9. Sollmann, T.: A Manual of Pharmacology and Its Applications to Therapeutics and Toxicology. Philadelphia, W. B. Saunders Co., 1957, pp. 1117–1128.

ONCHOCERCIASIS*

N. E. Robinson, EAST LANSING, MICHIGAN

Onchocerca cervicalis is a filarid nematode, the adult residing in the ligamentum nuchae, where it produces calcified nodules. Adult Onchocerca produces large numbers of microfilariae, which migrate via connective tissues to the superficial layers of the dermis. Ninety-five per cent of microfilariae are found within six in of the ventral midline, but in heavy infestations, microfilariae are found in other parts of the skin, including the eyelids, and may invade the eye (p. 382).

Investigations in several parts of the world have demonstrated that up to 90 per cent of horses have microfilariae of *O. cervicalis* in the skin. Transmission between horses is by insects, usually Culicoides sp, which feed on the skin of the horse. Because so many horses have microfilariae in the skin with little inflammatory response, it is difficult to know if Onchocerca is a cause of dermatitis or if the skin disease usually attributed to Onchocerca is a response to the bite of the vectors. It has been suggested that skin disease results only when microfilariae die and initiate a hypersensitivity reaction. Because of the uncertainty of the role of Onchocerca in causing dermatitis, other causes of dermatitis must be eliminated before a diagnosis of onchocerciasis is made.

CLINICAL SIGNS

A nonseasonal diffuse dermatitis is attributed to *O. cervicalis*. Lesions consist of alopecia and scaling and may be pruritic. They occur primarily on the unpigmented areas of the face. The ventral midline dermatitis and diffuse, intensely pruritic disease formerly attributed to Onchocerca are most probably responses to the bite of vectors (p. 558).

DIAGNOSIS

Because a high percentage of horses are infested with microfilariae, the demonstration of microfilariae does not confirm a diagnosis, but the absence of microfilariae in skin lesions makes Onchocerca an unlikely cause of the condition. Microfilariae can be demonstrated by mincing a small piece of skin on a glass slide, covering it with saline, and incubating it at room temperature for 5 to 10 min. Live microfilariae migrate from the skin and can be observed with the low-power objective of the microscope.

THERAPY

Diethylcarbamazine citrate,* 3 gm per day for 21 days, kills the microfilariae. The drug is given mixed with grain or sweet feed. Death of the microfilariae may provoke intense pruritus, which can be controlled by administration of corticosteroids for the first days of diethylcarbamazine therapy. Owners should also be warned that therapy may be accompanied by uveitis (p. 382).

Ivermectins, a group of anthelminthics currently undergoing clinical trials, destroy skin microfilariae. In one trial, ivermectin (22, 23-dihydroavermectin B_1) at a dose of 0.2 mg per kg reduced the microfilariae count in an 8 mm diameter biopsy from several hundred to less than one. Ivermectin may be preferable to diethylcarbamazine because pruritus does not occur during therapy.

If a good response to therapy is obtained, treatment should be repeated four times per year.

Supplemental Readings

1. Cello, R. M.: Ocular onchocerciasis in the horse. Equine Vet. J., 3:148, 1971.
2. Klei, T. R., Torbert, B. J., and Onchou, R.: Efficacy of Ivermectin (22, 23-dihydroavermectin B_1) against adult *Seratia equina* and microfilariae of *Onchocerca cervicalis* in ponies. J. Parasitol., 66:859, 1980.
3. Mellor, P. S.: Studies on *Onchocerca cervicalis* Raillet and Henry 1910: *Onchocerca cervicalis* in British Isles. J. Helminthol., 47:97, 1973.
4. Mellor, P. S.: Studies on *Onchocerca cervicalis* Raillet and Henry 1910: II: Pathology in the horse. J. Helminthol., 47:111, 1973.
5. Stannard, A. A.: The skin. *In* Catcott, E. J., and Smithcors, J. F. (eds.): Equine Medicine and Surgery, 2nd ed. Wheaton, IL, American Veterinary Pub., Inc., 1972, p. 386.
6. Stannard, A. A., and Cello, R. M.: *Onchocerca cervicalis* infection in horses from the Western United States. Am. J. Vet. Res., 36:1029, 1975.

*This article was not reviewed by Dr. Stannard.

*Caricide, American Cyanamid Co., Princeton, NJ 08540

SWEET OR QUEENSLAND ITCH*
(Culicoides Hypersensitivity)

N. E. Robinson, EAST LANSING, MICHIGAN

A recurrent, seasonal, intensely pruritic dermatitis has been described in many parts of the world under a variety of local names such as "sweet itch" (Britain), "Queensland itch" (Australia), and "kasen" (Japan). The disease was formerly ascribed to the presence of *Onchocerca cervicalis* microfilariae in the skin. Because microfilariae occur in many horses without accompanying dermatitis, it is now believed that the disease is a hypersensitivity response to the bite of insects, particularly Culicoides sp. A ventral midline dermatitis has been suggested to be a result of hypersensitivity to the bite of horn flies (*Lyperosia irritans*).

CLINICAL SIGNS

Lesions of sweet itch, which are intensely pruritic, occur in the dorsal lumbosacral and dorsal coccygeal regions. Initially numerous papules develop, the hair is tufted, and there is hyperesthesia. This is followed by localized alopecia and self-excoriation to the point that serous effusion occurs. Lesions are particularly severe over the nuchal crest, frontal bones, mane, shoulders, and rump. Recurrent attacks lead to complete loss of hair, particularly in the mane and dorsum of the tail, hyperkeratinization, scaling, and transverse ridges in the skin.

Sweet itch occurs sporadically in groups of horses, with sensitive individuals suffering recurrent attacks. The condition rarely occurs in horses under one year of age, and there is no breed or sex predilection. Affected individuals develop clinical signs in the spring, become worse during the summer, and recover in the fall. In subsequent years, clinical signs are more intense. This seasonal incidence coincides with the biting season of Culicoides sp.

Ventral midline dermatitis occurs primarily in summer in warm climates. It is commonest in horses over four years of age. Lesions up to 30 cm in diameter occur close to the midline of the abdomen and thorax. They consist of thickened skin with scaling, alopecia, leukoderma, ulceration, and crust formation. Pruritus occurs in some cases.

PATHOLOGY AND PATHOGENESIS

Sweet itch lesions are characterized by subepidermal edema with congestion and perivascular cuffing of dermal vessels. Many eosinophils are found throughout the dermis, which also is infiltrated with some neutrophils and fibroblasts. The epidermis is abraded and shows acanthosis and local parakeratosis.

Characteristic lesions are produced immediately in sensitive horses at the site of injection of Culicoides extract. Sensitivity can also be transferred to the skin of normal horses by intradermal injection of serum from a sensitive horse. The tissue eosinophilia is generally characteristic of an IgE reaction.

DIAGNOSIS

The seasonal incidence of this condition in sensitive horses is characteristic. *Oxyuris equi* causes rubbing only at the base of the tail (p. 288).

THERAPY AND CONTROL

Sweet itch is best controlled by housing sensitive horses in stalls screened with very fine mesh. Ordinary window screen is too coarse. Horses need not be housed all day but only when Culicoides sp are biting. This may vary with the species of midge but generally is in late evening and early morning, particularly on humid days.

Insect repellants may offer some protection. Suitable compounds and methods of application are described on pp. 530 and 533. Control of Culicoides by spraying of breeding sites is not economically feasible.

In severely affected animals, pruritus may need to be controlled by oral administration of prednisolone (0.5 mg per kg).

Ventral midline dermatitis lesions should be washed with mild soap to remove crusts, and petroleum jelly should be applied as a barrier to further fly bites. Insect repellants are also useful. The size of the lesion may be reduced by topical application of an antibiotic-corticosteroid ointment.*

Supplemental Readings

1. Baker, K. P.: The rational approach to the management of sweet itch. Vet. Ann., *18*:163, 1978.
2. Baker, K. P., and Quinn, P. J.: A report on clinical aspects and histopathology of sweet itch. Equine Vet. J., *10*:243, 1978.
3. Reik, R. F.: Studies on allergic dermatitis ("Queensland itch") of the horse. Aust. Vet. J., *29*:177, 185, 1953.
4. Reik, R. F.: Studies on allergic dermatitis (Queensland itch) of the horse: The aetiology of the disease. Aust. J. Agric. Res., *5*:109, 1954.

---

*This article was not reviewed by Dr. Stannard.

*Neo-predef, Upjohn Co., Kalamazoo, MI 49001

Section 12

URINARY TRACT DISEASES

Edited by Christopher M. Brown

EXAMINATION OF THE URINARY SYSTEM 561

RENAL DISEASES 564

BLADDER DISEASES 567

EXAMINATION OF THE URINARY SYSTEM

Christopher M. Brown, EAST LANSING, MICHIGAN

Diseases of the urinary system, particularly of the kidney, are considered rare in the horse. However, over 30 per cent of equine kidneys may have pathologic changes in them. Although this incidence does not reflect the number of clinically affected animals, it does indicate that primary renal disease occurs in horses and that a more thorough examination of the system may be indicated in some circumstances.

PHYSICAL EXAMINATION

Observation and external examination of a horse may often give valuable information about the urinary system. The presence of dried urine on the perineum, tail, and legs of a mare may indicate urinary incontinence, and constant dribbling may indicate the same in the male. Observing micturition allows assessment of normality of position, method of urination, signs of pain, and the volume and nature of the urine passed. Direct external manual examination may not give much useful information. Contrary to widely held views by trainers and owners, horses with kidney disease rarely have sore backs. In foals, abdominal palpation may be helpful in assessing the size of the bladder if it is filled.

Rectal examination is one of the most useful techniques for physical examination of the urinary system in the adult horse. In the majority of average-sized horses, the left kidney is the only one that is palpable. The major part lies ventral to the left transverse process of the first two lumbar vertebrae. The right kidney is usually out of reach, but it may be displaced caudally and may be palpable if enlarged. Gentle rectal palpation of the left kidney is not usually painful, although very firm pressure may elicit some signs of discomfort. The kidney is usually fairly mobile and can be brought to the left paralumbar fossa behind the 18th rib. The surface of the kidney is usually smooth. The ureters and renal vessels are often difficult to identify with any certainty when normal.

In the male, the bladder is usually easy to feel and varies in size and position with filling. In mares, the state of the uterus influences the ease with which the bladder can be palpated. The pelvic urethra in the male is often difficult to identify, as it is surrounded by the accessory sex glands and the urethral muscles. It can, however, be easily identified with a urinary catheter in situ. The female urethra is short and wide and difficult to identify on rectal examination.

CYSTOSCOPY

Cystoscopy is relatively easy in the mare, and after draining the bladder, standard fiberoptic instruments can be easily guided through the urethra and into the bladder for visual examination of its contents, the mucosa, and the ureteric orifices. In males, the length and diameter of the urethra often precludes the passage of many standard fiberoptic endoscopes. It is, however, possible to gain access to the urethra and occasionally the bladder by this route in some males using a 100 cm long, 0.5 cm diameter instrument.

CATHETERIZATION

Bladder catheterization is indicated in horses for a variety of reasons, including establishing the patency of the urethra, the collection of urine samples, and the introduction of medications. The technique is simple and safe in the mare, in which rigid catheters can be passed "blindly" into the bladder. In males, it is usually necessary to tranquilize the animal so that handling of the penis is not resented. In addition, tranquilization usually relaxes the retractor penis muscles, causing the penis to extrude, making cleaning of the glans and introduction of the catheter easier. Acepromazine maleate* is probably one of the best agents for this procedure, as penile relaxation is usually good. There have, however, been occasional reports of permanent paralysis of the retractor penis muscles following the use of promazine tranquilizers in male horses. Although this is rare, it leads to trauma and severe excoriation of the penis, which eventually may have to be amputated. In both sexes, bladder catheterization should be carried out aseptically to avoid iatrogenic cystitis.

RENAL BIOPSY

Percutaneous biopsy of the left kidney can be performed fairly easily in most adult horses, particularly if they are tranquilized. The technique usually requires two people, one to position the kidney in the left paralumbar fossa by manipulation per rectum, while the other passes a needle biopsy instrument through the body wall at a prepared anesthetized

---

*Acepromazine maleate, Fort Dodge Labs, Fort Dodge, IA 50501

561

site directly over the held kidney. The person holding the kidney can usually detect if a successful renal puncture has been made, and the biopsy is then taken. Two samples, one medullary and one cortical, will give a better evaluation of renal pathology than a single sample. Care should be taken to avoid penetrating the kidney too deeply and damaging the main renal vessels. In acute severe renal disease, manipulation of the kidney may be very painful and may prevent a biopsy being taken. The most common complication is the formation of a perirenal hematoma. These can be quite large but usually resolve without ill effect.

RADIOGRAPHY

This cannot be used in the evaluation of the urinary system in the adult, although the male urethra can be demonstrated by retrograde contrast studies. However, in the foal, it is possible to perform plain, contrast, and double-contrast studies to demonstrate various parts of the urinary system.

SERUM BIOCHEMICAL ASPECTS OF URINARY DISEASE

Azotemia can be caused by either renal, prerenal, or postrenal factors. The most common cause of prerenal azotemia in the horse is reduced renal perfusion associated with dehydration and shock. Typical examples would be the animal with acute severe gastrointestinal obstruction or with acute severe diarrhea. Generally speaking, if glomerular filtration rate (GFR) is reduced, then typical changes take place in certain serum constituents.

One of the most widely measured indices of renal function is the blood urea nitrogen (BUN). Urea is not really toxic itself but is easily measured, and its serum elevation is usually accompanied by an elevation in other more toxic nitrogenous waste products such as the guanadine derivatives and phenols. Urea is produced in the liver as a product of amino acid deamination. Thus, in liver disease, BUN can fall, and in increased catabolism or increased dietary nitrogen, the BUN can be elevated. Hence, this index, although useful, is not exclusively controlled by renal function. In fact, even in renal disease, about 75 per cent of nephrons have to be damaged before BUN rises in most mammals examined.

Creatinine is not such a labile serum constituent and is generally uninfluenced by dietary and hepatic factors. Unlike urea, creatinine is neither significantly absorbed nor excreted after filtration by the glomerulus. It is, therefore, a good index of GFR. This is of value in calculating clearance ratios.

Failure in renal control of serum electrolytes can lead to changes in their concentrations. In a horse with severe tubular disease with polydipsia and polyuria, sodium conservation may fail, and total body sodium will fall. Serum sodium may, however, be normal, as the loss is accompanied by water loss. In an acute situation with anuria or oliguria, hypernatremia may develop. However, these situations often develop secondarily to hypovolemic shock precipitated by acute gastrointestinal obstructions or diarrhea. Under these circumstances, the trend to hypernatremia is often counteracted by the loss of electrolytes into the lumen of the obstructed gut or in the fluid feces.

The kidney is the main site of potassium excretion. In anuric or oliguric patients, hyperkalemia may develop, and the toxic effects of potassium on the heart may often be a factor in the death of some of these horses. In animals with more chronic renal failure, serum potassium levels are often normal.

Serum chloride levels tend to follow serum sodium levels, and hyperchloremia or hypochloremia may develop in acute and chronic renal failure in the horse. Overall, the most constant finding in the horse is that animals with chronic renal failure tend to be hypochloremic.

The changes in serum calcium and phosphorus levels in horses with renal failure are different from those in the dog and cat. In the horse, the kidney seems to be the major site of body calcium regulation rather than the intestine. When horses have both kidneys removed, they become hypercalcemic and hypophosphatemic. This may also occur in horses with spontaneous renal failure. High levels of serum calcium are potentially nephrotoxic, and it is possible that the hypercalcemia of equine renal failure may promote further renal damage and compound the situation.

Disturbances in acid-base balance may occur in horses with renal disease if there is a failure to conserve bicarbonate and excrete hydrogen ions. The nonvolatile acids of protein breakdown are also retained, and metabolic acidosis ensues. This is partially offset by buffer systems, and as a result, measured serum bicarbonate is low. If the buffer systems fail to compensate adequately, then serum pH falls. The contribution that reduced renal function makes to the metabolic acidosis seen in some acutely, severely ill equine patients is unknown. Many are losing large amounts of bicarbonate into the gastrointestinal tract, and hypoperfusion of other organs may be causing significant anaerobic activity and increased production of lactic acid.

All of the preceding serum changes may occur if the reduction in renal function is due to primary renal disease or to renal hypoperfusion. Only by examining the urine, the product of renal function, will it be possible to determine whether the problem is prerenal or renal.

URINALYSIS

Equine urine is usually cloudy, strong-smelling, and often rather mucoid. It is usually alkaline in adults (pH 7.0 to 9.0), and the bulk of the cloudiness is due to precipitated calcium carbonate crystals. If the pH is below 6.0, then these crystals are not usually present. In renal failure, the changes in equine urine are very like those seen in other mammals. In hypovolemic states with prerenal uremia, a small volume of concentrated urine is produced. In the polyuric phase of renal failure, the urine will be dilute and of high volume.

Microscopic and biochemical analysis of urine can be helpful. Blood, either as free hemoglobin or erythrocytes, may indicate intravascular hemolysis, acute glomerular damage, or hemorrhage in the ureters, bladder or urethra. Protein, usually albumin, is usually present in significant amounts when glomeruli are damaged. Protein may also be present when there is tubular failure to absorb it from the glomerular filtrate. Glucose may be present either when the renal threshold is exceeded in hyperglycemic states, about 150 mg per dl in horses, or when renal tubules are damaged and fail to absorb filtered glucose. If an equine urine sample contains measurable glucose, then serum glucose should be measured to determine the cause. Pituitary neoplasia and subsequent hypoadrenocorticosteroidism are the most likely causes of polydipsia, polyuria with hyperglycemia, and glucosuria, whereas polydipsia-polyuria with glucosuria and normal blood glucose is indicative of renal tubular disease. The hyperglycemia associated with strenuous exercise may also cause a transient postexercise glucosuria. Horses do not usually produce ketones even when severely starved, so routine urinalysis is usually negative for ketones.

Urinary sediment is often difficult to evaluate in horses owing to large amounts of calcium carbonate crystals. These may be cleared by acidifying the urine. Occasionally, oxalate crystals may also be found in normal equine urine. Hyaline casts are often seen in urine from horses with a variety of systemic diseases and are not indicative of renal disease. On the other hand, granular and epithelial casts are formed in diseased tubules and often include the cellular debris from the tubular lining. They are found in large numbers when urine flow is low in acute tubular disease. They are still significant when there is polyuria, as high flow rates will tend to inhibit their production, even when there are damaged tubules.

ASSESSMENT OF GLOMERULAR FILTRATION AND RENAL CLEARANCE

The calculation of the clearance into the urine from the plasma for various substances can be used to assess renal function. However, for their accurate determination, timed urine collection is required. Although this is feasible in the horse, it is impractical. This can be overcome by the use of creatinine clearance ratios. In the horse, creatinine clearance parallels inulin clearance, and it approximates GFR.

The ratio of the clearance of a substance from plasma to urine to the clearance of creatinine from plasma to urine indicates the extent to which that substance is being excreted or conserved by the tubules. This is so because creatinine clearance is a constant relative to GFR; once filtered, it is neither significantly excreted nor absorbed by the tubules.

Clearance ratios are calculated by the following equation:

$$\frac{C_x}{C_{cr}} = \frac{[X]_u}{[X]_p} \times \frac{[Cr]_p}{[Cr]_u}$$

where C_{cr} = clearance of creatinine, C_x = clearance of x, $[X]_p$ = concentration of x in plasma, $[X]_u$ = concentration of x in urine, $[Cr]_p$ = concentration of creatinine in plasma, $[Cr]_u$ = concentration of creatinine in urine. When multiplied by 100, they are the percentage ratios, and in horses, for sodium the normal range is 0.2 to 1.0 per cent, for potassium 16 to 65 per cent, and for phosphate 0.0 to 1.0 per cent. Usually in tubular failure these values will be elevated.

The sodium sulfanilate clearance test can also be used to assess GFR in the horse. In the dog, it can detect renal disease before azotemia develops. In horses, the agent is injected at 10 mg per kg intravenously, and heparinized blood samples taken at 30, 60, and 90 minutes. The concentration of sodium sulfanilate is measured colorimetrically and is plotted on semilogarithmic graph paper, and clearance half-time is calculated. This is 39.5 ± 4.4 min for normal horses.

Supplemental Readings

1. Behr, M. J., Hackett, R. P., Bentick-Smith, J., Hillman, R. B., King, J. M., and Tennant, B. C.: Metabolic abnormalities associated with rupture of the urinary bladder in neonatal foals. J. Am. Vet. Med. Assoc., *178*:263, 1981.
2. Brobst, D. F., Bramwell, K., and Kramer, J. W.: Sodium sulphanilate clearance as a method of determining renal function in the horse. J. Equine Med. Surg., *2*:500, 1978.
3. Brobst, D. F., Grant, B. D., Hilbert, B. J., Nickels, F. A., Wagner, P., and Waugh, S. L.: Blood biochemical changes in horses with prerenal and renal disease. J. Equine Med. Surg., *1*:171, 1977.
4. Chapman, D. I., Haywood, P. E., and Lloyd, P.: Occurrence of glycosuria in horses after strenuous exercise. Equine Vet. J., *13*:259, 1981.
5. Traver, D. S., Salem, C., Coffman, J. R., Garner, H. E., Moore, J. N., Johnson, J. H., Tritschler, L. G., and Amend, J. F.: Renal metabolism of endogenous substances in the horse: Volumetric vs. clearance methods. J. Equine Med. Surg., *1*:378, 1977.

RENAL DISEASES

M. A. Collier, ITHACA, NEW YORK

Christopher M. Brown, EAST LANSING, MICHIGAN

It is convenient to consider renal failure in two separate categories, acute and chronic. However, it is often difficult to establish such a clear distinction clinically. This is so because up to 75 per cent of the nephrons can be destroyed before clinical signs develop, and the acute onset of renal failure may indicate the sudden failure of chronically diseased kidneys.

ACUTE RENAL FAILURE

The majority of acute renal failure in horses is due to ischemic or toxic chemical nephrosis. Ischemic damage to the tubules occurs following renal hypoperfusion. This usually occurs as a result of peripheral hypotension, most frequently during shock. The hypotension may also occur during or may be compounded by general anesthesia. Surgical manipulation of abdominal viscera in the dog causes a reduction in renal blood flow, and this may also occur during abdominal surgery in the horse. Thus, the equine patient most likely to suffer from renal ischemia is the hypovolemic, endotoxic horse with an acute abdominal disorder requiring general anesthesia and surgery. Other patients, such as those with acute severe diarrhea and endotoxemia, are also at risk. The severity and duration of the renal ischemia determines the severity of the renal damage. The longer and more profound the hypoperfusion, the more severe and irreversible the lesions.

Patients with both shock and ischemic nephrosis have clinical and biochemical evidence of renal failure. However, it is usually impossible to determine how much of the derangement is due to renal factors per se and how much to prerenal factors.

Many substances are potentially nephrotoxic to horses, including plants (such as Quercus sp), heavy metals (such as mercury), and drugs (such as aminoglycosides and sulfonamides). A common cause of toxic nephrosis in horses is myoglobin and less commonly hemoglobin. In acute severe myopathies, significant amounts of myoglobin may be released. This is readily filtered by the glomeruli and is presented in a high concentration to the tubular epithelium. Both myoglobin and hemoglobin may precipitate within the lumina of the tubules. Diffuse tubular damage ensues.

CLINICAL SIGNS AND DIAGNOSIS

Both ischemic and toxic nephrosis will cause similar clinical signs. However, as both usually occur as a result of or in conjunction with other clinical problems, the resulting clinical signs may often be due to a combination of these problems. The renal failure is usually a mixture of renal and prerenal syndromes. The onset of signs may be delayed by up to 24 hours after the insult. Oliguria, or rarely anuria, will initially be present. If low urine flow is due to hypovolemia alone, then the urine will be very concentrated; normal flow and specific gravity will return when the animal is rehydrated. If, however, on rehydration the oliguria persists, then severe tubular damage should be suspected, particularly if there is no response to systemic diuretics, such as furosemide.

If the horse survives the peracute phase, then a period of diuresis develops and continues until the tubular epithelium has regenerated and matured. Tubules lined with immature and regenerating cells cannot concentrate urine. This period of polydipsia and polyuria can persist for many weeks.

On rectal examination, the left kidney may be swollen and painful when handled. In severe cases, the right kidney may be so enlarged that it is also palpable. Urinalysis usually shows granular and epithelial casts made up predominantly of sloughed tubular epithelial cells. The urine is often acidic. Serum biochemical and electrolyte values vary depending upon other coexisting diseases, but elevated BUN and creatinine are consistent findings.

A renal biopsy confirms the diagnosis and can be very helpful in the prognosis. In ischemic nephrosis, both tubular epithelial cells and their basement membranes may be damaged. In toxic nephrosis, only the epithelial cells tend to be damaged, and the basement membrane remains intact. The presence of an intact basement membrane is a good prognostic sign, as regeneration of tubular epithelium only occurs when the membrane is present. During the polyuric phase, repeated biopsies at one- to two-week intervals could be helpful in assessing progress and determining if continued support is justified.

TREATMENT

Initial therapy is directed toward correcting fluid, electrolyte, and acid-base imbalances as determined by laboratory analysis. If oliguria persists after rehydration has been achieved, great care should be taken to avoid overhydration. Administration should be controlled to meet those fluid losses arising from the lungs, skin, and the gastrointestinal system (p. 311). Diuretics, such as furosemide, may be administered to promote urine flow, but in severe tubular nephrosis, they will be ineffective.

If the horse survives the acute phase and enters the reparative phase of the disease, then the problems are (1) to maintain adequate fluid and electrolyte intake to counteract urinary loss, and (2) to reduce the nitrogenous excretion load of the kidney. If the horse remains azotemic and depressed, it may be reluctant to drink. It may then be necessary to give fluids and electrolytes either parenterally or via stomach tube. Lactated Ringer's solution is suitable in most cases for intravenous therapy. If the animal is eating and drinking well, then free choice water and mineralized salt should be available at all times. Food should have a low nitrogen content, such as grass-hay and cracked corn.

Many of these severely ill, azotemic, enterotoxemic, or myositic horses run a high risk of developing laminitis. Several drugs used in the management of this condition are potentially nephrotoxic, such as phenylbutazone and meclofenamic acid. It is important, therefore, that animals that have suffered a potential renal insult and that also run the risk of laminitis should not be given these nonsteroidal anti-inflammatory drugs.

Horses that suffer acute extensive renal tubular damage may recover apparently adequate renal function. This can take several weeks, and during this period, the animal will lose a considerable amount of weight. If serum analysis and urinalysis indicate that adequate renal function has returned, this does not mean that the horse has fully normal kidneys. It means that the remaining nephrons have repaired and compensated to control fluid electrolyte and acid-base balances. The animal possibly has a significantly reduced renal reserve.

CHRONIC RENAL DISEASE

PYELONEPHROSIS

This disease is not common in the horse and occurs more often in females than in males. It is usually a postparturient condition, most cases arising from ascending infections. Thus, most are associated with cystitis and ureteritis. Occasionally the disease arises hematogenously. The causative organisms vary, although in one series of eight cases, *Corynebacterium renale* was isolated from all. However, streptococci were also seen in the urine sediments of these horses, and this suggests that they possibly had mixed infections.

CLINICAL SIGNS AND DIAGNOSIS

The disease is chronic with anorexia, weight loss, and depression as nonspecific features. As cystitis is often present, pollakiuria and tenesmus may also be features. Urine may be blood-tinged or may contain blood clots. Early in the disease, there may be vague signs of abdominal discomfort. In well-advanced cases, large amounts of both kidneys may be destroyed, and clinical signs of renal failure may ensue.

Rectal examination may reveal a thickened bladder wall indicative of cystitis, and the ureters and left kidney may feel abnormal. It has been suggested that the ureters in the mare are more readily palpated per vagina than per rectum. They may be dilated and thickened. The kidney may be roughened and painful with adhesions to the body wall.

Hematologic findings are usually consistent with a chronic infection, and there may be a mild anemia. This may arise either from chronic infection or from reduced erythropoietin production or both. Urinalysis is consistent with an active purulent infection within the urinary tract, with inflammatory cells, protein, blood, and bacteria present. Urine culture may isolate the involved organisms.

TREATMENT

The disease is often well established, and severe renal damage has occurred by the time it is diagnosed. Based on culture and sensitivity testing, the appropriate antimicrobial therapy can be started. Although many antibiotics are concentrated by the kidney and reach high levels in the urine (for example, penicillin G and tetracycline), there are few data that describe intrarenal levels. High urinary levels of appropriate antibiotics will be helpful in treating bacilluria, and as a consequence, the source of reinfection for the kidney may be removed. However, if the infection is well established within the kidney, high urinary concentrations of antibiotics may be of little benefit. (Urinary levels are discussed under Cystitis, p. 567.) Limited data from experimental animals suggest that ampicillin achieves renal concentrations up to eight times those in serum. However, in pyelonephritis, the levels may be only half those in serum. Nitrofurantoin does not appear in the urine of people with severe renal failure and is contraindicated in azotemic patients. Therapy may halt further progression of the disease, but adequate repair will often not occur. The prognosis in all well-established cases is very guarded.

GLOMERULONEPHRITIS

This is an uncommon but regularly reported disease in horses. Both membranoproliferative and mesangioproliferative glomerulonephritis have been described. The acute phases have not been described, and most horses have been examined during the chronic stages. The etiology has not been established in the horse. In one series of 45 horses, 42 per cent were found to have immune complex–induced glomerulopathy. Some cases have been associated with equine infectious anemia antigens, and in others it has been suggested that streptococcal antigens may be involved in some cases. One case has been described with lesions similar to those seen in systemic lupus erythematosus in humans. In most clinically affected cases, both glomeruli and tubules are often damaged, and as a result, the clinical signs are related to abnormal function of both.

CLINICAL SIGNS AND DIAGNOSIS

Clinical signs are nonspecific. A history of chronic weight loss is common. Polydipsia, polyuria, and pollakiuria are not constant in all cases. Rectal examination may reveal a smaller firm left kidney, but this is not true in all cases. The nephrotic syndrome has been described in one horse with focal glomerulosclerosis.

Most animals when investigated will be azotemic and hypochloremic. Some may be hypercalcemic and hypophosphatemic. Several have nonregenerative mild anemias. Sodium sulfanilate clearance is often prolonged, up to five times the normal rate. Urine usually has a normal pH but is very dilute. Some cases have traces of blood in the urine, and most have some degree of proteinuria. Cellular debris and casts are not numerous (Liu et al., personal communication, 1981). Twenty-four–hour water deprivation usually only causes a slight increase in urine specific gravity. (This should not be performed if the animal is severely azotemic.)

A renal biopsy will often confirm the diagnosis.

TREATMENT

Supportive therapy, including fluids, electrolytes, and a low-nitrogen diet, is recommended. However, once diagnosed, the lesions are usually irreversible, and no specific therapy has been reported. The prognosis is unfavorable.

PARASITIC RENAL DISEASE

Renal coccidiosis associated with *Klossiella equi* has been described in the horse. A schizont generation develops in the endothelial cells of Bowman's capsule, and several further stages of development occur along the length of the tubules. Sporocysts are released in the urine, and the cycle is completed on ingestion, with hematogenous passage of sporozoites from the gut to the kidney.

All reports indicate that this organism does not cause sufficient damage to give clinical signs, although parasites may often be seen throughout the kidney. It is mentioned here, as it may be identified either by renal biopsy or at necropsy and clinical renal failure attributed to its presence. Such an attribution is not usually justified.

Micronema deletrix, a helminth parasite found occasionally in the horse, has been reported to cause multiple granulomas in equine kidneys. As with *Klossiella,* no clinical signs have been attributed to its presence.

NEOPLASMS

Neoplasms of the equine kidney are rare. Most reported cases have been necropsy findings and have been unrelated to clinical signs. Tumors that have been reported include adenocarcinoma and squamous cell carcinoma. Presumably if these occurred within the left kidney, their presence could be detected by rectal examination.

OXALATE NEPHROPATHY

The ingestion of oxalate-containing plants by horses can lead to a variety of signs, including renal disease. However, many equine urine samples contain a few oxalate crystals in the absence of clinical renal disease. Similarly, oxalate crystals may be found within renal tubules in horses showing clinical signs of renal disease. The crystals can be occasional or very common. The presence of the crystals has in the past been taken as evidence of oxalate poisoning, and a diagnosis of oxalate nephropathy has been made. There is often no evidence that these horses have been exposed to oxalates or their precursors. Frequently, these kidneys have glomerular changes as well. Currently, the significance of oxalate crystals within equine renal tubules is unknown. It is probable that they merely reflect an abnormality in renal tubular function rather than a cause of that malfunction.

RENAL CALCULI

These are rare and have been described at necropsy. No clinical data are available, but if advanced cases were encountered, then signs of pain and chronic renal disease would be expected.

Supplemental Readings

1. Andrews, E. J.: Oxalate nephropathy in a horse. J. Am. Vet. Med. Assoc., *154*:49, 1971.
2. Banks, K. L., and Henson, J. B.: Immunologically mediated glomerulitis of horses. I and II. Lab. Invest., 26:701, 1972.

3. Berggren, P. C.: Renal adenocarcinoma in a horse. J. Am. Vet. Med. Assoc., *176*:1252, 1980.
4. Boyd, W. L., and Bishop, L. M.: Pyelonephritis of cattle and horses. J. Am. Vet. Med. Assoc., *90*:156, 1937.
5. Jackson, O. F.: Renal calculi in a horse. Vet. Rec., *91*:7, 1972.
6. McCausland, I. P., and Milestone, B. A.: Diffuse mesangio-proliferative glomerulonephritis in a horse. N. Z. Vet. J., *24*:239, 1976.
7. Roberts, M. C., and Seiler, R. J.: Renal failure in a horse with chronic glomerulonephritis and renal oxalosis. J. Equine Med. Surg., 3:278, 1979.
8. Rubin, H. L., and Woodward, J. C.: Equine infection with *Micronema deletrix.* J. Am. Vet. Med. Assoc., *165*:256, 1974.
9. Vetterling, J. M., and Thompson, D. E.: *Klossiella equi.* Baumann, 1946 (Sporozoa: Eucoccidia: Adeleina) from equids. J. Parasitol., *58*:589, 1972.
10. Von Kidas, I., and Szazados, I.: Membrano-proliferative diffuse glomerulonephritis bei einem Pferd. Deutsch Tierartz. Wchshr., *24*:618, 1974.
11. Wimberly, H. C., Antonovych, T. T., and Lewis, R. M.: Focal glomerulosclerosis-like disease with nephrotic syndrome in a horse. Vet. Pathol., *18*:692, 1981.

BLADDER DISEASES

Christopher M. Brown, EAST LANSING, MICHIGAN
M. A. Collier, ITHACA, NEW YORK

CYSTITIS

This may be primary, arising from an ascending infection from the vagina or penis, or secondary to cystic calculi, bladder paralysis, or poor catheterization technique.

CLINICAL SIGNS AND DIAGNOSIS

In cases other than those secondary to bladder paralysis, the clinical signs are similar, irrespective of the cause. Pollakiuria and stranguria occur, often with pain and grunting. Pyelonephritis often develops as an ascending infection in chronic cases, and then the clinical signs will be combined with those of renal disease. The most common organisms associated with equine cystitis are streptococci, staphylococci, *Corynebacterium renale*, and various coliforms. The infections are often mixed.

Rectal examination of the bladder may suggest a primary cause, such as a calculus or paralysis, but in acute primary cases, the bladder may feel normal. Handling the bladder may be painful to the horse and may induce tenesmus. In more chronic cases, the bladder may well be thickened. Urine will contain inflammatory cells and often blood. Casts are not usually present in significant numbers if there is no renal involvement. Bacteria may be obvious on microscopic examination of the urine. Culture may identify the causative organism or organisms.

TREATMENT

Culture and sensitivity will indicate which antimicrobial therapy should be instituted. Agents should be selected that are excreted in high concentrations in the urine. The penicillins, cephalosporins, aminoglycosides, sulfonamides, trimethoprim, and nitrofurantoin are primarily excreted by the kidney in their active form. This is also true for most tetracyclines except chlortetracycline. When given at normal systemic levels, penicillin G may achieve urinary levels sufficiently high to be effective against *E. coli* and Proteus sp, which in other body fluids would not be true. Experimentally produced *Proteus mirabilis* cystitis in ponies was successfully treated with trimethoprim-sulfadiazine paste given orally for 13 days. In depressed animals with reduced water intake, it may be necessary to give oral fluids to maintain an adequate urine flow. If a primary problem such as calculi or paralysis is present, then appropriate action should be taken (see next sections). In chronic cases, the prognosis is guarded.

CYSTIC CALCULI

No predisposing causes have been identified for calculus formation in the horse. They are usually of calcium carbonate, but some also contain calcium oxalate and phosphate.

CLINICAL SIGNS AND DIAGNOSIS

In mares calculi can become very large before clinical signs of cystitis become obvious. In males they may cause problems earlier by wedging in the neck of the bladder and arresting urine flow. The animal may adopt the position to urinate and never pass any urine, or it may begin to urinate, and then the flow is suddenly arrested. Occasionally, a calculus will pass into the male urethra and will cause acute obstruction. Horses of either sex with cystic calculi may have a history of postexercise hematuria. Unlike the brownish urine passed by horses with exercise-induced myopathies, the urine passed by horses with cystic calculi contains fresh blood, often only in the last portion of the urine voided.

Rectal examination may confirm the presence of a large calculus, but if the bladder is full and the stone is small, then it may be missed. The bladder should, therefore, be catheterized and emptied, and the rectal examination should be repeated. Catheterization is also helpful in the male, as the calculus may be lodged in the urethra or bladder neck. Cystoscopy may be helpful; in addition to assessing the size and nature of the calculus, the state of the bladder wall can then be determined. Urinalysis is similar to that in cystitis.

TREATMENT

Surgical removal of the calculus is the only effective therapy. In the mare, the size of the stone may determine the approach. Extremely large ones will have to be removed via celiotomy and cystotomy. Smaller ones can be removed through the urethra, either intact or after being crushed into smaller pieces. In males, two choices are available, either via celiotomy or by subischial urethrotomy and then probing forward into the bladder to break up and retrieve the calculus. In addition to surgical treatment, all cases should be evaluated and treated for cystitis.

BLADDER PARALYSIS

Any lower spinal cord lesions could potentially lead to bladder paralysis. Two conditions in particular have been associated with this condition. They are neuritis of the cauda equina and poisoning with Sudan grass, both of which can cause additional signs, including ataxia, analgesia of the skin, and, in neuritis of the cauda equina, tail paralysis.

CLINICAL SIGNS AND DIAGNOSIS

Reflex emptying of the bladder is lost, and continued distention and stretching further reduce any active contractions. The bladder fills to its maximal capacity, and urine is discharged on a more or less continuous basis as the bladder overflows. In males, urine drips continually from the penis or runs out in spurts as the horse moves. In mares, the continuous incontinence causes severe scalding of the

thighs, which may be raw, ulcerated, and encrusted with dried urine. The inflammation of the vulva and vagina may cause continuous "winking" and some tenesmus.

On rectal examination, the bladder is found to be very distended and often displaced well over the pelvic brim. Large amounts of calcium carbonate crystals may settle in the atonic bladder, and several kilograms of sebulous material may be present. This further aggravates the situation, stretching the bladder and drawing it further ventrally into the abdomen. This sandlike concretion may be palpable per rectum. Secondary bacterial cystitis is often present.

TREATMENT

The underlying neurologic deficits are usually not treatable and are irreversible. If the cause is acute or secondary to acute obstruction, then it may be reversible. The bladder should then be emptied regularly, either by placement of an indwelling catheter or by repeated catheterizations. Emptying may be assisted by rectal massage of the bladder. If excessive amounts of crystals have accumulated, then repeated lavage may be helpful in breaking down the mass and flushing it out. Cases with bacterial cystitis should be treated appropriately as discussed earlier.

RUPTURE OF THE BLADDER

Although this can occur in any type and age of horse, it is more common by far in neonatal male foals. In these cases, it possibly occurs during parturition when the foal is passing through the mare's pelvis. Intravesicular pressure is increased, and the male urethra is long and narrow and possibly is being compressed ventrally. The bladder usually ruptures in the dorsal area. In female foals, presumably, the urine is easily expressed out of the short, wide urethra into the amniotic cavity.

CLINICAL SIGNS AND DIAGNOSIS

Affected foals appear normal for one or two days after birth. A failure to urinate or the passage of only small amounts of urine may go unnoticed. They become progressively duller and anorexic. The most striking feature is the development of abdominal distention. It is gradual, progressive, and on physical examination is found to be due to fluid. This is in direct contrast to those foals with acute intestinal obstruction, in which abdominal distention is rapid in onset and predominantly due to gas. Intestinally obstructed foals are usually very colicky; those with ruptured bladders may be mildly colicky or may have no apparent pain.

Progressive fluid accumulation in the peritoneum of a neonatal male foal is strongly suggestive of a ruptured bladder. Careful observation in an unbedded stall over a few hours will confirm that little or no urine is being passed. A urinary catheter can be easily passed into the bladder, but little if any urine is obtained.

Plain radiographs of the abdomen show the presence of fluid in the peritoneal cavity. Retrograde contrast cystography may help in demonstrating the tear. Abdominocentesis yields a free-flowing clear fluid, which may or may not smell like urine. Laboratory examination of the fluid will show a much higher urea nitrogen content than is found in plasma, sometimes as much as three times the normal amount.

Some serum biochemical and electrolyte values may be abnormal. Some foals have elevated urea levels, and most have elevated creatinine levels. Most are hyperkalemic, hyponatremic, hypochloremic, and dehydrated.

TREATMENT

Surgical repair of the defect is the only permanent solution. However, it is unwise to anesthetize these animals until their acid-base, fluid, and electrolyte status has been determined and any severe abnormalities corrected. This is best done by placing a peritoneal drain to slowly remove the fluid and administering appropriate fluids intravenously.

The prognosis is good if the diagnosis is made early and if severe life-threatening metabolic changes have not taken place.

PATENT URACHUS

This neonatal condition occurs when the urachus fails to close completely at birth. As a result, the bladder is connected to the navel via the urachus. Clinical signs are variable and depend to some extent upon the presence or absence of secondary complications. Simple uncomplicated cases may go unnoticed for several days.

CLINICAL SIGNS AND DIAGNOSIS

Urine may drip continuously or intermittently from the navel. Often it is only obvious when the foal attempts to urinate in the normal way. Urine then flows not only from the urethra but also from the urachus. Complications arise owing to urine scalding of the navel, causing a severe dermatitis. This may become infected, causing a localized abscess or, more seriously, an ascending infection along the remnants of the umbilical vessels. Infection may pass along the patent urachus and give rise to cystitis.

A permanently moist navel or the squirting of fluid from the navel are strongly suggestive signs. Gently probing the navel with a cotton-tipped applicator may identify the patent urachus. Retrograde contrast cystography will confirm the patency of the urachus and will give an impression of its diameter.

TREATMENT

Occasionally the urachus will close spontaneously, particularly if it is inflamed or infected. Those that do not can be treated in two ways, either by chemical cautery or surgically. The objective of chemical cautery is to promote a localized inflammatory response within the urachus and to achieve its closure with granulation tissue. Two agents are commonly used, either phenol or silver nitrate. Concentrated phenol solution is applied using cotton-tipped applicators, and silver nitrate is obtainable in pre-prepared applicators.* The foal should be firmly restrained or tranquilized when the cautery is performed. This prevents spillage of the agents on the abdominal skin and also reduces the risk of breaking the applicator within the urachus. A liberal coating of petroleum jelly or a similar barrier cream should be applied around the navel to prevent scalding, not only from urine but also from the chemical agents. Two applications daily for three to four days will often be enough to promote adequate granulation and closure. The foal should receive systemic antibiotic therapy for the duration of treatment and for two additional days after closure.

If chemical cautery fails to promote closure or if the urachus is considered too large to be treated by this method, surgery is indicated. This requires general anesthesia, celiotomy, and recognition and ligation of the urachus.

Supplemental Readings

1. Behr, M. J., Hackett, R. P., Bentick-Smith, J., Hillman, R. B., King, J. M., and Tennant, B. C.: Metabolic abnormalities with rupture of the urinary bladder in neonatal foals. J. Am. Vet. Med. Assoc., *178*;263, 1981.
2. Roberts, M. C.: Ascending urinary tract infection in ponies. Aust. Vet. J., 55:191, 1979.

*Silver Nitrate Applicators, Graham-Field Surgical Co., New Hyde Park, NY 11040

Section 13

TOXICOLOGY

Edited by F. W. Oehme and T. Tobin

TOXICOSES COMMONLY OBSERVED IN HORSES 573

GENERAL PRINCIPLES IN TREATMENT OF POISONING 577

INSECTICIDES 580

RODENTICIDES 584

SNAKE BITE 587

BLISTER BEETLE 588

CARBON TETRACHLORIDE 590

PHENOTHIAZINE 590

PETROLEUM PRODUCTS 591

LEAD 592

SELENIUM 593

PLANT TOXICITIES 595

WATER QUALITY 607

THE ETIOLOGIC DIAGNOSIS OF SUDDEN DEATH 611

TOXICOSES COMMONLY OBSERVED IN HORSES

Frederick W. Oehme, MANHATTAN, KANSAS

A knowledge of the common poisons in the practice area, the frequency of various toxicities, and the incidence of these poisonings during certain seasons of the year or during various activities helps the practitioner to narrow the potential range of poisonings from which a diagnosis may be made. In suspected poisoning, it is better to concentrate on common toxicities than to devote diagnostic and therapeutic efforts on a wide variety of potential toxins.

While each practitioner must learn the type and frequency of the chemical exposures possible in the practice area, certain groups of chemicals or toxin-containing materials frequently cause poisoning in horses. Tables 1 through 5 summarize the signs and therapy of the common toxicoses causing gastrointestinal, nervous system, and hematologic signs and those causing skin problems.

EMERGENCY TREATMENT

Urgency is of utmost importance in treating toxicoses. Three rules to follow are begin treatment promptly; retain samples of blood, urine, and feces for analysis; and keep the animal warm during therapy.

The practitioner must act to prevent further absorption of toxin. This can be simply accomplished by moving the horse to a different pasture or stall and supplying fresh food and water, i.e., preventing access to the toxin. In cases of skin exposure, a thorough washing with a mild detergent and plenty of water is necessary. In cases of ingested poisons a gastric lavage in the unconscious or anesthetized horse or a laxative of mineral oil (3 liters PO) should be used to empty the digestive tract.

Treatment should be followed by oral administra-

TABLE 1. PRIMARY CLINICAL SIGNS ARE GASTROINTESTINAL

Toxin	Signs	Treatment
Acids	Corrosion of mucous membrane of upper GI tract; colic and purgation followed by acute shock	Milk of magnesia, 20–30 ml PO Flush externally with water; apply paste of sodium bicarbonate
Alkalis	As for acids	4–6 egg whites to 1 l. tepid water followed by a cathartic Flush externally with water
Arsenic	Acute: abdominal pain, staggering gait, extreme weakness, trembling, salivation, diarrhea, fast, feeble pulse Subchronic: depression, anorexia, watery diarrhea, increased urination followed by anuria, dehydration, ataxia, trembling, stupor, cold extremities	Tannic acid, strong tea, or protein (egg white) to absorb; d-penicillamine, 11 mg/kg qid for 7–10 days PO; or sodium thiosulfate, 8–10 gm of 20% solution IV, and 20–30 gm plus 300 ml water PO; or dimercaprol (BAL), 3 mg/kg IM Repeat every 4 hours for 2 days, then qid on day 3, then bid until day 10 Supportive fluid and electrolyte therapy
Carbon tetrachloride	Loss of appetite, dullness, staggering gait, gastroenteritis, bloody feces, constipation followed by diarrhea, collapse, and death	Empty stomach, give high protein and carbohydrate diet; maintain fluid and electrolyte balance Do not give epinephrine
Petroleum distillates	Immediate bloat, shivering, and incoordination Anorexia	Mineral oil, 3 l. PO; after ½ hr, 20% sodium sulfate, 250–1000 gm PO
Phenols and creosols	Gastroenteritis, painful abdomen, weakness and depression, sternal recumbency	Wash skin, apply sodium bicarbonate (0.5%) dressing Mineral oil, 3 l. PO Activated charcoal, 250–500 gm PO
Plants: Oak (tannins)	Constipation, abdominal pain, hematuria, weakness	Symptomatic treatment, stimulants, blood transfusions, and fluid therapy
Ragwort (alkaloid)	Acute: dullness, weakness, abdominal pain, nervous excitement Chronic: prolonged poor condition, icterus, yawning, drowsiness, staggering gait	Symptomatic treatment

TABLE 2. PRIMARY CLINICAL SIGNS ARE CENTRAL NERVOUS SYSTEM STIMULATION

Toxin	Signs	Treatment
Alkaloids	Nervousness, difficult breathing, loss of muscular control, excess salivation, convulsions	Potassium permanganate, 2–4 ml/kg (1:10,000 solution) gastric lavage or PO Physostigmine salicylate, 30–120 mg SC or IM
Insecticides: Carbamates	Profuse salivation, diarrhea, muscle fasciculation, hyperactivity, followed by posterior paresis	Atropine sulfate, 0.5–1.0 mg/kg IV or to effect (dry mucous membranes), repeat dose as needed
Chlorinated hydrocarbons	CNS stimulation, violent excitation, muscle fasciculations, cranial to caudal convulsions	External: wash thoroughly with soap and water Barbiturates or chloral hydrate to control seizures Activated charcoal 250–500 gm PO with 20% sodium sulfate, 250–1000 gm PO
Organophosphates	As for carbamates	Atropine sulfate, 0.5–1.0 mg/kg IV or to effect (dry mucous membranes) followed by pralidoxime chloride (2-PAM, protopam chloride), 2% solution, 25–50 mg/kg by slow IV, repeat as needed, usually every 8–12 hrs
Lead	Blindness, muscle twitching, ataxia, head pressing, convulsions; often appears as GI involvement (diarrhea, salivation, anorexia)	Activated charcoal, 250–500 gm PO with 20% sodium sulfate, 250–1000 gm PO Calcium disodium EDTA, 28.5 mg/kg qid for 5 days Initial dose IV, then SC as 10 mg/ml in 5% dextrose
Plants: Larkspur (alkaloid)	Hypersensitivity, muscular trembling, collapse, prostration, convulsions Constipation, bloat, excessive salivation sometimes noted	Physostigmine (2.2 grains) plus pilocarpine (4.4 grains) plus strychnine (1.1 grains) in 20 ml water given SC per 500 kg, use with caution
Locoweed (selenium plus others)	Very excitable and irritable, abnormal gait, separate from herd, head held peculiarly, disturbed vision, chronic loss of weight, weakness, prostration, convulsions	Laxative, sedatives, quiet
Lupine (alkaloid)	Nervousness, loss of muscular control, frothing at the mouth, convulsions	Sedatives, laxatives, see alkaloids
Oleander (glycoside)	Overstimulation of the vagus, abdominal pain, diarrhea, tremors, progressive paralysis, coma	Atropine sulfate, gastric lavage Symptomatic treatment
Poison hemlock (alkaloid)	Incoordination, salivation, abdominal pain, weakness, shallow, irregular respiration, coma	Laxatives, tannic acid, stimulants Supportive treatment
Water hemlock (resinoid)	Violent spasms resulting in rapid respiration and heart rate, coma	Symptomatic treatment Artificial respiration
White snakeroot (tremetol)	Marked trembling, incoordination, weakness, inability to stand Partial throat paralysis	Laxatives, stimulants
Yellow star thistle (unknown)	Lip twitching, involuntary chewing, mouth open, inability to swallow or hold food in mouth, mechanical damage to lips	Symptomatic treatment

tion of an activated charcoal slurry (250 to 500 gm in 2 to 4 liters warm water). Administer a specific antidote, if known; otherwise treat the horse symptomatically. Assist the patient's respiration if necessary, keep the patient warm, and observe the initial signs carefully.

POISONOUS PLANTS

In horses other than those continually stabled and fed hay and commercial feed, the risk from injury due to poisonous or harmful weeds is a serious one. Pastures contain a variety of plants, often unrecognized, and plants growing along fences are often protected from mowing while still being accessible to the horse. Weather conditions may reduce the available pasture while weeds thrive. The clinical signs may be acute or subacute, but the effects are usually the result of animals consuming the plant material for several days and eventually showing the effects in one or more body systems.

Gastrointestinal problems, characterized by colic and diarrhea, may develop from plants such as castor bean (p. 604), oleander (p. 602), and bracken fern (p. 600). Damage to the liver, usually the result of continued plant ingestion for many weeks, produces an altered temperament, a dummy-like attitude, loss of weight, and hepatic cirrhosis. Fiddleneck (Amsinckia) (p. 596), groundsel (Senecio) (p.

TABLE 3. PRIMARY CLINICAL SIGNS ARE CENTRAL NERVOUS SYSTEM DEPRESSION

Toxin	Signs	Treatment
Mercury	Muscle incoordination, ataxia, hyperesthesia, tremor, convulsions, and coma Can appear as GI involvement (diarrhea, anorexia, emaciation)	Activated charcoal, 250–500 gm PO Dimercaprol (BAL), 3 mg/kg IM; repeat every 4 hrs for 2 days, then qid on 3rd day, then bid for 10 days until recovery Supportive fluid and electrolyte therapy

Plants:
  Black locust
  (glycoside)
	Anorexia, depression, weakness, posterior paresis, irregular pulse, labored breathing	Digitalis
		Symptomatic treatment

Crotolaria (alkaloid)	Acute: anorexia, gastric irritation, tenesmus, bloody feces Chronic: emaciation and depression	Supportive therapy
Death camas (steroid alkaloid)	Stiff-leggedness, hypersensitivity, anxious expressions, dyspnea, weakness, posterior paresis, convulsions	Atropine sulfate (4.4 mg) plus picrotoxin (17.6 mg) in 5 ml water given IV per 100 kg; repeat every 2 hrs for 2–3 injections
Horsetail (thiaminase plus unknown)	Weakness, diarrhea, rapid weight loss, incoordination, coma	Thiamine hydrochloride 100–200 mg SC daily for several days
Milkweed (resinoid)	Incoordination, depression, shallow respiration, inability to stand, coma	Symptomatic treatment
Bracken fern (thiaminase)	Emaciation, incoordination, marked progress to paralysis and inability to rise	Thiamine hydrochloride 100–200 mg SC daily for several days

TABLE 4. PRIMARY CLINICAL SIGNS ARE BLOOD ALTERATIONS

Toxin	Signs	Treatment
Chlorates, nitrites	Staggering, purging, abdominal pain, hematuria, hemoglobinuria, dyspnea, cyanosis Blood is dark brown	4% methylene blue 10 mg/kg IV; repeat at intervals of several hours
Cyanide Arrowgrass, corn, elderberry, prunus sp, sorghum sp	Initial excitement and muscle tremors followed by pronounced polypnea and dyspnea, salivation, lacrimation, and voiding of feces and urine Gasping for breath and clonic convulsions Blood is bright cherry red	20% sodium nitrite (10 ml) plus 20% sodium thiosulfate (30 ml), 0.09 ml/kg IV
Phenothiazine	Hemolysis, anemia, hemoglobinuria, weakness, anorexia, fever, icterus, colic, constipation, and diarrhea	Methylamphetamine 0.1–0.2 mg/kg IV for phenothiazine tranquilizers Symptomatic treatment

TABLE 5. PRIMARY CLINICAL SIGNS ARE EPITHELIAL DAMAGE

Toxin	Signs	Treatment
Plants: Horsebrush	Photosensitization	Topical ointments; symptomatic treatment Keep out of sun; graze at night
St. Johnswort	Photosensitization	See horsebrush
Foxtail	Mechanical injury	Symptomatic treatment
Cheatgrass	Mechanical injury	Symptomatic treatment
Needlegrass	Mechanical injury	Symptomatic treatment
Poverty grass	Mechanical injury	Symptomatic treatment
Crimson clover	Mechanical injury	Symptomatic treatment

596), and crotolaria (p. 596) are common plants that induce liver damage. Many horses with liver damage will exhibit central nervous system effects, assumed to result from the buildup of ammonia. This excitability and altered personality may be confused with direct central nervous system effects induced by another series of poisonous plants. Clinical signs of hyperexcitability, incoordination, paresis or paralysis, abnormal body movements or posturing, convulsions, and coma may result from yellow star thistle (p. 595), locoweed (p. 599), lupine, nicotine (p. 580), and the selenium-containing plants (p. 593). By the time central nervous system effects are observed, most horses are no longer treatable.

Sudden death may be due to cyanide-containing plants such as sorghums (p. 598) fed by owners unaware of the danger. A number of pasture plants contain awns and thistles that induce mechanical injury to the lips, gums, and tongues of consuming horses. Others, such as vines and coarse plants, may provide a digestive tract obstruction.

INSECTICIDES AND RODENTICIDES

The organophosphate insecticides (p. 582) and chlorinated hydrocarbon insecticides (p. 581) are common poisons of horses. Chlordane, heptachlor, aldrin, dieldrin, isodrin, endrin, toxaphene, lindane, methoxychlor, and the variety of organophosphate compounds that are continually growing in number and in ingenuity of naming are highly toxic compounds that horses are exposed to topically or via ingestion.

The rodenticides that may produce poisoning in horses include strychnine (p. 584), ANTU (p. 585), compound 1080 (p. 585), warfarin (p. 584), arsenic (p. 585), barium (p. 587), thallium (p. 586), phosphorus (p. 586), and zinc phosphide (p. 586).

MEDICATIONS

Because of the variety of "health products" provided to horses by their proud and enthusiastic owners, toxicoses due to drugs and chemical products intended for maintaining and improving equine health are not uncommon. Vitamins, stimulants, analgesics, anthelmintics, and tranquilizers may all cause problems due to misuse through overapplication or erroneous routes of administration. When several of these drugs are used concurrently, chemical interactions may occur, resulting in adverse drug reactions. The inherent sensitivity of the horse to foreign chemicals contributes further to the relatively high incidence of drug reactions in equine medicine.

SNAKE AND INSECT BITES

The sensitivity of horse skin and tissue, coupled with the environments in which many horses are housed or pastured, leads to a high incidence of insect (p. 558) or snake bites (p. 587). Localized and occasionally generalized reactions are common; fatalities occur if individual sensitivity is great or if bites evoke swelling that interferes with vital functions. Fortunately the incidence of snake and insect bite is seasonal and usually is restricted to specific regions.

MISCELLANEOUS TOXICOSES

Fungi are everywhere, and under appropriate conditions of moisture, temperature, and carbohydrate availability, they may grow in horse feeds. The presence of spoiled feed should remind the clinician of the possibility of fungal growth and the presence of mycotoxins. Aflatoxins produce pronounced liver damage, while other mycotoxins may induce colic, hemorrhagic gastroentertis, kidney dysfunction, blood coagulation defects, and interference with immune status.

Gases may be generated under a variety of housing or environmental conditions. Carbon monoxide, hydrogen sulfide, nitrogen dioxide, ammonia, sulfur dioxide, carbon disulfide, and hydrogen cyanide are all toxic to horses in confined and poorly ventilated situations.

Supplemental Reading

Galitzer, S., and Oehme, F. W.: Emergency procedures for equine toxicoses. Equine Prac., *1*:49, 1979.

GENERAL PRINCIPLES IN TREATMENT OF POISONING

Frederick W. Oehme, MANHATTAN, KANSAS

The treatment of any poisoning is based upon a sound diagnosis. Except in emergency treatments, in which case general antidotal therapy is employed, every attempt should be made to utilize the available diagnostic information to formulate the most specific treatment for the poisoning.

DIAGNOSIS

The diagnosis of poisoning is based upon an adequate history, clinical evaluation of the patient, and a necropsy if death occurs and other animals are still involved. Since few poisonings have pathognomonic clinical syndromes or necropsy lesions, the history is often a key to diagnosis. Observation, an adept questioning procedure, and utilization of the practitioner's knowledge of management practices and personality quirks of the client assist greatly in generating diagnostic clues. The clinical signs in poisoned horses may involve a variety of body systems, with the central nervous system, digestive tract, liver, and blood frequently being affected. General signs of poisoning are lack of appetite, depression, weight loss, dehydration, colic, and frequent and difficult respiration. Hyperexcitability, incoordination, muscular twitching, abnormal posturing and body movements, and convulsions leading to prostration and coma may be suggestive of primary central nervous system effects or can be secondary to liver or digestive tract disturbance.

Diagnosis is especially difficult in chronic, low-grade poisonings that may involve biochemical or metabolic "interference syndromes" or may reflect the gradual accumulation of chemicals in various body systems and the eventual expression of their toxicity. The history and general physical appearance of the patient will often suggest a long-term process that may be at variance with the client's insistence that the horse "just got sick."

Whenever possible, a complete postmortem examination should be performed on animals dying from poisons. Although very few poisonings provide pathognomonic necropsy findings, there are many horses thought to have been poisoned that upon necropsy have a strangulation or torsion of the digestive tract, a discovery that warrants the effort involved in performing field necropsies. Although laboratory studies are frequently expensive, they are often the only definitive procedures to identify the cause of an intoxication. Unfortunately, the laboratory is not able to perform an all-encompassing screening test, and the clinician must suggest the most likely or suspected poison for laboratory assay. Suggestions for sample collection are given in the article on the etiologic diagnosis of sudden death (p. 611). In the living patient, blood and urine, as well as samples of suspected contaminated material, may be submitted for analysis.

The clinician should not rely upon the laboratory assay and should not wait for histopathologic or laboratory results before initiating therapy and suggesting management changes. "Tincture of time" is applicable only if the patient can spontaneously deal with the disease process. In cases of overwhelming intoxications or in instances of continuing ingestion and accumulation of a toxic compound, not waiting even a matter of hours before initiating treatment may mean the difference between recovery or death. There will be numerous instances in which an absolute diagnosis is not confirmed, but circumstantial, clinical, and perhaps gross pathologic evidence suggests a general group of poisons or a specific intoxication. Treatment should then be initiated promptly to prevent further absorption. Apply specific antidotes where possible, hasten elimination of the circulating toxin, and provide supportive therapy to the animal.

TREATMENT PRINCIPLES

It is useful to follow a general set of objectives in dealing with poisonings in horses. These general steps are stabilization of the patient (if necessary), prevention of further exposure to or absorption of the toxin, application of specific antidotes or therapy, increasing elimination of the absorbed poison, and supportive therapy to counteract the specific organ effects of the poisoning. To respond to these objectives requires not only prompt action but also the availability of appropriate and necessary equipment and medications. Table 1 is a listing of the suggested components for an emergency poisoning kit. These items are fundamental to the treatment of equine poisonings and should always be available and fully stocked for immediate use by the clinician.

STABILIZATION OF THE PATIENT

Since a patient dying of respiratory failure is frequently not helped even by prompt administration of a specific antidote, it is most important to ensure

TABLE 1. EQUINE EMERGENCY POISONING KIT

Parenteral Solutions	Oral Medications	Equipment	Miscellaneous Items
Atropine sulfate	5% Acetic acid (vinegar)	Aspirator bulb	Mild detergent
Barbiturates (phenobarbital, pentobarbital)	Activated charcoal	Blankets	Oxygen
	Albumin (diluted egg white)	Endotracheal tubes, several sizes	Sodium bicarbonate paste
Calcium disodium EDTA	0.15% Calcium hydroxide		
23% Calcium gluconate	20% Magnesium sulfate solution	Enema kit	
Digitalis	Milk of magnesia	Gauze rolls and tape	
Dimercaprol (BAL)	Mineral oil	Intravenous catheters and stylets	
Lactated Ringer's	d-Penicillamine		
4% Methylene blue	1:10,000 Potassium permanganate solution	Mechanical respirator or compression bag	
Normal saline		Needles (hypodermic)	
Physostigmine	20% Sodium sulfate	Stethoscope	
Picrotoxin	Tannic acid	Stomach tubes, several sizes	
Pilocarpine	Vegetable oils, lard	Syringes	
Pralidoxine chloride (2-PAM, Protopam chloride)		Thermometers	
		Urinary catheters, various sizes	
Sedatives		Venotomy kit	
Thiamine hydrochloride			
1% Sodium nitrite			
20% Sodium nitrite			
20% Sodium thiosulfate			
Stimulants			
Strychnine			
Vitamin K_1			

that the horse does not die while the clinician is deciding upon the appropriate course of action. An adequate and patent airway should be ensured, and cardiac and respiratory function must be stabilized and maintained. Endotracheal intubation and artificial respiration may be coupled with cardiac stimulation to maintain these vital functions. Blood pressure should be adequate to ensure kidney perfusion and glomerular filtration. If in doubt, catheterization of the bladder should be performed and urinary flow monitored. Mechanical means may be used to stimulate vital signs and to maintain them, with drugs employed as necessary. Once the clinician has assured himself or herself that vital signs are stable, management of the poisoning may then continue.

PREVENTION OF FURTHER EXPOSURE AND/OR ABSORPTION

In a situation in which horses are being exposed to the toxic material, they should either be removed from that environment, or the toxic substance should be taken away from the patients. This may involve removal of the animals from a pasture or shed or may necessitate the cleaning of hay, grain, or water sources so that further consumption is halted. If the toxin has been applied to the skin, the animal should be washed with water and a mild detergent to remove the unabsorbed chemical. Abundant water should be used to wash the skin and to dilute any remaining toxin. Protective clothing

should be worn by the veterinarian or animal handler during this process.

Absorption of toxins in the digestive tract may be limited by the use of adsorbents, such as activated charcoal, preferably of vegetable origin, used at a minimum of ½ lb (250 gm) for a foal, with up to 1½ lb (750 gm) used for an adult horse. Up to 1 gal (4 l) of warm water (depending upon the animal's size) should be used to make a slurry of the activated charcoal, which is then administered by stomach tube. The activated charcoal adsorbs many organic toxins but is relatively ineffective against inorganic and heavy metal poisons. The slurry should be left in the stomach for 20 to 30 minutes and then should be followed with a laxative to hasten removal of the charcoal and adsorbed chemical from the patient. Unless evacuated from the digestive tract, the poison may dissociate from the adsorbent and eventually may be absorbed by the patient. Although activated charcoal is probably the most effective adsorbent, other compounds such as bentonite, fuller's earth, and tannic acid may also be utilized to adsorb various toxic agents.

If no adsorbent is available, laxatives should be utilized to remove the toxic material from the digestive tract as soon as possible. Mineral oil (1 to 1½ gal, 4 to 6 l), 500 gm of magnesium sulfate or 1 mg of lentin (carbachol) may be administered to a mature horse. The sulfate laxatives (sodium or magnesium) are probably the most effective agents for evacuation of the digestive tract. If mineral oil is used initially, the use of a saline cathartic 30 to 45 minutes after oil administration will be an effective purgative. If the patient already has diarrhea due to the toxic syndrome, further administration of a purgative may add to the risk of dehydration.

SPECIFIC ANTIDOTES

If the poisoning is identified early and an antidote available, it should be used early in the treatment regimen, immediately following stabilization of the patient and prevention of further exposure and absorption. There are, however, very few poisons with specific antidotes, and it is frequently not possible to identify the toxic syndrome until later in the management of the patient. The specific antidotes given in Table 1 may be applied for such poisonings as insecticides, arsenic, cyanide, nitrite, and others. In some cases, doses are critical, but in most the animal is being titrated with the antidote against the body burden of the toxin. For example, in insecticide poisonings, atropine is given to effect by intravenous administration. As the clinical signs abate, the rate of atropine administration is diminished. In the absence of specific antidotes, application of sound therapeutic principles and common sense in further managing the poisoned patient is critical.

INCREASED ELIMINATION OF THE ABSORBED POISON

General nonspecific detoxicants may be used in the absence of specific antidotes. Intravenous administration of 100 to 500 ml of 20 per cent calcium gluconate, 500 to 1000 ml of 10 to 50 per cent dextrose, or 150 to 500 ml of 25 per cent sodium thiosulfate solution is useful.

Since absorbed toxins are usually excreted by the kidneys, renal excretion may be enhanced by the use of large volumes of intravenous fluids (electrolytes, 5 per cent dextrose, or saline) or by the use of diuretics, which should be carefully managed to avoid dehydration. Adequate renal function and hydration of the patient are vital concerns. If a urinary flow of 0.1 ml per kg body weight per minute is not maintained by the patient, hydration of the affected horse should be improved.

SUPPORTIVE THERAPY

The final objective is to maintain the various body functions in a state compatible with detoxification of the poison and patient recovery. Central nervous system excitement may be managed by the use of sedatives, barbiturates, or combinations of tranquil-

izers, chloral hydrate, and magnesium sulfate. Convulsions are most effectively handled by pentobarbital administration, but care must be taken to ensure that respiration is not depressed. Although inhalation anesthetics are excellent for long-term management of central nervous system hyperactivity, prolonged anesthesia in horses is not without risk of gas exchange problems and muscle damage. Central nervous system depression is often complicated by respiratory depression, and both conditions must be managed. Artificial ventilation may support respiration while stimulants such as doxapram (5 to 10 mg per kg) pentylenetetrazol (6 to 10 mg per kg), or bemegride (10 to 20 mg per kg) may be administered intravenously to stimulate central nervous system activity. The action of the stimulants is of relatively short duration; hence, the clinician may wish to place more emphasis on artificial ventilation (p. 475), since adequate respiratory support frequently stimulates recovery from central nervous system depression.

Effective respiratory support requires an adequate patent airway, which may be obtained by an endotracheal tube or by performing a tracheostomy. A mechanical respirator is of great value, but manual compression of the bag of an anesthetic machine may also be utilized with equal efficiency. In the event of cyanosis, oxygen may be necessary, but under most conditions, environmental air is adequate. A mixture of 50 per cent oxygen and 50 per cent environmental air may also be employed.

Support of cardiovascular function requires adequate heart function, appropriate circulating blood volume, and appropriate acid-base balance. Fluid volume and cardiac activity are of most immediate concern. Heart rate may be aided by the use of closed-chest cardiac massage and by the administration of therapeutic agents intravenously or directly into the heart. The slow administration of calcium gluconate has been useful in some instances. Digoxin, 0.2 to 0.6 mg per kg intravenously, may also be effective. Clinical judgment is important to determine the type and extent of cardiac stimulation to be pursued.

For decreased circulating volume, whole blood administration is a valuable procedure. Hypovolemia due to water loss alone may be treated by administering lactated Ringer's solution, saline, or 5 per cent dextrose solutions. Administration of 2 to 10 mg dexamethasone per kg body weight intravenously is useful to prevent shock.

Acidosis is corrected by the administration of sodium bicarbonate, sodium lactate, or lactated Ringer's solution. Alkalosis is less commonly seen but may be reversed by the intravenous administration of physiologic saline (10 mg per kg) followed by 200 mg ammonium chloride per kg per day orally. Such therapy requires careful monitoring to ensure the administration of appropriate concentrations and volumes.

Animals with severe diarrhea may require very careful monitoring of water and electrolyte balance. Fluid requirements may be given via stomach tube or intravenously. Symptomatic care of gastrointestinal disturbances includes protectants such as Kaopectate* or bentonite.

Body temperature should be maintained within normal limits by protection from environmental cold or heat, by providing heat lamps to prevent hypothermia, or cold water enemas, cold water baths, or ice bags to reduce hyperthermia. Constant monitoring of the animal's body temperature is necessary to ensure that vital biochemical and physiologic detoxification processes are able to proceed at optimal physiologic temperatures. Since horses are ex-

tremely sensitive to pain, control of pain is important.

Although it is optimal to have all the suggested procedures operational in each poisoned individual, practicality dictates that the clinician select those measures most appropriate to the case being managed. Careful attention to the application of these objectives in the poisoned horse will ensure maximal therapeutic effectiveness.

Supplemental Readings

1. Bailey, E. M.: Management and treatment of toxicosis. *In* Howard, J. L. (ed.): Current Veterinary Therapy, Food Animal Practice. Philadelphia, W. B. Saunders Co., 1981, pp. 378–388.
2. Buck, W. B., Osweiler, G. D., and Van Gelder, G. A.: Clinical and Diagnostic Veterinary Toxicology, 2nd ed. Dubuque, IA, Kendall/Hunt, 1976.
3. Fowler, M. E.: Diagnosis and treatment of poisonings. *In* Catcott, E. J., and Smithcors, J. F. (eds.): Equine Medicine and Surgery, 2nd ed. Wheaton, IL, American Veterinary Pub., 1972, pp. 189–192.

*Kaopectate, Upjohn Co., Kalamazoo, MI 49001

INSECTICIDES

Frederick W. Oehme, MANHATTAN, KANSAS

Of all the chemicals to which horses might be exposed, insecticides constitute the largest and most potentially toxic group of compounds. They are chemicals that may either be intentionally applied for insect or parasite control in the animal, or they may be accidentally consumed via contamination of feed, forage, water, or the stable enviornment. These potentially hazardous situations make it imperative that the equine veterinarian be well informed of the dangers and safety of the various types of insecticides, and be prepared to diagnose and manage any instances of clinical intoxication.

There are three general groups of insecticide material to which horses may be routinely exposed: The plant-origin insecticides, the chlorinated hydrocarbon insecticides, and the organophosphorus and carbamate materials.

PLANT-ORIGIN INSECTICIDES

This group includes insect control agents derived from plant materials and some that are now synthesized rather than extracted from plants. Rotenone and pyrethrins are materials applied topically directly to the horse and are essentially nontoxic. Clinical cases of rotenone or pyrethrin poisoning are extremely rare and are always due to massive inges-

tion of these insecticides rather than topical application. The materials are not absorbed from the skin and may be clinically considered of no hazard.

NICOTINE

Nicotine is an extremely toxic chemical, but fortunately, it is used only for mite control in buildings. Nicotine sulfate is never directly applied to horses. Toxicity is, therefore, limited to accidental contamination of feeding materials or water or of horses being housed in recently sprayed stables.

CLINICAL SIGNS

If toxicity does result from nicotine sulfate contact, the signs of poisoning occur within a few minutes. They are characteristically those of central nervous system stimulation, producing marked excitement, rapid respiration and salivation. If the animal consumed the nicotine, irritation of the oral mucosa is seen, with increased peristalsis and diarrhea occurring with the ingestion of low to moderate doses. The initial stimulation period is followed by depression, with the horse becoming incoordinated and ataxic and having a rapid pulse with shallow and slow respiration. This leads rapidly to a flaccid paralysis, with coma and death occurring within a few hours. Death usually occurs during a terminal convulsive seizure from paralysis of the respiratory muscles. Recovery from sublethal doses is usually complete within four to six hours after exposure. No characteristic postmortem lesions are found with nicotine sulfate other than cyanosis and congestion of internal organs. With oral ingestion, congestion of the digestive tract mucous membranes, particularly the upper portion of the small intestine, may be seen.

THERAPY

Treatment of nicotine sulfate poisoning is usually not feasible because death occurs rapidly. However, spontaneous recovery may occur if only small amounts are ingested. Topical nicotine should be washed from the skin. The administration of laxatives, tannic acid, or potassium permanganate may help to eliminate ingested nicotine. General supportive care is aimed at prolonging life to allow biological detoxification.

CHLORINATED HYDROCARBON INSECTICIDES

Chlorinated hydrocarbon insecticides are slowly being removed from routine use as agricultural chemicals, but their application is still permitted on some non–food-producing animals, including horses. Although their environmental use has been reduced because of their biologic persistence, as a group these insecticides are effective agents. However, their slow metabolism and persistence in animal tissues causes biologic accumulation following repeated exposures. Horses may thus develop toxicity either from application of excessive concentrations or because of frequent, repeated applications of single recommended amounts. Because of their lipid solubility, all members of this class of insecticides are easily absorbed through the intact skin after topical application or close confinement of animals in recently sprayed housing areas.

CLINICAL SIGNS

The clinical signs of chlorinated hydrocarbon insecticide poisoning are intermittent, with colic and severe neurologic effects predominating. Hyperexcitability, hyperesthesia, and tonic-clonic convulsive seizures may alternate with periods of depression. The toxicity usually begins within an hour of application or exposure, with the animal initially being apprehensive. A period of hyperexcitability follows, characterized by exaggerated responses to stimuli and spontaneous muscle twitches and spasms. The

muscle tremors usually originate in the head area and progress posteriorly to involve the neck, shoulder, back, and rear leg muscles. Early in the syndrome, the horse may develop these spasms while standing, but as they become more severe, the animal will collapse into lateral recumbency. The horse may have chewing movements, may twist or elevate its head, and may undergo abnormal posturing prior to the development of convulsions. Body temperature may be elevated during seizures. Intermittent respiratory paralysis occurs during the convulsions. The convulsions may last several hours, and the patient either dies during a severe seizure or undergoes gradual recovery, with the severity of each subsequent convulsion decreasing until body control and posture are once more regained. Recovered horses may have minor neurologic problems for a few days following recovery, with depression and partial loss of appetite remaining for three to five days. Most fatally affected horses will die within 12 hours after the onset of seizures. No characteristic postmortem lesions are observed in fatal cases other than those resulting from terminal convulsions and trauma due to the seizures.

THERAPY

Although there is no specific treatment for chlorinated hydrocarbon poisoning, conscientious attempts should be made to remove all unabsorbed insecticide from the patient's body. Washing of the skin with soap and warm water is very important. In instances of oral ingestion of chlorinated hydrocarbon insecticide, large amounts of activated charcoal may given by stomach tube to bind the unabsorbed material. Oily laxatives should be avoided, but magnesium sulfate and similar cathartics can be given following the activated charcoal to empty the digestive tract of the contained insecticide. The neurologic effects may be diminished by the use of sedatives or anesthetics. Barbiturates seem to provide most effective control of the centrally originating seizures, but chloral hydrate and tranquilizers may also be used. Repeated dosing is required to control the seizures, and animals that recover need smaller doses as the severity of the convulsions diminishes. Intravenous fluids may be given in severe or prolonged cases to maintain hydration. Generally supportive care will hasten recovery.

Since a variety of chlorinated hydrocarbon insecticides are available, it may be important to determine the specific chemical involved in any poisoning and to establish its source so that future cases can be prevented. The most common chlorinated hydrocarbons used on horses are toxaphene and lindane. Benzene hexachloride, aldrin, endrin, dieldrin, methoxychlor, heptachlor, and chlordane are other chlorinated hydrocarbon insecticides that may be applied on and around horses. While each has its specific toxicity, individual horses may show hypersensitivity to the dose considered safe for the "average" horse. Young colts, weak and debilitated animals, and old horses with potential liver or kidney disease are especially at risk from exposure to the chlorinated hydrocarbon group of insecticides.

ORGANOPHOSPHORUS AND CARBAMATE INSECTICIDES

Unlike chlorinated hydrocarbons, the organophosphorus and carbamate insecticides have little environmental and biologic persistence and are, therefore, increasing in use. Their insecticidal properties depend upon an acute and overwhelming toxicity. Unfortunately, this same event often occurs in horses exposed to this group of chemicals.

As with the chlorinated hydrocarbon compounds, horses may be exposed by overzealous skin application, by spraying of the insecticide in confined areas containing horses, or by accidental contamination of forage, feed, or water. In addition, organophosphate compounds are also used for control of digestive tract parasites in horses, and toxicities occasionally result from this method of application. Horses with digestive tract lesions, animals with intestinal conditions that increase absorption (such as constipation or mucosal inflammation or irritation), or certain hypersensitive individuals are particularly likely to show clinical effects from the oral application of these compounds. The organophosphorus compounds include trichlorfon, dermeton, malathion, dichlorvos (DDVP), ronnel, Rulene, parathion, and diazinon. The carbamate group of insecticides is represented by carbaryl.

CLINICAL SIGNS

Both the organophosphorus and carbamate insecticides have their effect and cause their clinical signs by binding acetylcholinesterase, thereby permitting continuous cholinergic stimulation and excessive autonomic and muscular activity. Effects manifested within the first hour after exposure include frequent urination, increased peristalsis reflected as colic, and "patchy" sweating, particularly of the skin of the neck, shoulders, and rib cage of the affected horse. Salivation may be moderate to profuse, and the parasympathetic stimulation produces defecation, urination, and a general sense of anxiety or uneasiness in the patient. The heart rate is slow, respiratory efforts become exaggerated, and the animal may develop severe abdominal pains. A stiff-legged gait and muscle tremors of the face, neck, and other body muscles occur as the syndrome progresses. The muscular hyperactivity from organophosphorus

and carbamate insecticides never develops into convulsions, as is so typical of the chlorinated hydrocarbon insecticides. Rather, the hyperactivity of the skeletal muscles is generally followed by muscle weakness, incoordination and ataxia, and prostration.

Respiratory failure is a sign of severe toxicity. Bronchoconstriction and pulmonary edema complicate respiratory efforts, and weakness of the respiratory muscles leads to difficult, frequent, and shallow respiratory efforts. Death is due to anoxia. Death may occur within minutes to several hours after the initial signs develop. Except in cases of oral absorption, when continuing absorption prolongs clinical signs, horses that do not die within 12 hours after exposure have a good chance of spontaneous recovery.

Some of the newer organophosphorus and carbamate insecticides are capable of producing variations in this clinical syndrome. All the described clinical signs may not be seen in any one horse, but several of the signs are usually present. In all instances, however, terminal muscle weakness and respiratory dysfunction are severe, and death is due to interference with and paralysis of respiratory efforts. If the diagnosis is in doubt, low blood cholinesterase activity will confirm the toxicity.

Interactions of organophosphorus and carbamate insecticides with other chemicals affecting the same enzyme systems are possible. Drugs working by this mechanism will have additive and sometimes synergistic clinical effects. Phenothiazine derivatives, such as the promazine tranquilizers, potentiate the effects of these cholinesterase-inhibiting insecticides. The administration of succinylcholine, carbachol, physostigmine, or neostigmine is contraindicated if horses have recently been exposed to organophosphorus or carbamate insecticides. The acetylcholinesterase inhibition persists for at least 14 days following organophosphorus insecticide exposure, and at least 30 days or more are required before normal circulating levels of acetylcholinesterase return in organophosphorus-exposed horses. The effects of carbamate insecticides are much shorter, but interaction with other anticholinesterase compounds is still possible if exposures occur with three to five days of each other.

Postmortem lesions associated with organophosphorus or carbamate poisoning are nonspecific. Excessive pulmonary fluids and evidence of excessive fluids in the mouth and digestive tract are supportive but not confirmatory for organophosphorus or carbamate poisoning. In some horses, the excessive peristaltic activity will result in pooling of the blood in "bands" in the small intestinal tract mucosa, and 1 to 7 cm wide areas of the mucosa of the small intestine will appear hyperemic. The bladder may be empty owing to excessive urination, and liquid feces may be found in the rectum. Final confirmation of death due to organophosphorus or carbamate insecticides depends upon the detection of significant plasma, brain, liver, or kidney concentrations of the suspected chemical. Excessively depressed plasma and red blood cell cholinesterase activity may also support a diagnosis.

THERAPY

Fortunately for horses affected with organophosphorus or carbamate toxicity, an effective and specific treatment regimen is available. It involves providing respiratory assistance if death due to respiratory dysfunction is imminent, chemically antagonizing the signs produced by the excessive acetylcholine present at synapses, and aiding the dissociation of inhibited (complexed) acetylcholinesterase throughout the body.

All horses should be immediately treated intravenously with atropine sulfate. The approximate dosage of 1.0 mg per kg must be given to effect, with mydriasis and an absence of salivation used as end points. Since the atropine administered is being titrated against the absorbed organophosphorus or carbamate, the actual amount of atropine required in any case will be variable. After the initial atropine administration, repeated doses may be given every $1\frac{1}{2}$ to 2 hours as required. Additional doses of atropine may be administered subcutaneously. Intravenous atropine administration is also a useful diagnostic tool. Horses not showing decreased clinical effects (decreased anxiety and less evidence of dyspnea and colic) when atropine is administered are probably not suffering from organophosphorus or carbamate insecticide poisoning.

Although atropine dramatically counteracts the parasympathetic signs within a few minutes after administration, it will only minimally reduce the skeletal muscle and nervous system effects. It also will not counteract the insecticide-acetylcholinesterase binding, which is relatively resistant to spontaneous hydrolysis.

Oximes are utilized to increase release of the inhibited enzyme. These compounds (2-PAM, pralidoxime chloride, TMB-4, and the commercially available Protopam chloride) are effective in binding the organophosphorus compound and freeing it from the enzyme-phosphorus complex. This releases the previously inhibited acetylcholinesterase to return to its normal physiologic functions. At least 20 mg Protopam chloride per kg are required, but occasionally as much as 30 to 35 mg per kg may be necessary to secure lasting results. The compound is given intravenously and is repeated every four to six hours. It is important that early treatment with the oximes be instituted. After 18 to 20 hours of organophosphorus exposure, a stabilized enzyme-

insecticide complex has occurred. This complex is refractory to oxime therapy, which may need to be maintained for several days to be effective. The most effective results are observed with a combination of atropine and oxime treatment. In this way, the immediate clinical signs are treated, and the enzyme-organophosphorus complex is broken and directly antagonized.

Since oximes may have some deleterious effects in certain cases of carbamate poisoning, the routine use of oximes in cases not specifically known to be organophosphorus-produced is not recommended. In those instances, immediate treatment with atropine will provide life-saving effects. Since carbamate poisoning is short-lived owing to spontaneous dissociation of the complex and rapid biotransformation of the carbamate insecticide, repeated treatments with atropine are usually not necessary. Carbamate toxicity usually produces death within two hours, or spontaneous recovery occurs shortly thereafter. Provided that additional absorption of the carbamate insecticide does not occur through skin or the digestive tract, one or two treatments with atropine should be sufficient to manage carbamate toxicity. Rapid recovery should then follow.

To prevent additional absorption of the organophosphorus or carbamate insecticide, soap and water should be used to wash dermally exposed animals, and 1 to 2 lbs (0.5 to 1 kg) of activated charcoal should be administered orally in a water slurry to decontaminate the digestive tract of orally exposed horses. Osmotic laxatives should also be employed to empty the digestive tract.

The described specific therapy is usually quite adequate for routine cases of organophosphorus or carbamate toxicity. However, in severe instances or in episodes that are prolonged owing to delay in treatment or continuing exposure, clinical judgment must be used in the application of supportive therapy. Animals in life-threatening situations with severe respiratory embarrassment should be supported with artificial respiration where appropriate. Electrolyte and fluid therapy may be indicated in severely poisoned animals affected for several days. Whole blood and amino acid infusions may also be useful in ensuring the most effective management of these cases of insecticide toxicity.

Supplemental Readings

1. Carson, T. L., and Furr, A. S.: Insecticides. *In* Howard, J. L. (ed.): Current Veterinary Therapy, Food Animal Practice, Philadelphia, W.B. Saunders Co., 1981, pp. 475–477.
2. Clarke, M. L., Harvey, D. G., and Humphreys, D. J.: Veterinary Toxicology, 2nd ed. London, Bailliere Tindall, 1981, p. 97.
3. Fowler, M. E.: Chlorinated hydrocarbon parasiticides. *In* Catcott, E. J., and Smithcors, J. F. (eds.): Equine Medicine and Surgery, 2nd ed. Wheaton, Il, American Veterinary Pub., 1972, p. 194.

RODENTICIDES

Frederick W. Oehme, MANHATTAN, KANSAS

Rodenticide toxicity in horses is relatively uncommon because most owners ensure that rodenticides are not placed in their horse's proximity. Should horses be exposed to rodenticides, the method of packaging and placement of bait usually result in the animal receiving less than a toxic dose. Since many of the commonly used anticoagulant rodenticides require several days of exposure, the potential for toxicity is further reduced.

In instances of feed contamination with highly toxic rodenticides, not only may a sufficient dosage be received, but also continual daily ingestion may result in accumulation of the toxic chemical. If the feed is being given to several horses, more than one animal may become ill, and a classic "outbreak" of poisoning may be seen. Environmental or feed contamination has produced poisoning from such rodenticides as warfarin and other anticoagulants, strychnine, ANTU, arsenic, fluoroacetate, zinc phosphide, and Vacor. In addition, potential toxic effects from phosphorus, thallium, barium chloride, and Castrix must also be considered whenever rodenticide toxicity in horses is discussed.

WARFARIN, PIVAL, AND OTHER ANTICOAGULANTS

Single doses of 75 to 100 mg per kg are toxic, but a dose of 2 mg or less per kg on a repeated daily basis is more likely and effective in producing poisoning. The anticoagulants antagonize vitamin K and produce coagulation system defects. Vascular shock may be seen with single large doses, but more commonly, mild to massive hemorrhages occur throughout the body. Nose bleeds, diarrhea with free blood in the stool, and subcutaneous hematomas (particularly over bony prominences and points of contact with hard surfaces) are typical signs. Lameness may occur due to hemorrhage into joint capsules, and soreness may be seen due to muscle hematomas. Occasionally, affected animals are first recognized by continual bleeding following owner or veterinary parenteral medication, and anemia may be observed upon examination of the mucous membranes or the performance of blood counts. The diagnosis is usually obvious upon the finding of elevated prothrombin times and clinical evidence of anemia and diffuse hemorrhagic foci. Occasionally in horses, acute death is seen due to massive hemorrhage into the thorax, abdominal cavity, or around the brain; these are obvious upon postmortem examination.

THERAPY

Treatment involves removal from the source of the anticoagulant, replacement of the inhibited coagulation factors, and supplying vitamin K to competitively antagonize the presence of the anticoagulant rodenticide. The horse should be removed from its immediate environment to prevent further exposure, or the source of the bait should be detected and removed. If ingestion of the anticoagulant has occurred within 24 hours, saline cathartics and activated charcoal may be administered. Whole blood (p. 325) will reverse anemia, will immediately replace missing coagulation factors, and will stabilize the horse against immediate life-threatening situations. Vitamin K_1 should be administered (1 mg per kg twice daily for five days). Synthetic vitamin K (menadione) is considerably less effective and should be reserved for less severe cases or for follow-up therapy by the owner (10 to 20 mg per kg for seven days orally or parenterally) following alleviation of the acute stage of the crisis. During the early stages of recovery, the horse should be kept quiet and should be handled as little as possible. Undue excitement and the potential for trauma carry the risk of producing internal or external hemorrhage that may be severe.

STRYCHNINE

At a dose of 0.5 to 1 mg per kg, horses may be poisoned with a single oral dose of strychnine. The rodenticide antagonizes inhibitory spinal cord neurons and allows excess activity of the central nervous system to cause convulsions and seizures in the patient. Acute onset of tetanus-like seizures is characteristic. The animal is hyperexcitable and hyperreflexic, so that wind, noise, and skin contact produce an aggravated reaction, often leading to muscle seizures, prostration, and tetanic convulsions. The syndrome is violent, with seizures progressing from moderate to fatal with 15 to 45 minutes. The seizure pattern is characteristic, and no significant postmortem lesions are found. A rapid onset of rigor mortis suggests strychnine poisoning.

THERAPY

No specific antidote is available, but seizures can be controlled with central nervous system depressants such as pentobarbital, chloral hydrate–magnesium sulfate combinations, or glyceryl guaiacolate (5 per cent solution intravenously, 212 mg per kg). The seizures are controlled by administering these compounds to effect and as often as necessary to control muscle activity. Care must be taken to avoid depressing the respiratory center with the central nervous system depressant, and the availability of respiratory support may be vital to recovery. Activated charcoal (0.5 to 1 kg per animal) should be administered orally to bind unabsorbed strychnine in the digestve tract and to prevent continual absorption and recurrence of signs. A laxative should be administered upon clinical recovery to hasten digestive tract elimination of the charcoal-bound strychnine. Healthy horses usually recover within 24 hours if treatment is conscientiously applied.

ANTU (Alpha-Naphthyl ThioUrea)

Although toxicity is not seen frequently in horses owing to the limited availability of this agent, this rodenticide produces dramatic lethal effects if consumed. The toxic dose varies from 25 to 75 mg per kg and produces its toxicity by increased permeability of the lung capillaries. Pulmonary edema is the outstanding clinical sign. The affected horse develops moist rales, increased respiratory efforts, muscle weakness, and severe dyspnea as pulmonary edema and hydrothorax cause anoxia and rapidly developing cyanosis. As the condition progresses, foamy froth bubbles from the nose and mouth of the laboring animal. Death occurs within hours after the beginning of signs, with the animal prostrate and large volumes of white frothy foam emanating from the nose and mouth. Postmortem observations reveal hydrothorax, pulmonary edema, and frothy edematous fluid filling the air spaces of the lung, bronchioles, trachea, nose and mouth.

THERAPY

No antidote is available to treat this rapidly fulminating condition. The animal should be kept as quiet as possible to reduce tissue oxygen demands, and sedation may be used if necessary. Oxygen should be administered. Osmotic diuretics (such as 50 per cent glucose or mannitol) and atropine administration (0.05 mg per kg) have been suggested to reduce pulmonary edema, but their effectiveness in field cases is not proven. Fluid balance should be ensured by monitoring skin tone and hemoconcentration. Secondary infections may be avoided by supplying broad-spectrum antibiotics during the stressful period of digestive tract irritation and inflammation.

FLUOROACETATE (Compound 1080)

This rodenticide is one of the most lethal based on a milligram dosage. The toxic dose ranges from approximately 0.25 to 1.5 mg per kg. The compound is converted to a metabolite that blocks the energy production cycle of the cell, producing cellular death due to lack of energy. When this affects the neurons of the central nervous system, dramatic major organ and central nervous system effects result. The chemical initially induces cardiac arrhythmias, a rapid, weak pulse, anxiousness, and hyperexcitability, with ventricular fibrillation, sudden excitement, and convulsions and death following quickly with sudden collapse. Because of the small quantity of toxin required to produce death, horses may consume sufficient amounts through feed or environmental contamination to become ill. The use of this chemical in range country for coyote and predator animal control may cause exposure to horses grazing native pastures. No significant postmortem lesions are found, and the rapidity of this compound's action may lead the owner to report "sudden death" as the only observation.

THERAPY

No specific antidote is available, but seizures and excessive nervous activity should be controlled with short-acting barbiturates given to effect. Activated charcoal may be given orally to reduce further absorption of fluoroacetate. Glycerol monoacetate (0.1 to 0.5 mg per kg intramuscularly) may be given every hour for several doses, but its effectiveness has only been shown if given before or at the same time that clinical signs develop. The clinician must use common sense and knowledge of respiratory physiology to manage horses affected with ANTU poisoning. Recovery from this toxicity is not common once clinical signs have developed.

ARSENIC

This compound is used as a rodent and insect control agent, as well as being employed as a herbicide in agricultural weed programs. The toxic dose ranges from 2 to 7 mg per kg. Arsenic is a very irritating heavy metal and produces digestive tract irritation within hours after the ingestion of a toxic dose. Horses have signs of colic and excessive peristaltic activity and exhibit typical signs of digestive tract obstruction or irritation. After several hours, diarrhea develops, which is at first fluid and mucoid. After 12 hours, the diarrhea becomes blood-tinged owing to bleeding of the digestive tract. Affected horses may become rapidly dehydrated from arsenic toxicity and may often be misdiagnosed as having colitis or a digestive tract obstruction. A careful physical examination will reveal congestion of most mucous membranes and obvious pain upon external and rectal palpation. The continuing excessive peristaltic activity followed by the appearance of bloody feces may help in the diagnosis.

THERAPY

Dimercaprol (BAL) is the specific antidote for arsenic. It is given intramuscularly four times daily at the rate of 3 to 4 mg per kg. Sodium thiosulfate (20 per cent solution, 30 to 40 mg per kg intravenously) may be given two or three times daily in lieu of BAL. Since BAL is inherently nephrotoxic, it should only be given for three to four days. Sodium thiosulfate may then be administered until recovery. In severe acute cases, the combination of BAL and sodium thiosulfate may be valuable in providing additional sulfur for binding and detoxification of the arsenic. Since dehydration is a frequent complication of arsenic poisoning, the administration of electrolytes and glucose should be considered. Fluid balance should be ensured by monitoring skin tone and hemoconcentration. Secondary infections may be avoided by supplying broad-spectrum antibiotics during the stressful period of digestive tract irritation and inflammation.

ZINC PHOSPHIDE

With toxic doses of 20 to 40 mg per kg, zinc phosphide produces toxicity by being broken down in the acid of the stomach to phosphine. The toxicity of this compound is greater when the stomach is full owing to the additional acidity present during the digestive process. The phosphine generated produces irritation of the mucous membranes of the digestive tract, pulmonary edema, and cardiovascular collapse. The animal affected with toxicity becomes depressed, colicky and dyspneic. Occasionally horses will develop convulsive seizures. The digestive tract hyperemia is seen on postmortem examination together with excessive pulmonary fluid.

THERAPY

The acidity of the intestinal tract may be neutralized by administering 2 to 4 l of 5 per cent sodium bicarbonate. This should be repeated as needed together with laxatives to purge the digestive tract of the unabsorbed zinc phosphide. Supportive treatment may be utilized, but no specific antidote is available.

VACOR

This rodenticide was very popular during the past several years but has recently been removed from the market owing to unexpected chronic adverse effects in dogs, cats, and humans. The toxic dose is in the range of 300 mg per kg. The compound is a general metabolic toxin and produces effects in the gastrointestinal tract and nervous system by apparently affecting biologic oxidation-reduction reactions. Affected horses may show colic, mental confusion and uneasiness, increased peristalsis, and some difficulty in vision.

THERAPY

Because of the high dose required for lethal toxicity, most affected horses recover spontaneously, but affected animals should be treated with cathartics and supportive care to replace fluid loss and to control any nervous activity that might inflict damage to the horse or property. Nicotinamide is a specific antidote used in dogs and humans. It may be employed in horses by giving 1000 mg per kg every four hours for two days, followed by 1 gm of nicotinamide per day orally for seven more days.

PHOSPHORUS

Phosphorus is a systemic poison that has a toxic dose of 1 to 4 mg per kg. White and yellow phosphorus are the toxic forms capable of producing digestive tract, liver, and kidney damage. The early signs of toxicity are abdominal pain and a fluid, hemorrhagic diarrhea. After several days, generalized depression, icterus, and hepatorenal failure develop, followed shortly thereafter by death. A saline cathartic may be administered early in the syndrome to evacuate the digestive tract. Liver damage is obvious. Treatment is supportive and symptomatic, since no direct antidote is available. Glucose and lipotrophic agents (such as methionine) may be beneficial in hepatotoxic conditions (pp. 249 and 251).

THALLIUM

Although no longer used extensively as a rodenticide, thallium is notoriously toxic to all body systems. It has a toxic dose of 10 to 15 mg per kg, with about 50 mg per kg required to kill. Almost all body systems are affected, but the digestive tract, skin, and respiratory and nervous systems are the most severely involved. The clinical onset of signs is usually delayed 24 to 48 hours after ingestion, but once signs occur, the digestive tract becomes severely damaged. A hemorrhagic gastroenteritis is present, together with difficult respiration, fever, and inflammation of the gums and eyelids. Chronic skin lesions, hair loss, tremors, or muscular seizures develop later.

THERAPY

Evacuation of the digestive tract with laxatives and purgatives is indicated. Glucose, parenteral vitamins, antibiotics, and general supportive therapy are employed as needed. The use of dithizone, as recommended in small animals, has not been evaluated in horses, nor has the use of Prussian blue as an adsorbing agent in the digestive tract.

BARIUM CHLORIDE

This infrequently used rodenticide is a generalized poison that produces digestive tract irritation, generalized depression, and prostration following consumption of doses in excess of 150 mg per kg. The toxicity is sufficiently nonspecific to make diagnosis difficult. Symptomatic and supportive therapy may be utilized to counter the digestive tract irritation and the general toxicity of this compound.

CASTRIX

Castrix is a convulsive rodenticide that requires only 25 mg or less per kg to produce effects. Affected animals become anxious and then nervous, with muscular tremors leading to convulsions and prostration in extreme cases. Sedation of the affected horse with central nervous system depressants, as well as orally administered activated charcoal and purgatives to bind the unabsorbed rodenticide and flush the digestive tract, is recommended.

Supplemental Readings

1. Fowler, M. E.: Toxicity of rodenticides. *In* Catcott, E. J., and Smithcors, J. F. (eds.): Equine Medicine and Surgery, 2nd ed. Wheaton, IL, American Veterinary Pub., 1972, p.200.
2. Osweiler, G. E., and Hook, B. S.: Rodenticides. *In* Howard, J. L. (ed.): Current Veterinary Therapy, Food Animal Practice. Philadelphia, W. B. Saunders Co., 1981, pp. 478–480.

SNAKE BITE

Frederick W. Oehme, MANHATTAN, KANSAS

Probably several hundred horses are bitten by poisonous snakes in the United States each year with a mortality ranging from 10 to 30 per cent. The most dangerous snake for horses is the large rattlesnake of the genus Crotalus. Other pit vipers that may bite horses are copperheads and water moccasins. The venom from these three types of snakes is mainly hemotoxic and proteolytic and produces extreme local swelling with marked tissue and red blood cell destruction and a direct effect on the heart. The fourth poisonous snake seen in the United States is the coral snake, found primarily in the southeast. This snake is not a major source of equine snake bite because of its shy nature and its distribution in areas where horses are not used. The coral snake venom is essentially a rapidly acting neurotoxin.

CLINICAL SIGNS

Most snake bites in horses occur during the warm days of the spring and throughout the summer when snakes are out and active. Horses are bitten most frequently on the nose, head, and neck. They are less frequently bitten on the legs and chest, although exposure of the legs is common, especially if horses are moving through tall grass. Because of the lack of abundant muscle or connective tissue on the lower limbs, snake bites in those areas are occasionally not detected owing to minimal injection of venom and limited tissue swelling. Bites of the nose and head are extremely serious because of the rapid swelling that follows a bite. The bitten area becomes edematous, and the tissue reaction spreads throughout the head and neck. If the horse is bitten on the nose, the nose and nasal mucosa swells, and blood-stained exudate may drain from each nostril. The eyelids and ears may also swell, producing a deformed appearance. Swelling of the throat may produce audible dyspnea and life-threatening respiratory distress, which may require emergency tracheotomy. The effects of the bite may be sufficiently severe to cause depression and muscular weakness.

The severity of the snake bite is usually related

to the size of the snake involved, the size of the bitten horse, the amount of venom injected, the site of the bite, and prior physical condition of the horse. Most bitten horses will not die, but sometimes, swelling of the throat or a massive injection of venom by a large rattlesnake in a tissue site producing rapid absorption may produce a fatal outcome. However, even with limited mortality, the tissue necrosis and prolonged recovery period required for healing are of considerable concern.

THERAPY

A variety of treatments may be employed for bitten horses, depending upon the site and severity of the bite, the time elapsed since the horse was bitten, and the value of the individual animal. If the horse is in respiratory distress, tracheotomy or other respiratory assistance is required. Anti-inflammatory compounds, such as corticosteroids, are of considerable value in reducing tissue swelling and necrosis. Although no work has been reported using antihistamines in horses, studies in mice and dogs have indicated that antihistamines are contraindicated in snake bite. Antivenom specific for the snake thought to be involved may be used systemically or via injections at the site of the bite. The risk of anaphylactic reactions must be considered, since antivenom is made from horse serum. Antivenom is most useful when given early in the clinical course. Antibiotics, particularly broad-spectrum ones, are indicated because bacteria are injected during the bite. Tetanus antitoxin is always indicated in snake bites in horses.

Additional treatments that may be considered by the clinician, depending upon the circumstances, are fluids to combat shock or dehydration, epinephrine to reduce the risk of circulatory collapse, calcium gluconate to limit hemolysis of red blood cells, and the injection of proteolytic enzymes to reduce tissue swelling.

If the time between bite and initiation of treatment warrants, an incision may be made over the fang marks and suction applied. If the bite is on an extremity, a tourniquet may be placed above the bite area for 15- to 20-minute intervals. Cold water packs applied to the bite area may prevent swelling, but the direct application of ice or other frozen materials is contraindicated, as it causes additional tissue damage.

It is important that the animal be treated as soon as possible and that the veterinarian see the patient either by going to the location of the bitten horse or meeting the animal and owner at some mutually determined location. The time that elapses between the bite and initiation of treatment appears to be the most important factor in reducing tissue damage and the risk of mortality.

Supplemental Reading

Burger, C. H.: Snakebite poisoning. *In* Catcott, E. J., and Smithcors, J. F. (eds.): Equine Medicine and Surgery, 2nd ed. Wheaton, IL, American Veterinary Pub., 1972, pp. 213–214.

BLISTER BEETLE

Frederick W. Oehme, MANHATTAN, KANSAS

Blister beetles are small, striped insects that live in fields, feeding on other insect eggs, honey, grasses, and crops. They belong to the genus Epicauta and are found from the Midwest to the East Coast and south to the Gulf of Mexico. Adult beetles are found in pastures and hay fields throughout the summer and persist there until the first frost.

The toxicity of blister beetles is due to the cantharidin found in their body fluid. Cantharidin is a severe irritant; it produces vesicles or blisters when applied to the skin and severe mouth, throat, and digestive tract irritation when ingested. Upon absorption, the material is rapidly excreted through the kidneys, producing damage to the urinary system as it is being eliminated.

Blister beetle problems have developed with the development of equipment permitting rapid drying of cut forage. Since the beetles live in clusters in pastures and hay fields and move in swarms, patches of beetles occur in various areas of the fields. Under previous harvesting conditions, the beetles would move out of the cut hay after it was mowed and prior to baling. However, with the newer techniques of cutting and crimping the hay in one operation, the cluster of beetles is often crushed and killed before they have the opportunity to flee. The subsequent baling results in numerous insects in one small area of harvested forage. One bale of hay may contain many insects, while the next may have none. Alfalfa is the hay most commonly involved with blister beetle poisoning, probably because of the wide use of cutting and crimping operations.

CLINICAL SIGNS

The severity of the toxic effects depends on the number of blister beetles eaten by the horse. The cantharidin concentration varies from less than 1 per cent to greater than 5 per cent of the dry weight of the insect, and as little as 5 to 15 gm of dried beetles may be lethal to a horse. The simple digestive tract of the horse allows undiluted and direct contact of the toxic principle with mucous membranes.

Depending upon the dose of insects received, individual horses may show mild to severe digestive tract pain and colic, fever, diarrhea (ranging from watery feces to a mucoid, bloody discharge), congested mucous membranes, straining with frequent passing of blood-tinged urine, attempts to frequently drink small amounts of water, depression, anorexia, and muscle weakness leading to prostration and death. Occasionally, horses may die suddenly without showing any clinical signs, but most blister beetle cases are ill for several hours to days before becoming weak and prostrate and then dying. In acute cases, the massive doses received appear to result in profound shock and rapid death. Rapid respiration, dyspnea with abdominal breathing, and sweating (probably a result of the severe abdominal pain) may also be seen. Horses surviving for one or more days become dehydrated owing to the loss of fluid from the diarrhea and frequent urination. Total blood loss from the digestive tract and urinary system is minimal but in rare cases may be a serious complication. The erosion of the mucous membranes of the digestive and urinary tracts may allow secondary bacterial infections to become systemic. As the disease progresses, urinary function becomes compromised, and blood urea nitrogen and creatinine levels increase.

Necropsy examination confirms the mild to severe irritation of the digestive tract and urinary system. Hyperemia and sloughing of the mucosa of the esophagus, stomach, and gastrointestinal tract are common. The kidneys are pale and swollen, and hemorrhagic and inflamed mucosa are seen in the renal pelvis, ureters, bladder, and urethra. Some horses have areas of pale and degenerated cardiac muscle in the atrium and ventricle. Clinicians are often surprised at the extent of the damage produced by the poison, but the lesions explain why death is not uncommon with blister beetle toxicity.

An accurate and sensitive analytical procedure to detect cantharidin in blood, urine, or digestive tract contents from suspected cases of blister beetle poisoning has recently been developed. It is not widely available and is expensive, but its direct application will allow confirmation of poisoning suspected from the clinical signs and/or necropsy observations.

THERAPY

Because of the acuteness of this toxicity, successful treatment must be applied promptly and conscientiously. If one horse in a group is affected, all hay, particularly alfalfa hay, must be removed from the feeding areas. Substitute hay should be carefully examined for the presence of beetles. All exposed but unaffected horses should be provided with abundant fresh water and sufficient room to prevent any injury from unexpected colic. Horses showing signs of toxicity should be treated with digestive tract protectants and mild laxatives to promote complete but gentle emptying of the digestive tract. Fluid intake must be maintained, and if patients refuse water, intravenous fluid therapy should be instituted promptly. Urinary flow should be monitored to ensure that urination is abundant and frequent. Complications may be minimized by providing broad-spectrum antibiotic coverage and other organ-specific medication as indicated to prevent septicemia and renal and cardiac damage. Good nursing care, including conscientious observation, rapid response to changes in patient status, and thoughtful protection of the horses from mechanical injury due to colic, is important for successful recovery. Mild to moderate cases may recover in a matter of days, while horses with severe cases of poisoning may require longer periods for recovery. Occasionally, such patients have after effects from residual digestive tract or urinary system damage, resulting in sporadic diarrhea or colic and occasional episodes of hematuria and renal pain.

PREVENTION

Because of the prevalence of blister beetles in pastures and hay fields and particularly the high incidence of beetles in choice alfalfa hay used to feed horses, it is important that owners examine hay for possible blister beetle contamination before it is offered for consumption. All portions of the hay should be examined, since clustering of the insects may result in some of the bales being "clean," while others may contain sufficient blister beetles to produce acute and lethal poisoning in one or more horses.

Supplemental Readings

1. Oehme, F. W.: Blister beetles: Equine killers found in horse-bound hay. Kansas Horseman, 2:6, 1981.
2. Panciera, R. J.: Cantharidin (blister beetle) poisoning. *In* Catcott, E. J., and Smithcors, J. F. (eds.): Equine Medicine and Surgery, 2nd ed. Wheaton, IL, American Veterinary Pub., 1972, pp. 224–225.

CARBON TETRACHLORIDE

Frederick W. Oehme, MANHATTAN, KANSAS

Occasionally carbon tetrachloride enters the equine diet by accident or through its misuse as an anthelmintic. The compound is volatile and has a peculiar odor, which may result in horses rejecting feed containing this compound. Atmospheric concentrations of less than one part per million are detectable by the healthy horse's nose.

The toxicity of this drug may be expressed in several ways. Inhalation or absorption of large quantities of carbon tetrachloride can cause central nervous system depression and narcosis. Ingestion of carbon tetrachloride results in rapid absorption from the digestive tract and a toxic effect upon the liver cells, producing fatty degeneration in small quantities and centrilobular necrosis if larger amounts are absorbed. Because repeated administration of small quantities of carbon tetrachloride produces no toxic signs and since fatal cases of poisoning usually reveal kidney damage to a greater extent than liver pathology, the hepatic effects of carbon tetrachloride most likely must be accompanied by severe renal failure to produce clinical signs of toxicity and death. Local application of carbon tetrachloride, such as the parenteral injection of carbon tetrachloride in oil, produces localized tissue necrosis and may lead to lameness.

The toxic dose of carbon tetrachloride for horses is variable, with as little as 0.25 ml per kg producing serious liver damage in some animals, while 3 ml per kg may produce no signs in other individuals. Poisoning in horses, however, is usually acute, with signs manifesting themselves within the first 24 to 36 hours. Occasionally, severe signs may be delayed for another 48 hours, but eventually depression, muscle weakness, and ataxia follow the initial loss of appetite. Constipation is followed by diarrhea with the passage of blood-stained feces. Total collapse occurs terminally, with death usually occurring within 24 hours of the onset of severe signs. Gastroenteritis of the upper digestive tract is a consistent postmortem finding. The liver and kidneys are congested with gross evidence of degeneration and necrosis, hemorrhages, and focal areas of fatty degeneration. Microscopically, the liver has centrilobular necrosis, and the kidneys have cloudy swelling and necrosis of the tubular epithelium. Repeated administration of moderate doses of carbon tetrachloride may produce liver fibrosis and cirrhosis. This circumstance would be unusual in horses owing to the finicky appetite of this species.

A specific antidote for carbon tetrachloride is not available. The general principles of treating poisoning (p. 577) should be followed, with special attention to eliminating further exposure and reducing additional absorption by the use of activated charcoal adsorbent and the use of laxatives and saline purges to rapidly empty the digestive tract. General supportive and symptomatic care is useful in allowing the patient time to detoxify and excrete the absorbed carbon tetrachloride. Horses showing clinical signs of carbon tetrachloride toxicity are best given a guarded prognosis, since the extent of liver and/or kidney damage in individual cases is unpredictable based upon the known carbon tetrachloride exposure or the degree of clinical signs seen.

Supplemental Reading

Clarke, E. G. C., and Clarke, M. L.: Veterinary Toxicology. Baltimore, Williams and Wilkins, 1975.

PHENOTHIAZINE

Frederick W. Oehme, MANHATTAN, KANSAS

The use of phenothiazine as an anthelmintic is complicated by its toxicity, the mechanism of which is not understood. The toxicity of phenothiazine varies greatly between individuals, young and debilitated animals being most susceptible. Toxicity depends on absorption from the gastrointestinal tract, and, therefore, small particle size, digestive tract stasis, and other factors increasing absorption favor toxicity. Multiple small doses are less likely to be toxic than a single large dose. Horses receiving more than 30 gm are likely to exhibit toxic signs. In general, single doses should not exceed 67 mg per kg.

The urine of horses receiving phenothiazine is red. This is because some phenothiazine is absorbed from the digestive tract as phenothiazine sulfoxide, which is metabolized in the liver, and the metabolites are excreted in urine, where they turn red on exposure to air.

CLINICAL SIGNS

Toxic signs are usually seen within hours of drug administration but occasionally develop in one to two days. The most common signs are anorexia and depression of rapid onset followed by hindleg weakness and a staggering gait. Digestive tract pain and colic are also common. The absorbed phenothiazine and/or its metabolites may also induce hemolysis of red blood cells, leading to anemia, icterus, and hemoglobinuria. Extreme cases may progress to dyspnea, a weak, rapid pulse, and prostration. There may be no postmortem lesions, but if present, they usually are an enlarged liver, swollen kidneys and spleen, generalized icterus of subcutaneous tissues, and dark red urine in the bladder.

Phenothiazine photosensitivity, due to the metabolite phenothiazine sulfoxide, is uncommon in horses.

THERAPY

Oral administration of mineral oil and general symptomatic care of colic are important. Where red blood cell hemolysis is evident, whole blood transfusion should be employed. Corticosteroids may be employed, but other treatments, such as stimulants and intravenous glucose, have not been of value for treating the phenothiazine-induced hemolysis of red blood cells.

The photosensitization is best avoided by keeping affected horses in the shade and out of direct sunlight for three to five days after dosing. Eye or skin lesions may be treated with topical ointments or salves.

The general problem of phenothiazine toxicity in horses can best be avoided by not using phenothiazine in those situations producing a high risk of poisoning. Doses should be carefully calculated. Dosing of horses with digestive tract problems should be postponed, and use of phenothiazine in horses with conditions favoring increased digestive tract absorption of the drug should be avoided.

Supplemental Reading

Clarke, M. L., Harvey, D. G., and Humphreys, D. J.: Veterinary Toxicology, 2nd ed. London, Bailliere Tindall, 1981, pp. 98–99.

PETROLEUM PRODUCTS

Frederick W. Oehme, MANHATTAN, KANSAS

Horses generally avoid feed, forage, or water containing petroleum products. However, horses with a depraved appetite or those confined to areas containing petroleum products may ingest these materials. Various petroleum products may be applied by owners to control insects or to treat skin conditions with "home remedies."

Petroleum products include kerosene, gasoline, and other fuel oils, waste crankcase oil, and crude oil or partially refined petroleum materials. Petroleum distillates may also be used as vehicles for the application of insecticides or other environmental sprays. Waste oily materials are used to reduce dust in arenas. The used petroleum materials may contain contaminants, such as lead, pentachlorophenol (PCP), or tetrachlorodibenzodioxine (TCDD). Inhalation of spray may occur when stables are sprayed with petroleum products.

CLINICAL SIGNS

The clinical signs of petroleum product toxicity depend upon the type of product being applied, its contaminants, and the route of exposure. Ingestion of the petroleum products may produce blistering of the muzzle and mouth, salivation, colic, mild to moderate diarrhea, and one to three days of reduced appetite.

When petroleum products are applied to the skin, local irritation with some hair loss results. The horse may rub the involved area, producing additional inflammation and possibly bleeding. Inhalation of droplets of petroleum products will result in mild respiratory tract irritation. Coughing, sneezing, increased respiratory rate, and pulmonary congestion may develop following heavy exposure.

The application to the skin of petroleum products containing lead results in significant lead absorption. If repeatedly applied, lead accumulation in tissues may result in signs of lead poisoning. PCP- or TCDD-containing petroleum products will induce chronic weight loss and a rough hair coat. The usual exposure to such products is moderate, and only in extreme cases will permanent or lethal damage result.

THERAPY

The treatment for petroleum product toxicity varies with the type and extent of exposure. In many instances, conservative and supportive therapy is sufficient, while in other situations, such as aspiration pneumonia from petroleum product droplet inhalation, even the most vigorous antibiotic and supportive therapy is ineffectual. In general, the petroleum material should be removed from contact with the animal as soon as possible. Laxatives (particularly the osmotic variety) may be used to empty the digestive tract, and soap and water should be used on the skin to remove topically applied petroleum materials. Provision of soft feed will reduce irritation to the mouth and digestive tract. With severe gastrointestinal irritation, parenteral fluid therapy or nasogastric tube feeding may be necessary. Soothing ointments may be used topically to protect irritated skin, and antibiotics may be employed to reduce the potential for systemic infections. Although cases of petroleum product toxicity in horses are rare and most are minimally toxic, the clinician must always recognize the potential for more severe reactions and, therefore, should support the animal to hasten recovery.

Supplemental Reading

Rowe, L. D.: Crude oils, fuel oils, and kerosene. *In* Howard, J. L. (ed.): Current Veterinary Therapy, Food Animal Practice. Philadelphia, W. B. Saunders Co., 1981, pp. 517–520.

LEAD

Frederick W. Oehme, MANHATTAN, KANSAS

Lead poisoning in horses in uncommon. However, when horses are placed in environments where lead is available, toxicity can result. The equine clinician should therefore monitor the environment of patients to ensure that lead is not a factor in any neurologic disease.

Lead almost always enters the body via the digestive tract, although smaller amounts may be inhaled into the lung and by phagocytosis will enter the circulation. Reported cases of lead poisoning in horses have usually resulted from environmental contamination from industrial smelting operations. Effluents from such mining and ore-producing activities contain large amounts of lead that are distributed by prevailing wind patterns to contaminate surrounding pastures and animal holding areas. In addition, lead-base paints may be improperly used around horse facilities, and batteries, used motor oil, putty and caulking compounds, grease, or linoleum may provide additional sources for ingestion. Horse pastures near heavily traveled highways may develop high lead concentrations from automobile engine exhaust systems. In areas of hard water tending toward an acidic pH, lead water pipes or lead connections in water lines provide a source for lead in the water. In areas of marginal management, poor-quality pastures may allow animals access to dump sites, which could contain a variety of sources for lead. Except in instances of massive exposure to lead-containing materials (such as partially used containers of lead-base paint), chronic and continuing exposure to the lead is required for many days or weeks before toxicity is evident. Depending upon the method of exposure, as much as 500 gm may be required to produce fatalities, while daily exposure to 2.4 mg of lead per kg of body weight has been suggested as a chronic cumulative fatal dose.

CLINICAL SIGNS

Lead toxicity in horses is manifested by a variety of signs, mostly related to a peripheral neuritis. This is demonstrated by general weakness, a knuckling of the fetlocks and pharyngeal paralysis with laryngeal hemiplegia. Incoordination may be seen in advanced cases. In some horses, anemia with basophilic stippling of red blood cells is seen. Joint enlargement and stiff joints may also be observed, particularly in young horses, especially if there are complicating intoxications with other heavy metals.

The most characteristic and life-threatening effect of lead is laryngeal hemiplegia resulting from damage to the recurrent laryngeal nerve. Inspiratory dyspnea and respiratory sounds are easily detected upon moderate exercise. Affected horses may collapse and die of respiratory insufficiency after only minimal exertion. The presence of severe unexplained respiratory difficulties following mild exercise should suggest laryngeal damage and the possibility of lead intoxication. In extreme instances, food and water may be regurgitated from the nostrils following feeding.

DIAGNOSIS

Diagnosis is based upon blood lead analysis in the living animal. While clinical cases have been reported with blood lead concentrations as low as 0.3 parts per million (ppm), many horses with blood lead levels of 0.4 to 0.6 ppm or greater may exhibit no clinical signs. After death, liver or kidney lead concentrations of at least 15 ppm will support a lead poisoning diagnosis. Necropsy observations are usually nonspecific and are not helpful in the diagnosis.

THERAPY

Since almost all cases of lead poisoning in horses are chronic, removal of the animals from the source of the lead is an important first step in the treatment of poisoning. Removal of the source early enough in the syndrome may allow spontaneous improvement and eventual recovery. For severely affected animals, the intravenous administration of calcium disodium edetate (calcium EDTA or calcium versenate) is essential. Treatment is administered slowly in saline or 5 per cent dextrose at the rate of 75 mg calcium EDTA per kg daily for four to five days.

The dose may be divided into two or three administrations over a day's time. Treatment is then stopped for two days, and the sequence is then repeated for another four to five days.

Adequate nutritional intake should be ensured, and any anorexic horses should be fed by stomach tube until appetite returns. While treatment may be beneficial in early or mild cases of lead poisoning, the damage to the recurrent laryngeal and other peripheral nerves can be permanent in severe cases, and complete recovery may not always occur.

Supplemental Readings

1. Burrows, G. E.: Lead toxicosis in domestic animals: A review of the role of lead mining and primary lead smelters in the United States. Vet. Human Toxicol., 23:337, 1981.
2. Burrows, G. E., Sharp, J. W., and Root, R. G.: A survey of blood lead concentrations in horses in the North Idaho lead/silver belt area. Vet. Human Toxicol., 23:328, 1981.
3. Fowler, M. E.: Lead poisoning. *In* Catcott, E. J., and Smithcors, J. F. (eds.): Equine Medicine and Surgery, 2nd ed. Wheaton, IL, American Veterinary Pub., 1972, pp. 192–193.
4. Sexton, J. W., and Buck, W. B.: Lead. *In* Howard, J. L. (ed.): Current Veterinary Therapy, Food Animal Practice. Philadelphia, W. B. Saunders Co., 1981, pp. 498–500.

SELENIUM

Frederick W. Oehme, MANHATTAN, KANSAS

Selenium poisoning in horses occurs primarily in the Midwest Plains States. It is associated with the presence of naturally occurring selenium in soils. Because rainfall leaches much of the selenium from the native soils, selenium toxicity is largely seen in the region west of the Mississippi River to the western slope of the Rocky Mountains.

Selenium toxicity may be due to water supplies that contain 0.5 parts per million (ppm) or more of selenium, but more commonly it is due to the consumption of plants that are grown on soils containing selenium. The majority of cases of selenium toxicity are due to the consumption of secondary accumulator plants, which extract soil selenium normally unavailable to most range plants. These accumulator plants are found on seleniferous soils that contain greater than 5 ppm selenium and are less commonly found on soils with lower selenium content.

Plants that require high-selenium-content soils for survival are called "indicator plants" or "obligate accumulators" and generally build up 100 times or more of the selenium levels of other plants in the

same area. Facultative or "secondary selenium accumulators" do not require high-selenium-content soils for survival, but when growing on seleniferous soils, they accumulate selenium levels up to 10 times the selenium concentrations found in nonaccumulator plants in the same area.

While these accumulator plants may build up high concentrations of selenium that will induce relatively acute toxic syndromes in horses consuming them, plants such as cereal crops grown in seleniferous soils will passively build up soluble selenium in their plant matrices. These crop plants may contain more than 5 ppm selenium, the tolerance limit for selenium in the diet of livestock.

Plants of the species of Astragalus (vetch) are most commonly associated with selenium toxicity in horses. However, other plants of species of Xylorrhiza (woody aster), Oonopsis (goldenweed) and Stanleya (prince's plume) also contain members that can produce selenium poisoning. These seleniferous plants are toxic when consumed fresh as well as when they are foraged in the dormant or dry state.

They are, therefore, toxic during all seasons. Some plants have a higher selenium concentration when large than when small, but others seem to have smaller selenium concentrations as they mature in the growing season. Although horses generally avoid poisonous species of selenium-containing plants when good forage is available, moderate starvation may result in these plants being consumed. Once seleniferous plants are eaten, horses may subsequently seek them out even when adequate forage is made available.

CLINICAL SIGNS

Selenium poisoning may be acute or chronic. Ingestion of plants containing large concentrations of selenium results in death in several hours to a day. Signs indicate nervous, digestive, cardiovascular, and respiratory system involvement. Depression, diarrhea, labored breathing, rapid prostration, and death due to respiratory failure make this condition difficult to diagnose owing to its complexity of signs and rapidity of action.

The subacute form of toxicity results from the ingestion of moderate amounts of selenium-containing material and is characterized by signs of liver and brain involvement over several days to several weeks. A depressive mania that causes blindness, straying from a group of animals, muscle weakness, and finally paralysis is usually unresponsive to therapy and results in death. The blindness and central nervous system disturbance have led to this syndrome being called "blind staggers."

Chronic selenium poisoning, or the lay term "alkali disease," occurs if low doses somewhat in excess of 5 to 10 ppm selenium are consumed and accumulated in the body over a period of several weeks to several months. This chronic disease manifests the basic mechanism by which selenium interacts with biologic tissues, that is, binding of the selenium with sulfur-containing tissue compounds. The affected horses gradually lose weight and are only moderately depressed. Appetite may vary, but anorexia is not usual. There is loss of hair from the mane and tail, and the hoof wall on one or more feet develops a break at the coronary band. As this break grows out, the hooves become cracked and roughened, and the breaking off of portions of this weakened wall may give the hoof a ragged appearance. Affected animals are lame and tender in the feet. The loss of hair and breaks in the hoof wall are due to the altered chemical content of these sulfur-containing structures. Fatalities are rare with chronic selenium poisoning, but affected animals are often destroyed or sold because owners often become impatient and discouraged by the chronic and apparently unresponsive syndrome. Horses on selenium-containing water supplies (with as little as 0.1 to 2.0 ppm selenium) are especially sensitive to chronic selenium poisoning owing to the continued ingestion of low concentrations of the element.

Acute selenium poisoning produces only minor internal hemorrhages due to the terminal convulsions. Subacute selenium toxicity, because of its longer duration, induces internal congestion, moderate hyperemia of the digestive tract, and some fatty degeneration and focal necrosis of the liver. Lesions of chronic selenium poisoning are observed when one or more affected animals are sacrificed as an aid for diagnosis. Anemia, fatty atrophy of the heart, paleness and firmness of the liver with cirrhosis seen on microscopic examination, moderate and diffuse gastroenteritis, and joint erosions due to the disturbed gait are all characteristic of this long-term syndrome.

Selenium concentrations of 8 to 20 ppm in the hooves, 1 to 4 ppm in blood, and 11 to 45 ppm in hair are associated with chronic selenium poisoning. In more acute syndromes, the hoof and hair selenium concentrations are less than in the chronic syndrome, whereas concentrations in blood and liver are significantly greater.

THERAPY

There is no effective treatment for selenium poisoning, although animals seen before death should be managed symptomatically. In subacute cases, the administration of 4 to 6 mg strychnine sulfate per 600 to 800 lbs (275 to 375 kg) subcutaneously every two to three hours has been suggested as beneficial. However, the overall value of therapy must be carefully weighed against the low rate of eventual recovery, and the equine clinician is urged to balance any additional therapeutic expenditure against the low probability of recovery in this situation.

Chronic cases have a 50 per cent chance of recovery. The liver damage, as reflected in the weight loss and poor condition, and the damage to joints and hooves require long-term therapy. Arsenic in the form of sodium arsenite may be added to water or salt to biochemically protect the sulfur-containing structures in the body. Approximately 5 ppm of inorganic arsenic are recommended in drinking water, with salt containing 35 to 40 ppm arsenic recommended as a useful supplement. Naphthalene (4 to 5 gm orally per day) for five days has also been utilized for treating horses affected with chronic selenium poisoning. The dose is repeated for five additional days after a rest period of five days between dosing sequences.

The altered hoof conformation associated with chronic selenium poisoning requires corrective hoof trimming at frequent intervals. Acrylic may be used to support the weakened hoof wall or to replace damaged and nonfunctional portions of the wall.

Careful attention to the animal's hoof structure is necessary to avoid chronic damage to the sensitive laminae and to joint surfaces. Horses being treated for chronic selenium toxicity should be confined away from exposure to the responsible selenium-containing plant. A high-quality balanced ration must be made available to the recovering patient.

Supplemental Readings

1. Hulbert, L. C., and Oehme, F. W.: Plants poisonous to livestock, 3rd ed. Manhattan, KS, Kansas State University, 1980, pp. 56–57.
2. Hultine, J. D., Mount, M. E., Easley, K. J., and Oehme, F. W.: Selenium toxicosis in the horse. Equine Pract., *1*:57, 1979.

PLANT TOXICITIES

Ann A. Kownacki, ATASCADERO, CALIFORNIA

Thomas Tobin, LEXINGTON, KENTUCKY

This chapter reviews the toxic plants affecting horses, describing the clinical syndromes and suggesting the conditions under which the horse may encounter the plant. It is not meant to serve as a taxonomic key and, therefore, does not describe the plants. Descriptions can be found in several excellent references.[6, 11, 15, 19, 24]

The etiology of many toxic syndromes in horses is never determined. Plant poisoning should be considered in any sudden onset of illness, especially if it is accompanied by gastrointestinal disorders, nervous signs, sudden collapse, or death. In these cases, there may be a recent history of exposure to a toxic plant. Many of the chronic toxicities may also have sudden onset of signs, sometimes well after the animal stops eating the toxic plant. Determining the etiologic agent is often difficult. A good history is imperative in the diagnosis of plant poisoning. Where an animal has been, the changes in feed in the past six months, and the alterations in environment must all be carefully considered.

Many animals coexist with poisonous plants without harm, grazing the surrounding herbage with impunity. A stress such as introduction of a newcomer to the herd may precipitate the ingestion of unfamiliar plants, including toxic species. When forage is scarce or under conditions of overcrowding, animals may seek out any green plant, including those that are poisonous. A common link in the history of many acute poisonings is the introduction of plant clippings into the horse's pen by an unsuspecting gardener.

The age of the animal and the amount of plant consumed affect an animal's susceptibility. The time of year, soil type, and climatic conditions alter production of the plant toxin. Methods and times of harvesting of contaminated pastures will also affect the ultimate toxicity of the plant.

YELLOW STAR THISTLE (*Centaurea solstitialis*); RUSSIAN KNAPWEED (*C. repens*) (*C. picris*)

TOXIC PRINCIPLE

The toxic principle is an unidentified alkaloid.

LOCATION OF THE PLANT

C. solstitialis grows primarily in California, and the other Centaurea sp are a source of poisoning in the other Pacific Coast states and as far east as Colorado.[26, 43]

C. repens is more toxic than *C. solstitialis*, and a horse must consume 59 to 71 per cent and 86 to 200 per cent of its body weight, respectively, in fresh plant before signs of the disease occur.[22] Continuous ingestion over an average of 54 days for *C. solstitialis* and 30 days for *C. repens* is required to exceed the toxic threshold. Although ingestion of either the dried or fresh plant causes clinical signs, the majority of cases occur between October and November or in June and July. At these times in California, yellow star thistle may be the only available forage on dry pasture. Younger animals are said to be most commonly affected and seem to acquire a taste for the weed despite its spines.

Only horses are affected by the plant's toxin. Donkeys with access to the weed do not seem to be affected. Ruminants can eat the thistle without suffering any ill effect. Experimental attempts to reproduce the disease in other animal species have been unsuccessful.[7, 8, 30]

CLINICAL SIGNS

Signs develop acutely and are usually fully evident at the time of clinical presentation. Horses are at that time in good flesh. The primary clinical sign is an inability to hold or chew food with a concomitant inability to eat or drink and a characteristic facial dystonia.[13, 18] The upper lip is hypertonic, the cheeks are drawn tightly against the mandible, and the corners of the mouth may be held halfway open with the tongue moving awkwardly in an attempt to retain food in the mouth. Horses may immerse their heads up to their eyes and get water in this manner, as they can swallow if food or water is placed far enough back in the throat.[7] Chewing, yawning, or head tossing may be seen.

Most frequently, horses stand with their heads down in their frustrated attempts to get food. The development of severe facial edema is common. At other times, they may appear depressed or inattentive but can easily be aroused. Gait is not generally affected, although some horses may walk aimlessly or may show slight hypermetria[13] or stiffness in the walk.[7] Occasionally, central nervous system disorders such as head pushing, walking through obstacles, or excitement to the extent of self-induced trauma may be seen.

Signs are the most severe for the first day or two but thereafter subside to a static level. In a few cases, unilateral signs predominate, such as unidirectional circling or reluctance to be turned in one direction. Signs are irreversible, and if the animal is not destroyed, it will eventually die of dehydration, starvation, or aspiration pneumonia.

PATHOLOGY

Liquefactive necrosis of the substantia nigra and globus pallidus sections of the brain is the pathognomonic lesion of the disease, hence, the name equine nigropallidal encephalomalacia.[7] Prior to seven days of the clinical course, only discoloration of these brain areas may be seen. The specific lesions are most often bilateral, although any or all of the four sites may be affected. Other more subtle brain lesions have been demonstrated in experimental horses.[22] Traumatic lesions or signs of secondary complications may also be present.

TREATMENT

No treatment is available, although slight symptomatic relief has been obtained with massive doses of atropine.[18] Although horses have been kept alive for months by tube feeding, euthanasia is recommended.

RAGWORTS (Senecio sp); **STINKING WILLIE** *(S. jacobaea);* **COMMON GROUNDSEL** *(S. vulgaris);* **FIDDLENECK** (Amsinckia sp); **TARWEED** *(A. intermedia);* **RATTLEWEED** (Crotalaria sp); **SALIVATION JANE** *(Echium lycopsis)*

TOXIC PRINCIPLE

A variety of pyrrolizidine alkaloids are toxic principles.

LOCATION OF THE PLANT

Senecio is found throughout much of the southern United States, the Pacific Northwest, and parts of New England.[3, 19] Crotalaria is used extensively as a cover crop in the South as far west as Texas.[19, 24] Amsinckia is a common hay and pasture contaminant and is native to the Pacific Coast states.[24]

CONDITIONS OF TOXICITY

The majority of the pyrrolizidine alkaloid–containing plants are unpalatable and are only eaten when other forage is scarce or when baled or pelleted in hay.[3] The weeds grow in winter and early spring and are, therefore, found in first cutting hay.[6, 15] Owing to the management practices of hay making in California, it has been estimated that no more than 4 per cent of the state's total acreage is contaminated at any time.

The effects of the alkaloids are cumulative, and ingestion occurs over a period of weeks before the liver is damaged enough to cause clinical signs of disease.[24] Clinical cases are usually recognized in the late summer to early winter months.[19] If ingestion has been sporadic, animals may develop signs months after the first exposure, and the offending hay may no longer be available to aid in diagnosis. Hay with 15 per cent Amsinckia or Senecio content will kill a horse over a period of time, but perhaps 50 to 150 lbs of weed must be ingested before signs appear.[3]

Although most farm animals are susceptible to the pyrrolizidine alkaloids, there is some species variation. The horse is certainly the most sensitive to the effects of the toxin. The different plant genera cause a wide variety of signs in the different animal species.[22]

For the most part, the four plant genera that contain pyrrolizidine alkaloids cause a similar set of signs in the horse. Although clinical toxicities from *Echium lycopsis* have only been reported in Australia,[37] the plant's recent advent in a limited area of California makes exposure a possibility.[24]

CLINICAL SIGNS

In rare cases, ingestion of at least 20 lbs of pyrrolizidine alkaloid–containing plant at one time has caused acute toxicity characterized by extreme excitement and violence, gastrointestinal signs, pupillary dilation, and increased heart rate.[3, 29]

Toxicity from chronic ingestion of pyrrolizidine alkaloid–containing plants is much more common. Overt signs of chronic ingestion also appear abruptly, although weight loss and anorexia may have developed slowly over at least a month prior to clinical recognition of the disease.[15, 24]

The alkaloids damage the liver, and elevations in the icteric index, alkaline phosphatase, sorbitol dehydrogenase, and prothrombin time may all occur. Bromsulphthalein retention half time is consistently elevated, and liver biopsy is usually diagnostic. Neutrophilia with a toxic left shift has been seen.

Signs of hepatoencephalopathy due to increased blood ammonia level resulting from a malfunctioning liver are typical.[22, 24] A horse may be depressed or drowsy,[6, 22] may yawn,[4, 6] and may keep its head down or may press it against stationary objects.[4, 15, 35] The uncoordinated, staggering gait sometimes gives the disease the name "sleepy staggers."[6, 15] Circling or aimless walking is seen in 80 per cent of clinical cases.[24] Lack of obstacle avoidance and apparent blindness have also been noted.

Chronic liver damage may lead to the accumulation in the skin of phototoxic substances and signs of photosensitization in the lightly pigmented areas of the face or legs. Other signs related to liver disease are ascites or subcutaneous edema secondary to hypoalbuminemia and portal hypertension.[15] The mouth may be ulcerated and may have an offensive odor;[24] abdominal pain and diarrhea may be present.

In the last two weeks of life, the animal often goes through a rapid progression of signs. A hemolytic crisis may be clinically demonstrated by the presence of hemoglobinuria. Terminally, the mucous membranes may be congested, and icterus may no longer be recognizable as severe anemia develops.[15, 20] The horse commonly dies quietly but may undergo delirium, collapse, and convulsions before death.

PATHOLOGY

Pyrrolizidine alkaloid–intoxicated horses are often emaciated, have decreased muscle mass, and show jaundice. The liver is usually enlarged, weighing more than 7 kg, and has a mottled appearance with an accentuated lobular pattern. It is so firm that it cannot be crushed with the fingers. Occasional reports suggest a pale, small liver, but firmness is a consistent finding.[37] The kidneys may be enlarged and congested,[6] as are the adrenals. Widespread petechial and ecchymotic hemorrhages may be seen with subendocardial, gastrointestinal tract, mesenteric,[6] and urinary bladder hemorrhages. Edema is seen in the lungs[6, 15] or brain. Cytotoxic edema in the central nervous system is the basis for the neurologic signs seen with advanced liver disease; however, the central nervous system lesions in the horse are not as extensive as those in other animals with hepatoencephalopathy.

Liver histopathology is diagnostic. Megalocytosis with increased nuclear size, bile duct hyperplasia, and perilobular fibrosis are the classic findings.[6, 22, 37] The kidneys may show megalocytosis and mild nephrosis.[22, 37] Veno-occlusion has been reported in horses eating *Crotalaria* sp[24] but is thought to be just another manifestation of the general effects of pyrrolizidine alkaloids on the liver.[4] Proliferation of collagen and subendothelial swelling of central or hepatic veins lead to narrowing of the vessel walls. The veno-occlusion may lead to an increase in portal pressure and the congestion seen in the liver and gastrointestinal tract.

TREATMENT

Once clinical signs appear in a horse, the prognosis for survival is poor. The use of a methionine and dextrose saline drip was reported to be effective in two horses poisoned by ingesting *Senecio*[36] but was ineffective in cases of *Crotalaria retusa* poisoning.[22] Recent reports suggest that intravenous infusion of glucose and branched-chain amino acids may help considerably. Recovery rates of 30 to 40 per cent have been reported. Herbicides are useful when the plants are in the rapidly growing stages, and the cinnabar moth, *Tyria jacobalae*, has been reported as an effective control for ragwort.

CHOKECHERRY *(Prunus virginiana)*

TOXIC PRINCIPLE

Chokecherry contains the cyanogenic glycosides amygdalin in the fruit and prunasin in the leaves.[16]

LOCATION OF THE PLANT

Chokecherry is found in most of the United States in a variety of climates.[11, 19, 24]

CONDITIONS OF TOXICITY

Because the cyanogenic compounds are located in one part of the plant's cells and the enzymes needed for degradation are located in another part,[22] the cherry and other cyanogenic plants do not easily release free cyanide. Unusual field conditions such as drought, frost, wilting, or stunting of the plants combined with maceration by the animal are necessary to release lethal levels of cyanide. Great potential for toxicity occurs in immature or rapidly growing varieties.[5] Because the stomach acidity destroys the enzymes, liberating cyanide from the glycosides, monogastrics are more resistant than ruminants to the plant's effects.[4]

Once cyanide is released, animals can metabolize it, but if much of the plant is ingested, the cyanide blocks cytochrome oxidase, preventing oxygen uptake by tissues. Clinical signs are due to tissue anoxia despite adequate blood oxygen content, which gives the cherry red color of the blood.[5, 15]

CLINICAL SIGNS

Death occurs within minutes to an hour of ingestion of the offending plant. The progression of signs following the eating of large amounts of wild cherry leaves is as follows. Dyspnea with flaring of the nostrils occurs almost immediately. Lifting of the tailhead is seen, and involuntary micturition or defecation has been described. Central nervous system signs of agitation, including trembling, ataxia, and muscular contractions, are pronounced. Finally the horse becomes prostrate and kicks and flails its legs. Respiratory arrest occurs minutes before cardiac arrest.

PATHOLOGY

Mucous membranes often appear red and well oxygenated,[4] but this is not a consistent clinical finding. Hemorrhages in the heart and other organs are a result of violent death.[5]

TREATMENT

Although the veterinarian usually arrives too late to institute treatment, intravenous adminstration of 4 ml per 45 kg of body weight of a mixture of 1 ml of 20 per cent sodium nitrite and 3 ml of 20 per cent sodium thiosulfate can be effective. An additional 20 gm of sodium thiosulfate given orally will fix free cyanide in the stomach.[4]

Sodium nitrite forms methemoglobin, which reacts with free cyanide to form nontoxic cyanmethemoglobin. Thiosulfate reacts with cyanide and with enzymatic catalysis forms thiocyanate, which is eliminated in the urine.

Determination of cyanide-associated deaths in the field can be performed by testing suspect plants or abdominal contents.[5] The material should be crushed and placed in a jar with some water and a few drops of chloroform and sulfuric acid. Suspend strips of filter paper wetted with a preformed mixture of 4 gm sodium bicarbonate and 0.5 gm picric acid in 100 ml water in the jar without contacting the plant material. Heat for 5 to 10 minutes. If cyanide is present, the paper will turn a brick red color in a few minutes.

SORGHUM SP

TOXIC PRINCIPLE

The cyanogenic glycoside dhurrin, which can be hydrolyzed to free cyanide, is the toxic principle.

LOCATION OF THE PLANT

Sorghum is found in the Southwest and in much of the eastern United States.[1, 3, 11, 14, 24]

CONDITIONS OF TOXICITY

Milo and Sudan grass are both members of the Sorghum sp and are excellent forage plants. *S. halpense* or Johnson grass, though not unique in containing the glycoside, is the most toxic of the sorghums alone or in hybrid pastures and is often considered a weed. It is, however, used in some of the Southern states as a forage crop.[24] As with other cyanogenic-containing plant species, the sorghums may have increased toxic potential under certain environmental conditions (see Chokecherry).

Pastures rather than hays are most commonly associated with clinical toxicity,[11] as mature plants have far less toxic potential.[19] Many of the Sorghum sp have been bred for low cyanogenic potential.[5] Two syndromes seen in horses grazed on sorghum pastures bear similarities to the lathyrism syndrome in humans and may be related to chronic exposure to low levels of cyanide or the accumulation of lathyrogenic principles or both.

Lathyrism occurs in the underdeveloped countries, in people consuming poor-quality legumes, including Lathyrus sp, some peas, Vicia sp, and vetches. These plants are cyanogenic. With long-term ingestion, some cyanide is metabolized to neurolathyrogenic compounds, which cause focal axonal degeneration and demyelination of the lumbar and sacral parts of the spinal cord with a concomitant paresis or paralysis. Additionally, osteolathyrogenic compounds may be produced.

CLINICAL SIGNS

Several syndromes have been described in horses on sorghum pasture. The commonest syndrome is acute cyanide toxicity, which causes loss of livestock, especially on sorghum hybrid pastures, which are more toxic than the pure stands.[4] Signs of acute cyanide toxicity are described under chokecherry poisoning (p. 597).

A condition unique to horses grazing sorghum pastures has been recognized in the southwestern United States.[4, 5, 14] Equine sorghum cystitis ataxia is characterized by posterior ataxia with curious incoordination of the hindlegs, especially when the animal is backed, turned, or trotted. Urinary incontinence and cystitis with bladder atony are observed in 50 per cent of horses.[1] Urine scalds may cause loss of hair, and the urine may be thick and may puddle owing to the large amount of sediment. Death in adult horses is usually due to pyelonephritis. Pregnant mares grazing these pastures may abort or may give birth to deformed foals. Articular ankylosis or arthrogryposis in these foals may cause dystocia.[34]

A condition very similar to the sorghum cystitis ataxia syndrome has been reported following ingestion of baled hay containing caley pea (*Lathyrus hirsutis*) in California.[14] Initially the animals seem to be in pain and carry all their body weight on the forelegs with the hindlegs "camped under." The animals are uncoordinated but are not paretic and remain alert, retaining normal vital signs. Residual signs may be seen for years after the initial plant insult, and the horse may develop a "stringhalt-like gait" in which the hindlimbs are primarily affected. The leg is, however, held in prolonged flexion, and the gait abnormalities are most marked when the animal is moved out or backed. No pain is associated with this stage of the disease, and cystitis has not been observed.

PATHOLOGY

The lesions characteristic of the cystitis ataxia syndrome are acute fibrinopurulent cystitis, chronic ulcerative sclerosing cystitis with accumulation of bladder sediment, and degeneration of the spinal cord as described earlier for neurolathyrism.

TREATMENT

Treatment of acute cyanide poisoning is described under chokecherry poisoning (p. 597). There is no specific treatment for the chronic syndromes.

LOCOWEED (Astragalus sp and Oxytropis sp)

TOXIC PRINCIPLE

These plants contain locoine, an incompletely characterized extract with some alkaloidal properties.[24]

LOCATION OF THE PLANT

Astragalus sp that accumulate selenium are found throughout the Western United States, and those that produce locoism are found in most of the same states.[24] Oxytropis sp are more restricted to the central United States.

CONDITIONS OF TOXICITY

The "loco" syndrome is produced by many of the Astragalus and Oxytropis sp and affects all species of livestock. The entire plant is poisonous at any time of the year. Many of the greater than 300 Astragalus are toxic, but the toxicity of the plants varies among years and locations.[24]

Certain members of Astragalus grow only on seleniferous soils and accumulate selenium, causing a syndrome characteristic of selenium toxicity. A few Astragalus sp, known commonly as milkvetch, cause an acute syndrome in sheep evident when the animals are stressed or driven.[6, 24] The clinical signs are primarily related to damage to the respiratory system. Poisoning of this type in horses has not been reported in the United States but has been described in British Columbia.[24] Signs develop less than one week after ingestion of the plant and include roaring, staggering, salivation, and sudden death.

Horses are the species most susceptible to the "loco" syndrome. The ingestion of 30 per cent of their body weight in plants is required over 1½ months.[24] The most severe signs may not be noted until after the animal has ceased to ingest the plant.[17] Although animals are not usually attracted to the plant when better forage is available, once it is eaten, horses will seek out the plant, even when dry, to the exclusion of other plants.

CLINICAL SIGNS

In the early stages, "loco" syndrome may cause the animal to be unpredictable and dangerous to ride. Affected horses may separate themselves from other animals and may carry the head in abnormal ways, in part owing to the apparent visual distur-

bances and altered perception of spatial relationships, thereby running into objects or over cliffs.[14, 19]
Locomotor ataxia has been reported with staggering
or circling, incoordination, and abnormal or exaggerated movements of the limbs.[17] Unsuccessful attempts to rear may result in the horse falling back
on its haunches.[24] Although generally the horse is
listless and depressed, excitation aggravates these
locomotor signs and may precipitate nervousness,
trembling, and the classical description of wild behavior. The course of the disease is chronic, progressing to locomotor paralysis and difficulty in pre-
hension, causing weakness and starvation.[17]
Convulsive death may follow an episode of excitement.[19] Recovery in some cases is incomplete owing
to irreversible brain damage, and the animal is at
best suitable only for reproduction.[3]

A second syndrome associated with Astragalus
ingestion is known as "blind staggers" but is seen
more often in cattle. Straying, muscular weakness
or partial paralysis, and visual impairment have
been noted.

The selenium-accumulating species of Astragalus
have been referred to as poison vetches.[24] These
plants, as well as the woody aster (*Xylorrhiza pur-
ryi*) and others, are called "indicator" plants because
they grow only on selenium-containing soils.[22]
When these plants contain enough selenium to
make acute toxicity a possibility, they are generally
unpalatable. However, chronic selenium toxicity
can occur from eating forages grown on selenium-
rich land. Chronic selenium toxicity, "alkali disease," is characterized in horses by loss of mane and
tail hair and lameness caused by damage to the coronary band (p. 593).

PATHOLOGY

Generalized emaciation and hypertrophy of the
thyroid gland, kidney, liver,[22] and adrenal gland[17]
have been described. Transitory edematous vacu-
olization of brain cells and other organ systems occurs.[22, 24] In the central nervous system, these lesions are replaced in time by small eosinophilic
argyrophillic bodies called spheroids and may account for the residual neurologic effects.[22] The parenchymal organs can repair themselves if the animals are removed from exposure to the offending
plant before the onset of clinical signs. Most signs
of the disease can be explained by the brain lesions,
but damage to the other organs can account for
many of the problems with assimilation and metabolism of ingesta. Vacuoles in the retina and lacrimal
gland explain visual impairment and the decreased
lacrimation that gives the eye a dull appearance.

Acute selenium toxicity is characterized pathologically by hemorrhages and congestion in many organs. The liver and kidneys undergo degenerative
changes.

TREATMENT

There is no antidote for locoine. A clinical response to reserpine has been reported[38] but has not
been confirmed.

BRACKEN FERN (*Pteridium aquilinum*)

TOXIC PRINCIPLE

The toxic principle is thiaminase.[27]

LOCATION OF THE PLANT

Bracken fern is especially abundant in forested
areas, burns, or abandoned sandy fields throughout
the Northwest and northern United States to the
upper Midwest.[3, 19]

CONDITIONS OF TOXICITY

Toxicity can occur at any time of the year, depending on climatic conditions. Horses usually consume bracken fern in the late summer when other
forage is scarce,[19] although horses can acquire a taste
for the plant in pasture[10, 15] or when it is used as
bedding.[24] Toxicity due to ingestion of hay containing 20 per cent or more bracken is most common in
the winter months.[19] Levels of thiaminase in the
plant peak in the late summer. Thiaminase is destroyed by heat but not by drying. The entire plant
is toxic.[10]

CLINICAL SIGNS

Horses generally must consume bracken fern for
30 to 60 days before signs of toxicity are observed.[3]
Signs can appear even if horses have not ingested
bracken fern for two to three weeks. On presentation, blood thiamine levels are low.[15] Clinical signs
are due to myelin degeneration in peripheral
nerves; generalized weakness and muscle problems
are related to a buildup of pyruvates. Animals lose
weight progressively starting several days after exposure to the plant.

The first gait abnormality seen is an unsteady
walk[1] about 30 days after the first ingestion of
bracken.[19] This incoordination progresses over the
next week or so to overt staggering, hence, the
name "bracken staggers."[6] The animal stands pe-

culiarly with the back arched and the feet based widely in the back. There may be crossing of the front legs when the animal is in motion and wide action in the rear.[4] Severe muscle tremors and weakness appear, especially when animals are forced to work. Bradycardia with cardiac arrhythmias is not uncommon early in the course of the disease, but tachycardia occurs terminally, accompanied by a rise in temperature.[6] At this time, the animal usually becomes recumbent and may exhibit clonic spasms and the typical opisthotonus of thiamine deficiency.[6] Without treatment, death occurs within 2 to 10 days after the onset of clinical signs.[19] There has been a clinical report of a hemolytic crisis associated with bracken fern ingestion.[23]

PATHOLOGY

Although postmortem lesions are not diagnostic, enteritis with some pericardial and epicardial hemorrhages is observed.[19]

TREATMENT

The prognosis for full recovery is good if the disease is recognized before the animal becomes recumbent. Thiamine hydrochloride (0.25 to 0.5 mg per kg) should be administered daily either intravenously or intramuscularly.[11]

HORSETAIL, MARESTAIL, SCOURING RUSH (*Equisetum arvense*)

This plant is found in wetter and colder areas than bracken fern and over a wider geographic range.[3, 19] The toxic principle is the same, and signs are virtually identical to those of bracken fern poisoning. Cases are always associated with ingestion of the plant in hay.[3, 6, 15]

WATER HEMLOCK, COWBANE (Cicuta sp)

TOXIC PRINCIPLE

Cowbane contains cicutoxin, a resin.

LOCATION OF THE PLANTS

Found in wet areas and ditches, Cicuta sp are common from the upper Midwest westward to the Pacific.

CONDITIONS OF TOXICITY

Poisonings are most frequently seen in cattle, often when ground is reclaimed.[40] The majority of livestock deaths occur in the spring when the leaves are the most palatable and when the root can be easily pulled up and digested.[19] As the leafy plant matures in summer and fall and when found in hay, it has a lower toxicity. The roots are the most toxic part of the plant and remain so even when dried. Eight ounces of the root are lethal to mature horses.[19]

CLINICAL SIGNS

Signs occur between 10 and 60 minutes after ingestion and are due to the toxin's irritant action in nerve cells, which results in central nervous system stimulation. The horse shows signs of apprehension with pupillary dilation and slight muscle tics of the neck, which progress to contractions of major muscle groups. The animal thereafter has difficulty maintaining its balance and may back up. Breathing rapidly becomes labored, and the animal falls down and convulses. Death due to respiratory paralysis occurs less than 30 minutes after ingestion of a lethal dose of water hemlock.

PATHOLOGY

There are no characteristic lesions at necropsy.

TREATMENT

If a lethal dose is ingested, death is an inevitable consequence, but gastric lavage and anticonvulsive therapy (p. 347) may otherwise be helpful.[3] Livestock that survive for five to six hours seem to recover without ill effects.[11] The plant can be controlled with 2,4-D.[40]

POISON HEMLOCK (*Conium maculatum*)

TOXIC PRINCIPLE

A number of alkaloids, the most toxic being N-methyl conine,[11] are toxic principles.

LOCATION OF THE PLANT

Poison hemlock is a ubiquitous weed **found** throughout the United States.

CONDITIONS OF TOXICITY

The plant appears in early spring, and most toxicities occur at this time when the plant is palatable.[11] The level of *N*-methyl conine increases as the plant matures, and the root becomes toxic only later in the year. Drying seems to neutralize the toxic principle, and the plant is not a problem in hay. Four to five pounds of fresh leaves have been lethal to horses.[16]

CLINICAL SIGNS

Conine acts similarly to nicotine, causing first stimulation, then depression of the autonomic ganglia. Signs occur within about two hours of eating the plant. Horses may fall without signs of approaching paralysis and retain normal corneal reflexes but lack awareness.[27] Variable signs of apprehension with mydriasis and posterior muscle incoordination to the point of extensive trembling have preceded falling episodes. The clinical course may continue over several hours to a day or two, and the animal may be comatose for part of this time, but this in itself may not be fatal. Death in severe cases occurs within 5 to 10 hours of the onset of signs.[40]

PATHOLOGY

There are no diagnostic postmortem findings, although the toxin is eliminated via the kidneys and lungs, giving the urine and exhaled air a characteristic mousey odor.[6]

TREATMENT

Adequate nursing of recumbent animals and administration of laxatives may aid in successful recovery. Tannic acid can be used to neutralize the active principle, and stimulants such as strychnine, atropine, or metrazol have been reported to be effective.[6]

WILD JASMINE *(Cestrum diurnum)*

TOXIC PRINCIPLE

A steroidal glycoside[22] that acts like vitamin D is the toxic principle.

LOCATION OF THE PLANT

Cestrum is found in waste ground in Texas[24] and Florida.[25]

CONDITIONS OF TOXICITY

Cestrum diurnum produces a vitamin D–like factor that bypasses the usual feedback regulation of normal vitamin D metabolism in the horse.[25] When a horse ingests the plant and is also on a ration containing adequate calcium and phosphorus, more calcium is absorbed than can be physiologically accommodated.[41] Although hypercalcemia is moderate to severe, phosphorus levels are usually normal.[25] The elevated calcium levels cause sustained secretion of calcitonin, which contributes to osteopetrosis. Hypercalcemia also decreases parathyroid activity, which can be seen histologically.[25]

The exact amount of the plant required to cause toxicity is unknown, but Cestrum is toxic at all times of the year.[3]

The South American *Solanum malacoxylon* is associated with the disease enteque seca,[24] which causes signs very similar to those of jasmine poisoning.[41] Hyperphosphatemia occurs with hypercalcemia, and there is calcification of soft tissue, for example, in the lungs, diaphragm, and kidney. *Solanum sodomauim* in Hawaii has been implicated in a similar syndrome in cattle.[41] *Trisetum flavescens* in Germany has also been reported to cause vitamin D–like toxicity.[25]

CLINICAL SIGNS

Horses that have ingested *C. diurnum* retain normal appetites but invariably demonstrate weight loss over two to six months.[25] As the disease progresses, lameness increases in severity, and the animals develop a humped-up appearance and a short choppy gait. Animals lie down frequently. Pain around the flexors and suspensory ligaments with overextension of the fetlock joint has been observed.

PATHOLOGY

Dystrophic calcinosis of the elastic tissues of the heart, major arteries, tendons, and ligaments is seen.[25]

TREATMENT

Regression of the disease can occur when animals are moved to clean pastures and are carefully nursed.

OLEANDER *(Nerium oleander)*

TOXIC PRINCIPLE

Oleandrin and nerioside glycosides akin to digitoxin[6] are the toxic principles.

LOCATION OF THE PLANT

Oleander is found primarily in the southern United States from coast to coast.[19]

CONDITIONS OF TOXICITY

The entire plant is toxic. Toxicity may occur at any time of the year but is most likely when animals are given plant trimmings to eat. Horses will rarely eat the fresh plant,[15] though the wilted or dried leaves are less bitter and more palatable. Thirty or 40 green or dry leaves, about ¼ lb, are fatal. Death occurs less than 12 hours after ingestion.[3]

CLINICAL SIGNS

Depression and a profuse catarrhal, watery, or bloody diarrhea and colic occur within a few hours of ingestion. Alternating bradycardia and tachycardia are accompanied by a variety of arrhythmias and murmurs that cannot be localized to any heart area.[15] Peripheral vessel constriction may cause pallor of the mucous membranes and coldness of the extremities. Sweating may be profuse.[35] Muscle anoxia may give rise to tics. Ultimately, horses become comatose and die.

PATHOLOGY

There are no characteristic lesions. A mild gastroenteritis with hemorrhage into the gut lumen, onto various body organs, and on visceral pleura, the epicardium, and endocardium has been observed.[6] Ascites has been seen.[15]

TREATMENT

Horses may die without showing signs of sickness, making treatment impossible. Laxatives and enemas should be helpful in sublethal poisonings. Atropine in conjunction with propranolol has also been advocated.[6]

DEATH CAMAS (Zigadenus sp)

TOXIC PRINCIPLE

A steroidal glycosidal alkaloid, zygadenine,[3] is the toxic principle.

LOCATION OF THE PLANT

Zigadenus sp are found west of the Mississippi on sandy plains and in the foothills of the Rocky Mountains.

CONDITIONS OF TOXICITY

Although many Zigadenus sp are toxic, only Z. *nuttallii*, which is more geographically restricted, has been reported as a cause of toxicity in horses.[24] Colic and salivation in a group of pack mules in the California Sierras was, however, attributed to another Zigadenus sp.[15] Poisonings are most likely to occur in the spring on ranges where other forages are scarce, since the plant is unpalatable to horses. Less than 10 lbs of the plant need to be ingested to produce signs of a frequently fatal toxicity.[3]

CLINICAL SIGNS

Signs begin within several hours of ingestion, although death may not occur for up to several days.[24] Depression, staggering, profuse salivation, pupillary constriction, and decreased heart and respiratory rate have all been observed.[31]

PATHOLOGY

There are no distinctive lesions.[19]

TREATMENT

An effective treatment described for sheep is 2 mg atropine sulfate and 8 mg picrotoxin in 5 ml of water per 100 lbs of body weight subcutaneously as needed to ameliorate signs.[24] Atropine sulfate (33 mg) and carbachol (0.25 to 0.5 mg) have been recommended for horses.[3] Clinical success has been less effective than with sheep.

WHITE SNAKEROOT (Eupatorium rugosum)

TOXIC PRINCIPLE

The primary toxic component is the higher alcohol tremetol, which is incapable of producing the clinical disease when completely dried. Since excreted slowly, tremetol exerts a cumulative effect.[6]

LOCATION OF THE PLANT

Snakeroot is found throughout the Midwest and parts of the South.

CONDITIONS OF TOXICITY

Poisonings occur in the late summer and fall. Although toxicity decreases with drying, the plant in hay retains enough toxicity to cause problems. The lethal plant dose in the horse is 2 to 10 lbs.[3] Tremetol is accumulated in the milk, and this can be an indirect route for toxicity in suckling animals.[19] The rayless goldenrod (*Isocoma wrightii*), another North American plant, also contains tremetol and can produce a similar syndrome.[35]

CLINICAL SIGNS

The onset of signs varies from less than two days to three weeks after ingestion and may be precipitated by any type of stress.[24] If a toxic dose has been consumed, enzymatic damage to the heart muscle occurs, precipitating a bout of rapid shaking, especially in the flanks and rear legs, hence the name "trembles." If the animal is not stressed, the only signs are reluctance to move, sluggishness, stiffness of gait, or ataxia. Horses are the least likely of the domestic animals to tremble and may die without doing so.[24] Partial throat paralysis and severe sweating have been reported in horses.[35] The disease in horses tends to run a shorter clinical course than in other animals, with death occurring in about two days.[11]

PATHOLOGY

Hemorrhages in the heart, gastrointestinal tract, and other organs occur as a result of heart failure. The most consistent lesion is congestion of the liver, kidneys, or central nervous system. There is also fatty degeneration of the liver.

TREATMENT

Since the disease is usually recognized late in its clinical course, treatment is usually frustrating and ineffective. Mineral oil laxatives offer the best approach. Plants may be controlled with 2, 4-D.

CASTOR BEAN (*Ricinus communis*)

TOXIC PRINCIPLE

The seeds contain a phytotoxin, ricin.

LOCATION OF THE PLANT

The plant is grown in the Southwest and the Southeast.

CONDITIONS OF TOXICITY

Although unpalatable, the seeds or castor bean byproducts may be consumed when mixed with other feedstuffs.[16] The horse is very susceptible to ricin, and 25 gm of castor bean is a lethal dose.[15]

CLINICAL SIGNS

Phytotoxins are antigenic plant proteins that may act as potent proteolytic enzymes, causing signs of gastrointestinal irritation.[24] If enough of the toxin is absorbed, signs of anaphylaxis and shock predominate.[19] Usually a latent period of several hours to two days occurs before the onset of signs, which are rapidly progressive.[14, 16, 24] Initially there are dullness, slight incoordination, and profuse sweating, possibly with muscular spasms in the neck and shoulders. The respiratory and heart rates are increased. The heart contractions may be so strong that the entire body shakes, and the pounding of the heart against the thorax may be seen from 10 feet away. Usually a nonhemorrhagic watery diarrhea occurs and is accompanied by colic.[28]

Early signs are accompanied by a fever spike and a left shift in the hemogram. As the episode progresses, leukopenia and a progressive rise in hematocrit due to dehydration are observed.[12] Death occurs within 36 hours, and terminal convulsions are seen.

PATHOLOGY

Congestion of internal organs occurs.[15] Inflammation and hemorrhage in the gastrointestinal tract, epicardium, and endocardium[12] are common along with pooling of fluid in the intestine and engorgement of the right heart.[28]

TREATMENT

Treat the horse for shock and give sedatives.[16]

YEW (Taxus sp)

TOXIC PRINCIPLE

The alkaloid taxine is found in most Taxus sp.

LOCATION OF THE PLANT

The plant is found as an ornamental throughout most of the United States.

CONDITIONS OF TOXICITY

The plant is poisonous year-round, but toxicity occurs when animals are given access to the trimmings, usually in the spring or summer.[11] The horse is the species most susceptible to the alkaloid's toxicity, and one mouthful can be lethal.[3, 6] Drying or storage does not lessen toxicity.[6] One veterinary diagnostic laboratory attributed 50 per cent of horse deaths from toxic agents to the ingestion of Japanese yew *(Taxus caspictata).*[2]

CLINICAL SIGNS

Taxine depresses cardiac conduction.[2] Death in donkeys and horses can be so sudden that few abnormalities are noted before collapse and extensor rigidity or muscle spasms.[2] Animals are most often found lying next to the Taxus source, as death can occur within five minutes after ingestion.

PATHOLOGY

There are no characteristic lesions. Postmortem diagnosis is best confirmed by finding plant fragments within the stomach. This may be difficult in horses and requires the use of a dissection microscope owing to the complete mastication of plants by the horse.[2]

TREATMENT

Death comes so rapidly that there is no time to treat the animal symptomatically, and there is no known antidote.

BLACK NIGHTSHADE *(Solanum nigrum)*

TOXIC PRINCIPLE

The glycoalkaloid solanine[16] is the toxic principle.

LOCATION OF THE PLANT

The plant is found east of the Rocky Mountains.

CONDITIONS OF TOXICITY

Toxicity usually occurs in late summer and early fall when other forages are lacking. All parts of the plant are toxic, especially the berries.[16] The concentration of toxic alkaloid varies with soil, climate, season, and region. One to 10 lbs may be lethal.[3]

CLINICAL SIGNS

Although several poisoning syndromes are recognized, horses usually exhibit central nervous sys-tem signs of depression, dullness, weakness, and prostration.[6] In addition, the toxin has a direct irritant effect on the gastrointestinal mucosa, causing signs of colic and pain. Copious diarrhea is said to be a good prognostic sign.[6]

PATHOLOGY

The primary pathologic sign is a slight gastroenteritis.

TREATMENT

There is no antidote for solanine. Good nursing care is required. Plants should be controlled with herbicides.

ST. JOHN'S WORT *(Hypericum perforatum)*

TOXIC PRINCIPLE

The primary photosensitizing agent hypericin is the toxic principle.

LOCATION OF THE PLANT

St. John's wort is found as a pasture weed in parts of the Pacific Coast and the Atlantic Coast[19] toward the Southeast.[16]

CONDITIONS OF TOXICITY

Primary photosensitization is a rare occurrence in horses but is much more commonly reported in sheep and cattle. St. John's wort and others contain photodynamic agents that reach the skin after absorption from the digestive tract. When the animal is subsequently exposed to sunlight, the compounds cause cellular damage at the skin level. Species of clover (Trifolium), vetches (Vicia), and buckwheat (Fagopyrum) have all been incriminated in primary or contact photosensitivity. *Trifolium hybridum* may also cause liver disease in horses.[11]

Photosensitizing plants seem to cause the problem when they are in the lush green stage and are growing rapidly.[6] In the case of St. John's wort, large amounts need to be eaten, and the plant is not very palatable, so cases of toxicity are rare.

CLINICAL SIGNS

The first signs of photosensitivity may be seen within four to five days of ingestion.[6] Erythema and edema of the white or lightly pigmented areas occur first. The eyelids may be swollen, and keratitis and conjunctivitis may be present. Within a few days, the affected areas blister, and the skin sloughs, opening an avenue for secondary bacterial infection. The horse will seek out shade and may resent having the affected areas touched.

PATHOLOGY

There are no pathognomonic lesions.

TREATMENT

Horses will make a full recovery in one to two weeks if kept out of the sun and removed from the source of the plant. Corticosteroids may be helpful to decrease some of the inflammatory response. Antibiotics are useful to control bacterial infection. Open wounds should be given routine care.

MISCELLANEOUS PLANT TOXICITIES

A few other plant-related toxic syndromes deserve mention. Acorn poisoning has not been recorded in horses in the United States, but there have been several reports from England.[24, 42] Signs of colic and hematuria were noted in two horses about one week after they had access to clippings of oak leaves *(Quercus rubra)*.[9] Ingestion of wild onions *(Allium canadense)* has caused acute hemolytic anemia with hemoglobinuria and icterus.[33]

Very recently, a toxic syndrome has been recognized in horses in the summer and fall following the ingestion of leaves of the red maple *(Acer rubrum)* found in the Northeastern United States.[39] Abrupt onset of signs of lethargy, icterus, and hemoglobinuria were noted in all cases. Animals were often febrile and rapidly developed anemia with methemoglobinemia and Heinz bodies. Brown discoloration of all tissues was noted at necropsy with enlargement of the kidneys, liver, and spleen.

The black locust *(Robinia pseudoacacia)*, which is found in the eastern United States, contains a phytotoxin that is extremely toxic.[11, 24] Horses may become poisoned when tied to the tree and allowed to strip the bark. Horses usually show weakness, posterior paralysis, anorexia, and depression.[20] Mydriasis, mild colic, diarrhea, a rapid, irregular heartbeat, or diaphragmatic flutter may be noted. Animals may die in a few days or may survive, depending on the amount ingested.

Sleepy grass (Stipa sp) can cause mechanical damage to the mouth owing to the plant's physical characteristics. Ingestion of the New Mexico variety can produce a transient drowsiness that may last as long

as two days, making movement of the animals difficult.[22, 35]

Mild signs of central nervous system depression and increased urination are seen when horses ingest large amounts of Scottish broom *(Cytisus scoparius)*.[20]

References

1. Adams, L. G., Dollahite, J. W., Romane, W. M., Bullard, T. L., and Bridges, C. H.: Cystitis and ataxia associated with sorghum ingestion by horses. J. Am. Vet. Med. Assoc., 155:518, 1967.
2. Alden, C. L., Fasnaugh, C. J., Smith, J. B., and Mohan, R.: Japanese yew poisoning of large domestic animals in the midwest. J. Am. Vet. Med. Assoc., 170:314, 1977.
3. Bailey, E. M., et al.: The sky is blue, the plant is green, the horse is dead. Equus, 21:45, 1979.
4. Blood, D. C., Henderson, J. A., and Radostits, O. M.: Veterinary Medicine: A Textbook of the Diseases of Cattle, Sheep, Pigs and Horses, 5th ed. Philadelphia, Lea and Febiger, 1979.
5. Buck, W. B., Osweiler, G. D., and Van Gelder, G. A.: Clinical and Diagnostic Veterinary Toxicology, 2nd ed. Dubuque, Iowa, Kendall/Hunt Pub. Co., 1976.
6. Clarke, E. G. C., and Clarke, M. L.: Veterinary Toxicology. Baltimore, Williams and Wilkins, 1975.
7. Cordy, D. R.: Nigropallidal encephalomalacia in horses associated with ingestion of yellow star thistle. J. Neuropathol. Exp. Neurol., 13:330, 1954.
8. Cordy, D. R.: Nigropallidal encephalomalacia (chewing disease) in horses on rations high in yellow star thistle. Proc. 91st Annu. Meet. Am. Vet. Med. Assoc., 1954, pp. 149–154.
9. Duncan, C. S.: Oak leaf poisoning in two horses. Cornell Vet., 51:159, 1961.
10. Evans, W. C.: Thiaminases and their effects on animals. Vitam. Horm., 33:467, 1975.
11. Evers, R. A., and Link, R. P.: Poisonous plants of the midwest. Special Publication 24, Urbana, IL, College of Agriculture, University of Illinois, 1972.
12. Fowler, M. E.: Differential diagnostic problems in plant poisonings. Ann. NY Acad. Sci., 111:577, 1964.
13. Fowler, M. E.: Nigropallidal encephalomalacia in the horse. J Am. Vet. Med. Assoc., 147:607, 1965.
14. Fowler, M. E.: Diseases caused by chemical and physical agents. In Catcott, E. J., and Smithcors, J. F. (eds.): Equine Medicine Surgery, 2nd ed. Wheaton, IL, American Veterinary Pub., 1972.
15. Fowler, M. E.: Plant poisoning and biotoxins. Davis, CA, Dept. of Medicine, School of Veterinary Medicine Pub., 1978.
16. Garner, R. J.: Veterinary Toxicology, 2nd ed. London, Baillière Tindall, 1961.
17. Harries, W. N., Baker, F. P., and Johnston, A.: An outbreak of locoweed poisoning in horses in southwestern Alberta. Can. Vet. J., 13:141, 1972.
18. Holliday, T. A.: Clinical neurology for veterinarians. Davis, CA, Dept. of Surgery, School of Veterinary Medicine Pub., 1979, pp. 307–310.
19. Hulbert, L. C., and Oehme, F. W.: Plants Poisonous to Livestock, 2nd ed. Manhattan, KS, Kansas State University Press, 1965.
20. Kates, A. H., Davis, D. E., McCormack, J., and Miller, J. F.: Poisonous plants of the southern United States. Athens, GA, Georgia Cooperative Extension Service, 1980.
21. Keeler, R., James, L. F., Binns, W., and Shupe, J. L.: An apparent relationship between locoism and lathyrism. Can. J. Comp. Med. Vet. Sci., 31:334, 1967.

22. Keeler, R. F., Van Kampen, K. R., and James L. F.: Effects of Poisonous Plants on Livestock. New York, Academic Press, 1978.
23. Kelleway, R. A., and Geovjian, L.: Acute bracken fern poisoning in a 14-month-old horse. VM SAC, 73:295, 1978.
24. Kingsbury, J. M.: Poisonous Plants of the United States and Canada. Englewood Cliffs, NJ, Prentice-Hall, 1964.
25. Krook, L., Wasserman, R. H., Shively, J. N., Tashjian, A. H., Brokken, T. D., and Morton, J. F.: Hypercalcemia and calcinosis in Florida horses: Implication of the shrub *"Cestrum diurnum"* as the causative agent. Cornell Vet., 65:26, 1975.
26. Larson, K. A., and Young, S.: Nigropallidal encephalomalacia in horses in Colorado. J. Am. Vet. Med. Assoc., 156:626, 1970.
27. MacDonald, H.: Hemlock poisoning in horses. J. Am. Vet. Med. Assoc., 49:1211, 1937.
28. McCunn, J.: Castor bean poisoning in horses. Vet. J., 101:136, 1945.
29. McLintock, J., and Fell, B. F.: Clinical communication: a case of acute ragwort poisoning in the horse. Vet. Rec., 65:319, 1953.
30. Mettler, F. A., and Stern, G. M.: Observations on the toxic effects of yellow star thistle. J. Neuropathol., 22:164, 1963.
31. Morris, M. D.: Nuttall death camus poisoning in horses. Vet. Med., 39:462, 1949.
32. O'Sullivan, B. M.: Crofton weed (*Eupatorium adenophorum*) toxicity in horses. Aust. Vet. J., 55:19, 1979.
33. Pierce, K. R., Joyce, J. R., England, R. B., and Jones, L.
P.: Acute hemolytic anemia caused by wild onion poisoning in horses. J. Am. Vet. Med. Assoc., 160:323, 1972.
34. Pritchard, J. T., and Voss, J. L.: Fetal ankylosis in horses associated with hybrid Sudan pastures. J. Am. Vet. Med. Assoc., 150:871, 1967.
35. Radeleff, R. D.: Veterinary Toxicology, 2nd ed. Philadelphia, Lea and Febiger, 1970.
36. Retief, G. P.: The use of crystalline methionine as a treatment for liver damage in racehorses. J. S. Afr. Vet. Med. Assoc., 33:405, 1962.
37. Sharrock, A. G.: Pyrrolizidine alkaloid poisoning in a horse in New South Wales. Aust. Vet. J., 45:388, 1969.
38. Staley, E. E.: An approach to treatment of locoism in horses. VM SAC, 73:1205, 1978.
39. Tennant, B., Dill, S. G., Glickman, L. T., Murro, E. T., King, J. M., Polak, D. M., Smith, M. C., and Kradel, D. C.: Red maple poisoning in horses associated with acute hemolytic anemia and methemoglobinemia. Proc. 26th Annu. Conv. Am. Assoc. Eq. Pract., 1980, p. 243.
40. Tucker, J. M., et al.: Poisonous hemlocks: Their identification and control. California Agricultural Experiment Station Bulletin (Circular 530), Berkeley, CA, University of California, 1965.
41. Wasserman, R. H.: Active vitamin D–like substances in *Solanum malacoxylon* and other calcinigenic plants. Nut. Rev., 33:1, 1975.
42. Wharmby, M. J.: Acorn poisoning. Vet. Rec., 99:343, 1976.
43. Young, S., Brown, W. W., and Klinger, B.: Nigropallidal encephalomalacia in horses caused by the ingestion of weeds of the genus Centaurea. J. Am. Vet. Med. Assoc., 157:1602, 1970.

WATER QUALITY

Frederick W. Oehme, MANHATTAN, KANSAS

Good-quality water is an essential part of horse management, but because of the variable conditions under which horses are kept and the variety of sources from which horses receive their water, there are possibilities for deterioration in water quality and potential harm to the horses consuming it.

Water sources for horses may come from public water supplies originating from reservoirs or community or public deep wells, from open ponds, springs, or streams, from dug or drilled wells on the farm or premises where the horses are kept, or from local collections of rain or spring water in ponds, dirt-lined pools, or metal containers. In some cases, the water being collected and offered to horses is from heated springs originating deep in various layers of mineral-rich rocks or from water that has percolated through disrupted soils and mine tailings rich in minerals and metals. Superheated water from springs (geothermal water) is usually contaminated with underground elements in concentrations from a few hundred mg per l to many thousands of mg per l. The most common chemicals are

sodium, potassium, lithium, calcium, magnesium, ammonium, silica, chloride, fluoride, borate, sulfate, carbonate, bicarbonate, hydrogen sulfide, carbon dioxide, and some particularly toxic elements, such as arsenic, molybdenum, selenium, and a variety of other heavy metals. These substances may occur as suspended solids, in solution, or as combinations of the two forms.

In certain areas of the Rocky Mountain plateau and the Mississippi Valley, mining and ore recovery operations are common. Disrupted soils and processed rock are readily available to be leeched by rains, carrying dissolved chemicals to water collection basins or streams that might be used to water horses. Tailings are finely ground rock and minerals that have been processed to remove the commercially desirable ores. Excessive concentrations of soluble salts are present in many tailings and may also be leeched out of piles of tailings into horses' drinking water supplies. Most mine tailing materials contain various sulfides, which may oxidize to form acid and thus lower the water pH and increase solubility of heavy metals. The hazard of pollution of water supplies with heavy metals, therefore, increases as tailing waters age and oxidize.

The numerous sources of water for use by horses and the variable conditions under which it may be collected and stored result in numerous physical, chemical, and microbiologic contaminants potentially present in the final product offered to horses. Agricultural practices, particularly those used in intensive land use, increase the frequency with which agricultural chemicals appear in such waters. The most potentially hazardous contaminants in horses' water supplies are microorganisms, dissolved solids and salts, nitrates and nitrites, fluoride, heavy metals (such as arsenic, cadmium, copper, iron, lead, mercury, selenium, and zinc), and the variety of pesticides used in daily farming operations.

BACTERIAL MICROORGANISMS

The presence of potentially pathogenic microorganisms is usually tested by evaluating the degree of bacterial contamination from animal or human wastes. Laboratory tests examine for indicator organisms rather than for actual pathogens; the coliforms are the principal indicators of the suitability of a particular water supply. However, specific bacterial examinations for other disease-producing organisms may also be performed by appropriately equipped laboratories. The usual limitations placed on animal waters are that the coliform count should not exceed 5000 per 100 ml of water. Contamination of horses' water supplies is more likely to occur if fecal wastes are draining into the water supply or if wells receive water from nearby feedlots or animal holding areas. Surface waters open to sunlight and oxygen may present less of a hazard owing to the sterilizing effects of ultraviolet light.

DISSOLVED SOLIDS AND SALTS

Salinity is the concentration of solids in water and is an expression of the amount of dissolved salts in a particular water supply. The ions most commonly involved in high saline waters are calcium, magnesium, sodium, bicarbonate, chloride, and sulfate. Water hardness is the tendency of water to precipitate soap or form scale on heated surfaces. It is generally expressed as the sum of calcium and magnesium, but other cations, such as iron, strontium, aluminum, zinc, and manganese, also contribute to hardness. Although water with cation concentrations above 120 mg per l is classified as hard, the hardness of water in itself is not a problem in horses' drinking water. Rather, the concentration of dissolved salts (sodium, magnesium, calcium, bicar-

bonate, sulfate, and chloride) is of much greater concern. Soluble salt concentrations of less than 7000 mg per l in horses' drinking water are considered safe. Between 7000 and 10,000 mg soluble salts per l in drinking water present mild risks for pregnant or lactating horses and thus should be avoided if possible in those stress situations. Waters with soluble salt concentrations greater than 10,000 mg per l present greater risks and are not recommended for consumption by horses, although field experience suggests that in most cases the major effect is transient diarrhea. Soluble salt concentrations considerably greater than 10,000 mg per l (for example, greater than 12,000 mg per l) present considerably greater risks and should not be made available for consumption by horses.

NITRATES AND NITRITES

Nitrates and nitrites are extremely water-soluble and move easily with ground water. The most common source of contamination for horses' water supplies is surface water runoff from high organic matter–containing soils or grounds heavily fertilized with nitrogen. Nitrates are not significantly toxic to horses, since horses lack the ability to rapidly reduce nitrates to the more toxic nitrite. However, if water supplies have high levels of nitrite, this ion oxidizes the iron in hemoglobin to the trivalent state, forming methemoglobin. The result is acute methemoglobinemia and potentially rapid death. Levels of nitrite in water for horses should not exceed 10 mg per l. Some evidence suggests that low levels of nitrate in waters may produce chronic effects on mares stressed with late pregnancy or on foals beginning to supplement nursing with available water supplies. Among the suggested effects from low-level nitrate are infertility and late-term abortions, poor growth rate in young animals, vitamin A deficiency, interference with iodine metabolism, and increased susceptibility to infections. Although good experimental evidence substantiating these field observations is lacking, clinicians may wish to consider recommending alternate water sources in instances in which patients have one or more of these observed effects and nitrate levels in available waters exceed 90 mg per l. If other obvious etiologic factors have been ruled out, instances of rapid improvement have occurred in such circumstances two to three weeks after implementing a water change.

FLUORIDE

Fluoride in water at concentrations of 3 mg per l or more will cause mild fluorosis and mottling of developing teeth. In some areas of the country, horses' water supplies may considerably exceed this level, resulting in badly worn and discolored teeth and skeletal bone changes. Soreness of the teeth and sensitivity to heat and cold, quidding of feed, and intermittent lameness are effects of chronic exposure to fluoride. There is little fluoride accumulation in soft tissues. Following removal of the fluoride-containing water, the lameness problems will improve, but the bone and teeth changes are permanent.

HEAVY METALS

Heavy metals in water seldom present problems to horses because they usually do not occur at high levels. However, under unusual instances of chemical spills, drainage through dump sites, or leeching from mining operations, hazardous levels of certain heavy metals may appear in water offered to horses. Aluminum, beryllium, boron, chromium, cobalt, copper, iodide, iron, manganese, molybdenum, and zinc are examples of such potential metal contaminants. Suggested acceptable limits for these metals and other potential contaminants in livestock waters are listed in Table 1.

Some heavy metal elements may be of special hazard to horses because of their inherent toxicity or tissue accumulation. Arsenic may induce digestive tract irritation. Cadmium is potentially a nephrotoxic compound if high concentrations are consumed. Copper may induce liver damage owing to its biologic accumulation in that organ, with red blood cell destruction occurring during a "hemolytic crisis." Lead accumulates in all tissues, particularly the liver and kidneys, and the peripheral nervous system of horses is particularly sensitive to this metal. Respiratory distress on moderate exercise is an early indication of lead toxicity in horses. Mercury is more readily absorbed in the organic form than in the metallic state. Digestive tract irritation and later kidney and central nervous system effects may be seen, depending upon its form and concentration in consumed water supplies. Selenium is an essential element, but in some areas of the United States, it is present in water at concentrations sufficient to produce chronic selenium toxicity. Levels in excess of 0.5 parts per million (ppm) may induce weight loss, loss of long hair of the mane and tail, and changes in the hoof wall. Zinc is also an essential element but may induce digestive tract disturbances or arthritic problems in horses consuming abnormal amounts in water.

TABLE 1. RECOMMENDED LIMITS OF CONCENTRATION OF SOME POTENTIALLY TOXIC SUBSTANCES IN DRINKING WATER FOR LIVESTOCK*

| Substance | Safe Upper Limit of Concentration (mg/L) | | |
	(For Humans) U.S. EPA	(For Animals) U.S. EPA	NAS
Aluminum	—	5.0	—
Arsenic	0.05	0.2	0.2
Barium	1.0	—	NE
Beryllium	—	No Limit†	—
Boron	—	5.0	—
Cadmium	0.01	0.05	0.05
Chromium	0.05	1.0	1.0
Cobalt	—	1.0	1.0
Copper	—	0.5	0.5
Fluoride	—	2.0	2.0
Iron	—	No Limit	NE
Lead	0.05	0.1	0.1
Manganese	—	No Limit	NE
Mercury	0.002	0.001	0.01
Molybdenum	—	No Limit	NE
Nickel	—	—	1.0
Nitrate	45	100	440
Nitrite	—	33	33
Selenium	0.01	0.05	—
Vanadium	—	0.1	0.1
Zinc	—	25.0	25.0

*Modified from Carson, TL: Water quality for livestock. *In* Howard, J. L. (ed.): Current Veterinary Therapy, Food Animal Practice. Philadelphia, W. B. Saunders Co., 1981, pp. 420–424.

†No limit/not established (NE). Experimental data available are not sufficient to establish definite limits or recommendations.

EPA = Environmental Protection Agency

NAS = National Academy of Sciences

PESTICIDES

Agricultural chemicals, such as pesticides, enter water from soil runoff, spray drift, rainfall, direct application to ponds or lakes, accidental spills, or faulty waste disposal techniques. High levels present in water owing to accidental spills may produce acute toxicity, either nervous signs from the chlorinated hydrocarbon insecticides or excessive salivation and digestive tract activity with moderate peripheral nervous signs from organophosphate or carbamate insecticides. Levels in waters sufficient to produce intoxication in consuming horses will always produce fish kills, since fish are considerably more sensitive to insecticide concentrations than are horses. Chronic toxicity is infrequent, except in the instance of chlorinated hydrocarbon exposures, when persistent residues may accumulate in equine tissues. Biodegradation of the organophosphate and carbamate insecticide is rapid, and chronic exposures are unlikely. In general, water concentrations of pesticides less than 0.1 mg per l are acceptable for equine use.

CLINICAL SIGNS

The clinical effects likely to be seen in horses consuming poor-quality water vary considerably with the type and concentration of the contaminant. In some instances, one chemical entity may be responsible for a clinical syndrome. Acute toxicities may result from the release of large amounts of soluble pollutants as a result of pond failure or the washing of chemicals through rainfall from highly contaminated soils. In other instances, chemical spills will produce massive contamination and effects similar to those observed with direct application or consumption of specific compounds. Chronic intoxication may occur by small amounts of drainage from contaminated soils or through constant environmental pollution. The equine clinician must evaluate each situation critically and must relate the disease syndrome to water exposure and concentrations of hazardous materials in the equine water source.

TREATMENT AND PREVENTION

Until a definitive diagnosis is available, treatment of affected horses can only be symptomatic and supportive. Once an accurate diagnosis has been made, the most appropriate therapy and management should be employed. Such management should always include removal of horses from the contaminated water supply and determination that the replacement water supply does not present other hazards. Balanced and adequate mineral supplementation is imperative, since the intake of chemical elements via water often results in mineral imbalances. Salt hunger or depraved appetite due to mineral inadequacies may induce horses to seek out hazardous water supplies to satisfy cravings. In most instances, water quality hazards are a chronic management problem that develops over a period of many months. Their resolution may also require considerable effort and adequate time for patient recovery.

Preventing horses from having to utilize poor-quality water is important. In quality equine practices, the periodic chemical analysis of water supplies may be a useful safeguard against future health difficulties.

Supplemental Readings

1. Carson, T. L.: Water quality for livestock. *In* Howard, J. L. (ed.): Current Veterinary Therapy, Food Animal Practice. Philadelphia, W. B. Saunders Co., 1981, pp. 420–424.
2. Oehme, F. W.: Water quality as related to animal health. Quality Water for Home and Farm. St. Joseph, MO, American Society of Agricultural Engineers, Pub. 1-79, 1979, pp. 21–29.
3. Shupe, J. L., Peterson, H. B., and Olson, A. E.: Toxicants in geothermal waters and in mine tailings. *In* Howard, J. L. (ed.): Current Veterinary Therapy, Food Animal Practice. Philadelphia, W. B. Saunders Co., 1981, pp. 424–428.

THE ETIOLOGIC DIAGNOSIS OF SUDDEN DEATH

Frederick W. Oehme, MANHATTAN, KANSAS

The horse that dies quickly or is found dead with no premonitory signs is both an emotional and diagnostic problem. Reactions of disbelief, shock, or amazement may turn to guilt, defensiveness, anger, or an emotional demand for action and answers. The equine clinician may be confronted by an excited and anxious client.

A human tendency is for the clinician to grasp at the first opportunity to pacify the client. The "catch-all" diagnosis of "poisoning" may provide an easy way out until the client asks, "Poisoned how?" Since there are many possible reasons for horses dying suddenly, it is the ethical responsibility of every veterinarian to conscientiously inform clients of the potential causes of the situation. If the client is willing to stand the expense and effort, a thorough diagnostic program should be initiated to resolve the many questions raised by the sudden death. Much harm, both morally and professionally, has been done by hasty diagnoses being suggested and accepted by emotionally distraught clients.

The causes of sudden death must be explored in the same way that any other equine disease is investigated. Not only toxic but also nutritional, metabolic, infectious, and even accidental causes of death should be considered in a differential diagnosis. Circulatory collapse due to cardiovascular failure, lightning stroke or electrocution, anaphylaxis, trauma producing brain and spinal cord damage, acute digestive tract torsion or displacement, and even fatal gunshot wounds are just as viable initial possibilities for producing acute death as are infectious or chemical etiologies. The history surrounding the circumstance and the events leading up to the finding of the dead horse are critical. Because the owner is often upset, a history obtained by the owner's observations should be carefully reviewed. The "facts" may be inaccurate and should be considered suspect if the physical findings and observations of the clinician do not support the history provided by the client.

Following a detailed history and examination of the environment and circumstances of the incident, a thorough postmortem examination should be performed. Despite the awkwardness and frequent inconvenience of such examinations, all body systems and organs should be observed. Minor lesions in the digestive tract, central nervous system, or circulatory system may suggest conditions that further scrutiny will prove contributory to death. All abnormalities should be carefully recorded, and specimens of selected body tissues should be collected and preserved for microbiologic, histopathologic or chemical examination. Environmental samples of water, feed, pasture content, or other suspected etiologic sources should be collected for possible later laboratory study.

At the conclusion of the clinical investigation, the veterinarian should present his or her initial impressions to the client. If evidence is strong supporting one cause, the client may be satisfied and the issue may be resolved. In many instances, more than one potential cause of death is apparent, and the clinician should then provide the client with options for additional action. Costs involved (for toxicology examinations, these are significant) and the time interval before reasonable responses may be expected should be realistically presented and discussed. The client should also recognize that despite the expenditure of considerable time, money, and effort, the results of the laboratory examinations may not be conclusive and that an absolute final diagnosis may not be possible despite the best of intentions. At whatever point the client and veterinarian decide to cease further evaluations, all parties should feel confident that all practical options and alternatives have been considered. The veterinarian should also make sure that the client has had the best available opinion as to what caused the sudden death of the horse and that the client has also been offered recommendations to prevent this disaster in the future.

CHEMICAL CAUSES OF SUDDEN DEATH

Chemically caused sudden death in previously apparently healthy horses may be due to exposure to lethal amounts of highly toxic chemicals, exposure to single large doses of poisons, the misapplication of drugs and chemicals producing unusual exposure situations, or individual animal hypersensitivity or idiosyncrasies resulting in unique toxic reactions. The latter circumstances are especially popular diagnoses when routine examinations of individual sudden deaths produce negative results. In some cases, there is indeed foundation for suggesting such a cause-and-effect relationship, but an absolute diagnosis of such may be very difficult to confirm.

FAILURE OF OXYGEN TRANSPORT IN BLOOD

Toxins that produce an inability of the blood to properly oxygenate vital tissues produce dramatic and sudden death. Cyanide toxicity, produced by ingestion of plants such as sorghum (p. 598), wild cherry (p. 597), and arrowgrass, and nitrite and chlorate ingestion may cause death within 5 to 10 minutes. Cyanide poisoning produces bright cherry-red blood and tissues, while nitrite and chlorate poisoning produces chocolate-brown methemoglobinemia.

TOXIC GASES

Environments that favor the presence of toxic gases can induce fatalities within minutes after exposure. Some housing environments may result in fatalities overnight from faulty air circulation or the accumulation of waste gases. Carbon monoxide induces pink-red blood and results from exposure to heater or automobile exhaust fumes. Chloroform and hydrogen sulfide are central nervous system and cardiovascular depressants, producing sudden death by respiratory failure.

INSECTICIDES

The insecticides are all toxic in small quantities and are capable of inducing fatalities within minutes to hours after exposure. The organophosphate and carbamate insecticides are the most lethal (p. 582). Chlorinated hydrocarbon insecticides produce convulsions and violent death, which may not be observed (p. 581). Nicotine, applied as nicotine sulfate for insects in housing structures, is rapidly absorbed with fatality due to peripheral and central nervous system dysfunction (p. 580).

PLANT TOXINS

Of the numerous plant toxins, several are extremely lethal and are capable of producing almost immediate fatalities. Blue-green algae may induce sudden death in horses consuming water with algae in it. Japanese yew induces muscle weakness, tremors, and death minutes after consumption (p. 604). Cicuta (water hemlock) induces violent seizures and almost immediate fatality (p. 601). Oleander (Nerium) is a rapid cardiovascular toxin (p. 602). Castor bean (Ricinus) contains a plant protein that induces a shock reaction in horses that consume it (p. 604). The plants containing high levels of oxalates (Halogeton, Sarcobatus) dramatically lower circulating calcium levels, with sudden death due to hypocalcemia.

BACTERIAL TOXINS

Bacterial toxins, such as those formed by *E. coli*, may induce autointoxication and sudden death due to digestive tract absorption of ingested or digestive tract–formed bacterial poisons (p. 57). Dietary changes or excesses are important circumstances leading to such fatalities.

VENOMS

The venom of insects contains complex neurotoxins, and some contain irritating substances such as formic acid. Stings from bees, wasps, and ants induce not only local reactions but also a rapid and generalized effect producing collapse. Death may occur if repeated stings are received. Blister beetles (p. 588) may induce sufficient digestive tract irritation to cause shock and early death. Bites from snakes, such as the rattlesnake, produce massive tissue reaction. If this reaction interferes with respiration, death due to suffocation is possible (p. 587).

DRUGS

A variety of drugs are potentially fatal. Curare may induce immediate respiratory failure. Overdosage of intravenous antimicrobial agents can produce shock and death. Improper administration of parenteral medication (with drugs intended for intramuscular injection being given intravenously) is an unfortunate cause of prompt fatality. Individual horse hypersensitivity or allergy to therapeutic agents can produce sudden death. Fortunately, immediate administration of epinephrine is an effective emergency treatment for these situations.

FEED CONTAMINATION

Accidental or intentional contamination of feed with acutely toxic chemicals is a human factor that is occasionally responsible for sudden horse deaths. Arsenic and strychnine may be accidentally included in horse feeds or may be added maliciously. Rumensin is acutely toxic in small doses to horses and may be in cattle feeds that are later offered to horses.

SAMPLE COLLECTION AND SUBMISSION

Tissue selection and collection for chemical analysis and its proper submission to testing laboratories are important scientific and legal procedures to secure meaningful analytical results. Samples collected from horses dying suddenly from suspected poisoning should include liver, kidney, stomach or intestinal contents, urine, and whole blood. At least 10 ml of whole blood should be submitted together

TABLE 1. SPECIMENS REQUIRED FOR SELECTED TOXICOLOGIC TESTS

Analysis Requested	Specimen Required	Amount of Specimen Desired	Special Precautions
Aflatoxin	Food	200 gm	Keep dry and cool
Ammonia	Whole blood, urine	5 ml	Maintain air-tight
	Stomach contents	100 gm	Freeze until tested
ANTU	Stomach and intestinal contents, liver	200 gm	Must be tested 12–24 hours after ingestion
Arsenic	Liver, kidney	50 gm	
	Food, stomach contents	100 gm	
	Urine	50 ml	
Carbon monoxide	Whole blood	15 ml	
Chlorinated hydrocarbon insecticide	Whole blood	10 ml	Keep tissues separate and free of contamination; use only chemically clean glass jars to package
	Body fat, stomach contents	100 gm	
	Liver, kidney	50 gm	
Cholinesterase	Whole blood	10 ml	Keep refrigerated
Copper	Whole blood	10 ml	
	Liver, kidney	50 gm	
	Feces	100 gm	
Ethylene glycol	Serum, urine	10 ml	Fix in formalin for histopathologic examination
	Kidney	Both kidneys	
Fluoroacetate (1080)	Stomach contents	All available	Freeze until tested
	Kidney	One whole	
	Urine	50 ml	
	Liver	50 gm	
	Bait, source	100 gm	
Lead	Whole blood	10 ml	Use only heparin or citrate as anticoagulant
	Liver, kidney	50 gm	
Methemoglobin	Whole blood	10 ml	
Nitrate, nitrite	Water	50 ml	
	Source	100 gm	
Organophosphorus insecticide, carbamate insecticide	Body fat, stomach contents	50 gm	
	Whole blood	10 ml	Use only heparin as anticoagulant
	Urine	50 ml	
	Food	100 gm	
Oxalate	Kidney	Both kidneys	Fix in formalin for histopathologic examination
Phenothiazine or derivative	Food or other source	50 gm	
Strychnine	Stomach contents, urine	All available	
	Liver	50 gm	
Thallium	Urine	10 ml	
	Liver, kidney	50 gm	
Warfarin	Liver, food, source	100 gm	
Zinc	Liver, kidney	50 gm	
	Source	100 gm	

(Modified from Oehme, F. W.: Laboratory diagnosis of chemical intoxications. Vet. Clin. North Am., 6:723, 1976.)

with 50 ml or more of urine and at least 100 gm each of liver and kidney. At least 200 gm of digestive tract contents should be collected if available. In specific suspected intoxications, the collection of other selected organs may also be indicated. The entire brain, 100 gm or more of body fat and spleen, and generous samples of hair or hoof and bone may be of special value in certain circumstances.

Often overlooked is the submission of samples from suspected sources of the poison. Feed, water, weeds in the area, and suspected sources or baits are excellent samples for determining the possible origin of a toxicity. Generous portions (in excess of 200 gm and preferably 1 lb) of each sample should be provided. Table 1 lists the suggested specimens and amounts desired for the toxicologic tests likely to be considered in evaluating causes of sudden death in horses.

Specimens should be taken free of chemical contamination and debris and should not be washed because of the possibility of contaminating the specimen or removing residues of the toxic material. Clean glass or plastic containers that can be tightly sealed are excellent for collecting specimens. Each sample should be preserved separately in an individual container labeled with the owner's and animal's identification and the type of tissue or specimen in the container. Preservatives, such as formalin, should never be added unless there is a specific reason for doing so. In those cases, such information should be included on the specimen label. Samples of the preservative, if used, should also be submitted separately for possible analytical reference. Serum or blood samples should be kept refrigerated, while tissue specimens are best frozen. They should be packaged so that they arrive at the laboratory while still frozen.

The importance of supplying a complete account of history, signs, and lesions observed cannot be overemphasized. This should all be a part of the fundamental information supplied to the laboratory with the samples. The clinician's name and address, the owner's name and address, and the horse's breed, sex, age, and weight should be basic information. Additional facts should include the number of other horses in the field or on the farm, whether other animals were affected or died, the type of management, feeding program, history of past illness or problems, and immunization records. Other facts that would be helpful to the laboratory include the period of time that the horse had been eating the last batch of prepared feed, the type of pasture, the presence of trash, dumps, old motors, or farm machinery and their access to the animal, descriptions of the clinical signs and postmortem findings, including negative observations, length of time since the horse was last observed, its condition at the last observation, medications that were given before death, and any treatments for parasites. All such information is equally important when analyses originally requested are negative and the need for intelligently suggesting and selecting other analytical procedures becomes obvious. If adequate specimen material and a detailed history of circumstances, signs, necropsy lesions, and other appropriate history are available, the laboratory toxicologist is in an excellent position to provide alternatives for assay and to offer optimal assistance and service. The recording of this information also documents specific facts and responsibilities in the event that legal action is later taken.

If a concurrent histopathologic examination is requested, samples for histopathology should be preserved in 10 per cent buffered formalin and shipped in containers separate from those being used for the chemical analysis. Since the tissues for chemical assay are usually frozen, separate specimens and separate packages for the histopathologic studies should be provided so that the formalinized tissues do not also undergo freezing.

Plastic bags, cardboard, newspaper, and various forms of ice are good for packing specimens. Liquids should be shipped in leakproof containers and individually wrapped in packing material to prevent leakage and contamination of other specimens or accompanying mail. Ideally, the best method for submitting samples to a laboratory is by personal messenger. Often the owner of the deceased animal is sufficiently concerned to make the delivery. Bus and truck services may also be used, as well as the postal service. In all instances, delivery time should be anticipated so that holidays and weekends are avoided.

Proper interpretation of the laboratory test results is important for accurate assessment of the etiologic cause of sudden death. Frequently too much emphasis is placed on individual laboratory values when many factors in the patient's biology and the exposure circumstances are capable of producing variations. In addition, laboratory variations inherent in any procedure add to the variability of results. A competent laboratory should provide a normal range of values and comments indicating those results considered abnormal.

THE FINAL EVALUATION . . . POISONING?

All the available data and information must now be taken into consideration to evaluate whether a poisoning was the cause of the horse's sudden death. The mere presence of a suspected toxicant is not always sufficient to confirm poisoning, nor is a negative finding conclusive evidence that a toxicosis did not occur. The persistence of certain compounds, such as heavy metals and chlorinated hydrocarbon insecticides, and their common environmental occurrence ensure that these chemicals are usually detected in most horse tissues regardless of the cause of death. Other rapidly metabolized toxins, such as the organophosphate and carbamate insecticides, may not be detected on postmortem chemical analysis owing to postmortem decomposition or rapid biodegradation to metabolites. The clinician's previous experience with poisoning should help in evaluating the analytical results, but tissue levels of poisons must be related to concentrations normally found in healthy animals. Thus, it is important to establish that the chemical concentrations detected are meaningful and indeed dose-related to the specific sudden death. An experienced toxicologist is of potential value in helping to relate the field and laboratory data to the clinical circumstances. The clinician should not hesitate to contact such individuals for assistance at this crucial time.

Given a complete clinical and environmental history, the physical and pathologic observations from the horse, the results of clinical chemistry, histopathology, and chemical analysis, and perhaps the benefit of consultation, the clinician should be able not only to properly interpret the results of chemical analysis but also to put into focus the history, clinical signs, and other examination results. The responsibility for the definitive or most likely diagnosis (or alternative diagnoses) should be assumed by the equine clinician after all the circumstantial, clinical, postmortem, pathologic, and laboratory findings have been carefully and competently evaluated.

References

1. Barkan, B. A., and Oehme, F. W.: A classification of common Midwestern animal toxicoses. Vet. Toxicol., *17*:34, 1975.
2. Buck, W. B.: Use of diagnostic laboratories. *In* Howard, J. L. (ed.): Current Veterinary Therapy, Food Animal Practice. Philadelphia, W. B. Saunders Co., 1981, pp. 369–376.
3. Fowler, M. E.: Poisoning syndromes associated with sudden collapse and death. *In* Catcott, E. J., and Smithcors, J. F. (eds.): Equine Medicine and Surgery, 2nd ed. American Veterinary Pub., Wheaton, IL, 1972, p. 197.
4. Harvey, D. G.: Has it been poisoned? Br. Vet. J., *137*:317, 1981.
5. Oehme, F. W.: Laboratory diagnosis of chemical intoxication. Vet. Clin. North Am., 6:723, 1976.

Section 14
APPENDICES

Normal Clinical Pathology Data 619

Table of Common Drugs: Approximate Doses 621

Aging the Horse 625

NORMAL CLINICAL PATHOLOGY DATA

J. D. Krehbiel, EAST LANSING, MICHIGAN

The values presented here are primarily derived from our own laboratory. Variations will occur depending upon the methods used and the breed, age, sex, training, and emotional status of the horse.

More complete listings of normal data from horses of a variety of breeds and ages are available in the references listed at the end of this section.

TABLE 1. SERUM CHEMISTRY VALUES

Test	Units	Mean Value	Range
Blood urea nitrogen	mg/dl	16	10–25
Creatinine	mg/dl	1.7	1.0–2.4
Total protein	gm/dl	6.5	5.6–7.5
Albumin	gm/dl	3.4	2.7–3.7
Fibrinogen	mg/dl	—	94–294
Glucose	mg/dl	90	70–130
Total bilirubin	mg/dl	2.2	1.0–5.0
Cholesterol	mg/dl	135	100–189
Alkaline phosphatase	IU/l 30°	111	84–128
Serum glutamic oxaloacetic transaminase	IU/l 30°	198	157–253
Lactic dehydrogenase	IU/l 30°	140	100–191
Creatine phosphokinase	IU/l 30°	142	97–188
Hydroxybutyric dehydrogenase	IU/l 30°	409	257–544
Sorbitol dehydrogenase	IU/l 30°	3	1–6
Calcium	mg/dl	11.6	10.3–13.3
Chloride	mEq/l	102.5	98–109
Magnesium	mg/dl	2.5	2.2–2.8
Potassium	mEq/l	3.2	2.2–4.1
Phosphorus	mg/dl	3.4	1.8–5.2
Sodium	mEq/l	137	130–143
Osmolality	mOsm	278	276–282

TABLE 2. NORMAL BLOOD CELL VALUES

	Hot-Blooded Horses		Cold-Blooded Horses	
	Mean	*Range*	*Mean*	*Range*
Total erythrocytes ($\times 10^6$ per µl)	9.5	6–12	7.5	5.5–9.5
Packed cell volume (%)	41	32–52	35	24–44
Hemoglobin (gm/dl)	14.5	11–19	11.5	8–14
Mean corpuscular volume (fl)	45	34–58	44	40–48
Mean corpuscular hemoglobin concentration (%)	35	32–38	35	32–38
Total leukocytes ($\times 10^3$ per µl)	9.0	5.5–12.5	8.5	6–12
Segmented neutrophils (%)	52	30–65	54	30–75
Segmented neutrophils ($\times 10^3$ per µl)	—	2.7–5.8	—	2.5–6.2
Nonsegmented neutrophils (%)	0.5	0–1.0	1.0	0–2.0
Nonsegmented neutrophils ($\times 10^3$ per µl)	—	0–0.1	—	0–0.1
Lymphocytes (%)	39	17–68	35	15–50
Lymphocytes ($\times 10^3$ per µl)	—	1.5–6.0	—	1.2–5.0
Monocytes (%)	4	0.5–7.0	5	2–10
Monocytes ($\times 10^3$ per µl)	—	0–0.6	—	0.1–0.8
Eosinophils (%)	4	0–11	5	2–12
Eosinophils ($\times 10^3$ per µl)	—	0–0.9	—	0.1–1.0
Basophils (%)	0.5	0–3.0	0.5	0–3.0
Basophils ($\times 10^3$ per µl)	—	0–0.17	—	0–0.17
Platelets ($\times 10^5$ per µl)	—	1–3.5	—	1–3.5

TABLE 3. ACID-BASE AND BLOOD GAS VALUES

	Arterial (carotid)		Venous (jugular)	
	Mean	*SD*	*Mean*	*SD*
Blood pH	7.411	0.032	7.389	0.022
P_{O_2} torr	96	8.0	46	3.0
P_{CO_2} torr	41	3.0	43	3.0
HCO_3^- mEq/l	25.3	1.06	25.4	1.7
Base excess mEq/l	1.1	1.4	0.7	1.7

(From Blackmore, D. J., and Brobst, D.: Biochemical Values in Equine Medicine. Newmarket, England, Animal Health Trust, 1981.)

TABLE 4. BLOOD SAMPLES REQUIRED FOR ASSAYS

Albumin	1 ml serum	Differential white blood cell count	3 unstained smears
Alkaline phosphatase	1 ml serum*	Electrophoresis, serum protein	1 ml serum
Bilirubin, total and direct	1 ml serum	Eosinophil count	1 tube EDTA blood
Blood chemistry profile	2–3 ml serum	Glucose	1 ml plasma, NaFl anticoagulant
Blood parasites	unstained blood smears		
Blood urea nitrogen	1 ml serum	Hematocrit	1 tube EDTA blood
Bone marrow cytology	3–5 unstained thin smears	Hemoglobin	1 tube EDTA blood
Calcium	1 ml serum	Hydroxybutyric dehydrogenase	1 ml serum*
Complete blood count	1 tube EDTA blood plus 3 unstained blood smears	Lactic dehydrogenase	1 ml serum*
		Lipids	1 ml serum
Chloride	1 ml serum	Magnesium	1 ml serum
Cholesterol	1 ml serum	Osmolality, serum	1 ml serum
Creatine phosphokinase	1 ml serum*	Osmolality, urine	2 ml urine
Creatinine	1 ml serum	Phosphorus	1 ml serum
Cytology		Potassium	1 ml serum
Routine	2–3 ml fluid in EDTA and/or 3 unstained smears	Red blood cell count	1 tube EDTA blood
		Serum glutamic oxaloacetic transaminase	1 ml serum*
Total count	2–3 ml fluid in EDTA	Sorbitol dehydrogenase	1 ml serum*
Specific gravity/total protein	2–3 ml fluid in EDTA	Sodium	1 ml serum
Differential count	3 unstained smears	Total protein, serum	1 ml serum
Special stains	same as routine	White blood cell count	1 tube EDTA blood plus 3 unstained smears

*Serum enzymes may be thermolabile; samples must be refrigerated.

References

1. Archer, R. K., and Jeffcott, L. B.: Comparative Clinical Hematology. London, Blackwell Scientific Pub., 1977.
2. Benjamin, M. M.: Outline of Veterinary Clinical Pathology, 3rd ed. Ames, IA, Iowa State University Press, 1979.
3. Blackmore, D. J., and Brobst, D.: Biochemical Values in Equine Medicine. Newmarket, England, Animal Health Trust, 1981.
4. Coles, E. H.: Veterinary Clinical Pathology, 3rd ed. Philadelphia, W. B. Saunders Co., 1980.
5. Duncan, J. R., and Prasse, K. W.: Veterinary Laboratory Medicine. Ames, IA, Iowa State University Press, 1977.
6. Kaneko, J. J.: Clinical Biochemistry of the Domestic Animals, 3rd ed. New York, Academic Press, 1980.
7. Schalm, O. W., Jain, M. D., and Carroll, E. J.: Veterinary Hematology, 3rd ed. Philadelphia, Lea and Febiger, 1975.

TABLE OF COMMON DRUGS: APPROXIMATE DOSES

N. Edward Robinson, EAST LANSING, MICHIGAN

Name of Drug	Dose	Route
Acepromazine	0.04–0.10 mg/kg	IV or IM
Acetylsalicylic acid	30–100 mg/kg	PO
Adrenocorticotropic hormone gel	1 unit/kg	IV
Amikacin	6.6 mg/kg t.i.d.	IM or IV
Aminophylline	4–7 mg/kg t.i.d.	PO
Aminopropazine fumarate	0.5 mg/kg b.i.d.	IM or IV
Aminopyrine	2.5–10 mg/450 kg	IV or IM
Amphotericin B	0.3 mg/kg in 5% dextrose	IV
Ampicillin sodium	10–100 mg/kg q.i.d.	IV or IM
Ampicillin trihydrate	10–20 mg/kg b.i.d,	IM
Atropine	0.02–0.1 mg/kg	IV or IM
Atropine	1–4% solution	Topical
Aurothioglucose	1 mg/kg at weekly intervals	IM
Benzathine penicillin G	4000 U/kg every 2 days	IM
Bismuth subsalicylate	2–4 qts/450 kg b.i.d.	PO
Boldenone undecylenate	1 mg/kg repeated at 3-week intervals	IM
Bromhexine	30 mg/kg	PO
Calcium disodium edetate	1 ml 6.6% solution/kg daily in 3 divided doses	IV
Calcium gluconate	To effect	IV
Cambendazole	20 mg/kg (not in first trimester of pregnancy)	PO
Captan	3% solution	Topical
Carbon disulfide	24 ml/450 kg	PO
Cascara sagrada	10–20 ml 20% solution/450 kg	SQ
	4–8 mg/kg	IM
Cephalexin	25 mg/kg q.i.d.	PO
Charcoal (activated)	2–8 oz/450 kg b.i.d.	PO
Chloral hydrate	7% solution to effect (usually 50–100 ml)	IV
	50–60 gm/450 kg	PO
Chloramphenicol	10–50 mg/kg q.i.d.	PO
Chloramphenicol palmitate	20–50 mg/kg q.i.d.	PO
Chloramphenicol sodium succinate	20–50 mg/kg q.i.d.	IM
Cimetidine HCl	1000 mg divided b.i.d. or t.i.d. in foals	PO
Clenbuterol	0.8 μg/kg b.i.d.	PO or IV
Corticotropin	1 unit/kg	IM
Coumaphos	0.06% wash, 0.1% dust	Topical
Danthron	15–30 ml/450 kg	PO
Dantrolene	1–2 mg/kg	PO
Dexamethasone	0.2–4 mg/kg	IV or IM
Dextran	8 gm/kg as 6% solution daily for up to 3 days	IV
Diazepam	0.05–0.4 mg/kg (repeat in 30 min if necessary)	IV
Dichlorvos	35 mg/kg	PO
Dichlorvos	0.93% solution	Topical
Diethylcarbamazine	6.5 mg/kg	PO
Digitalis or digitoxin	0.03–0.06 mg/kg for digitalization 0.01 mg/kg maintenance	PO
Digitalis tincture	0.3–0.6 ml/kg for digitalization 0.05–0.1 ml/kg maintenance	PO
Digoxin	0.06–0.08 mg/kg for digitalization 0.01–0.02 mg/kg maintenance	PO

Table continued on following page

Name of Drug	Dose	Route
Dihydrostreptomycin	5–15 mg/kg t.i.d.	IM
Dimethyl sulfoxide	90% solution	Topical
Dinaprost tromethamine	10 mg/450 kg	IM
Dioctyl sodium sulfosuccinate	20–240 gm/450 kg	PO
Dioxathion	0.15% wash	Topical
Diphenylhydantoin	1–10 mg/kg q 2–4 hrs	IV, IM, or PO
Dipyrone	22 mg/kg	IV or IM
Dolophine HCl	0.2–0.4 mg/kg	IM
Doxapram	0.5 mg/kg	IV
Ephedrine sulfate	0.7 mg/kg b.i.d.	PO
Epinephrine 1:1000	10 ml/450 kg	IM or SC
Erythromycin	10 mg/kg t.i.d.	IV or IM
Estradiol cypionate	5–10 mg/450 kg	IM
Estrone sulfate	0.05–0.1 mg/kg for epistaxis prevention	IV
Ethylene diamine dihydriodide	0.5–1.5 gm/450 kg s.i.d.	PO
Febantel	6 mg/kg	PO
Fenbendazole	5 mg/kg	PO
Flumethasone	1.0–2.5 mg/450 kg	IV or IM
Flunixin meglumine	1 mg/kg s.i.d.	IV, IM, or PO
9-Fluoroprednisolone acetate	5–20 mg/450 kg	IM
Fluprostenol	250 µg/450 kg	IM
Follicle stimulating hormone	10–50 mg	IV, IM, or SC
Furazolidone	4 mg/kg t.i.d.	PO
Furosemide	1 mg/kg	IV
	0.3–0.6 mg/kg 60–90 min prior to racing for epistaxis prevention	
Gentamicin	1–3 mg/kg q.i.d.	IM
Glyceryl guaiacolate	3.0 mg/kg for expectoration	PO
	100 mg/kg for anesthesia combined with barbiturate in 5% dextrose (5% solution)	IV
Griseofulvin	10 mg/kg s.i.d.	PO
Heparin	50 U/kg added to intraperitoneal lavage fluid.	
	80 IU/kg b.i.d. for anticoagulation	SQ
Human chorionic gonadotrophin	2500 USP units	IV
	10,000 USP units	IM or SC
Hydrocortisone sodium succinate	1.0–4.0 mg/kg	IV drip
Insulin	0.4 U/kg	IM or SC
Insulin-protamine zinc	0.15 IU/kg b.i.d.	IM or SC
Iodinated casein	1–5 gm/450 kg s.i.d.	PO
Iodochlorhydroxyquin	10 gm/450 kg (repeat for 3–4 days, then gradually reduce dose if response is obtained)	PO
Isoniazid	5–20 mg/kg s.i.d.	PO
Isoproterenol HCl	0.4 µg/kg by slow infusion (discontinue when heart rate doubles)	IV
Kanamycin sulfate	5 mg/kg t.i.d.	IM
Kaopectate	2–4 qts/450 kg b.i.d.	PO
Ketamine	2 mg/kg	IV
Levallorphan tartrate	0.02–0.04 mg/kg	IV
Levamisole	2–5 mg/kg	PO or IM
Lidocaine	1–1.5 mg/kg bolus or slow drip	IV
Lindane	3% spray	Topical
Magnesium sulfate	20–100 gm/450 kg	PO
Malathion	0.5% wash, 5% dust	Topical
Mannitol	0.25–2.0 gm/kg as 20% solution by slow infusion	IV

Name of Drug	Dose	Route
Mebendazole	8.8 mg/kg	PO
	15–20 mg/kg s.i.d. for 5 days for lungworms	
Meclofenamic acid	2.2 mg/kg	PO
Meperidine HCL	2.2–4.0 mg/kg	IM
	0.5–1.0 mg/kg (may cause excitement)	IV
Methionine	10 gm/450 kg s.i.d.	PO
Methocarbamol	15–25 mg/kg slow infusion	IV
Methoxychlor	0.5% wash	Topical
Methylcellulose flakes	0.25–0.5 kg in 8–10 l water/450 kg	PO
Methylprednisolone	0.5 mg/kg	PO
Methylprednisolone acetate	20–40 mg	Subconjunctival
Methylprednisolone sodium succinate	0.5 mg/kg	IV or IM
	10–20 mg/kg for shock	IV
Miconazole	1–2% solution	Topical
Mineral oil	3–4 l/450 kg	PO
Morphine sulfate	0.2–0.4 mg/kg	IM
Naloxone	0.01–0.02 mg/kg	IV
Naproxen	10 mg/kg	PO
Neomycin	5–15 mg/kg s.i.d.	PO
Neostigmine	0.4–2 mg/100 kg	SC
Niclosamide	100 mg/kg	PO
Nitrofurantoin	4.5 mg/kg t.i.d.	PO
Ouabain	2.5–3.0 mg/450 kg q 1½ to 2 hrs until heart rate slows or intoxication develops. Do not exceed 10 gm total.	IV
Oxacillin	25–50 mg/kg b.i.d.	IM or IV
Oxfendazole	10 mg/kg	PO
Oxibendazole	10 mg/kg	PO
Oxymorphone	0.02–0.03 mg/kg	IM
Oxytetracycline	5–10 mg/kg b.i.d.	IV
Oxytocin	5–40 U/450 kg as bolus	IV
	80–100 U in 500 ml saline by slow infusion	IV
	20–150 U/450 kg	IM
Penicillin G, procaine	5000–20,000 IU/kg b.i.d.	IM
Penicillin G, potassium	5000–50,000 IU/kg q.i.d.	IV
	200,000 IU/kg q.i.d.	PO
Penicillin G, sodium	5000–50,000 IU/kg q.i.d.	IV
Pentabarbital	3–15 mg/kg	IV
Pentazocine	0.3 mg/kg slow injection	IV
	0.3 mg/kg	IM
Phenobarbital	1–10 mg/kg	IV
Phenothiazine	55 mg/kg	PO
	27.5 mg/kg with piperazine	
Phenylbutazone	2–4 gm/450 kg s.i.d.	PO
	1–2 gm/450 kg s.i.d.	IV
Phenylephrine	10% solution	Topical
Phenytoin	1–10 mg/kg q 2–4 hrs	IV, IM, or PO
Piperazine salts	88 mg base/kg	PO
	44 mg base/kg with CS$_2$	
	55 mg base/kg with thiabendazole	
Potassium iodide	0.5–5.0 mg/kg s.i.d.	IV
Potassium permanganate	1% solution for mouthwash	
Povidone-iodine	10% volume/volume solution	
Prednisolone acetate	0.25–1.0 mg/kg	IM
Prednisolone sodium succinate	0.25–1.0 mg/kg	IV
Prednisolone tabs	0.25–1.0 mg/kg	PO
Prednisone	0.25–1.0 mg/kg	IM
Primidone	1 gm/foal b.i.d.	PO

Table continued on following page

Name of Drug	Dose	Route
Progesterone	100 mg/450 kg/day in oil for prevention of abortion (p. 405)	IM
Progesterone	150–200 mg/450 kg/day in oil to inhibit follicular development Can be combined with 10 mg/450 kg estradiol 17β	IM
Progesterone	100 mg/450 kg/day in oil with 1 mg/450 kg estradiol 17β for 5 days to cause uterine involution	IM
Progesterone (repositol)	1000 mg/450 kg once weekly for prevention of abortion (p. 405)	IM
Promazine HCl	0.4–1.0 mg/kg	IV or IM
Propantheline bromide	0.014 mg/kg	IV
Propranolol	150–350 mg/450 kg t.i.d.	PO
	25–75 mg/450 kg b.i.d.	IV
Prostalene	2 mg/450 kg	SC
Pyrantel pamoate	6.6 mg (base)/kg	PO
	13.2 mg (base)/kg for cestodes	PO
Pyrilamine maleate	1 mg/kg	IV, IM, or SC
Pyrimethamine	1 mg/kg loading dose followed by 0.5 mg/kg b.i.d.	PO
Quinidine sulfate	5 gm test dose, then 10 gm b.i.d., increasing to 15 gm q.i.d. on day 10	PO
Ronnel	2.5% spray	Topical
Selenium (sodium selenite)	5.5 mg/450 kg	IM
Stilbestrol	30 mg/450 kg	IM
Sodium iodide	20% solution, 10–40 ml/day	IV
Spectinomycin	20 mg/kg t.i.d.	IM
Stanozolol	0.5 mg/kg, up to 4 doses 1–2 weeks apart	IM
Stirofos	1% wash	Topical
Streptomycin	5–15 mg/kg t.i.d.	IM
Sulfonamides	100–200 mg/kg on day 1 50–100 mg/kg subsequently Check individual products for specific dosage.	IV, SC, or PO
Terbutaline sulfate	3.3 μg/kg	IV
Tetramethrin	0.4% solution, wipe on	Topical
Theophylline	1.0 mg/kg q.i.d.	PO
Thiabendazole	44 mg/kg 440 mg/kg larvicidal	PO
Thiamine	100–200 mg/450 kg	
Thiamylal sodium	2–4 mg/kg	IV
Thiopental	8–12 mg/kg	IV
Toxaphene	0.5% wash	Topical
Triamcinolone acetonide	0.1–0.2 mg/kg	IM or SC
Trichlormethiazide	200 mg/450 kg	PO
Trichlorfon	35 mg/kg	PO
Trichlorfon	90% powder	Topical
Tripelennamine hydrochloride	1 mg/kg	IM
Trimethoprim-sulfamethoxazole	2 mg/kg trimethoprim b.i.d. 10 mg/kg sulfa	PO
Tylosin	10 mg/kg b.i.d.	IM
Vitamin E	50 mg/450 kg	IM
Vitamin K₁	40–50 mg/450 kg	SC
Warfarin	30–75 mg/450 kg	PO
Xylazine	0.5–1.0 mg/kg	IV

This table was composed primarily from doses recommended by authors. It is recommended that the manufacturer's literature be checked before a drug is used. Not all drugs have been approved for use in horses.

AGING THE HORSE

N. Edward Robinson, EAST LANSING, MICHIGAN

DENTAL FORMULAS

Deciduous teeth:

$$2(DI\frac{3}{3} \, DC\frac{0}{0} \, DP\frac{3}{3}) = 24$$

Permanent teeth:

$$2(I\frac{3}{3} \, C\frac{1}{1} \, P\frac{3 \text{ or } 4}{3} \, M\frac{3}{3}) = 40 \text{ or } 42$$

ERUPTION DATES

Deciduous incisors:	Centrals:	0–10 days
	Intermediates:	4–10 weeks
	Corners:	6–10 months
Deciduous premolars:		Both 2 weeks
Permanent incisors:	Centrals:	2½ years
	Intermediates:	3½ years
	Corners:	4½ years
Permanent canines (males only):		4–5 years
Permanent premolars:	P1 (wolftooth):	5–6 months
	P2:	2½ years
	P3:	3 years
	P4:	4 years
Permanent molars:	M1:	9–12 months
	M2:	2 years
	M3:	3½–4 years

WEAR OF INCISOR TEETH

Age	Wear pattern
1 year	Crowns of central deciduous incisors are in wear.
1½ years	Crowns of intermediate deciduous incisors are in wear.
2 years	All deciduous incisors are in wear.
5 years	All permanent incisors are in wear and infundibula are present in all incisors.
6 years	Infundibula are worn out of lower central permanent incisors.
7 years	Infundibula are worn out of lower intermediate permanent incisors. A hook develops on posterior edge of upper corner incisors.
8 years	Infundibula are worn out of all lower permanent incisors. Dental star appears rostral to the infundibulum on lower central incisors.
9 years	Infundibula are worn out of upper central permanent incisors. Dental star appears on upper central and lower intermediate incisors.

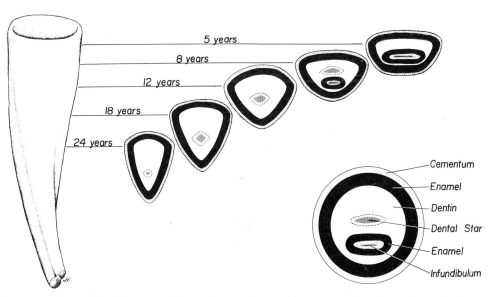

Figure 1. Schema of occlusal (table) surface of I₁ correlated with age of horse. From St. Clair, L. E.: Teeth. *In* Getty, R. (ed.): *Sisson and Grossman's The Anatomy of the Domestic Animals.* Philadelphia, W. B. Saunders Co., 1975.

10 years   Infundibula are worn out of upper intermediate permanent incisors. Dental star is present on all upper and lower incisors.

11 years   Infundibula are worn out of all upper and lower incisors. Dental star approaches center of incisors.

IDENTIFICATION OF DECIDUOUS AND PERMANENT INCISORS

Deciduous incisors, which are smaller and whiter than permanent incisors, have a characteristic "neck" or narrowing at the gum line. Permanent incisors are larger and darker-colored than deciduous incisors, and there is no neck at the gum line.

CHANGES IN INCISOR SHAPE WITH AGE

Permanent incisors change in shape with age. When viewed in profile, the permanent incisors meet in a gently curving arch in young horses. With age the incisors meet at an increasingly acute angle, the lower incisors projecting almost directly forward from the mandible in the aged horse.

The occlusal surfaces of the incisors also change shape with age (Fig. 1). In the young adult, the occlusal surfaces are elliptical with the long axis transverse. In the middle-aged horse, the occlusal surfaces form an almost equilateral triangle with one angle directed caudally. The triangular shape becomes more pronounced in the aged horse but is isosceles in form, with the short side of the triangle forming the rostral surface of the tooth.

GALVANE'S GROOVE

A longitudinal groove is present on the lateral (vestibular) surface of the upper corner incisor of horses between 10 and 30 years of age. It appears at the gum line in 10-year-olds, reaches halfway down the tooth at 15 years, and reaches the occlusal surface by 20 years. At 25 years, the groove extends from halfway down the tooth to the occlusal surface, and by 30 years it is no longer evident.

Supplemental Readings

1. Ensminger, M. A.: Determining the age and height of horses. *In* Ensminger, M. A.: Horses and Horsemanship. Danville, IL, The Interstate Publishers, Inc. 1977, p. 45.
2. St. Clair, L. E.: Teeth. *In* Getty, R. (ed.): Sisson and Grossman's The Anatomy of the Domestic Animals. Philadelphia, W. B. Saunders Co., 1975, p. 460.

Current Therapy in Equine Medicine

INDEX

Letters in *italics* refer to illustrations; letters followed by (t) refer to tables.

Abdomen, abscesses in, 38–39
diseases of, acute, blood pressure in, 130–131
Abdominocentesis, in chronic diarrhea, 216
in large bowel obstruction, 233
Abortion, bacterial, 420
causes of, 415–422
elective, 441–442
equine herpesvirus and, 4
fetal, 416
fetal anomalies and, 417–418
infectious, 419–422
mycotic, 420
noninfectious, 417
prevention of, 415–422
with progesterone, 406–407
twinning and, 417
viral, 420
Abscess(es), abdominal, 38–39
internal, 38–40
pulmonary, 500–504
subcutaneous, 39–40
Acer rubrum, toxicity of, 606
Acetylcysteine, for treatment of chronic airway disease, 510(t)
Acid(s), fatty, vs. bilirubin, *118*
gastrointestinal toxicity of, 573(t)
Acid-base balance, and fluid therapy, 316
disturbances of, in colitis-X, 203–204
in urinary disease, 562
normal values for, 620(t)
Actinobacillosis, 14–17
Actinobacillus, and bacterial endocarditis, 147
and foal pneumonia, 501
sensitivity of, to antibiotics, 51(t)
Adenoma, of thyroid, 160
Adenovirus, 5
Agammaglobulinemia, 324
Agar gel immunodiffusion (AGID) test, 8
Age, and body weight, 96(t)
and wear of teeth, 625–626, *625*
Aging, 625–626
Airway, diseases of, chronic, 505–512. See also *Chronic Airway Disease (CAD).*
smooth muscle tone of, therapeutic agents and, *508*
Albumin, normal values for, 619(t)
Alfalfa, protein content of, 68(t)
Alkali(s), gastrointestinal toxicity of, 573(t)
Alkali disease, 594
Alkaline phosphatase, normal values for, 619(t)
Alkaloid(s), central nervous system toxicity of, 574(t)

Alkaloid(s) (*Continued*)
gastrointestinal toxicity of, 573(t)
Allergen(s), skin tests with, for diagnosis of summer pasture–associated obstructive pulmonary disease, 514
Alpha-naphthyl ThioUrea (ANTU), toxicity of, 585
Amikacin, bacteria effective against, 471(t)
for treatment of bacterial endometritis, 413(t)
for treatment of respiratory diseases, 469(t), 472
Aminoglycoside(s), blood plasma concentrations of, 55(t)
for treatment of foal pneumonia, 503
for treatment of pleuritis, 526
side effects of, 49(t)
types of, 44(t)
Amphotericin B, dosage of, 53(t)
for treatment of bacterial endometritis, 413(t)
for treatment of mycotic diseases, 34
for treatment of phycomycosis, 550
for treatment of sinusitis, 485
side effects of, 34
Ampicillin, bacteria effective against, 471(t)
dosage of, 53(t)
for treatment of bacteremia, 37(t)
for treatment of bacterial endometritis, 413(t)
for treatment of respiratory diseases, 469(t), 470
for treatment of salmonellosis, 209(t)
for treatment of sinusitis, 484
incompatibility of, 48(t)
minimal inhibitory concentrations of, 52(t), 54(t)
Amsinckia sp, toxicity of, 596–597
Analgesic(s), for treatment of large bowel obstruction, 234–235
for treatment of small bowel obstruction, 228
for treatment of thromboembolic colic, 240
use in endotoxemia, 61
Anemia, 295–296
blood loss and, 297–299
copper deficiency and, 79
dyserythropoietic, 305
Heinz body, 300–301
hemolytic, 299–303
immune mediated, 301–303
infectious, 7–9
equine, 300
inflammatory disease and, 304
insufficient erythropoiesis and, 303–305
iron deficiency, 78, 304

Anemia (*Continued*)
responsive, 295
strangles and, 25
Anesthesia, and myopathy-neuropathy, 370–374
blood pressure in, 130
ventilation during, 476
Anestrus, behavioral, 400–401
Angioedema, 535–536
Anhidrosis, 170–171
Anoplocephala sp, and cestode infections, 287
Anorexia, gastrointestinal disease and, 175
Antagonism, of antibiotics, 46
Antagonists, narcotic, for treatment of respiratory depression, 475–476
Anthelmintic(s), 196–197
for management of colic, 221(t)
for treatment of chronic airway disease, 511–512
Anthrax, 17–18
vaccination program for, 42, 42(t)
Antibacterial agent(s), types of, 44(t)
Antibiotic(s), 43–57
additive effects of, 46
bacteria sensitive to, 50(t)
biologic half-lives of, 53(t)
blood plasma concentrations of, 55(t)
broad-spectrum, for treatment of bacteremia, 37, 37(t)
for treatment of small bowel obstruction, 229
characteristics of, 43
classification of, 43–44, 44(t)
clinical use of, 49–52
dosage of, 53(t)
fixed combinations of, 47
for management of colic, 221(t)
for treatment of chronic airway disease, 511
for treatment of colitis-X, 205
for treatment of cranial trauma, 343
for treatment of cystitis, 567
for treatment of dermatophilosis, 554
for treatment of large bowel obstruction, 236
for treatment of peritonitis, 242–243
for treatment of respiratory disease, 467–475
for treatment of thromboembolic colic, 239
for treatment of ulcerative keratitis, 389(t)
for treatment of uveitis, 385
incompatibilities of, 48(t)
intrauterine infusion of, for induction of abortion, 441
for treatment of bacterial endometritis, 412, 413(t)

627

Antibiotic(s) (*Continued*)
  mechanisms of action of, 43–44
  minimal inhibitory concentrations of, 52(t), 54(t)
  nebulization of, for treatment of respiratory diseases, 474
  selection of, 45(t)
    according to identified microorganism, 56(t)
  serum protein binding of, 468(t)
  side effects of, 47, 49(t)
  sites of action of, 45(t)
  use after removal of retained placenta, 427(t)
  use in endotoxemia, 61
Antibiotic sensitivity test(s), 45
Antibiotic therapy, guidelines for, 52
  reasons for failure of, 46–47
Anticholinergic drug(s), for treatment of chronic airway disease, 507–509
Anticoagulant(s), as rodenticides, toxicity of, 584
  use in blood transfusion, 326
Anticonvulsant(s), for treatment of seizure disorders, 347(t)
Antidote(s), 579
Antifungal agent(s), types of, 44(t)
Antihistamine(s), for treatment of chronic airway disease, 511
Anti-inflammatory agent(s), for treatment of pleuritis, 526
Antimicrobial agent(s), 43–57. See also *Antibiotic(s).*
Antiperistaltic(s), for management of colic, 221(t)
Antiprostaglandin(s), for management of colic, 222
  for treatment of large bowel obstruction, 235
  for treatment of uveitis, 384
Antithiamine factor(s), 90
Antitoxin, tetanus, 27–28
Antituberculous agent(s), types of, 44(t)
Aorta, diseases of, 152
Arteritis, viral, 6–7
  and abortion, 421–422
Aspergillosis, 32–33
Ascorbic acid, 88
  deficiency of, signs of, 89(t)
  functions of, 89(t)
  sources of, in feed, 89(t)
Arrhythmia(s), cardiac, 131–141
  detection of, 132–138
  electrocardiography in, 131–138, *132–138*
  murmurs associated with, 145
  sinus, 132, *133*
  supraventricular, 132–135
  treatment of, 138–141
  ventricular, 135, 137, *137*
Arsenic, toxicity of, 573(t), 585–586
Arteriosclerosis, aortoiliofemoral, 153–155
Arteritis, verminous, chemotherapy of, 224
  viral, 6–7
Artificial insemination, program for, evaluation of, 459–460. See also *Insemination, artificial.*
Arytenoepiglottic fold(s), and coughing, 465
Arytenoepiglottis, entrapment of, 494–495
Arytenoid cartilage(s), chondromas of, and coughing, 466
Arytenoidectomy, for treatment of laryngeal hemiplegia, 499
Ascariasis, 262–267
  control of, 266
  diagnosis of, 264
  pathogenesis of, 263
  treatment of, 264–266
Aspiration, tracheobronchial, for diagnosis of summer pasture–associated obstructive pulmonary disease, 513–514
Assay(s), blood samples required for, 620(t)
Astragalus sp, toxicity of, 599–600
Atrioventricular block, 134–135, *136*
Atrioventricular valve(s), diastolic murmurs associated with, 144–145

Atrioventricular valve(s) (*Continued*)
  systolic murmurs associated with, 143
Atrium, depolarization of, 127
Atropine, for treatment of cardiac arrhythmias, 140
  for treatment of chronic airway disease, 507–508, 508(t)
  for treatment of organophosphorus insecticide poisoning, 583
  for treatment of summer pasture–associated obstructive pulmonary disease, 515–516
Atropine test, intravenous, for diagnosis of summer pasture–associated obstructive pulmonary disease, 514
Aurothioglucose, for treatment of pemphigus foliaceus, 541
Auscultation, for diagnosis of chronic airway disease, 506
  in examination of cardiovascular system, 122–124
Autotransfusion, 328
Avermectin(s), for treatment of bots infections, 286
  for treatment of strongylosis, 276
Azotemia, 562

B cell(s), function of, in evaluation of immune system, 322
Babesia sp, and equine piroplasmosis, 300
Bacillus Calmette-Guérin (BCG), for treatment of sarcoid, 539–540
Bacteremia, 36–38
Bacteria, in water, 608
  isolated from horses, sensitivity of, to antibiotics, 51(t)
  sites of, 50(t)
Bait(s), for flies, 533(t)
BAL, for treatment of arsenic poisoning, 586
Barium chloride, toxicity of, 587
Barley, as energy source, 66
Basophil(s), normal values for, 619(t)
"Bastard strangles," 25
BCG, for treatment of sarcoid, 539–540
Beat(s), premature, atrial, *138*
  supraventricular, 132, *134, 138*
  ventricular, 135, 137, *137–138*
Behavior, abnormalities of, 335–339
  diseases affecting, 338
  disorders of, and fertility, 449–450
  medication and, 339
  normal variations in, 335–337
Benzimidazole(s), for treatment of ascariasis, 265
  for treatment of strongylosis, 274–275
  teratogenicity of, 274
  therapeutic doses of, 275(t)
β₂ stimulator(s), for treatment of summer pasture–associated obstructive pulmonary disease, 515
Bicarbonate, for treatment of colitis-X, 203
  sodium, use in fluid therapy, 312–313
Bilirubin, serum, fasting and, *117*
  total, normal values for, 619(t)
  vs. fatty acids, *118*
Bilirubinemia, 116–118
Biopsy, renal, 561–562
  uterine, for diagnosis of endometritis, 411
Bladder, calculi of, 567–568
  catheterization of, 561
  diseases of, 567–569
  paralysis of, 568
  rupture of, 568–569
    in neonates, 15(t)
    vs. retained meconium, 261
Blastomycosis, North American, 34
Blindness, central nervous system and, 395
  differential diagnosis of, 377(t)
  night, 393
  ocular fundus and, 393–395

Blister beetle(s), poisoning from, 588–589
Blood, administration of, 327–328
  components of, separation of, 327
  laboratory values for, nutrition and, 112
  loss of, and anemia, 297–299
  mineral concentration in, 73
  samples required for assays, 620(t)
  storage of, 327
  transfusion of, 325–328
    collection in, 325–326
    dosage in, 326
    laboratory tests in, 325–326
    selection of containers in, 327
    selection of donor in, 325
Blood cell(s), normal values for, 619(t)
  red, insufficient production of, and anemia, 303–305
Blood count, complete, in evaluation of immune system, 322
Blood gas(es), normal values for, 620(t)
Blood pressure, abdominal disease and, 130–131
  in anesthesia, 130
  in colic, 130
  indirect measurement of, 128–131
  normal values for, 129–130
Blood test(s), in chronic diarrhea, 217
Blood urea nitrogen (BUN), in urinary disease, 562
  normal values for, 619(t)
Blood value(s), normal, 293–295, 293(t)–294(t)
Blow fly(flies), control of, 534
Body pregnancy, 418
Body weight, age and, 96(t)
  and fluid therapy, 315, 315(t)
Bone, calcium deficiency and, 74
  growth of, vitamin A and, 85
Bone marrow, biopsy of, 296–297
Bordetella, sensitivity of, to antibiotics, 51(t), 471(t)
Bot fly(flies), control of, 534
Bots, 283–286
Botulism, syndromes with, 367–369
Bowel, large, obstruction of, 231–236. See also *Large bowel, obstruction of.*
  small, obstruction of, 224–231. See also *Small bowel, obstruction of.*
Bracken fern, toxicity of, 575(t), 600–601
Brain, trauma to, syndromes resulting from, 341(t)
Brain stem, injury of, signs of, 342(t)
Breed(s), light vs. heavy, hematologic values for, 294(t)
Breeding, artificial, 456–460
  ejaculate in, 457–458
  phantom mare in, 456–457
  semen collection in, 456–457
  artificial lighting and, 399
Bromhexine, for treatment of chronic airway disease, 510, 510(t)
Bronchodilator(s), diagnostic use of, in chronic airway disease, 507
  for treatment of chronic airway disease, 507, 508(t)
  for treatment of foal pneumonia, 504
  for treatment of summer pasture–associated obstructive pulmonary disease, 515
Brood mare(s), feeding programs for, 92–94, 92(t)
Brucellosis, 19–20
Buffer(s), in semen extenders, 458

Calcium, 73–77
  deficiency of, clinical signs of, 74–75
    diagnosis of, 75–76
    signs of, 82(t)
  for treatment of hyperparathyroidism, 163
  functions of, 74, 82(t)
  normal values for, 619(t)

Calcium (*Continued*)
  requirements for, 75, 75(t)
  sources of, in feed, 82(t)
  supplements with, 75
Calculi, cystic, 567–568
Cannon, keratosis of, 546
Carbamate(s), central nervous system toxicity of, 574(t)
Carbendazole, for control of strongyloidosis, 282
  for treatment of strongylosis, 275(t)
Carbenicillin, for treatment of bacterial endometritis, 413(t)
  incompatibility of, 48(t)
  minimal inhibitory concentration of, 54(t)
Carbon disulfide, for treatment of bots infections, 284
Carbon tetrachloride, toxicity of, 573(t), 590
Carcinoma, squamous cell, 259
Cardiac arrhythmia(s), 131–141. See also *Arrhythmia(s), cardiac.*
Cardiac defect(s), congenital, 146
  in neonates, 15(t)
Cardiac murmur(s), 141–146. See also *Murmur(s), cardiac.*
Cardiovascular system, diseases of, 119–155
  examination of, 121–125
    auscultation in, 122–124
    history in, 121
    palpation in, 121–122
    percussion in, 122
  pharmacologic support of, in colitis-X, 205
Carotene, and vitamin A, 85
Cartilage(s), chondromas of, and coughing, 466
Caslick's operation, for treatment of bacterial endometritis, 412
Castor bean, toxicity of, 604
Castrix, toxicity of, 587
Cataract(s), 390–393
  acquired, 392
  congenital, 391–392
Cathartic(s), for relief of large bowel obstruction, 234
  saline, for correction of impaction, 223
    for management of colic, 221(t)
Catheter(s), and thrombophlebitis, 151
  retention, nasolacrimal, 379–381, *381*
  subpalpebral, 379–381, *380*
Catheterization, cardiac, 124
  of bladder, 561
Cautery, for treatment of pharyngitis, 491–492
Centaurea sp, toxicity of, 595–596
Central nervous system, and blindness, 395
Cephalosporin(s), bacteria effective against, 471(t)
  for treatment of respiratory diseases, 474
  types of, 44(t)
Cephalothin, incompatibility of, 48(t)
  minimal inhibitory concentration of, 54(t)
Cerebrospinal fluid, analysis of, 332–335
  collection of, 331
    for diagnosis of seizure disorders, 348
    from recumbent horse, *332*
    from standing horse, *333*
  cytologic examination of, 333–334
  differential cell count in, 334, *334*
  physical appearance of, 334
  quantitative protein content of, 335
  refractive index of, 334
  total cell count in, 333–334
Cervical spine, arthrodesis of, 361–362
Cervical vertebral malformation, 359–362
  and stenosis, *360*
  pathogenesis of, 361
  treatment of, 361–362
Cervix, disorders of, 409–410
  examination of, 409
  laceration of, postpartum, 429
  relaxation of, and induction of parturition, 439
Cesarean section, 424–425
Cestode infection(s), 287–288

Cestrum diurnum, toxicity of, 602
Charcoal, activated, for treatment of toxicosis, 578
Cheatgrass, epithelial toxicity of, 575(t)
Chemotherapy, for treatment of retained placenta, 426–427
Chest, percussion of, 463–464
Chigger(s), and mange, 529
Chloral hydrate, for management of colic, 220
  for treatment of seizure disorders, 347(t)
Chloramphenicol, blood plasma concentrations of, 55(t)
  dosage of, 53(t)
  for treatment of bacteremia, 37(t)
  for treatment of bacterial endometritis, 413(t)
  for treatment of colitis-X, 205
  for treatment of peritonitis, 243
  for treatment of respiratory diseases, 469(t), 470
  for treatment of salmonellosis, 23
  incompatibility of, 48(t)
  minimal inhibitory concentrations of, 52(t), 54(t)
  side effects of, 49(t)
  types of, 44(t)
Chlorate(s), hematologic toxicity of, 575(t)
Chloride, 77–78
  deficiency of, in colitis-X, 202
    signs of, 82(t)
  functions of, 82(t)
  normal values for, 619(t)
  sources of, in feed, 82(t)
Chloromycetin, bacteria effective against, 471(t)
  for treatment of salmonellosis, 209(t)
Choke, 192
  diet in, 112
  treatment of, 194–195
Chokecherry, toxicity of, 597–598
Chondroma(s), of arytenoid cartilages, and coughing, 466
Chorioptes bovis, and mange, 529
Chronic airway disease (CAD), 500–512
  clinical signs of, 505
  diagnosis of, 506–507
  incidence of, 505
  pathogenesis of, 505–506
  treatment of, 507–512
Cicuta sp, toxicity of, 601
Cleft palate, 177–181
  postoperative feeding in, 180
  surgical approach to, *178–179*
Clenbuterol, for treatment of chronic airway disease, 508(t), 509
  for treatment of exercise-induced pulmonary hemorrhage, 519
Clindamycin, incompatibility of, 48(t)
  minimal inhibitory concentration of, 54(t)
Clostridiosis, intestinal, 210–212
Clostridium botulinum, and shaker foals, 367
Coagulant(s), for treatment of exercise-induced pulmonary hemorrhage, 517
Coagulation, disorders of, acquired, 308
  screening tests for, 307, *307*
  intravascular, disseminated, 309–311. See also *Disseminated intravascular coagulation.*
Cobalt, 80
Coccidioidomycosis, 33
Colic, blood pressure in, 130
  flatulent, 236–238
    rectal examination in, 237
  medical management of, 220–224
    drugs for, 221(t)
  pain relief in, 220–222
  retained meconium and, 261
  thromboembolic, 238–241
Colitis-X, 200–207
  acid-base imbalance in, 203–204
  and dehydration, 201–202
  antibiotic therapy in, 205

Colitis-X (*Continued*)
  antitoxic therapy in, 206
  cardiovascular failure in, 205
  colloid expansion in, 204–205
  diagnosis of, 201
  electrolyte therapy in, 202
    oral, 204, 204(t)
  etiology of, 200
  modification of fecal consistency in, 206
  modification of motility in, 206
  nutritional support in, 206
  pain control in, 206
  treatment of, 201–206
Colon, impaction of, diet in, 112
  thromboembolism of, 238–241
  trocarization of, in flatulent colic, 237
Colostomy, end-on, *258*
  for treatment of rectal tears, 257
  loop, *258*
Complete blood count (CBC), in evaluation of immune system, 322
Compound 1080, toxicity of, 585
Conception, twin, elimination of, 417
  prevention of, 417
Condom, for collection of semen, 443
Conium maculatum, toxicity of, 601–602
Conjunctivitis, 387
Convulsion(s), in foals, 349
Copper, 79
  deficiency of, signs of, 83(t)
  functions of, 83(t)
  sources of, in feed, 83(t)
Corn, as energy source, 66
Cornea, dystrophy of, 389
  opacities of, 388–390
    congenital, 388
    differential diagnosis of, 377(t)
Corpus luteum, persistence of, 401
Corticosteroid(s), for induction of parturition, 440
  for treatment of angioedema, 535–536
  for treatment of chronic airway disease, 510–511
  for treatment of contact dermatitis, 548
  for treatment of dermatophilosis, 554
  for treatment of habronemiasis, 551–552
  for treatment of large bowel obstruction, 235
  for treatment of malabsorption syndromes, 247
  for treatment of nodular collagenolytic granuloma, 545
  for treatment of pemphigus foliaceus, 541
  for treatment of small bowel obstruction, 229
  for treatment of urticaria, 535–536
  use in endotoxemia, 61
Corynebacterium equi, and foal pneumonia, 501
Corynebacterium pseudotuberculosis, and abortion, 420
  and subcutaneous abscesses, 39
Corynebacterium sp, antibiotic sensitivity of, 51(t), 471(t)
Coughing, 463–467
  clinical examination in, 463–464
  history of, 463
  pulmonary sources of, treatment of, 466–467
  upper respiratory causes of, 464–466
Cowbane, toxicity of, 601
Craniotomy, 343
Cranium, trauma to, pathophysiology of, 340
Creatine phosphokinase, normal values for, 619(t)
Creatinine, in urinary disease, 562
  normal values for, 619(t)
Creep feeding, 94
Creosol(s), gastrointestinal toxicity of, 573(t)
Cribbing, 181–183
  strap for prevention of, *182*
Cricoid cartilage, dorsal surface of, *500*
Crimson clover, epithelial toxicity of, 575(t)
Crotolaria, central nervous system toxicity of, 575(t)

Cryoprotective(s), for semen extenders, 458
Cryosurgery, for treatment of pharyngitis, 491–492
  for treatment of sarcoid, 538–539
  for treatment of warts, 537
Cryptococcosis, 33
Culex tarsalis, and western equine encephalomyelitis, 352
Culicoides, hypersensitivity to, 558
Cyanide, hematologic toxicity of, 575(t)
Cyproheptadine, for treatment of pituitary gland tumors, 168
Cyst(s), salivary, 184
  subepiglottal, 496
Cystitis, 567
Cystoscopy, 561

DDVP, for treatment of bots infections, 285
Death, sudden, chemical causes of, 611–612
  differential diagnosis of, 611–615
  poisoning and, 614
  sample collection after, 612–614, 613(t)
Death camus, central nervous system toxicity of, 575(t)
  toxicity of, 603
Decompression, nasogastric, for treatment of gastric dilatation, 198
  for treatment of small bowel obstruction, 228
Dehydration, assessment of, 201(t)
  clinicopathologic features of, 313(t)
  with colitis-X, treatment of, 201–202
Dehydrogenase, hydroxybutyric, normal values for, 619(t)
  lactic, normal values for, 619(t)
  sorbitol, normal values for, 619(t)
Demand valve, for administration of oxygen therapy, 481
  for emergency ventilation, 477
Demodicosis, 544–545
Depolarization, atrial, 127
Dermatitis, contact, 547–548
Dermatophilosis, 553–554
Dermatophytosis, and folliculitis, 543–544
Dermoid(s), congenital, 388
Dexamethasone, for treatment of spinal cord trauma, 357
  for treatment of summer pasture–associated obstructive pulmonary disease, 516
Dextrose, use in fluid therapy, 313
Diabetes mellitus, 169–170
  clinical signs of, vs. pituitary gland tumor, 170(t)
Diarrhea, chronic, 216–220
  abdominocentesis in, 216
  absorption studies in, 217
  differential diagnosis of, 218–220
  exploratory laparotomy in, 217
  fecal examination in, 216–217
  laboratory tests in, 217
  rectal examination in, 216
  treatment of, 218–220
  diet in, 112
  foal heat, 213–214
  rotavirus infections and, 11
  strongyloidosis and, 281
Diazepam, for treatment of seizure disorders, 347(t)
Dichlorvos, for treatment of ascariasis, 266
  for treatment of bots infections, 285
  for treatment of strongylosis, 275
Dictyocaulus arnfieldi, 520–522
Diestrus, prolonged, 401–402
Diet, and postanesthesia myopathy, 374
Diethylcarbamazine, for treatment of chronic airway disease, 512
  for treatment of onchocerciasis, 557
Digitalis glycoside(s), for treatment of cardiac arrhythmias, 140

Dihydroquinidine gluconate, for treatment of cardiac arrhythmias, 139
Dihydrostreptomycin, for treatment of respiratory diseases, 473
Dilantin, for treatment of seizure disorders, 348
Dilatation, gastric, 197–198
Dimercaprol, for treatment of arsenic poisoning, 586
Dimethyl sulfoxide, for treatment of cranial trauma, 342
  for treatment of spinal cord trauma, 358
Dinoprost, for treatment of prolonged diestrus, 402
Diphenylhydantoin, for treatment of seizure disorders, 348. See also *Phenytoin.*
Dipyrone, for treatment of large bowel obstruction, 235
Discharge, nasal, differential diagnosis of, 483
  ocular, differential diagnosis of, 377(t)
  in young horses, 385–388
Disease, hematologic response to, 295–296
  infectious, 1–62. See also specific diseases.
Disodium cromoglycate, for treatment of exercise-induced pulmonary hemorrhage, 518
Disseminated intravascular coagulation (DIC), 309–311
  causes of, 310(t)
  hematologic tests in, 310(t)
Distention, abdominal, 197–198
  correction of, 222–224
Diuretic(s), osmotic, for treatment of cranial trauma, 342
Drainage, pleural, for treatment of pleuritis, 525, *525*
Drug(s), and abortion, 419
  and sudden death, 612
  common, approximate doses of, 621(t)–624(t)
Dust, organic, and chronic airway disease, 506
Dysphagia, gastrointestinal disease and, 175
Dystocia, causes of, 423–424
Dystrophy, muscular, selenium deficiency and, 81

Eastern equine encephalomyelitis (EEE), 350–352
  vaccination program for, 41, 42(t)
Echium lycopsis, toxicity of, 596–597
Echocardiography, 124
Eclampsia, 111
Ectoparasite(s), control of, 529–535
  pesticides for, 530(t)–531(t)
Edema, malignant, 21–22
Ehrlichiosis, 13–14
  equine, 300
Ejaculate, in artificial breeding, 457–458
Electrocardiography, and prediction of performance, 148–149
  for diagnosis of arrhythmias, 131–138, *132–138*
  limitations of, 125–127
  multiple-lead tracing in, 126
  normal tracing in, *132*
  principles of, 125–126
  single-lead tracing in, 126
Electroencephalography, for diagnosis of seizure disorders, 348
Electrolyte(s), for tube feeding, 115(t)
  serum, in urinary disease, 562
Electrolyte balance, 314
Electrolyte therapy, for treatment of large bowel obstruction, 235
  in colitis-X, 202
  oral, in colitis-X, 204(t)
Electrophoresis, serum, 322
Embryo, loss of, 415–416
Empyema, and gluttural pouch disease, 485–487
Encephalomyelitis, equine, eastern, 350–352
  vaccination program for, 41, 42(t)
  Venezuelan, vaccination for, 41

Encephalomyelitis (*Continued*)
  equine, western, 352–355
    transmission to humans, 355
Endocarditis, bacterial, 147–148
Endocrine disease(s), 157–171
Endometritis, bacterial, 410–414
  treatment of, 413(t)
Endoscopy, for diagnosis of chronic airway disease, 506
  for diagnosis of sinusitis, 484
Endothelialitis, 390
Endotoxemia, 57–62
  clinical signs of, 57, 58(t)
  diagnosis of, 59–60, 59(t)
  fluid therapy in, 60–61
  pathophysiology of, 57–59
  treatment of, 60–62, 60(t)
Endotoxin, defense mechanisms invoked by, *58*
Endotracheal tube(s), sizes of, 477(t)
Enema, for treatment of retained meconium, 261
Energy, 65–68
  requirements for, 66(t)
  sources of, 65–68
    composition of, 66(t)
    in semen extenders, 458
Enteritis, anterior, 214–215
  granulomatous, 219
  Salmonella and, 207–210
Enterobacter, sensitivity of, to antibiotics, 51(t), 471(t)
Enterotoxemia, overfeeding and, 96
Entropion, 385–386
Environment, alteration of, in chronic airway disease, 507
  management of, for treatment of summer pasture–associated obstructive pulmonary disease, 515
Eosinophil(s), normal values for, 619(t)
Ephedrine, for treatment of chronic airway disease, 508(t), 509
Epiglottis, diseases of, 494–496
  hypoplasia of, 495
Epiphysitis, overfeeding and, 95
Equine herpesvirus type 1 (EHV-1), 4–5
  and abortion, 420–421
  and myeloencephalitis, 362–364
Equine herpesvirus type 2 (EHV-2), 5
Equine infectious anemia (EIA), 7–9, 300
Equine intestinal clostridiosis (EIC), 210–212
Equine papilloma virus (EPV), 536
Equine protozoal myeloencephalitis (EPM), 365–367
Equine rhinovirus (ERV), 6
Equine viral arteritis (EVA), 6–7
Equisetum arvense, toxicity of, 601
Erythrocyte(s), parameters for, in young horses, 294(t)
  total, normal values for, 619(t)
Erythromycin, bacteria effective against, 471(t)
  dosage of, 53(t)
  for treatment of respiratory diseases, 473
  incompatibility of, 48(t)
  minimal inhibitory concentrations of, 52(t), 54(t)
  side effects of, 49(t)
Erythropoiesis, insufficient, and anemia, 303–305
Escherichia coli, and abortion, 420
  antibiotic sensitivity of, 51(t), 471(t)
Esophagoscopy, 193
Esophagostomy, for tube feeding, 115
Esophagotomy, for treatment of food choke, 194–195
Esophagus, diseases of, 192–196
  clinical signs of, 192–193
  etiology of, 192
  treatment of, 194–195
  radiography of, 193–194
  stricture of, 195
  surgical approach to, 195
Estradiol, for synchronization of ovulation, 405

Estrogen(s), for treatment of exercise-induced
   pulmonary hemorrhage, 518
Estrous period, advance of ovulation within, 404
Estrus, advance of, 404
   and seizures, 349
   irregular, progesterone for treatment of, 406
   suppression of, with progesterone, 406
Eupatorium rugosum, toxicity of, 603–604
Exanthema, coital, 5
Exercise, and pulmonary hemorrhage, 516–519
   intolerance of, chronic airway disease and, 505
Exhaustion, clinical signs of, 319–320, 319(t)
   medical management of, 318–321
   prevention of, 318–319
Expectorant(s), for treatment of chronic airway
      disease, 509, 510(t)
   for treatment of foal pneumonia, 504
Extraction, of fetus, 424
Exudate, in respiratory disease, and antibiotics,
      468
   vs. transudate, 523
Eye(s), administration of medication to, 378–382
   systemic, 382
   topical, 378
   cloudy, differential diagnosis of, 377(t)
   discharge from, differential diagnosis of,
      377(t)
   in young horses, 385–388
   diseases of, 375–395. See also *Ocular
      disease(s).*
   inflamed, differential diagnosis of, 377(t)
   innervation of, 379, *379*
   red, 382–385
Eye drop(s), administration of, 378
Eyelid(s), innervation of, *379*
   swollen, differential diagnosis of, 377(t)
Eyelid block(s), 378–379

Face fly(flies), control of, 533
Face mask, for administration of oxygen, 479
Fasting, and hyperlipemia, 107
   and serum bilirubins, *117*
Febantel, for treatment of strongylosis, 276
Feces, examination of, in chronic diarrhea,
      216–217
   in diagnosis of strongylosis, 271–272
   leukocytes in, 217
Feed(s), calcium in, 76(t)
   commercial, 98, 99(t), 100
      nutrient requirements for, according to type
         of horse, 99(t)
   composition of, 66(t), 70(t)
      mineral, 76(t)
   contamination of, and sudden death, 612
   nonconcentrate, energy content of, 67(t)
   pelleted, 98
   phosphorus in, 76(t)
   relative weights of, 67(t)
   supplements for, in treatment of exercise-
      induced pulmonary hemorrhage, 519
   vitamin content of, 86(t)
Feeding, force, 113–115
   intravenous, 113–114
      in foals, solution for, 114(t)
   programs for, 91–97
      at racetracks, 98(t)
   tube, 114–115, 115(t)
      schedule for, 176(t)
Fenbendazole, for treatment of lungworm
      infections, 521
   for treatment of strongylosis, 275(t)
Fermentation, excessive, and distention, 223
Fertility, artificial insemination and, 459–460
   of stallions, disorders affecting, 449–455
      evaluation of, 442–448
      perineal injuries and, 437
      rectovestibular injuries and, 437
Fescue, and abortion, 419
Fetal membrane(s), removal of, 425–426, 426(t)

Fetotomy, partial, 424
Fetus, abortion of, 416
   extraction of, 424
Fibrillation, atrial, 133–134, *135*
   ventricular, 137–138, *138*
Fibrin degradation products (FDPS), 310
Fibrinogen, in young horses, 294(t)
   normal values for, 619(t)
Fiddleneck, toxicity of, 596–597
Filtration, glomerular, assessment of, 563
Floating, of teeth, 188–189
Flucytosine, for treatment of cryptococcal
      meningitis, 35
Fluid(s), intravenous, for treatment of
      exhaustion, 320
   replacement, polyionic, 312
Fluid balance, 314
Fluid therapy, 311–318
   clinical evaluation in, 314–317
   evaluation of deficit in, 313–314
   for treatment of exhaustion, 320–321
   for treatment of large bowel obstruction, 235
   in acute renal failure, 564–565
   in colitis-X, 201–202, 204
   in thromboembolic colic, 239
   packed cell volume in, 202(t)
   planning of, 317–318
   plasma protein in, 202(t)
   use of bicarbonate in, 312–313
Flumethasone, for induction of parturition, 440
Fluoride, in water, 608–609
Fluorine, 83–84
Fluoroacetate, toxicity of, 585
Fluorosis, 83–84
Fluprostenol, for induction of parturition, 440
   for treatment of prolonged diestrus, 402
Fly(flies), control of, 532–534
   pesticides for, 530(t)–531(t), 533(t)
Foal(s), adolescent, seizure disorders in, 349
   intravenous feeding in, solution for, 114(t)
   neonatal, drug therapy in, 52
      feeding programs for, 94
      seizure disorders in, 349
   orphan, feeding programs for, 94
   pneumonia in, 500–504
   rejection of, 336
   weakness in, differential diagnosis of, 15(t)
Foal heat diarrhea, 213–214
Foaling, gastrointestinal complications of, 430
Folliculitis, 542–545
Food choke, treatment of, 194–195
Forage, poisoning from, 369–370
Founder, 104–106
Foxtail, epithelial toxicity of, 575(t)
Fundus, ocular, and blindness, 393–395
Furadantin, bacteria effective against, 471(t)
Furazolidone, for treatment of salmonellosis,
      209(t)
Furosemide, for treatment of exercise-induced
      pulmonary hemorrhage, 518
Furunculosis, 542–545

Galvane's groove, in teeth, 626
Gas(es), toxic, and sudden death, 612
Gasterophilus sp, and bots, 283–286
Gastric disease(s), 196–200
Gastrointestinal tract, diseases of, 173–289
   clinical signs of, 175–177
   neoplasms of, 259–260
Genitalia, examination of, for evaluation of
      stallion fertility, 446
   infections of, 454–455
   injuries of, traumatic, 450–451
   tumors of, 451–452
Gentamicin, bacteria effective against, 471(t)
   dosage of, 53(t)
   for treatment of actinobacillosis, 16
   for treatment of bacteremia, 37(t)
   for treatment of bacterial endometritis, 413(t)

Gentamicin (*Continued*)
   for treatment of peritonitis, 243
   for treatment of respiratory diseases, 469(t),
      472
   for treatment of salmonellosis, 209(t)
   incompatibility of, 48(t)
   minimal inhibitory concentrations of, 52(t),
      54(t)
Gestation, length of, and induction of parturition,
      439
Glaucoma, 394
Glomerular filtration, assessment of, 563
Glomerulonephritis, 565–566
Glossitis, 185–186
Glucocorticoid(s), for treatment of cranial
      trauma, 342
   for treatment of summer pasture–associated
      obstructive pulmonary disease, 516
Glucose, normal values for, 619(t)
Glucose absorption test, 246
Glyceryl guaiacolate, for treatment of chronic
      airway disease, 510, 510(t)
Gnat(s), control of, 532, 534
   pesticides for, 530(t)
Goiter, 159
   iron deficiency and, 80
Gonadotrophin, chorionic, for induction of
      ovulation, 403
Grain(s), as energy source, 65–67
   mineral composition of, 76(t)
   minimum protein requirements in, 69(t)
   mixtures of, with protein, 93(t)
Granuloma, collagenolytic, nodular, 545
Granulosa-theca cell tumor(s), 408
Grass sickness, 244–245
Grease heel, 549
Great vessel(s), diseases of, 152
Griseofulvin, dosage of, 53(t)
Grooming, for control of bots infections, 286
Groundsel, common, toxicity of, 596–597
Guaifenesin, for treatment of seizure disorders,
      347(t)
Guttural pouch disease, 485–489
   and coughing, 464–465
   treatment of, infusion for, 486–487
      surgical, 487
      systemic, 487
Guttural pouch mycosis, 487–489

Habronemiasis, 452, 551–552
Hair, follicles of, inflammation of, 542–545
   mineral content of, 73
Harter's iodine, composition of, 465(t)
Hay(s), as energy source, 67–68, 67(t)
   harvesting of, proper times for, 68(t)
   requirements for, 91
Head, trauma to, 339–344
   management of, 343(t)
   medical therapy for, 342–343
   neurologic examination after, 341
   physical examination after, 340–341
   surgical management of, 343–344
Heart, catheterization of, 124
   congenital defects of, 146
      in neonates, 15(t)
   diseases of, 119–155. See also specific
      diseases.
   examination of, protocol for, 124–125
   murmurs of, 141–146. See also *Murmur(s),
      cardiac.*.
   valves of, acquired disease of, 141–142
      relationship to chest wall, *122*
Heart sound(s), and hemodynamic events, *123*
Heartbeat, premature, atrial, *138.* See also
   Beat(s), premature.
Heat bump(s), 110–111
Heinz body anemia, 300–301
Hematologic value(s), normal, for light breed
   horses, 293(t)

Hematologic value(s) (*Continued*)
  normal, for light vs. heavy breeds, 294(t)
Hematoma, intracerebral, 340
Hematopoietic system, 293–297
  diseases of, 291–328
  normal values for, 293–295, 293(t)
  response to disease, 295–296
Hemiplegia, laryngeal, 496–500
Hemlock, toxicity of, 574(t), 601–602
Hemoglobin, normal values for, 619(t)
Hemophilia, 309
Hemorrhage, and anemia, 297–298
  postpartum, 428–429
  pulmonary, exercise-induced, 516–519
Hemospermia, 452–453
Hemostasis, 306–309
  screening tests for, 308(t)
Heparin, for treatment of disseminated
    intravascular coagulation, 311
  for treatment of hyperlipemia, 109
Hepatitis, acute, 249–251
Herpesvirus, 4–5
  in neonates, 15(t)
  vaccination program for, 42(t)
Histoplasmosis, 33–34
Hoof(hooves), growth of, nutrition and, 100–109
Hormone(s), imbalance of, and abortion,
    418–419
Hormone test(s), for diagnosis of pituitary gland
    tumors, 166(t)
Horn fly(flies), control of, 532
Horse(s), adult, seizure disorders in, 349
  "cold-blooded," 293
  growing, improper nutrition of, problems
      associated with, 95–96
    nutritional requirements of, 95(t)–96(t)
  "hot-blooded," 293
  ill, nutrition of, 111–116
  mature, feeding programs for, 91
  working, feeding programs for, 91–92, 92(t)
Horse fly(flies), control of, 533–534
Horsebrush, epithelial toxicity of, 575(t)
Horsetail, toxicity of, 575(t), 601
House fly(flies), control of, 532
Human chorionic gonadotrophin (HCG), for
    induction of ovulation, 403
Hydroallantois, and abortion, 418
Hydrocarbon(s), chlorinated, central nervous
    system toxicity of, 574(t)
Hydroxybutyric dehydrogenase, normal values
    for, 619(t)
Hypercalcitonism, 159
Hypericum perforatum, toxicity of, 605–606
Hyperlipemia, 107-n110
  blood lipids in, and recovery rate, 109(t)
Hyperparathyroidism, secondary, nutritional,
    160–163
    calcium and phosphorus levels in, *162*
    pathology of, *162*
Hyperphosphatemia, 161
Hyperthermia, for treatment of sarcoid, 538
Hyperthyroidism, 160
Hypogammaglobulinemia, transient, 324
Hyposensitization, for treatment of summer
    pasture–associated obstructive pulmonary
    disease, 516
Hypothyroidism, 159

Icteric index, in young horses, 294(t)
Icterus, 116–118
  causes of, 117(t)
  hemolytic anemia and, 299
Idiopathic laryngeal hemiplegia (ILH), 496–500
IgM, deficiency of, 324
Ileus, treatment of, 198
Immune system, deficiency of, 323–324
  evaluation of, 322–323
Immune transfer, passive, 323–324

Immunodeficiency, combined, 324
Immunofluorescence, 322
Immunologic disease(s), 321–325
Impaction, colonic, diet in, 112
  correction of, 222–223
Incisor(s), deciduous vs. permanent,
    identification of, 626
  eruption schedule for, 625
  wear of, 625–626
Indifference, of antibiotics, 46
Infection, hematologic response to, 296
Infectious disease(s), 1–62
  in neonates, 15(t)
Inflammation, hematologic response to, 296
  in respiratory disease, and antibiotics, 468
Inflammatory disease, anemia in, 304
Influenza, 3–4
  vaccination program for, 42(t)
Injection(s), intraocular, 382
  retrobulbar, 382
  subconjunctival, 378
Insect bite, toxicity of, 576
Insecticide(s), and sudden death, 612
  for control of flies, 533(t)
  toxicity of, 574(t), 576, 580–583
Insemination, artificial, methods of, 459
  postovulation, 459
  program for evaluation of, 459–460
Insufflation, for administration of oxygen
    therapy, 479–481
  for emergency ventilation, 477
Insulin, with carbohydrates, for treatment of
    hyperlipemia, 109
Interval(s), electrocardiographic, duration of,
    132(t)
Intravenous fluid(s), composition of, 312(t)
Intubation, endotracheal, 476
Iodide(s), for treatment of chronic airway
    disease, 510, 510(t)
  for treatment of sporotrichosis, 556, 556(t)
Iodine, 80
  deficiency of, signs of, 82(t)
  functions of, 82(t)
  Harter's, composition of, 465(t)
  intrauterine infusion of, for induction of
    abortion, 441
  sources of, in feed, 82(t)
Iodochlorhydroxyquin (ICH), for treatment of
    chronic diarrhea, 218
Iron, 78–79
  deficiency of, and anemia, 78, 304
    signs of, 83(t)
  for treatment of blood loss anemia, 299
  functions of, 83(t)
Isoerythrolysis, neonatal, 15(t), 301–303
Isoniazid, dosage of, 53(t)
  for treatment of chronic airway disease, 511
  for treatment of respiratory diseases, 469(t),
    474
Isoproterenol, for treatment of chronic airway
    disease, 508(t), 509
Ivermectin(s), for treatment of onchocerciasis,
    557

Jasmine, toxicity of, 602

Kanamycin, bacteria effective against, 471(t)
  dosage of, 53(t)
  for treatment of bacteremia, 37(t)
  for treatment of bacterial endometritis, 413(t)
  for treatment of peritonitis, 243
  for treatment of respiratory diseases, 469(t),
    472
  incompatibility of, 48(t)
  minimal inhibitory concentrations of, 52(t),
    54(t)

Keratinization, abnormal, diseases of, 545–547
Keratitis, stromal, corneal, 390
  ulcerative, 389
Keratosis, linear, 546–547
  of cannon, 546
Ketoconazole, for treatment of fungal diseases,
    35
Kidney(s), biopsy of, 561–562
  neoplasms of, 566
Klebsiella, sensitivity of, to antibiotics, 51(t),
    471(t)

Labor, examination of mare during, 423
  restraint during, 423
Laboratory value(s), for blood cells, 619(t)
  for serum, 619(t)
Laminectomy, decompressive, subtotal dorsal,
    362
Laparotomy, exploratory, in chronic diarrhea,
    217
Large bowel, obstruction of, 231–236
  abdominocentesis in, 233
  clinical signs of, 232–233
  etiology of, 231, 231(t)
  history in, 232
  laboratory evaluation in, 233
  pathophysiology of, 231–232
  radiography in, 234
  rectal examination in, 232
  relief of, 234
  treatment of, 234–236
Larkspur, central nervous system toxicity of,
    574(t)
Larva(e), strongyle, migrating, chemotherapy of,
    278–279
Laryngitis, and coughing, 465
Laryngoplasty, complications of, 500
  for treatment of laryngeal hemiplegia, 498–499
Laryngoscopy, for diagnosis of hemiplegia,
    497–498
Larynx, hemiplegia of, 496–500
  surgical treatment of, results of, 499–500,
    499(t)
Lavage, peritoneal, for treatment of peritonitis,
    243–244
Laxative(s), for relief of large bowel obstruction,
    234
Lead, toxicity of, 574(t), 592–593
Leptospira pomona, and abortion, 420
Leukocyte(s), in young horses, 294(t)
  total, normal values for, 619(t)
Levallorphan, for treatment of respiratory
    depression, 476
Levamisole, for treatment of chronic airway
    disease, 511–512
  for treatment of lungworm infections, 522
Lice, control of, 532
  pesticides for, 530(t)
Lidocaine, for treatment of cardiac arrhythmias,
    140
Lighting, artificial, and reproduction, 399
Limb(s), positioning of, during surgery, and
    prevention of myopathy, 373–374
Lincomycin, incompatibility of, 48(t)
  minimal inhibitory concentration of, 54(t)
Lipemia, 107
Lipid(s), metabolism of, 107, *108*
Liver disease, chronic, 251–253
Locoweed, toxicity of, 574(t), 599–600
Locust, black, toxicity of, 575(t), 606
Lubricant(s), intestinal, for management of colic,
    221(t)
Lung(s), abscesses of, 500–504
  drainage of, for treatment of pleuritis, 525,
    525
  function of, tests of, in chronic airway disease,
    507
  hemorrhage of, exercise-induced, 516–519

Lung(s) (*Continued*)
  parasites in, 520–522
Lungworm, 520–522
Lupine, central nervous system toxicity of, 574(t)
Lymph node(s), biopsy of, 323
Lymphangitis, ulcerative, 31–32
Lymphatic system, diseases of, 291–328
Lymphocyte(s), in young horses, 294(t)
  normal values for, 619(t)
Lymphoma, malignant, 305
Lymphoproliferative disease(s), 305–306
Lymphosarcoma, intestinal, 259–260

Macrolide(s), types of, 44(t)
Magnesium, 77
  deficiency of, signs of, 82(t)
  functions of, 82(t)
  normal values of, 619(t)
  sources of, in feed, 82(t)
Malabsorption syndrome(s), 245–248
  diagnosis of, 246–247
  etiology of, 245–246
  treatment of, 247–248
Mane, seborrhea of, 546
Manganese, 81
Mange, mites and, 529
Mannitol, for treatment of cranial trauma, 342
  for treatment of spinal cord trauma, 357
Maple, red, toxicity of, 606
Mare(s), behavior of, variations in, 336
  feeding programs for, 92–94, 92(t)–93(t)
  lactating, sample rations for, 98(t)
  pregnant, protein requirements of, 93
    sample rations for, 98(t)
Marestail, toxicity of, 601
Mask, for administration of oxygen, 479
Mating, disorders of, 449–450
Mean corpuscular volume (MCV), normal values
    for, 619(t)
Mebendazole, for treatment of lungworm
    infections, 521, 521(t), *522*
  for treatment of strongylosis, 275(t)
Meconium, retained, 260–262
Medication, and behavior, 339
Mercury, central nervous system toxicity of,
    575(t)
Metal(s), heavy, in water, 609, 609(t)
Methicillin, incompatibility of, 48(t)
  minimal inhibitory concentration of, 54(t)
Methylxanthine(s), for treatment of summer
    pasture–associated obstructive pulmonary
    disease, 515
Metritis-laminitis-toxemia syndrome, 430–431
Miconazole, for treatment of fungal diseases, 35
Milkweed, central nervous system toxicity of,
    575(t)
Milo, as energy source, 66(t)
Mineral(s), 71–84
  deficiency of, areas of, in United States, *72*
    signs of, 82(t)–83(t)
  functions of, 82(t)–83(t)
  in plants and soil, alteration of, 73
  interrelationship of, 73
  micronutrient allowances for, 78(t)
  sources of, 71
    in feed, 82(t)–83(t)
  toxicity of, areas of, in United States, *72*
  trace, mixtures containing, 78(t)
Mineral oil, for correction of impaction, 222–223
Mineral supplement(s), calcium content of, 77(t)
  phosphorus content of, 77(t)
Minimal inhibitory concentration (MIC), 49
  of antibiotics, 49, 52(t), 54(t)
Mite(s), and mange, 529
  control of, pesticides for, 530(t)
Moisture, and contact dermatitis, 547
Molybdenum, 83
  functions of, 82(t)

Monocyte(s), normal values for, 619(t)
Morphine, derivatives of, for management of
    colic, 221
Mosquito(es), and eastern equine
    encephalomyelitis, 350–352
  and western equine encephalomyelitis, 352
  control of, 532, 535
    pesticides for, 530(t)
Mucocele(s), salivary, 184
Mucokinetic agent(s), for treatment of chronic
    airway disease, 510
Mucomyst, for treatment of chronic airway
    disease, 510(t)
Mud fever, 549
Murmur(s), cardiac, 141–146
  benign, 142
  classification of, 142–145
  clinical significance of, 145–146
  diastolic, 143–145
  grading of, 122–123
  systolic, 142–143
  with arrhythmias, 145
Muscle(s), function of, in botulism, 368
Mutation, obstetrical, 424
Mycobacterium tuberculosis, 30
Mycosis, guttural pouch, 487–489
  treatment of, surgical, 489
    systemic, 488–489
    topical, 487–488
Mycotic disease(s), 32–35
Mydriatic(s), for treatment of uveitis, 384
Myectomy, for treatment of cribbing, 181–182
Myeloencephalitis, equine herpesvirus-1 and,
    362–364
  protozoal, equine, 365–367
Myeloma, plasma cell, 306
Myelophthisis, 304
Myeloproliferative disease(s), 305–306
Myocardium, hypertrophy of, and performance,
    145
Myopathy, exertional, 101–104
  recumbency in, 103
Myopathy-neuropathy, postanesthesia, 370–374
Myositis, anesthesia and, 371

Nalorphine, for treatment of respiratory
    depression, 476
Naloxene, for treatment of respiratory depression,
    476
Narcotic(s), antagonists of, for treatment of
    respiratory depression, 475–476
Nasolacrimal duct, blocked, 386–387
Nebulization, for treatment of chronic airway
    disease, 510
  for treatment of foal pneumonia, 504
  for treatment of respiratory diseases, 474
Necrobiosis, nodular, 545
Needlegrass, epithelial toxicity of, 575(t)
Neomycin, bacteria effective against, 471(t)
  dosage of, 53(t)
  for treatment of bacteremia, 37(t)
  for treatment of bacterial endometritis, 413(t)
  for treatment of respiratory diseases, 473
Neonate(s), drug therapy in, 52
  weakness in, differential diagnosis of, 15(t)
Neoplasm(s), gastrointestinal, 259–260
  renal, 566
Neostigmine, for correction of impaction, 223
Nerium oleander, toxicity of, 602–603
Nervous system, disease(s), of 329–374. See also
    Neurologic disease(s).
Neurectomy, of spinal accessory nerves, for
    treatment of cribbing, 182, *182*
Neurologic disease(s), 329–374
Neutrophil(s), in young horses, 294(t)
  normal values for, 619(t)
  toxic, characteristics of, 296(t)
Nicotine, toxicity of, 580–581

Night blindness, 393
Nightshade, black, toxicity of, 605
Nitrate(s), in water, 608
Nitrite(s), hematologic toxicity of, 575(t)
  in water, 608
Nitrofurantoin, minimal inhibitory concentration
    of, 54(t)
Nitrogen, nonprotein, toxicity of, 71
  utilization of, 70–71
Nutrition, 63–118
  and abortion, 419
  and hoof growth, 100–101
  of ill horses, 111–116
  status of, assessment of, 112
Nutritional therapy, for treatment of
    malabsorption syndromes, 248
Nystatin, dosage of, 53(t)

Oak, gastrointestinal toxicity of, 573(t)
Oats, as energy source, 65
Obstetrics, 422–425
Ocular disease(s), 375–395
  approach to, 377
  diagnosis of, 377(t)
Ocular insert(s), 378
Ocular therapy, administration of, 378–382
Ointment(s), ocular, administration of, 378
Oleander, toxicity of, 574(t), 602–603
Onchocerciasis, 557
OP'-DDD, for treatment of pituitary gland
    tumors, 168
Optic nerve, atrophy of, 394
  dysfunction of, 395
Oral cavity, surgical approach to, *178*
Orchitis, 455
Organophosphate(s), central nervous system
    toxicity of, 574(t)
  for treatment of habronemiasis, 551–552
  for treatment of strongylosis, 275
Osmolality, of serum, normal values for, 619(t)
Outflow tract(s), cardiac, murmurs associated
    with, 142–144
Ovary(ies), tumors of, 408–409
Overfeeding, 65
Ovulation, advance of, within estrous period, 404
  control of, 404–405
  group, 404
  induction of, 402–403
  synchronization of, 404–405
Oxacillin, dosage of, 53(t)
  incompatibility of, 48(t)
  minimal inhibitory concentration of, 54(t)
Oxalate(s), and nephropathy, 566
Oxfendazole, for treatment of strongylosis,
    275(t)
Oxibendazole, for treatment of strongylosis,
    275(t)
Oxime(s), for treatment of organophosphorus
    insecticide poisoning, 583
Oxygen, toxicity of, 481
  transport of, in blood, failure of, 611–612
Oxygen cage, 479
Oxygen therapy, 478–481
  indications for, 478
Oxytetracycline, dosage of, 53(t)
  for treatment of anthrax, 18
  for treatment of bacteremia, 37(t)
  for treatment of ehrlichiosis, 13–14
  for treatment of respiratory diseases, 469(t),
    473
  incompatibility of, 48(t)
  minimal inhibitory concentrations of, 52(t)
Oxytocin, after removal of retained placenta,
    427(t)
  for induction of parturition, 439–440
  for removal of fetal membranes, 426
Oxytropis sp, toxicity of, 599–600
Oxyuris infection(s), 288–289

Pacemaker, atrial, wandering, 132–133, *133*
Packed cell volume, and electrolyte therapy, 315
  normal values for, 619(t)
Pain, abdominal, gastric dilatation and, 196
  and behavior, 338
  control of, in colic, 220–222
  in colitis-X, 206
Palate, cleft, 177–181. See also *Cleft palate.*
  soft, diseases of, 493–494
  dorsal displacement of, and coughing, 466
Palpation, in examination of cardiovascular
  system, 121–122
Pancreas, secretions of, 253
Pancreatitis, chronic, 253–254
Pancytopenia, aplastic, 304
Pandy test, for analysis of cerebrospinal fluid,
  334
Papillomatosis, 536–537
Paranoplocephala mamillana, and cestode
  infections, 287
Parascaris equorum, 522
  and ascariasis, 262–267
Parasitism, 196–197
  and coughing, 466
  pulmonary, 520–522
Parasympatholytic agent(s), for treatment of
  summer pasture–associated obstructive
  pulmonary disease, 515–516
Parathyroid hormone, biosynthesis of, *161*
  increased secretion of, 161
Pars intermedia, tumors of, 164–169
  laboratory tests for, 165–167, 165(t)–166(t)
  pathology of, 167
  treatment of, 168
Parturition, complications after, 428–431
  induction of, 438–442
    indications for, 438–439
    methods of, 439–441
    site for, 438
  normal, 422–423
Pasteurella, sensitivity of, to antibiotics, 51(t),
  471(t)
Pellet(s), feed, 98
Pemphigus foliaceus, 541–542
Penicillin(s), bacteria effective against, 471(t)
  blood plasma concentrations of, 55(t)
  dosage of, 53(t)
  for treatment of actinobacillosis, 16
  for treatment of anthrax, 18
  for treatment of bacteremia, 37(t)
  for treatment of bacterial endometritis, 413(t)
  for treatment of foal pneumonia, 503
  for treatment of intra-abdominal abscesses, 39
  for treatment of peritonitis, 243
  for treatment of pleuritis, 526
  for treatment of respiratory diseases, 469–470,
    469(t)
  for treatment of sinusitis, 484
  for treatment of strangles, 26
  incompatibility of, 48(t)
  minimal inhibitory concentrations of, 52(t),
    54(t)
  side effects of, 49(t)
  types of, 44(t)
Penis, injuries of, traumatic, 450–451
  neoplasms of, 451–452
  paralysis of, 451
Pentazocine, for treatment of large bowel
  obstruction, 235
Pentobarbital, for treatment of seizure disorders,
  347(t)
Percussion, for diagnosis of chronic airway
  disease, 506
  in examination of cardiovascular system, 122
Performance, prediction of, electrocardiography
  and, 148–149
Pergolide, for treatment of pituitary gland
  tumors, 168
Pericardiocentesis, 150
Pericarditis, 149–151

Perineum, injuries of, and fertility, 437
  parturient, 431–437
    repair of, operative technique in, 433–436,
      434–435
  lacerations of, degrees of, 432–433
Periodontal disease, 190
Peritoneal fluid, analysis of, 227(t)
  evaluation of, in thromboembolic colic, 239
  normal, composition of, 233(t), 242(t)
Peritoneal lavage, for treatment of peritonitis,
  243–244
Peritonitis, 241–244
  rectal tears and, 257
Pesticide(s), for control of ectoparasites,
  530(t)–531(t)
  in water, 610
Petroleum, toxicity of, 591–592, 573(t)
Phantom mare, 456–457
Pharyngeal lymphoid hyperplasia (PLH),
  490–493
Pharyngitis, 490–493
Pharynx, ulcers of, and coughing, 465
Phenobarbital, for treatment of seizure disorders,
  347(t)
Phenol(s), gastrointestinal toxicity of, 573(t)
Phenothiazine, for treatment of strongylosis,
  272–273
  toxicity of, 590–591, 575(t)
Phenylbutazone, and gastric ulcer, 199
  for treatment of founder, 105
  use of removal of retained placenta, 427(t)
Phenylguanidine(s), for treatment of ascariasis,
  265
Phenytoin, for treatment of seizure disorders,
  347(t)
Phonocardiography, 124
Phosphatase, alkaline, normal values for, 619(t)
Phosphate(s), organic, for treatment of ascariasis,
  265
Phosphodiesterase inhibitor(s), for treatment of
  chronic airway disease, 509
Phosphorus, 73–77
  deficiency of, clinical signs of, 74–75, 82(t)
    diagnosis of, 75–76
  functions of, 74, 82(t)
  normal values for, 619(t)
  requirements for, 75, 75(t)
  sources of, in feed, 82(t)
  supplements containing, 75
  toxicity of, 586
Phycomycosis, 550–551
Picadex, for treatment of bots infections, 285
Pinocytosis, 323
Pinworm(s), 288–289
Piperazine(s), for treatment of ascariasis,
  264–265
  for treatment of strongylosis, 273
Piroplasmosis, equine, 300
Pituitary gland, extracts of, for induction of
  ovulation, 403
  tumors of, 160, 164–169
    clinical signs of, 165(t)
    vs. diabetes mellitus, 170(t)
    laboratory tests for, 165–167, 165(t)–166(t)
    pathology of, 167
    treatment of, 168
Pival, as rodenticide, toxicity of, 584
Placenta, anomalies of, and abortion, 417–418
  retained, 425–427
    removal of, supportive therapy after, 427(t)
Placentitis, ascending, and abortion, 420
Plant(s), toxicity of, 574, 576, 595–607
  and sudden death, 612
  central nervous system, 574(t)–575(t)
  epithelial, 575(t)
  gastrointestinal, 573(t)
  minerals, in alteration of, 73
Plasma, mineral concentration in, 73
  protein in, and fluid therapy, 315, 315(t)
  in young horses, 294(t)

Plasma (*Continued*)
  transfusion of, 325
Platelet(s), disorders of, screening tests for, 307
  normal values for, 619(t)
Pleuritis, 523–526
  chronic, and coughing, 466–467
Pneumocystis carinii, and foal pneumonia, 501
Pneumonia, in foals, 500–504
  hematologic findings in, 502
Poisoning, 571–615. See also *Toxicology* and
  Toxicosis.
  and sudden death, 614
  emergency kit for, 578(t)
  prevention of further exposure in, 578–579
  supportive therapy in, 579–580
  treatment of, principles of, 577–580
Polyionic solution(s), for treatment of small
  bowel obstruction, 228
Polymyxin B, minimal inhibitory concentration
  of, 54(t)
Potassium, 78
  concentration of, and fluid therapy, 316
  deficiency of, in colitis-X, 203
    signs of, 82(t)
  functions of, 82(t)
  normal values for, 619(t)
  sources of, in feed, 82(t)
Poverty grass, epithelial toxicity of, 575(t)
Povidone-iodine, uterine infusion of, for removal
  of fetal membranes, 426
  for treatment of bacterial endometritis,
    413
  for treatment of pyometra, 415
Pregnancy, twin, elective abortion in, 441
  management of, progesterone for, 407
Prematurity, and weakness, 15(t)
Premolar(s), deciduous, retained, 189
  eruption schedule for, 625
Prepuce, injuries of, traumatic, 450–451
Presentation, and dystocia, 423–424
Primidone, for treatment of seizure disorders,
  347(t)
Progesterone, clinical uses of, 406–407
  for induction of ovulation, 404
  for management of twin pregnancy, 407
  for prevention of abortion, 406–407
  for suppression of estrus, 406
  for treatment of irregular estrus, 406
  for treatment of uterine involution, 406
  therapy with, 405–407
Prolapse, rectal, 254–255
Propranolol, for treatment of cardiac arrhythmias,
  139–140
Propylene glycol, for treatment of chronic airway
  disease, 510(t)
Prostaglandin(s), for advance of estrus, 404
  for induction of abortion, 441
  for induction of parturition, 441
  for treatment of prolonged diestrus, 402
Protein, 68–71
  crude, 68
  deficiency of, 69
    and hoof growth, 101
  grain mixtures with, 93(t)
  in cerebrospinal fluid, 335
  in plasma, and fluid therapy, 315, 315(t)
    in young horses, 294(t)
  requirements for, 66(t), 69, 69(t)
  sources of, 69–70
    composition of, 70(t)
  supplements with, mineral composition of,
    76(t)
  total, normal values for, 619(t)
  toxicity of, 70
Proteus mirabilis, sensitivity of, to antibiotics,
  51(t)
Proteus vulgaris, sensitivity of, to antibiotics,
  471(t)
Prunus virginiana, toxicity of, 597–598
Pruritus, and behavior, 338

Pseudomonas sp, antibiotic sensitivity of, 51(t), 471(t)
Psoroptes equi, and mange, 529
Pteridium aquilinum, toxicity of, 600–601
Ptyalism, 183
Pulmonary disease, chronic, diet in, 112
    obstructive, and coughing, 466
        summer pasture–associated, 512–516
Pupil(s), cranial trauma and, 341
Pupillary membrane(s), persistent, 388
Purpura hemorrhagica, 307–308
Pyelonephrosis, 565
Pyometra, 414–415
Pyrantel, for treatment of strongylosis, 276
Pyrimethamine, for treatment of equine protozoal myeloencephalitis, 368
Pyrrolizidine alkaloid(s), and liver disease, 251

Queensland itch, 558
Quinidine, for treatment of cardiac arrhythmias, 139

Rabies, 9–10
    differential diagnosis of, 10
    vaccination program for, 42(t)
Racetrack(s), feeding programs at, 98(t)
Radiation, for treatment of sarcoid, 538
Radiography, for diagnosis of chronic airway disease, 507
    for diagnosis of foal pneumonia, 502–503, 503(t)
    for diagnosis of seizure disorders, 348
    for diagnosis of sinusitis, 483
    thoracic, 124
Ragwort, gastrointestinal toxicity of, 573(t)
    toxicity of, 596–597
Ranula(e), 184
Ration(s), creep, 99(t)
    sample, 97–98, 98(t)
Rattleweed, toxicity of, 596–597
Reagent strip(s), urinary, for analysis of cerebrospinal fluid, 334
Rectal examination, for evaluation of urinary tract, 561
Rectovestibular fistula(s), 436–437, *436–437*
Rectovestibular injury(ies), and fertility, 437
    parturient, 431–437
    postpartum, 429–430
    repair of, operative technique in, 433–436, *434–435*
Rectum, examination of, in chronic diarrhea, 216
    prolapse of, 254–255
    tears of, 256–259
        classification of, 256–257
Recumbency, exertional myopathy and, management of, 103
Refractive index, of cerebrospinal fluid, 334
Regurgitation, causes of, 193(t)
Renal clearance, 563
Renal disease(s), 564–567
    chronic, 565–566
    parasitic, 566
Renal failure, acute, 564–565
Renal function, and fluid therapy, 316–317
Repolarization, ventricular, 127
Reproduction, 397–460
    artificial lighting and, 399
Respiratory disease(s), 461–526
    antibiotic treatment of, 467–475
        and drug interactions, 468–469
        routes of administration of, 467
    bacteria causing, antibiotic sensitivity of, 471(t)
    host factors in, 468
Respiratory tract, viral infections of, 464
Retina, degeneration of, 394

Retina (*Continued*)
    detachment of, 394
    dysfunction of, 393–394
Rhinopneumonitis, 4–5
    equine, vaccine for prevention of, 41
Rhinosporidiosis, 35
Rhinovirus, 6
Rhizoctonia leguminicola, and ptyalism, 183
Rhythm, cardiac, 126
Riboflavin, 90
    deficiency of, signs of, 89(t)
    functions of, 89(t)
    sources of, in feed, 89(t)
Ricinus communis, toxicity of, 604
Rickets, vitamin D deficiency and, 86–87
Robinia pseudoacacia, toxicity of, 606
Rodenticide(s), toxicity of, 584–587
Rotavirus infection(s), 11–12
Roughage, mineral composition of, 76(t)
Russian knapweed, toxicity of, 595–596

Sacrosciatic ligament(s), relaxation of, and induction of parturition, 439
St. John's wort, toxicity of, 575(t), 605–606
Saline, intrauterine infusion of, for induction of abortion, 441
    use in fluid therapy, 312
Saliva, increased secretion of, 183
Salivary cyst(s), 184
Salivary gland(s), diseases of, 183–184
    inflammation of, 183
    neoplasia of, 184
Salivation, excessive, gastrointestinal disease and, 175
Salivation Jane, toxicity of, 596–597
Salmonella, sensitivity of, to antibiotics, 51(t)
    shedding of, in feces, 219
Salmonellosis, 22–24
    control of, 210
    enteric, 207–210
        treatment of, 208–210
            antimicrobial agents for, 209(t)
Sarcoid, BCG therapy for, 539–540
    surgical treatment of, 537–539
    verrucous, vs. warts, 536
Sarcoptes scabiei, and mange, 529
Salt(s), in water, 608
    requirements for, 77–78
Scours, 213–214
Scouring rush, toxicity of, 601
Scratches, 549
Screwworm(s), control of, pesticides for, 530(t)
Screwworm fly(flies), control of, 534
Seborrhea, 546–547
Sedative(s), for management of colic, 221(t)
Seizure(s), causes of, 345, 346(t)
    description of, 344–345
    disorders with, 344–349
        history in, 345
        physical examination in, 346
        treatment of, 345–349
Selenium, 81–83
    deficiency of, and abortion, 419
        areas of, in United States, 72
        signs of, 82(t)
    functions of, 82(t)
    sources of, in feed, 82(t)
    toxicity of, 593–595
        areas of, in United States, 72
Self-mutilation, 337
Semen, blood in, 452–453
    collection of, 443–446
        in artificial breeding, 456–457
        preparation of stallion for, 444
    color of, 446
    evaluation of, 444–446
    pH of, 445, 447
    quality of, tests of, 446–448

Semen (*Continued*)
    stored, 458
    urine in, 453–454
Semen extender(s), 458–459
    formula for, 453(t), 459
Senecio sp, toxicity of, 596–597
Septicemia, actinobacillosis and, 16
    in neonates, 15(t)
Serum, chemical values in, 619(t)
Serum glutamic oxaloacetic transaminase (SGOT), normal values for, 619(t)
Shaker foal(s), 367–369
Shampoo, for treatment of seborrhea, 546
Shigellosis, 14–17
Shock, endotoxin, 57–62
    and leukocyte numbers, *59*
    clinical signs of, 58(t)
    fluid therapy in, 60–61
    treatment of, 60–62, 60(t)
Sialoadenitis, 183
Sialocele(s), 184
Sialolith(s), 183–184
Sialosis, gastrointestinal disease and, 175
Single radial immunodiffusion (SRID), 322
Sinus(es), anatomy of, 481
    paranasal, *482*
Sinusitis, 481–485
    diagnosis of, 482–483
    etiology of, 481–482
    treatment of, 484–485
Skin, bacteria isolated from, 543(t)
    diseases of, 527–558
    fungi isolated from, 543(t)
    infections of, bacterial, and folliculitis, 543
Skin test(s), allergen, for diagnosis of summer pasture–associated obstructive pulmonary disease, 514
"Sleeping sickness," 352–355
Small bowel, obstruction of, 224–231
    abdominal evaluation in, 227
    classification of, 225(t)
    clinical signs of, 226
    diagnosis of, 225–226
    hematologic evaluation in, 227
    history in, 226
    prevention of, 229
    rectal examination in, 227
    rupture of, ascariasis and, 263
    treatment of, 227–229, 230(t)
Snake bite, 587–588
    toxicity of, 576
Snakeroot, white, toxicity of, 603–604, 574(t)
Sodium, 77–78
    concentration of, and fluid therapy, 315, 315(t)
    deficiency of, clinical signs of, 314
        in colitis-X, 202
        signs of, 82(t)
    functions of, 82(t)
    normal values for, 619(t)
    sources of, in feed, 82(t)
Sodium bicarbonate, use in fluid therapy, 312–313
Sodium gluconate, for treatment of aortoiliofemoral arteriosclerosis, 155
Soft palate, diseases of, 493–494. See also *Palate, soft.*
Soil, minerals in, alteration of, 73
Solanum nigrum, toxicity of, 605
Sorbitol dehydrogenase, normal values for, 619(t)
Sorghum sp, toxicity of, 598–599
"Sour milk," for treatment of intestinal clostridiosis, 212
Spasm, intestinal, correction of, 222–224
Spectinomycin, for treatment of respiratory diseases, 474
Sperm, counting of, methods of, 458
    number of, in ejaculate, testicular size and, 447
Sperm cell(s), morphology of, 445, 447–448
"Sperm count," 457

Spermatozoa, concentration of, 445
motility of, 447
Spinal cord, trauma to, 355–359
medical therapy in, 357–358
neurologic examination in, 356–357
nursing management in, 358
pathophysiology of, 356
surgical treatment of, 358
Spinal tap, 331
Sporotrichosis, 555–556
treatment of, medications for, iodine content of, 556(t)
Spray(s), for control of flies, 533(t)
Stable fly(flies), control of, 532
Stallion(s), behavior of, variations in, 336
feeding programs for, 94
fertility of, disorders affecting, 449–455
evaluation of, 442–448
use in artificial breeding, 456
Staphylococci, antibiotic sensitivity of, 51(t), 471(t)
Stenosis, atrioventricular, 144
Steroid(s), for treatment of uveitis, 384
ovarian, for synchronization of ovulation, 405
Stimulant(s), intestinal, for management of colic, 221(t)
respiratory, for treatment of respiratory depression, 475
Stinking Willie, toxicity of, 596–597
Stomach, dilatation of, 197–198
diseases of, 196–200
ulcers of, 199–200
Stomatitis, vesicular, 12
Strangles, 24–27
vaccination program for, 42, 42(t)
Streptococcus, and abortion, 420
and bacterial endocarditis, 147
and foal pneumonia, 501
and strangles, 24
antibiotic sensitivity of, 51(t), 471(t)
Streptomycin, bacteria effective against, 471(t)
dosage of, 53(t)
for treatment of anthrax, 18
for treatment of respiratory diseases, 473
minimal inhibitory concentration of, 54(t)
Stress, and abortion, 418–419
and salmonellosis, 23
Stricture, esophageal, 195
Strongyloides westeri, 281
Strongyloidosis, 281–283
Strongyle(s), small, 271
Strongylosis, 267–280
clinical signs of, 272
control of, 276–278
diagnosis of, 271–272
hematologic findings in, 272
pathogenesis of, 268–271
treatment of, 272–276
Strongylus edentatus, 270
Strongylus equinus, 270–271
Strongylus vulgaris, 269–270
and thromboembolic colic, 238
Strychnine, toxicity of, 584–585
Sulfamethazine, dosage of, 53(t)
for treatment of bacteremia, 37(t)
for treatment of respiratory diseases, 469(t)
Sulfamethylphenazole, dosage of, 53(t)
Sulfasalazine, for treatment of malabsorption syndromes, 247
Sulfonamide(s), blood plasma concentrations of, 55(t)
for treatment of respiratory diseases, 474
minimal inhibitory concentration of, 54(t)
Sulfur, 81
"Summer sore," 551–552
Superinfection, uterine, 412
Supplement(s), calcium, 75, 76(t)–77(t)
phosphorus, 75, 76(t)
protein, mineral composition of, 76(t)
Surgery, for treatment of large bowel obstruction, 236

Surgery (Continued)
positioning during, for prevention of myopathy, 373–374
Sweet feed bumps, 110–111
Sweet itch, 110–111, 558
Swelling, suprapharyngeal, and coughing, 466
Sympathomimetic agent(s), for treatment of chronic airway disease, 509
Synergism, of antibiotics, 46

T cell(s), function of, in evaluation of immune system, 323
T lymphocyte(s), evaluation of, 323
Tachycardia(s), 133, 134
atrial, 138
ventricular, 137, 138
Tail, seborrhea of, 546
Tannin, gastrointestinal toxicity of, 573(t)
Tapeworm(s), 287
Tarweed, toxicity of, 596–597
Taxus sp, toxicity of, 604–605
Teasing, 400
Teeth, care of, 186–192
deciduous, formulas for, 187(t)
eruption schedule for, 187(t), 625
examination of, 187–191
restraint in, 187
floating of, 188–189
number of, 625
permanent, formulas for, 187(t)
wear of, age and, 625–626, 625
anatomic factors in, 186
wolf, removal of, 188
Tendon(s), contracted, overfeeding and, 95–96
Teratoma(s), ovarian, 408
Testicle(s), neoplasms of, 452
size of, and number of sperm, 447
torsion of, 452
trauma to, 451
Tetanospasmin, 27
Tetanus, 27–29
complications of, 29
malignant edema and, 21
vaccination programs for, 41, 42(t)
Tetany, transit, 77
Tetracycline, and intestinal clostridiosis, 212
bacteria effective against, 471(t)
blood plasma concentrations of, 55(t)
incompatibility of, 48(t)
minimal inhibitory concentration of, 54(t)
side effects of, 49(t)
types of, 44(t)
Tetrahydropyrimidine(s), for treatment of ascariasis, 265
Thallium, toxicity of, 586–587
Theophylline, for treatment of chronic airway disease, 508(t), 509
Thiabendazole, for treatment of lungworm infections, 522
for treatment of strongylosis, 275(t)
for treatment of strongyloidosis, 282
for treatment of thromboembolic colic, 240
Thiamine, 88, 90
deficiency of, signs of, 89(t)
sources of, in feed, 89(t)
Thistle, yellow star, toxicity of, 574(t), 595–596
Thoracentesis, for treatment of pleuritis, 524
Thorax, radiography of, in foals, 503(t)
Throat spray(s), for treatment of pharyngitis, 492
Thromboembolism, of colon, 238–241
Thrombophlebitis, 151–152
Thyroid, adenoma of, 160
diseases of, 159–160
Ticarcillin, for treatment of bacterial endometritis, 413(t)
Tick(s), 529–532
control of, pesticides for, 530(t)–531(t)
species of, 531
Timothy, protein content of, 68(t)

Tobramycin, minimal inhibitory concentration of, 54(t)
Tongue, inflammation of, 185–186
Torsion, testicular, 452
Toxicology, 571–615
tests in, specimens required in, 613(t)
Toxicosis, central nervous system signs of, 574(t)–575(t)
common, 573–576
emergency treatment of, 573–574
epithelial signs of, 575(t)
gastrointestinal signs of, 573(t)
hematologic signs of, 575(t)
Toxin(s), and abortion, 419
and behavior, 338
bacterial, and sudden death, 612
elimination of, in botulism, 368
tetanus, neutralization of, 27–28
Trauma, and cataracts, 392
and glossitis, 185
cranial, 339–344
management of, 343(t)
pathophysiology of, 340
syndromes resulting from, 341(t)
vertebral, types of, 355–356
Tracheitis, and coughing, 465
Tracheostomy tube(s), sizes of, 477(t)
Tranquilizer(s), for management of colic, 221, 221(t)
Transfaunation, for treatment of chronic diarrhea, 218
Transfusion, of blood, 325–328. See also Blood, transfusion of.
Transudate, vs. exudate, 523
Trephine, diagnostic, for diagnosis of sinusitis, 484
sites for, 483
Trichlorfon, for treatment of ascariasis, 266
for treatment of bots infections, 285
for treatment of strongylosis, 275
Trimethoprim, for treatment of bacteremia, 37(t)
side effects of, 49(t)
Trimethoprim-sulfa, for treatment of equine protozoal myeloencephalitis, 368
for treatment of foal pneumonia, 503
for treatment of respiratory diseases, 469(t), 473–474
for treatment of salmonellosis, 23, 209(t)
Trocarization, for treatment of thromboembolic colic, 240
in flatulent colic, 237
Tube feeding, 114–115(t)
schedule for, 176(t)
Tuberculosis, 29–31
Tumor(s), granulosa-theca cell, 408
ovarian, 408–409
Twinning, 417
abortion and, 417, 441
Tylosin, for treatment of respiratory diseases, 474

Udder(s), enlargement of, and induction of parturition, 439
Ulcer(s), gastric, 199–200
pharyngeal, and coughing, 465
Umbilical cord, anomalies of, 418
Underfeeding, 65
Urachus, patent, 569
Urethra, trauma to, 451
Urethritis, bacterial, 455
Urinalysis, 563
Urinary tract, diseases of, 559–569
serum biochemical aspects of, 562
examination of, 561–563
Urospermia, 453–454
Urticaria, 535–536
Uterus, biopsy of, for diagnosis of endometritis, 411
culture of, for diagnosis of endometritis, 411

Uterus (*Continued*)
infusion of antibiotics into, for treatment of endometritis, 412
involution of, progesterone for treatment of, 406
prolapsed, postpartum, 428
rupture of, postpartum, 428
Uveitis, 382–385
and cataracts, 392
causes of, 383(t)
treatment of, 384(t)

Vaccination, programs for, 42(t), 40–48
Vaccine(s), for preventation of anthrax, 18
for prevention of botulism, 367
for prevention of eastern equine encephalomyelitis, 41, 351
for prevention of herpesvirus, 4
for prevention of influenza, 3
for prevention of rabies, 10
for prevention of rhinopneumonitis, 41
for prevention of strangles, 26
for prevention of tetanus, 29, 41
for prevention of Venezuelan equine encephalomyelitis, 41
for prevention of viral abortion, 421
for prevention of western equine encephalomyelitis, 41, 354
for treatment of brucellosis, 20
Vacor, toxicity of, 586
Vagina, artificial, 443
preparation of, 456
rupture of, postpartum, 429
Valve(s), atrioventricular, diastolic murmurs associated with, 144–145
systolic murmurs associated with, 143
cardiac, acquired disease of, 141–142
Vascular system, diseases of, 119–155. See also *Cardiovascular disease(s).*
Vasodilator(s), use in endotoxemia, 61
Venezuelan equine encephalomyelitis, vaccination for, 41
Venom, and sudden death, 612

Ventilation, emergency, 475–478
mechanical, 476–477
Ventricle(s), repolarization of, 127
Ventriculectomy, for treatment of laryngeal hemiplegia, 498
Vertebra(e), cervical, malformation of, 359–362
stenosis of, 359
trauma to, types of, 355–356, 356(t)
Vesicular stomatitis virus (VSV), 12
Vestibular disease, and behavior, 338
Vetaspirator, for emergency ventilation, 477
Vice(s), 336
treatment of, 337(t)
Vision, and behavior, 338
loss of, cataracts and, 391
Vitamin(s), 84–90
deficiency of, signs of, 89(t)
functions of, 89(t)
in feeds, 86(t), 89(t)
requirements for, 87(t)
Vitamin A, 84–86
deficiency of, signs of, 89(t)
sources of, in feed, 89(t)
Vitamin B₁₂, 90
deficiency of, signs of, 89(t)
sources of, in feed, 89(t)
Vitamin C, 88
Vitamin D, 86–87
deficiency of, signs of, 89(t)
sources of, in feed, 89(t)
Vitamin E, 87–88
deficiency of, signs of, 89(t)
sources of, in feed, 89(t)
Vitamin K, 88
deficiency of, and coagulation disorders, 308
signs of, 89(t)
sources of, in feed, 89(t)
Vulva, laceration of, postpartum, 430

Warfarin, toxicity of, 308, 584
Wart(s), 536–537
Water, bacteria in, 608
dissolved solids in, 608

Water (*Continued*)
fluoride in, 608–609
heavy metals in, 609, 609(t)
nitrates and nitrites in, 608
pesticides in, 610
quality of, 607–610
salts in, 608
toxic substances in, 609(t)
Water saline, for treatment of chronic airway disease, 510(t)
Waveform(s), electrocardiographic, duration of, 132(t)
Weakness, in neonates, differential diagnosis of, 15(t)
Weaning, early, 96–97
Weanling(s), feeding programs for, 95
rations for, 99(t)
Weight, age and, 96(t)
and fluid therapy, 315, 315(t)
loss of, gastrointestinal disease and, 176
Western equine encephalomyelitis (WEE), 352–355
vaccine for prevention of, 41, 354
White muscle disease, 81
Wolf teeth, removal of, 188

Xylazine, for treatment of colic, 221
for treatment of large bowel obstruction, 235
for treatment of seizure disorders, 347(t)
Xylose absorption test, 246

Yew, toxicity of, 604–605

Zigadenus sp, toxicity of, 603
Zinc, 79–80
deficiency of, signs of, 83(t)
sources of, in feed, 83(t)
Zinc phosphide, toxicity of, 586